THE BREAST

Comprehensive Management of Benign and Malignant Disorders

THIRD EDITION

THE BREAST

COMPREHENSIVE MANAGEMENT OF
BENIGN AND MALIGNANT DISORDERS

Volume One

EDITED BY

KIRBY I. BLAND, MD
Fay Fletcher Kerner Professor and Chairman
Department of Surgery
Deputy Director University of Alabama Comprehensive Cancer Center
University of Alabama School of Medicine
Birmingham, Alabama

EDWARD M. COPELAND III, MD
Edward R. Woodward Professor and Chairman Emeritus
Department of Surgery
University of Florida College of Medicine
Gainesville, Florida

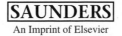
SAUNDERS
An Imprint of Elsevier

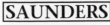

SAUNDERS
An Imprint of Elsevier

11830 Westline Industrial Drive
St. Louis, Missouri 63146

THE BREAST: COMPREHENSIVE MANAGEMENT   0-7216-9490-X
OF BENIGN AND MALIGNANT DISORDERS

Previous editions copyrighted 1998, 1991

Library of Congress Cataloging-in-Publication Data
The breast : comprehensive management of benign and malignant disorders / edited by
    Kirby I. Bland, Edward M. Copeland III. – 3rd ed.
        p. ; cm.
    Includes bibliographical references and index.
    ISBN 0-7216-9490-X
        1. Breast–Cancer–Treatment.   2. Breast–Diseases–Treatment.   I. Bland, K. I. II.
Copeland, Edward M.
    [DNLM: 1. Breast Diseases–therapy.   2. Breast Neoplasms–therapy. WP 900 B828 2004]
    RC280.B8B674 2004
    618.1'906–dc22

                                                                            2003060826

Acquisitions Editor: Joe Rusko
Developmental Editor: Arlene Chappelle
Publishing Services Manager: Peggy Fagen
Designer: Amy Buxton

Printed in the United States of America

Last digit is the print number: 9   8   7   6   5   4   3   2   1

To our wives,
Lynn and Martha,
in appreciation for the generous support they provided to our careers
which allowed the development of this book,
and to our mentors,
Edward R. Woodward, Jonathan E. Rhoads, and Richard G. Martin, Sr.,
and to physicians and nurses of all oncologic disciplines
who care for patients with diseases of the breast

ASSOCIATE EDITORS

Nancy E. Davidson, MD
Professor of Oncology
Breast Cancer Research Chair in Oncology
The Sidney Kimmel Comprehensive Cancer Center at
  Johns Hopkins
Bunting/Blaustein Cancer Research Building
Baltimore, Maryland

David L. Page, MD
Professor of Pathology and Epidemiology
Vanderbilt University Medical Center
Nashville, Tennessee

Abram Recht, MD
Associate Professor
Department of Radiation Oncology
Harvard Medical School
Senior Radiation Oncologist and Deputy Chief
Department of Radiation Oncology
Beth Israel Deaconess Medical Center
Boston, Massachusetts

Marshall M. Urist, MD
Champ Lyons Professor and Vice Chairman
Department of Surgery
University of Alabama at Birmingham
Birmingham, Alabama

CONTRIBUTORS

Thomas Aversano, MD
Associate Professor of Medicine
Johns Hopkins Medical Institutions
Baltimore, Maryland
73 *Management of Pericardial Metastases in Breast Cancer*

Sunil Badve, MD, FRCPath
Assistant Professor of Pathology and Laboratory
  Medicine
Division of Surgical Pathology
Indiana University School of Medicine
Indianapolis, Indiana
24 *Steroid Hormone Receptors*

Glen C. Balch, MD
Senior Resident, Department of Surgery
Vanderbilt University Medical Center
Nashville, Tennessee
53 *Intraoperative Evaluation of Surgical Margins
  in Breast-Conserving Therapy*

Abdalla Z. Bandak, MD
Assistant Professor, Division of Plastic and
  Reconstructive Surgery
Department of Surgery
Medical College of Virginia
Richmond, Virginia
43 *Breast Reconstruction following Mastectomy*

Alfred A. Bartolucci, PhD
Professor, Department of Biostatistics
University of Alabama at Birmingham
Birmingham, Alabama
36 *Design and Conduct of Clinical Trials for Breast Cancer*

Lawrence W. Bassett, MD
Iris Cantor Professor of Breast Imaging
David Geffen School of Medicine at UCLA
Los Angeles, California
31 *Breast Imaging*

Elisabeth K. Beahm, MD
Associate Professor, Department of Plastic and
  Reconstructive Surgery
The University of Texas M.D. Anderson Cancer Center
Houston, Texas
63 *Surgical Procedures for Advanced Local and Regional
  Malignancies of the Breast*

Isabelle Bedrosian, MD
Fellow, Department of Surgical Oncology
The University of Texas M.D. Anderson Cancer Center
Houston, Texas
80 *General Considerations for Follow-Up*

Samuel W. Beenken, MD
Professor, Department of Surgery
University of Alabama at Birmingham
Birmingham, Alabama
1 *History of the Therapy of Breast Cancer*
6 *Gynecomastia*
9 *Evaluation and Treatment of Benign Breast Disorders*

Rashmi K. Benda, MD
Assistant Professor of Radiation Oncology
University of Florida Health Science Center
Gainesville, Florida
65 *Radiotherapy for Locoregional Failure*
68 *Radiotherapy for Palliation*

Kirby I. Bland, MD
Fay Fletcher Kerner Professor and Chairman
Department of Surgery
Deputy Director University of Alabama
  Comprehensive Cancer Center
University of Alabama School of Medicine
Birmingham, Alabama
1 *History of the Therapy of Breast Cancer*
2 *Anatomy of the Breast, Axilla, Chest Wall, and Related
  Metastatic Sites*
3 *Breast Physiology: Normal and Abnormal Development
  and Function*
6 *Gynecomastia*
8 *Congenital and Acquired Disturbances of Breast
  Development and Growth*
9 *Evaluation and Treatment of Benign Breast Disorders*
20 *Assessment and Designation of Breast Cancer Stage*
37 *Evolution of Surgical Principles and Techniques for the
  Management of Breast Cancer*
38 *Indications and Techniques for Biopsy*
39 *General Principles of Mastectomy: Evaluation and
  Therapeutic Options*
40 *Halsted Radical Mastectomy*
41 *Modified Radical Mastectomy and Total (Simple)
  Mastectomy*
42 *Breast Conservation Therapy in Invasive Breast Cancer*
45 *Wound Care and Complications of Mastectomy*
64 *Level I Lymph Node Dissection*
80 *General Considerations for Follow-Up*

Patrick I. Borgen, MD
Chief, Breast Service
Co-Director, Breast Cancer Disease Management Team
Memorial Sloan-Kettering Cancer Center
New York, New York
52 *The Detection and Significance of Axillary Lymph Node
  Micrometastases*

Malcolm V. Brock, MD
Assistant Professor of Surgery
Division of Thoracic Surgery
Johns Hopkins University School of Medicine
Baltimore, Maryland
71 *Diagnosis and Management of Pleural Metastases in Breast Cancer*

Heather M. Brown, MD
Assistant Professor, Department of Pathology, Immunology and Laboratory Medicine
University of Florida
Gainesville, Florida
34 *Cytologic Needle Samplings of the Breast: Techniques and End Results*

Blake Cady, MD
Director, Breast Health Center
Women and Infants Hospital of Rhode Island
Providence, Rhode Island
50 *Selective Management of the Axilla in Minimally Invasive and Small Invasive Ductal Carcinoma*
54 *Surgical Management of "Early" Breast Cancer*

Susan W. Caro, RNC, MSN
Director, Family Cancer Risk Service
Vanderbilt-Ingram Cancer Center
Nashville, Tennessee
79 *Management of the Patient at High Risk*

G. Scott Chandler, MD
Surgical Resident, Department of Surgery
UCLA
Los Angeles, California
41 *Modified Radical Mastectomy and Total (Simple) Mastectomy*

Helena R. Chang, MD, PhD
Professor of Surgery
Director, Revlon/UCLA Breast Center
Los Angeles, California
41 *Modified Radical Mastectomy and Total (Simple) Mastectomy*

Maureen Chung, MD, PhD
Rhode Island Hospital
Brown University
Providence, Rhode Island
50 *Selective Management of the Axilla in Minimally Invasive and Small Invasive Ductal Carcinoma*
54 *Surgical Management of "Early" Breast Cancer*

Hiram S. Cody III, MD
Attending Surgeon
Breast Service, Department of Surgery
Memorial Sloan-Kettering Cancer Center
Professor of Clinical Surgery
The Weill Medical College of Cornell University
New York, New York
52 *The Detection and Significance of Axillary Lymph Node Metastases*
74 *Bilateral Breast Cancer*

Edward M. Copeland III, MD
Edward R. Woodward Professor and Chairman Emeritus
Department of Surgery
University of Florida College of Medicine
Gainesville, Florida
39 *General Principles of Mastectomy: Evaluation and Therapeutic Options*
40 *Halsted Radical Mastectomy*
41 *Modified Radical Mastectomy and Total (Simple) Mastectomy*
64 *Level I Lymph Node Dissection*
76 *Local Recurrence, the Augmented Breast, and the Contralateral Breast*

Charles E. Cox, MD
Professor of Surgery
University of South Florida
Director, Comprehensive Breast Cancer Program
H. Lee Moffitt Cancer Center and Research Institute
Tampa, Florida
46 *Lymphedema in the Postmastectomy Patient: Pathophysiology, Prevention, and Management*

Anne Cramer, MD
Assistant Professor, Department of Plastic Surgery
University of Kansas School of Medicine
Director, Gene and Barbara Burnett Burn Center
Kansas City, Kansas
43 *Breast Reconstruction following Mastectomy*

David T. Curiel, MD, PhD
Professor of Medicine
Division of Human Gene Therapy
Director, Gene Therapy Center
University of Alabama
Birmingham, Alabama
27 *Gene Therapy of Breast Cancer*

Michele G. Cyr, MD
Director, General Internal Medicine
Rhode Island Hospital
Associate Professor of Medicine
Brown Medical School
Providence, Rhode Island
81 *Menopausal Hormone Therapy: Benefits, Risks, and Alternatives*

Nancy E. Davidson, MD
Professor of Oncology
Breast Cancer Research Chair in Oncology
The Sidney Kimmel Comprehensive Cancer Center at Johns Hopkins
Bunting/Blaustein Cancer Research Building
Baltimore, Maryland
62 *Adjuvant Systemic Therapy of Breast Cancer*

Jorge I. de la Torre, MD, FACS
Assistant Professor of Surgery
Division of Plastic Surgery
University of Alabama at Birmingham School of Medicine
Chief, Plastic Surgery Section
Birmingham VA Medical Center
Director, Center for Advanced Surgical Aesthetics
Birmingham, Alabama
43 *Breast Reconstruction following Mastectomy*
44 *Macromastia and Reduction Mammaplasty*

Jennifer F. De Los Santos, MD
Assistant Professor, Radiation Oncology
Wallace Tumor Institute
Birmingham, Alabama
42 *Breast Conservation Therapy in Invasive Breast Cancer*

Marvin A. Dewar, MD, JD
Associate Professor, Community Health and Family Medicine
Vice President, Affiliations and Provider Relations
Shands HealthCare
University of Florida
Gainesville, Florida
86 *Legal Issues in Breast Disease*

Robert B. Dickson, PhD
Lombardi Cancer Center
Washington, DC
25 *Molecular Oncology of Breast Cancer*

William C. Dooley, MD, FACS
Professor, Department of Surgery
Institute for Breast Health
Oklahoma City, Oklahoma
35 *Breast Ductoscopy*

Toby J. Dunn, MD
Chief Resident in Surgery
Washington University School of Medicine/Barnes-Jewish Hospital
St. Louis, Missouri
29 *Immunology and the Role of Immunotherapy in Breast Cancer*

William D. Dupont, PhD
Professor of Biostatistics
Department of Preventive Medicine
Vanderbilt University Medical Center
Nashville, Tennessee
23 *Risk Factors for Breast Carcinoma in Women with Proliferative Breast Disease*
79 *Management of the Patient at High Risk*

Philip L. Dutt, MD
Novato, California
13 *Extent and Multicentricity of In Situ and Invasive Carcinoma*

Timothy J. Eberlein, MD
Bixby Professor and Chairman, Department of Surgery
Washington University School of Medicine
Surgeon-in-Chief, Barnes-Jewish Hospital
Olin Distinguished Professor and Director,
The Alvin J. Siteman Cancer Center at Washington University and Barnes-Jewish Hospital
St. Louis, Missouri
29 *Immunology and the Role of Immunotherapy in Breast Cancer*

Mary Edgerton, MD, PhD
Assistant Professor, Departments of Pathology and Biomedical Informatics
Vanderbilt University Medical Center
Nashville, Tennessee
13 *Extent and Multicentricity of In Situ and Invasive Carcinoma*

Mahmoud El-Tamer, MD
Columbia University
New York, New York
19 *Patterns of Recurrence in Breast Cancer*

Franklin P. Flowers, MD
University of Florida
Gainesville, Florida
15 *Epithelial Neoplasms and Dermatologic Disorders*

M. Judah Folkman, MD
Department of Surgery
Children's Hospital and Harvard Medical School
Boston, Massachusetts
28 *Angiogenesis in Breast Cancer*

Barbara Fowble, MD
Senior Member Emeritus
Fox Chase Cancer Center
Philadelphia, Pennsylvania
61 *Breast-Conserving Therapy for Early-Stage Invasive Cancer*

Gary M. Freedman, MD
Fox Chase Cancer Center
Philadelphia, Pennsylvania
61 *Breast-Conserving Therapy for Early-Stage Invasive Cancer*

Eric R. Frykberg, MD
Professor of Surgery
University of Florida Health Sciences Center
Jacksonville, Florida
37 *Evolution of Surgical Principles and Techniques for the Management of Breast Cancer*

Thomas A. Gaskin III, MD, FACS
Director of Breast Care Center, Princeton Baptist Medical Center
The Surgeon's Group
Birmingham, Alabama
82 *Rehabilitation*

Edward P. Gelmann, MD
William M. Scholl Professor of Oncology and Medicine
Lombardi Cancer Center
Georgetown University
Washington, DC
25 *Molecular Oncology of Breast Cancer*

Sharon Hermes Giordano, MD
Assistant Professor, Department of Breast Medical Oncology
The University of Texas M.D. Anderson Cancer Center
Houston, Texas
66 *Locally Advanced Breast Cancer: Role of Medical Oncology*

Armando E. Giuliano, MD
John Wayne Cancer Institute
Saint John's Health Center
Clinical Professor of Surgery
UCLA
Santa Monica, California
51 *Lymphatic Mapping and Sentinel Lymphadenectomy for Breast Cancer*

Peter S. Goedegebuure, PhD
Department of Surgery
Washington University School of Medicine
St. Louis, Missouri
29 *Immunology and the Role of Immunotherapy in Breast Cancer*

William H. Goodson III, MD
California Pacific Medical Center Research Institute
San Francisco, California
4 *Discharges and Secretions of the Nipple*

William J. Gradishar, MD, FACP
Director, Breast Medical Oncology
Associate Professor of Medicine, Robert H. Lurie Comprehensive Cancer Center
Northwestern University Feinberg School of Medicine
Chicago, Illinois
24 *Steroid Hormone Receptors*
70 *Endocrine Therapy of Breast Cancer*

Baiba J. Grube, MD
Associate Director, Joyce Eisenberg Keefer Breast Center
John Wayne Cancer Institute
Santa Monica, California
51 *Lymphatic Mapping and Sentinel Lymphadenectomy for Breast Cancer*

Wael Harb, MD
Clinical Assistant Professor of Medicine
Indiana University Medical Center
Indianapolis, Indiana
69 *Chemotherapy for Metastatic Breast Cancer*

Seth P. Harlow, MD
Associate Professor of Surgery
University of Vermont College of Medicine
Burlington, Vermont
67 *Detection and Clinical Implications of Occult Systemic Micrometastatic Disease*

Ronda S. Henry-Tillman, MD
Associate Professor, Department of Surgery
Director of Women's Oncology Clinic
Women's Breast Cancer CAVHS
University of Arkansas for Medical Sciences
Little Rock, Arkansas
10 *Etiology and Management of Breast Pain*

Gabriel N. Hortobagyi, MD, FACP
Professor of Medicine
Nellie B. Connally Chair in Breast Cancer
Chairman, Department of Breast Medical Oncology
Division of Cancer Medicine
The University of Texas M.D. Anderson Cancer Center
Houston, Texas
66 *Locally Advanced Breast Cancer: Role of Medical Oncology*

Virginia Huang, MD
Staff Physician
Southern California Permanente Medical Group
Plastic Surgery Department
Fontana, Californai
43 *Breast Reconstruction following Mastectomy*

Kelly K. Hunt, MD
Associate Professor
Chief, Surgical Breast Section
Department of Surgical Oncology
The University of Texas M.D. Anderson Cancer Center
Houston, Texas
63 *Surgical Procedures for Advanced Local and Regional Malignancies of the Breast*
80 *General Considerations for Follow-Up*

Roy A. Jensen, MD
Associate Professor of Pathology, Cell and
Developmental Biology, and Cancer Biology
Vanderbilt University Medical Center
Nashville, Tennessee
11 *In Situ Carcinomas of the Breast: Ductal Carcinoma In Situ, Paget's Disease, Lobular Carcinoma In Situ*

Joyce E. Johnson, MD
Department of Pathology
Vanderbilt University School of Medicine
Nashville, Tennessee
13 *Extent and Multicentricity of In Situ and Invasive Carcinoma*

V. Craig Jordan, OBE, PhD, DSc
Diana, Princess of Wales Professor of Cancer Research
Director, Lynn Sage Breast Cancer Research Program
Robert H. Lurie Comprehensive Cancer Center
Northwestern University Feinberg School of Medicine
Chicago, Illinois
70 *Endocrine Therapy of Breast Cancer*

Rena Kass, MD
University of Arkansas for Medical Sciences
Arkansas Cancer Research Center
Little Rock, Arkansas
3 *Breast Physiology: Normal and Abnormal Development and Function*

Mark C. Kelley, MD
Associate Professor of Surgery
Chief, Division of Surgical Oncology and Endocrine Surgery
Vanderbilt University Medical Center
Nashville, Tennessee
53 *Intraoperative Evaluation of Surgical Margins in Breast-Conserving Therapy*

Kenneth A. Kern, MD
Clinical Professor of Surgery and Surgical Oncology
Hartford Hospital and the University of Connecticut School of Medicine
Hartford, Connecticut
87 *The Delayed Diagnosis of Symptomatic Breast Cancer*

Larry Kestin, MD
Staff Physician, Department of Radiation Oncology
William Beaumont Hospital
Royal Oak, Michigan
58 *Radiotherapy and Ductal Carcinoma In Situ*

Kristin M. Kilbourn, PhD, MPH
Assistant Professor, Department of Psychology
Northern Arizona University
Flagstaff, Arizona
84 *Psychosocial Interventions for Breast Cancer Patients*

Christina J. Kim, MD
Assistant Professor, Section of Surgical Oncology
Arizona Cancer Center, University of Arizona
Tucson, Arizona
20 *Assessment and Designation of Breast Cancer Stage*

Eileen B. King, MD
University of California at San Francisco
Larkspur, California
4 *Discharges and Secretions of the Nipple*

V. Suzanne Klimberg, MD
Professor of Surgery and Pathology
Arkansas Cancer Research Center
University of Arkansas for Medical Sciences
Central Arkansas Veteran Health Services
Little Rock, Arkansas
3 *Breast Physiology: Normal and Abnormal Development and Function*
10 *Etiology and Management of Breast Pain*

Kara C. Kort, MD
Assistant Professor of Surgery
SUNY Upstate Medical University
Syracuse, New York
5 *Subareolar Breast Abscess: The Penultimate Stage of the Mammary Duct–Associated Inflammatory Disease Sequence*

David N. Krag, MD
SD Ireland Professor of Surgery
University of Vermont College of Medicine
Burlington, Vermont
67 *Detection and Clinical Implications of Occult Systemic Micrometastatic Disease*

Helen Krontiras, MD
Assistant Professor of Surgery
University of Alabama at Birmingham
Birmingham, Alabama
42 *Breast Conservation Therapy in Invasive Breast Cancer*
45 *Wound Care and Complications of Mastectomy*

Joy Kunishige, MD
St. Luke's Roosevelt Hospital Center
New York, New York
15 *Epithelial Neoplasms and Dermatologic Disorders*

Michael D. Lagios, MD
Breast Cancer Consultation Service
Tiburon, California
11 *In Situ Carcinomas of the Breast: Ductal Carcinoma In Situ, Paget's Disease, Lobular Carcinoma In Situ*

Gregory E. Lakin, BA
Ponce School of Medicine
Ponce, Puerto Rico
77 *Carcinoma of the Breast in Pregnancy and Lactation*

Andrew Laman, MD
Hematology/Medical Oncology
UPMC Cancer Centers
Pittsburgh, Pennsylvania
17 *Primary Prevention of Breast Cancer*

Laura Liberman, MD, FACR
Attending Radiologist
Memorial Sloan-Kettering Cancer Center
New York, New York
52 *The Detection and Significance of Axillary Lymph Node Micrometastases*

D. Scott Lind, MD
Professor, Department of Surgery
University of Florida College of Medicine
Gainesville, Florida
76 *Local Recurrence, the Augmented Breast, and the Contralateral Breast*

Marc E. Lippman, MD
John G. Searle Professor and Chair
Department of Internal Medicine
University of Michigan School of Medicine
Ann Arbor, Michigan
25 *Molecular Oncology of Breast Cancer*

Minetta C. Liu, MD
Assistant Professor of Medicine and Oncology
Lombardi Cancer Center
Georgetown University Hospital
Washington, DC
25 *Molecular Oncology of Breast Cancer*

Henry T. Lynch, MD
Chairman, Preventive Medicine and Public Health
Professor of Medicine
Director of Creighton's Hereditary Cancer Institute
Creighton University School of Medicine
Omaha, Nebraska
18 *Breast Cancer Genetics: Heterogeneity, Molecular Genetics, Syndrome Diagnosis, and Genetics Counseling*

Jane F. Lynch, BSN
Instructor, Department of Preventive Medicine
Creighton University School of Medicine
Omaha, Nebraska
18 *Breast Cancer Genetics: Heterogeneity, Molecular Genetics, Syndrome Diagnosis, and Genetics Counseling*

Anne T. Mancino, MD, FACS
Associate Professor of Surgery
University of Arkansas for Medical Services
Chief, General Surgery
Central Arkansas Veterans Healthcare System
Little Rock, Arkansas
3 *Breast Physiology: Normal and Abnormal Development and Function*

John C. Mansour, MD
Department of Surgery
University of Wisconsin Hospital and Clinics
Madison, Wisconsin
32 *The Kinetics of Neoplastic Growth and Interval Breast Cancer*

Joseph N. Marcus, MD
Department of Pathology
Missouri Baptist Medical Center
St. Louis, Missouri
18 *Breast Cancer Genetics: Heterogeneity, Molecular Genetics, Syndrome Diagnosis, and Genetics Counseling*

Lawrence B. Marks, MD
Professor, Department of Radiation Oncology
Duke University Medical Center
Durham, North Carolina
56 *Radiotherapy Techniques*

Scot A. Martin, MD
Las Cruces, New Mexico
43 *Breast Reconstruction following Mastectomy*

Alvaro Martinez, MD, FACR
Chairman, Department of Radiation Oncology
William Beaumont Hospital
Royal Oak, Michigan
58 *Radiotherapy and Ductal Carcinoma In Situ*

Shahla Masood, MD
Department of Pathology
University of Florida Health Sciences Center
Jacksonville, Florida
34 *Cytologic Needle Samplings of the Breast: Techniques and End Results*

Marlene C. McCarthy, HLD
Chair, Rhode Island Breast Cancer Coalition
Providence, Rhode Island
85 *Patient and Family Resources*

John B. McCraw, MD
Department of Surgery
University of Mississippi Medical Center
Jackson, Mississippi
39 *General Principles of Mastectomy: Evaluation and Therapeutic Options*
43 *Breast Reconstruction following Mastectomy*

Ann McMellin, CST
Patient Care Specialist
Virginia Beach Plastic Surgery
Virginia Beach, Virginia
43 *Breast Reconstruction following Mastectomy*

Michael M. Meguid, MD, PhD
Professor, Department of Surgery and Neuroscience
  Program
Upstate Medical University
University Hospital
Syracuse, New York
5 *Subareolar Breast Abscess: The Penultimate Stage of the*
  Mammary Duct–Associated Inflammatory Disease
  Sequence

Nancy Price Mendenhall, MD
Professor and Chairman, Department of Radiation
  Oncology
Shands Cancer Center
University of Florida
Gainesville, Florida
65 *Radiotherapy for Locoregional Failure*
68 *Radiotherapy for Palliation*

Carolyn Mies, MD
Associate Professor of Pathology and Laboratory
  Medicine
Director, Breast Pathology Subspeciality Service
University of Pennsylvania
Philadelphia, Philadelphia
14 *Mammary Sarcoma and Lymphoma*

Suhail K. Mithani, MD
Resident, General Surgery
Johns Hopkins Hospital
Baltimore, Maryland
53 *Intraoperative Evaluation of Surgical Margins*
  in Breast-Conserving Therapy

Monica Morrow, MD
Professor of Surgery
Northwestern University Feinberg School of Medicine
Director, Lynn Sage Breast Program
Northwestern Memorial Hospital
Chicago, Illinois
49 *Therapeutic Value of Axillary Lymph Node Dissection*

Anne W. Moulton, MD
General and Internal Medicine
Rhode Island Hospital
Providence, Rhode Island
81 *Menopausal Hormone Therapy: Benefits, Risks, and*
  Alternatives

Diane Mullins, MD
Mountain Area Pathology Group
Asheville, North Carolina
15 *Epithelial Neoplasms and Dermatologic Disorders*

Neal Naff, MD
Assistant Professor of Neurosurgery
Johns Hopkins
Baltimore, Maryland
72 *Management of Central Nervous System Metastases*
  in Breast Cancer

John E. Niederhuber, MD
Professor
Departments of Surgery and Oncology
University of Wisconsin–Madison
Madison, Wisconsin
32 *The Kinetics of Neoplastic Growth and Interval Breast*
  Cancer

Patricia J. Numann, MD
Professor of Surgery
Director, Comprehensive Breast Care Program
Medical Director University Hospital
Syracuse, New York
5 *Subareolar Breast Abscess: The Penultimate Stage of the*
  Mammary Duct–Associated Inflammatory Disease
  Sequence

Albert Oler, MD, PhD
Formerly Assistant Professor of Pathology
State University of New York Health Science Center
Syracuse, New York
5 *Subareolar Breast Abscess: The Penultimate Stage of the*
  Mammary Duct–Associated Inflammatory Disease
  Sequence

Ruth M. O'Regan, MD
Assistant Professor of Hematology/Oncology
Director, Translational Breast Cancer Research
Winship Cancer Institute
Emory University
Atlanta, Georgia
24 *Steroid Hormone Receptors*

David L. Page, MD
Professor of Pathology and Epidemiology
Vanderbilt University Medical Center
Nashville, Tennessee
6 *Gynecomastia*
7 *Benign, High-Risk, and Premalignant Lesions of the*
  Breast
11 *In Situ Carcinomas of the Breast: Ductal Carcinoma In*
  Situ, Paget's Disease, Lobular Carcinoma In Situ
13 *Extent and Multicentricity of In Situ and Invasive*
  Carcinoma
23 *Risk Factors for Breast Carcinoma in Women with*
  Proliferative Breast Disease
78 *The Unknown Primary Presenting with Axillary*
  Lymphadenopathy
79 *Management of the Patient at High Risk*

Christoph Papp, MD
Professor, Department of Plastic, Aesthetic, and
  Reconstructive Surgery
Krankenhaus der Barmherzigen Brüder
Salzburg, Austria
43 *Breast Reconstruction following Mastectomy*

Lori Pierce, MD
Associate Professor, Department of Radiation Oncology
University of Michigan
Ann Arbor, Michigan
60 *Postmastectomy Radiotherapy*

Raphael E. Pollock, MD, PhD
Head of Division of Surgery
Professor and Chairman Department of Surgical
  Oncology
The University of Texas M.D. Anderson Cancer Center
Houston, Texas
63 *Surgical Procedures for Advanced Local and Regional
  Malignancies of the Breast*

Janet E. Price, DPhil
The University of Texas M.D. Anderson Cancer Center
Houston, Texas
26 *Concepts and Mechanisms of Breast Cancer Metastasis*

Christopher A. Puleo, PA-C
H. Lee Moffitt Cancer Center and Research Institute at
  The University of South Florida
Tampa, Florida
46 *Lymphedema in the Postmastectomy Patient:
  Pathophysiology, Prevention, and Management*

Abram Recht, MD
Associate Professor
Department of Radiation Oncology
Harvard Medical School
Senior Radiation Oncologist and Deputy Chief
Department of Radiation Oncology
Beth Israel Deaconess Medical Center
Boston, Massachusetts
57 *Radiotherapy for Locally Advanced Disease*
59 *Radiotherapy and Regional Nodes*

Douglas S. Reintgen, MD
Director, Lakeland Regional Cancer Center
Lakeland, Florida
46 *Lymphedema in the Postmastectomy Patient:
  Pathophysiology, Prevention, and Management*

David S. Robinson, MD
Professor of Surgery
Paul G. Koontz, MD, Endowed Chair of Breast Disease
University of Missouri at Kansas City
Kansas City, Missouri
Comprehensive Breast Center
Coral Springs, Florida
33 *Stereotactic Imaging and Breast Biopsy*
77 *Carcinoma of the Breast in Pregnancy and Lactation*

Lynn J. Romrell, PhD
Professor, Anatomy and Cell Biology
Associate Dean, Medical Education
University of Florida College of Medicine
Gainesville, Florida
2 *Anatomy of the Breast, Axilla, Chest Wall, and Related
  Metastatic Sites*
8 *Congenital and Acquired Disturbances of Breast
  Development and Growth*

Ernest L. Rosato, MD
Thomas Jefferson Medical College
Philadelphia, Philadelphia
30 *Examination Techniques: Roles of the Physician
  and Patient in Evaluating Breast Diseases*

Francis E. Rosato, MD
Professor of Surgery
Thomas Jefferson Medical College
Philadelphia, Philadelphia
30 *Examination Techniques: Roles of the Physician
  and Patient in Evaluating Breast Diseases*

Arlan L. Rosenbloom, MD
Division of Pediatric Endocrinology
University of Florida
Gainesville, Florida
3 *Breast Physiology: Normal and Abnormal Development
  and Function*

Wendy S. Rubinstein, MD, PhD, FACMG
Medical Director, Evanston Northwestern Healthcare
  Center for Medical Genetics
Assistant Professor of Medicine
Northwestern University Feinberg School of Medicine
Chief, Division of Genetics
Evanston Hospital
Evanston, Illinois
18 *Breast Cancer Genetics: Heterogeneity, Molecular
  Genetics, Syndrome Diagnosis, and Genetics Counseling*

Gordon Francis Schwartz, MD, MBA
Professor of Surgery
Jefferson Medical College
Attending Surgeon, Thomas Jefferson University
  Hospital
Consultant Surgeon, Pennsylvania Hospital
Philadelphia, Philadelphia
47 *Biology and Management of Lobular Carcinoma In Situ
  of the Breast*

Mark Shiroishi, MD
Resident, Department of Radiological Sciences
David Geffen School of Medicine at UCLA
Los Angeles, California
31 *Breast Imaging*

Melvin J. Silverstein, MD
University of Southern California
Norris Comprehensive Cancer Center
Los Angeles, California
48 *Ductal Carcinoma In Situ: Diagnostic and Therapeutic Controversies*

Rache M. Simmons, MD
Associate Professor of Surgery
Weill Medical School of Cornell University
New York, New York
55 *Image-Guided Ablation of Breast Tumors*

Jean F. Simpson, MD
Department of Pathology
Vanderbilt School of Medicine
Nashville, Tennessee
7 *Benign, High-Risk, and Premalignant Lesions of the Breast*
12 *Malignant Neoplasia of the Breast: Infiltrating Carcinomas*

Karan P. Singh, PhD
Department of Biostatistics
University of Alabama at Birmingham
Birmingham, Alabama
36 *Design and Conduct of Clinical Trials for Breast Cancer*

S. Eva Singletary, MD
Professor of Surgical Oncology
Department of Surgical Oncology
The University of Texas M.D. Anderson Cancer Center
Houston, Texas
22 *Investigational and Molecular Prognostic Factors for Breast Carcinoma*

George W. Sledge, Jr., MD
Professor of Medicine
Indiana University Medical Center
Indianapolis, Indiana
69 *Chemotherapy for Metastatic Breast Cancer*

Nicolas Slenkovich, MD
University of Alabama at Birmingham
Birmingham, Alabama
43 *Breast Reconstruction following Mastectomy*

Carrie L. Snyder, RN, BSN, OCN
Department of Preventive Medicine
Creighton University
Omaha, Nebraska
18 *Breast Cancer Genetics: Heterogeneity, Molecular Genetics, Syndrome Diagnosis, and Genetics Counseling*

Vered Stearns, MD
Assistant Professor of Oncology
The Sidney Kimmel Comprehensive Cancer Center at Johns Hopkins
Baltimore, Maryland
62 *Adjuvant Systemic Therapy of Breast Cancer*

Theresa V. Strong, PhD
Associate Professor, Department of Medicine
Gene Therapy Center
Birmingham, Alabama
27 *Gene Therapy of Breast Cancer*

Toncred M. Styblo, MD
Associate Professor of Surgery
Emory University School of Medicine
Atlanta, Georgia
21 *Clinically Established Prognostic Factors in Breast Cancer*

Magesh Sundaram, MD, FACS
Division of Surgical Oncology
Roger Williams Medical Center
Providence, Rhode Island
33 *Stereotactic Imaging and Breast Biopsy*
77 *Carcinoma of the Breast in Pregnancy and Lactation*

Daniel W. Tench, MD
Athens Regional Medical Center
Athens, Georgia
78 *The Unknown Primary Presenting with Axillary Lymphadenopathy*

Marshall M. Urist, MD
Champ Lyons Professor and Vice Chairman, Department of Surgery
University of Alabama at Birmingham
Birmingham, Alabama
38 *Indications and Techniques for Biopsy*

Luis O. Vásconez, MD
Division Director, Plastic Surgery
University of Alabama at Birmingham
Birmingham, Alabama
39 *General Principles of Mastectomy: Evaluation and Therapeutic Options*
43 *Breast Reconstruction following Mastectomy*
44 *Macromastia and Reduction Mammaplasty*

Frank A. Vicini, MD
Department of Radiation Oncology
William Beaumont Hospital
Royal Oak, Michigan
58 *Radiotherapy and Ductal Carcinoma In Situ*

Victor G. Vogel, MD, MHS, FACP
Director, Magee/UPCI Breast Cancer Prevention Program
University of Pittsburgh Cancer Institute
Professor of Medicine and Epidemiology
University of Pittsburgh School of Medicine
Magee-Womens Hospital
Pittsburgh, Philadelphia
16 *Epidemiology of Breast Cancer*
17 *Primary Prevention of Breast Cancer*

Frederick B. Wagner, Jr., MD, LHD
Grace Revere Osler Professor Emeritus of Surgery
Jefferson Medical College of Thomas Jefferson
  University
Honorary Doctor of Humane Letters
Thomas Jefferson University
Philadelphia, Pennsylvania
1 *History of the Therapy of Breast Cancer*

Edward J. Wilkinson, MD
Professor and Vice Chairman, Department of
  Pathology
University of Florida College of Medicine
Gainesville, Florida
12 *Malignant Neoplasia of the Breast: Infiltrating
Carcinomas*
34 *Cytologic Needle Samplings of the Breast: Techniques
and End Results*

David J. Winchester, MD, FACS
Associate Professor of Surgery
Northwestern University Feinberg School of Medicine
Evanston, Illinois
75 *Cancer of the Male Breast*

David P. Winchester, MD
Chairman, Department of Surgery
Evanston Northwestern Healthcare
Evanston, Illinois
75 *Cancer of the Male Breast*

Antonio C. Wolff, MD
Assistant Professor of Oncology
The Sidney Kimmel Comprehensive Cancer Center
  at Johns Hopkins
Baltimore, Maryland
62 *Adjuvant Systemic Therapy of Breast Cancer*

Carol Woo, MD
Breast Surgery
Fellowship Trained
Mid-Hudson Oncology, PLLC
Dyson Center for Cancer Care
Vassar Brothers Hospital
Poughkeepsie, New York
48 *Ductal Carcinoma In Situ: Diagnostic and Therapeutic
Controversies*

William C. Wood, MD
Joseph Brown Whitehead Professor and Chairman,
  Department of Surgery
Emory University School of Medicine
Atlanta, Georgia
21 *Clinically Established Prognostic Factors in Breast
Cancer*

Timothy J. Yeatman, MD
H. Lee Moffitt Cancer Center
Tampa, Florida
20 *Assessment and Designation of Breast Cancer Stage*

Rex C.W. Yung, MD
Assistant Professor of Medicine
Division of Pulmonary and Critical Care Medicine
Johns Hopkins University School of Medicine
Baltimore, Maryland
71 *Diagnosis and Management of Pleural Metastases
in Breast Cancer*

James R. Zabora, ScD, MSW
Dean, National Catholic School of Social Service
The Catholic University of America
Washington, DC
83 *Psychosocial Consequences of Breast Cancer*

Richard Zellars, MD
Assistant Professor of Oncology
Johns Hopkins Oncology Center
Baltimore, Maryland
72 *Management of Central Nervous System Metastases
in Breast Cancer*

Robert A. Zlotecki, MD, PhD
Department of Radiation Oncology
University of Florida
Gainesville, Florida
68 *Radiotherapy for Palliation*

FOREWORD

"In the world of surgical oncology: Biology is King, Selection is Queen, Technical manoeuvre is the Prince." Blake Cady

The third edition of *The Breast: Comprehensive Management of Benign and Malignant Diseases* again establishes itself as the premier textbook in this area. Consisting of 23 sections and 87 chapters, Bland and Copeland have brought together under this umbrella the foremost authorities on breast diseases. The contributors to the third edition are multinational and multidisciplinary, including a unique combination of basic scientists and clinicians whose synergistic efforts contribute to an outstanding edition.

As early as 3000 BC, the medical literature reflects an interest in tumors of the breast. Hippocrates, Celsus, and Galen made it clear in their writings that "up to and through the Middle Ages, use of the knife was shunned and decried" in preference to the use of ointments, caustic materials, salves, and vitriol. Special historical reference should be made to St. Agatha, the patron saint of "the breast, wet nurses and bell founders whose aid was sought in many diseases of the breast and in fire, colic and dysentery." In 1973 Haagensen stated that "we have taken a great leap backwards in the treatment of carcinoma of the breast."

Fisher, in contrast, ushered in a new era in studying breast cancer when he remarked that "breast cancer is a heterogeneous, systemic disease involving a complexity of host-tumor inter-relationships; variations in locoregional therapy are unlikely to affect survival substantially."

For generations, the breast has been the focal point of great emotion, increasing lay dialogue, scientific investigation, and diagnostic innovations. The diagnosis, treatment, and etiology of breast cancer have geometrically escalated, and for the better. Although public interest in this subject (the breast industry) is not of recent vintage, the medical literature graphically illustrates the continuing research efforts across many disciplines. All too often, physicians themselves do not possess the level of awareness and knowledge necessary to keep pace with consumer interest and demands, particularly with the advent of computers. Bland and Copeland have greatly assisted in bridging this deficit.

During the last decade, each year approximately 4500 to 5000 articles were published on breast diseases in the medical and surgical literature. Textbooks of this vintage are rare and a labor of love. Yokefellows Kirby Bland and Ted Copeland have combined their efforts to bring pride and knowledge to the discipline of surgery. The depth of this edition reflects their experience and the hands-on involvement of well-known clinicians. Information contained in these chapters represents a state-of-the-art knowledge in our understanding of bimolecular events involving the breast. The National Institutes of Health funding for research has doubled in the last decade. Their increased support for research, particularly translational investigations, has been important.

The Breast: Comprehensive Management of Benign and Malignant Diseases is a tour de force, including pertinent information regarding the history of the breast, its anatomy and physiology, congenital abnormalities, mastodynia, the heterogeneous expressions of breast cancer, counseling and psychosocial implications, the influence of hormones on the breast, immunotherapy, the application of biostatistics to clinical trials, and improved techniques in breast reconstruction.

This edition covers an increasing array of emerging diagnostic and therapeutic techniques in breast diseases. Of particular interest is the concentration in Sections III through V regarding benign diseases, an area receiving increasing attention in recent years. Improved diagnostic imaging, lymphatic mapping, and other technical changes have led to an earlier diagnosis of breast cancer with improved results. This up-to-date review of currently available diagnostic techniques and treatment patterns has affirmatively affected survivability. This is an excellent reference and is a must for your library.

Claude H. Organ, MD, FACS
Emeritus Professor
University of California, San Francisco–East Bay
President-Elect, American College of Surgeons

PREFACE

Universally, industrialized societies readily acknowledge the impact of breast disease in human society as a major epidemiologic issue that continues to expand exponentially. The biometry branch of the National Cancer Institute in the United States continues to recognize breast cancer as the most frequent carcinoma occurring in women. Furthermore, 1 of every 3 American women will consult a physician for breast diseases, and approximately 1 of every 4 women will undergo a breast biopsy. Of critical demographic importance, the lifetime risk for 1 of every 8 American women to develop an invasive carcinoma of the breast is significant and continues to enlarge. Moreover, current estimates suggest that the rapidly evolving diagnosis of ductal carcinoma in situ may represent as great as one fourth of all breast cancers diagnosed within the next two decades. All these demographic features support the concern of the epidemiologic increase for diagnosis of this neoplasm.

The first edition of *The Breast*, published in 1991, placed the diagnosis and therapy of breast disease in a working perspective, integrating contemporary, multidisciplinary oncologic principles and therapeutic approaches. The latter included surgery, radiation oncology, pathology, medical oncology, radiology, pharmacokinetics, genetics, transplantation, and biostatistics. These disciplines are synergistic in that they support the mission of hospice, social services, and psychosocial support teams to holistically treat all aspects of breast disease. Moreover, each medical discipline has pursued an evolutionary process as new therapeutic modalities were added, which has enhanced clinical outcomes and patient care.

Since the second edition was published in 1998, unprecedented progress in the therapy of breast diseases has been evident. Surgery and medicine have, in general, evolved very rapidly as a consequence of notable scientific events: (1) an enlargement for the identification of breakthrough molecular and genetic subdisease process understanding with expansion of the knowledge base for phenotypically normal and abnormal (proliferative) disease processes (e.g., cancer genetics, cellular regulatory events in carcinogenesis, carcinoma initiation and disease progression, invasion and metastasis, molecular diagnostic and prognostic markers); (2) DNA sequencing of the human genome with identification of mutational variance that affects genetic progression and phenotypic expression; (3) innovative therapeutic advents such as immunotherapy, gene therapy, bone marrow transplantation, angiogenesis inhibitors, and other technical approaches that employ (and exploit) new knowledge of biology; (4) an emerging perspective that properly guides clinical outcomes research; and (5) advances in surgical techniques and technology. At present, no other human organ system has had the integration of multimodal diagnostic and therapeutic approaches that are as recognized, focused, and successful as those that have been developed for breast neoplasms.

The third edition of *The Breast* represents a comprehensive reference that was developed with the intent of being highly readable for all medical researchers and clinicians and that reviews the basic tenets essential for diagnosis and therapy of the various benign and malignant disorders of the breast. The Editors have sought to develop the proper address of many recognized abnormalities presenting in the diagnosis and therapy of metabolic, physiologic, and neoplastic derangements of the organ. When we compare this edition with the first and second editions, we consider the present text to be even more thorough, inclusive, and relevant to scientific and clinical achievements.

Moreover, it is our considered opinion that the current edition will meet the requirements of young clinicians and scientists to acquire fundamental knowledge of basic, clinical, and laboratory concepts and techniques that will complement their oncology training. Integration of these principles with advancements in technologic, molecular, cellular, and biologic sciences represents the twenty-first century definition of each specialty involved with the care of breast disease. However, the ultimate measure of professional skill and effectiveness expected of us as clinicians in the management of breast diseases will be the quality that this text brings to bear upon patient outcomes, as well as emotional and physical morbidity.

The third edition is not intended to replace standard textbooks of surgery and medicine, nor is this edition considered an encyclopedic recitation of the myriad of pathologic permutations that exist with various disorders of this organ site. This edition of *The Breast*, however, should coexist with, and not substitute for, other major medical and surgical reference books. Each chapter is selectively organized and supported with notations of carefully selected journal articles, monographs, or chapters within major reference texts that the contributors of these specific subjects consider a valuable resource. Thus this work represents a distillation of the herald contributions of innumerable physicians, physiologists, anatomists, geneticists, clinical scientists, and noted health-related workers who have devoted their careers and research to the management of various disorders of the breast.

The third edition represents 23 sections and 87 chapters, with at least 30% more information than the second edition. The opening section documents the historical aspects of breast disease, incorporating the major scientific contributions of investigators and surgeons of the nineteenth and twentieth centuries. This section follows with pertinent physiology, anatomy, pathology, genetics, molecular biology, pharmacokinetics, surgery, radiation biology, medical oncology, and biostatistics. Throughout the third edition, authors and co-authors have sought to supplement the text with supportive history of the evolution and chronology of therapeutic principles. In addition, special sections are dedicated to the management of unusual and advanced presentations of the disease.

Additional chapters provide new approaches to the management of breast pain and the risk for carcinoma of the breast following hormonal replacement therapy; a chapter is included that defines patterns of recurrence. The significant evolution of precise staging evident with lymphatic mapping and sentinel lymph node biopsy has been addressed in depth and provides a new level of precise documentation of technique and outcomes as a consequence of the international experience with the technique since the completion of the second. The authors also have strived to incorporate new approaches for gene therapy and counseling for genetic mutations, angiogenesis, immunology, and the evolving role for the immunotherapy of breast cancer. Furthermore, applications of nutritional management and evolving psychologic principles are incorporated in the text. Two chapters, again, are dedicated to addressing legal issues that relate to the management of breast disease. An additional chapter documents the nationwide resources available to both patients and practitioners. Chapters are also dedicated in this edition to covering the psychologic considerations of breast disease and its implications, which affect patient, spouse, and family members.

Inevitably, overlap will continue to exist among several chapters as a consequence of the dynamic interplay and expectations of medical and surgical practitioners involved with the diagnostic and therapeutic management of the cancer patient. However, the Editors have made every effort to minimize repetitious remarks and dedicated comments except where controversial or "state-of-the art" issues for management exist.

A salient attribute of the text includes the integration of basic science with translational research to emphasize efforts at transfer of knowledge from the bench laboratory to the bedside and the clinic. Only with evolving applications of phase II and phase III trials can the clinician objectively assess the therapeutic value of evolving technical and therapeutic management strategies. These translational research objectives will continue to evaluate promising chemotherapeutics, immunologic agents, inhibitors of angiogenesis, and additional molecularly engineered products that have promise to inhibit neoplastic progression in this organ.

The authors, again, are hopeful that the third edition of *The Breast* has achieved its developmental and scientific goals for assimilating and collating contemporary basic and clinical scientific data to provide clinicians and researchers with multidisciplinary principles used in practice for the treatment of diseases of the breast. We gratefully acknowledge the opportunity provided by the immense challenge that has been entrusted to us by the publisher and are, again, hopeful that our diligence to task has been properly served.

Kirby I. Bland
Edward M. Copeland III

ACKNOWLEDGMENTS

The Editors are deeply indebted to the authors and their co-authors who have contributed to the third edition of *The Breast: Comprehensive Management of Benign and Malignant Diseases*. It is the view of the Editors and Associate Editors that this most recent edition is the most comprehensive international reference on diseases of the breast. Both the Editors and Associate Editors have strived to embellish pertinent clinical trials with basic and translational surgical science that has appropriate outcomes when applied in the clinics. Therefore we are deeply indebted to the Associate Editors and to all contributors for their efforts toward the completion of this comprehensive work.

The untold hours essential to properly prepare this treatise represent time taken from busy clinical practices, research laboratories, and our families. Thus the diligent efforts of the contributors to provide insightful state-of-the art presentations are gratefully acknowledged. Furthermore, the updating of proper scientific knowledge by these contributors is therefore praiseworthy, with their choice of selective illustrations, tables, and references to bring this text to its readable state of completeness and comprehensiveness.

The Editors further wish to pay tribute to the diligent work by the staff members of the W.B. Saunders Company, who have made publication of the third edition possible. Special appreciation should also be paid to Louis Reines, former President of W.B. Saunders, who always provided strong encouragement and support for initiation of the first, second, and now, the third editions of this tome. Lisette Bralow, former Vice President and Editor-In-Chief for medical books of W.B. Saunders, provided strong support for completion of this edition, which has currently been supervised in an extraordinary and skillful manner by Mr. Joe Rusko. Arlene Chappelle, developmental editor for the book, was instrumental in organizing oversight of the editorial process, procurement of manuscripts, and scheduling.

For these noteworthy contributions, the Editors and Associate Editors are most appreciative.

We further thank our editorial staff: Carol Ann Moore, Donna Manning, Connie Weldon, and Cindy deSa, who examined materials to ensure they were as flawless as possible. I am also grateful to all editorial assistants in the Departments of Surgery at the University of Alabama at Birmingham, as well as our (KIB, EMC) former secretary and editorial assistant, Ervene Katz, of the University of Florida, who has retired since the publication of this edition. We also express gratitude to Louis Clark and Jonathan Bland, the principal artists who skillfully prepared the illustrations and line drawings used throughout various chapters of the text.

The Editors and Associate Editors are all deeply appreciative for our Residents and Research Fellows in Surgery, Medicine, Pathology, and Radiation Oncology for their intellectual stimulation and their continual encouragement to proceed with development of the third edition. To the faculty and residents who have reviewed manuscripts, rendered opinions, and offered suggestions, we gratefully acknowledge their critiques, enlightening commentary, and sustained interest.

Finally, to all who were involved with the development of this text, inclusive of our immediate families and friends who expressed interest and encouragement in the completion of this textbook, we greatly appreciate your indulgence for the time allowed for us to pursue the ambitious goal of preparing what we consider to be a readable, comprehensive text that properly embraces the tenets essential for the diagnosis and therapy of breast diseases. The Editors and Associate Editors further realize that the goals organized and accomplished by the editorial staff and the publisher for the third edition could have been achieved only with the immense dedication to task that is evident in the contributions of the authors of each chapter, the artists, and our dedicated editorial assistants.

Kirby I. Bland
Edward M. Copeland III

CONTENTS

THE BREAST

Comprehensive Management of
Benign and Malignant Disorders

I

HISTORY OF THE THERAPY OF BREAST CANCER

CHAPTER

1

History of the Therapy of Breast Cancer

SAMUEL W. BEENKEN
FREDERICK B. WANGER, JR.
KIRBY I. BLAND

Chapter Outline

Cancer of the breast, with its uncertain cause, has captured the attention of physicians throughout the ages. Despite centuries of theoretical meanderings and scientific inquiry, breast cancer remains one of the most dreaded of human diseases. The story of efforts to cope with breast cancer is complex, and there is no happy ending as in diseases for which cause and cure have been found. However, progress has been made in lessening the horrors that formerly devastated the body and psyche.

This chapter records some of the key milestones in the development of our current understanding of the biology and therapy of breast cancer, which is based on the achievements and contributions of many doctors and scientists over many hundreds of years. Although the milestones listed here are important ones, the list is by no means comprehensive. This chapter is meant to be a useful reference to all those who would like to know more about the historical background of breast cancer and about the development of modern breast cancer therapy.

Ancient Civilizations

CHINESE

Huang Di, the Yellow Emperor, was born in 2698 BCE and subsequently wrote the *Nei Jing*, the oldest treatise of medicine, which gives the first description of tumors and documents five forms of therapy: spiritual care, pharmacology, diet, acupuncture, and the treatment of specific diseases.

EGYPTIAN

Imhotep, an Egyptian physician, architect, and astrologer, was born in 2650 BCE. He designed the first pyramid at Saqqara and was deified as the god of healing. The early Egyptians documented many cases of breast tumors, which were treated with cautery. To preserve their findings, the Egyptians etched their cursive script on thin sheets of papyrus leaf and also engraved or painted hieroglyphics on stone. Among six principal papyri, the most informative one with respect to diseases of the breast is that acquired by Edwin Smith (b. 1822) in 1862 and presented to the New York Historical Society at the time of his death. Dating to about 1600 BCE, it is a papyrus roll 15 feet long, with writing on both sides.[1] The front contains 17 columns describing 48 cases devoted to clinical surgery. References are made to diseases of the breast such as abscesses, trauma, and infected wounds. Case 45 is perhaps the earliest recording of breast cancer, with the title *Instructions Concerning Tumors on His Breast* (Figure 1-1). The examiner is told that a breast with bulging tumors, very cool to the touch, is an ailment for which there is no treatment.

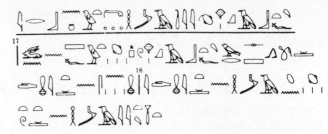

FIG. **1-1** Recording of the earliest known case of breast cancer (1600 BCE). (*From the* Edwin Smith Papyrus. *Published in facsimile and hieroglyphic transliteration with translation and commentary by James Henry Breasted. Birmingham, AL, The Classics of Medicine Library, 1984. Reprinted with permission.*)

BABYLONIAN

The Code of Hammurabi (ca. 1750 BCE) was commissioned in Babylon. Its 282 clauses provided the first laws that regulated medical practitioners and dealt with physicians' responsibilities and fees. At that time, internal medicine consisted mainly of a recitation of litanies and incantations against the demons of the earth, air, and water. Surgery consisted of opening an abscess with a bronze lancet. If the patient died or lost an eye during treatment, the physician's hands were cut off.

CLASSIC GREEK PERIOD (460 TO 136 BCE)

Medicine in Europe had its origins in ancient Greece. The scientific method and clinical advancement of medicine is credited to Hippocrates (b. 460 BCE), who also defined its ethical ideals. His basic philosophy was the linkage of four cardinal body humors (blood, phlegm, yellow bile, and black bile) with four universal elements (earth, air, water, and fire). Perfect health depended on a proper balance in the dynamic qualities of the humors. It was generally believed that blood was in the arteries and veins, phlegm in the brain, yellow bile in the liver, and black bile in the spleen. Hippocrates divided diseases into three general categories: those curable by medicine (most favorable), those not curable by medicine but curable by the knife, and those not curable by the knife but curable by fire. The *Corpus Hippocraticum* deals with the treatment of fractures, tumors, surgery, asthma, allergies, and diseases of the skin. A well-documented case history of Hippocrates describes a woman with breast cancer associated with bloody discharge from the nipple. Hippocrates associated breast cancer with cessation of menstruation, leading to breast engorgement and indurated nodules.

Alexandria on the Nile, founded by Alexander the Great in 332 BCE, became the focal point of Greek science during the third and second centuries BCE. More than 14,000 students studied various elements of Hellenistic knowledge there. This knowledge was contained in

700,000 scrolls in the largest library in antiquity, which was subsequently destroyed by Julius Caesar. Rudimentary anatomic studies were conducted and led to progress in the tools and techniques of surgery.

GRECO-ROMAN PERIOD (150 BCE TO 500 AD)

Following the destruction of Corinth in 146 BCE, Greek medicine migrated to Rome. During the preceding six centuries, the Romans had lived without physicians. They depended on medicinal herbs, assorted concoctions, votive objects, religious rites, and superstitions (Figure 1-2).

Aurelius Celsus, a Roman born in 25 BCE, described the cardinal signs of inflammation (calor, rubor, dolar, and turgor). He wrote *De Medicina* around 30 AD, which contains an early clinical description of cancer. In it he mentions the breasts of women as one of the sites of cancer and describes a fixed irregular swelling with dilated tortuous veins and ulceration. He also delineates four clinical stages of cancer: early cancer, cancer without ulcer, ulcerated cancer, and ulcerated cancer with cauliflower-like excrescences that bled easily. Celsus opposed treatment of the last three stages by any method, because aggressive measures irritated the condition and led to inevitable recurrence.

The Greek physician Leonides is credited with the first operative treatment for breast cancer in the first century AD. His method consisted of an initial incision into the uninvolved portion of the breast, followed by applications of cautery to stop the bleeding. Repeated incisions and applications of cautery were continued until the entire breast and tumor had been removed and the underlying tissues were covered with an eschar. With Roman influence and support, surgical instruments became highly specialized, as witnessed by the finding of more than 200 different instruments in the excavations of Pompei and Herculaneum (Figures 1-3 and 1-4).

The greatest Greek physician to follow Hippocrates was Galen (b. 131 AD). He was born on the Mediterranean coast of Asia Minor, studied in Alexandria, and practiced medicine for the rest of his life in Rome. He is credited as the founder of experimental physiology, and his system of pathology followed that of Hippocrates.

Galen considered black bile, especially when it was extremely dark or thick, to be the most harmful of the four humors and the ultimate cause of cancer. He described breast cancer as a swelling with distended veins resembling the shape of a crab's legs. To prevent accumulation of black bile, Galen advocated the patient be purged and bled. He claimed to have cured the disease in its early stage when the tumor was on the surface of the body and all the "roots" could be extirpated at surgery. The roots were not derived from the tumor but were dilated veins filled with morbid black bile. When removing the tumor, the surgeon had to be aware of the danger of profuse hemorrhage from large blood vessels. On the other hand, the surgeon was advised to allow the blood to flow freely for a while to allow the black blood to escape.

Middle Ages

The Middle Ages may be considered the period between the downfall of Rome and the beginning of the Renaissance. The doctrine of the four humors, which formed the basis of Hippocratic medicine, was endowed with authority by Galen and governed all aspects of medical thinking throughout and beyond the Middle Ages. This influence can be traced in the Christian, Jewish, and Arabic traditions.

CHRISTIAN

From the Christian standpoint, the monks and clerics who constituted the educated class maintained medicine in the Middle Ages. In 529, with the founding by Saint

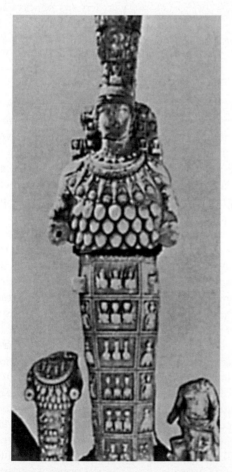

FIG. **1-2** Statue of Diana of Ephesus, a fertility deity invoked by Roman women, displaying 20 accessory pectoral breasts. (*From Haagensen CD: Diseases of the breast, ed 2, Philadelphia, 1971, WB Saunders.*)

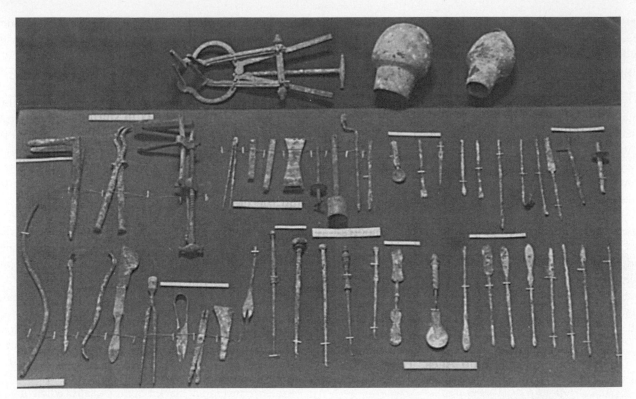

FIG. **1-3** Surgical instruments (79 AD) from excavations of Pompei and Herculaneum. (*Courtesy Archives of Thomas Jefferson University, Philadelphia, PA.*)

Benedict of the Monastery on Monte Cassino in central Italy, there arose a heightened interest in medicine in the scattered cloisters of the Roman Church. Monte Cassino fostered the teaching and practice of medicine, along with the copying and preserving of ancient manuscripts. Many satellite monasteries developed throughout Christendom in which the monks treated the sick and copied medical manuscripts. Subsequently, monastic schools spread under the Benedictines to England,

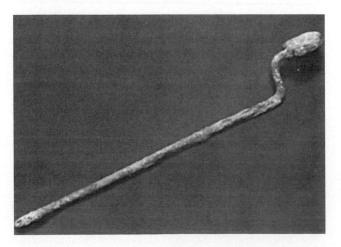

FIG. **1-4** Roman cautery (79 AD) depicted from Figure 1-3.

Scotland, Ireland, France, Switzerland, and most of the European continent. The patron saint for breast disease was Saint Agatha. She had been a martyr in Sicily in the middle of the third century when her two breasts were torn off with iron shears because of resistance to the advances of the governor Quinctianus (Figure 1-5). On Saint Agatha's day, two loaves of bread representing her breasts are carried in procession on a tray.

The Council of Rheims (1131) excluded monks and the clergy from the practice of medicine. From that time on, laymen increasingly carried on medical teaching and practice. Cathedral schools, although in clerical hands, profited from greater freedom than the monasteries had provided and enjoyed the intellectual contacts of the large cities. Further growth of cities in the eleventh and twelfth centuries led to the rise of universities, which led to the removal of medicine from monastic influence.

Paul of Aegina (b. 625) was an Alexandrian physician and surgeon famed for his *Epitomae Medicae Libri Septem*, which contained descriptions of trephining, tonsillotomy, paracentesis, and mastectomy. Lanfranc of Milan (b. 1250) was an Italian surgeon who worked in Paris and wrote *Chirurgia Magna*, which contained sections on anatomy, embryology, ulcers, fistulas, and fractures, as well as sections on herbs and pharmacy and on cancer of the breast.

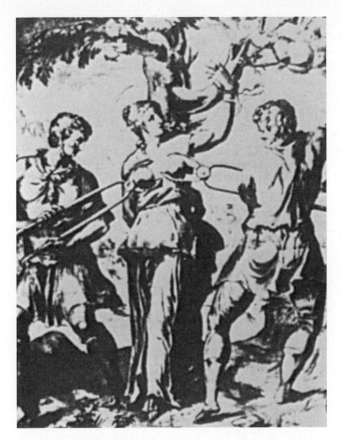

FIG. **1-5** Martyrdom of Saint Agatha. (*From Robinson JO: Am J Surg 151:318, 1986.*)

JEWISH

Jewish physicians were active at Salerno, Spain, as early as the ninth century. They achieved great distinction not only in the art of healing but also in their literary efforts. Popes, kings, and noblemen sought their services. In a time when poisoning of enemies and rivals was common, the Jews were considered the safest medical advisers. The Arabian rulers and Egyptian caliphs also preferred them to their Mohammedan doctors, who practiced magic and astrology in their treatment of disease.

Under the tolerant Moors of Spain and the early Christian rulers of Spain and Portugal, the Jews became leaders in the medical profession. The foremost among them was Moses Maimonides. Born in Cordova, Spain, in 1135, he studied medicine at Cairo and became the physician to Saladin, the Sultan of Egypt. In addition to his own medical treatise, he translated from Arabic into Hebrew the five volume *al-Quanum fil-Tibb* of the Iranian physician Avicenna (b. 980), which was the authoritative encyclopedia of medicine during the Middle Ages. Maimonides also made a collection of the aphorisms of Hippocrates and Galen.

Jewish physicians remained prominent in Spain under the Western Caliphate until they were banished from the country in 1492. The Salerno School exploited them as teachers until it had enough indigenous talent to proceed without them. Even at Montpellier in southern France the Jews were excluded in 1301. It would not be until the onset of the modern industrial age that they would again be admitted to citizenship throughout Europe and given university freedom, which once more liberated their brilliant medical talent.

ARABIC

Western society is indebted to Arabic scholars and physicians who valued and preserved the teachings and writings of their Greek predecessors. Without the intervention of the Arabs, the writings of the Greek physicians might have been lost. Baghdad, the capital of the Islamic Empire in Iraq, became the center for translation of the Greek authors. The library at Cordova had 600,000 manuscripts, and the one at Cairo had 18 rooms of books. The Tartars raided the library in Baghdad in 1260 and threw the books into the river.

Rhazes (b. 860), one of the great Arabic physicians, condoned excision of breast cancer only if it could be completely removed and the underlying tissues cauterized. He warned that incising a breast cancer would produce an ulceration. Haly ben Abbas, a Persian who died in 994, authored an encyclopedic work in medicine and surgery based on Rhazes and the Greek sources. He endorsed the removal of breast cancers with allowance for bleeding to evacuate melancholic humors, which were widely believed to predispose to cancer. He did not tie the arteries and made no mention of cautery. Avicenna was the successor to Haly ben Abbas and was known as the "Prince of Physicians." He was chief physician to the hospital at Baghdad and was the author of a vast scientific and philosophical encyclopedia, *Kitab-ash-shifa*, as well as the *al-Quanum fil-Tib*, both of which remained authoritative references for centuries.

The Renaissance

The transition from the medieval to the modern era occurred in the latter part of the fifteenth century, with the introduction of gunpowder into warfare, the discovery of America, and the invention of the printing press. During this period, medical teaching flourished in universities in Montpellier, Bologna, Padua, Paris, Oxford, and Cambridge.

Andreas Vesalius (b. 1514) was a Flemish physician who revolutionized the study of medicine with his detailed descriptions of the anatomy of the human body, based on his own dissection of cadavers. While at the University of Padua, he wrote and illustrated the first comprehensive textbook of anatomy, *De Humani*

Corporis Fabrica Libri Septem (1543). He recommended mastectomy for breast cancer and the use of sutures rather than cautery to control bleeding.

Ambrose Paré (b. 1510) studied medicine in Paris and through his war experience became the greatest surgeon of his time. His conservative surgical approach to cancer was detailed in *Oeuvres Complètes* (1575). He encouraged the use of vascular ligatures and avoidance of cautery and boiling oil. He condoned the excision of superficial breast cancers but attempted to treat other breast cancers through application of lead plates, which were intended to compress the blood supply and arrest tumor growth. He made the important observation that breast cancer often caused swelling of the axillary "glands." Michael Servetus (b. 1509), a Spaniard who studied in Paris, was burned at the stake for his heretical discovery that blood in the pulmonary circulation passes into the heart after having been mixed with air in the lungs. For cancer of the breast, Servetus suggested that the underlying pectoralis muscles be removed as well as the axillary glands described by Paré.

Wilhelm Fabry (b. 1560) is held in esteem as the "Father of German Surgery." His name was honored by the placement of a wreath at his statue in Hilden near Düsseldorf, Germany, by members of the International Society of the History of Medicine in 1986 (Figure 1-6). He devised an instrument (Figure 1-7) that compressed and fixed the base of the breast so that a knife could amputate it more swiftly and less painfully.[2] His text, *Opera,* included clear descriptions of breast cancer operations and illustrations of amputation forceps. He stipulated that the tumor should be mobile so that it could be removed completely, with no remnants being left behind. The other famous German surgeon of this period was Johann Schultes (b. 1595), known as Scultetus, who was an illustrator of surgery and inventor

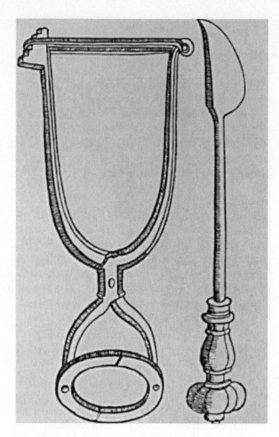

FIG. **1-7** Mastectomy instruments of Fabry von Hilden in late sixteenth century. (*From Robinson JO:* Am J Surg *151:319, 1986.*)

of surgical instruments. His book, *Armamentarium Chirurgicum,* which was published posthumously in 1653, contained illustrations of surgical procedures, one of which represented amputation of the breast. He used heavy ligatures on large needles, which transfixed the breast so that traction would facilitate its removal by the knife. Hemostasis was secured by cauterization of the base of the tumor (Figure 1-8).

Because of the morbidity and mortality of breast cancer surgery and a paucity of competent surgeons, few breast amputations were actually performed. Nonsurgical remedies for breast cancer appeared in rudimentary scientific journals that were published toward the end of the century (Figure 1-9).

Eighteenth Century

The 1700s were slow to develop significant new concepts in pathology and physiology. The arbitrary separation of scirrhus and breast cancer in the doctrine of Galen was still held. Scirrhus was considered by most to be a benign growth that under adverse circumstances could undergo malignant degeneration, whereas others

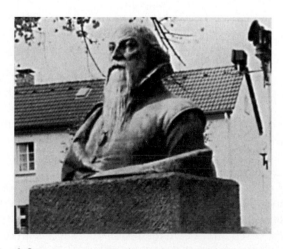

FIG. **1-6** Statue of Wilhelm Fabry in Hilden, Germany. (*Courtesy Dr. Ellen Wiederhold, Burgermeister of Hilden.*)

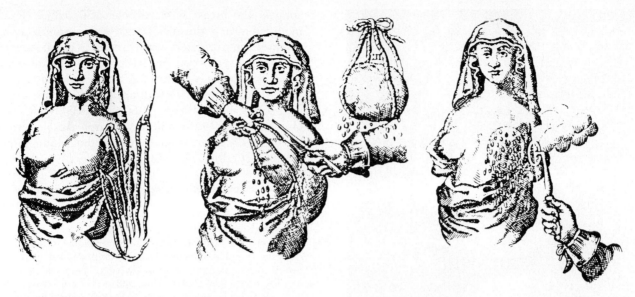

FIG. **1-8** Mastectomy procedure of Scultetus in the seventeenth century. (*Courtesy Robinson JO:* Am J Surg *151:320, 1986.*)

regarded it as an existing stage of cancer. Most believed that scirrhus originated in stagnation and coagulation of body fluids within the breast (local cause). Others believed it to occur from a general internal derangement of the body juices (systemic cause). In accepting both causes, some authors wrote that the local cause could be a precipitating factor in a predisposed patient. Hermann Boerhaave (b. 1668) taught that Galen's yellow bile was blood serum rather than bile itself, that phlegm was serum that had been altered by standing, and that black bile was a part of a clot that had separated off and become a darker color. Thus the four humors of Galen were only different components of the blood. Pieter Camper (b. 1722) described and illustrated the internal mammary lymph nodes, and Paolo Mascagni (b. 1752) did the same for the pectoral lymph nodes. Death caused by metastasis from breast cancer was not yet understood. If death was not caused by hemorrhage, it was ascribed to a general decomposition of the humors.

In Edinburgh, Scotland, which was strongly oriented to university teaching, the separation of surgeons from

For blood of the breasts.
Take two dramms of Leeks-feed, and yrrhe, it stancheth the blood that cometh out of the breast by spitting, although it bee grief to the teeth and roat.

FIG. **1-9** Home remedy "for blood of the breasts" (1664).

barbers was accomplished by 1718. In London, where barber-surgeon guilds had existed, the separation occurred in 1745. A new era of British surgery was instituted when William Cheselden (b. 1688), surgeon to St. Thomas' and St. George's Hospitals, first established private courses in anatomy and surgery. The Hunter brothers, John (b. 1728) and William (b. 1718), followed suit. These courses attracted students from all over the country, the continent, and America. John Hunter is credited as being the founder of experimental surgery and surgical pathology.

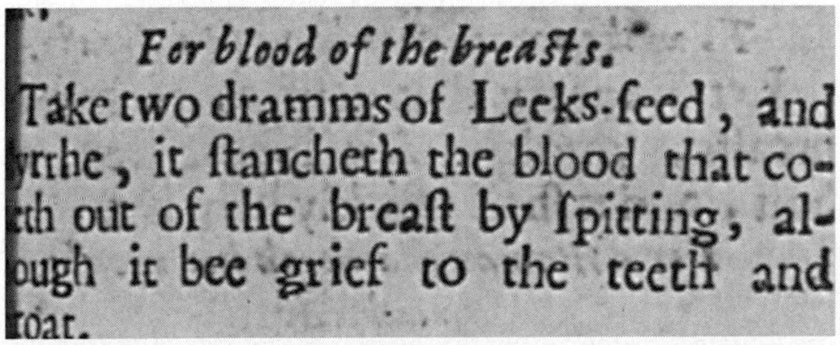

Henri le Dran (b. 1685) of France (Figure 1-10) concluded that cancer was a local disease in its early stages and that its spread to the lymphatic system signaled a worsened prognosis.[3] This was a courageous contradiction to the humoral theory of Galen, which had persisted for a thousand years and was to be upheld by many for two centuries to come. A colleague of le Dran, Jean Petit (b. 1674), first Director of the French Academy of Surgery, supported these principles. He advocated removal of the breast, the underlying pectoral muscle, and the axillary lymph nodes.[4] Another French surgeon, Bernard Pehrilhe, attempted to transmit cancer by injecting human breast cancer tissue into dogs.

The German surgeon Lorenz Heister (b. 1683) favored the use of a guillotine machine for breast tumors using the traction strings of Scultetus. This not only was rapid but also removed all the skin of the breast. Heister described the patient-surgeon relationship as follows: "Many females can stand the operation with the greatest courage and without hardly moaning at all. Others, however, make such a clamour that they may

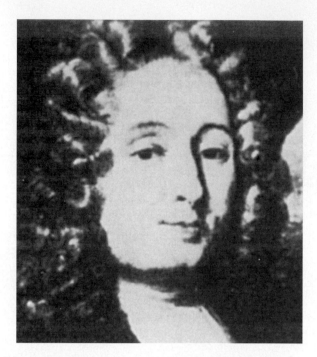

FIG. **1-10** Henri François le Dran (1685-1770) noted that lymphatic spread worsened the prognosis of breast cancer. (*From Robinson JO: Am J Surg 151:321, 1986.*)

dishearten even the most undaunted surgeon and hinder the operation. To perform the operation, the surgeon should therefore be steadfast and not allow himself to become disconcerted by the cries of the patient."

Large numbers of mastectomies were performed during the early eighteenth century, but this number decreased during the second half of the century because of poor results and the indiscriminate mutilation that occurred with improper patient selection and with physician bias. In 1757 it was reported that in Amsterdam, a densely populated town with 200,000 inhabitants, "not six times a year a breast was amputated with reasonable chance of a cure."

Nineteenth Century

Breast surgery changed dramatically in the 1800s: William Morton introduced anesthesia in the United States in 1846, while Joseph Lister introduced the principle of antisepsis in England in 1867.

EUROPEAN SURGERY

At the beginning of the nineteenth century, the treatment for breast cancer remained in confusion. In 1811 Samuel Young in England revived the method of Paré, in which compression was used to cut off the blood supply of the tumor.[5] Nooth, another English surgeon, sprayed the breast with carbolic acid, which was a modified form of the ancient practice of cauterization.

James Syme (b. 1799) was a famous Scottish surgeon. His daughter married Sir Joseph Lister. Much of his breast surgery was performed before the use of anesthesia.[6] His third surgical apprentice, John Brown (b. 1810), wrote *Rab and His Friends* (1858), which contains a vivid description of breast surgery as performed by the then 28-year-old Syme in the Minto House Hospital of Edinburgh, Scotland.

The operating theater is crowded; much talk and fun and all the cordiality and stir of youth. The surgeon with his staff of assistants is there. In comes Allie (the patient): one look at her quiets and abates the eager students. Allie stepped upon a seat, and laid herself on the table, as her friend the surgeon told her; arranged herself, gave a rapid look at James (her husband), shut her eyes, rested herself on me (Brown), and took my hand. The operation was at once begun; it was necessarily slow; and chloroform—one of God's best gifts to his suffering children—was then unknown. The surgeon did his work. The pale face showed its pain, but was still and silent. Rab's (a mastiff) soul was working within him; he saw that something strange was going on—blood flowing from his mistress, and she suffering; his ragged ear was up, and importunate; he growled and gave now and then a sharp impatient yelp; he would have liked to have done something to that man. But James had him firm, and gave him a glower from time to time, and an intimation of a possible kick—all the better for James, it kept his eye and his mind off Allie. It is over: she is dressed, steps gently and decently down from the table, looks for James; then turning to the surgeon and the students, she curtsies—and in a low, clear voice, begs their pardon if she has behaved ill. The students—all of us—wept like children; the surgeon helped her up carefully—and resting on James and me, Allie went to her room, Rab following. Four days after the operation what might have been expected happened. The patient had a chill, the wound was septic, and she died.[7]

Later in life Syme was able to operate with the patient under anesthesia. He felt it incumbent on the surgeon to search very carefully for axillary glands in the course of the operation but stated that the results were almost always unsatisfactory when the glands were involved, no matter how perfectly they seemed to have been removed. Sir James Paget (b. 1814) reported an operative mortality of 10% in 235 patients and among survivors, recurrence within 8 years. In 139 patients with scirrhus carcinoma, those who did not undergo surgery lived longer than those who did.[8] In 1874 Paget published *On Disease of the Mammary Areola Preceding Cancer of the Mammary Gland,* which described cancer of the nipple accompanied by eczematous changes and cancer of the lactiferous ducts (Paget disease of the breast).[9]

Charles Moore (b. 1821) of the Middlesex Hospital in London championed the belief that the only possibility of cure for breast cancer was through wider and more extensive surgery, despite the frequent disastrous results (Figure 1-11). His famous paper, *On the Influence of Inadequate Operation on the Theory of Cancer* (1867), was widely accepted.[10] He stressed that the tumor should not

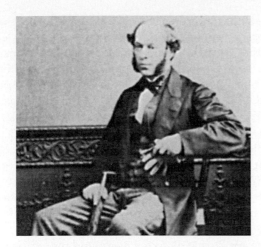

FIG. **1-11** Charles Moore, British surgeon of the mid-nineteenth century, advocated wider and more extensive breast surgery. (*From Robinson JO:* Am J Surg *151:323, 1986.*)

be cut and that recurrences originated as a result of dispersion from the primary growth and were not independent in origin. His operation called for removal of the entire breast, with special attention to removal of the skin in continuity with the main mass of the tumor. Moore did not advocate removal of the pectoralis major muscle.

The father of surgical antiseptic technique and one of England's most respected surgeons, Sir Joseph Lister (b. 1827), agreed with Moore's principles and advocated division of the origins of both pectoral muscles to gain better exposure of the axilla for the axillary gland dissection. His contribution of carbolic acid spray was not widely accepted for 15 to 20 years.[11] In 1877 Mitchell Banks of Liverpool, England, advocated removal of the axillary glands in all cases of surgery for breast cancer. He washed the wound with carbolic acid solution but avoided the spray because of its cooling effect on the patient.

Alfred-Armand-Louis-Marie Velpeau (b. 1795) of France, originally apprenticed to the blacksmith trade, rose to become professor of clinical surgery at the Paris Faculty, which was established in 1834. In his *Treatise on Diseases of the Breast* (1854), he claimed to have seen more than 1000 benign or malignant breast tumors during a practice of 40 years.[12] In those times once the cancer had been excised, the patient and surgeon parted company and follow-up was scanty. In 1844 Jean-Jacques-Joseph Leroy d'Etiolles (b. 1798) conducted a study of 1192 patients with breast cancer. He concluded that mastectomy was more harmful than beneficial. The 1854 Congress of the Académie de Médecine discussed whether cancer should be treated at all.

New practices developed in Germany in 1875, when Richard von Volkmann (b. 1830) removed the entire breast, no matter how small the primary tumor, as well as the pectoral fascia, with an occasional thick layer of the underlying muscle, and the axillary nodes. Theodor Billroth (b. 1829) also removed the entire breast but wondered whether local excision of the tumor with a surrounding zone of normal tissue would not be adequate for small lesions. In fixed tumors, however, his resection included the pectoral fascia, along with a thick layer of the underlying muscle.[13] Ernst Kuster (b. 1839) of Berlin, Germany, recommended that the axillary fat be removed along with the axillary glands. Lothar Heidenhain (b. 1860), a pupil of Volkmann, recommended removal of the superficial portion of the pectoralis major muscle even if the tumor was freely mobile, but he also recommended that the entire muscle, with its underlying connective tissue, be removed if the tumor was fixed.[14] Concerning benign breast disease, Sir Astley Cooper (b. 1768), an eminent English surgeon, published *Illustrations of the Diseases of the Breast* in 1829, which clearly differentiated fibroadenomas from chronic cystic mastitis.

Other important milestones of the nineteenth century are as follows. In 1829 French gynecologist and obstetrician Joseph Récalmier introduced the term *metastasis* to describe the spread of cancer. In 1830 the English surgeon Everard Home (b. 1756) published a book on cancer, which contained the first illustrations of the appearance of cancer cells under the microscope. Heinrich von Waldeyer-Hartz (b. 1836) developed a histologic classification of cancers showing that carcinomas come from epithelial cells, whereas sarcomas come from mesodermal tissue. In 1865 Victor Cornil (b. 1837) described malignant transformation of the acinar epithelium of the breast. In 1893 the first description of loss of differentiation by cancer cells ("anaplasia") was made by David von Hensemann, a German pathologist.

AMERICAN SURGERY

In the nineteenth century, Philadelphia was the medical center of the United States. It harbored the country's oldest medical college, the University of Pennsylvania (founded in 1765), the Jefferson Medical College (founded in 1824), and more than 50 other medical schools. It had a permanent medical college for women, as well as one in homeopathy and one in osteopathy.

Joseph Pancoast (b. 1805) was a dexterous surgeon-anatomist, who in the flowery language of his era, was said "to have an eye as quick as a flashing sunbeam and a hand as light as floating perfume." His *Treatise on Operative Surgery*,[14] published in 1844 in the preanesthetic and preantiseptic era, illustrates a mastectomy (Figure 1-12). The patient is awake, with eyes open, and is semireclining. An assistant compresses the subclavian artery above the clavicle with the thumb of one hand. Larger vessels in the wound are compressed with the thumb and index finger of the assistant's other

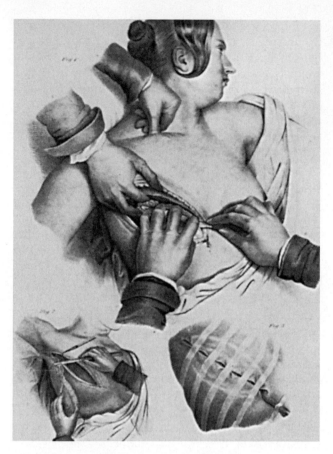

FIG. **1-12** Mastectomy (1844) of Dr. Joseph Pancoast in the preanesthetic and preantiseptic era. En bloc removal with axillary lymphatic drainage.

hand. Ligatures are left long and brought through the lower pole of the wound, where they act as a drain and can be pulled out later as they slough off. In one of the smaller sketches, the axillary glands are shown in continuity with the breast, visualized through a single incision that extended into the axilla. This was the first illustration of en bloc removal of the breast with its axillary lymphatic drainage. Skin removal was scanty, with easy approximation of the wound using five wide adhesive strips.

Samuel D. Gross (b. 1805) was designated as "the greatest American surgeon of his time." His approach to cancer of the breast, however, was more conservative than that of Pancoast, his colleague. He described extirpation of the breast as "generally a very easy and simple affair." Using a small elliptical incision, he attempted to save enough skin for easy approximation of the edges of the wound. He aimed for healing by first intention, which was less likely if the wound were permitted to gape. In dealing with inordinately vascular tumors, he ligated each vessel but generally considered this as awkward and unnecessary. Glands in the axilla were removed only if grossly involved, in which case they were removed through the outer angle of the incision or through a separate one. The glands were enucleated with the finger or handle of the scalpel. It was his rule not to approximate the skin until 4 or 5 hours after the operation, "lest secondary hemorrhage should occur, and thus necessitate the removal of the dressings." In the sixth edition of his *System of Surgery* (1882), he devoted 30 pages to diseases of the breast.[15]

Samuel W. Gross (b. 1837) took a much more aggressive approach than that of his eminent father. He stated in 1887 that "no matter what the situation of the tumor may be, or whether glands can or cannot be detected in the armpit, the entire breast, with all the skin covering it, the paramammary fat, and the fascia of the pectoral muscle are cleanly dissected away, and the axillary contents are extirpated. It need scarcely be added that aseptic precautions are strictly observed."[16] Removal of all the skin of the breast led to its designation as the "dinner plate operation." Against the criticism that an open large wound resulted in granulations from which cancer would again develop, he said, "When fireplugs produce whales, and oak trees polar bears, then will granulations produce cancer, and not until then."

The younger Gross personally examined all the tumors he removed under the microscope. In 1879 he helped his father found the Philadelphia Academy of Surgery, the oldest surgical society in the United States. Following his premature death in 1889, his widow married William Osler. In her will of 1928, Lady Osler bequeathed an endowment for a lectureship at the Jefferson Medical College in honor of her first husband and his special interest in tumors.

D. Hayes Agnew (b. 1818) of the University of Pennsylvania wrote *Principles and Practice of Surgery* (1878), which endorsed Listerian antisepsis.[17] He shared the pessimistic view of many eminent surgeons of the time that few cancers were ever cured with surgery. *The Agnew Clinic* by Thomas Eakins (b. 1844) is a masterpiece of American art depicting a mastectomy performed in 1889 under conditions that would have been considered ideal for the time (Figure 1-13).

Toward the later part of the nineteenth century, Philadelphia had to share its limelight with a number of other cities throughout the country, especially with Baltimore, where the recently organized Johns Hopkins Hospital Medical School produced a revolution in medical education and research. At that institution, William Halsted (b. 1852) recommended, "the suspected tissues [breast cancer] be removed in one piece lest the wound become infected by the division of tissue invaded by the disease, or by division of the lymphatic vessels containing cancer cells, and because shreds of cancerous tissue might be readily overlooked in a piecemeal extirpation." He advocated such wide removal of the skin that a graft would be required and recommended that the

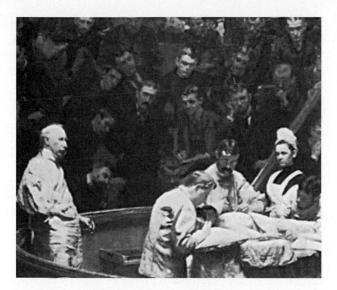

FIG. **1-13** Eakins' Agnew Clinic (1889) depicting mastectomy under ideal conditions of the time. (*Courtesy University of Pennsylvania School of Medicine, Philadelphia, PA.*)

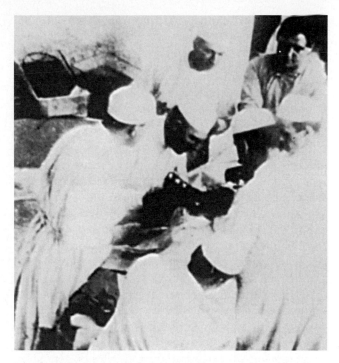

FIG. **1-14** Dr. William S. Halsted performing a radical mastectomy. Note the absence of masks. (*Courtesy College of Physicians of Philadelphia, Philadelphia, PA.*)

pectoralis major muscle be part of the en bloc specimen regardless of the size of the tumor.[18] Later, he went on to favor removal of the sheaths of the upper portion of the rectus abdominis, serratus anterior, subscapularis, latissimus dorsi, and teres major muscles.[19] Although there was nothing dramatically new in Halsted's operation, he placed it on a logical and scientific basis, spelled out the exact technique, and dispersed his principles widely throughout the profession (Figure 1-14).

Another scholar of breast cancer and mastectomy techniques, Willie Meyer (b. 1854) of the New York Graduate School of Medicine, described a similar technique only 10 days after Halsted's published paper.[20] He advocated removal of the pectoralis minor muscle in addition to the major. His operation has been referred to as the *Willie Meyer modification of the Halsted procedure.* At the close of the nineteenth century, the Halsted radical mastectomy had been established as state-of-the-art for surgical treatment of breast cancer. This procedure was unchallenged for 70 years, until the advent of breast conservation methods.

In 1895 I. Cullen credited William Welch (b. 1850), a pathologist at Johns Hopkins, as being the first to use frozen section in the diagnosis of breast lesions.[21] Welch is stated to have used this procedure in 1891 on a patient who was found to have a benign breast tumor.

Twentieth Century

At the beginning of the twentieth century, it was evident that a higher cure rate for breast cancer would not be achieved through surgery alone. This lowering of surgical expectations stimulated scientific inquiry through epidemiologic studies, laboratory research, and statistical analysis of practical experiences with breast cancer surgery in its various pathologic stages.

SURGERY

The radical mastectomy described simultaneously by Halsted and Meyer, although extensive, did not include the supraclavicular and internal mammary nodes. In 1907 Halsted reported the removal of supraclavicular nodes in 119 patients.[22] In 44 patients with metastatic deposits, only 2 were alive and well after 5 years. In 1910 C. Westerman reported surgery involving a patient with local recurrence in which he disarticulated the arm and resected three ribs.[23] The thoracic wall defect was repaired with a pedicled flap. In two other cases he carried out a partial excision of the thoracic wall and closed the defect with tissue from the contralateral healthy breast. These last two patients died within weeks, and the follow-up on the first was only for 1½ years. The surgeons discontinued these extensive operations within a few years because of the increased operative mortality and poor survival rates.

The internal mammary nodes were neglected until the third decade of the century. In 1927 William Handley (b. 1872) of the Middlesex Hospital directed attention to the frequency of internal mammary node involvement, especially when axillary lymph nodes were enlarged.[24] He reported the removal of internal mammary nodes as an extension of the radical mastectomy. After World War II, Jerome Urban and Owen Wangensteen, among others, advocated a "supraradical mastectomy," in which the dissection was carried into the mediastinum and the neck.[25,26]

The late Cushman Haagensen (Figure 1-15) of Columbia-Presbyterian Medical Center in New York City dedicated his life to the surgical and pathologic study of breast diseases. He classified breast cancers in his patients according to size, clinical findings, and nodal status while establishing a breast unit where comprehensive data were maintained.[27] He was the first to propose self-examination of the breast and to suggest that lobular neoplasia (lobular carcinoma in situ) was not actual cancer. He distinguished this "marker of risk" from ductal carcinoma in situ.

In 1937, London surgeon Geoffrey Keynes demonstrated that less radical surgery was needed in breast cancer, with radiation giving equally good results. However, at the close of World War II, radical mastectomy remained the standard operation for breast cancer. In 1948 two reports appeared that were destined to change the management of breast cancer and become accepted as general principles in the management of localized disease. The first was the concept of modified radical mastectomy by D. Patey and W. Dyson from the Middlesex Hospital in London.[28] The second was treatment with simple mastectomy and radiotherapy, introduced by R. McWhirter of the University of Edinburgh.[29] Subsequent studies of patients treated with simple, radical, and modified radical mastectomies with or without radiotherapy revealed a striking similarity in survival rates. The contemporary trend (since 1970) has been breast conservation surgery followed by irradiation. Axillary dissection was confined to level I and II lymph nodes.

In the later years of the twentieth century, Donald Morton (Figure 1-16) and associates at the John Wayne Cancer Center in Santa Monica, California, developed the sentinel lymph node biopsy technique. It was originally proposed as an alternative to elective lymph node dissection for staging regional lymphatics in patients with cutaneous melanoma.[30] Subsequently, A. Giuliano investigated its use as an alternative to elective axillary lymph node dissection in patients with breast cancer.[31] Sentinel lymph node biopsy is now revolutionizing breast cancer staging and is redefining the indications for axillary dissection. In this application the technique uses lymphoscintigraphy and blue dye to localize the "sentinel" axillary lymph node, which is the node most likely to contain breast cancer metastases.

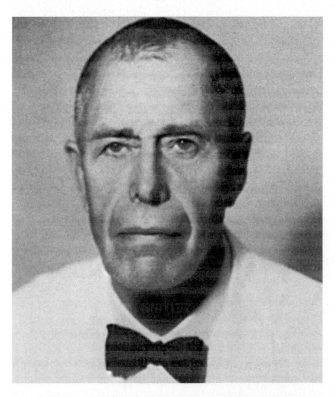

FIG. **1-15** Dr. Cushman D. Haagensen, a strong advocate of radical mastectomy, who classified and analyzed breast cancer for half a century. (*Courtesy Dr. Gordon Schwartz.*)

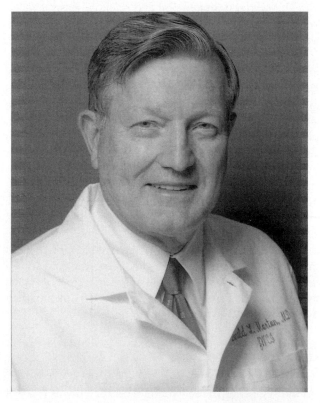

FIG. **1-16** Dr. Donald L. Morton, John Wayne Cancer Center, Santa Monica, CA.

RADIOTHERAPY

Two months after the discovery of x-rays in 1895 by Wilhelm Roentgen (b. 1845), Emile Grubbe (b. 1875), a second-year medical student in Chicago, irradiated a patient with cancer of the breast. He protected the skin surrounding the lesion with tinfoil. He subsequently became the first professor of roentgenology at the Hahnemann Medical College of Philadelphia. In 1896 Hermann Gocht (b. 1869) of Hamburg, Germany, irradiated two advanced cases of breast cancer while protecting the adjacent skin with flexible lead.[32] In 1898 Marie Curie and her husband Pierre discovered and isolated the radioactive elements polonium and radium. Their skin was burned as a result of working near these compounds, and in 1904 it was demonstrated that radium rays destroyed human cells.

In 1902 Guido Holzknecht (b. 1872) of Vienna, Italy, introduced a practical dosimeter. The therapeutic application of ionizing radiation soon followed. In 1902 Russian physician S. Goldberg successfully used radium in the treatment of cancer. In 1903 one of the first departments of radiotherapy for cancer was established at the Cancer Hospital in London, under the direction of J. Pollock. Georg Perthes (b. 1869), professor of surgery in Leipzig, Germany, in 1903 ascribed the "curative effect" of x-rays secondary to their inhibition of cell division.[33] Postoperative radiotherapy was initiated in many hospitals in America and Europe in the years before World War I. The equipment of the day permitted a maximum voltage of only 150 kV. Immediately after the war, the voltages used increased, ranging from 170 to 200 kV.

In 1929 S. Harrington of the Mayo Clinic reported his follow-up of 1859 breast cancer cases irradiated between 1910 and 1923.[34] After analyzing his results, he expressed doubts about the value of ancillary radiotherapy. Even with improved equipment, controversy continued between enthusiasts and opponents of radiotherapy. George Pfahler (b. 1874) of Philadelphia recommended postoperative radiotherapy in all cases of breast cancer, starting 2 weeks after surgery. In his report of 1022 cases, he found no significant improvement in survival with stage I disease but did document an improved 5-year survival rate for patients with stage II disease.[35]

Radiotherapy as the sole therapeutic modality for breast cancer had been used for inoperable cases since the beginning of the twentieth century, but it was not until 1922 that a claim was made for its sole use in operable cases. William Stone (b. 1867) of New York City claimed the superiority of radiotherapy over radical surgery for the treatment of operable breast cancer. He based his conclusions on his experience with 10,000 cases. Geoffrey Keynes (b. 1887) of St. Bartholomew's Hospital in London reported in 1932 that radium can be used as a source of therapeutic irradiation.[36] After experience with this modality as an adjunct to surgery for breast cancer, he extended its use to being the sole treatment. He claimed a 5-year survival rate of 77% in the absence of enlarged axillary nodes and 36% with axillary involvement.

Supervoltage x-rays became available in the 1930s. At that time, François Baclesse (b. 1896) of Paris championed local excision of breast cancer, followed by radiotherapy. He reported cases studied between 1937 and 1953 at the Curie Foundation and concluded that for stage I and stage II cancers, his results were equal to those of radical mastectomy. In 1948 Robert McWhirter (b. 1904) proposed simple mastectomy followed by radiotherapy.[29] He argued that radical mastectomy for stage I disease was an overkill but was often inadequate for stage II disease, in which distant metastatic disease commonly developed. In the 1960s, even higher voltage x-rays were developed, along with the cobalt beam. In the late 1970s the development of the linear accelerator allowed the delivery of whole-breast radiotherapy of 4000 to 5000 cGy, with focal boost to the tumor bed to 6000 to 7000 cGy.

During the later part of the twentieth century, partial mastectomy ("lumpectomy"), axillary node dissection, and adjuvant breast irradiation played an increasingly important role in the therapy of early-stage breast cancer. The validity of breast conservation therapy was demonstrated through a series of carefully designed and controlled clinical trials coordinated through the National Surgical Adjuvant Breast and Bowel Project (NSABP). An American surgeon, Bernard Fischer (Figure 1-17), served as chairman of the NSABP from 1967 to 1994 and since 1995 has been its scientific director. Fisher's systematic analyses brought breast cancer therapy into a new era and has set a standard for the investigation of therapies for other solid tumors.[37]

HORMONAL THERAPY

Hormonal treatment for breast cancer was considered even before the beginning of the twentieth century. In 1889 Albert Schinzinger (b. 1827) of Freiburg, Germany, proposed oophorectomy before mastectomy to produce "early aging" in menstruating women. This was based on his belief that the prognosis of breast cancer was worse in younger patients. In 1896 and again in 1901, George Beatson (b. 1848) of Glasgow, Scotland, reported three cases of advanced breast cancer that responded favorably to oophorectomy.[38] In 1900 S. Boyd performed the first combined oophorectomy and mastectomy for breast cancer. In 1905 a series of 99 patients with breast cancer treated by oophorectomy was presented at the Royal Medical and Chirurgical Society by a surgeon at the London Hospital, Hugh Lett.

In 1953 the late Nobel laureate and surgeon/urologist Charles Huggins (Figure 1-18) of the University of Chicago advocated oophorectomy and adrenalectomy to remove the major sources of estrogens in the body.[39]

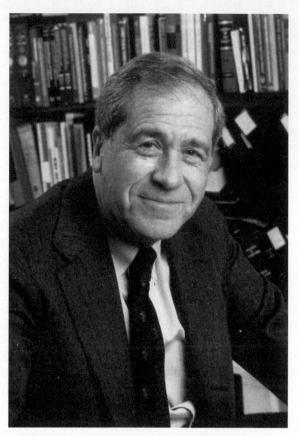

FIG. **1-17** Dr. Bernard Fisher, National Surgical Adjuvant Breast and Bowel Project (NSABP), Pittsburgh, PA.

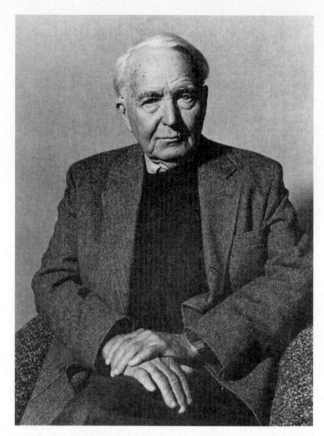

FIG. **1-18** Dr. Charles B. Huggins, Nobel Laureate, University of Chicago, Chicago, IL.

Some cases of breast cancer responded with dramatic remissions, whereas others remained unaffected. In the early 1950s hypophysectomy for advanced breast cancer was recommended, with results similar to those of adrenalectomy. Clinical administration of hormones started in 1939, when P. Ulrich reported the beneficial effect of testosterone in two cases of breast cancer.[40] In 1944 Alexander Haddow (b. 1912) of Edinburgh, Scotland, and his collaborators observed a favorable effect of synthetic estrogen in advanced breast cancer.[41] Edward Dodds of London synthesized stilbestrol in 1938.[42] I. Nathanson reported its effect on advanced breast cancer in 1946.[43] In the 1950s and 1960s estrogens and androgens remained in active use. In 1973 W. McGuire demonstrated estrogen receptors in human breast tumors.[44] In 1975 K. Horowitz identified progesterone receptors in hormone-dependent breast cancer.[45] Since the 1980s tamoxifen and other selective estrogen receptor modulators (SERMs) have been used for the treatment and prevention of breast cancer.

CHEMOTHERAPY

The use of chemical compounds, especially arsenic, in the treatment of breast cancer dates to ancient times. However, Paul Ehrlich (b. 1854) is credited as being the "father of chemotherapy." He coined the designation *chemotherapy* and by 1898 had isolated the first alkylating agent. In a series of historic experiments, he methodically studied a group of compounds that led to the discovery of salvarsan in 1910, which successfully treated syphilis in rabbits.[46] It was not until just after World War II that his work was applied to the treatment of cancers.

During World War II, the U.S. Office of Scientific Research produced nitrogen mustard, an alkylating agent. A ship containing this substance blew up in the Naples, Italy, harbor, and the sailors who were exposed developed marrow and lymphoid hypoplasia. Experimental work with nitrogen mustard for the treatment of lymphosarcoma began at Memorial Hospital in New York City, but the results were withheld until the war secrecy ban was lifted in 1946. In that same year Frederick Phillips and Alfred Gilman demonstrated that nitrogen mustards could cause regression of certain lymphomas and leukemias.

Other antineoplastic drugs brought into clinical use were the purine and pyrimidine antagonists. In 1957 C. Heidelberger and collaborators reported the action of 5-fluorouracil, which has remained useful in the treatment of breast cancer.[47] In addition, the National

Institutes of Health organized a cancer and chemotherapy national service. In 1958 patients were entered into a randomized, double-blind study using thiotriethylenephosphoramide, an alkylating agent. In 1963 E. Greenspan and his group in New York City were some of the first to engage in multidrug trials, using the antimetabolite methotrexate in combination with the alkylating agent thiotepa.[48]

MAMMOGRAPHY

Before and after World War I, early diagnosis of breast cancer was difficult. Patients sought advice only when they felt a hard lump. Surgeons looked for skin retraction and inversion of the nipple and palpated the breast and axilla for masses. In 1913 a German surgeon, A. Salomon, used mammography to study 3000 amputated breasts and was able to differentiate scirrhus forms of breast cancer from nodular types.[49] He noted the microcalcifications in intraductal carcinomas but failed to appreciate their significance. In 1927 O. Kleinschmidt wrote a book in which he described mammography as an aid in diagnosis.[50]

Jacob Gershon-Cohen of Philadelphia studied x-ray mammary patterns from 1937 to 1948 and made notable progress in the accurate diagnosis of breast cancer. He tirelessly advocated the use of x-rays as an aid to clinical diagnosis and in 1948 was the first to demonstrate the feasibility of detecting occult carcinomas.[51] In 1962 at the M.D. Anderson Hospital and Tumor Institute, R. Egan described imaging of the breast with only two radiographic views. He reported a study of 2522 mammograms in which differentiation between benign and malignant tumors was made without the aid of clinical findings.[52] Since then, mammography has become the most important diagnostic tool for breast cancer.

CANCER BIOLOGY

The twentieth century saw unprecedented growth in our understanding of cancer biology, especially breast cancer biology. In the first part of the century, numerous observations were made concerning the development and behavior of cancer. In 1900 Leo Loeb experimentally transmitted cancer through several generations of animals. In 1911 Jean Clunet of France demonstrated the experimental production of cancer using x-rays. In 1920 an American pathologist, Albert Borders, classified cancers with regard to malignant potential on the basis of the state of differentiation of cancer cells. In 1932 the French physician Antoine Lacassagne demonstrated that breast cancer could be produced in animals with estrone benzoate. In 1944 P. Denoix of the Institut Gustav-Roussy in France proposed the tumor, node, metastasis (TNM) classification for cancer. In 1959 M. Macklin performed a comprehensive analysis of the role of hereditary factors in the predisposition to breast cancer.

The latter part of the twentieth century saw the development of molecular biology and the explanation of breast cancer development and behavior in terms of human genetics. In 1926 American geneticist Hermann Müller exposed fruit flies to x-rays and produced mutations and hereditary changes. He demonstrated that the mutations were the result of breakages in chromosomes and changes in individual genes. Hugh Cairns (b. 1922), a molecular biologist and virologist from Oxford University, showed that cancer developed from a single abnormal cell as a result of DNA mutation. Peter Vogt (b. 1932), a German-born American microbiologist from the University of South California, discovered oncogenes, which play a role in the normal growth of mammalian cells but can cause cancer through mutation. In 1970 David Baltimore, a New York City oncologist, announced his discovery of the enzyme reverse transcriptase, which can transcribe RNA into DNA, contributing greatly to our understanding of how viruses participate in the development of cancer. In 1978 David Lane, a professor of oncology at Dundee, Scotland, discovered the tumor-suppressor gene p53. Bert Vogelstein (b. 1949), a Baltimore oncologist and a pioneer in the study of the molecular basis of cancer, analyzed DNA from colon cancer cells and described mutation of three tumorsuppressor genes: APC, DCC, and p53. Judith Folkman (b. 1933), an American surgeon, elucidated the importance of angiogenesis and opened the way for new therapy. In 1994 the first breast cancer gene, *BRCA1*, was identified, and in 1996 *BRCA2* was discovered. Building on these and other discoveries, the twenty-first century will undoubtedly see the development of genetically based therapies for breast cancer that will complement or replace the empirical therapies of the past.

REFERENCES

1. Breasted JH: *The Edwin Smith surgical papyrus. Classics of med lib,* vol III, Chicago, 1930, University of Chicago Press.
2. Fabry W: *Observationum et curationum chirurgicarum centuriae: cent II,* IA Huguetan, 1641.
3. le Dran F: Mémoire avec une précis de plusieurs observations sur le cancer, *Mem Acad Roy Chir Paris* 3:1, 1757.
4. Petit JL: *Oeuvres completes, section VII,* Limoges, 1837, R. Chapoulard.
5. Young S: *Minutes of cases of cancer and cancerous tendency successfully treated, with a preparatory letter addressed to the Governors of the Middlesex Hospital by Samuel Whitbread,* London, 1815, E Coxe & Son.
6. Syme J: *Principles of surgery,* London, 1842, H Balliere.
7. Brown J: *Horae Subsecivae,* ed 2, London, 1910, Adam & Charles Black.
8. Paget J: On the average duration of life in patients with scirrhus cancer of the breast, *Lancet* 1:62, 1856.
9. Paget J: On disease of the mammary areola preceding cancer of the mammary gland, *St Bart Hosp Rep* 10:87, 1874.

10. Moore C: On the influence of inadequate operations on the theory of cancer, *R Med Chir Soc Lond* 1:244, 1867.

11. Lister J: On the antiseptic principle in the practice of surgery, *Lancet* ii:95, 353, 668, 1867.

12. Velpeau AALM: *Traité des Maladies du Sein et de la Region Mammaire*, Paris, 1854, V Masson.

13. Volkmann R: *Beitrage zur Chirurgie*, Leipzig, 1875, Breitkopf & Hartel.

14. Heidenhain L: Ueber die Ursachen der localen Krebsrecidive nach Amputation Mammae, *Arch Klin Chir* 39:97, 1889.

15. Gross SD: *System of surgery*, vol II, ed 5, Philadelphia, 1872, Henry C Lea's Son.

16. Gross SW: An analysis of two hundred and seven cases of carcinoma of the breast, *Med News* 51:613, 1887.

17. Agnew DH: *The principles and practice of surgery*, vol III, Philadelphia, 1883, JB Lippincott.

18. Halsted WS: The results of operations for the cure of cancer of the breast performed at the Johns Hopkins Hospital from June 1889 to January 1894, *Johns Hopkins Hosp Rep* 4:297, 1894-1895.

19. Halsted WS: A clinical and histological study of certain adenocarcinomata of the breast, *Ann Surg* 28:557, 1898.

20. Meyer W: An improved method of the radical operation for carcinoma of the breast, *Med Rec* 46:746, 1894.

21. Cullen IS: A rapid method of making permanent specimens from frozen sections by the use of formalin, *Bull Johns Hopkins Hosp* 6:67, 1895.

22. Halsted WS: The results of radical operations for cure of cancer of the breast, *Ann Surg* 46:1, 1907.

23. Westerman CWG: Thoraxexcisie bij recidief van carcinoma mammae, *Geneesk Med Lydschr* 54:1681, 1910.

24. Handley WS: Parasternal invasion of the thorax in breast cancer and its suppression by the use of radium tubes as an operative precaution, *Surg Gynecol Obstet* 45:721, 1927.

25. Urban JA, Baker HW: Radical mastectomy in continuity with en bloc resection of the internal mammary lymph chain, *Cancer* 5:992, 1952.

26. Wangensteen OH: Discussion to Taylor and Wallace: carcinoma of the breast, fifty years' experience at the Massachusetts General Hospital, *Ann Surg* 132:839, 1950.

27. Haagensen CD: *Diseases of the breast*, ed 3, Philadelphia, 1986, WB Saunders.

28. Patey DH, Dyson WH: The prognosis of carcinoma of the breast in relation to the type of operation performed, *Br J Cancer* 2:7, 1948.

29. McWhirter R: The value of simple mastectomy and radiotherapy in the treatment of cancer of the breast, *Br J Radiol* 21:599, 1948.

30. Morton DL et al: Technical details for intraoperative lymphatic mapping for early stage melanoma, *Arch Surg* 127:392, 1992.

31. Giuliano AE et al: Lymphatic mapping and sentinel lymphadenectomy for breast cancer, *Ann Surg* 220:391, 1994.

32. Gocht H: Therapeutische Verwendung der Rontgenstrahlen, *Fortschr Geb Roentgenstr* 1:14, 1897.

33. Perthes GC: Ueber den Einfluss der Roentgenstrahlen auf epitheliale Gewebe, insbesondere auf das Carcinom, *Langenbecks Arch Klin Chir* 7:955, 1903.

34. Harrington SW: Carcinoma of the breast; surgical treatment and results, *JAMA* 92:280, 1929.

35. Pfahler GE: Results of radiation therapy in 1,022 private cases of carcinoma of the breast from 1902 to 1928, *AJR Am J Roentgenol* 27:497, 1932.

36. Keynes GL: The radium treatment of carcinoma of the breast, *Br J Surg* 19:415, 1932.

37. Fisher B, Redmons C, Fisher ER: The contribution of recent clinical trials of primary breast cancer therapy to an understanding of tumor biology, *Cancer* 46:1009, 1980.

38. Beatson GT: The treatment of cancer of the breast by oophorectomy and thyroid extract, *BMJ* 2:1145, 1901.

39. Huggins C, Doa TLY: Adrenalectomy and oophorectomy in the treatment of advanced carcinoma of the breast, *JAMA* 151:1388, 1953.

40. Ulrich P: Testosterone et son role possible dans le traitement de certains cancers du sein, *Int Union Against Cancer* 4:377, 1939.

41. Haddow A, Watkinson JM, Patterson D: Influence of synthetic estrogen upon advanced malignant disease, *BMJ* 2:393, 1944.

42. Dodds EC: Significance of synthetic estrogens, *Acta Med Scand* 90(suppl):141, 1938.

43. Nathanson IT: The effect of stilboestrol in advanced cancer of the breast, *Cancer Res* 6:484, 1946.

44. McGuire WL, De La Garza M: Similarity of estrogen receptors in human and rat mammary carcinoma, *J Clin Endocrinol Metab* 36:548, 1973.

45. Horowitz KB: Progesterone receptors and hormone dependent breast cancer, doctoral dissertation, Dallas, 1975, University of Texas Southwestern Medical School.

46. Ehrlich P: *Closing notes on experimental chemotherapy of spirillosco*, Berlin, 1910, J Springer.

47. Heidelberger C et al: Fluorinated pyrimidines, a new class of tumor inhibitory compounds, *Nature* 179:663, 1957.

48. Greenspan EM et al: Response of advanced breast carcinoma to the combination of the antimetabolic methotrexate and the alkylating agent thio-TEPA, *Mt Sinai J Med* 33:1, 1963.

49. Salomon A: Beitrage zur Pathologic und Klinik der Mammar-Carcinom, *Arch Klin Chir* 105:573, 1913.

50. Kleinschmidt O: Brustdruse. In Zweife P, Payr E (eds): *Die Klinik der Bosartigen Geschwulste*, vol III, Leipzig, 1927, S Hirzel.

51. Gershon-Cohen J: *Atlas of mammography*, New York, 1970, Springer-Verlag.

52. Egan RL: Experience with mammography in a tumor institution, *Radiology* 25:894, 1960.

SUGGESTED READINGS

Bordley J III, Harvey AM: *Two centuries of American medicine, 1776-1976*, Philadelphia, 1976, WB Saunders.

de Moulin D: *A short history of breast cancer*, The Hague, 1983, Martinus Nijhoff.

Garrison FH: *An introduction to the history of medicine*, Philadelphia, 1929, WB Saunders.

Grubbe EH: *X-ray treatment: its origin, birth and early history*, St Paul, 1949, Bruce Publishing.

King LS: *The medical world of the eighteenth century*, Huntington, NY, 1971, RE Krieger.

Lee HSJ: *Dates in oncology. Landmarks in medicine series*, New York, 2000, The Parthenon Publishing Group.

Levens P: *The pathway to health*, London, 1664. In special collections of Thomas Jefferson University Library, Philadelphia.

Pancoast J: *Treatise on operative surgery*, Philadelphia, 1844, Carey & Hart.

Riesman D: *Medicine in the Middle Ages*, New York, 1935, Paul B Hoeber.

II

ANATOMY AND PHYSIOLOGY OF THE NORMAL AND LACTATING BREAST

CHAPTER

2

Anatomy of the Breast, Axilla, Chest Wall, and Related Metastatic Sites

LYNN J. ROMRELL

KIRBY I. BLAND

Chapter Outline

Mammary glands, or breasts, are a distinguishing feature of mammals. They have evolved as milk-producing organs to provide nourishment to the offspring, which are born in a relatively immature and dependent state. The act of nursing the young provides physiologic benefit to the mother by aiding in postpartum uterine involution and to the young in transferring passive immunity. The nursing of the young is also of significance in the bonding between the mother and her offspring.

During embryologic development, there is growth and differentiation of the breasts in both sexes (for a review see Morehead[1]). Paired glands develop along paired lines, the milk lines, extending between the limb buds from the future axilla to the future inguinal region. Among the various mammalian species, the number of paired glands varies greatly and is related to the number of young in each litter. In humans and most other primates, normally only one gland develops on each side in the pectoral region. An extra breast (polymastia) or nipple (polythelia) may occur as a heritable condition in about 1% of the female population. These relatively rare conditions also may occur in the male. When present, the supernumerary breast or nipple usually forms along the milk lines; about one third of the affected individuals have multiple extra breasts or nipples.

In the female the breasts undergo extensive postnatal development, which is correlated with age and regulated by hormones that influence reproductive function. By about 20 years of age, the breast has reached its greatest development, and by the age of 40, it begins atrophic changes. During each menstrual cycle, structural changes occur in the breast under the influence of ovarian hormone levels. During pregnancy and lactation, striking changes occur not only in the functional activity of the breast but also in the amount of glandular tissue. The actual secretion and production of milk is induced by prolactin from the pituitary and somatomammotropin from the placenta. With the changes in the hormonal environment that occur at menopause, the glandular component of the breast regresses, or involutes, and is replaced by fat and connective tissue.[2]

Gross Anatomic Structure—Surface Anatomy

FORM AND SIZE

The breast is located within the superficial fascia of the anterior thoracic wall. It consists of 15 to 20 lobes of glandular tissue of the tubuloalveolar type. Fibrous connective tissue forms a framework that supports the lobes, and adipose tissue fills the space between the lobes.[3] Subcutaneous connective tissue surrounds the gland and extends as septa between the lobes and lobules, providing support for the glandular elements, but it does not form a distinctive capsule around the components of the breast. The deep layer of the superficial fascia, which lies on the posterior (deep) surface of the breast, rests on the pectoral (deep) fascia of the thoracic wall. A distinct space, the *retromammary bursa*, can be identified surgically on the posterior aspect of the breast between the deep layer of the superficial fascia and the deep investing fascia of the pectoralis major and contiguous muscles of the thoracic wall (Figure 2-1). The retromammary bursa contributes to the mobility of the breast on the thoracic wall. Fibrous thickenings of the connective tissue interdigitate between the parenchymal tissue of the breast, extending from the deep layer of the superficial fascia (hypodermis) and attaching to the dermis of the skin. These suspensory structures, called *Cooper's ligaments*, insert perpendicular to the delicate superficial fascial layers of the dermis, or corium, permitting remarkable mobility of the breast while providing support.

At maturity, the glandular portion of the breast has a unique and distinctive protuberant conical form. The base of the cone is roughly circular, measuring 10 to 12 cm in diameter and 5 to 7 cm in thickness. Commonly, breast tissue extends into the axilla as the axillary tail (of Spence). There is tremendous variation in the size of the breast. A typical nonlactating breast weighs between 150 and 225 g, whereas the lactating breast may exceed 500 g.[4,5] In a study of breast volume in 55 women, Smith and colleagues[6] reported that the mean volume of the right breast was 275.46 ml (SD = 172.65, median = 217.7, minimum = 94.6, maximum = 889.3) and the left breast was 291.69 ml (SD = 168.23, median = 224.0, minimum = 106.9, maximum = 893.9).

The breast of the nulliparous female has a typical hemispheric configuration with distinct flattening above the nipple.[7] The multiparous breast, which has experienced the hormonal stimulation associated with pregnancy and lactation, is usually larger and more pendulous. As noted, during pregnancy and lactation, the breast increases dramatically in size and becomes more pendulous. With increasing age, the breast usually decreases in volume, becomes somewhat flattened and pendulous, and is less firm.

EXTENT AND LOCATION

The mature female breast extends inferiorly from the level of the second or third rib to the inframammary fold, which is at about the level of the sixth or seventh rib, and laterally from the lateral border of the sternum to the anterior or midaxillary line. The deep or posterior surface of the breast rests on portions of the deep

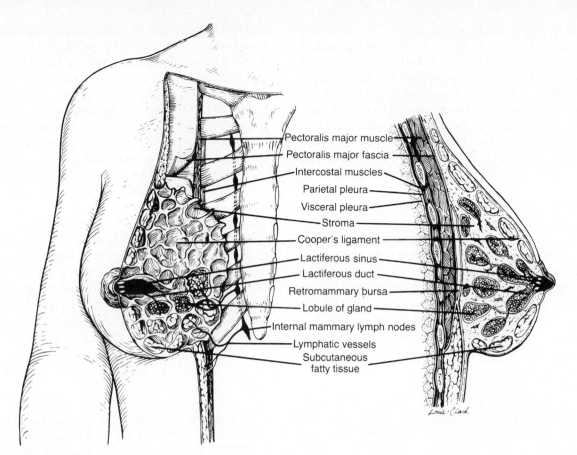

FIG. 2-1 A tangential view of the breast on the chest wall and a sectional (sagittal) view of the breast and associated chest wall. The breast lies in the superficial fascia just deep to the dermis. It is attached to the skin by the suspensory ligaments of Cooper and is separated from the investing fascia of the pectoralis major muscle by the retromammary bursa. Cooper's ligaments form fibrosepta in the stroma that provide support for the breast parenchyma. From 15 to 20 lactiferous ducts extend from lobules comprised of glandular epithelium to openings located on the nipple. A dilation of the duct, the lactiferous sinus, is present near the opening of the duct in the subareolar tissue. Subcutaneous fat and adipose tissue distributed around the lobules of the gland give the breast its smooth contour and, in the nonlactating breast, account for most of its mass. Lymphatic vessels pass through the stroma surrounding the lobules of the gland and convey lymph to collecting ducts. Lymphatic channels ending in the internal mammary (or parasternal) lymph nodes are shown. The pectoralis major muscle lies adjacent to the ribs and intercostal muscles. The parietal pleura, attached to the endothoracic fascia, and the visceral pleura, covering the surface of the lung, are shown.

investing fasciae of the pectoralis major, serratus anterior, and external abdominal oblique muscles and the upper extent of the rectus sheath. The axillary tail (of Spence) of the breast extends into the anterior axillary fold. The upper half of the breast, and particularly the upper outer quadrant, contains more glandular tissue than does the remainder of the breast.

Microscopic Anatomic Structure

NIPPLE AND AREOLA

The epidermis of the nipple and areola is highly pigmented and somewhat wrinkled. It is covered by keratinized, stratified squamous epithelium. The deep surface of the epidermis is invaded by unusually long dermal papillae that allow capillaries to bring blood close to the surface, giving the region a pinkish color in young, fair-skinned individuals. At puberty, the pigmentation of the nipple and areola increases and the nipple becomes more prominent. During pregnancy, the areola enlarges and the degree of pigmentation increases. Deep to the areola and nipple, bundles of smooth muscle fibers are arranged radially and circumferentially in the dense connective tissue and longitudinally along the lactiferous ducts that extend up into the nipple. These muscle fibers are responsible for the erection of nipple that occurs in response to various stimuli (for a review of the anatomy of the nipple and areola, see Giacometti and Montagna[8]).

The areola contains sebaceous glands, sweat glands, and accessory areolar glands (of Montgomery), which are intermediate in their structure between true mammary glands and sweat glands. The accessory areolar glands produce small elevations on the surface of the areola. The sebaceous glands (which usually lack associated hairs) and sweat glands are located along the margin of the areola. Whereas the tip of the nipple contains numerous free sensory nerve cell endings and Meissner's corpuscles in the dermal papillae, the areola contains fewer of these structures.[9] In a review of the innervation of the nipple and areola, Montagna and Macpherson[10] reported observing fewer nerve endings than described by other investigators. They reported that most of the endings were at the apex of the nipple. Neuronal plexuses are also present around hair follicles in the skin peripheral to the areola, and pacinian corpuscles may be present in the dermis and in the glandular tissue. The rich sensory innervation of the breast, particularly the nipple and areola,[11] is of great functional significance. The suckling infant initiates a chain of neural and neurohumoral events, resulting in the release of milk and maintenance of glandular differentiation that is essential for continued lactation.

INACTIVE MAMMARY GLAND

The adult mammary gland is composed of 15 to 20 irregular lobes of branched tubuloalveolar glands. The lobes, separated by fibrous bands of connective tissue, radiate from the *mammary papilla,* or *nipple,* and are further subdivided into numerous lobules. Those fibrous bands that connect with the dermis are the *suspensory ligaments of Cooper.* Abundant adipose tissue is present in the dense connective tissue of the interlobular spaces. The intralobular connective tissue is much less dense and contains little fat.

Each lobe of the mammary gland ends in a *lactiferous duct* (2 to 4 mm in diameter) that opens through a constricted orifice (0.4 to 0.7 mm in diameter) onto the nipple (see Figure 2-1). Beneath the areola, each duct has a dilated portion, the *lactiferous sinus.* Near their openings, the lactiferous ducts are lined with stratified squamous epithelium. The epithelial lining of the duct shows a gradual transition to two layers of cuboidal cells in the lactiferous sinus and then becomes a single layer of columnar or cuboidal cells through the remainder of the duct system. Myoepithelial cells of ectodermal origin lie within the epithelium between the surface epithelial cells and the basal lamina.[12] These cells, arranged in a basketlike network, are present in the secretory portion of the gland but are more apparent in the larger ducts. They contain myofibrils and are strikingly similar to smooth muscle cells in their cytology.

In light microscopy, epithelial cells are characteristically seen to be attached to an underlying layer called the *basement membrane.* With electron microscopy, the substructure of the basement membrane can be identified.

The inner layer of the basement membrane is called the *basal lamina.* In the breast, the parenchymal cells of the tubuloalveolar glands, as well as the epithelial and myoepithelial cells of the ducts, rest on a basement membrane or basal lamina. The integrity of this supporting layer is of significance in evaluating biopsy specimens of breast tissue. Changes in the basement membrane have important implications in immune surveillance, transformation, differentiation, and metastasis.[13-16]

The morphology of the secretory portion of the mammary gland varies greatly with age and during pregnancy and lactation (Figure 2-2). In the inactive gland, the glandular component is sparse and consists chiefly of duct elements (Figure 2-3). Most investigators believe that the secretory units in the inactive breast are not organized as alveoli and consist only of ductules. During the menstrual cycle, the inactive breast undergoes slight cyclical changes. Early in the cycle, the ductules appear as cords with little or no lumen. Under estrogen stimulation, at about the time of ovulation,

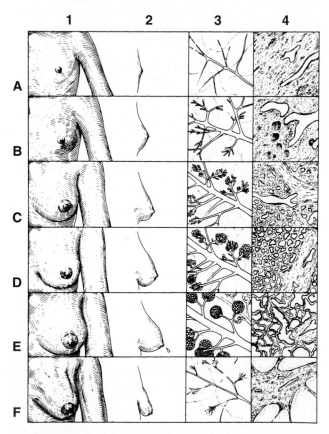

FIG. 2-2 Schematic drawing illustrating mammary gland development. Anterior and lateral views of the breast are shown in columns 1 and 2. The microscopic appearances of the ducts and lobules are illustrated in columns 3 and 4, respectively. Panels: **A,** prepubertal (childhood); **B,** puberty; **C,** mature (reproductive); **D,** pregnancy; **E,** lactation; **F,** postmenopausal (senescent) state. *(From Copeland EM III, Bland KI: The breast. In Sabiston DC Jr [ed]: Essentials of surgery, Philadelphia, 1987, WB Saunders.)*

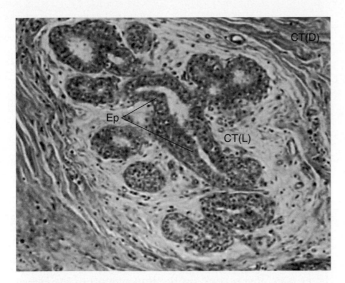

FIG. **2-3** Inactive or resting human mammary gland. The epithelial *(Ep)* or glandular elements are imbedded in loose connective tissue *[CT(L)]*. Within the lobule the epithelial cells are primarily duct elements. Dense connective tissue *[CT(D)]* surrounds the lobule. ×160. *(Courtesy Michael H. Ross, Ph.D., University of Florida College of Medicine, Gainesville, FL.)*

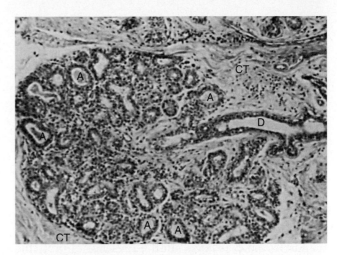

FIG. **2-4** Proliferative or active (pregnant) human mammary gland. The alveolar elements of the gland become conspicuous during the early proliferative period (compare with Figure 2-3). Within the lobule of the breast, distinct alveoli *(A)* are present. The alveoli are continuous with a duct *(D)*. The alveoli are surrounded by highly cellular connective tissue *(CT)*. The individual lobules are separated by dense connective tissue septa. ×160. *(Courtesy Michael H. Ross, Ph.D., University of Florida College of Medicine, Gainesville, FL.)*

secretory cells increase in height, lumens appear as small amounts of secretions accumulate, and fluids and lipid accumulate in the connective tissue. Then, in the absence of continued hormonal stimulation, the gland regresses to a more inactive state through the remainder of the cycle.

ACTIVE MAMMARY GLANDS: PREGNANCY AND LACTATION

During pregnancy, in preparation for lactation, the mammary glands undergo dramatic proliferation and development. These changes in the glandular tissue are accompanied by relative decreases in the amount of connective and adipose tissue. Plasma cells, lymphocytes, and eosinophils infiltrate the fibrous component of the connective tissue as the breast develops in response to hormonal stimulation. The development of the glandular tissue is not uniform, and variation in the degree of development may occur within a single lobule. The cells vary in shape from low columnar to flattened. As the cells proliferate by mitotic division, the ductules branch and alveoli begin to develop. In the later stages of pregnancy, alveolar development becomes more prominent (Figure 2-4). Near the end of pregnancy, the actual proliferation of cells declines and subsequent enlargement of the breast occurs through hypertrophy of the alveolar cells and accumulation of their secretory product in the lumens of the ductules.

The secretory cells contain abundant endoplasmic reticulum, a moderate number of large mitochondria, a supranuclear Golgi complex, and a number of dense lysosomes.[17,18] Depending on the secretory state of the cell, large lipid droplets and secretory granules may be present in the apical cytoplasm. Two distinct products produced by the cells are released by different mechanisms.[19] The protein component of the milk is synthesized in the granular endoplasmic reticulum, packaged in membrane-limited secretory granules for transport in the Golgi apparatus, and released from the cell by fusion of the granule's limiting membrane with the plasma membrane. This type of secretion is known as *merocrine secretion*. The lipid, or fatty, component of the milk arises as free lipid droplets in the cytoplasm. The lipid coalesces into large droplets that pass to the apical region of the cell and project into the lumen of the acinus prior to their release. As they are released from the cell, the droplets are invested with an envelope of plasma membrane. A thin layer of cytoplasm is trapped between the lipid droplet and plasma membrane as lipid is being released. It should be emphasized that only a very small amount of cytoplasm is lost during this secretory process, classically known as *apocrine secretion*.

The milk released during the first few days after childbirth is known as *colostrum*. It has a low lipid content but is believed to contain considerable quantities of antibodies that may provide the newborn with some degree of passive immunity. The lymphocytes and plasma cells that infiltrate the stroma of the breast during its proliferation and development are believed to be, in part, the source of the components of the colostrum. As the plasma cells and lymphocytes decrease in number, the production of colostrum stops and lipid-rich milk is produced.

HORMONAL REGULATION OF THE MAMMARY GLAND

Production of estrogens and progesterone by the ovary at puberty stimulates and influences the initial growth of the mammary gland (see Chapter 3). Subsequent to this initial development, slight changes occur in the morphology of the glandular tissue with each ovarian, or menstrual, cycle. During pregnancy, the corpus luteum and placenta continuously produce estrogens and progesterone, which stimulate proliferation and development of the mammary gland. The growth of the glands is also dependent on the presence of prolactin, produced by the adenohypophysis; somatomammotropin (lactogenic hormone), produced by the placenta; and adrenal corticoids.

The level of circulating estrogens and progesterone drops abruptly at parturition with the degeneration of the corpus luteum and loss of the placenta. The secretion of milk is then brought about by increased production of prolactin and adrenal cortical steroids. A neurohormonal reflex regulates the high level of prolactin production and release. The act of suckling by the infant initiates impulses from receptors in the nipple that regulate cells in the hypothalamus. The impulses also cause the release of oxytocin in the neurohypophysis. The oxytocin stimulates the myoepithelial cells of the mammary glands, causing them to contract and eject milk from the glands.[20] In the absence of suckling, secretion of milk ceases and the glands regress and return to an inactive state.

After menopause, the gland atrophies, or involutes. As the release of ovarian hormones is diminished, the secretory cells of the alveoli degenerate and disappear, but some of the ducts remain. The connective tissue also demonstrates degenerative changes, marked by a decrease in the number of stromal cells and collagen fibers.

Thoracic Wall

The thoracic wall is composed of both skeletal and muscular components. The skeletal components include the 12 thoracic vertebrae, the 12 ribs and their costal cartilages, and the sternum. The spaces between the ribs, the *intercostal spaces*, are filled with the *external, internal,* and *innermost intercostal muscles* and the associated *intercostal vessels* and *nerves* (Figure 2-5). Some anatomists refer to the innermost layer as the *intima* of the *internal intercostal muscle*. The terminology chosen is of no particular consequence; the relationship that should be appreciated is that the intercostal veins,

arteries, and nerves pass in the plane that separates the internal intercostal muscle from the innermost (or intimal) layer. The *endothoracic fascia*, a thin fibrous layer of connective tissue forming a fascial plane continuous with the most internal component of the investing fascia of the intercostal muscles and the adjacent layer of the periosteum, marks the internal limit of the thoracic wall. The parietal pleura rests on the endothoracic fascia.

It is important to recognize that the muscles and skeletal girdles of the upper extremities almost completely cover the thoracic wall anteriorly, laterally, and posteriorly. For the surgeon concerned with the breast, a knowledge of the anatomy of the axilla and pectoral region is essential.

The 11 pairs of *external intercostal muscles* whose fibers run downward and forward form the most superficial layer (see later section on the innervation of the breast and Figure 2-11). The muscle begins posteriorly at the tubercles of the ribs and extends anteriorly to the costochondral junction. Between the costal cartilages, the muscle is replaced by the *external intercostal membrane*. The fibers of the 11 pairs of *internal intercostal muscles* run downward and posteriorly. The muscle fibers of this layer reach the sternum anteriorly. Posteriorly, the muscle ends at the angle of the ribs and then the layer continues as the *internal intercostal membrane*. The *innermost intercostal muscles (intercostales intimi)* form the most internal layer and have fibers that are oriented more vertically but almost in parallel with the internal intercostal muscle fibers. The muscle fibers of this layer occupy approximately the middle half of the intercostal space. This is the least well developed of the three layers. It can best be distinguished by the fact that its fibers are separated from the internal intercostals by the intercostal vessels and nerves.

The *subcostalis* and *transversus thoracis muscles* are located on the internal surface of the thoracic wall. They occur in the same plane as the innermost intercostal muscles and are considered anterior and posterior extensions of this layer. The subcostal muscles are located posteriorly and have the same orientation as the innermost intercostal muscles. They are distinct because they pass to the second or third rib below (i.e., they pass over at least two intercostal spaces). Anteriorly, the *transversus thoracis muscles* form a layer that arises from the lower internal surface of the sternum and extends upward and laterally to insert on the costal cartilages of the second to sixth ribs (Figure 2-6). These fibers pass deep to the internal thoracic artery and accompanying veins.

All of these muscles are innervated by the intercostal nerves associated with them. These nerves also give branches to the overlying skin. In a similar fashion, the intercostal vessels supply intercostal muscles and give branches to the overlying tissues. The intercostal nerves

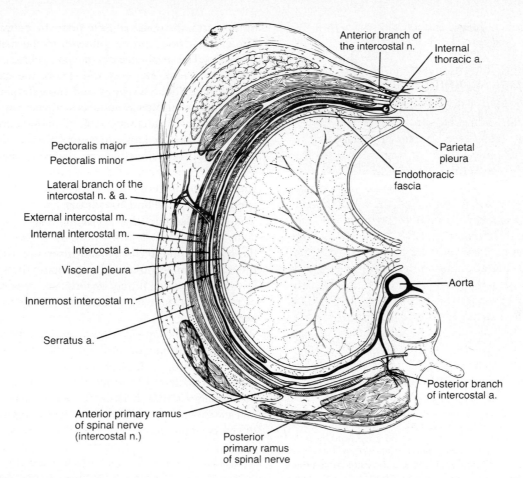

Anterior branch of
the intercostal n.

Internal
thoracic a.

Pectoralis major

Pectoralis minor

Parietal
pleura

Endothoracic
fascia

Lateral branch of the
intercostal n. & a.

External intercostal m.

Internal intercostal m.

Intercostal a.

Visceral pleura

Innermost intercostal m.

Aorta

Serratus a.

Posterior branch
of intercostal a.

Anterior primary ramus
of spinal nerve
(intercostal n.)

Posterior
primary ramus
of spinal nerve

FIG. **2-5** Cross section of the breast and chest wall illustrating the layers of the thoracic wall and paths of blood vessels and nerves. The intercostal muscles occur in three layers: external, internal, and innermost. The intercostal vessels and nerves pass between the internal and innermost layers. The posterior intercostal arteries arise from the aorta and pass anterior to anastomose with the anterior intercostal arteries that are branches of the internal thoracic artery. The veins are not shown but basically follow the course of the arteries. The intercostal nerves are direct continuations of the anterior primary rami of thoracic spinal nerves. They supply the intercostal muscles and give anterior and lateral branches that supply the overlying skin, including that of the breast. The breast lies superficial to the pectoralis major muscle and the underlying pectoralis minor muscle. The serratus anterior muscle originates from eight or nine fleshy digitations on the outer lateral surface of the ribs and inserts on the ventral surface of the medial (vertebral) border of the scapula. Parietal pleura attaches to the endothoracic fascia that lines the thoracic cavity. Visceral pleura covers the surface of the lungs. The thin channels in the substance of the lung represent lymphatic channels that convey lymph to pulmonary lymph nodes located in the hilum of the lung. Lymphatic channels draining the thoracic wall and overlying skin and superficial fascia are not illustrated but follow the path of the blood vessels that supply the region (see text).

are direct continuations of the ventral primary rami of the upper 11 thoracic spinal nerves. As the nerves pass anteriorly, they give branches to supply the intercostal muscles. In addition, each nerve gives a relatively large lateral cutaneous branch, which exits the intercostal space along the midaxillary line near the attachment sites of the serratus anterior muscle on the ribs. The lateral cutaneous nerves then give branches that extend anteriorly and posteriorly. As the intercostal nerve continues anteriorly, it gives additional branches to the intercostal muscles. Just lateral to the border of the sternum the upper five intercostal nerves pierce the internal intercostal muscle and the external intercostal membrane to end superficially as the *anterior cutaneous*

nerves of the chest. These nerves give rise to medial and lateral branches that supply the overlying skin. The lower six intercostal nerves continue past the costal margin into the anterior abdominal wall and are therefore identified as *thoracoabdominal nerves.*

The *intercostal arteries* originate in two groups: the anterior and posterior intercostal arteries. The *posterior intercostal arteries,* except for the first two spaces, arise from the thoracic aorta. The posterior intercostals for the first two spaces arise from the superior intercostal artery, which is a branch of the costocervical trunk. The anterior intercostals are usually small paired arteries that extend laterally to the region of the costochondral junction. The anterior intercostal arteries of the upper

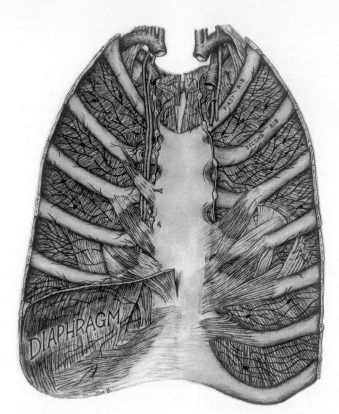

FIG. **2-6** The anterior thoracic wall as viewed internally. The internal thoracic arteries and veins can be seen as they pass parallel to and about 1 cm from the sternal margin. Except in the upper two or three intercostal spaces, the transversus thoracic muscle lies deep to these vessels. The internal thoracic lymphatic trunks and associated parasternal lymph nodes accompany these vessels. Lymphatic channels located in the intercostal spaces convey lymph from the thoracic wall anteriorly to the parasternal nodes or posteriorly to the intercostal nodes.

five intercostal spaces arise from the internal thoracic (or mammary) artery; those of the lower six intercostal spaces arise from the musculophrenic artery. The anterior and posterior intercostal veins demonstrate a similar distribution. Anteriorly, they drain into the musculophrenic and internal thoracic veins. Posteriorly, the intercostal veins drain into the azygos and hemiazygos systems of veins.

The superficial muscles of the pectoral region include the *pectoralis major* and *minor muscles* and the *subclavius muscle*. The *pectoralis major muscle* is a fan-shaped muscle with two divisions. The clavicular division (or head) originates from the clavicle and is easily distinguished from the larger costosternal division that originates from the sternum and costal cartilages of the second through sixth ribs. The fibers of the two divisions converge laterally and insert into the crest of the greater tubercle of the humerus along the lateral lip of the bicipital groove. The *cephalic vein* serves as a convenient landmark defining the separation of the upper lateral border

of the pectoralis major muscle from the deltoid muscle. The cephalic vein can be followed to the deltopectoral triangle, where it pierces the *clavipectoral fascia* and joins the axillary vein. The pectoralis major muscle acts primarily in flexion, adduction, and medial rotation of the arm at the shoulder joint. This action brings the arm across the chest. In climbing, the pectoralis major muscles, along with the latissimus dorsi muscles, function to elevate the trunk when the arms are fixed. The pectoralis major muscle is innervated by both the medial and the lateral pectoral nerves, which arise from the medial and lateral cords of the brachial plexus.

Located deep to the pectoralis major muscle, the *pectoralis minor muscle* arises from the external surface of the second to the fifth ribs and inserts on the coracoid process of the scapula. Although its main action is to lower the shoulder, it may serve as an accessory muscle of respiration. It is innervated by the medial pectoral nerve.

The *subclavius muscle* arises from the first rib near its costochondral junction and extends laterally to insert into the inferior surface of the clavicle. It functions to lower the clavicle and stabilize it during movements of the shoulder girdle. It is innervated by *the nerve to the subclavius muscle,* which arises from the upper trunk of the brachial plexus.

Axilla

A knowledge of the anatomy of the axilla and its contents is of paramount importance to the clinician. It is also essential that the surgeon be thoroughly familiar with the organization of the deep fascia and neurovascular relationships of the axilla.

BOUNDARIES OF THE AXILLA

The axilla is a pyramidal compartment between the upper extremity and the thoracic walls (Figure 2-7). It is described as having four walls, an apex, and a base. The curved *base* is made of axillary fascia and skin. Externally, this region, the *armpit,* appears dome-shaped (and covered with hair after puberty). The *apex* is not a roof but an aperture that extends into the posterior triangle of the neck through the *cervicoaxillary canal.* The cervicoaxillary canal is bounded anteriorly by the clavicle, posteriorly by the scapula, and medially by the first rib. Most structures pass through the cervical axillary canal as they course between the neck and upper extremity. The *anterior wall* is made up of the pectoralis major and minor muscles and their associated fasciae. The *posterior wall* is composed primarily of the subscapularis muscle, located on the anterior surface of the scapula, and to a lesser extent by the teres major and

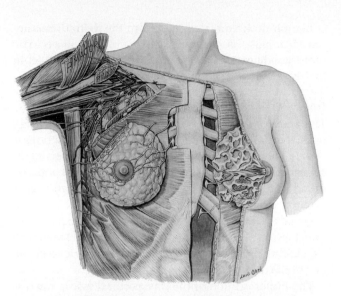

FIG. 2-7 The anterior chest illustrating the structure of the chest wall, breast, and axilla. See text for details of the structure of the axilla and a description of its contents. On the right side, the pectoralis major muscle has been cut lateral to the breast and reflected laterally to its insertion into the crest of the greater tubercle of the humerus. This exposes the underlying pectoralis minor muscle and the other muscles forming the walls of the axilla. The contents of the axilla, including the axillary artery and vein, components of the brachial plexus, and axillary lymph node groups and lymphatic channels, are exposed. On the left side, the breast is cut to expose its structure in sagittal view. The lactiferous ducts and sinuses can be seen. Lymphatic channels passing to parasternal lymph nodes are also shown.

latissimus dorsi muscles and their associated tendons. The *lateral wall* is a thin strip of the humerus, the bicipital groove, between the insertions of the muscles of the anterior and posterior walls. The *medial wall* is made up of serratus anterior muscle that covers the thoracic wall in this region (over the upper four or five ribs and their associated intercostal muscles).

CONTENTS OF THE AXILLA

The axilla contains the great vessels and nerves of the upper extremity. These, along with the other contents, are surrounded by loose connective tissue. Figure 2-7 illustrates many of the key relationships of structures within the axilla. The vessels and nerves are closely associated with each other and are enclosed within a layer of fascia, the *axillary sheath*. This layer of dense connective tissue extends from the neck and gradually disappears as the nerves and vessels branch.

The axillary artery may be divided into three parts within the axilla: (1) The first segment, located medial to the pectoralis minor muscle, gives one branch—the supreme thoracic artery that supplies the thoracic wall over the first and second intercostal spaces. (2) The

second part, located posterior to the pectoralis minor muscle, gives two branches—the thoracoacromial trunk and the lateral thoracic artery. The thoracoacromial trunk divides into the acromial, clavicular, deltoid, and pectoral branches. The lateral thoracic artery passes along the lateral border of the pectoralis minor on the superficial surface of the serratus anterior muscle. Pectoral branches of the thoracoacromial and lateral thoracic arteries supply both the pectoralis major and minor muscles and must be identified during surgical dissection of the axilla. The lateral thoracic artery is of particular importance in surgery of the breast because it supplies the *lateral mammary branches*. (3) The third part, located lateral to the pectoralis minor, gives off three branches—the anterior and posterior circumflex humeral arteries, which supply the upper arm and contribute to the collateral circulation around the shoulder, and the subscapular artery. Although the latter artery does not supply the breast, it is of particular importance in the surgical dissection of the axilla. It is the largest branch within the axilla, giving rise after a short distance to its terminal branches, the subscapular circumflex and the thoracodorsal arteries, and it is closely associated with the central and subscapular lymph node groups. In the axilla the thoracodorsal artery crosses the subscapularis and gives branches to it and to the serratus anterior and the latissimus dorsi muscles. A surgeon must use care in approaching this vessel and its branches to avoid undue bleeding that obscures the surgical field.

The *axillary vein* has tributaries that follow the course of the arteries just described. They are usually in the form of venae comitantes, paired veins that follow an artery. The *cephalic vein* passes in the groove between the deltoid and pectoralis major muscles and then joins the axillary vein after piercing the clavipectoral fascia.

Throughout its course in the axilla, the axillary artery is associated with various parts of the *brachial plexus* (Figure 2-8). The cords of the brachial plexus—medial, lateral, and posterior—are named according to their relationship with the axillary artery. A majority of the branches of the brachial plexus arise in the axilla. The *lateral cord* gives four branches, namely, the *lateral pectoral nerve*, which supplies the pectoralis major; a branch that communicates with the medial pectoral nerve, which is called the *ansa pectoralis*[21]; and two terminal branches, the *musculocutaneous nerve* and the *lateral root of the median nerve*. Injury to the medial or lateral pectoral nerves, or the ansa pectoralis,[21] which joins them, may lead to loss of muscle mass and fatty necrosis of the pectoralis major or minor muscles,[22] depending of the level of nerve injury. The ansa pectoralis lies anterior to the axillary artery, making it vulnerable to injury during lymph node dissection in the axilla.

The *medial cord* usually gives five branches, the *medial pectoral nerve* (which supplies both the pectoralis major

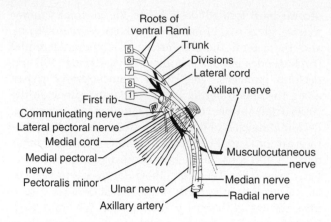

FIG. **2-8** Schematic drawing of the brachial plexus illustrating its basic components. The cords are associated with the axillary artery and lie behind the pectoralis minor muscle. The names of the cords reflect their relationship to the artery. Compare with Figure 2-7 to identify the course of these structures in more detail.

and minor), the *median brachial cutaneous nerve*, the *medial antebrachial cutaneous nerve*, and two terminal branches—the *ulnar nerve and the lateral root of the median nerve*. The *posterior cord* usually has five branches. Three of these nerves arise from the posterior cord in the superior aspect of the axilla—the *upper subscapular*, the *thoracodorsal*, and the *lower subscapular*; the cord then divides into its two terminal branches—the *axillary* and *radial* nerves.

Two additional branches of the brachial plexus, the *long thoracic* and *intercostobrachial nerves*, are of particular interest to surgeons because they are vulnerable to injury during axillary dissection. The *long thoracic nerve* is located on the medial wall of the axilla. It arises in the neck from the fifth, sixth, and seventh roots of the brachial and then enters the axilla through the cervicoaxillary canal. It lies on the surface of the serratus anterior muscle, which it supplies. The long thoracic nerve is covered by the serratus fascia and is sometimes accidentally removed with the fascia during surgery. This results in paralysis of part or all of the serratus anterior muscle. The functional deficit is an inability to raise the arm above the level of the shoulder (or extreme weakness when one attempts this movement). A second nerve, the *intercostobrachial*, is formed by the joining of a lateral cutaneous branch of the second intercostal nerve with the medial cutaneous nerve of the arm. This nerve supplies the skin of the floor of the axilla and the upper medial aspect of the arm. Sometimes, a second intercostobrachial nerve may form an anterior branch of the third lateral cutaneous nerve. This nerve is commonly injured in axillary dissection, resulting in numbness of the skin of the floor of the axilla and the medial aspect of the arm.

Lymph nodes are also present in the axilla. They are found in close association with the blood vessels. The lymph node groups and their location are described in the section on the lymphatic drainage of the breast.

AXILLARY FASCIAE

The anterior wall of the axilla is composed of the pectoralis major and minor muscles and the fascia that covers them. The fasciae occur in two layers: (1) a superficial layer investing the pectoralis major muscle, called the *pectoral fascia*, and (2) a deep layer that extends from the clavicle to the axillary fascia in the floor of the axilla, called the *clavipectoral (or costocoracoid) fascia*. The clavipectoral fascia encloses the subclavius muscle located below the clavicle and the pectoralis minor muscle (Figure 2-9).

The upper portion of the clavipectoral fascia, the *costocoracoid membrane*, is pierced by the cephalic vein, the lateral pectoral nerve, and branches of the thoracoacromial trunk. The medial pectoral nerve does not pierce the costocoracoid membrane but enters the deep surface of the pectoralis minor supplying it and passes through the anterior investing layer of the pectoralis minor to innervate the pectoralis minor. The lower portion of the clavipectoral fascia, located below the pectoralis minor muscle, is sometimes called the *suspensory ligament of the axilla* or the *coracoaxillary fascia*.

Halsted's ligament, a dense condensation of the clavipectoral fascia, extends from the medial end of the clavicle and attaches to the first rib (see Figures 2-7 and 2-9, *A*). The ligament covers the subclavian artery and vein as they cross the first rib.

Fascial Relationships of the Breast

The breast is located in the superficial fascia in the layer just deep to the dermis, the *hypodermis*. In approaching the breast, a surgeon may dissect in a bloodless plane just deep to the dermis. This dissection leaves a layer 2 to 3 mm in thickness in thin individuals in association with the skin flap. The layer may be several millimeters thick in obese individuals. The blood vessels and lymphatics passing in the deeper layer of the superficial fascia are left undisturbed.

Anterior fibrous processes, the *suspensory ligaments of Cooper*, pass from the septa that divide the lobules of the breast to insert into the skin. The posterior aspect of the breast is separated from the deep, or investing, fascia of the pectoralis major muscle by a space filled with loose areolar tissue, the *retromammary space* or *bursa* (see Figure 2-1). The existence of the retromammary space and the suspensory ligaments of Cooper allows the breast to move freely against the thoracic

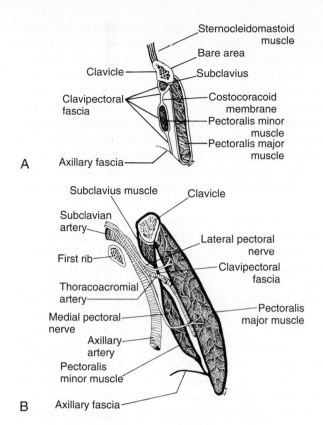

A

Sternocleidomastoid muscle
Bare area
Clavicle
Subclavius
Clavipectoral fascia
Costocoracoid membrane
Pectoralis minor muscle
Pectoralis major muscle
Axillary fascia

B

Subclavius muscle
Clavicle
Subclavian artery
First rib
Thoracoacromial artery
Medial pectoral nerve
Axillary artery
Pectoralis minor muscle
Axillary fascia
Lateral pectoral nerve
Clavipectoral fascia
Pectoralis major muscle

FIG. **2-9** Sagittal sections of the chest wall in the axillary region. **A,** The anterior wall of the axilla. The clavicle and three muscles inferior to it are shown. **B,** Section through the chest wall illustrating the relationship of the axillary artery and medial and lateral pectoral nerves to the clavipectoral fascia. The clavipectoral fascia is a strong sheet of connective tissue that is attached superiorly to the clavicle and envelops the subclavius and pectoralis minor muscles. The fascia extends from the lower border of the pectoralis minor to become continuous with the axillary fascia in the floor of the axilla.

wall. The space between the well-defined fascial planes of the breast and pectoralis major is easily identified by the surgeon removing a breast. Connective tissue thickenings, called *posterior suspensory ligaments,* extend from the deep surface of the breast to the deep pectoral fascia. Because breast parenchyma may follow these fibrous processes, it has been common practice to remove the adjacent portion of the pectoralis major muscle with the breast.

It is important to recognize, particularly with movements and variation in the size of the breast, that its deep surface contacts the investing fascia of other muscles in addition to the pectoralis major. Only about two thirds of the breast overlies the pectoralis major muscle. The lateral portion of the breast may contact the fourth through seventh slips of the serratus anterior muscle at its attachment to the thoracic wall. Just medial to this,

the breast contacts the upper portion of the abdominal oblique muscle, where it interdigitates with the attachments of the serratus anterior muscle. As the breast extends to the axilla, it has contact with deep fascia present in this region.

BLOOD SUPPLY OF THE BREAST

The breast receives its blood supply from (1) perforating branches of the internal mammary artery; (2) lateral branches of the posterior intercostal arteries; and (3) several branches from the axillary artery, including highest thoracic, lateral thoracic, and pectoral branches of the thoracoacromial artery (Figure 2-10). For reviews of the blood supply of the breast, see Cunningham,[23] Maliniac,[24] and Sakki.[25]

Branches from the second, third, and fourth anterior perforating arteries (Figures 2-10 and 2-11) pass to the breast as *medial mammary arteries.* These vessels enlarge considerably during lactation. The lateral thoracic artery gives branches to the serratus anterior muscle, both pectoralis muscles, and the subscapularis muscle. The lateral thoracic artery also gives rise to *lateral*

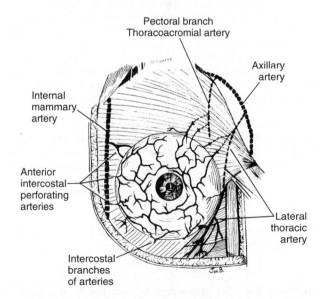

Pectoral branch Thoracoacromial artery
Axillary artery
Internal mammary artery
Anterior intercostal perforating arteries
Lateral thoracic artery
Intercostal branches of arteries

FIG. **2-10** Arterial distribution of blood to the breast, axilla, and chest wall. The breast receives its blood supply via three major arterial routes: (1) medially from anterior perforating intercostal branches arising from the internal thoracic artery, (2) laterally from either pectoral branches of the thoracoacromial trunk or branches of the lateral thoracic artery (the thoracoacromial trunk and the lateral thoracic arteries are branches of the axillary artery), and (3) from lateral cutaneous branches of the intercostals arteries that are associated with the overlying breast. The arteries indicated with a dashed line lie deep to the muscles of the thoracic wall and axilla. Many of the arteries must pass through these muscles before reaching the breast.

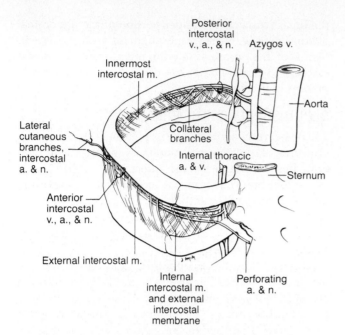

FIG. **2-11** A segment of the body wall illustrating the relationship of structures to the ribs. Two ribs are shown as they extend from the vertebrae to attach to the sternum. The orientation of the muscle and connective tissue fibers is shown. The external intercostal muscle extends downward and forward. The muscle layer extends forward from the rib tubercle to the costochondral junction, where the muscle is replaced by the aponeurosis, called the *external intercostal membrane.* The internal intercostal muscle fibers with the opposite orientation can be seen through this layer. The innermost intercostal muscle fibers are present along the lateral half of the intercostal space. The intercostal nerve and vessels pass through the intercostal space in the plane between the internal and innermost (or intima of the internal) intercostal muscle layers. Anterior intercostal arteries arise from the internal thoracic artery; anterior intercostal veins join the internal thoracic vein. Posterior intercostal arteries arise from the aorta; posterior intercostal veins join the azygos venous system on the right and the hemiazygos system on the left. Lymphatics follow the path of the blood vessels. Anteriorly, lymphatics pass to parasternal (or internal mammary) nodes that are located along the internal mammary vessels; posteriorly, they pass to intercostal nodes located in the intercostal space near the vertebral bodies.

mammary branches that wrap around the lateral border of the pectoralis major muscle to reach the breast. In the second, third, and fourth intercostal spaces, the posterior intercostal arteries give off *mammary branches;* these vessels increase in size during lactation.

The thoracodorsal branch of the subscapular artery is not involved in the supply of blood to the breast but it is important to the surgeon who must deal with this artery during the dissection of the axilla. The central and scapular lymph node groups are intimately associated with this vessel. Bleeding that is difficult to control may result from cutting of branches of these vessels.

A fundamental knowledge of the pattern of venous drainage is important because carcinoma of the breast may metastasize through the veins and because lymphatic vessels often follow the course of the blood vessels. The veins of the breast basically follow the path of the arteries, with the chief venous drainage toward the axilla. The superficial veins demonstrate extensive anastomoses that may be apparent through the skin overlying the breast. The distribution of these veins has been studied by Massopust and Gardner[26] and Haagensen[27] using photographs taken in infrared light. Around the nipple, the veins form an anastomotic circle, the *circulus venosus.* Veins from this circle and from the substance of the gland transmit blood to the periphery of the breast and then into vessels joining the internal thoracic, axillary, and internal jugular veins.

Three principal groups of veins are involved in the venous drainage of the thoracic wall and the breast: (1) perforating branches of the internal thoracic vein, (2) tributaries of the axillary vein, and (3) perforating branches of posterior intercostal veins. Metastatic emboli traveling through any of these venous routes will pass through the venous return to the heart and then be stopped as they reach the capillary bed of the lungs, providing a direct venous route for metastasis of breast carcinoma to the lungs.

The *vertebral plexus of veins (Batson's plexus)* may provide a second route for metastasis of breast carcinoma via veins.[28-30] This venous plexus surrounds the vertebrae and extends from the base of the skull to the sacrum. Venous channels exist between this plexus and veins associated with thoracic, abdominal, and pelvic organs. In general, these veins do not have valves, making it possible for blood to flow through them in either direction. Furthermore, it is known that increases in intraabdominal pressure may force blood to enter these channels. These vessels provide a route for metastatic emboli to reach the vertebral bodies, ribs, and central nervous system. (The spread of carcinoma of the prostate to the vertebral bodies and central nervous system occurs through these venous communications.) These venous communications are of particular significance in the breast, where the posterior intercostal arteries are in direct continuity with the vertebral plexus.

Innervation of the Breast

Miller and Kasahara[31] have described the microscopic anatomic features of the innervation of the skin over the breast. They suggest that the specialization of the innervation of the breast, areola, and nipple is associated with the erection of the nipple[11] and flow of milk mediated through a neurohormonal reflex. As was explained previously, the act of suckling initiates impulses from receptors in the nipple that regulate cells in the hypothalamus. In response to the impulses, oxytocin is released in the neurohypophysis. The oxytocin stimulates the myoepithelial cells of the mammary glands, causing them to contract and eject milk from the glands. In the dermis of the nipple, Miller and Kasahara[31] found large numbers of multibranched free nerve endings; in the dermis of the areola and peripheral, Ruffini-like endings and Krause end-bulbs. The latter two receptor types are associated with tactile reception of stretch and pressure.

Sensory innervation of the breast is supplied primarily by the *lateral and anterior cutaneous branches of the second through sixth intercostal nerves* (see Figure 2-11). Although the second and third intercostal nerves may give rise to cutaneous branches to the superior aspect of the breast, the nerves of the breast are derived primarily from the fourth, fifth, and sixth intercostal nerves. A limited region of the skin over the upper portion of the breast is supplied by nerves arising from the cervical plexus, specifically, the anterior, or medial, branches of the *supraclavicular nerve*. All of these nerves convey sympathetic fibers to the breast and overlying skin and therefore influence flow of blood through vessels accompanying the nerves and secretory function of the sweat glands of the skin. However, the secretory activity of the breast is chiefly under the control of ovarian and hypophyseal (pituitary) hormones.

The lateral branches of the intercostal nerves exit the intercostal space at the attachment sites of the slips of serratus anterior muscle. The nerves divide into anterior and posterior branches as they pass between the muscle fibers. As the anterior branches pass in the superficial fascia, they supply the anterolateral thoracic wall; the third through sixth branches, also known as *lateral mammary branches*, supply the breast. The lateral branch of the second intercostal nerve is of special significance because a large nerve, the *intercostal brachial*, arises from it. This nerve, which can be seen during surgical dissection of the axilla, passes through the fascia of the floor of the axilla and usually joins the medial cutaneous nerve of the arm. However, it is of limited functional significance. If this nerve is injured during surgery, the patient will have loss of cutaneous sensation from the upper medial aspect of the arm and floor of the axilla.

The anterior branches of the intercostal nerves exit the intercostal space near the lateral border of the sternum. These nerves send branches medially and laterally over the thoracic wall. The branches that pass laterally reach the medial aspect of the breast and are sometimes called *medial mammary nerves*.

Lymphatic Drainage of the Breast

LYMPH NODES OF THE AXILLA

The primary route of lymphatic drainage of the breast is through the axillary lymph node groups (see Figures 2-7 and 2-12). Therefore it is essential that the clinician understand the anatomy of the grouping of lymph nodes within the axilla. Unfortunately, the boundaries of groups of lymph nodes found in the axilla are not well demarcated. Thus there has been considerable variation in the names given to the lymph node groups. Anatomists usually define five groups of *axillary lymph nodes*[32,33]; surgeons usually identify six primary groups.[27] The most common terms used to identify the lymph nodes are indicated as follows:

1. The axillary vein group, usually identified by anatomists as the lateral group, consists of four to six lymph nodes that lie medial or posterior to the axillary vein. These lymph nodes receive most of the lymph draining from the upper extremity (Figure 2-13). The exception is lymph that drains into the deltopectoral lymph nodes, a lymph node group sometimes called infraclavicular. The deltopectoral lymph nodes are not considered part

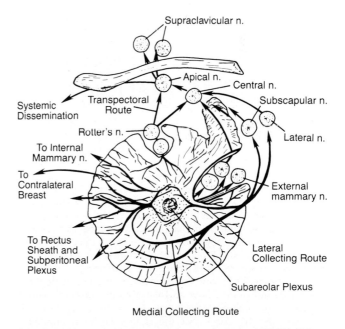

FIG. **2-12** Schematic drawing of the breast identifying the position of lymph nodes relative to the breast and illustrating routes of lymphatic drainage. The clavicle is indicated as a reference point. See the text and Figure 2-14 to identify the group or level to which the lymph nodes belong. Level I lymph nodes include the external mammary (or anterior), axillary vein (or lateral), and scapular (or posterior) groups; level II, the central group; and level III, the subclavicular (or apical). The arrows indicate the routes of lymphatic drainage (see text).

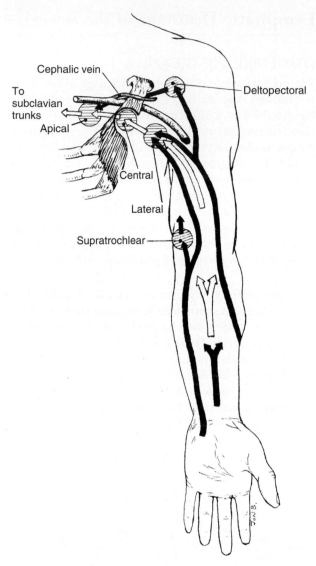

FIG. **2-13** Schematic drawing illustrating the route of lymphatic drainage in the upper extremity. The relationship of this drainage to the major axillary lymph node groups is indicated by the arrows. All the lymph vessels of the upper extremity drain directly or indirectly through outlying lymph node groups into the axillary lymph nodes. The outlying lymph nodes are few in number and are organized into three groups: (1) supratrochlear lymph nodes (one or two, located above the medial epicondyle of the humerus adjacent to the basilic vein), (2) deltopectoral lymph nodes (one or two, located beside the cephalic vein where it lies between the pectoralis major and deltoid muscle just below the clavicle), and (3) variable small isolated lymph nodes (few and variable in number; may be located in the cubital fossa or along the medial side of the brachial vessels). Note that the deltopectoral lymph node group drains directly into the subclavicular, or apical, lymph nodes of the axillary group.

of the axillary lymph node group but rather are outlying lymph nodes that drain into the subclavicular (or apical) lymph node group (see later discussion).

2. The *external mammary group,* usually identified by anatomists as the *anterior* or *pectoral group,* consists of four or five lymph nodes that lie along the lower border of the pectoralis minor in association with the lateral thoracic vessels. These lymph nodes receive the major portion of the lymph draining from the breast. Lymph drains primarily from these lymph nodes into the central lymph nodes. However, lymph may pass directly from the external mammary nodes into the subclavicular lymph nodes.

3. The *scapular group,* usually identified by anatomists as the *posterior* or *subscapular group,* consists of six or seven lymph nodes that lie along the posterior wall of the axilla at the lateral border of the scapula in association with the subscapular vessels. These lymph nodes receive lymph primarily from the inferior aspect of the posterior neck, the posterior aspect of the trunk as far inferior as the iliac crest, and the posterior aspect of the shoulder region. Lymph from the scapular nodes passes to the central and subclavicular nodes.

4. The *central group* (both anatomists and surgeons use the same terminology for this group) consists of three or four large lymph nodes that are embedded in the fat of the axilla, usually posterior to the pectoralis minor muscle. They receive lymph from the three preceding groups and may receive afferent lymphatic vessels directly from the breast. Lymph from the central nodes passes directly to the subclavicular (apical) nodes. This group is often superficially placed beneath the skin and fascia of the midaxilla and is centrally located between the posterior and anterior axillary fold. This nodal group is commonly palpable because of its superficial position and allows the clinical estimation of metastatic disease.[27,34]

5. The subclavicular group, usually identified by anatomists as the apical group, consists of 6 to 12 lymph nodes located partly posterior to the upper border of the pectoralis minor and partly superior to it. These lymph nodes extend into the apex of the axilla along the medial side of the axillary vein. They may receive lymph directly or indirectly from all the other groups of axillary lymph nodes. The efferent lymphatic vessels from the subclavicular lymph nodes unite to form the subclavian trunk. The course of the subclavian trunk is highly variable. It may directly join the internal jugular vein, the subclavian vein, or the junction of these two; likewise, on the right side of the trunk, it may join the right lymphatic duct, and on the left side, it may join the thoracic duct. Efferent vessels from

the subclavicular lymph nodes may also pass to deep cervical lymph nodes.

6. The *interpectoral* or *Rotter's group*,[35] a group of nodes identified by surgeons[27] but usually not by anatomists, consists of one to four small lymph nodes that are located between the pectoralis major and minor muscles in association with the pectoral branches of the thoracoacromial vessels. Lymph from these nodes passes into central and subclavicular nodes.

Surgeons also define the axillary lymph nodes with respect to their relationship with the pectoralis minor muscle (Figure 2-14).[34,36] These relationships are illustrated schematically in Figure 2-15. Lymph nodes that are located lateral to or below the lower border of the pectoralis minor muscle are called *level I* and include the external mammary, axillary vein, and scapular lymph node groups. Those lymph nodes located deep or posterior to the pectoralis minor muscle are called *level II*

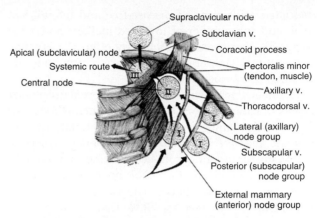

FIG. **2-15** Schematic drawing illustrating the major lymph node groups associated with the lymphatic drainage of the breast. The Roman numerals indicate three levels or groups of lymph nodes that are defined by their location relative to the pectoralis minor. Level I includes lymph nodes located lateral to the pectoralis minor; level II, lymph nodes located deep to the muscle; and level III, lymph nodes located medial to the muscle. The arrows indicate the general direction of lymph flow. The axillary vein and its major tributaries associated with the pectoralis minor are included.

and include the central lymph node group and possibly some of the subclavicular lymph node group. Those lymph nodes located medial or superior to the upper border of the pectoralis minor muscle are called *level III* and include the subclavicular lymph node group.

Surgeons use the term *prepectoral* to identify a single lymph node that is only rarely found in the subcutaneous tissue associated with the breast or in the breast itself in its upper outer sector.[27] Haagensen reports finding only one or two prepectoral nodes each year among the several hundred mammary lesions studied.

SENTINEL LYMPH NODE BIOPSY

Several recent reviews[37-49] have discussed the potential benefits and risks of sentinel lymph node (SLN) identification and biopsy in breast cancer surgery and treatment. The basic principle of SLN biopsy is that the first lymph node which receives drainage from a tumor will be the first site of lymphatic metastasis. The status of the SLN reflects the status of the more distal lymph nodes along the lymphatic chain. Lee and colleagues[43] report on several studies that have shown that if only one lymph node has metastatic involvement, it is almost always the SLN; furthermore, it is often the only site of metastasis.

The three most important pathologic determinants of the prognosis of early breast cancer are the status of the axillary lymph nodes, histologic grade, and tumor size. For the past century, axillary lymph node dissection (ALND) has been an integral part of breast cancer management. The presence of axillary metastasis is

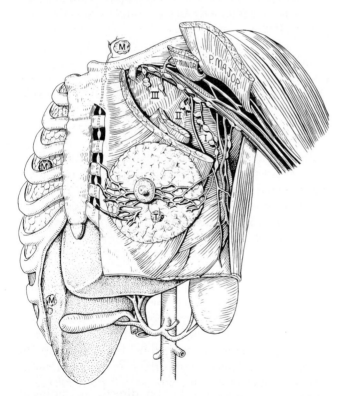

FIG. **2-14** Lymphatic drainage of the breast. The pectoralis major and minor muscles, which contribute to the anterior wall of the axilla, have been cut and reflected. This exposes the medial and posterior walls of the axilla, as well as the basic contents of the axilla. The lymph node groups of the axilla and the internal mammary nodes are depicted. Also shown is the location of the long thoracic nerve on the surface of the serratus anterior muscle (on the medial wall of the axilla). The scapular lymph node group is closely associated with the thoracodorsal nerve and vessels. The Roman numerals indicate lymph node groups defined in Figure 2-15.

associated with reduced disease-free and overall survival, and the number of involved axillary nodes has prognostic significance. SLN biopsy offers the possibility of optimal sampling of the axillary lymph nodes for the staging of breast cancer.

A number of techniques have been reported to optimize the identification of the SLN. The two main methods used are blue dye and/or radiolabeled material. In both methods the dye or radiolabeled material is injected around the tumor or deep in the overlying skin. With the blue dye, the location of the SLN is not known preoperatively and the blue stained lymphatics are followed intraoperatively to find the SLN. Use of radiolabeled material allows the tracer to be detected preoperatively with lymphoscintigraphy, or intraoperatively with γ probe, or a combination of the two. Lee and colleagues[43] report that in recent large studies, the SLN was identified 93% to 99% of the time. They also report that in the larger series of studies, the false-negative SLN with metastasis elsewhere in the axilla is in the range of 1% to 11%.

Before SLN biopsy can be used to determine specific surgical approaches and the extent of adjuvant chemotherapy and regional radiation therapy, there must be consensus on the sensitivity of the method and the accepted false-negative rates. In his review, Von Smitten[49] reports rates of detection of sentinel nodes ranging from 66% to 100% and false-negative rates of 17% to 0% have been reported. Von Smitten[49] suggests a theoretical false-negative rate of 2% to 3% may be acceptable; Cody[37] suggests a goal for surgeons and institutions using SLN biopsy to be at least 90% successful in finding the SLN with no more than 5% to 10% false-negative findings. In the case of SLN biopsy, as is true in most areas of medicine, the skill, expertise, and thoroughness of the pathologist who reads the specimen is of utmost importance.

LYMPH FLOW

A conceptualization of lymphatic drainage of the breast is essential to the student of this organ's pathophysiology. Metastatic dissemination of breast cancer occurs predominantly by lymphatic routes that are rich and extensive and arborize in multiple directions through skin and mesenchymal (intraparenchymal) lymphatics. The delicate lymphatics of the corium are valveless; flow encompasses the lobular parenchyma and thereafter parallels major venous tributaries to enter the regional lymph nodes. This unidirectional lymphatic flow is pulsatile as a consequence of the wavelike contractions of the lymphatics to allow rapid transit and emptying of the lymphatic vascular spaces that interdigitate the extensive periductal and perilobular network. As a consequence of obstruction to lymph flow by inflammatory or neoplastic diseases, a reversal in lymphatic flow is evident and can be appreciated microscopically as endolymphatic

metastases of the dermis or breast parenchyma. This obstruction of lymphatic flow accounts for the neoplastic growth in local and regional sites remote from the primary neoplasm.

Lymphatic flow is typically unidirectional, except in the pathologic state, and has preferential flow from the periphery toward larger collecting ducts. Lymphatic capillaries begin as blind-ending ducts in tissues from which the lymph is collected; throughout their course these capillaries anastomose and fuse to form larger lymphatic channels that ultimately terminate in the thoracic duct on the left side of the body or the smaller right lymphatic duct on the right side. The thoracic duct empties into the region of the junction of the left subclavian and internal jugular veins, whereas the right lymphatic duct drains into the right subclavian vein near its junction with the internal jugular vein.

Haagensen emphasized that lymphatics of the dermis are intimately associated with deeper lymphatics of the underlying fascial planes, which explains the multidirectional potential for drainage of superficial breast neoplasms. Preferential lymphatic flow toward the axilla is observed in lesions of the upper anterolateral chest. In addition, at the level of the umbilicus, tributaries diverge such that chest and upper anterior and lateral abdominal wall lymph also enter channels of the axilla. Thus carcinomatous involvement of skin, even of the inframammary region, has preferential flow to the axilla rather than to the groin.[27]

Anson and McVay[34] and Haagensen[27] acknowledged two accessory directions for lymphatic flow from breast parenchyma to nodes of the apex of the axilla: the *transpectoral* and *retropectoral routes* (see Figure 2-12). Lymphatics of the transpectoral route (i.e., interpectoral nodes) lie between the pectoralis major and minor muscles and are referred to as *Rotter's nodes*. The transpectoral route begins in the loose areolar tissue of the retromammary plexus and interdigitates between the pectoral fascia and breast to perforate the pectoralis major muscle and follow the course of the thoracoacromial artery and terminate in the subclavicular (level III) group of nodes.

The second accessory lymphatic drainage group, the retropectoral pathway, drains the superior and internal aspects of the breast. Lymphatic vessels from this region of the breast join lymphatics from the posterior and lateral surface of the pectoralis major and minor muscles. These lymphatic channels terminate at the apex of the axilla in the subclavicular (level III) group. This route of lymphatic drainage is found in approximately one third of individuals and is a more direct mechanism of lymphatic flow to the subclavicular group. This accessory pathway is also the major lymphatic drainage by way of the external mammary and central axillary nodal groups (levels I and II, respectively).[27,34]

The recognition of metastatic spread of breast carcinoma into internal mammary nodes as a primary route of systemic dissemination is credited to the British surgeon R.S. Handley.[50] Extensive investigation confirmed that central and medial lymphatics of the breast pass medially and parallel the course of major blood vessels to perforate the pectoralis major muscle and thereafter terminate in the internal mammary nodal chain.

The internal mammary nodal group (see Figures 2-6 and 2-14) is anatomically situated in the retrosternal interspaces between the costal cartilages approximately 2 to 3 cm within the sternal margin. These nodal groups also traverse and parallel the internal mammary vasculature and are invested by endothoracic fascia. The internal mammary lymphatic trunks eventually terminate in subclavicular nodal groups (see Figures 2-6, 2-12, and 2-15). The right internal mammary nodal group enters the right lymphatic duct, and the left enters the main thoracic duct (Figure 2-16). The presence of supraclavicular nodes (stage IV disease) results from lymphatic permeation and subsequent obstruction of the inferior, deep cervical group of nodes of the jugular-subclavian confluence. In effect, the supraclavicular nodal group represents the termination of efferent trunks from subclavian nodes of the internal mammary nodal group. These nodes are situated beneath the lateral margin of the inferior aspect of the sternocleidomastoid muscle beneath the clavicle and represent common sites of distant metastases from mammary carcinoma.

Cross-communication from the interstices of connecting lymphatic channels from each breast provides ready access of lymphatic flow to the opposite axilla. This observation of communicating dermal lymphatics to the contralateral breast explains occasional metastatic involvement of the opposite breast and axilla. Structures of the chest wall, including the internal and external intercostal musculature (see Figure 2-11), have extensive lymphatic drainage that parallels the course of their major intercostal blood supply. As expected, invasive neoplasms of the lateral breast that involve deep musculature of the thoracic cavity will have preferential flow toward the axilla. Invasion of medial musculature of the chest wall allows preferential drainage toward the internal mammary nodal groups, whereas bidirectional metastases may be evident with invasive central or subareolar cancers.

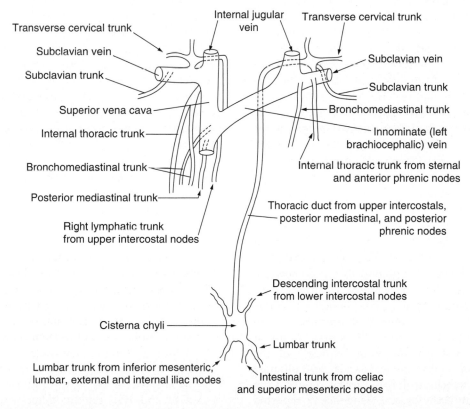

Internal jugular vein

Transverse cervical trunk

Transverse cervical trunk

Subclavian vein

Subclavian vein

Subclavian trunk

Subclavian trunk

Superior vena cava

Bronchomediastinal trunk

Internal thoracic trunk

Innominate (left brachiocephalic) vein

Bronchomediastinal trunk

Internal thoracic trunk from sternal and anterior phrenic nodes

Posterior mediastinal trunk

Thoracic duct from upper intercostals, posterior mediastinal, and posterior phrenic nodes

Right lymphatic trunk from upper intercostal nodes

Descending intercostal trunk from lower intercostal nodes

Cisterna chyli

Lumbar trunk

Lumbar trunk from inferior mesenteric, lumbar, external and internal iliac nodes

Intestinal trunk from celiac and superior mesenteric nodes

FIG. **2-16** Schematic of the major lymphatic vessels of the thorax and the root of the neck. The thoracic duct begins at the cisterna chyli, a dilated sac that receives drainage from the lower extremities and the abdominal and pelvic cavities via the lumbar and intestinal trunks. Lymph enters the systemic circulation via channels that join the great veins of the neck and superior mediastinum. The lymphatic vessels demonstrate considerable variation as to their number and pattern of branching. A typical pattern is illustrated here. Most of the major trunks, including the thoracic and right lymphatic ducts, end at or near the confluence of the internal jugular with the subclavian.

The lymphatic vessels that drain the breast occur in three interconnecting groups[51]: (1) A primary set of vessels originates as channels within the gland in the interlobular spaces and along the lactiferous ducts; (2) vessels draining the glandular tissue and overlying skin of the central part of the gland pass to an interconnecting network of vessels located beneath the areola, called the *subareolar plexus*[52]; and (3) a plexus on the deep surface of the breast communicates with minute vessels in the deep fascia underlying the breast. Along the medial border of the breast, lymphatic vessels within the substance of the gland anastomose with vessels passing to parasternal nodes.

Using autoradiographs of surgical specimens, Turner-Warwick[51] demonstrated that the main lymphatic drainage of the breast is through the system of lymphatic vessels occurring within the substance of the gland and not through the vessels on the superficial or deep surface. The main collecting trunks run laterally as they pass through the axillary fascia in the substance of the axillary tail. The subareolar plexus plays no essential part in the lymphatic drainage of the breast.[51] Using vital dyes, Halsell and co-workers[53] demonstrated that this plexus receives lymph primarily from the nipple and the areola and conveys it toward the axilla. The lymphatics communicating with minute vessels in the deep fascia play no part in the normal lymphatic drainage of the breast and provide an alternative route only when the normal pathways are obstructed. More than 75% of the lymph from the breast passes to the axillary lymph nodes (see Figure 2-12). Most of the remainder of the lymph passes to parasternal nodes. Some authorities have suggested that the parasternal nodes receive lymph primarily from the medial part of the breast. However, Turner-Warwick[51] reported that both the axillary and the parasternal lymph node groups receive lymph from all quadrants of the breast, with no striking tendency for any quadrant to drain in a particular direction.

Other routes for the flow of lymph from the breast have been identified. Occasionally, lymph from the breast reaches intercostal lymph nodes, located near the heads of the ribs (see later discussion). Lymphatic vessels reach this location by following lateral cutaneous branches of the posterior intercostal arteries. Lymph may pass to lymphatics within the rectus sheath or subperitoneal plexus by following branches of the intercostal and musculophrenic vessels. Lymph may pass directly to subclavicular, or apical, nodes from the upper portion of the breast. Haagensen[27] reported treating a patient who had apparently demonstrated direct metastasis from the breast to the supraclavicular nodes.

The skin over the breast has lymphatic drainage via the *superficial lymphatic vessels*, which ramify subcutaneously and converge on the axillary lymph nodes. The anterolateral chest and the upper abdominal wall above the umbilicus demonstrate striking directional flow of lymph toward the axilla. Below the umbilicus (the umbilicus establishing a "watershed"), superficial lymphatics carry lymph to the inguinal lymph node groups. It is important to recognize that the skin of the inframammary region drains into the axillary lymph nodes and not into the inguinal nodes. Lymphatic vessels near the lateral margin of the sternum pass through the intercostal space to the *parasternal lymph nodes*, which are associated with the internal thoracic vessels. Some of the lymphatic vessels located on adjacent sides of the sternum may anastomose in front of the sternum. In the upper pectoral region, a few of the lymphatic vessels may pass over the clavicle to *inferior deep cervical lymph nodes.*

The SLN identification is also providing better evidence of the paths of axillary lymphatic drainage of the breast. This technique is especially useful in identifying the lymphatic drainage into the parasternal or internal mammary lymph nodes.[38] The lymphatic vessels from the deeper structures of the thoracic wall drain primarily into parasternal, intercostal, or diaphragmatic lymph nodes (see later discussion).

LYMPH NODES OF THE THORACIC WALL

The lymphatic drainage of the skin and superficial tissues of thoracic and anterior abdominal walls is described in the section on the lymphatic drainage of the breast. Three sets of lymph nodes and associated vessels—*parasternal, intercostal,* and *diaphragmatic*—are involved in the lymphatic drainage of the deeper tissues of the thoracic wall:

1. *The parasternal, or internal thoracic, lymph nodes* consist of small lymph nodes located about 1 cm lateral to the sternal border in the intercostal spaces along the internal thoracic, or mammary, vessels (see Figures 2-1 and 2-6). The parasternal nodes lie in the areolar tissue underlying the endothoracic fascia that borders the space between the adjacent costal cartilages. The distribution of the nodes in the upper six intercostal spaces has been the subject of several studies since Stibbe's report in 1918 of an average total of 8.5 internal mammary nodes per subject, including both sides.[54] Stibbe reported that they usually occurred in the pattern of four on one side and five on the other. Each of the three upper spaces usually contained one lymph node, as did the sixth space. Often, there were no lymph nodes in the fourth or fifth space; an extra node usually was found in one of the upper three spaces on one of the sides. Soerensen[55] reported finding an average of seven nodes of minute size

per subject in 39 autopsies, with an average of 3.5 on each side. Ju (as reported by Haagensen[27]) studied 100 autopsy subjects and found an average of 6.2 parasternal nodes per subject, with an average of 3.1 per side. A majority was found in the upper three spaces. However, in contradiction to Stibbe's findings, a lower but similar frequency of nodes was seen in all three of the lower intercostal spaces. Putti[56] studied 47 cadavers and found an average of 7.7 nodes per subject—again, with a majority of the nodes in the upper three spaces and many fewer in the lower spaces. Arão and Abrão[57] studied 100 autopsy specimens and found a much higher frequency of lymph nodes than had been previously reported. They found an average total of 16.2 per subject, with an average of 8.9 on the right side and 7.3 on the left. In 56.6% of the subjects, they found retromanubrial nodes between the right and left lymphatic trunks at the level of the first intercostal space. An average of 6.6 nodes were seen when the retromanubrial nodes were present.

2. The *intercostal lymph nodes* consist of small lymph nodes located in the posterior part of the thoracic cavity within the intercostal spaces near the head of the ribs (see Figure 2-11). One or more may be found in each intercostal space in relationship with the intercostal vessels. These lymph nodes receive the deep lymphatics from the posterolateral thoracic wall, including lymphatic channels from the breast. Occasionally, small lymph nodes occur in the intercostal spaces along the lateral thoracic wall. Efferent lymphatics from the lower four or five intercostal spaces, on both the right and the left sides, join to form a trunk that descends to open into either the cisterna chyli or the initial portion of the thoracic duct. The upper efferent lymphatics from the intercostal nodes on the left side terminate in the thoracic duct; the efferent lymphatics from the corresponding nodes on the right side end in the right lymphatic duct.

3. The *diaphragmatic lymph nodes* consist of three sets of small lymph nodes (anterior, lateral, and posterior) located on the thoracic surface of the diaphragm.

The *anterior set of diaphragmatic lymph nodes* includes two or three small lymph nodes (also known as *prepericardial lymph nodes*) located behind the sternum at the base of the xiphoid process, which receive afferent lymphatics from the convex surface of the liver, and one or two nodes located on each side near the junction of the seventh rib with its costal cartilage,

which receive afferents from the anterior aspect of the diaphragm. Afferent lymphatics also reach the prepericardial nodes by accompanying the branches of the superior epigastric blood vessels that pass from the rectus abdominis muscle and through the rectus sheath. Efferent lymphatics from the anterior diaphragmatic nodes pass to the *parasternal nodes.* This lymphatic channel is a potential route by which metastases from the breast may invade the parasternal region, with the potential for spread to the liver. As Haagensen[27] suggests, metastasis via this (rectus muscle) route most likely occurs only when the internal mammary lymphatic trunk is blocked higher in the upper intercostal spaces. When blockage occurs, the flow of lymph may be reversed and carcinoma emboli from the breast may reach the liver. It is significant to note that the autopsy subjects studied by Handley,[58] who demonstrated this route of metastasis, had locally advanced breast carcinoma. Handley and Thackray[50] described the importance of the parasternal lymph nodes in carcinoma of the breast. Clearly, as Haagensen[27] and others have suggested, this route is not of importance in early cancer of the breast unless the primary tumor is located in the extreme lower inner portion of the breast where it overlies the sixth costal cartilage.

The *lateral set of diaphragmatic lymph nodes* consists of two or three small lymph nodes on each side of the diaphragm adjacent to the pericardial sac where the phrenic nerves enter the diaphragm. On the right side, they are located near the vena cava; on the left side, near the esophageal hiatus. Afferent lymphatic vessels reach these nodes from the middle region of the diaphragm; on the right side, afferent lymphatics from the convex surface of the liver also reach these nodes. Efferent lymphatics from the lateral diaphragmatic nodes may pass to the parasternal nodes via the anterior diaphragmatic nodes, to posterior mediastinal nodes, or to anterior nodes via vessels that follow the course of the phrenic nerve.

The *posterior set of diaphragmatic lymph nodes* consists of a few lymph nodes located adjacent to the crura of the diaphragm. They receive lymph from the posterior aspect of the diaphragm and convey it to posterior mediastinal and lateral aortic nodes.

LYMPH NODES OF THE THORACIC CAVITY

Three sets of nodes are involved in the lymphatic drainage of the thoracic viscera—*anterior mediastinal (brachiocephalic), posterior mediastinal,* and *tracheobronchial.* Although a knowledge of the lymphatic drainage of the thoracic viscera may not be particularly significant in treating carcinoma of the breast, it is important that one understand the system of collecting lymphatic trunks in this region (see Figure 2-16), which all empty into the confluence of the internal jugular and subclavian veins.

For better comprehension of the pattern of lymphatic drainage in this region, a brief description of the regions and organs drained by the three thoracic lymph node groups is provided. The *anterior mediastinal group* consists of six to eight lymph nodes located in the upper anterior part of the mediastinum in front of the brachiocephalic veins and the large arterial trunks arising from the aorta. These correspond to the *retromanubrial nodes* as identified by Arão and Abrão.[57] The anterior mediastinal nodes receive afferent lymphatics from the thymus, thyroid, pericardium, and lateral diaphragmatic lymph nodes. Their efferent lymphatic vessels join with those from the tracheobronchial nodes to form the *bronchomediastinal trunks.*

The *posterior mediastinal group* consists of 8 to 10 nodes located posterior to the pericardium in association with the esophagus and descending thoracic aorta. They receive afferent lymphatics from the esophagus, the posterior portion of the pericardium, the diaphragm, and the convex surface of the liver. Most of their efferent lymphatic vessels join the thoracic duct, but some pass to *tracheobronchial nodes.*

The *tracheobronchial group* consists of a chain of five subgroups of lymph nodes—tracheal, superior tracheobronchial, inferior tracheobronchial, bronchopulmonary, and pulmonary—located adjacent to the trachea and bronchi, as is indicated by the descriptive names. The bron-chopulmonary nodes are found in the hilus of each lung; the pulmonary nodes are found within the substance of the lung in association with the segmental bronchi. The tracheal nodes receive afferent lymphatics from the trachea and upper esophagus. The remaining nodes within this group form a continuous chain with boundaries of lymphatic drainage that are not well defined. The pulmonary and bronchopulmonary nodes receive afferent lymphatic vessels from the lungs and bronchial trees. The inferior and superior tracheobronchial nodes receive afferent lymphatic vessels from the lungs and bronchial trees. The inferior and superior tracheobronchial nodes receive afferent lymphatic vessels from the bronchopulmonary nodes; the inferior tracheobronchial nodes also receive some afferent lymphatic vessels from the heart and posterior mediastinal organs. Efferent vessels from the subgroups of the tracheobronchial group pass sequentially to the level of the tracheal nodes. Efferents from the latter

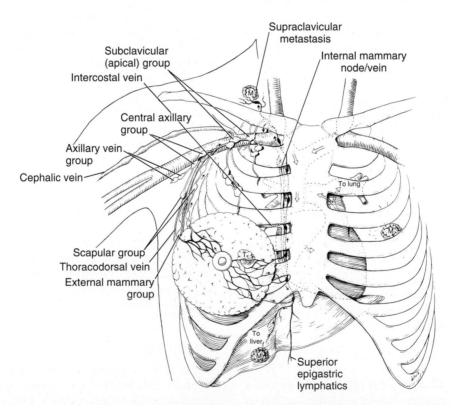

FIG. **2-17** Venous drainage of the breast and its relationship to the lymphatics. Lymphatic vessels parallel the course of the three major groups of veins serving the breast and provide routes for metastasis: intercostal, axillary, and internal mammary veins. Visceral metastases to the liver or lungs are possible via vessels providing venous or lymphatic drainage of the breast because these structures communicate with the major venous trunks. *(From Copeland EM III, Bland KI: The breast. In Sabiston DC, Jr [ed]: Essentials of surgery, Philadelphia, 1987, WB Saunders.)*

unite with efferents from parasternal and anterior mediastinal nodes to form the *right* and *left bronchomediastinal lymphatic trunks*. The left trunk may terminate by joining the thoracic duct, and the right trunk may join the right lymphatic duct. However, it is more common for the right and left trunks to open independently into the junction of the internal jugular and subclavian veins, each on their own side (see Figure 2-16).

Venous Drainage of the Mammary Gland

Lymphatic drainage of the epithelial and mesenchymal components of the breast is the primary route for metastatic dissemination of adenocarcinoma of this organ. However, the vascular route for tumor embolization via venous drainage systems has a major role for dissemination of neoplasms to the lung, bone, brain, liver, and so forth. The three groups of deep veins that drain the breast (Figure 2-17) and serve as vascular routes include the following:

1. The *intercostal veins*, which traverse the posterior aspect of the breast from the second to the sixth intercostal spaces and arborize to enter the vertebral veins posteriorly and the azygos vein centrally to terminate in the superior vena cava.
2. The *axillary vein*, which may have variable tributaries that provide segmental drainage of the chest wall, pectoral muscles, and the breast.
3. The *internal mammary vein perforators*, which represent the largest venous plexus to provide drainage of the mammary gland. This venous network traverses the rib interspaces to enter the brachiocephalic (innominate) veins. Thus perforators that drain the parenchyma and epithelial components of the breast allow direct embolization to the pulmonary capillary spaces to establish metastatic disease.[27,34]

References

1. Morehead JR: Anatomy and embryology of the breast, *Clin Obstet Gynecol* 25:353, 1982.
2. Helminen HJ, Ericsson JLE: Studies on mammary gland involution. I. On the ultrastructure of the lactating mammary gland, *J Ultrastruct Res* 25:193, 1968.
3. Cowie AT: Overview of mammary gland, *J Invest Dermatol* 63:2, 1974.
4. Spratt JS: Anatomy of the breast, *Major Probl Clin Surg* 5:1, 1979.
5. Spratt JS Jr, Donegan WL: Anatomy of the breast. In Donegan WL, Spratt JS Jr (eds): *Cancer of the breast*, ed 3, Philadelphia, 1979, WB Saunders.
6. Smith DJ Jr et al: Breast volume and anthropomorphic measurements: normal values, *Plast Reconstr Surg* 78:331, 1986.
7. Montagu A: Natural selection in the form of the breast in the female, *JAMA* 180:826, 1962.
8. Giacometti L, Montagna W: The nipple and areola of the human female breast, *Anat Rec* 144:191, 1962.
9. Sykes PA: The nerve supply of the human nipple, *J Anat (Lond)* 105:201, 1969.
10. Montagna W, Macpherson EA: Some neglected aspects of the anatomy of the human breasts, *J Invest Dermatol* 63:10, 1974.
11. Cathcart EP, Gairns FW, Garven HSD: The innervation of the human quiescent nipple, with notes on pigmentation, erection, and hyperneury, *Trans R Soc Edinb* 61:699, 1948.
12. Radnor CJP: Myoepithelium in the prelactating and lactating mammary glands of the rat, *J Anat (Lond)* 112:337, 1972.
13. Hoffman S et al: Functional characterization of antiadhesion molecules, *Perspect Dev Neurobiol* 2:101, 1994.
14. Stampfer MR, Yaswen P: Culture systems for study of human mammary epithelial cell proliferation, differentiation and transformation, *Cancer Surv* 18:7, 1993.
15. Thompson EW et al: Collagen induced MMP-2 activation in human breast cancer, *Breast Cancer Res Treat* 31:357, 1994.
16. Verhoeve D, Van-Marck E: Proliferation, basement membrane changes, metastasis and vascularization patterns in human breast cancer, *Pathol Res Pract* 189:851, 1993.
17. Tobon H, Salazar H: Ultrastructure of the human mammary gland. I. Development of the fetal gland throughout gestation, *J Clin Endocrinol Metab* 39:443, 1974.
18. Waugh D, Van Der Hoeven E: Fine structure of the human adult female breast, *Lab Invest* 11:220, 1962.
19. Wellings SR, Grunbaum BW, DeOme KB: Electron microscopy of milk secretion in the mammary gland of the C3H/Crgl mouse, *J Natl Cancer Inst* 25:423, 1960.
20. Linzell JL: The silver staining of myoepithelial cells particularly in the mammary gland, and their relation to ejection of milk, *J Anat (Lond)* 86:49, 1952.
21. Grife RM, Sullivan RM, Colborn GL: *The ansa pectoralis: anatomy and applications*, Gainesville, FL, 2002, American Association of Clinical Anatomists.
22. Moosman DA: Anatomy of the pectoral nerves and their preservation in modified mastectomy, *Am J Surg* 139:883, 1980.
23. Cunningham L: The anatomy of the arteries and veins of the breast, *J Surg Oncol* 9:71, 1977.
24. Maliniac JW: Arterial blood supply of the breast, *Arch Surg* 47:329, 1943.
25. Sakki S: Angiography of the female breast, *Ann Clin Res* 6(suppl 12):1, 1974.
26. Massopust LC, Gardner WD: Infrared photographic studies of the superficial thoracic veins in the female, *Surg Gynecol Obstet* 91:717, 1950.
27. Haagensen CD: Anatomy of the mammary glands. In Haagensen CD (ed): *Diseases of the breast*, ed 3, Philadelphia, 1986, WB Saunders.
28. Batson OV: The function of the vertebral veins and their role in the spread of metastases, *Ann Surg* 112:138, 1940.
29. Batson OV: The role of the vertebral veins and metastatic processes, *Ann Intern Med* 16:38, 1942.
30. Henriques C: The veins of the vertebral column and their role in the spread of cancer, *Ann R Coll Surg Engl* 31:1, 1962.
31. Miller MR, Kasahara M: Cutaneous innervation of the human breast, *Anat Rec* 135:153, 1959.

32. Gray H: The lymphatic system. In Clemente CD (ed): *Anatomy of the human body*, ed 30, Philadelphia, 1985, Lea & Febiger.

33. Mornard P: Sur deux cas de tumeurs malignes des mammelles axillaires aberrantes, *Bull Mem Soc Chir Paris* 21:487, 1929.

34. Anson BJ, McVay CB: Thoracic walls: breast or mammary region. In *Surgical anatomy*, vol 1, Philadelphia, 1971, WB Saunders.

35. Grossman F: *Ueber die Axillaren Lymphdrusen Inaug Dissert*, Berlin, 1986, C. Vogt.

36. Copeland EM III, Bland KI: The breast. In Sabiston DC Jr (ed): *Essentials of surgery*, Philadelphia, 1987, WB Saunders.

37. Cody HS III: Clinical aspects of sentinel node biopsy, *Breast Cancer Res* 3:104, 2001.

38. Cserni G, Szekeres JP: Internal mammary lymph nodes and sentinel node biopsy in breast cancer, *Surg Oncol* 10:25, 2001.

39. Gemignani ML, Borgen PI: Is there a role for selective axillary dissection in breast cancer? *World J Surg* 25:809, 2001.

40. Gulec SA et al: Gamma probe guided sentinel node biopsy in breast cancer, *Q J Nucl Med* 41:251, 1997.

41. Keshtgar MRS, Baum M: Axillary dissection over the years: where to from here? *World J Surg* 25:761, 2001.

42. Kiricuta IC: Sentinel node concept in breast cancer, *Strahlenther Onkol* 176:307, 2000.

43. Lee AHS et al: Pathological assessment of sentinel lymph-node biopsies in patients with breast cancer, *Virchows Arch* 436:97, 2000.

44. Mariani G et al: Radioguided sentinel lymph node biopsy in breast cancer surgery, *J Nucl Med* 442:1198, 2001.

45. Nieweg OE et al: Is lymphatic mapping in breast cancer adequate and safe? *World J Surg* 25:780, 2001.

46. Noguchi M: Sentinel lymph node biopsy and breast cancer, *Br J Surg* 89:21, 2002.

47. Noguchi MM, Taniya T: Biology and surgical management of breast cancer, *Breast Cancer* 8:16, 2001.

48. Tanis PJ et al: Anatomy and physiology of lymphatic drainage of the breast from the perspective of sentinel node biopsy, *J Am Coll Surg* 192:399, 2001.

49. Von Smitten K: Sentinel node biopsy in breast cancer, *Acta Oncol* 13:33, 1999.

50. Handley RS, Thackray AC: The internal mammary lymph chain in carcinoma of the breast, *Lancet* 2:276, 1949.

51. Turner-Warwick RT: The lymphatics of the breast, *Br J Surg* 46:574, 1959.

52. Grant RN, Tabah EJ, Adair FF: The surgical significance of subareolar lymph plexus in cancer of the breast, *Surgery* 33:71, 1953.

53. Halsell JT et al: Lymphatic drainage of the breast demonstrated by vital dye staining and radiography, *Ann Surg* 162:221, 1965.

54. Stibbe EP: The internal mammary lymphatic glands, *J Anat* 52:527, 1918.

55. Soerensen B: Recherches sur la localisation des ganglions lymphatiques parasternaux par rapport aux espaces intercostaux, *Int J Chir* 11:501, 1951.

56. Putti F: Richerche anatomiche sui linfonodi mammari interni, *Chir Ital* 7:161, 1953.

57. Arão A, Abrão A: Estudo anatomico da cadeia ganglionar mamaria interna em 100 casos, *Rev Paul Med* 45:317, 1954.

CHAPTER

3

Breast Physiology: Normal and Abnormal Development and Function

RENA KASS

ANNE T. MANCINO

ARLAN L. ROSENBLOOM

V. SUZANNE KLIMBERG

KIRBY I. BLAND

Chapter Outline

The mammary gland is composed of an epithelial system of ducts and lobuloalveolar secretory units embedded in a mesenchymally derived fat pad. The growth and morphogenesis of the epithelial structures of the breast occur in various stages and are associated with concomitant hormonal changes and affected by genetic mutations. Each stage reflects the effects of systemic hormones on the glandular epithelium as well as the paracrine effects of locally derived growth factors and other regulatory products produced in the stroma. Appreciating the relationship of epithelium to mesenchyme in normal growth is essential for understanding developmental abnormalities and factors that may lead to disease.

This chapter discusses the morphologic, hormonal, paracrine, and genetic changes and the clinical correlates of the various stages of development, including that of the embryo, infancy and childhood, puberty, pregnancy, lactation, and menopause.

Embryology to Childhood

MORPHOLOGY

The breast of the human newborn is formed through 10 progressive fetal stages that begin in the sixth week of fetal development.[1] The mammary gland originates from the milk streaks, bilateral ectodermal thickenings that extend from the axilla to the groin. The ectoderm over the thorax invaginates into the surrounding mesenchyme, with subsequent epithelial budding and branching.[2] During the later part of pregnancy this fetal epithelium further canalizes and ultimately differentiates to the end-vesicle stage seen in the newborn.[1] At term birth, the breast has 6 to 10 ducts that empty at the nipple. These ducts contain one layer of epithelium with vacuolated cytoplasm and one layer of myoepithelial cells, terminating in a dilated blind sac. These so-called ductules are the precursors of future lobuloalveolar structures, which ultimately are the milk-producing units of the breast. Similar to the development of the ductal system, the subareolar lymphatic plexus also develops from the ectoderm.[3]

From birth until 2 years of age, there is wide individual variability in the morphologic and functional stages in the breast, with some neonates having more well-developed lobular structures and others with more secretory epithelial phenotypes. (Lobular structures are further delineated in the morphology of puberty section.) The degree of morphologic differentiation does not correlate with functional ability. The ability of the entire ductal structure to respond to secretory stimuli may even occur in the rudimentary ductal systems.[4] Ultimately, in normal infant development the differentiated glandular structures involute, and only small ductal structures are left remaining within the stroma.[5]

During childhood the ductal structures and stroma grow isometrically at a rate similar to that of the rest of the body until puberty.[6] The lymphatics grow simultaneously with the duct system, maintaining connection with the subareolar plexus.[3] As in the fetal stage, there are no morphologic differences between the sexes.[4]

HORMONES

The initial fetal stages of breast development are relatively independent of sex steroid influence. At birth the withdrawal of maternal steroids results in secretion of neonatal prolactin (PRL) that stimulates newborn breast secretion.

REGULATORY FACTORS AND POTENTIAL GENES

It is currently accepted that epithelial ductal proliferation into the mesenchyme is modulated by local factors, which regulate the epithelial-mesenchymal interaction. Although a multitude of genes have been expressed in either the epithelium or mesenchyme during mammary embryogenesis, including fibroblast growth factor-7 (FGF-7),[7] tenascin-C,[8] syndecan-1,[9] t-box family of transcription factors,[10] androgen receptor,[11] estrogen receptor,[9] transforming growth factor-α (TGF-α), and the epidermal growth factor (EGF) receptor,[4] only the Lef-1,[12] parathyroid hormone–related protein (PTHrP),[13] and the type 1 parathyroid hormone (PTH)/PTHrP receptor (PTHR-1)[13] are required for mammary development. A deletion in any one of these three can result in a failure of mammogenesis.

CLINICAL CORRELATES

During fetal development the extrathoracic milk streak typically regresses. Failure to completely regress can result in accessory nipple (*polythelia*) and mammary tissue (*polymastia*). The accessory mammary tissue, most often located in the axilla, may swell during pregnancy and if associated with a nipple may function during lactation.[14] It is more common, however, to see *polythelia* on the thorax below healthy breasts. Mutations in the t-box family of transcription factors, normally activated during mammary embryogenesis, can result in *ulnar mammary syndrome* in humans. This may appear as mammary *hypoplasia, amastia* (lack of breasts), or an extra breast. These and other congenital abnormalities are further described in Chapter 8.

As previously described, PRL stimulates newborn breast secretion. This secretion, called *witch's milk,* contains water, fat, and debris; it occurs in 80% to 90% of infants, regardless of sex.[15,16] The secretion dissipates within 3 to 4 weeks as the influence of maternal sex hormones and PRL decreases. It should not be mechanically expressed, which could predispose to staphylococcal infection and result in breast bud destruction. The secretion may sequester at the nipple epithelium and resemble a pearl. This is called a *lactocele* and will resolve with time.[16]

Premature thelarche is breast development before the age of 8 years without concomitant signs of puberty. Usually bilateral, it is most commonly seen within the first 2 years of life. It is believed to be the result of the persistence or increase in the breast tissue present at birth, and it resolves within 3 to 5 years with no adverse sequelae.[17] It has been suggested that although the initial stimulation of the infant breast may be secondary to maternal influences, the persistence of breast tissue may be related to infant hormones that may support breast growth. Persistent elevations of follicle-stimulating hormone (FSH), luteinizing hormone (LH), and estradiol in infants support this hypothesis[18] (Figures 3-1 and 3-2).

A second period of *premature thelarche* may occur after 6 years of age.[19] The reason for breast bud formation is unclear; it can occur before the rise in estrogen levels, making it unlikely that estrogen is the key signal. Serum androgen levels,[20] free estrogen level,[21] and altered FSH secretion[22] have been implicated as potential factors. The breast tissue may persist or regress, but puberty occurs at the usual time and progresses normally. If assessment of bone age reveals no evidence of precocious puberty, no further evaluation is needed.[19]

Breast development before 8 years of age that is accompanied by other signs of puberty defines *precocious puberty*. Altered or premature gonadotropin–releasing hormone (GnRH) secretion may cause central precocious puberty (Figure 3-3). Although more commonly idiopathic, central precocious puberty can be caused by cerebral infections and granulomatous conditions. Certain tumors, in particular hypothalamic hamartomas can contain GnRH, disrupt the inhibition of GnRH, or

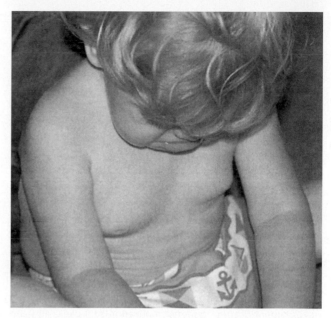

FIG. **3-2** Fifteen-month-old boy with mostly right breast enlargement with galactorrhea. Prolactin levels varied from 58 to 100 ng/ml and were unrelated to the cessation of galactorrhea and reduction in breast size by 18 months. Magnetic resonance imaging of the brain was unremarkable at 15 and 21 months of age. Bromocriptine therapy suppressed prolactin levels and was associated with breast regression.

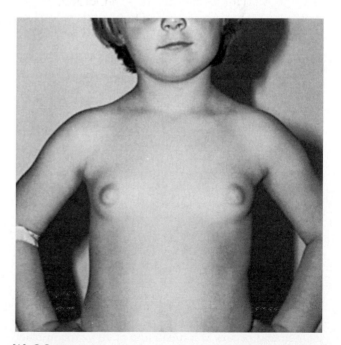

FIG. **3-3** Three-and-a-half-year-old girl with central precocious puberty (adolescent levels of gonadotropins and estrogen). Breast development had been present for only a few months but included nipple maturation. Facial maturation was that of a 5- to 6-year-old child. Height age was 4½ years, and osseous maturation was 5 years, 9 months.

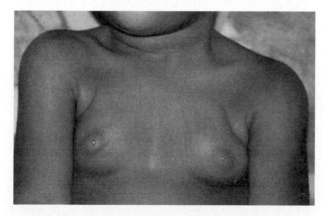

FIG. **3-1** Premature thelarche. Fourteen-month-old child with breast development from birth. Height was at the 50th percentile without acceleration, and no other signs of sexual maturation were present. Breast development was considered Tanner stage 3 without nipple maturation. There had been some regression over the several months before this picture was taken.

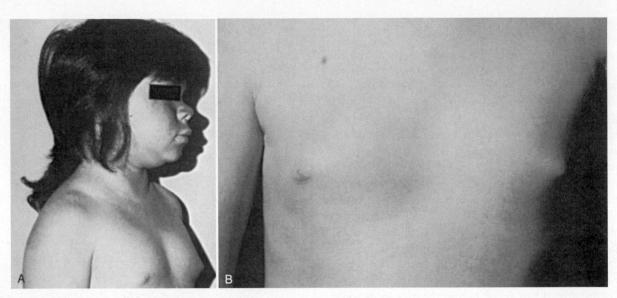

FIG. **3-4 A,** Thirteen-year-old girl with acquired hypothyroidism of approximately 5 years' duration, with Tanner stage 2 breast development despite osseous maturation of 8 years and comparable height age. **B,** Regression of breast development occurred within months of treatment with thyroid hormone. *(Courtesy Dr. A. Rosenbloom, Division of Pediatric Endocrinology, University of Florida, Gainesville, FL.)*

release TGF-α (a stimulant of GnRH), resulting in precocious puberty. Peripheral precocious puberty may result from the effects of estrogen from food,[23] from ovarian cysts, from constitutionally activated ovaries in McCune-Albright syndrome (a triad of café-au-lait spots, long-bone fibrous dysplasia, and precocious puberty), or in primary hypothyroidism (Figure 3-4).[16] In addition to a history and physical examination, serum gonadotropin and sex steroid levels should be obtained in the workup of precocious puberty. High levels of both gonadotropins and sex steroids indicate central precocious puberty. Magnetic resonance imaging (MRI) or computed tomography (CT) scanning of the head can be performed to rule out a central lesion before treatment with GnRH analogs. Suppressed (low) levels of gonadotropins and high levels of sex steroids are consistent with peripheral precocious puberty.[24]

Puberty

MORPHOLOGY

Thelarche, the beginning of adult breast development, marks the onset of puberty in the majority of white women and occurs at a mean age of 10 years; in black women it occurs at 8.9 years and is usually preceded by the appearance of pubic hair.[25] Changes in the breast contour and events in nipple development characterize the milestones in the staging system detailed by Tanner (Figure 3-5).[26] However, these outward changes in the breast do not necessarily correlate with underlying structural events occurring with the new hormonal milieu of puberty.

The immature ductal system before puberty is believed to undergo a sequential progression to a mature lobuloalveolar system during adolescent development (Figure 3-6). First, in the *ductal growth phase,* ducts elongate, ductal epithelium thicken, and periductal connective tissue increases. Stem cells in the ductal tree form club-shaped terminal end buds (TEBs), which are the site of the greatest rate of epithelial proliferation.[27,28] These TEBs are the lead point of advancement from the nipple into the peripheral mammary fat pad (mesenchyme). In the lobuloalveolar phase these TEBs further divide and form alveolar buds. Within a few years after menarche, most likely with the onset of ovulation, clusters of 8 to 11 of these alveolar buds empty into terminal ductal lobular units (TDLUs). In early puberty the TDLU is termed a *virginal lobule* or *lobule type 1* (Lob 1).[29] Lob 1 is the predominant lobule found at this stage of development. Under the cyclic influence of ovarian hormones, some of the Lob 1 will undergo further division and differentiate into a lobule type 2 (Lob 2). In Lob 2 the alveolar buds become smaller but four times more numerous than those in Lob 1; these buds are termed *ductules* or *alveoli.* Lob 2 are present in moderate numbers during the late teens but then decline after the midtwenties.[30] Ultimately, the greatest

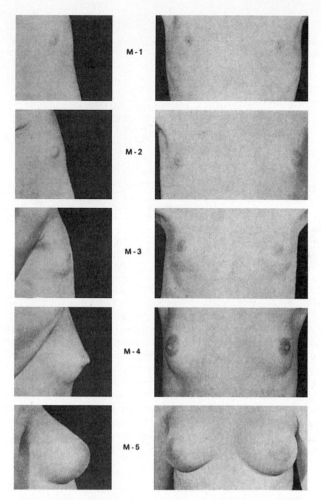

FIG. **3-5** Stages of breast development.[26] Stage 1 is preadolescent, with slight elevation of the papilla. In stage 2, there is elevation of the breast and papilla as a small mound, with an increase in size of the areola. Stage 3 is characterized by further enlargement of the breast, and in stage 4 the areola and papilla form a secondary mound above the level of the breast. In stage 5, the areola recedes into the general contour of the breast. *(From van Wieringen JD et al: Growth diagrams 1965 Netherlands, Second National Survey on 0-24 year olds. Netherlands Institute for Preventive Medicine TNO. Groningen, Netherlands, Wolters-Noordoff, 1971.)*

number of lobules will be found in the upper outer quadrant.[31,32]

In the mature breast, the subareolar lymphatic plexus contains communications with both deep and superficial intramammary lymphatics and provides a high volume of lymphatic outflow to regional lymph nodes. In lymphatic studies there appears to a consistent channel that originates from the subareolar plexus and extends to the regional lymph nodes, termed the *sentinel lymphatic channel.*[3]

During the human menstrual cycle the breast progresses through five histologic phases: *early follicular,* *follicular, luteal, secretory,* and ultimately *menstrual phase,* according to the characterizations of Vogel and colleagues[33] (Figure 3-7). The *early follicular phase* occurs from day 3 to day 7 in a 28-day cycle. The alveoli are compact, with poorly defined lumina, and sit within a dense stroma. There appears to be only one epithelial cell type at this point. According to some, minimum volume is seen 5 to 7 days after menses.[14] However, a pilot study using MRI demonstrated the minimum volume to occur at day 11.[34] The *follicular phase* follows from day 8 through day 14 and marks the progression of epithelial stratification into three cell types: the luminal, basal myoepithelial cell, and an intermediate cell. *Ovulation* initiates the *luteal phase,* which lasts from day 15 to day 29. In this phase there is an overall increase in the size of the lobules resulting from alveoli luminal expansion with secretory products, an increase in the number of alveoli, ballooning of the myoepithelial cells with increased glycogen content, and stromal loosening. The maximum size of the lobules and number of alveoli within each lobule is reached in the *secretory phase,* from day 21 to day 27. This is consistent with MRI breast-volume data.[34] During this phase there is active protein synthesis and apocrine secretion from the luminal epithelial cells. Peak mitotic activity occurs near day 22 to 24, after the progesterone peak and second estrogen peak.[35,36] The *menstrual phase* occurs on days 28 through 32 and is associated with the withdrawal of estrogen and progesterone. Apocrine secretion lessens and the lobules decrease in size, with fewer alveoli. Russo and Russo[30] suggest that each menstrual cycle fosters new budding that never fully returns to the baseline of the previous cycle. This positive proliferation continues until the midthirties and plateaus until menopause, when regression begins.

HORMONES

The pattern of release of GnRH from the hypothalamus initiates and regulates the release of FSH and LH seen with puberty. The initial immaturity of the hypothalamic-pituitary axis results in anovulatory cycles for the first 1 to 2 years after menses begin, subjecting the breast and the endometrium to the effects of unopposed estrogen. It is during this period of unopposed estrogen stimulation, considered an "estrogen window,"[37] that *the ductal growth phase* occurs (see Figure 3-6).

Estrogen is the major hormonal influence on the breast at the onset of puberty. Estrogen, a potent mammogen, primarily stimulates ductal growth but also increases fat deposition and contributes to later phases of development. Estrogen receptors have been identified in both the epithelium and the stroma.[38] Impaired ductal growth has been demonstrated in

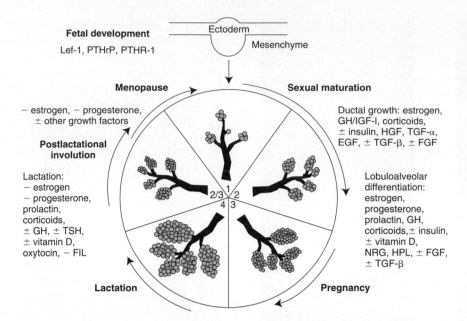

FIG. **3-6** Regulatory influences on breast development. Numbers (1, 2, 3, etc.) correspond to lobule type (1, 2, 3, etc.). Ectoderm invaginates into mesenchyme during fetal development. Sexual maturation begins with the onset of puberty through periods of ductal and lobuloalveolar growth and is reflected in the formation of lobules type 1 and 2. Pregnancy initiates the formation of lobule type 3. Lactation, which follows, is associated with lobule type 4. Postlactational involution follows, with regression of lobules. Menopause is characterized by a majority of lobules type 1 and 2, similar to the virgin state. *EGF,* Epidermal growth factor; *FGF,* fibroblast growth factor; *FIL,* feedback inhibitor of lactation; *GH,* growth hormone; *HGF,* hepatocyte growth factor; *HPL,* human placental lactogen; *IGF-I,* insulin-like growth factor-I; *Lef-1,* transcription factor Lef-1; *NRG,* neuregulin; *PTH,* parathyroid hormone; *PTHR-1,* PTH/PTHrP receptor type 1; *PTHrP,* parathyroid hormone–related peptide; *TGF-α,* transforming growth factor-α; *TGF-β,* transforming growth factor-β; *TSH,* thyroid-stimulating hormone. *(Modified from Russo*[49] *and Dickson R, Russo J: Biochemical control of breast development. In Harris J et al [eds]:* Diseases of the breast, *Philadelphia, 2000, Lippincott Williams & Wilkins.)*

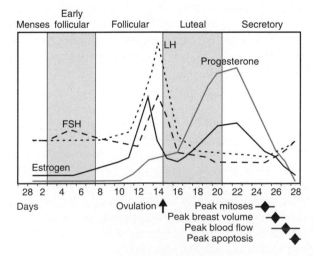

FIG. **3-7** Hormonal and histologic changes of the breast during the menstrual cycle. Maximal number of mitosis, breast volume, blood flow, and apoptosis follow the peak in progesterone. *FSH,* Follicle-stimulating hormone; *LH,* luteinizing hormone. *(Modified from Speroff L, Glass R, Kase N: Regulation of the menstrual cycle, Clinical Gynecologic Endocrinology and Infertility, Baltimore, 1999, Lippincott Williams & Wilkins; and Simpson.*[52]*)*

both mice lacking the functional gene for the estrogen receptor and mice treated with tamoxifen, an estrogen receptor modulator.[39] Despite its influential role, estrogen is unable to work independently. Lyon's classic experiments using oophorectomized, adrenalectomized, and hypophysectomized rodents demonstrated that a minimum combination of estrogen, growth hormone (GH), and corticoids are necessary to induce ductal growth.[40]

The effects of GH may be mediated by enhancing stromal secretion of insulin-like growth factor-I (IGF-I). IGF-I synergizes with estrogen to increase elongation and growth at the TEB[41] in a paracrine manner. In some reviews, glucocorticoids contribute to the maximal growth of ducts, but extensive ductal growth can occur in its absence.[42] Progesterone does not appear to be essential in early ductal growth.[43]

The exact trigger for ovulation is unclear, but it is postulated to be a combination of critical estrogen levels from the ovaries and alterations in FSH, LH, and gonadotropin levels.[44] The subsequent monthly progesterone secretion from the corpus luteum exposes the breast to the complete cyclic hormonal milieu of adulthood and facilitates the second phase of glandular growth, *lobuloalveolar growth*. Progesterone, working through the progesterone receptor (PR), is essential for lobuloalveolar development.[43] However, progesterone cannot independently bring the gland to maturity. Lyons, Li, and Johnson[40] demonstrated that prolactin, GH, estrogen, and glucocorticoids, in addition to progesterone, are necessary for full lobuloalveolar development.

PRL, a member of a multigene family including homologous GH and human placental lactogen (HPL), is also integral to lobuloalveolar development.[45] PRL-deficient knockout mice with adequate progesterone levels exhibited incomplete lobule formation.[46] PRL also works indirectly by facilitating progesterone's actions on the breast. PRL increases progesterone secretion from the corpus luteum by inhibiting progesterone's degradation enzyme, 20α-hydroxysteroid dehydrogenase.[47] In addition, PRL upregulates the PR in the mammary epithelium.[48] Estrogen contributes to lobuloalveolar development by upregulating PRs.[49] Insulin can bind to IGF-I receptors and may contribute to ductal or lobuloalveolar development, but it is not essential.[42,50,51]

Estrogen rises throughout the first half of the menstrual cycle and peaks at midcycle. After the LH surge, ovulation occurs with subsequent production of progesterone by the corpus luteum in the latter half of pregnancy. Progesterone peaks at the end of the third week, concurrently with a smaller second estrogen peak (see Figure 3-7).

Recent meta-analysis of studies of mammary gland changes during the menstrual cycle reflects a trend of peak physiologic and histologic changes that chronologically follow the peak in progesterone. These changes include a peak in mitosis within 24 hours of the progesterone peak and estimated peaks of breast volume, epithelial volume, and surface temperature within 2 to 4 days after the progesterone peak.[52] These changes may in part explain the clinical signs and symptoms of fullness and tenderness that occur premenstrually. Apoptosis peaks just before menses, approximately 5 days after the progesterone peak[53] (see Figure 3-7).

REGULATORY FACTORS AND POTENTIAL GENES

The continued importance of the mesenchyme in epithelial proliferation and differentiation is evident in ductal and lobuloalveolar growth during puberty. The effects of the aforementioned systemic hormones may be mediated through production of local growth factors (see Figure 3-2), which can act in a paracrine manner on the glandular tissue. Hepatocyte growth factor (HGF)/Scatter Factor (SF) stimulates proliferation of luminal cells and induces branching morphogenesis in myoepithelial cells, resulting in enhanced

ductal growth.[54,55] The mammary fibroblast in the mesenchyme is the likely source of HGF/SF in the breast, whereas its receptor, c-met, is localized to the ductal epithelium, illustrating its potential paracrine role.[56] Adhesion molecules, in particular $\alpha_2\beta_1$ integrins, may facilitate HGF-induced branching.[55,57] Hydrocortisone, possibly through induction of the c-met receptor, enhances the tubulogenic effect of HGF and also enhances luminal formation.[54] This may partially explain the finding of Lyons, Li, and Johnson[40] that corticoids are necessary for ductal growth. Tubulogenic activity is not restricted to HGF. TGF-α and EGF induce an increase in duct length, but to a lesser degree.[58] Several members of the FGF family have been implicated in ductal growth.[59] In low concentrations TGF-β stimulated elongation and branching of epithelial cords in vitro, but in high concentrations TGF-β was inhibitory.[58]

The vitamin D receptor (VDR), expressed in low levels in the mouse pubertal gland, is upregulated in pregnancy and lactation,[60] the time of lobuloalveolar development in mice, and is upregulated in response to cortisol, prolactin, and insulin.[61] Vitamin D, acting through its receptor, appears to be essential in lobuloalveolar development because VDR knockout mice had higher numbers of undifferentiated TEBs.[62] Diet may influence the composition of the mammary fat pad and may also affect glandular growth. Diets deficient in essential fatty acids result in impaired ductal growth and alveolar regression; in contrast, diets rich in unsaturated fat promote parenchymal growth and tumorigenesis and enhance the proliferative effects of EGF.[63-65] Neuregulins (NRGs) are members of the EGF family of growth factors also secreted from the stroma. A specific NRG, Heregulin (HRG), can activate the EGF receptor and contribute to lobuloalveolar growth[66,67] and secretory activity.[66]

The progression of the ductal epithelium through the mesenchymal stroma is also modulated by a constantly changing ratio of metalloproteinases (MMPs) that degrade the extracellular matrix (ECM) and tissue inhibitors of metalloproteinase (TIMPs) that inhibit degradation of the ECM. MMPs may facilitate branching morphogenesis by releasing growth factors sequestered in the matrix. MMP can process TGF-α[68] and cleave IGF,[69] increasing their bioavailability. Continual basement membrane and stromal matrix remodeling are necessary to allow for ductal growth and lobuloalveolar expansion.

CLINICAL CORRELATES

Several *normal variants* may occur during pubertal development that may cause embarrassment or unnecessary concern. Development may be initially unilateral and may mimic an isolated breast mass. This is normal, and a biopsy should not be performed because of the likelihood of permanent breast damage. It is also normal that final breast size may be asymmetric, with one breast slightly larger than the other, possibly related to handedness.[19] Rapid growth of the breast may result in skin striae. These pink or white marks should not be confused with the purple striae of Cushing's syndrome, particularly if other classic signs of Cushing's syndrome are lacking. Periareolar hair is common but should not be removed, because infection and irritation may ensue.[19]

Adolescent, juvenile, or *virginal hypertrophy* is a postpubertal continuation of epithelial and stromal growth that results in breasts that can weigh 3 to 8 kg. The diagnosis should be limited to severe breast enlargement that results in skin ulceration or physical limitations. Although usually postpubertal, this type of hypertrophy can also be seen with pregnancy or severe obesity.[70] It usually involves both breasts but can be unilateral, suggesting the role of local factors in its cause. There is an association with ancillary breast tissue in the axilla.[71] Penicillamine has been implicated as a cause, although hypertrophy may not regress after withdrawal of the drug.[72] Workup should include serum estradiol, prolactin, FSH, LH, cortisol, and somatomedin C levels and thyroid and liver function tests, as well as urine 17-keto and hydroxysteroid levels. Usually no systemic hormonal imbalances are seen. Ultrasound may provide information on discrete palpable lesions, but MRI is most useful for defining architecture and occult disease. Reduction mammaplasty is a treatment option, but hypertrophy may recur and total mastectomy with reconstruction may ultimately be needed. There has been limited experience with pharmaceuticals, including bromocriptine, tamoxifen, danazol, and medroxyprogesterone.[73,74]

In the adolescent male, *gynecomastia* occurs at age 13 to 14, when male pubertal changes and the sex hormones have established the male pattern.[75] It occurs in 70% of pubertal boys but rarely exceeds the Tanner B2 stage (elevation of the breast and papilla as a small mound).[18,24,76] Pubertal gynecomastia is usually resolved within several months to 2 years.[19] Generalized obesity can sometimes mimic gynecomastia. The primary complaint is concentric enlargement of breast tissue, but breast and nipple pain can occur in 25% of cases, with tenderness found in 40%. This histopathology of adolescent gynecomastia is proliferation of the ductal and stromal tissue without evidence of lobuloalveolar formation.[4] There is rarely a pathologic cause. An initial rise in estrogen levels, altered ratios of peripheral and central androgens to estrogens, increased diurnal periods of estrogen excess, and peripheral aromatization of androgen have been considered

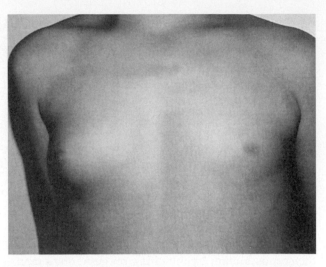

FIG. **3-8** Nine-year-old boy with a 1-year history of right-sided gynecomastia. Health, growth, and hormone profile were all normal. Mastectomy was performed for psychologic reasons, and there was no recurrence of problems.

causal (Figure 3-8).[18] Marijuana can cause gynecomastia, and its use should be ruled out.[77] Endocrinopathies, including *testosterone deficiency, LH receptor deficiency,* and *incomplete androgen insensitivity,* may result in breast formation (Figure 3-9). Rarely, when treated with glucocorticoids, a genetic female completely virilized by congenital adrenal hyperplasia and raised as a male, will undergo adrenal androgen-directed release of suppression of gonadotropins and have breast development (Figure 3-10).[16] Diagnosis begins with a good breast examination; this is best performed in the supine position. Breast lipomas, neurofibromas, and carcinomas are more typically nonpainful and eccentrically located. Pubescent gynecomastia may also be the first sign of gonadal tumors[78,79]; therefore an examination of the testes should also be performed. Serum levels of human chorionic gonadotropin, LH, testosterone, and estrogen can be obtained, with additional levels of prolactin and thyroid function tests if initial tests are abnormal. However, laboratory evaluation is typically reserved for prepubertal or postpubertal males. Cosmetic concerns may lead to consideration of a subcutaneous mastectomy but should be performed only after any underlying organic cause has been ruled out.

Failure of estrogen production leads to insufficient development of the ductal system. Lack of estrogen can be related to primary ovarian failure or absence or may result from hypogonadotropism. Primary ovarian failure may be the result of direct injury or torsion or may be associated with certain genetic syndromes (Table 3-1). The decreased estrogen level results in abnormal elevation of gonadotropin levels.

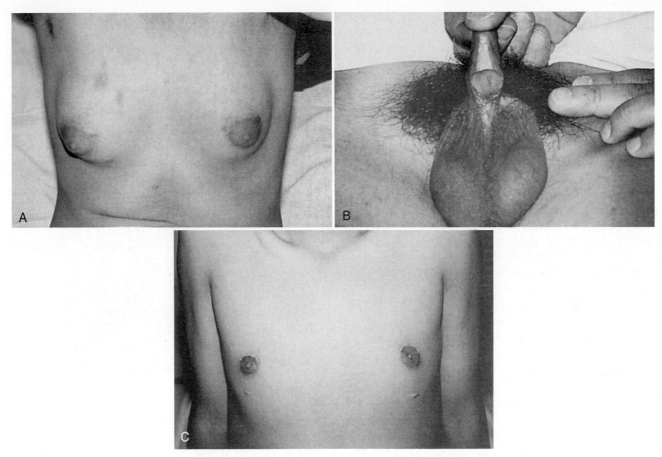

FIG. **3-9** Gynecomastia developing at adolescence in a 16-year-old boy with high testosterone and estrogen levels as a result of partial androgen resistance. **A,** Tanner stage 5 breast development. **B,** Penoscrotal hypospadias with relatively small phallus and normal size testicles (this condition has been referred to in the past as *Reifenstein's syndrome*). **C,** One year after mastectomy. Complete mastectomy is necessary to avoid regeneration of breast tissue.

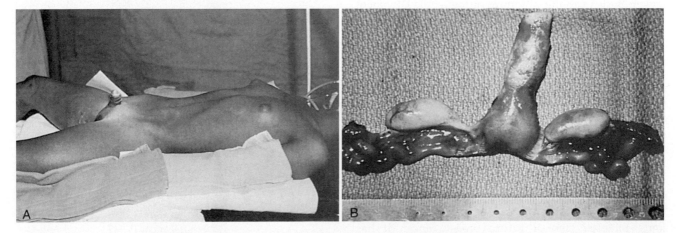

FIG. **3-10** Ten-year-old boy with congenital adrenal hyperplasia (CAH) resulting from P-450$_{c21}$–hydroxylase deficiency. Diagnosed at age 3 as a male with CAH, he developed breasts at approximately 6 years of age, when his bone age was sufficiently advanced for normal sexual maturation. He was finally recognized to have no testicular tissue at 10 years of age; despite complete virilization of the urethra, it was realized that the patient was a genetic female. **A,** Appearance at age 10 years. **B,** Normal female internal genitalia removed at age 10 years. This was followed by dramatic loss of breast tissue. The patient was subsequently treated with testosterone replacement therapy and given testicular prostheses.

| TABLE 3-1 | Failure of Estrogen Production |

PRIMARY OVARIAN FAILURE
Direct injury
  Chemotherapy
  Radiation
  Autoimmune oophoritis
  Galactosemia
Genetic syndromes
  Turner syndrome—loss of portion X chromosome
  Gonadal dysgenesis with normal chromosomes

HYPOGONADOTROPISM
Direct injury
  Brain tumors
  Radiation therapy to brain
Genetic syndromes
  Kallmann syndrome—midline facial, hyposmia
  Histocytosis X
  Bardet-Biedl—autosomal recessive syndrome
  Prader-Willi—may get menarche with weight loss
Functional hypogonadotropism
  Chronic illness
  Malnutrition
  High-performance athlete

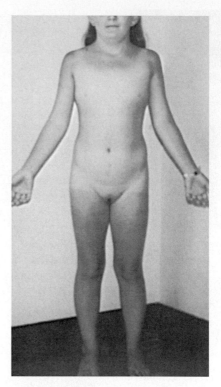

FIG. **3-11** Fifteen-year-old girl with Turner syndrome (XO) demonstrating a shieldlike chest with widely separated hypoplastic nipples and lack of sexual maturation.

The most common cause of primary ovarian failure is the Turner syndrome of gonadal dysgenesis. To prevent osteopenia and psychologic problems from sexual infantilism, cyclical estrogen therapy should not be unduly delayed (Figures 3-11 and 3-12).[80] Intrinsic errors may also occur in aromatase activity and adrenal steroid biosynthesis resulting in failure of female development and virilization; this is most commonly caused by the P-450$_{c21}$–hydroxylase deficiency (Figure 3-13).[80,81]

Hypogonadotropism may be caused by isolated gonadotropin insufficiency, brain tumors, and several genetic abnormalities. Chronic illness such as diabetes, hypothyroidism, Cushing's syndrome, or hyperprolactinemia can cause a functional hypogonadotropism. Malnutrition or low weight, such as that seen in high-performance athletes, can also cause a functional hypogonadotropism and delayed onset of puberty[82] (see Table 3-1).

Recent studies have demonstrated a positive correlation between tallness in pubertal girls (age 7 to 15) and increased risk of future breast cancer. It has been suggested that this may be related to persistently high serum IGF levels in tall women.[83] Conversely, overweight children seem to have a decreased risk of breast cancer. It is possible that the fat-derived estrogens cause an earlier differentiation of the breast, decreasing malignant potential.[83]

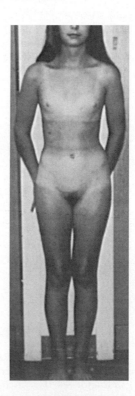

FIG. **3-12** Nineteen-year-old girl with Turner syndrome caused by mosaicism (XO/XX) demonstrating hypoplastic widely spaced nipples and some breast development as a result of estrogen therapy.

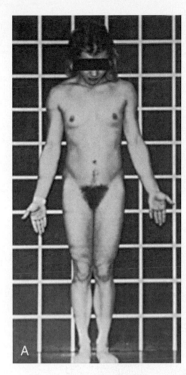
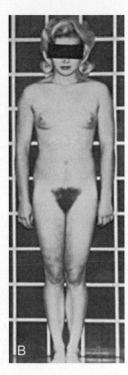

FIG. **3-13 A,** Sixteen-year-old girl with P-450$_{c21}$–hydroxylase deficiency not previously recognized. This young woman had a large clitoris removed at age 3 years. She is muscular and has frontal temporal hairline recession, masculine fascial features, and hair growth along the linea alba. She is hyperpigmented as a result of high adrenocorticotropic hormone levels. **B,** Following 10 months of hydrocortisone replacement therapy, with association of adrenal androgen production, which had been suppressing pituitary gonadotropin release. With gonadotropic stimulation of the ovaries, she underwent rapid breast development, with marked changes in subcutaneous fat and skin texture.

Pregnancy

MORPHOLOGY

Two phases occur during pregnancy to ultimately prepare the gland for lactation. The first phase, which occurs during early pregnancy, is the proliferation of the distal ducts to create more lobules and more alveoli within each lobule. There is considerable heterogeneity within the pregnant breast. Some lobular units may be resting while others expand with proliferative activity. This proliferation leads to the formation of more differentiated forms of lobules, lobule type 3 (Lob 3) and lobule type 4 (Lob 4). Lob 3 outnumbers the more primitive lobules by the end of the first trimester and can have up to 10 times the alveoli per lobules compared with Lob 1.[84] If the first term pregnancy occurs before the third decade of life, the number of Lob 3 significantly increases.[1] Lob 3 remains the dominant structure

in all parous women until the fourth decade of life, after which they start to decline and involute to Lob 1 and 2 after menopause (see Figure 3-6).

By the midpoint of pregnancy, the lobuloalveolar framework is in place and differentiation of the lobular units into secretory units begins. Cell proliferation and formation of new alveoli are minimized, and the alveoli differentiate into acini. During the last trimester the epithelial cells are filled with fat droplets, the acini distend with colostrum (an eosinophilic and proteinaceous secretion), and fat and connective tissue have largely been replaced by glandular proliferation. The increase in breast size during this period is secondary to distention of acini and increased vascularity.[85,86]

HORMONES

In pregnancy, estrogen, progesterone, and PRL work in concert to prepare the breast for lactation (Figure 3-14). As in puberty, PRL plays a continued role in lobuloalveolar differentiation. PRL increases beginning at 8 weeks and continues to rise throughout gestation and postpartum.[87,88] HPL, a member of the PRL family, is secreted during the second half of pregnancy. Although it has less bioactivity than prolactin, HPL concentration by the end of gestation is approximately 30 times the concentration of PRL.[87] This suggests that HPL may contribute to the prolactin effects on lobuloalveolar development and final maturation of the gestational gland.[44]

The estrogen increase during gestation parallels that of PRL.[88,89] Estrogen is believed to be a direct and indirect modulator of prolactin secretion. First, estrogen induces the differentiation of anterior pituitary lactotrophs, which secrete prolactin. Second, estrogen, through interaction with an estrogen-responsive element and an adjacent transcription factor–binding site, enhances prolactin gene expression.[89-92] Finally, estrogen suppresses the secretion of the PRL inhibitory factor (PIF) dopamine.[93]

During pregnancy, PRL primes the breast for lactation; however, initiation of lactogenesis is inhibited by the presence of progesterone. Although estrogen and progesterone are necessary for PRL receptor expression, paradoxically, progesterone reduces the binding and antagonizes the positive effects of PRL at its receptor.[94-96] Progesterone can directly suppress production of the milk protein casein by stimulating the production of a transcription inhibitor.[97]

REGULATORY FACTORS AND POTENTIAL GENES

As seen in puberty, NRG is expressed in the stroma of the mouse mammary gland during pregnancy.[66] In some in vivo models, NRG stimulated alveoli development and secretory activity, suggesting a potential role in mediating PRL. In other models (MMTV mice), however, NRG halted the progression

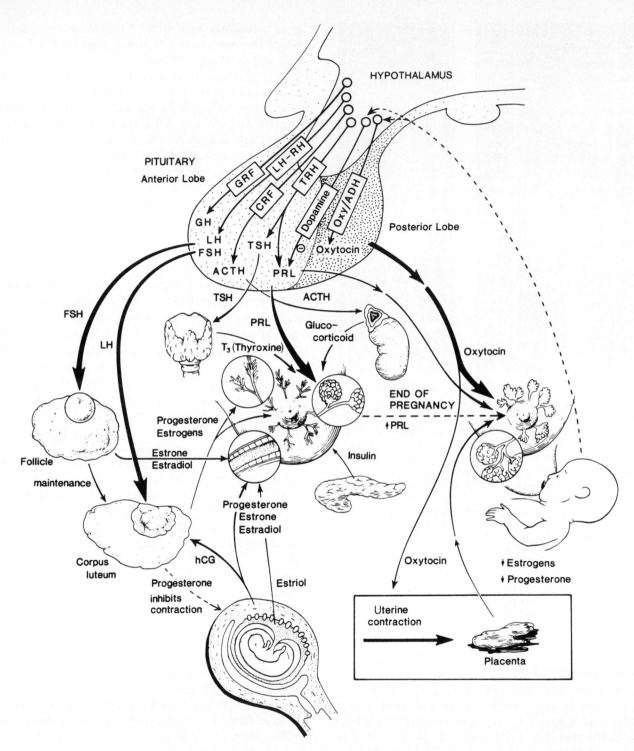

FIG. 3-14 Neuroendocrine control of breast development and function. Luteinizing hormone–releasing hormone *(LH-RH)*, also known as *gonadotropin-releasing hormone (GnRH)*, from the hypothalamus stimulates the pituitary secretion of luteinizing hormone *(LH)* and follicle-stimulating hormone *(FSH)*. Thyrotropin-releasing hormone *(TRH)* from the hypothalamus stimulates the release of prolactin *(PRL)*, against the inhibitory control of dopamine from the hypothalamus. The pituitary gonadotropins stimulate ovarian synthesis and the release of progesterone and estrogen, which have mammotrophic effects. Pregnancy enhances the secretion of estrogen and progesterone from the corpus luteum during the first 12 weeks and subsequently from the placenta. After delivery, PRL secretion increases. Neural stimuli from suckling stimulates prolactin and oxytocin release. Milk let-down occurs. Other hormones are depicted that contribute to the growth and function of the mammary gland, including glucocorticoid, growth hormone *(GH)*, insulin, and thyroxin. *ACTH,* Adrenocorticotropic hormone; *ADH,* antidiuretic hormone; *CRF,* corticotropin-releasing factor; *GRF,* growth hormone–releasing factor; *hCG,* human chorionic gonadotropin; *TSH,* thyroid-stimulating hormone.

of the lobuloalveolar system at the TEB stage, consistent with prolactin deficiency.[66,98] Activins and inhibins, members of the TGF-β family, may also play a role in modulating glandular development. Mutations in these factors result in an inhibition of alveolar development during pregnancy.[99] Certain intracellular signaling molecules, including the transcription factors A-myb, c-erbB, hox9a, hox9b, hox9d, and cell cycle protein cyclin D1, may play a role in the regulation of lobuloalveolar development. Deletions of the genes coding for these factors have caused impairment of lobuloalveolar development.[100-103]

In a similar fashion to that seen in puberty, proper balance between matrix-MMP[104,105] and its inhibitor TIMP-1[106] plays an important role in lobuloalveolar development during pregnancy and subsequent ability to lactate. For example, overexpression of TIMP caused a reduction in extracellular matrix remodeling and resulted in inhibition of lobuloalveolar development during pregnancy.[106]

CLINICAL CORRELATES

Gravid hypertrophy is the rapid and massive enlargement of the breast during pregnancy. Clinically and histologically it resembles that of *juvenile hypertrophy* discussed earlier. It may appear during a second pregnancy, after a normal first gestation, and its appearance is a risk factor for recurrence during future pregnancies.[74]

It has been shown that early parity has a protective effect against breast cancer. In an attempt to explain the protective effect of parity, the proliferative activity, steroid receptors, angiogenic index (AI), and protease inhibitors, Serpin and MDGI were measured in the three types of lobules, Lob 1, Lob 2, Lob 3, in parous and nulliparous women.[107,108] Lob 1, the most undifferentiated lobule, had the highest rate of proliferation and highest percentage of cells that expressed both estrogen receptors (ERs) and PRs. Of note, the cells that were highly proliferating were not the same population that expressed ER/PR receptors.[108] Lob 1 also had the highest AI, the number of blood vessels in relation to number of alveoli, and no expression of the protease inhibitors. As one progresses to Lob 3, proliferation, the percentage that are receptor positive, and the AI decreases, and there is expression of the protease inhibitors. Postmenopausal women who were parous ultimately had the same percentage of Lob 1 as the nulliparous women, but the proliferative index of Lob 1 in nulliparous women was higher than that of parous women. This difference persisted through menopause.[109-111] As it has been suggested that cancer initiation involves the interaction of a carcinogen with undifferentiated, highly proliferating mammary epithelium,[1] the Lob 1 of the nulliparous woman would seem to be a prime target.

Lactation

MORPHOLOGY/PRODUCT

Whereas the first half of pregnancy is marked by significant ductal and lobuloalveolar proliferation and formation of Lob 3 structures and some Lob 4 structures, the second half of gestation involves the final maturation of the gland into the secretory organ of lactation. The ability to synthesize and secrete the milk product is termed *lactogenesis*. This is composed of two stages. Lactogenesis I is the synthesis of unique milk components. This portion of the phase is accompanied by morphologic changes in the alveolar epithelial cell with an increase in protein synthetic structures (i.e., rough endoplasmic reticulum, mitochondria, and Golgi apparatus). Complex protein, milk fat, and lactose synthetic pathways are activated, but minimal secretion into the alveoli lumina occurs.[15,86] Studies measuring urine lactose, an index of the breast's synthetic activity, have confirmed that this stage begins, in most mothers, between 15 and 20 weeks of gestation.[112] The alveoli distend with colostrum, an immature milk product, and along with increased vascularity contribute to the increase in breast volume seen in the latter part of gestation. Lob 4, formed during pregnancy, persists throughout lactation (see Figure 3-6).[49]

Lactogenesis II is the initiation of significant milk secretion at or just after parturition[112] and is marked by a rise in citrate and α-lactalbumin.[42] The initial product is colostrum, which combines both nutritional elements and passive immunity for the baby. Transitional milk follows with less immunoglobulin and total protein. The ultimate product is mature milk that is composed of fat and protein suspended in a lactose solution. The fat, lactose, and protein are secreted in an apocrine fashion. Lactose and protein are also secreted in a merocrine fashion (Figure 3-15).[15] Mature milk secretion begins 30 to 40 hours postpartum[112] and averages 1 to 2 ml/g of breast tissue per day. The rate of lactation remains constant for the first 6 months of lactation.[113-115] During lactation the *stromal lymphatics* increase in comparison to other periods. Interepithelial gaps widen, allowing for more direct uptake of particles and fluids and improved clearance from the breast.[116]

After weaning occurs, the breast involutes and returns to a state resembling that of prepregnancy. The lobules decrease in size, with a decrease in the number of alveoli per lobule. The ducts are not involved, in contrast with menopausal involution when both the lobules and ducts are reduced in number. There are two phases of postlactational involution. The first phase is reversible and is associated with the accumulation of milk. It is triggered by either physical distortion of the luminal epithelial cells or by accumulation of apoptosis-inducing factors in

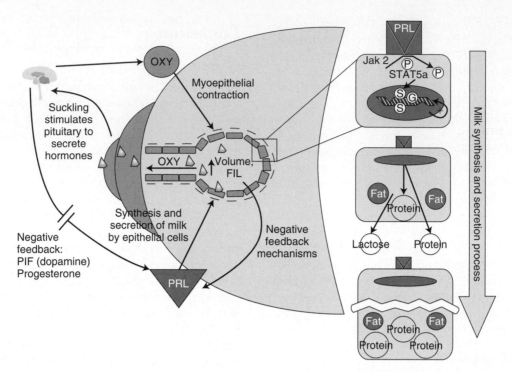

FIG. **3-15** Control of lactation. Suckling stimulates the pituitary to secrete oxytocin *(OXY)*, which causes myoepithelial contraction and milk release, and prolactin *(PRL)*, which promotes synthesis and secretion of milk. Increased alveolar intraluminal volume, milk levels of feedback inhibitor of lactation *(FIL)*, and systemic hormone (dopamine and progesterone) levels inhibit prolactin action. Expanded view details PRL action on the epithelial cell. PRL binds its transmembrane receptor, activating the Jak-STAT pathway with resultant phosphorylation of STAT5a. A ternary complex of a STAT5a dimer (S-S) with a glucocorticoid receptor (G) forms and binds DNA in the nucleus, stimulating production of milk proteins. The mRNA of certain milk proteins can positively feedback on further gene expression. Complex protein, milk fat, and lactose synthetic pathways are activated. Lactose and some milk proteins can be secreted in a merocrine fashion. Other milk proteins and fats are stored in vesicles in the apex of the luminal epithelial cell. The proteins and fats are then secreted into the lumen along with the apical portion of the cell (apocrine secretion). *PIF,* PRL inhibitory factor.

the milk.[117] The second phase is characterized by active tissue remodeling, including destruction of basement membranes and alveolar structure and irreversible loss of the differentiated function of the mammary gland.[118,119]

HORMONES

The continued importance of prolactin and related peptides in mammary gland growth and differentiation is seen with lactation, the terminal state of differentiation of the mature mammary gland (see Figures 3-14 and 3-15). PRL is the principal hormone for the synthesis of milk proteins and the maintenance of lactation.[6] Production of casein, the primary milk protein, will not occur in the absence of prolactin.[44] This hormone is secreted in increasing amounts throughout pregnancy and peaks before delivery. However, the presence of the PIF, luteal, and placental sex steroids, especially progesterone, prohibits PRL from achieving its full lactational effect.

Glucocorticoids work along with prolactin to differentiate mammary epithelium and stimulate milk synthesis and secretion. Both glucocorticoids and their receptors are increased in late pregnancy and lactation. Progesterone binds the glucocorticoid receptor and acts as a glucocorticoid antagonist.[86]

After birth, in the background of dissipating progesterone, prolactin, in concert with glucocorticoids, is able to initiate lactogenesis II. Neural stimuli from suckling enhance the release of PRL from the anterior pituitary gland. PRL then binds its membrane receptor. An intracellular portion of the receptor associates with Jak2, a tyrosine kinase, which ultimately phosphorylates STAT5a.[120] Isolated disruptions of STAT5a in mice have resulted in failure to lactate.[121] A dimeric complex of STAT5a couples with the glucocorticoid receptor, forming a ternary complex that then translocates to the nucleus and alters mRNA synthesis.[6] The mRNA of certain milk proteins can positively feedback on further gene expression (see Figure 3-15).[122]

Several stimulatory secretagogues of prolactin have been enumerated, including estrogen,[123] hypothalamic peptides, thyrotropin-releasing hormone (TRH) and vasoactive intestinal peptide (VIP),[124,125] and local factors EGF[126] and FGF.[127] Oral TRH may have benefits in improving lactation in women who occasionally breastfeed by increasing prolactin levels. In these women, their baseline prolactins were lower than that of average fully breastfeeding women.[128] Extrapituitary synthesis of prolactin occurs in the mammary gland and contributes to the high levels of the hormone secreted into the milk. Maturation of the newborn and fetal hypothalamic neuroendocrine system may be modulated by both prolactin in the milk and prolactin secreted into the amniotic fluid by the uterine decidua.[129]

Oxytocin is responsible for release of stored milk, commonly referred to as *milk let-down*. Oxytocin is secreted from the posterior pituitary by a sensory stimulation from the nipple/areola complex, via T4, T5, and T6 sensory afferent nerve roots. Uniquely, it can be secreted in anticipation of nursing in the presence of a crying infant[44] and can be inhibited by pain and embarrassment.[16] Oxytocin stimulates contraction of the myoepithelial cells surrounding the acini and small ducts, resulting in an expulsion of milk into the lactiferous sinuses.

GH, prolactin, and placental lactogen are structurally related hormones and may, to some extent, be interchangeable in function. Deficiency in one of them is not sufficient to cause lack of mammary gland development and function. For example, women with pituitary dwarfism who lack detectable GH, women who have had a pituitary adenoma removed with no subsequent rise in prolactin during pregnancy or lactation,[130] and women with low levels of human placental lactogen[130] had normal pregnancies and were able to breastfeed.

Glucocorticoid and systemic lactogenic hormones act as survival factors both during lactation and through the phase of involution.[131] Decreasing levels of systemic hormones allow for increasing apoptosis and progression into the second phase of involution.

REGULATORY FACTORS AND POTENTIAL GENES

Cell-cell interactions play a regulatory role in lobuloalveolar development and milk synthesis. Alterations in the expression of E-cadherin in luminal epithelial cells and P-cadherin in myoepithelial cells[132] alter the onset of lobuloalveolar development and milk synthesis.[133,134]

It has been noted that each breast has an independent rate of milk synthesis, suggesting a more important role for local factors in modulating function. Systemic factors, particularly PRL, do not appear to regulate the rate of milk synthesis. Luminal volume may contribute to

synthesis rate by altering the interaction between the basement membrane and the lactocyte, leading to an inhibition of the prolactin receptor.[135,136] Breast volume, however, is not the primary control of milk synthesis. Lactating goats, whose full breasts demonstrated a decrease in milk synthesis, had a resurgence of milk production when the milk was emptied and replaced isovolumetrically with a sucrose solution, suggesting that a compound within the milk was providing negative feedback. This intrinsic milk factor, the feedback inhibitor of lactation (FIL), is now thought to modulate local control of milk synthesis. This compound has been noted in many species, including women, and has been found to inhibit lactocyte differentiation, disrupt Golgi vesicle secretion, and inhibit protein synthesis in lactocytes.[137]

Involution requires active gene expression. During stage 1, there is upregulation of SGP-2, Stat 3, Fas antigen, WDNM1, and other TIMPs[138,139] and downregulation of milk protein and STAT5a and STAT5b.[139] During this first phase, local factors are sufficient to induce alveolar cell death, even in the presence of systemic lactogenic hormones. Insulin, dexamethasone, prolactin, and their combinations did not affect expression of WDNM1 and SGP-2 genes. EGF, however, strongly inhibited the expression of WDNM1 and SGP2 in cell culture, and the addition of EGF with insulin completely protected the cells in culture from apoptosis.[140] Thus EGF acts like a survival factor[140]; it is possible that loss of EGF induces gain of a death signal and leads to stage 1 of involution.

The second stage is characterized by the upregulation of MMPs gelatinase A and stromelysin-1 and serine protease urokinase-type plasminogen activator and downregulation of the inhibitor TIMP-1 and activation of proteinase-dependent pathways.[118] This change in ratio of MMP to TIMP, favoring MMP, is thought to correlate with the loss of expression of B-casein, a marker for milk production. The addition of TIMP-1 to change the ratio in the opposite direction favors cell survival and maintenance of secretory phenotype.[141]

CLINICAL CORRELATES

Chapman and Perez-Escamilla[142] have identified risk factors for *delayed onset of lactation*. These factors include lack of infant suckling, unscheduled cesarean delivery or vaginal delivery with prolonged stage 2 labor, and obesity. In these women, delay of lactogenesis II may be more than 72 hours postpartum. They should be encouraged to have frequent nursing sessions to potentially enhance the onset of lactation.[142] Progesterone, as described previously, inhibits the onset of lactogenesis II. Women who have portions of *retained placenta* may continue to have sufficient progesterone levels to inhibit their milk synthesis. The delay persists until the fragments are removed.[143,144] As described earlier, the exact role of insulin in lactogenesis is unclear; however, it has been observed that patients with *type 1 insulin-dependent diabetes mellitus* have a 24-hour delay in the onset of lactogenesis II. With assurance and prior knowledge of this information, these mothers can have success with breastfeeding.[143,144]

Although it was once concluded that women with smaller breasts had *inadequate milk production* and less success with breastfeeding, this has now been disproved. New computerized topographical techniques (computer breast measurement [CBM]) have allowed breast physiologists to study breast growth during pregnancy, short-term milk synthesis (between feeding intervals), and the degree of fullness without interrupting normal breastfeeding patterns.[112] Women with smaller-capacity breasts achieved lactational success by increasing the frequency of feedings and the degree of breast emptying with each feeding. Women with larger-capacity breasts have more flexibility in scheduling their feedings and can go longer at night without compromising their synthesis capabilities.[112]

Women who have minimal breast growth during pregnancy should not be dissuaded from breastfeeding. Women who had only small breast growth during pregnancy, with only a small increase in lactose in their urine, had compensatory growth during the first month postpartum. The growth during this month was equivalent to the growth of other women from conception to delivery.[112] Vigorous aerobic exercise should not be a deterrent to breastfeeding because it affects neither the volume nor the composition of breast milk.[145]

In the small subset of women who have lactational insufficiency secondary to low levels of prolactin, drugs such as metoclopramide have been shown to increase the secretion of prolactin. Low levels of prolactin should be documented and need to be measured 45 minutes after suckling. As mentioned, oral TRH may improve lactation in insufficient women noted to have low levels of prolactin, although hyperthyroidism in the mother may be a side effect.[128] Lactational failure may be the first sign of Sheehan's syndrome (infarction of the pituitary gland with ensuing insufficiency of prolactin and other hormones). Other rarer causes of lactational failure include lymphocytic hypophysitis, isolated hypoprolactinemia, or hypoprolactinemia as part of a generalized pituitary deficiency.[16]

Galactorrhea is the inappropriate secretion of milky fluid in the absence of pregnancy or breastfeeding for more than 6 months. The amount varies from minimal to excessive and may be produced spontaneously or require manual expression. White, clear, or yellowish fluid is produced from multiple ducts and may involve one or both breasts. Amenorrhea is often associated with galactorrhea,[146,147] but menses may be normal even in serious hormonal disorders. A variety of endocrine and nonendocrine disorders produce galactorrhea, involving either elevation of serum prolactin levels or altered responsiveness to normal prolactin levels.[148] In women, galactorrhea is usually seen when prolactin levels reach 200 ng/ml, but in males it is rare to see galactorrhea even with much higher levels.[149]

Stress from exercise, surgery, sexual intercourse, or sleep can inhibit PIF release, leading to an increase in PRL.[150] Drugs can stimulate PRL secretion either through direct stimulation of lactotrophs or by decreasing dopamine availability.[149,150] Drug-induced galactorrhea should resolve within 3 to 6 months after the drug is discontinued. Pituitary tumors and hypothalamic lesions may cause galactorrhea.[151] In hypothyroidism, excess TRH acts on the pituitary as a prolactin-releasing factor and increases prolactin secretion. Galactorrhea may also be associated with adrenal insufficiency,[152] Cushing's syndrome,[153] acromegaly,[154] renal failure,[155] or lung/renal tumors (ectopic prolactin secretion).[156] The afferent neural pathways normally stimulated by suckling may also be stimulated with mastectomy, thoracotomy, spinal lesions, or herpes zoster.

The workup should include a detailed history and a fasting serum prolactin level. If prolactin levels are elevated and physiologic or pharmacologic causes are excluded, further workup is needed. A serum thyroid-stimulating hormone level should be measured and if elevated treated with thyroxin. High-resolution CT[157] or MRI should be obtained to exclude a pituitary tumor.

In patients with prolactin levels less than 100 ng/ml and no evidence of a pituitary tumor, no treatment is needed. These patients should be followed with measurement of yearly prolactin levels. If the patient wishes to become pregnant or desires cessation of galactorrhea, bromocriptine may be used. Of note, the presence of a prolactinoma does not contraindicate the use of oral contraceptives or pregnancy.[44]

Menopause

MORPHOLOGY

As women approach menopause, there is an increased number of Lob 1 and a decline in Lob 2 and Lob 3, with all women by the end of the fifth decade having mostly Lob 1. Independent of age, nulliparous women have 65% to 80% Lob 1, 10% to 35% Lob 2, and 0% to 5% Lob 3. Parous women, from postlactational involution to the fourth decade, have 70% to 90% of Lob 3. After the fourth decade their breasts start to involute, and after menopause the breakdown of lobular percentages are equivalent to those of nulliparous women (see Figure 3-6).

Menopause otherwise progresses in much the same manner in both parous and nulliparous women. The climacteric phase from age 45 to 55 has a moderate decrease in glandular epithelium. This is followed by the postmenopausal phase, which typically occurs after age 50. During the postmenopausal phase, the glandular epithelium undergoes apoptosis, the interlobular stomal tissue regresses, and there is replacement by fat. The intralobular tissue is replaced by collagen. Menopausal involution results in reduction of the number of ducts and lobules. Fat intercalates the fibrous separations, so there are no well-defined quadrants or fascial planes. Lymphatic channels are also reduced in number.[3] Only residual islands of ductal tissue remain scattered throughout the fibrous tissue and fat.[15]

HORMONES

The ovarian hormones, estrogen and progesterone, have declined, and the ovarian androgens, androstenedione, testosterone, and dehydroepiandrosterone, become predominant.

REGULATORY FACTORS AND POTENTIAL GENES

Interestingly, little is known about factors responsible for this process.

CLINICAL CORRELATES

Age is a well-known risk factor for the development of breast cancer, and most breast cancers are seen in postmenopausal women. As discussed previously, postmenopausal women return to a high percentage of Lob 1, and in nulliparous women these Lob 1 cells have a higher proliferative index than that of parous women. Thus all postmenopausal women are more susceptible to interaction with carcinogens. The more highly proliferative cells in nulliparous women add to their risk. Diminished lymphatic capacity in postmenopausal women may impair localization of the sentinel lymph nodes and limit the utility of this technique in this higher risk group of women.[3]

REFERENCES

1. Russo J et al: Cancer risk related to mammary gland structure and development, *Microsc Res Tech* 52:204, 2001.
2. Cardiff RD, Wellings SR: The comparative pathology of human and mouse mammary glands, *J Mammary Gland Biol Neoplasia* 4:105, 1999.
3. Kern KA: Sentinel lymph node mapping in breast cancer using subareolar injection of blue dye, *J Am Coll Surg* 189:539, 1999.
4. Howard BA, Gusterson BA: Human breast development, *J Mammary Gland Biol Neoplasia* 5:119, 2000.
5. Anbazhagan R et al: Growth and development of the human infant breast, *Am J Anat* 192:407, 1991.
6. Horseman ND: Prolactin and mammary gland development, *J Mammary Gland Biol Neoplasia* 4:79, 1999.
7. Cunha GR, Hom YK: Role of mesenchymal-epithelial interactions in mammary gland development, *J Mammary Gland Biol Neoplasia* 1:21, 1996.
8. Chiquet-Ehrismann R et al: Tenascin: an extracellular matrix protein involved in tissue interactions during fetal development and oncogenesis, *Cell* 47:131, 1986.
9. Robinson GW, Karpf AB, Kratochwil K: Regulation of mammary gland development by tissue interaction, *J Mammary Gland Biol Neoplasia* 4:9, 1999.
10. Bamshad M et al: Mutations in human TBX3 alter limb, apocrine and genital development in ulnar-mammary syndrome, *Nat Genet* 16:311, 1997.
11. Sakakura T: Mammary embryogenesis. In Neville MC, Daniel CW (eds): *The mammary gland: development, regulation and function,* New York, 1987, Plenum Press.
12. Ven Genderen C et al: Development of several organs that require inductive epithelial-mesenchymal interactions is impaired in LEF-1 deficient mice, *Genes Dev* 8:2691, 1994.
13. Dunbar ME et al: Parathyroid hormone-related protein signaling is necessary for sexual dimorphism during embryonic mammary development, *Development* 126:3485, 1999.
14. Osborne M: Breast development and anatomy. In Harris JR LM, Morrow M, Osborne CK (eds): *Diseases of the breast,* New York, 2000, Lippincott Williams & Wilkins.
15. McCarty KS Jr, Nath M: Breast. In Sternberg S (ed): *Histology for pathologists,* Philadelphia, 1997, Lippincott-Raven.
16. Rosenbloom A: Breast physiology: normal and abnormal development and function. In Bland K, Copeland EM (eds): *The breast: comprehensive management of benign and malignant diseases,* vol 1, Philadelphia, 1998, WB Saunders.
17. Mills JL et al: Premature thelarche: natural history and etiologic investigation, *Am J Dis Child* 135:743, 1981.
18. Laurence DJ, Monaghan P, Gusterson BA: The development of the normal human breast, *Oxf Rev Reprod Biol* 13:149, 1991.
19. Sloand E: Pediatric and adolescent breast health, *Prim Care Pract* 2:170, 1998.
20. Murakami M et al: [Correlation between breast development and hormone profiles in puberal girls], *Nippon Sanka Fujinka Gakkai Zasshi* 40:561, 1988.
21. Radfar N, Ansusingha K, Kenny FM: Circulating bound and free estradiol and estrone during normal growth and development and in premature thelarche and isosexual precocity, *J Pediatr* 89:719, 1976.
22. Stanhope R et al: Studies of gonadotrophin pulsatility and pelvic ultrasound examinations distinguish between isolated premature thelarche and central precocious puberty, *Eur J Pediatr* 145:190, 1986.
23. Bongiovanni AM: An epidemic of premature thelarche in Puerto Rico, *J Pediatr* 103:245, 1983.
24. Styne D: Puberty. In Greenspan F, Gardner D (eds): *Basic and clinical endocrinology,* New York, 2001, McGraw-Hill.
25. Herman-Giddens ME et al: Secondary sexual characteristics and menses in young girls seen in office practice: a study from the Pediatric Research in Office Settings Network, *Pediatrics* 99:505, 1997.
26. Marshall WA, Tanner JM: Variations in pattern of pubertal changes in girls, *Arch Dis Child* 44:291, 1969.
27. Daniel C, Silberstein G: Postnatal development of the rodent mammary gland. In Neville M, Daniel C (eds): *The mammary gland: development, regulation, and function,* New York, 1987, Plenum Press.

28. Russo I, Medado J, Russo J: Endocrine influences on the mammary gland. In Jones T, Mohr U, Hunt E (eds): *Integument and mammary glands,* Berlin, 1989, Springer-Verlag.

29. Soderquist AM, Todderud G, Carpenter G: Elevated membrane association of phospholipase C-gamma 1 in MDA-468 mammary tumor cells, *Cancer Res* 52:4526, 1992.

30. Russo J, Russo IH: Development of human mammary glands. In Neville M, Daniel CW (eds): *The mammary gland,* New York, 1987, Plenum Press.

31. Shlykov IP, Chumachenko PA, Anokhina MA: [Development of the female mammary gland during young age (morphometric data)], *Arkh Anat Gistol Embriol* 85:54, 1983.

32. Hutson SW, Cowen PN, Bird CC: Morphometric studies of age related changes in normal human breast and their significance for evolution of mammary cancer, *J Clin Pathol* 38:281, 1985.

33. Vogel PM et al: The correlation of histologic changes in the human breast with the menstrual cycle, *Am J Pathol* 104:23, 1981.

34. Hussain Z et al: Estimation of breast volume and its variation during the menstrual cycle using MRI and stereology, *Br J Radiol* 72:236, 1999.

35. Longacre TA, Bartow SA: A correlative morphologic study of human breast and endometrium in the menstrual cycle, *Am J Surg Pathol* 10:382, 1986.

36. Ferguson DJ, Anderson TJ: Morphological evaluation of cell turnover in relation to the menstrual cycle in the "resting" human breast, *Br J Cancer* 44:177, 1981.

37. Korenman SG: The endocrinology of breast cancer, *Cancer* 46:874, 1980.

38. Pelletier G, El-Alfy M: Immunocytochemical localization of estrogen receptors alpha and beta in the human reproductive organs, *J Clin Endocrinol Metab* 85:4835, 2000.

39. Shyamala G: Progesterone signaling and mammary gland morphogenesis, *J Mammary Gland Biol Neoplasia* 4:89, 1999.

40. Lyons W, Li C, Johnson R: The hormonal control of mammary growth and lactation, *Rec Prog Horm Res* 14:219, 1958.

41. Kleinberg DL: Early mammary development: growth hormone and IGF-1, *J Mammary Gland Biol Neoplasia* 2:49, 1997.

42. Topper YJ, Freeman CS: Multiple hormone interactions in the developmental biology of the mammary gland, *Physiol Rev* 60:1049, 1980.

43. Lydon JP et al: Mice lacking progesterone receptor exhibit pleiotropic reproductive abnormalities, *Genes Dev* 9:2266, 1995.

44. Speroff L, Glass RG, Kase NG: *The breast: clinical gynecologic endocrinology and infertility,* Philadelphia, 1999, Lippincott Williams & Wilkins.

45. Moore DD, Conkling MA, Goodman HM: Human growth hormone: a multigene family, *Cell* 29:285, 1982.

46. Ormandy CJ et al: Null mutation of the prolactin receptor gene produces multiple reproductive defects in the mouse, *Genes Dev* 11:167, 1997.

47. Albarracin C et al: Identification of a major prolactin-regulated protein as 20 alpha-hydroxysteroid dehydrogenase; coordinate regulation of its activity, protein content, and messenger ribonucleic acid expression, *Endocrinology* 134:2453, 1994.

48. Ormandy CJ et al: The effect of progestins on prolactin receptor gene transcription in human breast cancer cells, *DNA Cell Biol* 11:721, 1992.

49. Russo IH, Russo J: Role of hormones in mammary cancer initiation and progression, *J Mammary Gland Biol Neoplasia* 3:49, 1998.

50. Friedberg SH, Oka T, Topper YJ: Development of insulin-sensitivity by mouse mammary gland in vitro, *Proc Natl Acad Sci USA* 67:1493, 1970.

51. Forsberg JG, Jacobsohn D, Norgren A: Modifications of reproductive organs in male rats influenced prenatally or pre- and postnatally by an "antiandrogenic" steroid (Cyproterone), *Z Anat Entwicklungsgesch* 127:175, 1968.

52. Simpson H et al: Meta-analysis of sequential luteal-cycle-associated changes in human breast tissue, *Breast Cancer Res Treat* 63:171, 2000.

53. Dyrenfurth I et al: Temporal relationships of hormonal variables in the menstrual cycle. In Ferin M et al (eds): *Institute for the study of human reproduction conference proceedings,* New York, 1974, Wiley.

54. Soriano JV et al: Hepatocyte growth factor stimulates extensive development of branching duct-like structures by cloned mammary gland epithelial cells, *J Cell Sci* 108:413, 1995.

55. Berdichevsky F et al: Branching morphogenesis of human mammary epithelial cells in collagen gels, *J Cell Sci* 107:3557, 1994.

56. Niranjan B et al: HGF/SF: a potent cytokine for mammary growth, morphogenesis and development, *Development* 121:2897, 1995.

57. Saelman EU, Keely PJ, Santoro SA: Loss of MDCK cell alpha 2 beta 1 integrin expression results in reduced cyst formation, failure of hepatocyte growth factor/scatter factor-induced branching morphogenesis, and increased apoptosis, *J Cell Sci* 108:3531, 1995.

58. Soriano JV et al: Roles of hepatocyte growth factor/scatter factor and transforming growth factor-beta1 in mammary gland ductal morphogenesis, *J Mammary Gland Biol Neoplasia* 3:133, 1998.

59. Coleman-Krnacik S, Rosen JM: Differential temporal and spatial gene expression of fibroblast growth factor family members during mouse mammary gland development, *Mol Endocrinol* 8:218, 1994.

60. Colston KW et al: Mammary gland 1,25-dihydroxyvitamin D3 receptor content during pregnancy and lactation, *Mol Cell Endocrinol* 60:15, 1988.

61. Mezzetti G, Barbiroli B, Oka T: 1,25-Dihydroxycholecalciferol receptor regulation in hormonally induced differentiation of mouse mammary gland in culture, *Endocrinology* 120:2488, 1987.

62. Narvaez CJ, Zinser G, Welsh J: Functions of 1alpha,25-dihydroxyvitamin D(3) in mammary gland: from normal development to breast cancer, *Steroids* 66:301, 2001.

63. Abou-el-Ela SH et al: Eicosanoid synthesis in 7,12-dimethylbenz(a)anthracene-induced mammary carcinomas in Sprague-Dawley rats fed primrose oil, menhaden oil or corn oil diet, *Lipids* 23:948, 1988.

64. Welsch CW, O'Connor DH: Influence of the type of dietary fat on developmental growth of the mammary gland in immature and mature female BALB/c mice, *Cancer Res* 49:5999, 1989.

65. Bandyopadhyay GK et al: Role of polyunsaturated fatty acids as signal transducers: amplification of signals from growth factor receptors by fatty acids in mammary epithelial cells, *Prostaglandins Leukot Essent Fatty Acids* 48:71, 1993.

66. Yang Y et al: Sequential requirement of hepatocyte growth factor and neuregulin in the morphogenesis and differentiation of the mammary gland, *J Cell Biol* 131:215, 1995.

67. Riese DJ II et al: The cellular response to neuregulins is governed by complex interactions of the erbB receptor family, *Mol Cell Biol* 15:5770, 1995.

68. Gearing AJ et al: Matrix metalloproteinases and processing of pro-TNF-alpha, *J Leukoc Biol* 57:774, 1995.

69. Fowlkes JL et al: Matrix metalloproteinases as insulin-like growth factor binding protein-degrading proteinases, *Prog Growth Factor Res* 6:255, 1995.

70. Strombeck J: Types of macromastia, *Acta Chir Scand Suppl* 1964.

71. Frantz A, Wilson JD: Endocrine disorders of the breast. In Wilson JD et al (eds): *Williams textbook of endocrinology,* Philadelphia, 1998, WB Saunders.

72. Finer N, Emery P, Hicks BH: Mammary gigantism and D-penicillamine, *Clin Endocrinol (Oxf)* 21:219, 1984.

73. Lafreniere R, Temple W, Ketcham A: Gestational macromastia, *Am J Surg* 148:413, 1984.

74. Baker SB et al: Juvenile gigantomastia: presentation of four cases and review of the literature, *Ann Plast Surg* 46:517, 2001.

75. Lee PA: The relationship of concentrations of serum hormones to pubertal gynecomastia, *J Pediatr* 86:212, 1975.

76. Braunstein G: Testes. In Greenspan F, Gardner D (eds): *Basic and clinical endocrinology,* New York, 2001, McGraw-Hill.

77. Thompson DF, Carter JR: Drug-induced gynecomastia, *Pharmacotherapy* 13:37, 1993.

78. Kuhn JM et al: Evaluation of diagnostic criteria for Leydig cell tumours in adult men revealed by gynaecomastia, *Clin Endocrinol (Oxf)* 26:407, 1987.

79. Kirschner MA, Cohen FB, Jespersen D: Estrogen production and its origin in men with gonadotropin-producing neoplasms, *J Clin Endocrinol Metab* 39:112, 1974.

80. Grumbach M, Conte F: Disorders of sex differentiation. In Wilson J, Foster D (eds): *Williams textbook of endocrinology,* Philadelphia, 1992, WB Saunders.

81. Morishima A et al: Aromatase deficiency in male and female siblings caused by a novel mutation and the physiological role of estrogens, *J Clin Endocrinol Metab* 80:3689, 1995.

82. Grumbach M, Styne D: Puberty: ontogeny, neuroendocrinology, physiology, and disorders. In Wilson J, Foster D (eds): *Williams textbook of endocrinology,* Philadelphia, 1992, WB Saunders.

83. Hilakivi-Clarke L et al: Tallness and overweight during childhood have opposing effects on breast cancer risk, *Br J Cancer* 85:1680, 2001.

84. Russo J, Rivera R, Russo IH: Influence of age and parity on the development of the human breast, *Breast Cancer Res Treat* 23:211, 1992.

85. McGreevy J, Bland K: The breast. In O'Leary JP, Capote LR (eds): *Physiologic basis of surgery,* Baltimore, 1996, Williams & Wilkins.

86. Kaplan CR, Schenken R: Endocrinology of the breast. In Mitchell G, Bassett L (eds): *The female breast and its disorders,* Baltimore, 1990, Williams & Wilkins.

87. Tyson JE et al: Studies of prolactin secretion in human pregnancy, *Am J Obstet Gynecol* 113:14, 1972.

88. Kletzky OA et al: Prolactin synthesis and release during pregnancy and puerperium, *Am J Obstet Gynecol* 136:545, 1980.

89. Tyson JE, Friesen HG: Factors influencing the secretion of human prolactin and growth hormone in menstrual and gestational women, *Am J Obstet Gynecol* 116:377, 1973.

90. Boockfor FR, Hoeffler JP, Frawley LS: Estradiol induces a shift in cultured cells that release prolactin or growth hormone, *Am J Physiol* 250:E103, 1986.

91. Maurer RA: Estradiol regulates the transcription of the prolactin gene, *J Biol Chem* 257:2133, 1982.

92. Barberia JM et al: Serum prolactin patterns in early human gestation, *Am J Obstet Gynecol* 121:1107, 1975.

93. Cramer OM, Parker CR Jr, Porter JC: Estrogen inhibition of dopamine release into hypophysial portal blood, *Endocrinology* 104:419, 1979.

94. Kelly PA et al: The prolactin/growth hormone receptor family, *Endocr Rev* 12:235, 1991.

95. Murphy LJ et al: Modulation of lactogenic receptors by progestins in cultured human breast cancer cells, *J Clin Endocrinol Metab* 62:280, 1986.

96. Simon WE, Pahnke VG, Holzel F: In vitro modulation of prolactin binding to human mammary carcinoma cells by steroid hormones and prolactin, *J Clin Endocrinol Metab* 60:1243, 1985.

97. Lee CS, Oka T: Progesterone regulation of a pregnancy-specific transcription repressor to beta-casein gene promoter in mouse mammary gland, *Endocrinology* 131:2257, 1992.

98. Krane IM, Leder P: NDF/Heregulin induces persistence of terminal end buds and adenocarcinomas in the mammary glands of transgenic mice, *Oncogene* 12:1781, 1996.

99. Robinson GW, Hennighausen L: Inhibins and activins regulate mammary epithelial cell differentiation through mesenchymal-epithelial interactions, *Development* 124: 2701, 1997.

100. Toscani A et al: Arrest of spermatogenesis and defective breast development in mice lacking A-myb, *Nature* 386:713, 1997.

101. Robinson GW et al: The C/EBPbeta transcription factor regulates epithelial cell proliferation and differentiation in the mammary gland, *Genes Dev* 12:1907, 1998.

102. Chen F, Capecchi MR: Paralogous mouse Hox genes, Hoxa9, Hoxb9, and Hoxd9, function together to control development of the mammary gland in response to pregnancy, *Proc Natl Acad Sci USA* 96:541, 1999.

103. Sicinski P et al: Cyclin D1 provides a link between development and oncogenesis in the retina and breast, *Cell* 82:621, 1995.

104. Sympson CJ et al: Targeted expression of stromelysin-1 in mammary gland provides evidence for a role of proteinases in branching morphogenesis and the requirement for an intact basement membrane for tissue-specific gene expression, *J Cell Biol* 125:681, 1994.

105. Witty JP, Wright JH, Matrisian LM: Matrix metalloproteinases are expressed during ductal and alveolar mammary morphogenesis, and misregulation of stromelysin-1 in transgenic mice induces unscheduled alveolar development, *Mol Biol Cell* 6:1287, 1995.

106. Alexander CM et al: Rescue of mammary epithelial cell apoptosis and entactin degradation by a tissue inhibitor of metalloproteinases-1 transgene, *J Cell Biol* 135:1669, 1996.

107. Russo J et al: Biological and molecular basis of human breast cancer, *Front Biosci* 3:D944, 1998.

108. Russo J et al: Pattern of distribution of cells positive for estrogen receptor alpha and progesterone receptor in relation to proliferating cells in the mammary gland, *Breast Cancer Res Treat* 53:217, 1999.

109. Russo J, Russo I: Estrogens and cell proliferation in the human breast, *J Cardiovasc Pharmacol* 28:19, 1996.

110. Russo J, Russo I: Role of differentiation in the pathogenesis and prevention of breast cancer, *Endocr Rel Cancer* 4:7, 1997.

111. Russo J, Russo I: Role of hormones in human breast development: the menopausal breast. In Wreo B (ed): *Progress in the management of menopause,* London, 1997, Parthenon Publishing.

112. Cregan MD, Hartmann PE: Computerized breast measurement from conception to weaning: clinical implications, *J Hum Lact* 15:89, 1999.

113. Kent JC et al: Breast volume and milk production during extended lactation in women, *Exp Physiol* 84:435, 1999.

114. Cox DB, Owens RA, Hartmann PE: Blood and milk prolactin and the rate of milk synthesis in women, *Exp Physiol* 81:1007, 1996.

115. Hartmann P, Sherriff J, Kent J: Maternal nutrition and the regulation of milk synthesis, *Proc Nutr Soc* 54:379, 1995.

116. Ohtani O et al: Lymphatics of the rat mammary gland during virgin, pregnant, lactating and post-weaning periods, *Ital J Anat Embryol* 103:335, 1998.

117. Marti A et al: Milk accumulation triggers apoptosis of mammary epithelial cells, *Eur J Cell Biol* 73:158, 1997.

118. Lund LR et al: Two distinct phases of apoptosis in mammary gland involution: proteinase-independent and -dependent pathways, *Development* 122:181, 1996.

119. Feng Z et al: Glucocorticoid and progesterone inhibit involution and programmed cell death in the mouse mammary gland, *J Cell Biol* 131:1095, 1995.

120. Bole-Feysot C et al: Prolactin (PRL) and its receptor: actions, signal transduction pathways and phenotypes observed in PRL receptor knockout mice, *Endocr Rev* 19:225, 1998.

121. Liu X et al: Stat5a is mandatory for adult mammary gland development and lactogenesis, *Genes Dev* 11:179, 1997.

122. Altiok S, Groner B: Beta-casein mRNA sequesters a single-stranded nucleic acid-binding protein which negatively regulates the beta-casein gene promoter, *Mol Cell Biol* 14:6004, 1994.

123. Seyfred MA, Gorski J: An interaction between the 5' flanking distal and proximal regulatory domains of the rat prolactin gene is required for transcriptional activation by estrogens, *Mol Endocrinol* 4:1226, 1990.

124. Yan GZ, Pan WT, Bancroft C: Thyrotropin-releasing hormone action on the prolactin promoter is mediated by the POU protein pit-1, *Mol Endocrinol* 5:535, 1991.

125. Bredow S et al: Increase of prolactin mRNA in the rat hypothalamus after intracerebroventricular injection of VIP or PACAP, *Brain Res* 660:301, 1994.

126. Pickett CA, Gutierrez-Hartmann A: Ras mediates Src but not epidermal growth factor-receptor tyrosine kinase signaling pathways in GH4 neuroendocrine cells, *Proc Natl Acad Sci USA* 91:8612, 1994.

127. Porter TE, Wiles CD, Frawley LS: Stimulation of lactotrope differentiation in vitro by fibroblast growth factor, *Endocrinology* 134:164, 1994.

128. Tyson JE, Perez A, Zanartu J: Human lactational response to oral thyrotropin releasing hormone, *J Clin Endocrinol Metab* 43:760, 1976.

129. Ben-Jonathan N et al: Extrapituitary prolactin: distribution, regulation, functions, and clinical aspects, *Endocr Rev* 17:639, 1997.

130. Franks S, Kiwi R, Nabarro JD: Pregnancy and lactation after pituitary surgery, *BMJ* 1:882, 1977.

131. Li M, Liu X, Robinson G, et al.: Mammary-derived signals activate programmed cell death during the first stage of mammary gland involution, *Proc Natl Acad Sci USA* 94:3425, 1997.

132. Daniel CW, Strickland P, Friedmann Y: Expression and functional role of E- and P-cadherins in mouse mammary ductal morphogenesis and growth, *Dev Biol* 169:511, 1995.

133. Delmas V et al: Expression of the cytoplasmic domain of E-cadherin induces precocious mammary epithelial alveolar formation and affects cell polarity and cell-matrix integrity, *Dev Biol* 216:491, 1999.

134. Radice GL et al: Precocious mammary gland development in P-cadherin-deficient mice, *J Cell Biol* 139:1025, 1997.

135. Streuli CH et al: Laminin mediates tissue-specific gene expression in mammary epithelia, *J Cell Biol* 129:591, 1995.

136. Streuli CH, Edwards GM: Control of normal mammary epithelial phenotype by integrins, *J Mammary Gland Biol Neoplasia* 3:151, 1998.

137. Daly SE, Owens RA, Hartmann PE: The short-term synthesis and infant-regulated removal of milk in lactating women, *Exp Physiol* 78:209, 1993.

138. Chapman RS et al: Suppression of epithelial apoptosis and delayed mammary gland involution in mice with a conditional knockout of Stat3, *Genes Dev* 13:2604, 1999.

139. Baik MG, Lee MJ, Choi YJ: Gene expression during involution of mammary gland, *Int J Mol Med* 2:39, 1998 (review).

140. Merlo GR et al: p53-dependent and p53-independent activation of apoptosis in mammary epithelial cells reveals a survival function of EGF and insulin, *J Cell Biol* 128:1185, 1995.

141. Talhouk RS, Bissell MJ, Werb Z: Coordinated expression of extracellular matrix-degrading proteinases and their inhibitors regulates mammary epithelial function during involution, *J Cell Biol* 118:1271, 1992.

142. Chapman DJ, Perez-Escamilla R: Identification of risk factors for delayed onset of lactation, *J Am Diet Assoc* 99:450, 1999.

143. Neubauer SH et al: Delayed lactogenesis in women with insulin-dependent diabetes mellitus, *Am J Clin Nutr* 58:54, 1993.

144. Arthur PG, Kent JC, Hartmann PE: Metabolites of lactose synthesis in milk from diabetic and nondiabetic women during lactogenesis II, *J Pediatr Gastroenterol Nutr* 19:100, 1994.

145. Dewey KG et al: A randomized study of the effects of aerobic exercise by lactating women on breast-milk volume and composition, *N Engl J Med* 330:449, 1994.

146. Sharp E: Historical review of a syndrome embracing utero-ovarian atrophy with persistent lactation, *Am J Obstet Gynecol* 30, 1935.

147. Forbes A et al: A syndrome, distinct from acromegamenorrhea, and low follicle-stimulating hormone excretion, *J Clin Endocrinol* 1951.

148. Archer DF: Current concepts of prolactin physiology in normal and abnormal conditions. *Fertil Steril* 28:125, 1977.

149. Frantz A: Prolactin secretion in physiologic and pathologic human conditions measured by bioassay and radioimmunoassay. In Josimovich J, Reynolds M, Cobo E (eds): *Lactogenic hormones, fetal nutrition, and lactation.* New York, 1974, Wiley.

150. Frantz AG: Prolactin, *N Engl J Med* 298:201, 1978.
151. Blackwell RE: Diagnosis and management of prolactinomas, *Fertil Steril* 43:5, 1985.
152. Kelver M, Nagamani M: Hyperprolactinemia in primary adrenocortical insufficiency, 44:423, 1985.
153. Mahesh VB, Pria SD, Greenblatt RB: Abnormal lactation with Cushing's syndrome: a case report, *J Clin Endocrinol Metab* 29:978, 1969.
154. Nabarro JD: Acromegaly, *Clin Endocrinol (Oxf)* 26:481, 1987.
155. Sievertsen GD et al: Metabolic clearance and secretion rates of human prolactin in normal subjects and in patients with chronic renal failure, *J Clin Endocrinol Metab* 50:846, 1980.
156. Turkington RW: Ectopic production of prolactin, *N Engl J Med* 285:1455, 1971.
157. Syvertsen A et al: The computed tomographic appearance of the normal pituitary gland and pituitary microadenomas, *Radiology* 133:385, 1979.

CHAPTER

4

Discharges and Secretions of the Nipple*

WILLIAM H. GOODSON III

EILEEN B. KING

Chapter Outline

*Supported by research grant CA 13556-17 from the National Cancer Institute, Bethesda, MD.

The frequency of discharges and secretions of the nipple necessitates a comprehensive discussion in the management of breast diseases. The purpose of this chapter is threefold: first, to inform the reader about nipple aspirate fluid (NAF) findings related to breast physiology, pathology, and risk for cancer; second, to describe cytologic findings in NAF and ductal lavage fluid (DLF) in assessing risk for breast cancer risk; and third, to discuss nipple discharge in diagnosis and management of breast disease, especially cancer and its precursors. This chapter concludes by describing methods for sample collection and preparation needed for optimum quality and best diagnostic results.

The terms *discharges* and *secretions* of the nipple are defined as follows: *Discharge* is fluid that escapes spontaneously from the nipple. *Secretion* is fluid present in the ducts that must be collected by nipple aspiration or by other means such as conventional breast pump or gentle massage and expression from the ducts (nonspontaneous secretion). *DLF* is a saline washing from individual breast ducts obtained with a microcatheter device.

Secretion in the Nonlactating Breast

The secretory activity of the female breast is manifested at varying levels throughout life—at birth, after puberty, and well into menopause. Secretion of this modified apocrine gland exhibits milklike characteristics, and lactation represents the ultimate secretory product. Nipple secretion is usually not clinically appreciated in nonlactating women because dense keratotic material plugs the openings of the lactiferous sinuses (Figure 4-1). Such secretion is observed, however, in duct lumens displayed in histologic sections of breast tissue (Figure 4-2). By removing the keratotic plugs and using a simple nipple aspirator device, the physician can easily obtain fluid from a large proportion of women (Figure 4-3).[1-4] Researchers have also obtained secretions by using a breast pump or with gentle manual expression.[5-9]

Both secretory and absorptive activities appear to be inevitable components of breast physiology. Reabsorption has been studied in rabbits by injecting breast ducts with various substances and observing their distribution in tissue, lymphatics, and blood.[10,11] Suspensions of India ink could be traced to these sites, and diphtheria antitoxin injected into ducts was subsequently measured in blood. Sartorius and co-workers[3] performed ductography using a water-soluble contrast medium in humans and noted that reabsorption occurred at different rates, depending on the presence of lesions.

FLUID AVAILABILITY RELATED TO AGE, RACE, AND OTHER FACTORS

In a study of 606 healthy nonlactating women, the availability of NAF was examined by race, age, menstrual history, menopausal status, and use of oral contraceptives or estrogen replacement therapy.[2] Samples of NAF were collected by a modified Sartorius technique. This procedure is noninvasive, simple, and well tolerated by the patient. Fluid availability was defined as one or more drops; on average, 20 to 30 µL was obtained. Fluid was most often obtained from white and Filipino women (70%) and was less frequently

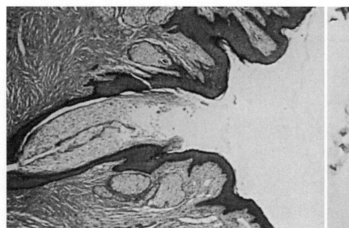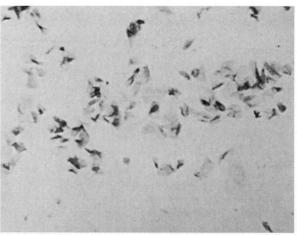

A   B

FIG. 4-1 A, Sagittal section of nipple duct opening demonstrates the usual plug of keratotic plaques obstructing the duct (hematoxylin and eosin stain; original magnification ×25). B, Nipple aspirate fluid sample contains abundant anucleate keratotic plaques from duct opening (Papanicolaou stain; original magnification ×25).

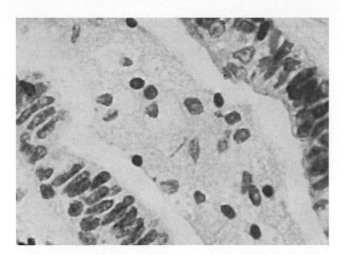

FIG. **4-2** Breast duct with lumen containing secretory material and exfoliated lining cells (hematoxylin and eosin stain; original magnification ×250).

available from black, Mexican-American, Japanese, and Chinese women (Table 4-1). Age was a significant factor, regardless of race, and women older than 50 years were less likely to yield fluid (Table 4-2). Phase of the menstrual cycle and history of pregnancy did not significantly affect the availability of NAF. Similarly, oral contraceptives and estrogen replacement therapy had little effect, although in postmenopausal women there was some increase in the amount of NAF obtained from those receiving estrogen replacement therapy. A comparison of secretory and menopausal status in white and Chinese women showed that significantly more premenopausal than postmenopausal women yielded fluid and that the difference was most striking in Chinese women (Table 4-3). The mammary and

ceruminous glands are both apocrine in type. A relatively high frequency of fluid availability in white women corresponded to a high incidence of the genetically determined wet earwax in these women.[12,13] This is particularly interesting because the international mortality and frequency rates for breast cancer seem to be associated with the frequency of the alleles for wet earwax.

In an additional study of 103 women with suspicious breast lesions, a higher frequency of NAF (88.4%) was observed than in healthy women, suggesting an association between NAF availability and breast disease.[2] Of 22 women in this study later found to have carcinoma, 16 (72%) had yielded NAF. Theoretically, breast epithelium, if displaying more secretory activity, would be more likely to be exposed to endogenous and exogenous carcinogens than would epithelium that displays less evidence of secretory activity.

Wynder and colleagues[4] evaluated NAF in relation to various epidemiologic factors associated with breast disease. Their findings are very similar to those described in other studies using the Sartorius technique, with breast disease status being among the most important.[2,4,14]

BIOCHEMICAL AND CYTOLOGIC COMPOSITION

NAF has many of the characteristics of colostrum or milk. Chemical analyses show that it is a secretion of both endogenous and exogenous substances. The fluid varies in color and appearance related to its composition. Like colostrum and milk, it contains exfoliated epithelial cells and nonepithelial cells of hematogenous and immune system origin. These components may vary in relation to the functional aspects of the breast, its pathology, and risk factors for breast cancer.

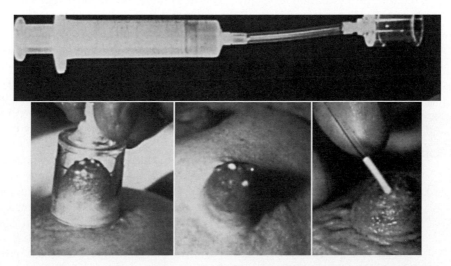

FIG. **4-3** Nipple aspirator is a cup-shaped plastic device fitted with tubing to connect with a syringe. The negative pressure created by the syringe causes drops of fluid to appear at each duct opening. The drops are then collected in a capillary tube.

TABLE 4-1   Nipple Aspirate Fluid (NAF) Availability among Various Racial Groups

GROUP	NUMBER WITH NAF	NUMBER ATTEMPTED (%)
White	158/225	(70.2)
Filipino	7/10	(70.0)
Black	23/37	(62.2)
Mexican American	37/71	(52.1)
Asian	65/263	(24.7)

TABLE 4-3   Nipple Aspirate Fluid (NAF) Availability and Menopausal Status in White and Chinese Women

| AGE GROUP | NUMBER WITH NAF/NUMBER ATTEMPTED (%) | |
	WHITES*	CHINESE†
Premenopausal	112/138 (81.2)	47/156 (30.1)
Postmenopausal	46/77 (59.7)	3/80 (3.8)

*$\chi^2 = 24.7$, $p < .001$.
†$\chi^2 = 20.4$, $p < .001$.

Biochemical Composition. The biochemical composition of NAF has been studied using micromethods to analyze the small volumes of available ductal secretion. The NAF contains lactose, β-lactalbumin, immunoglobulin, cholesterol, fatty acids, a number of steroids, and other endogenous substances.[15] Substances from exogenous sources are also secreted into the fluid. Examples are technetium, barbiturate, fatty acid, caffeine, pesticides, and nicotine and cotinine related to cigarette smoking. Approximately 10% of NAF samples demonstrate mutagenic activity with the Ames salmonella test. These findings demonstrate that breast fluid is a true secretory product. Detailed analysis has been made of many of these components, and their concentrations in breast secretion have been compared with those in plasma. Other studies have considered differences in composition of secretions among women with different risk factors for breast cancer. Among compounds of particular interest, because of their possible role in the pathogenesis of benign and malignant breast disease, are the estrogens and cholesterol with its epoxides and triol.

In a study of estrogen (estrone and estradiol) levels in serum and NAF, Petrakis and colleagues[16] evaluated samples from one or both breasts in 104 women and found estrogen levels to be 5 to 45 times higher in NAF

than in serum. They also found that NAF estrogen levels were lower in parous than in nulliparous women. This finding suggests that prolonged levels of estrogen in breast fluid after full-term delivery and lactation may in part explain the relative reduction in breast cancer risk in parous as compared with nulliparous women. In contrast, the serum estrogen levels were not related to parity.

Cholesterol and its oxidation products, 5, 6-α and β epoxides and their common hydrolysis product cholestane triol, were measured in NAF by Gruenke and associates.[17] Both of these epoxides have been implicated in oncogenic behavior in a number of different studies demonstrating induction of sarcomas, in vitro transforming of embryo hamster cell lines, chromosome damage and inhibition of DNA repair, and mutagenic activity.[18-21] In a study of 105 women without breast disease, levels of cholesterol and its β epoxide were found to increase with age but were reduced in parous women. The lower levels persisted for a minimum of 2 years after childbirth or lactation. As a result, parous women have less cumulative exposure to these biochemical substances with carcinogenic potential.[17]

That the color of NAF varies greatly is easily observed clinically. Excluding bloody fluids, the colors range from clear to black, with gradations classified as white, pale yellow, dark yellow, brown, and green. In a retrospective study of NAF from 2343 women, the colors of the samples were compared with their biochemical compositions.[22] Each sample had been coded at the time of collection in one of the seven color categories before biochemical analysis. Cholesterol, cholesterol 5, 6-α and β epoxides, cholestane triol, lipid peroxide, estradiol and estrone, and immunoglobulin levels were measured. The results were transformed into natural logarithms, and the means and standard deviations were determined for each breast fluid color group. Statistical significance was tested with a one-way analysis of variance. The mean concentrations of cholesterol and its epoxides and triol were strongly related to

TABLE 4-2   Nipple Aspirate Fluid (NAF) Availability and Age

| AGE GROUP (yr) | NUMBER WITH NAF/NUMBER ATTEMPTED (%) | |
	ALL RACES	WHITES
≤20	9/18 (50.0)	4/6 (66.6)
21-30	66/121 (54.5)	36/48 (75.0)
31-40	77/145 (53.1)	44/57 (77.2)
41-50	70/125 (56.0)	37/47 (78.7)
51-60	30/78 (38.5)	21/35 (60.0)
≥60	23/86 (26.7)	16/32 (50.0)
TOTAL	266/555 (47.9)	158/225 (70.2)

darker colorations. Higher concentrations of these substances were also associated with the darker colorations. Similar relationships were obtained for lipid peroxides, estrone, and estradiol. However, the immunoglobulin concentrations showed no relation to color. Although the exact mechanism of color production is unknown, the association with biochemical properties of the NAF is of clinical interest and will be discussed further later in this chapter.

Cytologic Composition. The cytology of breast fluid was first reported by Donne,[23] who in 1838 described the presence of foam cells in colostrum. The main attention remained focused on studies of colostrum, milk, and spontaneous nipple discharge. In an early study of nonspontaneous secretion, Jackson and Severance[5] and Jackson and colleagues[6] routinely attempted to express fluid from both breasts during the course of breast examination. They described the presence of red blood cells, vacuolated epithelial cells, and dark-staining epithelial cells, usually in clusters in air-dried smears on Wright's stain. Papanicolaou and colleagues[8] made a thorough and systematic study of the cytology of nonspontaneous breast secretions using a hand breast pump to obtain the specimen. More than 50% of the 1600 patients they examined yielded fluid by this method. These investigators emphasized that cytology of abnormal breast conditions could not be properly evaluated without adequate knowledge of what was normal, and they provided a description of the benign cell findings.

They noted that the two cell types most often encountered were foam cells and duct epithelial cells. A few small histiocytes and lymphocytes were also frequently present. Ringrose[9] achieved similar results and noted the same type of cytologic findings in fluid from asymptomatic women.

The cytologic findings in NAF from women without breast disease are primarily of interest for providing knowledge of "normal." Such knowledge is essential for comparisons of findings related to benign and malignant breast lesions and to ensure accurate interpretation of clinically significant disease. Benign findings have been evaluated microscopically by determining total cellularity and identifying cell types and the percentage of each type.[24] The samples from women without breast symptoms contain an average of $16,200 \pm 6500$ cells of all types. The cellularity varies with age and is increased in samples from women in the fourth decade of life, as compared with those of younger and older women. It must be emphasized, however, that there is a wide range in cellularity among individuals regardless of age. The timing of greater average cellularity in NAF samples can be considered fortuitous for the study of breast cancer precursors developing in women aged 30 to 50 years.

Benign epithelial cells, when present, consist of a few ductal cells; only rarely are apocrine metaplastic cells found in the absence of breast symptoms (Figures 4-4 and 4-5). Occasionally, squamous epithelial cells and transitional cell forms from the ampullary and distal portions of the duct are found within the nipple

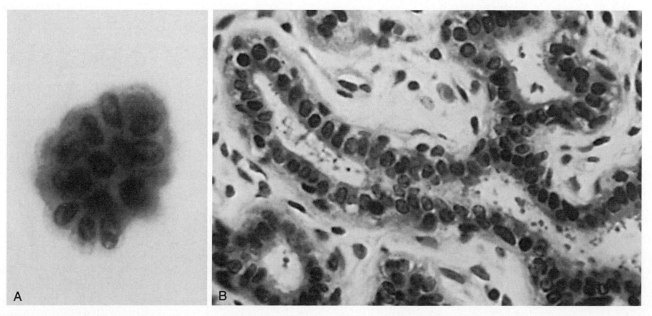

FIG. **4-4 A,** Benign duct epithelial cells in nipple aspirate fluid sample have uniform small oval nuclei and columnar shape (Papanicolaou stain; original magnification ×250). **B,** These cells correspond with the normal ductal lobular epithelium depicted in this section of benign breast tissue (hematoxylin and eosin stain; original magnification ×250).

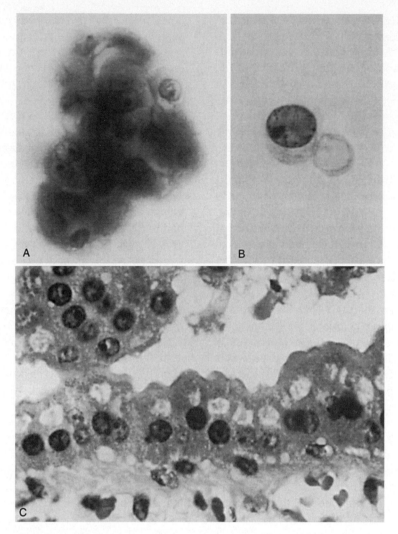

FIG. **4-5 A,** A group of apocrine metaplastic cells in nipple aspirate fluid have abundant granular and sometimes vacuolated cytoplasm. **B,** An apocrine bleb containing a large vacuole with a thin cytoplasmic envelope is separating from the border of this single cell (**A** and **B,** Papanicolaou stain; original magnification ×250). **C,** Multilayered apocrine metaplastic epithelium with tufts of cells separating into the duct lumen are depicted in this tissue section (hematoxylin and eosin stain; original magnification ×250).

(Figure 4-6). Duct openings often yield anucleate keratotic plaques that may be abundant when preparation before nipple aspiration has been inadequate (see Figure 4-1).

Foam cells are most often present and may be abundant. They show predominantly histiocytic characteristics when evaluated cytochemically with monoclonal antibodies or by other conventional means (Figure 4-7). The abundant, finely vacuolated cytoplasm of foam cells may contain yellow-brown pigment granules. Some granules have morphologic, electron microscopic, and staining features of lipofuscin and ceroid contained in lysosomes (Figure 4-8). Other pigmented granules represent hemoglobin and its products staining positively for iron (see Figure 4-8). Other cells are of hematogenous and immune system origin and consist of neutrophils, lymphocytes, and small histiocytes.

The mean percentage of various cell types in NAF from asymptomatic women and those with benign cytology and pathology is illustrated in Figure 4-9. In summary, "normal" cellular findings consist of few or no duct epithelial cells, a preponderance of foam cells, and moderate numbers of cells of hematogenous origin in samples of modest cellularity.

MENSTRUAL CYCLE CHANGES

Menstrual cycle effects on breast could potentially change the availability and composition of NAF. If there were cyclical changes in breast secretory activity, these changes would be reflected by the presence or absence of fluid at different times in the cycle. Particularly essential would be knowledge of any ductal lobular epithelial proliferative activity related to the cycle. Cyclical changes would affect the accuracy of

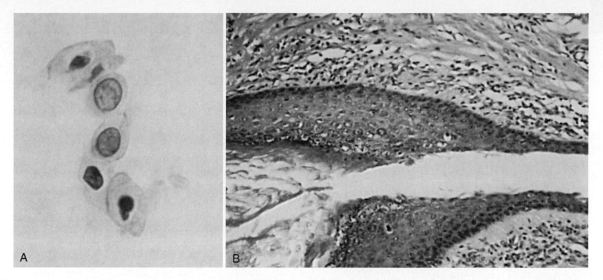

FIG. **4-6 A,** A group of squamous epithelial cells from ducts within the nipple have nuclei of variable size and staining with pyknosis in one (Papanicolaou stain; original magnification ×250). **B,** Note the parabasal squamous maturation of epithelium in the duct lining from which these cells are derived (hematoxylin and eosin stain; original magnification ×25).

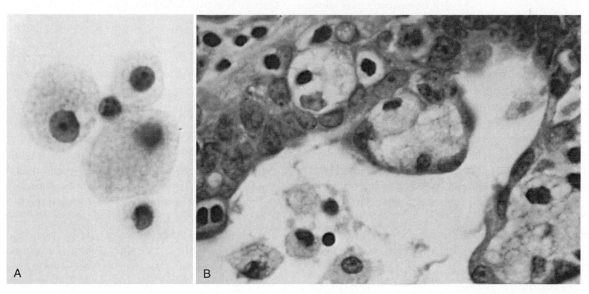

FIG. **4-7 A,** Typical large spherical foam cells with abundant finely vacuolated cytoplasm in nipple aspirate fluid. Nuclei are isodiametric and have prominent nucleoli (Papanicolaou stain; original magnification ×250). **B,** In the tissue section, the duct foam cells appear intraepithelial and also within the duct lumen (hematoxylin and eosin stain; original magnification ×250).

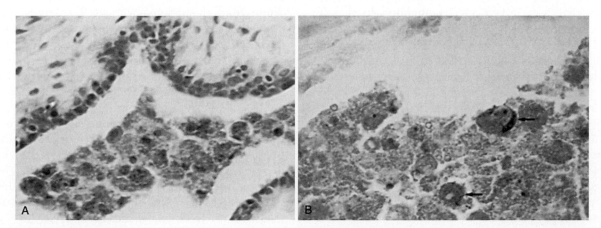

FIG. **4-8 A,** Foam cell containing golden brown pigment granules (hematoxylin and eosin stain; original magnification ×160); **B,** Iron-staining particles in foam cells (Prussian blue stain at arrows; original magnification ×250).

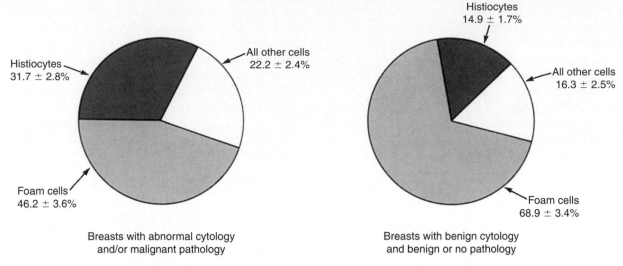

FIG. **4-9** Comparison of percentage of foam cells in two clinical groups.

diagnosis and interpretation of the cytologic findings in both NAF and nipple discharge. Current knowledge about histologic changes during the menstrual cycle suggests cyclical variations in NAF.

Breast tissue studies have shown cyclical changes related to follicular and luteal phases. Similar observations on changes in histologic pattern, cellular morphology, mitoses, and DNA content have been made.[25-28] Ductal lobular proliferative activity is demonstrated by increased numbers of mitoses and DNA synthesis in the luteal phase corresponding to the combination of estrogen and progesterone influences. Vogel and associates[29] found similar histologic changes, except that mitoses were observed early in the follicular phase. Some disagreement among such studies may be a result of inherent problems: heterogeneity of lobular development within the individual breast, variability between subjects, and inaccuracy in cycle data. Some of these problems have been addressed in more recent studies that have given special attention to sample selection and size and to statistical methods. Longacre and Bartlow[30] found excessive lymphocytes, duct epithelial degenerative changes, and sloughing into duct lumens in the late secretory and early menstrual phases. Ferguson and Anderson[25] also found cell depletion through a process of apoptosis in this time interval, which peaked on day 28. Some reports indicate that both breasts were examined and that no significant differences were found in morphologic changes.

Objective measures of breast epithelial cyclical changes are provided by DNA quantitative cytochemistry previously described in tissue sections and by image cytometry of fine-needle aspiration (FNA) samples. In FNA biopsies, image cytometry using five nuclear features—area, circumference, boundary fluctuation, chromatin granularity, and stain intensity—successfully discriminated samples from women in follicular phase and those in luteal phase.[31] This approach, applied to the individual woman, was 100% correct in identifying the phase of the cycle. Concerned by the proliferative changes that mimic atypia or malignancy in the postovulatory phase, the authors recommended that FNA be done only in the preovulatory phase.

Papanicolaou and associates[7] provided the first report of the cytology of nonspontaneous secretion related to the menstrual cycle. In 1958[8] they reported on fluid availability with a technique of gentle massage and breast pump application on the breasts of nonlactating women. From 46 of 129 women, aged 20 to 39 years, who yielded breast fluid, the fluid was most often obtained during the fourth (55%) or the first (40%) week of the cycle. Duct epithelial cells were scant or absent, and foam cells were the most common constituent. These researchers noted some cell enlargement and clusters of cells with cytoplasmic vacuolization that appeared different from small, undifferentiated duct epithelial cells. They proposed that these differences were related to the endocrine status of the individual; however, the findings were not analyzed with respect to the day or week of the menstrual cycle.

In our studies of NAF, there are some differences in fluid availability and cellularity associated with the phase of the menstrual cycle; however, these differences do not appear to be significant. In a study of 117 white women, 70.8% yielded fluid in the first week, 83.9% in the second week, 75.8% in the third week, and 82.8% in the fourth week of the menstrual cycle.[2] No significant differences were noted in cellularity or types of cells present. A group of 38 NAF samples from different women were selected for approximately equal distribution among the 4 weeks of a 28-day cycle. The samples were analyzed for total cellularity and cell types. Duct epithelial cells occurred singly and in groups, accompanied occasionally by apocrine metaplastic cells; foam cells were almost always present and abundant; and there were a few histiocytes, lymphocytes, and neutrophils. Although the measure of total cellularity, percentage of single duct cells, histiocytes, and lymphocytes have demonstrated trends toward elevation in the fourth week of the menstrual cycle, the results were not significant on discriminant analysis.

Complete cycles sampled at weekly intervals were evaluated in 14 women. Serum and NAF estrone and estradiol were determined at each examination and serum hormonal levels were compared with the menstrual history. In women whose serum hormonal patterns were consistent with a normal ovulatory cycle, no cytologic changes suggesting proliferation or degeneration were noted and there were no significant variations in cellularity or cell types. However, some increase in total cellularity and in percentage of lymphocytes did occur in the late postovulatory and early preovulatory phases.

Our studies of menstrual cycle changes in NAF cytology have revealed no significant differences that might affect the accuracy or diagnostic value of these findings. The sample size is small, and more data are needed before definitive conclusions can be drawn.

Pregnancy and Lactation-Associated Secretions

Responding to a variety of hormonal influences during pregnancy and lactation, the breast becomes fully developed anatomically and functionally. Development of the terminal ductal lobular unit involves proliferation of ductal and lobular epithelium and the manufacturing of secretory products, colostrum, and milk. The anatomic and physiologic features of the breast and its secretory products have been widely studied and amply discussed elsewhere (see Chapters 2 and 3). However, histologic studies in humans are limited by the availability of tissue from biopsies.[32,33] In lieu of human tissue, animal studies have provided some insights into breast changes during pregnancy and lactation.[34]

During pregnancy, the ductal lobular system undergoes extensive hyperplasia with rapid proliferation of epithelial linings as they form new ductules. These are arranged in close proximity with scant supporting stroma. This process is most marked in the first half of the pregnancy and is followed by some development of

the stromal component and infiltration of lymphocytes, plasma cells, and eosinophils. Evidence of secretory activity appears in the late months of pregnancy with the presence of protein-rich fluid in dilated duct lumens. The epithelial lining varies from flat to low columnar and exhibits merocrine secretory activity typical of glandular epithelium in other organs. The so-called apocrine secretion consists of lipid droplets that are free within the cytoplasm, become oriented at the free margin of the cell, and separate from the cell bounded by a thin envelope of cytoplasm.[35]

The "normal" cytology of breast secretions during pregnancy is characterized by increased cellularity compared with the resting breast. This is especially true in the late months of pregnancy. Cell types are the same as those found in the absence of pregnancy but show some differences in the proportions of various cells. Epithelial cell clusters are numerous and sometimes have a configuration suggesting papillary structure. In the late third trimester and after childbirth, neutrophils are abundant. Postpartum cellular patterns vary depending on the presence or suppression of lactation.[24-36]

An interesting point of view about the importance of breast cytology during pregnancy and lactation was expressed by Holmquist and Papanicolaou[36] and by Papanicolaou and colleagues.[8] They proposed that cytologic studies of breast secretion offer a noninvasive way of studying the effects of altered hormonal stimuli on breast epithelium during pregnancy and lactation. Such studies may also be relevant in demonstrating epithelial changes that might predate development of neoplastic disease of the breast. In their study of 20 antepartum and 39 postpartum women with clinically normal breasts, all of the subjects had full-term deliveries and their mean age was 27.2 (17 to 43) years. The cytologic samples were generally more cellular than those from nonpregnant women. The cell appearance and predominant cell type varied among individuals, sometimes between the right and left breast of the same individual, and among trimesters. Cell types were the same as those found in the absence of pregnancy or lactation; however, definite alterations in structure were noted. The cell types listed were foam cells, leukocytes, histiocytes, and gland epithelial cells consisting of single cells and cell clusters. *Foam cells* were found to have the same appearance as cells referred to as *colostrum bodies*, which have been described in "normal" breast fluid samples from nonpregnant women. Among the pregnant patients, Holmquist and Papanicolaou[36] note that the foam cells exhibited nuclear enlargement, binucleation, multinucleation, and increased cytoplasmic vacuolization as compared with those from nonpregnant women. They found an unexpectedly large number of ductal epithelial cells during pregnancy and lactation. The groups of cells were papillary in structure and similar to papillary fronds from intraductal papilloma. Differences were also noted in the cytology of postpartum smears from lactating patients compared with those of secretion following estrogen suppression of lactation. The former became virtually acellular at the end of the first week postpartum, whereas the latter exhibited cellularity and various types of cell clusters characteristic of those found during pregnancy.

Kline and Lash[37] studied the cytology of breast secretions obtained during the third trimester from 50 pregnant women 16 to 39 years old. This study was stimulated by the erroneous interpretation of cytologic findings during pregnancy based on the papillary groupings and changes similar to those described by Holmquist and Papanicolaou.[36] In the Kline and Lash study,[37] 43 of the 50 women had papillary groupings, whereas the remaining seven had only foam cells and leukocytes. Tissue from four biopsies obtained in the third trimester of pregnancy revealed tufts of cells forming "spurs" or invaginations into duct and alveolar lumens and similar structures that were desquamated into lumens and were suggestive of groups of cells found in the breast secretions. These investigators noted that the "spurs" were closely associated with the formation of new alveoli, and this offered a mechanism for their origin. Delicate capillary networks within these tufts of cells could be easily traumatized and could result in blood escaping into the breast secretion. Bloody secretion without significant breast pathology occurs in pregnant and postpartum patients. In a later study, these authors reported persistence of the antepartum cellular findings in 31 of 72 postpartum women; however, no information was provided on lactation or estrogen suppression of lactation.[38] Changes persisted beyond 2 months postpartum in only five women. Additional histologic studies of eight breast biopsies demonstrated findings similar to those described during pregnancy and lasting up to 2 months postpartum.

King and colleagues[24] also found increased cellularity associated with pregnancy. The occurrence of duct epithelial cells was compared in 136 samples, 68 from 34 pregnant women and 68 from 48 women who were not pregnant. From 1 to 80 groups of duct cells were found in 82 of the 136 individual samples. The total number of cells per group tended to be greater in pregnant and premenopausal nonpregnant women than in postmenopausal women. However, in comparing all the data from the three groups (using the Kolmogorov-Smirnov test), the only significant difference was between pregnant and postmenopausal patients. Recent studies of pregnancy effects were made on NAF from 27 women selected for equal distribution according to trimester and age. In this analysis, the cellularity was quite variable among women and trimesters; the mean cellularity was moderately increased compared with that of healthy women who were not pregnant (Table 4-4).

Breast fluid cytology during pregnancy and lactation reveals increased cellularity that is most marked in the late months of pregnancy and varies in the postpartum period. Increased numbers of duct epithelial cells in groups were reported by some to have changes like those associated with intraductal papilloma or papillary hyperplasia.[36-38] In addition, blood may be found in secretions from pregnant and lactating patients in the absence of clinically evident lesions.[37,38] These findings justify cautious interpretation of secretions from pregnant or lactating women.

Secretions Associated with Breast Disease

Nonspontaneous secretions or NAF display cellular patterns related to a variety of disease processes in the breast. Evaluation of duct fluid for screening or diagnostic purposes has met with varying degrees of success. Significant problems are caused by the limitations in sample availability and cellularity. Despite these considerations, cytologic abnormalities in NAF and nonspontaneous secretion have significant association with breast lesions of clinical and prognostic importance. The following discussions summarize the NAF patterns and histologic correlates for benign breast disease with and without increased risk for cancer and those associated with malignancy.

TABLE 4-4   Nipple Aspirate Fluid Availability in Pregnant and Nonpregnant Women

GROUP	CELLULARITY			AGE	
	NO. × 10³	MEAN	RANGE	MEAN	RANGE
First trimester	8	79.4	5.7-304	31	23-41
Second trimester	9	52.7	16.6-104	29	23-35
Third trimester	9	90.4	40.9-218	29	23-35
Nonpregnant	6	21.8	0.9-64	30	23-45

TABLE 4-5 Terminology and Criteria for Histologic Classification of Breast Disease in Tissue Sections

Nonproliferative lesions: Lesions such as adenosis, apocrine metaplasia, cysts, duct ectasia, fibroadenoma, inflammation, and squamous metaplasia

Hyperplasia (mild): Increase in layers of duct lining cells to three or four without cytologic atypia

Moderate hyperplasia: Multilayering of duct linings, sometimes papillary; bridging of duct lumen forming new irregular lumens; cellular and nuclear variability and minimal atypia

Atypical hyperplasia (ductal or lobular): Ductal changes appear more advanced than those of moderate hyperplasia; increasing monotony of the cell population suggestive of modal distribution; some, but not all, features of carcinoma in situ; *lobular* changes are increases in number of cells, expanding the ductule diameter but not completely filling the lumen

Carcinoma in situ (ductal or lobular): Ductal lesions may be subclassified as solid large cell, comedo, papillary, or cribriform; nuclear and cellular features of malignancy range from low to high grade; *lobular* lesions composed of monotonous population of small discohesive cells that completely fill and expand the ductules

BENIGN DISEASE WITHOUT INCREASED RISK FOR BREAST CANCER

Cytologic findings in NAF previously described as "normal" and those referred to as "hyperplasia" of minimal degree have no apparent association with increased risk for breast cancer. The histologic correlates are those defined in the Consensus Meeting article, "Is Fibrocystic Disease of the Breast Precancerous?"[39] Lesions not associated with increased risk for cancer were apocrine metaplasia, cyst, duct ectasia, fibroadenoma, fibrosis, mastitis, periductal mastitis, squamous metaplasia, and mild hyperplasia. Cytologic patterns in NAF are nonspecific and inadequate for definitive diagnosis of most benign lesions in this category. The histologic lesion referred to as *mild hyperplasia* is in concordance with changes of Welling's type ALA 1 or 2 and Black and Chabon's grade 2 lesions. It is described by the Consensus Meeting[39] as a lesion with three to four layers of cells without significant atypia lining breast ducts.[18,40-42] King and co-workers[40] note cytologic findings in NAF that correlate with this mild degree of hyperplasia (Tables 4-5 and 4-6; Figure 4-10).

Significant differences between cytologic findings in NAF from "normal" breasts and those with benign breast disease include increased average total cellularity and slightly greater prevalence of duct epithelial cells and groups of duct cells (Table 4-7). Apocrine metaplastic cells are also more likely to be seen in these samples. Proportionately, fewer foam cells are found in samples from women with cytologic abnormality or breast lesions (see Figure 4-9). Although there are distinct differences between "normal" samples and those associated with benign breast disease, the only cytologic features that correlate with specific lesions are those associated with hyperplasia and papilloma.

BENIGN DISEASE ASSOCIATED WITH INCREASED RISK FOR CANCER

Cytologic findings in NAF referred to as *moderate hyperplasia* or *atypical hyperplasia*, and in some studies grouped in one category called *atypical hyperplasia*, have shown a close association with histologic changes in these same categories. These histologic lesions are associated with increased risk for breast cancer.[39-44]

TABLE 4-6 Terminology and Criteria for Cytologic Classification of Nipple Aspirate Fluid, Secretion, or Discharge Samples

Benign, nonproliferative changes: Duct epithelial or apocrine metaplastic cells within normal limits

Hyperplasia (mild): Minimal cellular changes, slight cellular and nuclear enlargement; cell distribution predominantly in groups; papillary or apocrine metaplastic changes are subcategorized

Moderate hyperplasia: Moderate cellular changes; cell and nuclear enlargement disproportionate with N/C ratio increase; chromatin granularity becomes distinctive

Atypical hyperplasia: Cellular abnormalities are similar but more marked than with moderate hyperplasia; increased coarseness of chromatin; tendency for more single cells as well as groups of cells

Malignant cells: Single cells and groups of cells with unequivocal nuclear features of malignancy

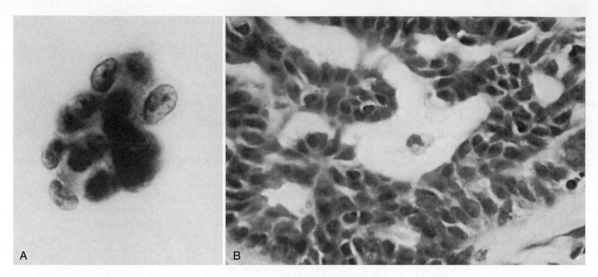

FIG. **4-10** **A,** Hyperplasia in nipple aspirate fluid represented here by a multilayered ball-like epithelial cell cluster with some nuclear enlargement and variability in size and staining (Papanicolaou stain; original magnification ×250). **B,** In mild hyperplasia, the duct lining cells are three or four layers in thickness and show some luminal bridging (hematoxylin and eosin stain; original magnification ×250).

Compared with similar women with no biopsy, the risk for breast cancer increased 1.5 to 2 times for those with moderate hyperplasia, and 5 times for those with atypical hyperplasia.[39] The histologic changes are defined in Table 4-5 and are illustrated in Figures 4-11 and 4-12. Also included in those with 1.5 to 2 times increased risk are women with papilloma with a fibrovascular core.

The significance of NAF cytology was evaluated by Petrakis and associates[44] in a preliminary follow-up study of women examined between 1972 and 1980. Among 5206 women without diagnosed breast cancer, there were 3194 (61%) with adequately cellular NAF. Atypical hyperplasia (moderate and atypical hyperplasia combined) was found in samples from 420 women (13%). Matching for age and race, follow-up data from 335 of these women were compared with findings from an equal number of women whose samples did not reflect atypical hyperplasia. Records of the San Francisco Bay Area Cancer Registry were used for the follow-up

8 to 15 years after the original NAF examination. During this period, breast cancer developed in 19 of the women with atypical hyperplasia and 6 of those without this cytologic abnormality ($p < .01$, chi-squared).

In 1988, Wrensch and colleagues[14] used a postal survey to contact 2701 of the women from the Petrakis study. They received replies from 2343 (87%) with 10 to 18 years of follow-up. Even the presence of nipple fluid was associated with increased risk for developing breast cancer. When compared with women from whom no fluid could be obtained, women with normal breast cytology were 1.8 times more likely to develop breast cancer (95%; confidence interval [CI] 0.9 to 3.9). Breast cancer was 2.5 times more likely to develop in women with hyperplasia (95%; CI 1.1 to 5.5) and 4.9 times as likely to develop in women with atypical hyperplasia (95%; CI 1.7 to 13.9; Figure 4-13). The relative risk for breast cancer was even higher when there was a family history of breast cancer. Most of this increased risk was in women 25 to 54 years old at the time NAF was studied. Risk for cancer did not significantly increase for the 547 women who were 55 years or older at the time NAF was studied.[14]

These findings were independently confirmed by extending the follow-up of the original study group ($n = 4046$) and an initial follow-up of a second group of women ($n = 3627$). The median years of follow-up for the original and the second group of women were 21 and 9 years, respectively. NAF with abnormal cytology was again found to be predictive of an increased risk for breast cancer.[45]

TABLE **4-7** Nipple Aspirate Fluid Cellularity in Benign Breast Disease		
	"NORMAL"* (×10³)	**BENIGN BREAST DISEASE** (×10³)
Average cellularity	6.2 ± 6.5	24.9 ± 13.1
Average number of duct cell groups per sample	4.2 ± 1.5	10.8 ± 3.2
Single duct cells	3.1 ± 1.7	10.5 ± 7.5

*Asymptomatic.

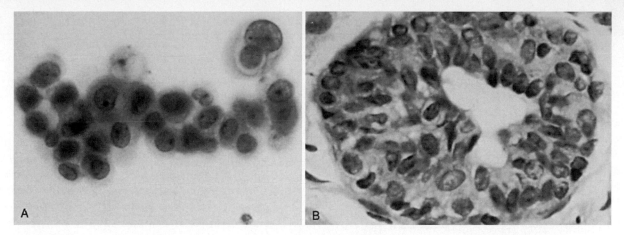

FIG. **4-11** **A,** Moderate hyperplasia depicted in a group of cells that have some enlargement of nuclei as well as variability in nuclear and cell sizes. The granularity is both fine and coarse, and nucleoli are evident in some (Papanicolaou stain; original magnification ×250). **B,** The tissue section has similar cytologic changes evident in the moderately hyperplastic ductal lining (hematoxylin and eosin stain; original magnification ×250).

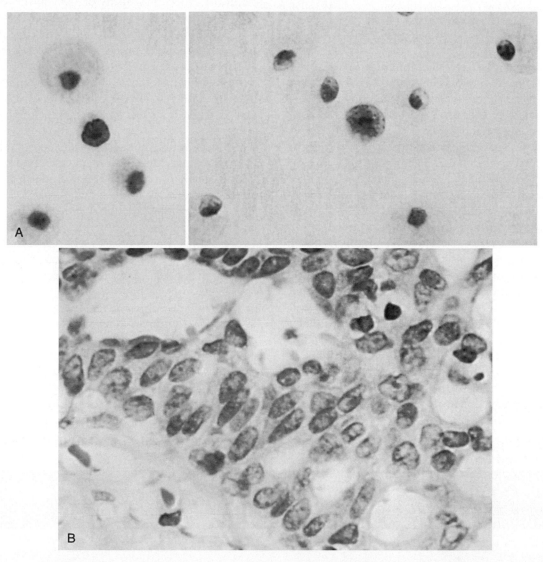

FIG. **4-12** **A,** Atypical hyperplasia shown here in single cells in nipple aspirate fluid samples. They are distinguished by disproportionate nuclear enlargement, irregular chromatinic membranes, and distinct granularity or hyperchromasia of chromatin (Papanicolaou stain; original magnification ×250). **B,** Atypical hyperplasia in tissue section with similar disproportionate nuclear/cytoplasmic ratio and somewhat monotonous cell population (hematoxylin and eosin stain; original magnification ×250).

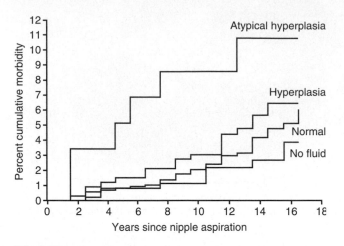

FIG. **4-13** The occurrence of breast cancer in relation to the findings on cytology of nipple aspiration fluid. *(From Wrensch MR et al: Am J Epidemiol 135:130, 1992.)*

The increased risk for subsequent breast cancer associated with the cytologic abnormality referred to as *atypical hyperplasia* appears similar to that found by Page and associates (see Chapter 7) in breast tissue lesions defined as moderate and atypical hyperplasia.[44]

NAF samples from moderate and atypical hyperplasia exhibit duct epithelial cells in cohesive groupings of nonpapillary or papillary pattern as well as isolated duct epithelial cells; however, they make up a very small proportion of cells in a sample. The individual cells within groups and isolated cells also show increasing degrees of nuclear enlargement, altered N/C ratio, and nuclear hyperchromasia. Nucleoli may be obscured or distinct and sometimes are enlarged. As the cytologic features become more monotonous and present a modal pattern, there also tends to be a loss of cohesiveness and an increase in single cells and smaller, loosely arranged groups. Calcific material or typical psammoma bodies have been found in central portions of cell clusters or within the cell cytoplasm.[46] The most significant changes that determine classification of moderate and atypical hyperplasia are in the nuclear and chromatin

structure. In correlating the NAF cytology findings with *benign breast biopsies*, 54% of those biopsies with histologic lesions of atypical hyperplasia also had cytologic findings of atypical hyperplasia (Table 4-8).[40]

Although there is a significant relationship of atypical hyperplasia with NAF and the subsequent changes in tissue, it is apparent that NAF cytology does not have sufficient predictive value to be useful for screening or diagnostic purposes. However, the NAF collection technique is simple and noninvasive and the results do warrant consideration for use as an adjunct to other procedures for evaluation of the breast and in the context of risk factor assessment.

Biochemical and cytologic findings in NAF are associated with atypical hyperplasia and increased risk for breast cancer. In a study of 135 control women and 68 women with benign breast disease, Wrensch and associates[47] found that cholesterol and its β epoxide in NAF increased in women with a first-degree relative with breast cancer. In that study, benign breast disease was classified histologically by the most marked ductal lobular epithelial abnormality. Increased cholesterol and β epoxide levels were significantly associated with proliferative breast disease. Progressively increasing concentrations of these substances were found with increasing degrees of histologic abnormalities. As already noted, the color of breast fluid is a good indicator of biochemical composition. Dark colors such as green and brown are associated with high cholesterol, cholesterol epoxides, and estrone and estradiol. Observations of dark breast fluid can be considered in combination with other factors in assessing the risk for atypical hyperplasia and breast cancer.

Proteins in NAF have also been studied. Mori and colleagues[48] measured carcinoembryonic antigen (CEA) using a dot-immunobinding assay that responds differentially to specific ranges of CEA concentration. Higher CEA concentrations (400 to 1000 ng/ml) were more common in NAF from women with breast cancer; however, high levels also occurred in some women without breast cancer.[48] Kawamoto[49] found that the

TABLE **4-8** Nipple Aspirate Fluid Cytology Related to Histologic Diagnosis in Breasts in the Presence and Absence of APD

| | HISTOLOGIC CLASSIFICATION | | | |
| | BENIGN (%) | | MALIGNANT (%) | |
CYTOLOGIC CLASSIFICATION	APD (n = 39)	NO APD (n = 60)	APD (n = 27)	NO APD (n = 7)
Benign	20.5	59.0	22.2	28.6
Hyperplasia	25.6	16.4	7.4	14.3
Atypical hyperplasia*	53.9	24.6	70.4	57.1

APD, Atypical proliferative disease.
*APD and atypical hyperplasia refer to moderate hyperplasia and atypical hyperplasia classifications combined.

lactic dehydrogenase isoenzyme five (LDH_5) is more common in NAF from women with breast cancer. LDH_5 is associated with anaerobic metabolism, and Kawamoto observed that malignant cells are thought to depend on anaerobic metabolism.[49]

BENIGN DISEASE WITH UNKNOWN RISK FOR CANCER

Referring again to histologic risk categories for benign breast disease as described by the Consensus Meeting,[39] two benign lesions—radial scar and lactiferous sinus solitary papilloma—were not included in risk categories because of insufficient data. Papilloma with a fibrovascular core was associated with a slightly increased risk for carcinoma compared with women with no breast biopsy.

Radial scar may have varying degrees of atypical proliferative change in the ductal epithelium. NAF cytologic findings in association with this lesion have not yet been evaluated.

The NAF cytology of papillary lesions is sufficiently distinctive to warrant further comment. In a study of 1309 asymptomatic women, Jackson and associates[6] obtained breast secretions that were diagnostic of a papillary lesion in 160 women. Intraductal or intracystic papilloma was confirmed in breast tissue examinations. It was noted that 46% were detected with cytologic examination as the initial finding. A complete description of cytologic findings associated with papilloma was provided by Papanicolaou and associates.[8] It is based on a study of 73 cases with histologic diagnosis of papilloma or papillomatosis. Only two of the papillomas were found in asymptomatic women from whom breast secretion was obtained with a breast pump. The remainder had a mass or nipple discharge. In 48% of the 73 cases, the diagnosis of papilloma was suggested by cytology. Most characteristic was the finding of many large groups of epithelial cells. The groups were long and branching and occasionally had a fibrovascular core. Borders of the groups tended to be scalloped, and cells sometimes cupped around each other. Although cytoplasm was homogeneous, vacuolization was not uncommon. Nuclei were small and hyperchromatic—rarely "active" and undergoing mitosis. Occasionally the cells were binucleate or multinucleate. A background of blood, macrophages, and foam cells was typical. The authors emphasized that similar findings in secretions during pregnancy and postpartum did not have the same diagnostic significance and should not be relied on for diagnosis of papilloma.

In our study of women with papilloma, the cytologic findings in NAF were correlated with histologic and clinical findings in 110 cases. The diagnosis of papilloma was suggested on cytology in 60% of these cases. In 32%

there was bloody discharge and/or an impression of papilloma based on the clinical findings. Distinctive papillary groupings were noted in 91% and heavy or moderate cellularity in 89% of cases. Blood was present in 64% of cases. Papillary groupings of duct epithelial cells with an identifiable fibrous or hyaline stalk were the most distinctive diagnostic finding. Other papillary groups of cells, apocrine metaplastic cells, foam cells along with hemosiderin-laden macrophages, and red blood cells are a frequent cellular accompaniment. Often, the cytologic findings represent only a few of these components and, although not entirely diagnostic of the lesion, can be correlated with the clinical presentation.

CARCINOMA IN SITU AND INVASIVE CARCINOMA

The cytologic patterns of malignancy in breast secretions are interpreted in terms of the anticipated histologic patterns to the extent that this is possible. The two major categories of breast carcinoma are ductal and lobular. These terms are applied to histologic and cytologic patterns and not necessarily to the anatomic site of origin. The tumors may be in situ or invasive. Subclassification of these main categories depends on variations in histologic pattern and cytologic differentiation. Terms applied to the subclassifications include *tubular, alveolar, signet-ring cell, medullary, mucoid,* and *papillary (cribriform)*. Paget's disease of the nipple is readily accessible for cytologic sampling and presents with or without clinical carcinoma of the breast. See Chapters 11 to 13 for complete descriptions of the histologic patterns of breast carcinoma.

Papanicolaou and associates[8] described and analyzed in detail the cytologic findings and their significance in breast secretions from 171 (18.5%) of 917 asymptomatic women. They concluded that, despite its limitations, cytology of breast secretions was valuable in differential diagnosis of mammary diseases and carcinoma. The sensitivity and specificity of the cytologic findings in benign breast disease were not mentioned; however, a cytologic diagnosis of malignancy was highly reliable. The criteria for diagnosis of malignant cells were based primarily on nuclear abnormalities. In secretions from 613 breasts of 438 asymptomatic women, one unsuspected carcinoma in situ was found. In 510 symptomatic women, 27 (60%) of 45 subsequently proven carcinomas were diagnosed on cytologic examination and there were no false-positive diagnoses. The differences in cytologic pattern associated with various types of mammary carcinoma are clearly described and illustrated. The generally recognized criteria of malignancy characterized the cells, and they were found either isolated or in small clusters. In groups of cells, the nuclei were often crowded and overlapped. Difficulty in identifying the malignant cells was sometimes associated with a background of predominantly inflammatory cells or of red blood cells and blood pigment.

The introduction of a more effective method for breast fluid collection from asymptomatic women led to recent reports on the cytology of NAF.[3,20] Cytologic patterns of carcinoma in NAF are described in limited terms by Sartorius and colleagues.[3] They reported seven carcinomas detected in cytology of NAF samples from asymptomatic women. An additional 11 women had cytologic evidence of carcinoma in the NAF; however, their results were also positive by palpation or mammography.

Cytologic diagnosis of malignancy in NAF samples examined by King and co-workers[40] was positive in only 20.6% of cases. When malignant cells are present, they are associated with a highly cellular sample compared with samples from breasts with benign diseases and from normal breasts.[50] Cells are distributed in small, loosely cohesive clusters, and there are increased numbers of isolated cells. The size of the cells and nuclei depends on the histologic lesion from which they are derived; however, diagnostic features representative of specific histologic patterns have not been identified because of the limited number of cases available for evaluation in this material. Nuclei show the chromatin changes generally considered representative of malignancy: hyperchromasia, coarse granularity, and condensation at the chromatinic membrane. A nucleolus is usually present and may be large, or there may be more than one. Cytoplasm varies in amount, is usually blue-green, and may contain vacuoles. N/C ratio is often altered because of disproportionate nuclear enlargement. The background findings are a disproportionate increase in histiocytes compared with foam cells; lymphocytes, neutrophils, red blood cells,

and protein precipitate are also part of the diathesis (Figure 4-14).

The low yield of positive cytologic diagnoses in NAF samples appears to be related to the unusual histopathology in this consecutive series of breast carcinomas. The selection was based on NAF sample availability and adequacy (defined as ≥10 duct epithelial cells). In this series, 26.6% of the lesions were carcinoma in situ. Nipple duct involvement within 1 cm of the surface of the nipple is infrequent (8%) in such tumors with an extent of less than 2.5 cm.[51] The better results in other series, some including symptomatic women, correspond with a higher frequency (50%) of nipple duct involvement within 1 cm of the surface associated with invasive lesions.

NAF samples are valuable in identifying the cytologic patterns associated with atypical hyperplasia in the presence of breast cancer. Atypical hyperplasia is much more prevalent in association with breast carcinoma and is uncommon in the absence of carcinoma (see Table 4-8).

Abnormal NAF cytology is predictive of increased risk for breast cancer. Assessment of breast cancer risk should include consideration of NAF evaluation despite limitations regarding fluid availability and cellularity. The NAF collection procedure is simple, easy to perform, and noninvasive.

Cytology of Ductal Lavage Fluid. Microcatheters have been developed for collection of epithelial cells from breast duct linings and for evaluating breast ducts radiographically using contrast media. Dooley and colleagues[52] have described excellent cellular samples using a saline lavage technique. They enrolled 507 women in a comparison study of NAF and DLF and found the lavage procedure to be safe and well

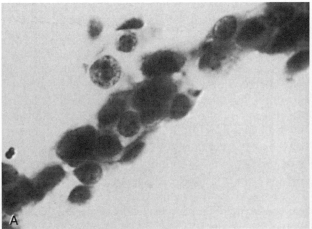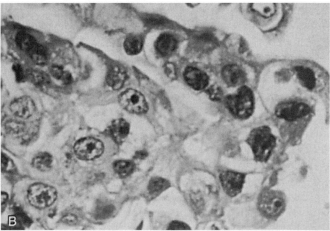

FIG. **4-14** **A,** Malignant cells in a group from a nipple aspirate fluid (NAF) sample exhibit nuclear hyperchromasia, coarse granularity, and irregularity in configuration (Papanicolaou stain; original magnification ×250). **B,** Cytologic features of ductal carcinoma are similar to those in the NAF sample (hematoxylin and eosin stain; original magnification ×250).

tolerated. Moreover, a median of 13,500 epithelial cells (range, 43,000 to 492,000 cells) was collected in DLF samples compared with a median of 120 epithelial cells (range, 10 to 74,300) in NAF samples. NAF was performed initially and DLF procedure was then carried out individually on each fluid-yielding duct. DLF samples displayed both increased cellularity and more frequent abnormal cells compared with NAF. Abnormal epithelial cells were found 3.2 times more often in DLF than in NAF. The increased number of cells in the DLF included both well-preserved isolated cells and groups of cells representing fragments of duct lining architectural features. The DLF sample is a valuable adjunct to NAF in assessing breast cancer risk.[52]

Spontaneous Nipple Discharge Associated with Breast Disease

Nipple discharge has been reported in 10% to 15% of women with benign breast disease and in 2.5% to 3% of those with carcinoma.[53,54] The discharge is often classified according to its appearance as milky, green, brown, bloody, serous, cloudy, or purulent. The significance of bloody discharge is its association with intraductal papilloma and other papillary lesions or carcinoma; however, it is also commonly found in the absence of such lesions. In a review of 386 nipple discharges without associated mass, 177 (46%) were bloody. Of patients with benign disease, 38% had bloody discharge, compared with 69% among women with carcinoma. Kilgore and associates[55] classify serous or bloody discharge as *pathologic* and discharge with evidence of secretory products as *physiologic*. Funderburk and Syphax[56] found serous or bloody fluid in 63% (106 of 167) and milky, colored, or clear fluid in 37% (61 of 167) of samples. The serous or bloody fluids were associated with carcinoma, papilloma, or other papillary lesions in 74% (78 of 106); fibrocystic change in 22%; and duct ectasia, drugs, and other conditions in 4% of samples. The majority (94%) of fluids with secretory components were associated with fibrocystic change and other nonproliferative

breast lesions; only 6% (4 of 61) were associated with papilloma. These findings are similar to those of other investigators.

The clinical significance of nipple discharge and appropriate management choices become most important when there is no palpable mass. Kilgore and colleagues[55] found 35% of carcinoma associated with nipple discharge that had no palpable mass, whereas Funderburk and Syphax[56] noted 82% of nipple discharge without palpable mass.

The cytologic diagnosis of nipple discharge samples has been most successful in association with breast cancer, Paget's disease of the nipple, and benign papilloma or papillary disease. Some examples of diagnostic results with nipple discharge appear in Table 4-9.[8,27,56-58] Uei and associates[58] analyzed the cytomorphology in NAF from both benign and malignant lesions. They noted some distinctive features in the structure of cell groups that improved the accuracy of diagnosis of breast cancer (41% to 66.3%) but also increased the false-positive interpretations from 0.9% to 3.6% (see Figure 4-14). The cellular characteristics associated with breast carcinoma are the same as those described for cytology of nonspontaneous nipple secretions. Of interest is the finding of a disproportionate number of cases of ductal carcinoma in situ and the unusual papillary carcinoma in the presence of malignant nipple discharge.[8,40,56]

Papilloma was diagnosed cytologically by Papanicolaou and associates[8] in 79% (34 of 43) of cases and was confirmed on tissue biopsy. Others have reported similar success with the cytologic diagnosis of intraductal papilloma.[55]

In a consecutive series of 212 nipple discharge samples, we encountered three (1.4%) with malignant cells (Figure 4-15). Follow-up of these three revealed infiltrating ductal carcinoma. In one of the three, the discharge occurring on a single occasion was the only clinical finding and the mammogram was unremarkable. Ductography was not performed; however, intraductal carcinoma was located by obtaining a biopsy at a depth of 1.0 to 1.5 cm below the nipple.

TABLE 4-9 Reported Results with Cytologic Examination of Nipple Discharge

AUTHOR	YEAR	NO.	WITH CA	POSITIVE CYTOLOGY NO.	(%)	FALSE-POSITIVE CYTOLOGY NO.	(%)
Papanicolaou[8]	1958	495	45	45	(60)	3	(1)
Kjellgren[57]	1964	216	25	21	(89)	15	(8)
Masukawa[27]	1966	94	16	6	(43)	1	(1)
Funderburk[56]	1969	182	7	6	(86)	—	—
Uei[58]	1980	190	80	53	(66)	4	(4)

The initial biopsy revealed borderline atypical hyperplasia and ductal carcinoma in situ. Node sampling revealed metastatic disease, and subsequent mastectomy provided evidence of microinvasive ductal carcinoma. A second case was similar in that the patient had no palpable mass and the lesion was located within 1 cm of the nipple surface. Thus, in two of the three patients with carcinoma, there was neoplastic involvement of a major duct at the nipple base, and in the remaining case, malignant cells were found freefloating in a duct within routine sections of the nipple (see Figure 4-15).

Hou and colleagues[59] reported an improvement in results with cytology of single duct discharge in absence of a mass when they used an intraductal aspiration method. Adequate samples were obtained from 96.6% (141 of 146 women) with intraductal aspiration compared with 76% collected by the conventional method using pressure. Among 27 cancers in the series, 24 (88.9%) were correctly diagnosed with the aspiration

sample compared with 9 (33.3%) using the conventional method.

These cases illustrate the clinical usefulness of cytology for evaluation of spontaneous nipple discharge in the absence of a palpable mass or significant mammographic findings. Cytology is indicated when the discharge is bloody or serous and there is no clinically evident mass.

Clinical Evaluation and Management of the Patient with Nipple Discharge

Localization of the source of the discharge, followed by biopsy of that source to diagnose/rule out cancer, is *the* principle for clinical care of nipple discharge. Reliability of nonsurgical approaches is not yet established.

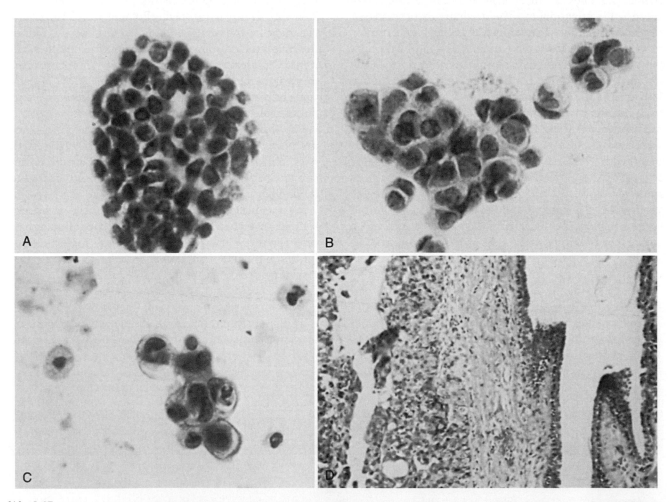

FIG. **4-15** Cellular features of malignancy in nipple discharge. **A,** Spherical multilayered group of malignant cells. **B,** Slightly discohesive sheet of malignant cells with prominent nuclear molding. **C,** Cluster of malignant cells with cellular detritus in the background. (**A** to **C,** Papanicolaou stain; original magnification ×250). **D,** Major duct involvement by tumor at base of nipple and adjacent uninvolved duct (hematoxylin and eosin stain; original magnification ×40).

Spontaneous nipple discharge is the chief complaint in 3% to 6% of women coming to breast specialty services. However, nipple discharge is often ignored. Newman and co-workers[60] found spontaneous discharge in 10% of 2685 women seen for routine examination. Cancer rarely presents as an *isolated* discharge: Chaudary and associates[61] reported that only 16 of 2476 cancers presented with isolated discharge; in our series of 516 cancers, less than 1% presented with discharge; Devitt,[62] however, reported discharge *associated* with 2% of all breast cancers.

ETIOLOGY

The majority of nipple discharges are caused by benign conditions; malignancy is found in only a small percentage. Benign papillomas and duct ectasia are more common in young women, and cancer is more common in older women (Figure 4-16).[63]

Ectasia is a dilation of ducts with loss of elastin in duct walls and chronic inflammatory cells, especially plasma cells, around duct walls. Theories of causation range from transudation of secretions sequestered in ducts dilated from previous pregnancy to primary periductal inflammation. Up to 60% of nipple discharges in duct ectasia contain bacteria (*Enterococcus*, anaerobic *Streptococcus*, *Staphylococcus aureus*, and *Bacteroides*), but whether infection is the primary cause or a secondary supercontamination is unknown.[64] Duct ectasia does not indicate predisposition to cancer.

Papillomas are benign epithelial lesions, with supporting stroma, growing within ducts, independent of the walls. Most common is solitary intraductal papilloma located in the major ducts near the nipple. A single papilloma is rarely associated with cancer.

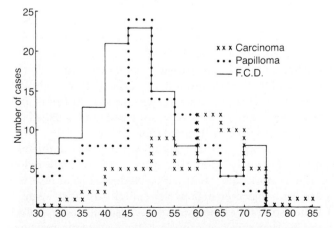

FIG. **4-16** Age distribution of patients with nipple discharge. Cancer is much more common in women older than 50 years. *F.C.D.*, Fibrocystic disease. *(From Murad TM et al: Ann Surg 195:259, 1982.)*

Less common are peripheral papillomas. Ohuchi and colleagues[65] reported that 6 of 25 patients with multiple peripheral papillomas had associated ductal carcinoma in situ. It has been suggested that peripheral papillomas are uncommon because they are an intermediate step in the formation of invasive cancer and often progress to cancer before they are diagnosed.[63]

Papillary-type lesions are also seen at the confluence of major ducts late in pregnancy and the early postpartum period and probably account for the bloody secretions sometimes seen during pregnancy.[38] They have no association with cancer.

Nipple discharge can be associated with cancer, although most such cases have an abnormality on physical examination or mammography. Occult carcinoma presenting with discharge is usually ductal carcinoma in situ or papillary carcinoma. In the presence of microinvasion, discharge is less common.[66] Drugs and hormonal disorders are rare causes of discharge but should be considered.

HISTORY

The most important point in the history is whether the discharge is spontaneous or elicited. Evaluation is required only if a discharge occurs in the absence of breast manipulation. For example, evaluation is required when a discharge makes a spot on a patient's clothes. Although literature from various cancer societies stresses that discharge may be a sign of cancer, one or more drops of liquid can be expressed from about half of women during their reproductive years and elicited-only discharge does not require further evaluation.

Breast discharge can be a response to a variety of stimuli other than underlying breast disease. Disordered hormone production as with anovulatory syndromes[67] may induce pathophysiologic responses in the breast.

Prolactinemia from pituitary adenoma may cause nipple discharge. It has been reported in up to 47% of cases in some series, but the 2.2% reported by Newman's group is probably more representative of the frequency of prolactin tumors in patients with discharge.[60] Normal serum prolactin levels are 20 µg/ml. If values are repeatedly elevated, thin-section computed tomography of the sella turcica is indicated. Patients with only moderate elevation often have normal radiologic results, but they should be followed closely. With advanced prolactin tumors, patients may show visual field loss or may have a history of infertility.

Because the breast is "a gland without feedback mechanisms, prolonged secretory response may follow short, often unrecognized surges in circulating prolactin."[65] These transient rises in prolactin may explain the nipple discharge in situations such as breast stimulation (especially sucking at the nipple), chest trauma, or after thoracotomy.

Large doses of tranquilizers (e.g., phenothiazines, reserpine, methyldopa) can induce lactation. Hooper and colleagues[68] noted galactorrhea in 24 of 100 psychiatric inpatients; 23 of the 24 were taking major tranquilizers. Lactation ceases after the drug is discontinued and may not return with smaller doses.[67] Inquiries should be made regarding possible industrial or agricultural exposure to estrogens.[69]

EXAMINATION

Examination should seek the duct or ducts producing the discharge, its color and nature, and other signs of breast pathology. The number of ducts producing discharge is almost as useful a guide as spontaneous discharge. Discharges from multiple ducts are rarely malignant, whereas single-duct discharge indicates a genuine risk for malignancy. Ciatto and co-workers[70] report that single-duct discharge has a relative risk of 4.07 (CI 2.7 to 6) of malignancy compared with an asymptomatic population, whereas multicentric or bilateral discharges have risks similar to those of the general population. Murad and colleagues[63] report that none of their patients with cancer had bilateral discharges.

Leis and associates[71] describe four types of discharge—serous, serosanguineous, sanguineous, and watery—that in ascending frequency (6.3%, 11.9%, 24.0%, and 45.5%, respectively) are more likely to be associated with cancer. However, although only 24% of bloody discharges were from cancer, clear discharge was so uncommon that 45% of all of their cancers did have a bloody discharge.

Chaudary's group[61] tested for heme with laboratory test sticks (as used for urine dip testing). Test sticks detect as few as 5 to 15 red blood cells per milliliter, which would not be visible as bloody fluid. All 16 patients with cancer had hemoglobin in nipple secretions; however, positive predictive value is low because 107 of 132 intraductal papillomas and 67 of 94 duct ectasias also had hemoglobin in the discharge. Blood is also present in nipple secretions from up to 20% of women during normal pregnancy.[37,72]

Single-duct discharges typically have a trigger point on the breast where pressure induces a discharge. This trigger point should be identified before planning surgery (see later discussion). The patient is examined in a standard position, preferably supine with the ipsilateral hand behind the head. Direct pressure is then applied at sequential points around the areola until the point where pressure causes the maximum discharge is found. It is useful to confirm this point on a separate examination before surgery.

Clinical breast examination is important because discharge with cancer often has a mass. Devitt[62] found in his series of patients with discharge that 8 of 10 women with cancer had palpable masses; 1 patient had nipple distortion but no mass. Leis and colleagues[71] report palpable masses in 88.1% of 67 patients with nipple discharge and cancer. However, discharge with mass is still more likely to be benign. Florio and colleagues[73] report cancer in only 10% of women with discharge and a mass; and King and colleagues[74] report cancer in only three of 11 women with discharge and an abnormal mammogram.

ROUTINE STUDIES

Mammography should be ordered for all patients with nipple discharge to seek a focal lesion and/or to estimate the extent of the abnormality if examination found a mass.

Exfoliative cytologic examination (examination of NAF discussed earlier) is useful when it shows cancer or abnormal cytology. However, the high false-negative rate precludes using NAF cytology to exclude cancer.

Carty and co-workers[75] proposed use of a "triple" test for evaluation of nipple discharge, similar to the triple test used with FNA cytology of palpable masses. They do not perform biopsy if clinical examination, mammography, and NAF cytologic examination are benign. In a series of 56 women, 17 required biopsy using these criteria and 5 had malignancy. The authors followed 38 of the other 39 women for a minimum of 5 years, with no further breast disease. Only 17 had nipple discharge on follow-up.

Diagnostic Tests Based on Duct Access Via the Nipple

The nipple can provide access to breast ducts for contrast injection, visualization, or lavage. Technical issues common to the three techniques are anesthesia and duct cannulation. Topical anesthetic agents, such as a cream with 2.5% lidocaine and 2.5% prilocaine (EMLA), anesthetize the nipple in 45 to 60 minutes. Judicious injection of local anesthesia near the base of the nipple also works (taking care not to cause distortion or hemorrhage in the nipple). Duct cannulation is achieved with recognition that the duct in the base of the nipple is tortuous and must be alternately gently stretched and pushed to allow passage of instrumentation.

Galactography (or ductography) involves cannulation of a previously identified duct with a small nylon catheter or needle (often with a 90-degree bend near the tip) and injection of a water-soluble contrast agent.[76] Water solubility is important because oil-based contact can be damaging or cause a serious systemic reaction; 0.10 to 1.5 ml is injected. Pain or discomfort marks the absolute time to cease injection. Mammograms are made immediately while the contrast material is in the breast.

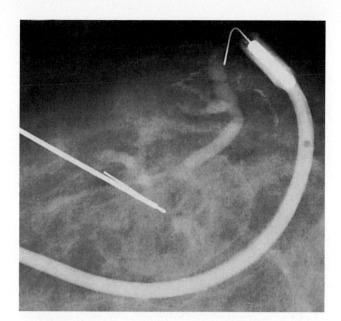

FIG. **4-17** Galactography combined with wire localization biopsy. The duct has an abrupt cutoff at the site of the lesion. The guide wire was placed while contrast media was within the duct. The contrast was not present at the time of the biopsy and could not be seen on the specimen radiograph. The lesion was a benign papilloma. *(Courtesy Edward A. Sickles, M.D.)*

Woods and colleagues[77] supplemented galactography with wire localization. A localization wire is placed while the contrast is still in the duct. Because water-soluble contrast medium does not usually persist in the duct, the specimen radiogram does not usually show any abnormality (i.e., there is no intraoperative means to verify removal of the correct tissue; Figure 4-17).

Tabar and associates[76] reported that 18 of 18 women with cancer were identified by galactography but that only half of them had a mass lesion on routine mammograms. Burni and de Guili,[78] however, report only 79% accuracy, based on patients who went on to surgical biopsy after galactography.

Dinkel and colleagues[79] support the latter view that galactography should be used primarily to estimate the extent of a lesion rather than to presume to rule out cancer. They correlated preoperative galactography with pathology for 143 duct excisions, which included 11 women with cancer. Most commonly, cancer caused a filling defect or cutoff on galactography; but still only 6 of 90 cases with filling defects had cancer. Two cancers caused duct compression, and one was associated with duct ectasia. Most important, 2 of 11 cancers had normal galactography.

Others have combined cytologic examination and galactography to select patients for biopsy.[73,80,81] They confirm that combined abnormal cytology results and abnormal galactography results indicate a high likelihood of either malignancy or a papilloma. However,

they provide minimal information on patients followed without biopsy.

Tiny fiberoptic scopes have made duct visualization possible.[82,83] With appropriate anesthesia, sequentially larger lacrimal duct probes are used to dilate the duct that produces the discharge. A tiny scope is introduced into the dilated nipple orifice, manipulated through the tortuous section of the duct in the nipple, and advanced into the ducts. As with other endoscopy techniques, fluid is gently introduced through the scope as it is advanced. Newer scopes can be introduced through a plastic sleeve, which serves both as a dilator and to provide access to obtain washings. In a darkened room, the light of the scope can be seen through breast tissue. If a point of interest is identified, the skin can be marked over the spot of light to guide subsequent biopsy. The role of this technique in diagnosis of discharge and other lesions is under active investigation.

Ductal lavage is a technique to improve cell retrieval and thereby improve on analysis of NAF.[52,59] Small amounts of fluid are washed into the duct using a catheter similar to that used for galactography. Fluid is collected as it drains; and cells are isolated and evaluated as for NAF.

DIAGNOSIS

Definitive diagnosis is based on biopsy that should first be directed to any area identified by physical examination, mammography, or other studies. If no specific lesion is identified, duct excision should be undertaken based on the pressure point described earlier.

Duct excision is an outpatient procedure done with the patient under local anesthesia, with or without sedation. Most patients can be made quite comfortable with conversation.

Long-acting anesthetic is infiltrated at the site of the proposed incision, under the areola, and around the nipple. Injection into the nipple is quite painful and unnecessary, because anesthetic will diffuse from surrounding tissue.

A circumareolar incision encompasses approximately 50% of the circumference of the areola, but not more lest the areolar skin by devascularized. The incision centers on the trigger point or the pathology located by galactography or other study. Meticulous hemostasis is maintained. Using small, blunt scissors (e.g., tenotomy scissors) allows gentle dissection, precludes large cuts, and reduces pain. The edge of the areola is elevated with a skin hook held with the thumb and two fingers of the nondominant hand while the ring finger of the same hand everts the skin of the areola to provide gentle tension.

There are three ways to find the duct: (1) Pass a small lacrimal duct probe through the skin opening

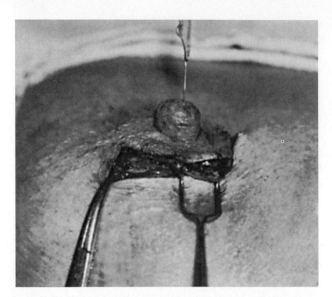

FIG. **4-18** Use of lacrimal duct probe to identify duct producing discharge. This procedure was performed using local anesthesia (see text). A small carcinoma was identified adjacent to the duct producing the discharge in this patient.

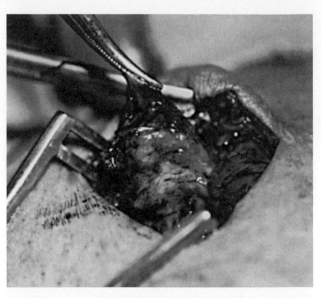

FIG. **4-20** Following separation of the duct from the nipple, gentle traction is maintained to identify the segment of breast to be removed. This procedure may be done with the patient under local anesthesia (see text).

(Figure 4-18), (2) identify the dilated duct by gentle dissection behind the nipple (Figure 4-19), and (3) inject the duct with methylene blue before making the skin incision. First, the duct is dissected superficially to the dermis of the nipple and removed, usually with a tiny fragment of skin. It is often useful to divide the duct under the nipple between hemostats to facilitate

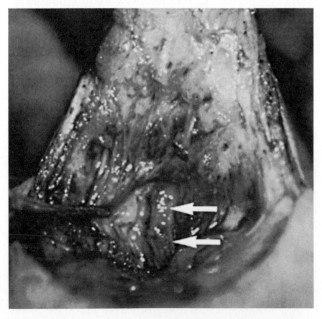

FIG. **4-19** Dilated duct is identified behind the nipple *(arrows)*. This procedure may be performed with the patient under local anesthesia (see text).

complete excision from within the nipple. Lesions may be found within the nipple.

Next, the duct leading deeper into the breast is grasped and, with gentle traction, dissected free from the breast with a small cone of surrounding tissue (Figure 4-20).[84] One duct usually identifies a specific segment of the breast that is denser than immediately adjacent tissue, often surrounded by either loose connective tissue or fatty tissue. The specimen increases in diameter as dissection extends into the breast. If a duct containing discharge is transected during dissection, it should be secured with a hemostat for later identification; after completion of the initial dissection, it should also be excised.

If methylene blue has been injected into the duct, all blue-stained areas are removed. Van Zee and colleagues[85] found that preoperative injection of dye facilitated excision. With methylene blue, they found pathology to explain the discharge in 100% of cases; without dye, they found pathology to account for only 67% of discharges.

In general, minimal local anesthesia is required for this part of the dissection *if* the surgeon uses minimal tension, small instruments that force slow progress and judiciously applies anesthetic to blood vessels.

Hemostasis must be meticulous. The outer edge of the breast gland tissue is approximated with small, absorbable sutures. A purse-string of absorbable suture is placed loosely under or behind the nipple to prevent inversion. Skin is then closed with subcuticular, absorbable suture and tape skin closures.

The patient is advised to wear her brassiere for support for 72 hours and to avoid vigorous activity during that time. To preserve platelet function, she is directed to avoid aspirin and nonsteroidal antiinflammatory drugs for 7 days before and after surgery.

PROGNOSIS

The prognosis after the diagnosis of nipple discharge seems good if cancer is not found in the initial evaluation. McPherson and Mackenzie[86] found recurrence of discharge in 5 of 72 patients between 2 weeks and 9 years after surgery. Cancer subsequently developed in 3 of the 72 patients, but 2 of the 3 lesions were in the contralateral breast and none of the 3 patients had recurrent discharge.

Sample Collection, Preparation, and Examination

An adequate sample for breast cytologic examination helps ensure good results with this method. The preparatory methods for breast cytologic examination include direct smears from spontaneous nipple discharge and membrane filtration of NAF samples. Cytologic examination needs to be systematic and thorough, and a classification system should use terminology related to the anticipated histopathology.

SAMPLE COLLECTION

Spontaneous nipple discharge is expressed directly onto the glass slide, which is held at the opening of the duct and moved across the drop of fluid and the surface of the nipple to make a thin spread. A specimen bottle of 95% ethanol should be held close to the breast so that the slide can be immediately placed in the fixative. It is suggested that four to six smears be prepared from each discharge, because the material is often more cellular in the last drops of fluid. If blood-tinged fluid is observed to be coming from one duct, its location should be noted and an attempt should be made to keep the sample from that duct separate from the remaining discharge. This can be accomplished by using a capillary pipette to collect the sample directly from the duct opening.[87]

NAF samples are collected using a suction cup device placed over the nipple and attached to a 10-ml syringe with a short length of plastic tubing (see Figure 4-3). Negative pressure to the cup over the nipple is achieved by withdrawing the plunger 5 to 6 ml and maintaining the pressure until fluid appears at the nipple or for 15 seconds. The amount of negative pressure achieved is 100 to 175 mm Hg, similar to the negative pressures developed by suckling infants.[15]

The steps in the NAF collection procedure are summarized as follows:

1. To remove any accumulated secretory material and exfoliated squamous cells from the nipple surface and duct openings, the nipple is first cleaned with a moist gauze or plastic sponge.
2. Then the nipple is soaked with Cerumenex (3%) to loosen plugs.
3. Subsequent gentle squeezing expresses the plugs, and the nipple is wiped dry.
4. Using suction combined with gentle hand pressure, the physician is able to obtain the nipple aspirate specimen. The suction device is placed over the nipple, and negative pressure is applied by withdrawing the plunger of the attached syringe. During aspiration, gentle hand pressure is applied to the breast, starting at the base and extending toward the nipple.
5. Generally, one or more beads of fluid appear on the surface of the nipple.
6. The specimen is then removed from the nipple into capillary tubes, suspended in 2 ml physiologic salt solution, and transported at once to the laboratory, or refrigerated when this is not possible.

or

7. If direct smears are to be prepared from the nipple, the patient should hold a bottle of fixative to one side of her breast. Smear the fluid lengthwise on a microscope slide and immerse *immediately* in the fixative.

The steps in the DLF collection procedure are as follows[52]:

1. DLF is collected immediately after NAF from all ducts yielding fluid on NAF.
2. Skin in the nipple area is cleaned with alcohol. A fenestrated sterile drape is placed over the nipple.
3. If necessary, ductal orifices are enlarged with dilators.
4. A separate microcatheter is used for each duct and each sample is labeled and identified on a 64-square nipple grid system as it is collected. The microcatheter is inserted 1.5 cm.
5. Sometimes a 2% lidocaine jelly is used on the microcatheter tip; a total of 1 to 3 ml 1% lidocaine without epinephrine is usually infused.
6. Approximately 2 to 6 ml normal saline is infused and is breast compressed to recover the fluid. This is repeated multiple times using a total of 10 ml normal saline per duct and recovering approximately 5 ml.

7. Each DLF sample is placed in a tube half filled with CytoLyt solution.

SAMPLE PREPARATION

Two important aspects of specimen preparation are concentration of cells and recovery of cells. *Cell concentration* refers to increasing the number of cells per unit volume or area. *Cell recovery* is the efficiency of collecting cells per unit volume of sample or the percentage of total cells in a sample. In NAF samples, cell recovery is especially important because of the scant cellularity. If concentration techniques lead to a differential loss of cells, the preparation method may interfere with the diagnostic value of the sample.

Direct smears require no special laboratory preparation other than appropriate staining with Papanicolaou stain or other stains preferred by the laboratory.

NAF samples are concentrated and recovered on membrane filters. Millipore filters are preferred because of the high rate of cell recovery (approximately 80% of cells per sample) and because of good-quality cytomorphology.[88] The following steps in membrane filtration are recommended to produce a filter of optimum quality with well-preserved cellular morphology:

1. Label the edge of a 46-mm Millipore filter (5-micron pore size) with a laundry ink pen and preexpand the filter for 10 seconds in 95% ethanol.
2. Assemble Millipore filtration apparatus using the glass base and a stainless steel screen.
3. Moisten screen and glass base with physiologic saline, allowing it to pool on the surface.
4. Place the preexpanded filter on the pooled saline.
5. Clamp on glass funnel and add 25 to 30 ml physiologic salt solution.
6. Adjust suction to a gentle drip.
7. Pour the entire well-mixed sample into the funnel. Allow filtration to proceed until the solution just covers the surface of the filter; never allow the filter to dry.
8. When the last saline product has been suctioned through the filter and a small amount of solution still covers the filter, add 95% ethanol. This ethanol should be added without disrupting the filter surface.
9. Discontinue suction and, adding more ethanol above the filter, allow the cells to fix for 2 minutes before completing the suctioning. Never let the filter dry.
10. Remove the filter and store in 95% ethanol until staining is done.

Precautions

1. Do not overload the filter. If filtration stops, immediately stop the vacuum and aspirate the remaining unfiltered specimen out of the funnel. Add 95% ethanol to the funnel, just covering the filter.
2. Never allow the filter to dry.
3. Bloody specimens can be treated with 50% ethanol after washing with physiologic salt solution and before fixation with 95% ethanol.

Staining of Millipore filter preparations can be accomplished by carrying the filter through the solutions on a clamp-style paper clip of a plastic filter holder. This method allows uniform diffusion of stains and solutions, providing consistently even staining. Filters should not be clipped to glass slides because uneven staining occurs.

Mounting Millipore filters requires special attention because of the thickness of the filter (130 ± 10 μm). Excess clearing solvent (xylene or toluene) should be removed before mounting by placing the filter, cell side up, on an absorbent paper towel. The filter must not be allowed to dry. Sufficient mounting medium (Permount, Fisher Permount, Fair Lawn, NJ; Eukitt, Electron Microscopy Sciences, Fort Washington, PA; or Kleermount, Carolina Biological Supply Co., Burlington, NC) should be spread evenly across a glass slide and the filter floated, cell side up, on the mounting medium. An additional drop of mounting fluid should be dropped on the filter surface before applying a no. 1 thickness coverslip.

CYTOLOGIC EXAMINATION

A complete and systematic examination of NAF, DLF, and breast discharge cytology by a cytotechnologist and pathologist with training and experience in this specialized area of cytopathology is required. Epithelial cells in NAF and breast discharge are often few and tend to be small; significant cells or groups of cells can easily be missed. Qualitative assessment is made of the cellular composition including types of cells and degree of cellularity. Cytologic evaluation is based on the changes in epithelial cells and accompanying cellular findings, and the final interpretation is considered in correlation with the clinical information.

Diagnostic terminology used for the cellular findings in NAF, DLF, and nipple discharge conforms to the expected lesion in subsequent biopsy. Morphologic terminology that is universally understood and consistent with standard nomenclature is preferred rather than systems that use numbers of nonspecific terms that are subject to a variety of interpretations.

Recommendation for further breast examination requires full knowledge of clinical information, and it should be emphasized that negative cytology does not exclude malignancy.

REFERENCES

1. Buehring GC: Screening for breast atypias using exfoliative cytology, *Cancer* 43:1788, 1979.
2. Petrakis NL, Mason L, Lee R: Association of race, age, menopausal status, and cerumen type with breast fluid secretion in nonlactating women, as determined by nipple aspiration, *J Natl Cancer Inst* 54:829, 1975.
3. Sartorius OW et al: Cytologic evaluation of breast fluid in the detection of breast disease, *J Natl Cancer Inst* 59:1073, 1977.
4. Wynder EL et al: Nipple aspirates of breast fluid and the epidemiology of breast disease, *Cancer* 56:1473, 1985.
5. Jackson D, Severance AO: Cytological study of nipple secretions: an aid in the diagnosis of breast lesions, *Tex State J Med* 41:512, 1946.
6. Jackson D, Todd DA, Gorsuch PL: Study of breast secretion for detection of intramammary pathologic change and of silent papilloma, *J Int Coll Surg* 15:552, 1951.
7. Papanicolaou GN et al: Cytologic evaluation of breast secretions, *Ann NY Acad Sci* 63:1409, 1956.
8. Papanicolaou GN et al: Exfoliative cytology of the human mammary gland and its value in the diagnosis of cancer and other diseases of the breast, *Cancer* 11:377, 1958.
9. Ringrose CA: The role of cytology in early detection of breast disease, *Acta Cytol* 10:373, 1966.
10. Bonser GM, Dossett SA, Jull SW: *Human and experimental breast cancer*, Springfield, IL, 1961, CC Thomas.
11. Keynes G: Chronic mastitis, *Br J Surg* 11:89, 1923.
12. Petrakis NL: Cerumen genetics and human breast cancer, *Science* 173:347, 1971.
13. Petrakis NL: Genetic cerumen type, breast secretory activity and breast cancer epidemiology. In Mulvihill JJ, Miller RW, Fraumeni JF Jr (eds): *Genetics of human cancer*, New York, 1977, Raven Press.
14. Wrensch MR et al: Breast cancer incidence in women with abnormal cytology in nipple aspirates of breast fluid, *Am J Epidemiol* 135:130, 1992.
15. Petrakis NL: Physiologic, biochemical, and cytologic aspects of nipple aspirate fluid, *Breast Cancer Res Treat* 8:7, 1986.
16. Petrakis NL et al: Influence of pregnancy and lactation on serum and breast fluid estrogen levels: implications for breast cancer risk, *Int J Cancer* 40:587, 1987.
17. Gruenke LD et al: Breast fluid cholesterol and cholesterol epoxides: relationship to breast cancer risk factors and other characteristics, *Cancer Res* 47:5483, 1987.
18. Bischoff F: Carcinogenic effects of steroids, *Adv Lipid Res* 7:165, 1969.
19. Kelsey MI, Pienta RJ: Transformation of hamster embryo cells by neutral sterols and bile acids, *Toxicol Lett* 9:177, 1981.
20. Kelsey MI, Pienta RJ: Transformation of hamster embryo cells by cholesterol-alpha-epoxide and lithocholic acid, *Cancer Lett* 6:143, 1979.
21. Parsons PG, Goss P: Chromosome damage and DNA repair induced in human fibroblasts by UV and cholesterol oxide, *Aust J Exp Biol Med Sci* 56:287, 1978.
22. Petrakis NL et al: Coloration of breast fluid related to concentration of cholesterol, cholesterol epoxides, estrogen and lipid peroxides, *Am J Clin Pathol* 89:117, 1988.
23. Donne A: *Die Milch und insbesondere die Milch der Ammen.* Weimar, 1838, Landes Industrie Komptoir.
24. King EB et al: Cellular composition of the nipple aspirate specimen of breast fluid: the benign cells, *Am J Clin Pathol* 64:728, 1975.
25. Ferguson DJP, Anderson TJ: Morphological evaluation of cell turnover in relation to the menstrual cycle in the "resting" human breast, *Br J Cancer* 44:177, 1981.
26. Masters JRW, Drife JO, Scarisbreck JJ: Cyclical variations of DNA synthesis in human breast epithelium, *J Natl Cancer Inst* 58:1263, 1977.
27. Masukawa T, Lewison EF, Frost JK: The cytologic examination of breast secretions, *Acta Cytol* 10:261, 1966.
28. Meyer JS: Cell proliferation in normal human breast ducts, fibroadenomas, and other duct hyperplasias, measured by nuclear labelling with tritiated thymidine: effects of menstrual phase, age, and oral contraceptive hormones, *Hum Pathol* 8:67, 1977.
29. Vogel PM et al: The correlation of histologic changes in the human breast with the menstrual cycle, *Am J Pathol* 104:23, 1981.
30. Longacre TA, Bartlow SA: A correlative morphologic study of human breast and endometrium in the menstrual cycle, *Am J Surg Pathol* 10:382, 1986.
31. Malberger E et al: Cellular changes in the mammary gland epithelium during the menstrual cycle: a computer image analysis study, *Acta Cytol* 31:305, 1987.
32. Dawson EK: A histological study of the normal mamma in relation to tumor growth, II: the mature gland in pregnancy and lactation, *Edinb Med J* 42:569, 1935.
33. Engels S: An investigation of the origin of the colostrum cells, *J Anat* 87:362, 1953.
34. Cole HA: The mammary gland of the mouse during the oestrous cycle, pregnancy and lactation, *Proc R Soc Lond B Biol Sci* 114:136, 1933.
35. Bloom W, Fawcett DW: *A textbook of histology*, ed 9, Philadelphia, 1968, WB Saunders.
36. Holmquist DG, Papanicolaou GN: The exfoliative cytology of the mammary gland during pregnancy and lactation, *Ann NY Acad Sci* 63:1422, 1956.
37. Kline TS, Lash SR: Nipple secretion in pregnancy: a cytologic and histologic study, *Am J Clin Pathol* 37:626, 1962.
38. Kline TS, Lash SR: The bleeding nipple of pregnancy and postpartum period: a cytologic and histologic study, *Acta Cytol* 8:336, 1964.
39. Consensus Meeting: Is "fibrocystic disease" of the breast precancerous? *Arch Pathol Lab Med* 110:171, 1986.
40. King EB et al: Nipple aspirate cytology for the study of breast cancer precursors, *J Natl Cancer Inst* 71:1115, 1983.
41. Rogers LW, Page DL: Epithelial proliferative disease of the breast: a marker of increased cancer risk in certain age groups, *Breast* 5:2, 1979.
42. Wellings SR, Jensen HM, Marcum RG: An atlas of subgross pathology of the human breast with special reference to possible precancerous lesions, *J Natl Cancer Inst* 55:231, 1975.
43. Black MM, Chabon AB: In situ carcinoma of the breast, *Pathol Annu* 4:185, 1969.
44. Petrakis NL et al: Prognostic significance of atypical epithelial hyperplasia in nipple aspirates of breast fluid, *Lancet* 2:505, 1987.
45. Wrensch MR et al: Breast cancer risk in women with abnormal cytology in nipple aspirates of breast fluid, *J Natl Cancer Inst* 93:1791, 2001.

46. Zimmerman AL, Barrett DL, Petrakis NL: The incidence and significance of intracytoplasmic calcifications in nipple aspirate specimens, *Acta Cytol* 21:685, 1977.

47. Wrensch MR et al: Breast fluid cholesterol and cholesterol beta-epoxide concentrations in women with benign breast disease, *Cancer Res* 49:2168, 1989.

48. Mori T et al: Evaluation an improved dot-immunobinding assay for carcinoembryonic antigen determination in nipple discharge in early breast cancer: results of a multicenter study, *Jpn J Clin Oncol* 22:371, 1992.

49. Kawamoto M: Breast cancer diagnosis by lactate dehydrogenase isozyme nipple discharge, *Cancer* 73:1836, 1994.

50. King EB et al: Cytopathology of abnormal mammary duct epithelium. In Nieburgs HE (ed): *Prevention and detection of cancer, part II, Detection*, vol 2, *Cancer detection in specific sites*, New York, 1976, Marcel Dekker.

51. Lagios MD, Westdahl PR, Rose MR: The concept and implications of multicentricity in breast carcinoma, *Pathol Annu* 16:83, 1981.

52. Dooley WC et al: Ductal lavage for detection of cellular atypia in women at high risk for breast cancer, *J Natl Cancer Inst* 93:1624, 2001.

53. Leis HP Jr, Dursi MD, Mersheimer WL: Nipple discharge: significance and treatment, *NY State J Med* 67:3105, 1967.

54. Urban JA, Egeli RA: Non-lactational nipple discharge, *CA Cancer J Clin* 28:130, 1978.

55. Kilgore AR, Fleming R, Ramos MM: The incidence of cancer with nipple discharge and the risk of cancer in the presence of papillary disease of the breast, *Surg Gynecol Obstet* 96:649, 1953.

56. Funderburk WW, Syphax B: Evaluation of nipple discharge in benign and malignant diseases, *Cancer* 24:1290, 1969.

57. Kjellgren O: The cytologic diagnosis of cancer of the breast, *Acta Cytol* 8:216, 1964.

58. Uei Y et al: Cytologic diagnosis of breast carcinoma with nipple discharge: special significance of the spherical cell cluster, *Acta Cytol* 24:522, 1980.

59. Hou M-F et al: A simple intraductal aspiration method for cytodiagnosis in nipple discharge, *Acta Cytologica* 44:1029, 2000.

60. Newman HF et al: Nipple discharge: frequency and pathogenesis in an ambulatory population, *NY State J Med* 83:928, 1983.

61. Chaudary MA et al: Nipple discharge: the diagnostic value of testing for occult blood, *Ann Surg* 196:651, 1982.

62. Devitt JE: Management of nipple discharge by clinical findings, *Am J Surg* 149:789, 1985.

63. Murad TM, Contesso G, Mouriesse H: Nipple discharge from the breast, *Ann Surg* 195:259, 1982.

64. Bundred NJ et al: Are the lesions of duct ectasia sterile? *Br J Surg* 72:844, 1985.

65. Ohuchi N, Abe R, Kasai M: Possible cancerous change of intraductal papillomas of the breast, *Cancer* 54:605, 1984.

66. Schuh ME et al: Intraductal carcinoma: analysis of presentation, pathologic findings, and outcome of disease, *Arch Surg* 121:1303, 1986.

67. Barnes AB: Diagnosis and treatment of abnormal breast secretions, *N Engl J Med* 275:1184, 1966.

68. Hooper JH, Welch VC, Shackelford RT: Abnormal lactation associated with tranquilizing drug therapy, *JAMA* 178:506, 1961.

69. Mills JL, Jeffreys JL, Stolley PD: Effects of occupational exposure to estrogen and progestogens and how to detect them, *J Occup Med* 26:269, 1984.

70. Ciatto S, Bravetti P, Cariaggi P: Significance of nipple discharge: clinical patterns in selection of cases for cytologic examination, *Acta Cytol* 30:17, 1986.

71. Leis HP et al: Breast biopsy and guidance for occult lesions, *Int Surg* 70:115, 1985.

72. Scott-Conner CEH, Schorr SJ: The diagnosis and management of breast problems during pregnancy and lactation, *Am J Surg* 170:401, 1995.

73. Florio MG et al: Surgical approach to nipple discharge: a ten-year experience, *J Surg Oncol* 71:235, 1999.

74. King TA et al: A simple approach to nipple discharge, *Am Surg* 66:960, 2000.

75. Carty NJ et al: Prospective study of outcome in women presenting with nipple discharge, *Ann Royal Coll Surg Engl* 76:387, 1994.

76. Tabar L, Dean PB, Penetek Z: Galactography: the diagnostic procedure of choice for nipple discharge, *Radiology* 149:31, 1983.

77. Woods ER et al: Solitary breast papilloma: comparison of mammographic galactographic, and pathologic findings, *AJR Am J Roentgenol* 159:487, 1992.

78. Berni D, de Guili E: The value of ductogalactography in the diagnosis of intraductal papilloma, *Tumori* 69:539, 1983.

79. Dinkel H-P et al: Predictive value of galactographic patterns for benign and malignant neoplasms of the breast for patients with nipple discharge, *Br J Radiol* 73:706, 2000.

80. Dinkel H-P et al: Galactography and exfoliative cytology in women with abnormal nipple discharge, *Obstet Gynecol* 97:625, 2001.

81. Ohuchi N, Furuta A, Mori S: Management of ductal carcinoma in situ with nipple discharge, *Cancer* 74:1294, 1994.

82. Dooley WC: Endoscopic visualization of breast tumors, *JAMA* 284:1518, 2000.

83. Shen K-W et al: Fiberoptic ductoscopy for patients with nipple discharge, *Cancer* 89:1512, 2000.

84. Jardines L: Management of nipple discharge, *Am Surg* 62:119, 1996.

85. Van Zee KJ et al: Preoperative galactography increases the yield of major duct excision for nipple discharge, *Cancer* 82:1874, 1998.

86. McPherson VA, Mackenzie WC: Lesions of the breast associated with nipple discharge: prognosis after local excision of benign lesions. *Can J Surg* 5:6, 1962.

87. Masukawa T: Improved cell collection technique in breast cytology, *Cytotech Bull* 7:4, 1970.

88. Barrett DL, King EB: Comparison of cellular recovery rates and morphological detail obtained using membrane filter and cytocentrifuge techniques, *Acta Cytol* 20:174, 1976.

III

BENIGN AND PREMALIGNANT LESIONS

5

Subareolar Breast Abscess: The Penultimate Stage of the Mammary Duct–Associated Inflammatory Disease Sequence

MICHAEL M. MEGUID

KARA C. KORT

PATRICIA J. NUMANN

ALBERT OLER

Chapter Outline

Historical Perspective and Terminology

The rational management of subareolar breast abscess, based on the understanding of its pathogenesis, has evolved over a long time. The vast array of terminology that has evolved over the years to describe both the clinical and histologic manifestations of this disease may have delayed an understanding of its pathogenesis. Terms such as *mastitis obliterans*,[1,2] *varicocele tumor of the breast*,[3] *periductal mastitis*,[4] *comedomastitis*,[5] *secretory cystic disease*,[6] *chronic pyogenic mastitis*,[7] and *plasma cell mastitis*[8] refer to the same disease process, each emphasizing a different perspective, and these, together with more recent terms, are summarized in Table 5-1.

Birkett, in 1850, described a "morbid condition of the lactiferous ducts" (see Table 5-1).[9] Bloodgood, in 1921, first documented the chronicity of this condition and its association with duct ectasia, blue-domed cyst, and periductal inflammation.[20] This disease was reported from different perspectives, based on clinical and microscopic observations (see Table 5-1). In 1951 two milestone reports unified this clinical entity. In the first, Zuska, Crile, and Ayres[14] emphasized the presence of a chronic, draining periareolar fistula associated with a breast abscess and proposed the pathogenesis to be (1) stasis of secretion in the duct, (2) dilation of lactiferous mammary duct, (3) ulceration of mammary duct epithelium with abscess formation, and (4) rupture of the abscess to form a draining sinus with a resulting fistula. They recommended excision of the tract with the involved "intranipple" portion of the duct. Their report established this to be a benign, noncancerous surgical condition that occurs frequently, is troublesome to both patient and surgeon, and is often mistaken for a recurrent primary inflammatory condition of the breast.[21,22]

The second report in 1951 was by Haagensen, who correlated clinical and pathophysiologic findings.[15] He proposed an evolutionary disease process and coined the descriptive term *mammary duct ectasia* for the benign condition of the breast characterized by dilation of the subareolar terminal ducts, with lumen filled with desquamated cellular debris and associated periductal fibrosis and inflammation. He proposed stages in the pathogenesis of subareolar abscess, starting with dilation of major subareolar mammary ducts, followed by accumulation of cellular debris and material containing lipid. During this stage, the ductal epithelium was normal and there was no evidence of inflammation. As the disease progressed, the duct dilation extended into the peripheral breast tissue from the central subareolar region, and fibrosis and a periductal lymphocytic infiltrate were observed. The epithelium became atrophic and discontinuous; lipid material permeated the stroma; and an inflammatory reaction with necrosis, polymorphonuclear leukocytes, histiocytes, lymphocytes, and plasma cells supervened. Multiple ducts could be affected. Haagensen concluded that the preceding historical descriptions were all expressions of the same disease process at various stages.

TABLE **5-1**	Nomenclature of Mammary Duct-Associated Inflammatory Disease*
TERM/PATHOGNOMONIC FACTOR	**INVESTIGATORS**
Morbid condition of lactiferous duct	Birkett, 1850[9]
Mastitis obliterans	Ingier, 1909[10] Payne et al, 1943[2]
Chronic pyogenic mastitis	Deaver and McFarland, 1917[7]
Stale milk mastitis	Cromar, 1921[11]
Varicocele tumor of the breast	Bloodgood, 1923[3]
Plasma cell mastitis	Adair, 1933[8]
Involutional mammary duct ectasia with periductal mastitis	Foote, 1945[12]
Comedomastitis	Tice et al, 1948[5]
Periductal mastitis	Geschickter, 1948[4]
Chemical mastitis	Stewart, 1950[13]
Fistulas of lactiferous ducts	Zuska et al, 1951[14]
Mammary duct ectasia	Haagensen, 1951[15]
Squamous metaplasia	Patey and Thackray, 1958[16]
Secretory cystic disease of the breast	Ingleby, 1942[6] Ingleby and Gershon-Cohen, 1960[17]
Periductal mastitis/duct ectasia	Dixon, 1989[18]
Mammary duct-associated inflammatory disease sequence (MDAIDS)	Meguid et al, 1995[19]

*Terms used to describe the major conceptual milestones from early literature to current times. These terms reflect the different stages at which the pathology was described.

In the 1960s, Bonser, Dossett and Jull[23] and Dossett[24] challenged this pathogenesis and suggested that the periductal inflammation was responsible for the subsequent development of duct ectasia. Azzopardi,[25] in his monograph *Problems in Breast Pathology,* reiterated this view and favored the term *periductal mastitis.*

In the 1980s, Dixon and co-workers[26] introduced the term *periductal mastitis/duct ectasia,* and in agreement with Dossett and Azzopardi, they described the periductal inflammation as the primary event and the duct ectasia as a secondary phenomenon. They suggested that the hypothesis that infection follows stasis of secretions was incorrect.[18,26] They viewed mammary duct ectasia as an ill-conceived umbrella term for unrelated conditions that might lead to major surgery.

During the course of this intellectual struggle to come to terms with a condition often described as a nuisance by clinicians, the key observation of squamous metaplasia of a lactiferous duct was not given its due recognition. Patey and Thackray[16] noted that in 6 of their 7 patients treated for mammary duct fistula, the portion of the associated duct from the fistulous tract to the nipple was partly or totally lined by squamous epithelium. The fistulous tract itself consisted of nonepithelialized granulation tissue. In the seventh patient the duct was lined by granulation tissue. Subsequently, Toker[27] reported the presence of a squamous lining in multiple ducts in a patient with a fistulous tract and concluded that the disease was the result of downward growth of squamous epithelium from the nipple into the subareolar mammary ducts. In 1970, Habif and colleagues[28] also observed squamous metaplasia in subareolar abscess.

Recent views put forward by Bundred and colleagues[29] and Dixon and co-workers[30] concerning the pathogenesis of this benign disease process propose that periductal inflammation is secondary to smoking and that duct ectasia is most likely an unrelated phenomenon. In contrast, our discussion of the pathogenesis of what we term the *mammary duct–associated inflammatory disease sequence* (MDAIDS) considers the interaction of various putative causal factors unifying the disease process while recognizing varied clinical expression. We see common elements in the spectrum of changes noted in MDAIDS. Furthermore, we believe in the original proposal by Haagensen that some form of mechanical obstruction, with associated retention of secretions, is at the core of the disease process, because (Table 5-2) the

| TABLE **5-2** | Frequency of Dilated Ducts as Incidental Findings at Operation or Autopsy and Frequency of Symptomatic Women and Men with MDAIDS |

INVESTIGATORS	FREQUENCY (%)	ALL PATIENTS WITH BREAST DISEASE (*n*)	AVERAGE AGE (yr)	TISSUE TYPE
ASYMPTOMATIC (INCIDENTAL AND AUTOPSY)				
Foote and Stewart, 1945[12]	38	200	42	Benign
	26	300	50	Carcinoma
Frantz et al, 1951[31]	25	225	62	"Normal breasts" postmortem
Sandison, 1957[32]	72*	800	75% <80	Postmortem
Sandison, 1962[33]	6	500	No data	Postmortem
Tedeschi et al, 1963[34]	60	20	Postmenopausal	"Normal breasts" postmortem
Davies, 1971[35]	38	208	No data	Postmortem
Browning et al, 1986[36]	8.2	1,256	46	Benign and malignant
Average = 29%		*n* = 3,509		
SYMPTOMATIC MDAIDS				
Geschickter, 1948[4]	2.3	3,107	40+	Benign
Sandison and Walker, 1962[37]	4.1	390	20-70	Benign
Bonser et al, 1961[23]	36.0	351	No data	Benign and malignant
Walker and Sandison, 1964[38]	12	283	48	Benign
Abramson DJ, 1969[39]	2.1	857	No data	Benign and malignant
Frischbier and Lohbeck, 1977[40]	10.8	1,256	No data	Benign and malignant
Thomas et al, 1982[41]	5.5	732	43	Benign
Dixon et al, 1983[26]	5.5	1,963	All ages (<30-89)	Benign and malignant
Browning et al, 1986[36]	4.1	1,256	47	Benign and malignant
Average = 5.9%		*n* = 10,195		

MDAIDS, Mammary duct–associated inflammatory disease sequence.
*Includes duct ectasia and cysts. Includes 11% with duct ectasia observed on gross examination.

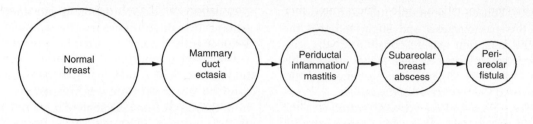

FIG. **5-1** The evolutionary stages of the mammary duct–associated inflammatory disease sequence (MDAIDS), from normal breast to its presentation of subareolar breast abscess and its sequela—periareolar fistula.

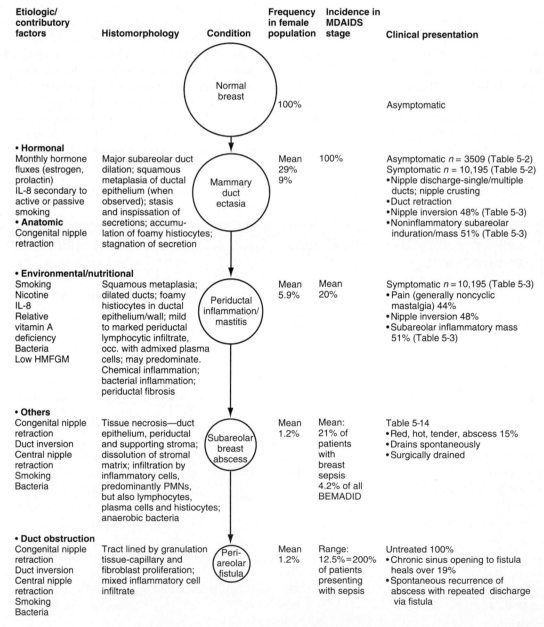

FIG. **5-2** Correlation between etiologic factors, histomorphologies, and clinical presentations of the mammary duct–associated inflammatory disease sequence *(MDAIDS)*. Also, shown is the estimated frequency of MDAIDS in the general female population and the calculated incidence of the different stages of MDAIDS as derived from the current literature.

frequency of asymptomatic dilatated ducts found incidentally in patients or at autopsy far exceeds the frequency of symptomatic duct dilation or ectasia.

Figure 5-1 depicts our conceptualization of the disease process, from normal breast to a subareolar abscess and its sequelae, periareolar fistulas. *MDAIDS* is a more inclusive term that comprehensively describes the phases of this disease. This term encompasses the antecedent benign disease process (i.e., mammary duct ectasia), periductal inflammation/mastitis, the abscess, and its sequelae.

On the basis of our own histomorphologic observations[19] and those of others,[16,27,28] we postulate that squamous metaplasia of mammary duct epithelium, in association with duct ectasia, has a major role in this obstruction. Because the breast is a modified sweat gland, the presence of squamous metaplasia affects the accumulation of the continuously produced secretions and facilitates infection. This metaplasia initiates a cascade of changes whose molecular bases are beginning to be understood and that lead to the MDAIDS shown schematically in Figures 5-1 and 5-2. Also shown in Figure 5-2 and Table 5-3 are the estimated frequency of MDAIDS in the general female population and the calculated incidence of the different disease phases of MDAIDS, based on data from the literature.

Depending on a number of variables—the location and extent of the squamous metaplasia; the degree of impediment to secretion flow; the impact of hormonal (estrogen, prolactin), environmental (smoking), and local paracrine effects of cytokines secondary to smoking (active or passive); and the impact of nutritional factors (relative vitamin A deficiency), anatomic factors (congenital nipple retraction), and no doubt other factors yet to be defined—in one or more major subareolar and transnipple mammary ducts (or on occasion minor ducts in the peripheral breast tissue) varying degrees of duct ectasia, a primary chemically induced inflammatory reaction, and secondary bacterial growth, subsequently followed by infection and periductal inflammation occur. This concept is supported by the increased recognition and consensus that proper management of this disease entails use of a combination of antibiotics to cover aerobes and anaerobes and surgical excision of the involved duct and the periductal inflammation. On the basis of this evidence, we therefore believe the term *MDAIDS* is appropriate and correct.

TABLE 5-3 Frequency of Symptoms and Signs in Patients with MDAIDS as Summarized from the Literature

SPECIFIC CONDITION	PATIENTS WITH MDAIDS (*n*)	PATIENTS WITH SPECIFIC CONDITION (*n*)	SYMPTOMATIC (%) OCCURRENCE	RANGE OF OCCURRENCE	REFERENCES
Nipple discharge					
Asymptomatic	103	8	8	—	36,
Symptomatic	577	238	41	21-84	26,36,38,41,42,43, 44,45,46,47
Nipple inversion/retraction					
Asymptomatic	103	7	7	—	36
Symptomatic	668	319	48	13-100	22,28,36,41,42,43,44,46,48, 49,50,51,52,53,54,55
Pain and tenderness					
Asymptomatic	103	12	12	—	36
Symptomatic	183	84	44	11-106	36,38,44,47,56,57
Mass (periareolar)					
Asymptomatic	103	33	32	—	36
Symptomatic	399	203	51	5-100	36,37,38,39,41,42,43, 44,46,47
Abscess					
Asymptomatic	103	1	1	—	36
Symptomatic	803	124	15	8-28	36,44,45,46,58,59,60
Fistula					
Asymptomatic	103	0	0	—	36
Symptomatic	176	34	19	12-67	36,39,44,58,61
Bilaterality					
Symptomatic	495	114	23	5-100	14,17,19,28,38,44,48,49, 51,52,58,59,62

Pathogenesis and Its Clinical Correlations

To fully appreciate the pathogenic process leading to subareolar abscess and its sequelae, familiarity with the normal structure and histologic appearance of the major subareolar lactiferous ducts, the ampulla, and the transnipple ducts is helpful. The breast is a modified sweat gland and thus produces a continuous, imperceptible discharge from the numerous orifices of the mammary ducts onto the nipple. This discharge is normally so small that it dries into a scarcely discernible crust on the nipple and is brushed away by the clothes.

As depicted in Figure 5-3, the secretory acini of the lobular tissue in the periphery of the breast open into small (minor) intralobular ducts, which then drain into the major lobar ducts. Some 16 to 18 major mammary ducts draining acini are organized in lobular groupings surrounded by fibrofatty tissue, each separated by Cooper's ligaments. As each major mammary duct converges centrally onto and traverses the base of the nipple, it dilates to form a secretion-storing lactiferous ampulla, situated beneath the nipple areolar complex. From the ampulla, situated beneath the nipple/areola complex, each duct transverses the nipple and opens via a separate opening at the apex of the nipple. Thus, if there are 18 lobules with major ducts, there will be 18 separate openings for the major mammary ducts that open onto the apex of the nipple. Occasionally there are two major ducts draining the lobules, which converge into one ampulla.

As shown in the low-power view of a longitudinal section of the nipple (Figure 5-4), each duct is lined by a double layer of cells (inner cuboidal or low columnar epithelium) and an outer myoepithelial layer, whereas the ampulla and the final few millimeters of the intranipple duct terminating on the surface are lined by stratified squamous epithelium. The average frequency of dilated ducts found incidentally at surgery or autopsy is 29% (see Tables 5-2 and 5-3 and Figure 5-2). This far exceeds the average frequency of 5.9% in

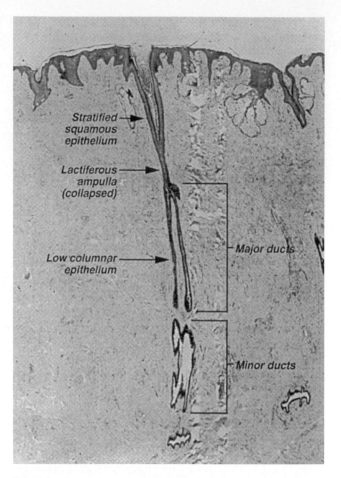

FIG. **5-4** Low-power longitudinal section of the nipple shows two major lactiferous ducts emptying into an ampulla (collapsed because of pathologic preparation) and then opening onto the surface of the nipple. *(Modified from Meguid MM et al:* Surgery *118:775, 1995.)*

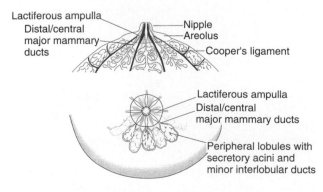

FIG. **5-3** Gross anatomic layout of normal breast structure.

symptomatic females and males (see Table 5-2) and suggests that a factor such as the relative imbalance of monthly hormone fluxes contributes to the development of early mammary duct ectasia.

In the literature on MDAIDS related to the pathologic process, several studies attribute ductal obstruction to squamous metaplasia or epidermalization of ductal columnar epithelium.[16,19,27,28] Based on these findings, our view of the evolution of MDAIDS, as postulated to correspond with the different histomorphologic changes, is shown schematically in Figure 5-2.

Figure 5-5, *A*, shows epidermalization of mammary duct epithelium. The squamous aplasia has progressed and has developed a granular layer (darkly stained subcorneal zone), which matures into keratin. This area of epidermalization is surrounded on either side by normal columnar epithelium consisting of a double layer of lining epithelial cells: the inner columnar and the outer flattened myoepithelial cells. At this stage, the symptoms may be discharge from one or more ducts, duct or nipple retraction, and/or subareolar induration

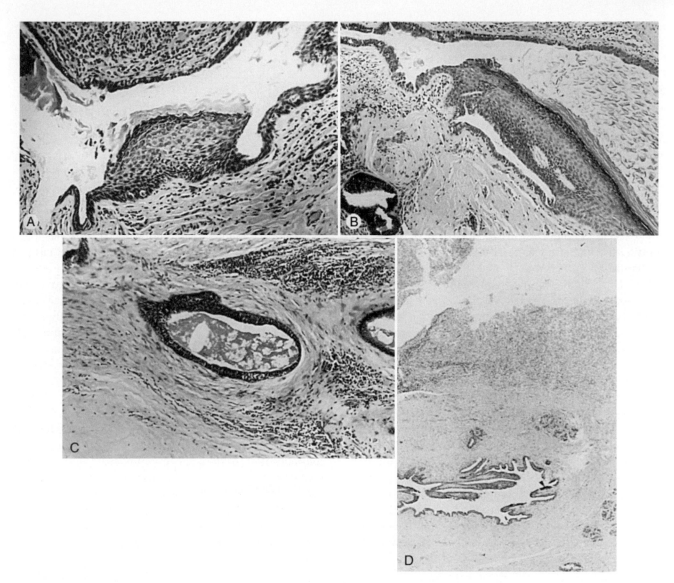

FIG. **5-5** Microscopic process of squamous metaplasia of major lactiferous duct in series of patients. Epidermalization-metaplasia with granular layer and keratin production **(A)**; production of copious keratin **(B)**, leading to keratin plugs **(C)** with ultimately acute and chronic inflammation (breast abscess) **(D)**. Abscess shown above a normal duct. *(From Meguid MM et al:* Surgery *118:775, 1995.)*

(see Figure 5-2). As the disease progresses, the active granular layer (Figure 5-5, *B*) produces copious amounts of keratin, leading to obstruction of the major ducts by keratin plugs (Figure 5-5, *C*). Following obstruction with keratin and cell debris, dilation of the duct and ampulla occurs because of the accumulation and stasis of secretory material from the acini. Clinically, the presenting symptom would be consistent with noncyclic mastalgia, nipple retraction, and/or subareolar induration (see Figure 5-2).

Finally, there is discontinuity or rupture of the thinned epithelial lining of the major duct, exposing the surrounding supporting stroma to the luminal contents and initiating chemically induced inflammation. In the process, the duct wall is permeated with lipid material, foamy histiocytes, and mild to marked periductal lymphocytic infiltrate, at times admixed with plasma cells (which may predominate). The keratin and the lipids of the secretions induce an inflammatory response—periductal inflammation, which presents clinically with symptoms of a subareolar inflammatory mass (see Figure 5-2). This milieu also serves as an excellent source for bacterial growth. The bacteria may be anaerobic or aerobic, from skin, endogenous breast flora, or oral contamination of the nipple.[63,64] Bacteria, both aerobic and anaerobic, can be cultured in more than 90% of breast tissue samples obtained at the time of augmentation or reduction mammoplasty.[63] Whether tissue samples are obtained from deep in the mammary gland or superficially, the main aerobic and anaerobic organisms cultured are coagulase-negative staphylococci and propionibacteria, respectively.[63,64] Endogenous breast flora is similar to that present on the skin[64] and is reflected in the incidence of bacteria cultured in nonpuerperal subareolar breast abscess specimens (see later in this chapter).[65] Colonization of the tissue leads to an abscess beneath the areola (Figure 5-5, *D*). Clinically, the patient may present with an early subareolar abscess (see Figure 5-2) or, if the process is more advanced and fluctuant, a spontaneously draining abscess opening onto the vermilion border of the areola. As the disease progresses, the abscess eventually presents as a chronic sinus lined by granulation tissue. On histologic examination, at varying distances from the opening of the fistula, the tract lined by granulation tissue communicates with the main subareolar duct lined by squamous or epidermalized epithelium, usually packed behind the obstruction by desquamated keratin, debris that interferes with the normal drainage of secretion.[28]

The obstruction associated with epidermalization and the associated keratin debris is more severe and more rapid than that of squamous metaplasia or hormone imbalance (see following discussion). As a consequence, epidermalization of the mammary duct would induce changes that are more likely to be symptomatic earlier. In this rapidly changing mammary duct environment, as ectasia evolves with the presence of desquamated keratin flakes, epithelial injury and discontinuity are more likely. By its nature, keratin is very irritating and readily elicits an inflammatory response. The presence of keratin flakes in the retained secretions, in contact with the subepithelial stroma, greatly accentuates the periductal inflammation. Although this implies that these events occur in this sequence, as suggested by several studies,[16,27,28] the process probably occurs simultaneously but to different degrees in different large subareolar mammary ducts. Thus the presenting symptoms may not always follow the sequence depicted in Figure 5-2.

Causes of the Mammary Duct–Associated Inflammatory Disease Sequence

A schema of the interactions of the putative causal factors on the three basic disease phases of MDAIDS—namely, duct ectasia, squamous metaplasia, and abscess—is presented in Figure 5-6. The molecular basis whereby ductal epithelium undergoes squamous metaplasia has been revealed via use of a knockout mice model. Initially, in 1958 Patey and Thackray[16] postulated that squamous metaplasia of the lactiferous ducts occurred secondary to a congenital anomaly of the duct system, because 6 of 7 patients studied had congenital nipple inversion. However, today, it is well recognized that vitamin A is necessary for preserving the cellular differentiation of columnar epithelia. Vitamin A deficiency promotes squamous metaplasia/epidermalization, a development also associated with smoking. Increased interleukin 8 (IL-8) in alveolar capillary wall macrophages in lung tissue of smokers, as compared with controls, with its paracrine action stimulating polymorphonuclear cell migration, may contribute to the acute inflammatory response.[66] The course and evolution of the disease process leading to subareolar abscess, with its underlying histomorphologic alterations and clinical expression as MDAIDS (see Figure 5-2), depend on the impact of these two factors. Smoking shifts the metabolism of estrogen away from

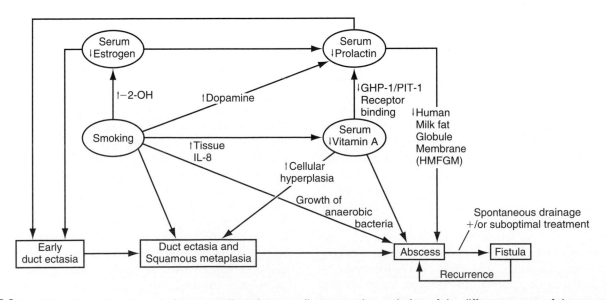

FIG. **5-6** Interplay of putative etiologic factors attributed as contributory to the evolution of the different stages of the mammary duct–associated inflammatory disease sequence *(MDAIDS)*.

active metabolites[67] and induces lower serum prolactin levels.[68] Retinoic vitamin A promotes prolactin secretion,[69] implying that a deficiency of this vitamin could have an inhibitory effect on prolactin secretion.

HORMONAL INFLUENCES

Healthy infants often have transient breast enlargement of a few weeks' duration, and transient duct ectasia has been observed in some of these infants. The ectasia is attributed to transplacental passage of maternal hormones.[33] Symptomatic MDAIDS associated with bloody nipple discharge has been documented in infants and young children.[70-72] Of interest is the observation of a 100% increase in serum prolactin in a 3-year-old boy that was associated with MDAIDS.[72]

Prolactin. Prolactin is essential for lactation. It participates in mammary growth through sensitization of the ductal epithelium to mitogenic synergism.[73] Prolactin secretion is stimulated by estrogen and inhibited by drugs such as dopamine, the prolactin inhibitory factor.[62]

In several studies, MDAIDS has been reported to be associated with increased serum prolactin. The association of MDAIDS and prolactinemia has been seen in the setting of prolactin-secreting pituitary chromophobe adenoma,[74] breast cancer,[75] and treatment with phenothiazine,[74] whose long-term use can lead to hyperprolactinemia.[76] Phenothiazine can induce breast enlargement, lactation, amenorrhea, and gynecomastia.

Shousha and co-workers[74] considered three possibilities for the association of MDAIDS with increased serum prolactin: (1) a direct relationship, (2) unrelated events, and (3) a process secondary to sudden decrease in serum prolactin. A decrease in serum prolactin has also been associated with smoking and may follow vitamin A deficiency.[68,69]

The impact of smoking on prolactin secretion has been investigated mainly with use of nicotine. This has biphasic effects depending on the dose and frequency of administration. One or two doses of nicotine can stimulate prolactin secretion.[77] However, repeated doses inhibit prolactin secretion[77] because of desensitization. Berta and co-workers[68] evaluated the effect of smoking on the serum prolactin levels of fertile women who had not smoked for at least 12 hours and observed significantly lower serum prolactin levels in smokers than in nonsmokers. Male smokers also have a lower serum prolactin value than nonsmokers.[68]

Smoking acts via dopamine and serum prolactin levels on estrogen metabolism. Estrogen stimulates prolactin secretion.[67] Smoking induces a shift in estrogen metabolism that results in a decrease in peripherally active estrogen metabolites (see following discussion), possibly reducing prolactin secretion.[78]

A third pathway to lower serum prolactin levels may be a vitamin A deficiency or smoking (see later in this chapter). Recent studies in vitro suggest that retinoic acid activates the promoter responsible for the pituitary-specific GHP-1/Pit-1 transcription factor necessary for the expression of the prolactin gene.[69] Low serum levels of vitamin A would result in less receptor binding and thus less transcription of GHP-1/Pit-1.

Permanent decreases in serum prolactin or fluctuation to a subnormal physiologic concentration may be secondary to dopamine release, altered estrogen metabolism, or decreased serum binding of vitamin A receptor. This decrease in serum prolactin could promote MDAIDS, as proposed by Shousha and co-workers.[74] As to the mechanisms by which decreased serum prolactin would induce MDAIDS, we believe them to be alterations in secretions (composition and/or viscosity), resulting in stasis or affecting adhesion molecules.

Prolactin deficiency may also play a role in the initial stages of infection. As stated earlier, prolactin stimulates lactation. Breast milk contains lipid globules enclosed by fragments of the apical membrane of mammary secretory cells, referred to as *human milk fat globule membrane* (HMFGM).[79] These membrane fragments are not present in infant formulas; the addition of HMFGM inhibits adhesion of bacteria such as *Escherichia coli* to epithelial cells, and their absence facilitates sepsis.[80,81] It may be postulated that with decreased levels of prolactin, breast secretions of a nonlactating woman would also contain less HMFGM, thus facilitating adhesion of endogenous or exogenous bacteria to mammary epithelial cells and onset of infection.

Estrogen. Michnovicz and co-workers[67] showed that in persons who smoked at least 20 cigarettes per day, smoking stimulated the metabolic pathway of estradiol, leading to 2α-hydroxylation rather than to 16α-hydroxylation. 2α-Hydroxylated compounds are virtually devoid of peripheral estrogen activity. This increase in 2α-hydroxylation may result from the altered metabolism of steroid hormones following stimulation of hepatic P-450 microsomal enzymes by nicotine or other components of cigarette smoke.[82] Low levels of serum estrogen caused by nicotine and cotinine, its major metabolite, contribute to the conversion of testosterone to estradiol by aromatase.[83] From the results of these studies, we postulate that decreased estrogen activity impairs the hormonally controlled integrity of the breast duct epithelium.

NUTRITIONAL FACTORS

Vitamin A. Vitamin A deficiency induces keratinizing squamous metaplasia on multiple mucosal surfaces, including those of the head and neck region, bronchi, uterus, and cervix.[84] In the cervix, reserve cell proliferation, the precursor to squamous metaplasia, has been shown to be under the control of retinoids.[85]

There is increasing epidemiologic and experimental evidence that vitamin A or retinoids have a significant biologic effect on mammary duct epithelial cell proliferation and differentiation, of which insufficient levels result in the development of squamous metaplasia, possibly a pivotal event leading to MDAIDS (see Figure 5-6).

Vitamin A deficiency is implicated as a contributing factor in the development of infection. Vitamin A deficiency impairs blood clearance of bacteria and results in decreased phagocytic activity in vitro.[86] Increased bacterial binding to epithelial cells is observed with vitamin A deficiency.[87] For sepsis associated with MDAIDS, we postulate that the HMFGM is altered (see Figure 5-6). The apical surface of normal mammary duct epithelial cells consists of microvilli,[88] which are altered in various conditions.[89] In respiratory epithelium, this surface alteration induced by vitamin A deficiency can be observed by scanning electron microscopy before the appearance of squamous metaplasia, evident by optical microscopy.[90]

SMOKING

In 1988 Schafer, Furrer, and Mermillod[91] demonstrated the association between cigarette smoking and recurrent subareolar breast abscess. The relative risk of a recurrent subareolar breast abscess increased directly between light and heavy cigarette smokers, and 90% of all patients with recurrent breast abscess had been exposed to cigarette smoke for many years before the breast disorder was manifested.[91]

Various studies[29,30,92] have shown that severe periductal inflammation was more often associated with heavy smoking (>10 cigarettes per day) and younger age (Figure 5-7). These studies also noted an increased incidence of mammary duct squamous metaplasia in smokers. Dixon and colleagues[30] performed a prospective analysis of 14,225 women, 4715 of whom were smokers. A prevalence of 2.28% (325 patients) of MDAIDS-related clinical symptoms was observed, and 54% of the patients were smokers.[30] When the severity of the disease process was correlated with smoking, only 28% of smokers had mammary duct ectasia. A significant increase in the percentage of smokers accounted for the subareolar abscess (87%) and periductal mastitis (88%) groups. The group with mammary duct fistula had the highest percentage of smokers (94%).[30] They also noted that an inflammatory response and its sequelae were associated with a younger age group.[30] On the basis of these analyses they postulated that clinical duct ectasia is likely to be totally unrelated to periductal mastitis.[30]

Conversely, the prospective data collected by Thomas, Williamson, and Webster[92] on 12,688 Welsh women did not uncover a significant difference in the percentage of smokers between patients with mammary duct ectasia (37%) and those with periductal mastitis (37.9%). In our smaller study of patients with recurrent subareolar breast abscesses, we found that 92% of them smoked, a percentage similar to that noted by Dixon's group.[30]

The molecular mechanisms by which smoking induces squamous metaplasia have yet to be identified, although their association is strong. Smoking-related squamous metaplasia of the bronchial mucosa is related to the intensity of tobacco use (packs per day) rather than to pack-years.[93] In the breast, within 30 minutes of smoking, nicotine and its metabolite cotinine are detected in the milk of lactating women.[94] In the nonlactating breast, glandular secretions are more concentrated, and in about 7% of women these secretions are mutagenic in the Ames tests and contain oxidized steroids and lipid peroxides.[95] These metabolites might be responsible for direct cellular injury leading to reactive squamous metaplasia.[95] Smoking reduces bioavailability of estrogen at target tissues by means of 2α-hydroxylation of estradiol, which may affect ductal cellular integrity.[67] In addition, nicotine and cotinine inhibit the aromatase-catalyzed conversion of testosterone to estrogen. A special class of estrogen derived from this reaction in humans is estradiol-17-sulfate and its metabolites, which originate from testosterone sulfate.[96] The metabolites 2-hydroxy- and 4-hydroxy-estrogen-17-sulfate are potent lipid peroxidation antagonists.[96] The serum levels of these two metabolites may well be reduced during smoking. This would facilitate the cytotoxic injury induced by smoking and the development of reactive hyperplasia and squamous metaplasia.

Smoking may also directly facilitate the development of the infection associated with MDAIDS. In vitro, smoke

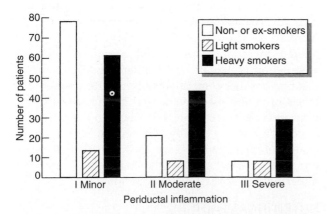

FIG. **5-7** Periductal inflammation and cigarette smoking in periductal mastitis ($p<.05$) *(Modified from Bundred NJ et al: In Recent developments in the study of benign breast disease. Proceedings of the 5th International Symposium on Breast Disease, London, 1993).*

inhibits the growth of gram-positive cocci more than it does gram-negative rods. Smokers tend to have heavy gram-negative colonization of the mouth.[97] Those not infection-prone included more current smokers and persons with longer smoking experience.[98] Nevertheless, in a study of anaerobic respiratory infection,[99] heavy smoking and chronic lower airway infection were deemed to be pathogenic factors in the absence of aspiration; however, smoking does not appear to predispose significantly to breast infection following mammary prosthesis.[100] Although the question has not been totally resolved, the possibility still exists that smoking may alter the composition of the endogenous flora in the mammary ducts and thus, in association with the previously discussed aberrations induced by prolactin and vitamin A deficiency, promote a bacterial infection.

Although the exact cause of MDAIDS is still unknown, certain contributing factors are becoming clearer. The repeated finding of squamous metaplasia has been well described in the literature.[28] Our own histomorphologic observations have also confirmed this finding.[19] Although it continues to make sense that squamous metaplasia and keratin plugging of lactiferous ducts may lead to obstruction and abscess formation, why the aforementioned process occurs remains unclear. Recent work by Li and colleagues[100a] suggests that a genetic alteration may explain the predisposition of certain women to this difficult clinical problem. At least in animal models, alterations in many genes have been shown to alter mammary gland development and tumor formation.[101-103] More specifically, transforming growth factor-β (TGF-β) has been shown to play a role in mammary development and tumor formation.[104-106] The role of TGF-β in the development of mammalian mammary abscess has also been described by Li and colleagues. TGF-β signals are known to be regulated by a group of serine kinases known as Smad4 (a central mediator for transforming growth factor-β [TGF-β]).[78] Specifically, with use of a Smad4 knockout mouse model, it has been shown that disruption of this gene repeatedly results in formation of mammary abscesses. This appears to be caused by transdifferentiation of normal mammary epithelium to squamous epithelium as a result of loss of TGF-β responsiveness. Histologic cross sectioning of these mice clearly showed increased proliferation of epithelial cells, keratinization, and squamous metaplasia associated with mammary abscess. This correlates almost precisely with the histologic picture seen in women with MDAIDS.

The preceding findings, although thus far shown only in a mouse model, promote a better understanding of the pathophysiology of human breast abscess as it relates to MDAIDS. It is hoped that further investigations will show a possible link between smoking or hormonal changes and these genetic alterations, which appear to be causally related to squamous metaplasia of the lactiferous duct.

Pathology of the Mammary Duct–Associated Inflammatory Disease Sequence

The least symptomatic stage consists of the earliest morphologic changes and includes mild mammary duct ectasia, foamy histiocytes with filling of duct lumens, and some degree of secretion stasis as granular flocculent intraluminal material distal to an area of squamous metaplasia. This can be quite focal and difficult to find histologically. In some of our more recent cases of early MDAIDS, this was present in only one or two serial histologic sections and was observed only by chance. In our more advanced MDAIDS cases the histologic evidence of squamous metaplasia and epidermalization was focal and not adjacent to the terminal end of the major mammary ducts.[19] The duct ectasia phase of MDAIDS is associated with changes in the periductal stroma, consisting of periductal fibrosis and fragmentation and disarray of (now) irregularly thick elastic fibers.[107] These stromal changes are found regardless of whether the duct ectasia occurs in the presence of periductal inflammation.[107] The presence of iron deposits suggests that intramural hemorrhage may have a role in the evolution of the disease process.

As the disease progresses, different degrees of histomorphologic changes are noted in association with the major and minor ducts. The major ducts exhibit increased ectasia and may contain dense inspissation of secretions and more pronounced periductal fibrosis. The minor ducts situated in the periphery of the breast tissue and the proximal parts of the lobules are dilated with foamy histiocytes or with homogeneous or granular secretions. Foamy histiocytes are seen permeating the ductal epithelium and surrounding stroma, which at first contains a mild lymphocytic inflammatory infiltrate. Less commonly, ducts are obliterated by fibrous tissue and even recanalized. Calcifications may occur. The presence of lipids in the stroma induces formation of lipid granulomas.

Subsequently, especially with infection, an abscess with a predominant acute inflammatory infiltrate may be observed. If the inflammation is more of the subacute or chronic type, the inflammatory exudate contains not only polymorphonuclear leukocytes but also lymphocytes, plasma cells, histiocytes, cell debris, and keratin. Although keratin was present in the intraluminal debris in most of our patients with abscesses, the inflamed segment of the duct was damaged so extensively that the foci of squamous metaplasia and epidermalization could no longer be found, even on examination of serial sections. This led us to conclude that if squamous metaplasia/epidermalization and ectasia affect only one inflamed duct, these changes may not be observed.

Clinical Overview of the Mammary Duct–Associated Inflammatory Disease Sequence

The incidence of MDAIDS is on the rise. It is closely associated with the consumption of tobacco, which is on the increase among women,[108] a circumstance that may explain the increase in frequency. Currently, symptomatic MDAIDS represents approximately 20% of all benign conditions of the breast.[109]

Figure 5-8 shows the age distribution of 186 patients with the clinical MDAIDS, combined from a couple of studies in the literature[18,41] in which this information was available and, for comparison, the age distribution of 1205 patients with operable breast cancer.[110] MDAIDS causes symptoms over a large age range, with the overall peak incidence between 40 and 49 years, although each symptom tends to peak at a different age (see following discussion).

The true incidence of the duct ectasia phase of MDAIDS can only be estimated because in most women it is subclinical or asymptomatic and is discovered only by chance at surgery (incidental) or autopsy. A degree of dilation of the major subareolar ducts is often seen during biopsy performed for both benign and malignant conditions of the breast. Thus asymptomatic duct ectasia of MDAIDS exists, but its clinical significance is uncertain. It is recognized, however,

that many women have asymptomatic dilation of the major subareolar mammary ducts that becomes symptomatic only when infection supervenes and becomes part of the broad clinical syndrome of MDAIDS.

On the basis of the findings of several postmortem studies and incidental findings in histologic sections examined for other breast diseases (see Table 5-2), the mean incidental frequency of MDAIDS appears to be approximately 30%. The mean incidence of symptomatic MDAIDS, based on a series of published studies, is approximately 6%. The pathologic process occasionally involves both breasts (usually with equal frequency).

Table 5-4 summarizes the major reported literature on the occurrence of MDAIDS in infants and males. Mammary duct ectasia also occurs in the breasts of elderly men who smoke (Table 5-4).[92] Consequently, mammary duct ectasia is not an involutionary disease as Haagensen asserted.[15] Clearly, this pathophysiologic condition is not limited to the female breast, a characteristic suggesting commonalities of etiologic and pathologic origin affecting mammary duct tissue.

The most common clinical presentation of the duct in MDAIDS is nipple discharge (see Figure 5-2 and Table 5-5). The reported prevalence averages 36% and ranges from 8% to 84%, depending on whether the patients are asymptomatic or symptomatic (see Table 5-3), and the syndrome accounts for 11% of bloody and 13% of serous nipple discharges.[117] Bilateral symptoms occur in one third to one half of patients.[36] The discharge may come from one or more ducts. The color varies, often between ducts in the same breast. The discharge is sometimes grossly tinged or tests positive for occult blood. From studies of nipple discharge, the calculated frequency of bloody discharge is 64%.[26,117-119]

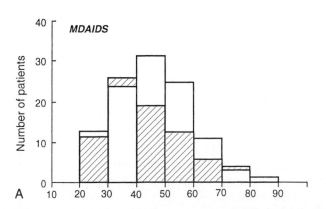
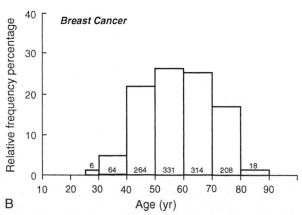

FIG. **5-8 A,** Age distribution of 186 patients with clinical symptoms of the mammary duct–associated inflammatory disease sequence (MDAIDS). *(Combined data: open bar from Thomas WG et al: Br J Surg 69:423, 1982; hatched bar from Dixon JM: World J Surg 13:715, 1989).* **B,** Age distribution of 1205 patients with operable breast cancer. *(Data from the Yorkshire Breast Cancer Group: Br J Surg 1983.)*

| TABLE **5-4** | Males and Infants with MDAIDS Culled from World Literature |

INVESTIGATORS	PATIENT NO.	AGE (yr)	CLINICAL FEATURES	COMMENTS
Tedeschi and McCarthy, 1974[111]	1	57	Left breast tenderness, 3-cm indurated mass; discharge—0, adenopathy—0	No history of meds; excision biopsy; simple mastectomy; smoking history not noted
Mansel and Morgan, 1979[112]	2	62	Painful left subareolar breast mass; bloody nipple discharge; bilateral, painless nipple retraction during previous 2 yr; presented with draining Left breast abscess	Total duct excision; smoking history not noted
	3	47	12-yr history recurrent right subareolar breast abscess with periareolar fistula; left breast and nipple normal	Simple mastectomy; smoking history not noted
	4	52	8-wk history tender left subareolar breast mass with intermittent discharge from periareolar fistula; right breast/nipple normal	No meds; antibiotics; subcutaneous mastectomy; smoking history not noted
Chan and Lau, 1984[113]	5	34	Right breast pain 1 wk; right nipple retracted with 2-cm, hard, tender subareolar mass; no nipple discharge; left breast normal	No meds; excision biopsy; smoking history not noted
McClure et al, 1985[114]	6	28	5-yr history swelling and occasional discomfort right breast; right breast enlarged; left breast normal	Phenotypically and karyotypically normal male; simple mastectomy; smoking history not noted
Ashworth et al, 1985[115]	7	50	2-mo history right subareolar breast mass; tender; no discharge; right subareolar abscess; left breast normal	No meds; major duct excision; smoking history not noted
Stringel et al, 1986[72]	8	3	Persistent bloody discharge right nipple; 1 yr later, bloody nipple discharge left breast	Normal endocrine work-up, prolactin elevated; no meds; right subcutaneous mastectomy, then left subcutaneous mastectomy
	9	5 mo	Bloody nipple discharge left breast; intermittent for 3 mo; then stopped spontaneously	No meds
Thomas et al, 1993[92]	10	66	Breast abscess	20 cigarettes/day
	11	62	Bilateral periductal mastitis/breast abscess	15-20 cigarettes/day
	12	52	Periductal mastitis/mammary fistula	15 g tobacco/day
	13	51	Breast abscess	20 cigarettes/day
	14	44	Periductal mastitis/breast abscess	10 cigarettes/day
Lambert et al, 1986[116]	15		Fistula in male	Data not provided
Ekland and Ziegler, 1973[52]	16 and 17		Two males with subareolar breast abscess	Data not provided

MDAIDS, Mammary duct–associated inflammatory disease sequence.

TABLE 5-5	Predominant Symptoms of the Mammary Duct Ectasia Component of MDAIDS	
	SYMPTOMATIC (n = 51)	INCIDENTAL (n = 103)
Nipple		
No discharge	13 (25%)	89 (86%)
Discharge	21 (41%)	7 (7%)
Inversion	5 (10%)	6 (6%)
Inversion + discharge	12 (24%)	1 (1%)
Pain		
None	17 (33%)	55 (53%)
Cyclical	21 (41%)	36 (35%)
Noncyclical	13 (25%)	12 (12%)
Lump		
None	21 (41%)	5 (5%)
Periareolar	23 (45%)	33 (32%)
Peripheral	7 (14%)	65 (65%)
Sepsis		
None	41 (81%)	102 (99%)
Abscess	4 (8%)	1 (1%)
Fistual	6 (12%)	0

Modified from Browning J et al: *J R Soc Med* 79:715, 1986.
MDAIDS, Mammary duct–associated inflammatory disease sequence.

The other clinical symptoms are related primarily to the periductal inflammation and mastitis component of MDAIDS, which presents as noncyclic mastalgia and tenderness and occurs in approximately 44% of women with symptomatic MDAIDS (see Table 5-3). Shown in Figures 5-2, 5-6, and 5-16 are the factors thought to predispose to infection and to lead to the periductal mastitis component of MDAIDS. The presentation of the periductal inflammation and mastitis component spans a spectrum. At its minimum, the presentation is a subareolar tender mass, which occurs in 51% of women (see Table 5-3). This mass may resolve spontaneously after 3 to 4 days but then recur at intervals of a few months or longer, a time sequence rarely seen with other breast conditions (see Figure 5-2). The inflammatory process is associated with foreshortening of the ducts, which results in partial or total nipple inversion. The reported incidence of nipple retraction/inversion varies widely, but the condition occurs in approximately 48% of symptomatic patients (see Table 5-3). Often, patients present with multiple manifestations of MDAIDS. Thus, in one study with a 10% prevalence of nipple inversion, the condition was associated with a discharge in 24%.[36] Pain of a noncyclic nature is associated with the inflammatory process and in various studies has occurred in approximately 44% of patients. At its worst presentation, the inflammation has progressed to a later stage of the MDAIDS, presenting as an obvious, large, florid red, hot, tender, fluctuant subareolar abscess that points at the vermilion border. Before the abscess either drains spontaneously or is drained surgically, it can be associated with pain, fever, and other signs of systemic sepsis. After spontaneous drainage, a persistent periareolar mammary duct fistula appears. Fistulas have been reported to occur in 12% to 67% of patients presenting with symptomatic MDAIDS (see Table 5-3).[36,39] This is followed by the hallmark of this disease process—a recurrent subareolar abscess at a later date, either at the same site or in an adjacent segment of the breast. The frequency of treated recurrent breast abscess or fistula depends on the management of the disease but is estimated to occur in about one third of women. The study of Browning, Bigrigg, and Taylor[36] comparing symptomatic and incidental mammary duct ectasia tends to support these concepts. Many women have asymptomatic mammary duct ectasia. Symptomatic duct ectasia is secondary to infection that gives rise to sepsis, nipple changes, pain, and a subareolar mass (see Figure 5-2). These were the predominant features in patients in the study (see Table 5-5), which included 51 who had symptoms of duct ectasia and 103 in whom the duct ectasia component of MDAIDS was found incidentally. This is the only study of its kind in the literature.

The term *MDAIDS* gives cohesion to a variety of conditions of the breast that until now appeared to be unrelated. The surgeon needs to be familiar with the pathophysiology of these conditions to avoid unnecessary surgery and to provide the patient with effective treatment.

Clinical Features Related to Management of the Mammary Duct–Associated Inflammatory Disease Sequence

NIPPLE DISCHARGE

Nipple discharge may be an early manifestation of MDAIDS. Table 5-6 shows the causes of nipple discharge in 204 patients, based on the report by Tabar, Dean, and Pentek.[117] Physical examination revealed an ipsilateral palpable mass together with the discharge in only 29 of 204 patients. None of the patients with mammary duct ectasia had palpable masses or significant mammographic changes. Most of the women (88%) who had bloody discharge did not have cancer. Exfoliative cytologic examination was positive for only 11% (2 of 18) of patients with carcinoma. As in other series, the age distribution for patients with the mammary duct ectasia component of MDAIDS was 20 to 73 years; the median age was not given. Patients with cancer were older (see Figure 5-8 and Table 5-6).

TABLE 5-6 | General Causes and Frequency of Nipple Discharge, Palpable Mass, and Age Distribution in 204 Patients

| | | TYPE OF SECRETION (*n*) | | | | | PALPABLE | AGE (yr) | |
HISTOLOGIC DISEASE	CASES	MILKY	GREENISH	SEROUS	BLOODY	TOTAL	TUMOR (*n*)	RANGE	MEAN
Fibrocystic disease	65	3	24	16	22	65 (32%)	14	20-58	43
Mammary duct ectasia	23		3	7	13	23 (11%)		20-73	53
Papilloma	68			20	48	68 (33%)	5	28-81	51
Papillomatosis	30			8	22	30 (15%)	3	36-77	53
Carcinoma	18	—	—	3	15	18 (9%)	7	40-78	59
TOTAL	204	3	27	54	120	204 (100%)	29		

Modified from Tabar L et al: *Radiology* 149:31, 1983.

Clinical Features. The age distribution of 45 women presenting with intermittent nipple discharge, combined from three studies, is shown in Figure 5-9; the peak age at which discharge occurred was the midforties.[118-120] In general, most women with nipple discharge have benign disease. Although nipple discharge may be an early manifestation of MDAIDS, other causes include mammary dysplasia, intraductal papilloma, intraductal carcinoma, and invasive carcinoma. Only 4% of women with nipple discharge have breast cancer,[108] although reports of incidence vary in the literature.[8,55,121-123]

Intermittent nipple discharge occurs in 8% to 84% of patients with MDAIDS, most of them young, premenopausal women (see Table 5-3). In Browning's study, nipple discharge occurred in only 8% of women with incidental duct ectasia but in 65% of symptomatic

patients. The secretions vary from yellow, brown, or red to dark green, and the consistency varies from serosanguineous to toothpaste-like.[119,123,124] In the early stages, it may involve one ductal opening or one segment of the breast (Figure 5-10). At times, it may involve many ducts (Figure 5-11) and may be bilateral. Clinically, patients notice a stain on their clothes or bedsheets or expression of a discharge during routine breast self-examination. The occurrence of bilateral or multiple-duct, greenish or multicolored sticky discharge simultaneously with burning pain, itching, and swelling in the region of the nipple as the underlying disease process[123] strongly suggests the duct ectasia component of MDAIDS (see Figure 5-2). There is no relation to menstrual history, parity, or breastfeeding and no distinguishing factors as it relates to age at first pregnancy or menopause.

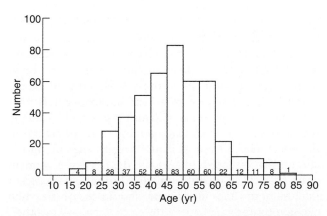

FIG. **5-9** Age distribution of 452 women with nipple discharge in nonmalignant breast disease culled from the literature. *(Data from Fischermann K et al: Acta Chir Scand 135:403, 1969; Rimsten A et al: Acta Chir Scand 142:513, 1976; and Chaudary MA et al: Ann Surg 196:651, 1982.)*

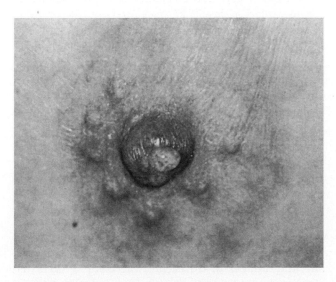

FIG. **5-10** Discharge from a single serosanguineous duct in a smoker. It was negative for occult blood.

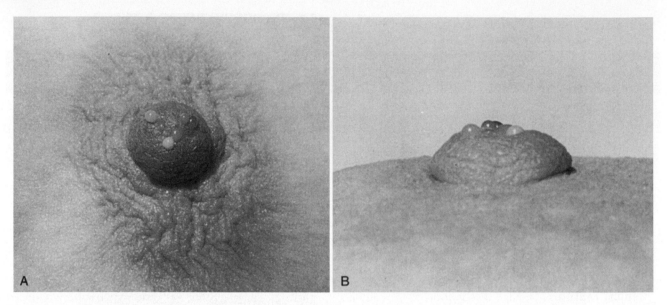

FIG. **5-11 A** and **B,** Multiple-duct nipple discharge, varying from green to yellow. It was sticky and negative for occult blood. Patient was a heavy smoker and complained of persistent subareolar nipple burning.

Investigation. A history should be obtained. The nature and quantity of the discharge, its spontaneity, and its relation to menstrual cycle, pregnancy, and occurrence of trauma should be determined. A number of medications, including agents for hormone replacement therapy, psychotropics, and antihypertensive drugs, as well as thyroid disorders and states of hyperprolactinemia, can cause nipple discharge. A persistent nipple discharge may be caused by hyperprolactinemia that is more often related to medications than to a pituitary adenoma (rare in clinical practice). Such physiologic discharges tend to be bilateral and multiductal in origin, and the secretion is clear to serous to milky and negative for occult blood. In such cases, serum prolactin should be measured, and if the value is elevated an appropriate endocrine workup should be initiated. If it is normal, the patient should be observed with monthly follow-ups. The patient's smoking habits should be addressed because of the relationship of MDAIDS and heavy smoking (see Figures 5-6 and 5-7).

The breast should be examined, and if a mass is identified, the duct or ducts from which the discharge comes should also be examined for masses. If a mass is identified, its management should be in accordance with that of a breast mass. In the absence of a mass, even if the nipple looks healthy, it should be inspected carefully while pressure is applied around the areola. Usually, pressure close to the areola and over the dilated subareolar mammary duct expresses the discharge. The site, the number of ducts, and the color of each discharge should be noted and recorded. The patient should express the nipple discharge to corroborate the physician's findings. Multiduct discharge indicates diffuse breast disease, often bilateral.

The clinical status of the subareolar ducts, as they course through the nipple, is assessed by gently palpating the ducts with the "finger-and-thumb" test, in which the intranipple and subnipple ducts are rolled between the tips of the finger and thumb (Figure 5-12, *A*). The normal feel can be described as a "grooved sensation," in which each mammary duct is clearly palpable as a thin cord. In ectasia, the mammary ducts are thickened with various degrees of duct inflammation. If the nipple discharge is associated with significant periductal inflammation, axillary lymphadenopathy may be found.[47]

With progressive degrees of mammary duct inflammation and fibrosis, the finger-and-thumb test becomes progressively more positive, because the digits cannot be approximated below the nipple, indicating thickening of the mammary ducts or the presence of a blue-domed cyst. Eventually, as the disease progresses, the fingertips are separated by a firm, nontender mass that appears to be continuous with and inseparable from the nipple (Figure 5-12, *B*). Such a mass is either central to the subareolar area or deviated toward the side of the chronically diseased mammary ducts. For a woman older than 35 years with unilateral nipple discharge, a mammogram and ultrasound should be obtained to exclude cancer.

Several investigations should be done. First should be exfoliative cytologic evaluation of the discharge by Papanicolaou smear and Romanowsky's stain

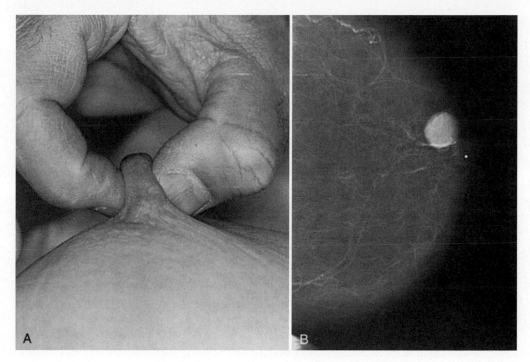

F I G. **5-12 A,** The finger-and-thumb test to assess degree of inflammatory involvement and dilation of subareolar mammary ducts. **B,** Craniocaudal mammogram view of left breast. Small white dot is nipple marker. Large round lesion is a blue-domed cyst of a major subareolar mammary duct. The finger-and-thumb test was grossly positive.

(methylene blue and eosin). Normal cytologic findings do not exclude an ongoing benign pathologic process or cancer. Typically, epithelial atypia is noted. A second study is bacteriologic culture of expressed discharge, a sample of which is obtained after cleaning of the nipple and surrounding areola with isopropyl alcohol. Two bacteriologic swab specimens should be taken: one for anaerobic culture and the other for aerobic culture.[58] In most cases (about 60%) involving nipple discharge associated with the duct ectasia component of MDAIDS, anaerobic bacteria are isolated from the nipple discharge and the ratio of anaerobes to aerobes is about 3:1.[58,65] Finally, the discharge should be tested for occult blood; in 64% of cases the test is positive.[26,63,117,118] An occult blood–positive discharge does not necessarily indicate cancer but suggests intraductal disease, whereas a clear discharge does not rule out cancer.[8,55,121-123,125]

If the cytologic analysis of a unilateral duct discharge is not contributory or if the discharge tests positive for occult blood, ductography should be performed (Figure 5-13, A). Ductography is a relatively simple technique whereby a small amount (0.1 to 1.5 ml) of sterile water-soluble contrast medium is injected into the discharging duct and the duct architecture is displayed mammographically. It is one way to rule out and determine the nature, extent, and location of intraductal lesions other than squamous metaplasia that are causing a discharge. It is particularly valuable when there are no other symptoms and neither physical examination nor mammography reveals the underlying cause. Successful visualization of duct lesions requires a skilled radiologist. Ductography repeated shortly before surgery with use of a mixture of 1% methylene blue dye and contrast medium, demonstrates to the surgeon the status of the duct at operation, facilitating more precise and less radical surgery. Ultrasound is useful for visualizing the dilated ducts, their points of obstruction, and associated cysts (Figure 5-13, B). In more advanced cases, fine-needle aspiration (FNA) cytologic examination of the indurated mass should reveal foamy macrophages and inflammatory cells, and FNA of a mass for bacteriologic studies will reveal mixed flora with a major anaerobic component.[53,65,126,127]

Treatment Plan. In the absence of a subareolar induration or mass and in the presence of a normal mammogram, if a single duct is involved and if the discharge is purulent or green and sticky, the patient should be treated with antibiotics. These should cover both aerobes and anaerobes.[58,65,128] A suitable

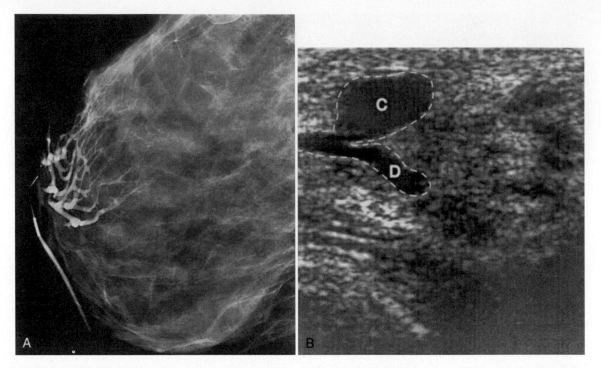

FIG. **5-13** **A,** Ductogram that was occult blood positive for a heavy smoker, showing multiple dilated and varicosed ducts. Pathology showed squamous metaplasia. **B,** Sonographic image showing a dilated duct *(D)* with obstruction and communicating cyst *(C)*. *(Courtesy Beverly Spirt, M.D., Department of Radiology, Breast Care Program, SUNY Health Science Center at Syracuse, NY.)*

combination includes a cephalosporin and metronidazole, each at a dosage of 500 mg by mouth three times a day for 10 days. It is anticipated that the infection will improve, and thereafter the patient is observed. However, recurrent infection after antibiotic therapy alone is not infrequent; to avoid disappointment, this possibility should be communicated to the patient. Recurrence should be expected because the underlying disease process has not been eradicated and this process is not covered by the antibiotics. If the discharge is not cleared by antibiotic therapy, a second 10-day course of antibiotics should be prescribed.

If the discharge is from multiple ducts and is persistent, is occult blood positive, and has not responded to antibiotic treatment, then on the basis of clinical judgment, surgery may be indicated. If during surgery the duct system as a whole is considered abnormal (Figure 5-14) or the presence of a blue-domed cyst (Figure 5-15) is noted, then the major subareolar mammary duct system should be excised.[44] A summary of the clinical evaluation and treatment is shown in Figure 5-16.

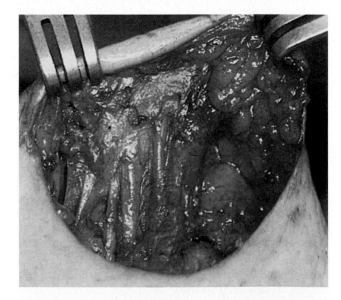

FIG. **5-14** Multiple dilated subareolar mammary ducts in a previous heavy smoker complaining of nipple discharge and pain. Pathologic analysis showed duct ectasia, periductal fibrosis, mild ductal epithelial hyperplasia, and chronic inflammatory infiltrate. Patient initially presented with multiple breast abscesses of the opposite breast 2 years previously while she was a smoker. Thereafter, she had stopped smoking.

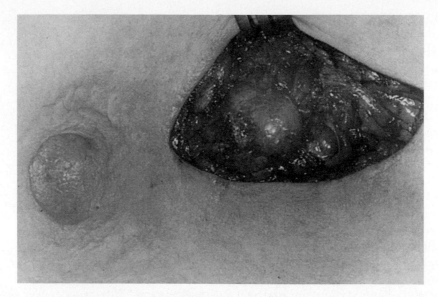

FIG. **5-15** Blue-domed cyst situated in lateral aspect subareolarly of the left breast. Pathologic analysis showed apocrine metaplasia, microcalcification, and papillomatosis.

Condition	Incidence of MDAIDS stage	Clinical presentation	Clinical evaluation	Treatment
Mammary duct ectasia	100%	Asymptomatic n = 3509 (Table 5-2) • Nipple discharge-single/ multiple ducts; nipple crusting • Duct retraction • Nipple inversion • Noninflammatory subareolar induration/mass (Table 5-3)	History Physical examination Cytology of discharge Occult blood of discharge Mammogram if mass/ induration present Ductogram FNA cytology	Antibiotics: metronidazole and a cephalosporin 500 mg tid for 10 days; duct excision; duct plate excision
Periductal inflammation/ mastitis	Mean 20%	Symptomatic n = 10,195 (Table 5-2) • Pain (noncyclic mastalgia) 44% • Nipple inversion 48% • Subareolar inflammatory mass 57%	History/physical examination FNA cytology Mammogram Ductogram	Discontinue smoking, antibiotics (as above); duct excision; duct plate excision; retinoic acid (future)
Subareolar breast abscess	Mean: 21% of patients with breast sepsis 4.2% of all BEMADID	(From Table 5-11) • Red, hot, tender, abscess 15% • Spontaneously drained; surgically drained	History/physical examination FNA cytology to rule out cancer C&S for origin	Antibiotics (as above); incision and drainage; excise duct(s); retinoic acid (future)
Peri- areolar fistula	Mean: 4.2% of patients with sepsis	Untreated 100% Sinus opening to fistula heals over; spontaneous recurrence of abscess with repeated discharge via fistula		Excise fistula and duct; close 2nd intention

FIG. **5-16** Clinical evaluation and treatment of the mammary duct–associated inflammatory disease sequence (MDAIDS), showing incidences of the stages of MDAIDS.

MDAIDS-RELATED BREAST PAIN AND TENDERNESS

Continuous noncyclic breast pain and tenderness may also be an early manifestation of MDAIDS. It need not present after a mammary duct discharge in the sequence of MDAIDS-related symptoms (see Figures 5-2, 5-6, and 5-16). On occasion, it may be the presenting symptom. A comprehensive discussion of mastalgia and its management is included in Chapter 10.

Clinical Features. The age distribution of 272 women who presented with noncyclic mastalgia in two studies is shown in Figure 5-17.[123,129] The peak symptoms occur in the midthirties. Breast pain falls into three broad groups: costochondral pain, lateral chest wall pain, and cyclic or noncyclic breast pain (Figure 5-18). Two thirds of women with mastalgia have cyclic pain, and one third have noncyclic pain.[130] Noncyclic breast pain is a recognized symptom of the mammary duct ectasia phase of MDAIDS.[41] It appears to be related to periductal inflammation. In a study by Preece and colleagues,[131] 25% of 232 patients with mastalgia had pain related to the duct ectasia and the periductal inflammatory components of MDAIDS.

The pain is quite exquisite. It is not a referred pain but arises from the breast itself. It is often continuous, characterized by burning, usually behind the nipple. It is characterized by aching of both breasts and tenderness. It is unpredictable in occurrence and does not vary with the menstrual cycle.[132] In a study by Maddox of 33 patients, the mean duration of pain was about 36 months (range, 5 to 156 months).[133] Similarly, in the study by Preece and colleagues[131] of the 62 patients with noncyclic pain related to mammary duct ectasia and periductal inflammation of MDAIDS, two thirds had had symptoms for 12 months or longer and only 5 of the 62 had had pain for less than 5 months on

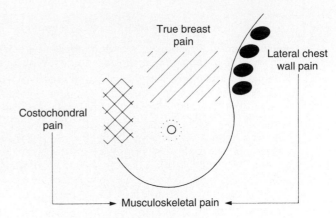

FIG. **5-18** Site of noncyclic breast pain. *(From Maddox PR et al: Br J Surg 76:901, 1989.)*

presentation. This pain comes on abruptly, is often worse in cold weather, is at the same site with serial visits, and disappears as suddenly as it appeared. Often, the history notes that the breast is "supersensitive." The patient's smoking habits should always be ascertained because of the evidence that noncyclic breast pain of MDAIDS is associated with heavy smoking (see Figures 5-6 and 5-7).

MDAIDS-related noncyclic breast pain can be distinguished from cyclic breast pain by recording the type of pain for 3 months on charts. Cyclic breast pain is typically poorly localized and in most instances is bilateral. The pain is usually described as heavy, increasing in severity from midcycle onward and improving with menstruation yet varying in severity from cycle to cycle. The breast is tender to touch.

Noncyclic breast pain related to MDAIDS can be distinguished from chest wall pain by either tender costochondral junctions (Tietze's syndrome) or tenderness along the ribs (musculoskeletal pain). Musculoskeletal pain is unilateral in more than 90% of the cases and is localized along the chest wall and costochondral junction. In contrast with noncyclic breast pain of MDAIDS, the mean duration of symptoms with musculoskeletal pain is shorter: 14.7 months (range, 2 to 48 months).[133] This type of pain responds well to a combination of lidocaine and hydrocortisone injected into the musculoskeletal site.

Investigation. A detailed history of the pain should be obtained: its clinical features, character, relationship to menstruation, site, radiation, and duration and factors that exacerbate or relieve it. Through physical examination, costochondral pain and lateral chest wall pain should be ruled out. The breast should be palpated gently for intramammary lesions, nipple discharge, or a trigger point. Mammography should be performed. Radiographic features that can be

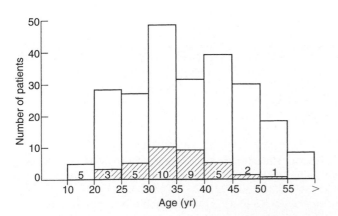

FIG. **5-17** Distribution by age of patients presenting with noncyclic breast pain. *(Data from Maddox PR et al: Br J Surg 76:901, 1989; and Preece PE: Practitioner 226:1373, 1982.)*

| TABLE **5-7** | General Management of Mastalgia |

1. Exclude cancer: Physical examination, mammography, and biopsy where indicated. For unremitting localized pain, follow frequently for at least 1 yr with repeat studies to exclude early cancer.

2. Adequate reassurance that the condition is benign will allow at least 85% of patients to accept and tolerate their pain. Those who require active treatment after reassurance are given a pain chart so that the pattern and severity of the pain can be monitored over the next 3 mo.

3. Noncyclic mastalgia can be treated with the expectation of an overall response rate of 44%. Individual drugs are no better than placebo, overall, but each drug appears to help a different group of patients. At present, there are no guidelines for predicting success for an individual drug. To reduce disappointment, patients should be warned before treatment of the low response rate. Most patients in this group, however, are willing to try any therapy with even a small chance of improvement, and they appreciate a frank assessment of the outcome.

4. Relapse is treated by recommencing the drug that was previously effective. With danazol, relapse may occur while the dose is being reduced or while the patient is taking maintenance doses. If the relapse is mild, a return to the previous dose may be sufficient to control the pain, but if symptoms are severe, return to the initial dose of 100 mg twice daily is usually necessary. Once the pain has been controlled, the dose can be reduced at monthly or 6-wk intervals to the maintenance dose for that patient. Symptoms are often exacerbated by emotional upheavals—bereavement and divorce in particular—although there is good evidence that the primary basis of the symptom is not psychologic in most cases.

5. Patients must be given adequate contraceptive advice, because drug treatment may interfere with the contraceptive pill and some patients' fertility may be enhanced by bromocriptine. Should pregnancy occur, the treatment must be discontinued immediately to avoid any untoward effects on the fetus.

Modified from Pye JK et al: *Lancet* 2:373, 1985.

associated with MDAIDS are coarse calcifications and the flame-shaped shadows of active periductal mastitis.[61,134,135]

In most patients, these findings are confined to the site of complaint. In addition, dilated ducts may be seen elsewhere in the breast or in the contralateral gland. For analysis of breast pain, ductography is seldom useful, and FNA cytology is neither rewarding nor cost effective.

Treatment Plan. After obvious pathologic causes of pain have been excluded and the patient has been assured that there is no cancer, usually no active treatment is needed, but wearing a firm supporting bra 24 hours a day and taking a nonsteroidal antiinflammatory drug or a mild analgesic for the duration of the pain often provides comfort (Table 5-7).[130,132,136,137] Overall, 44% of patients with noncyclic mastalgia reported a lasting response (i.e., no return of symptoms within 6 months of finishing therapy).

If this fails, some women with noncyclic MDAIDS-related breast pain respond to drugs used for cyclic mastalgia (Table 5-8). If their pain returns when treatment is stopped or the dose is reduced, these patients

| TABLE **5-8** | Drugs Used to Treat Cyclic Mastalgia |

AGENT	ACTION	DOSE	PREVALENCE OF SIDE EFFECTS
Danazol	Antigonadotropin: acts on pituitary-ovarian axis	200 mg/day for 2-4 mo; discontinued or decreased to 100 mg/day for 2 mo; then 100 mg on alternate days for 2 mo	22% abnormal menstrual cycle; headache; nausea; weight gain (6% severe)
Bromocriptine	Inhibits prolactin secretion	1.25 mg/day, increasing 1.25 mg every 7 day to a maximum of 2.5 mg/day for 2-4 mo, then stopped	33%: nausea; headaches; postural hypotension; constipation; depression (15% severe)
Evening primrose oil (rich in essential fatty acids)	Via prostaglandin pathways	6 capsules/day for 3-6 mo	2%: bloating; vague nausea

Data from Pye JK et al: *Lancet* 2:373, 1985.

should undergo treatment again with the drug to which the original response was good. If the initial response was poor or if troublesome side effects occurred, the patient should be treated with a different drug. For a few patients with sufficiently severe noncyclic MDAIDS-related breast pain, excision of all the major subareolar mammary duct systems is warranted.

NIPPLE RETRACTION AND SUBAREOLAR MASS AS RELATED TO MDAIDS

A change in nipple contour and retraction of an isolated opening of a nipple duct are among the early clinical features of MDAIDS. As the disease progresses, duct dilation and squamous metaplasia are accompanied by inflammatory changes and infiltration with lymphocytes. Periductal fibrosis with duct wall thickening occurs during chronic inflammation, and as ducts are destroyed and repaired, this leads to shortening of ducts and subsequent changes in nipple contour, flattening and retraction of the nipple, or deviation of the nipple (Figure 5-19). Although it is consistently publicized as an early sign of breast cancer, in most cases, nipple retraction is benign.

Mammary duct ectasia of MDAIDS is the most common pathologic cause of nipple inversion seen in well-breast clinics. In the series by Browning, Bigrigg, and Taylor,[36] the incidence varies from 10% to 24% in symptomatic MDAIDS patients, depending on the presence of discharge. Nipple inversion was reported to be noted in 7% of women in whom the mammary duct ectasia component of MDAIDS was found incidentally.[36] Nipple retraction tends to be slowly progressive, with the retraction becoming more marked with time. The process continues until it is complete and the whole nipple becomes inverted. The contralateral nipple may show similar changes, often lagging months or years in the development of retraction. In patients with mammary duct retractions, the incidence of bilaterality is approximately 15%.[137]

When the continuity of the duct epithelium is broken, lipoid material escapes through the duct wall, leading to a marked yellowish gray induration of the surrounding tissue. The mass, with or without obvious inflammation, is firm and circumscribed. At this stage, nipple retraction and dimpling are often present, and consequently the lesion is frequently misdiagnosed as carcinoma. Pain and tenderness with repeated inflammatory changes, both occurring over a long period, tend to rule out such a diagnosis; however, this should be confirmed pathologically via biopsy.

In addition to the usual atrophic epithelial changes in the duct epithelium and inflammatory reaction in the duct wall, there may be a marked cellular inflammatory response. The inflammatory cells consist chiefly of lymphocytes and plasma cells or almost entirely of plasma cells (plasma cell mastitis). Phagocytic giant cells surround the lipoid material, and an infiltration of histiocytes occurs in the breast stroma.

Clinical Features. Nipple retraction is painless and of little consequence to the patient, except to rule out cancer. Presenting symptoms range from minor nipple abnormalities to complete nipple retraction. Minor degrees of nipple retraction occur early in disease[138] and in one study were present in up to 75% of patients presenting with periareolar inflammation.[139] When the degree of retraction is slight, it can be missed unless carefully sought. Marked retraction or nipple inversion occurs later and develops during the course of repeated periductal inflammation.[1] The earliest change detected is characterized by retraction of the central portion of the nipple, showing a slight elliptical pattern in a horizontal plane. Nipple retraction is commonly associated with slight spontaneous nipple discharge, which at this stage of the disease process is usually multiductal and multicolored, consistent with duct ectasia.

Investigation. A correct diagnosis of MDAIDS can be made on the basis of history and examination. Length of history and onset of symptoms is of great importance. The time course of the observed changes should be elicited and is critical for a correct diagnosis, as is obtaining a history of episodes of inflammation.

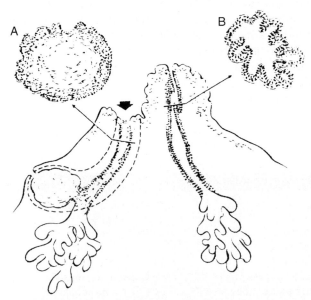

FIG. 5-19 Squamous metaplasia *(A)* often coexists with retraction of the nipple and plugging of the lactiferous duct with epithelial debris. Resulting suppuration breaks out at areolar margin. Dotted line designates margin of dissection recommended in core excision. In the normal situation *(B)*, cuboidal epithelium and ductal continuity are maintained. Note pleating in lactiferous sinus. *(From Powell BC et al: South Med J 70:935, 1977.)*

Both point to an ongoing subclinical inflammatory process consistent with MDAIDS, because nipple retraction can develop after one or two inflammatory episodes. Long-standing nipple inversion arising at puberty or during pregnancy and lactation is always benign and is easily recognized. Usually it is bilateral, but not invariably, with a significant slitlike appearance and no deformity of the areolas or surrounding skin.

A surgical opinion is generally sought when nipple retraction is first noticed. Alternatively, patients are not aware of these long-standing nipple changes unless they are accompanied by discharge, pain, or a mass. Typically, the duration of retraction is long. Rees, Gravelle, and Hughes[138] reported on a series of 30 patients (aged 25 to 75 years; mean, 52 years) with nipple retraction associated with the mammary duct ectasia phase of MDAIDS. The duration of retraction was 3 months to 16 months. The patient's smoking habits are important because of the evidence that nipple retraction of MDAIDS is associated with heavy smoking (see Figures 5-6 and 5-7).

Next, the breast should be examined carefully and in different positions to characterize the pattern of nipple retraction and to assess features that favor the diagnosis of mammary duct ectasia/periductal inflammation or cancer.[138] On physical examination, a typical transverse central inversion of the nipple is seen (Figure 5-20). In MDAIDS the nipple can usually be everted manually. The ability to evert the nipple, the presence of palpable ectatic mammary ducts felt as cords just beneath the nipple when performing the finger-and-thumb test (see Figure 5-12, *A*), and the absence of a mass help exclude a diagnosis of cancer. The breast is examined for nipple discharge and to

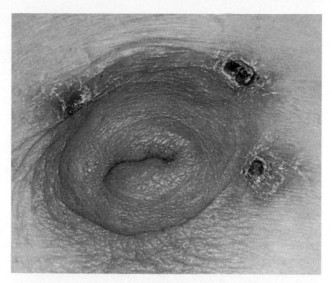

FIG. **5-21** Complete inversion of the central portion of the nipple, resulting in characteristic transverse nipple inversion with surrounding edema but without deformity of the remaining nipple. Patient also has signs of three periareolar fistulas.

rule out other causes of nipple inversion. If a mass is present, its size and location should be determined. In patients with long-standing and repeated episodes of subareolar inflammation, the central portion of the nipple becomes inverted and edematous (Figure 5-21).

Diagnostic difficulty arises in women who present usually in their fifties to seventies, with recent retraction of the nipple. Women older than age 40 years who present with sudden unilateral nipple retraction should be presumed to harbor a malignancy until proved otherwise. In MDAIDS, retraction of the nipples commonly precedes the development of the inflammatory reactions, especially in young women. With an acute breast abscess, the retraction is usually asymmetric. In contrast, with carcinoma the retraction is usually complete with distortion of the areolas, and there is seldom a serous or blood-stained discharge. Nipple retraction caused by carcinoma is a result of involvement of breast ducts by cancer, resulting in distortion because the cancer is commonly to one side, producing tilting or distortion of the nipple toward the tumor. The differences between nipple retraction of the mammary duct ectasia and periductal inflammation components of MDAIDS and that of carcinoma are detailed in Table 5-9. Mammography and ultrasound are necessary to exclude carcinoma in the retroareolar area in all patients.

Treatment. Treatment depends on the presence or absence of a mass.

Patient with No Mass. Younger patients with mammographically dense breasts are reassessed every 3 months. Older patients with fatty, atrophic breasts who have a negative mammogram are confidently

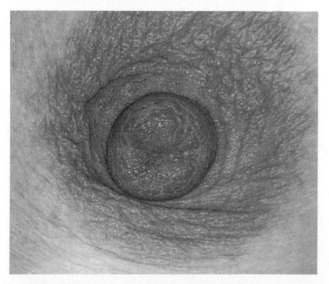

FIG. **5-20** Early central nipple inversion that developed during the previous 2 years in a smoker who was otherwise asymptomatic.

| TABLE 5-9 | Differential Diagnosis of Nipple Retraction of the MDAIDS Phase with Mammary Duct Ectasia and Carcinoma (Conditions Could Coexist) |

CLINICAL/INVESTIGATIVE FEATURE	MAMMARY DUCT ECTASIA OF MDAIDS	CARCINOMA
History	>1 yr (present since puberty)	<1 yr
Pain (%)	33	<10
Discharge	Creamy, green	Serous, blood stained
Nipple (examine carefully)	Partial, central, symmetrical retraction, often bilateral	Complete unilateral retraction with deformity of areola
Mass	Tender, firm lesion with discrete outline	Nontender, hard lesion with ragged outline
Mammography	Excludes cancer; minor ductal dilatation; in multiparas, atrophic fatty, premenopausal or postmenopausal; seen as tubular densities, sometimes beaded, extending from base of nipple fanning out into breast disk; in younger patients, breast disk is dense, breast ducts are transradiant tubular shadows; smooth, coarse calcification, rounded or branched; within ducts; unilateral or bilateral nipple retraction	
Cytology	Foam cells	Malignant glandular cells
Ductography	Ectatic ducts	Intraluminal mass
Fine-needle aspiration	Cystic lesion, no residual mass, no blood on aspiration	Hard lesion; malignant glandular cells
Mass	Biopsy	Biopsy
Follow-up	No mass: reexamine every 4 mo and take annual mammogram	

MDAIDS, Mammary duct–associated inflammatory disease sequence.

assured that there is no serious disease and are seen every 6 months, with a repeat mammogram at 1 year.

Patient with Palpable Mass. FNA cytologic analysis of the mass should be performed to rule out carcinoma. In MDAIDS, FNA cytologic examination shows foamy macrophages and inflammatory cells. If the mass is cystic, the fluid should be removed, tested for occult blood, and sent for cytologic examination. If the cytologic analysis is negative, the fluid contains no blood, and the mass disappears completely, management is similar to that for patients without a palpable mass. If there is a residual mass, excision biopsy is recommended. The subsequent management is based on the biopsy results. If the biopsy is negative for cancer, the patient should be followed up with repeat examinations and mammograms, initially at 4 months. The clinical evaluation and treatment are summarized in Figure 5-16.

SUBAREOLAR BREAST ABSCESS AND RECURRENT SUBAREOLAR BREAST ABSCESS AS RELATED TO MDAIDS

In the sequence of the pathophysiology of MDAIDS outlined in Figures 5-1, 5-2, and 5-16, the introduction of bacteria to the histopathologic stage of subareolar periductal inflammation leads to infection, manifesting ultimately as a subareolar breast abscess. Subareolar abscess is a challenging clinical entity. There are ample comments in the literature on the high incidence of persistence, recurrence, and bilaterality.[21,28,51,140]

Most reports on breast abscess identify mixed organisms with a major anaerobic component as the predominant bacterial flora in this disease. Table 5-10 typifies the spectrum of bacteria isolated from 29 women with breast abscesses.[65] Many of the anaerobic bacteria isolated are also commonly found in the vaginal vault, and prior vaginal manipulation leads to a hematogenous spread of these bacteria in a fashion comparable to the hematogenous, transient bacteremia that occurs with mastication. It has been reported that 10% of bacteremias that occur in the hospital are caused by anaerobes[127] and that even simple procedures such as sigmoidoscopy may lead to the presence of transient *Bacillus fragilis* in the blood.[141] The transient bacteremia following vaginal manipulation has been documented to be associated with anaerobic breast abscess.[142] In addition, facultative and obligate anaerobic microorganisms are also normal inhabitants of the oropharynx, and in smokers the flora of the oropharynx is predominantly anaerobic. This may be a source for subareolar mammary duct inoculation following oral stimulation

TABLE **5-10** Spectrum of Bacteria Isolated from 29 Women with a Breast Abscess

GENUS	ORGANISMS (n)
Aerobes	
Staphylococcus*	24
Streptococcus	4
Bacillus	2
Corynebacterium	1
Escherichia	1
Proteus	1
Pseudomonas	2
Anaerobes	
Actinomyces	3
Clostridium	2
Fusobacterium	1
Mitsuokella	1
Bacteroides*	8
Lactobacillus	3
Eubacterium	3
Propionibacterium*	16
Peptostreptococcus*	34
Veillonella	2

From Walker AP et al: *Arch Surg* 123:908, 1988.
*Predominant genus.

of the breast,[65] and stagnant mammary duct secretions form an ideal medium for bacterial infection.

Finally, coagulase-negative staphylococci, normally present on the skin, adhere to the squamous epithelial cells derived from the galactophores or colonize the nipple skin and may be yet another source of the infection.[143] All of these sites may contribute to the endogenous bacterial flora of the normal breast.[63,64] Finally, as shown in Table 5-4, these abscesses are not limited to females but also tend to occur in men who are heavy smokers, presumably also via hematogenous spread of oral bacteria secondary to mastication.

Anaerobic breast abscesses are usually seen in women of childbearing age with an inverted nipple and are due to underlying duct ectasia or chronic breast disease that provides a suitable nidus for the adhesion of these anaerobes.

Subareolar breast abscesses in the spectrum of MDAIDS are found in about 20% of patients with symptomatic MDAIDS undergoing surgery (see Table 5-11 and Figure 5-16). Both breasts are affected equally.[36] In approximately 10% of patients with subareolar abscess, the process is bilateral at presentation. Less frequent is the finding of multiple abscesses in one breast (see Figure 5-21) or an active small, acute, subareolar abscess with other areas of induration around the same

TABLE **5-11** Frequency of Recurrence or Subareolar Breast Abscess after Operation for MDAIDS

INVESTIGATORS	PATIENTS WITH LOCAL BREAST SEPSIS*/TOTAL "OPERATED PATIENTS"	SURGICAL PROCEDURE	RECURRENCE/OUTCOME
Hadfield, 1960 and 1968[44,45]	30/99	Excision major duct system	No recurrence (follow-up,1-7 yr)
Urban, 1963[54]	19/113	Excision major duct system	No recurrence (follow-up, ½-14 yr)
Ekland and Zeigler, 1973[52]	38/—	Incision and drainage, 27; duct excision, 11	Total recurrence, 15 (40%); incision and drainage, 11/27 (41%); duct excision, 4/11 (36%)
Thomas et al, 1982[41]	9/78	Incision and drainage	Recurrence, 7/9 (78%); abscess and one fistula, 7 (78%) (2 [22%] eventually had simple mastectomy)
Browning et al, 1986[36]	11/51	Excisional biopsy, 51% Formal duct excision, 41% Nipple retraction, 6% Mastectomy, 1%	Needed further operation, 12 (24%) Reoperated for sepsis, 11 (45%)
Scholefield et al, 1987[60]	28/—	Incision and drainage, 28 Hadfield procedure (secondary operation), 6	Further problems, 21 (75%), including 9 (32%) with fistulas No recurrence
Watt-Boolsen et al, 1987[22]	34/—	Incision and healing by granulation	Recurrence, 11/32 (34%) (10/11 fistulas; two patients lost to follow-up)
Hughes, 1989[144]	—/122	Subareolar dissection	Complication, 34 (28%)
Hartley et al, 1991[46]	13/46	Subareolar dissection	Recurrent sepsis, 8 (62%), including one fistula

MDAIDS, Mammary duct–associated inflammatory disease sequence.
*Abscess and/or fistula.

| TABLE 5-12 | Surgical Procedure and Frequency of Recurrence of Subareolar Breast Abscess or Fistula |

SURGICAL PROCEDURE	INVESTIGATOR	PATIENTS WITH LOCAL SEPSIS* (n)	RECURRENCE/OUTCOME
Excision of major duct system (Hadfield ductectomy)	Hadfield, 1960[44,45]	30	No recurrence
	Urban, 1963[54]	19	No recurrence
	Thomas et al, 1982[41]	7[†]	2 (29%) recurrences
	Browning et al, 1986[36]	21[‡]	1 (4%) required further surgery
	Scholefield et al, 1987[60]	6[†]	"Took care of problem"
	Meguid et al, 1995[19]	11	No recurrence
Incision and drainage	Ekland and Zeigler, 1973[52]	27	15 (41%) recurrences
	Thomas et al, 1982[41]	9	7 (78%) recurrences
	Scholefield et al, 1987[60]	28	21 (75%) further problems, including 9 (32%) fistulas
	Watt-Boolsen et al, 1987[22]	32	11 (34%) recurrences, including 10 fistulas
Duct excision	Ekland and Zeigler, 1973[52]	11	4 (36%) recurrences
	Browning et al, 1986[36]	26[‡]	11 (42%) repeat surgery
Subareolar dissection	Hartley et al, 1991[46]	13	8 (62%) recurrences, including 1 fistula

*Local sepsis (abscess and/or fistula).
†Secondary surgery after recurrence following incision and drainage.
‡Symptomatic (51 patients, including 10 with local sepsis).

nipple. Initially, a lesion can be a discrete tender lump with reddening of the skin that subsides spontaneously without drainage. In about half of the cases, however, there will be recurrence with eventual pointing, followed by either spontaneous or surgical drainage. Following only incision and drainage, the reported recurrence rate, as shown in Table 5-12, varies from 34% to 78%.[22,41]

Recurrence reflects the inadequacy of the operative treatment provided for the initial presentation of a subareolar breast abscess (i.e., merely surgical incision and drainage), because it is not based on a conceptual understanding of the underlying disease process and abnormality, which persist after the local operative procedure.

Clinical Features. As shown in Figures 5-1, 5-2, and 5-16, the penultimate stage in the pathophysiology of MDAIDS is a subareolar abscess, but there is considerable overlap in the sequence of the presenting symptoms. It is the ongoing active infection with an abscess that brings many patients with MDAIDS to the surgeon's attention; the antecedent disease process may have been sufficiently subclinical to have gone unnoticed or been forgotten by the patient except in hindsight. Subareolar breast abscess in relation to MDAIDS is a different lesion from a peripheral breast abscess or an abscess associated with lactation (Figure 5-22). Among 50 women with breast abscess,

Acute Peripheral Breast Abscess

Age: <40 yr
Etiology: Lactating/puerperium blocked duct
Site: Peripheral wedge
Organism: *Staphylococcus aureus*
Resolution: Invariable after drainage

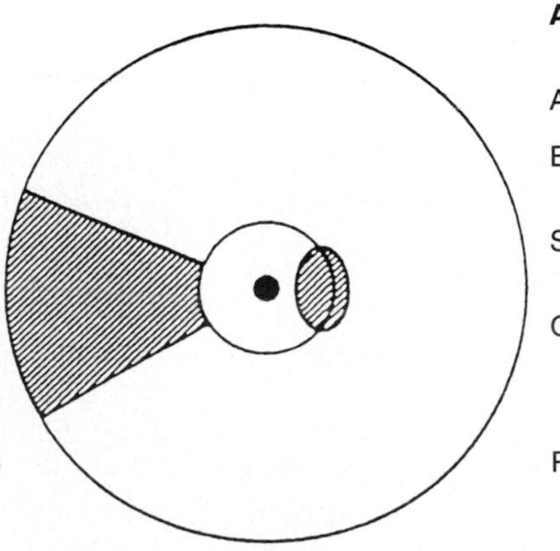

Acute Subareolar Breast Abscess Associated with Duct Ectasia

Age: Mean, 34 yr*
Etiology: Ectatic ducts, areas of squamous metaplasia of duct lining, with periductal inflammation
Site: Periareolar (preexisting nipple inversion and discharge)
Organism: *Staphylococcus aureus*
Bacteroides
Streptococcus (aerobes and anaerobes)
Enterococci (Table 5-10)
Resolution: Chronic local ongoing sepsis common despite incision and drainage, and often after subareolar dissection (Table 5-12)

*Mean of ages given in refs. 4, 43, 52, and 142.

FIG. 5-22 The main differences between an acute peripheral abscess and a subareolar abscess related to the mammary duct–associated inflammatory disease sequence (MDAIDS) are summarized. *(Modified from Benson EA: World J Surg 13:753, 1989.)*

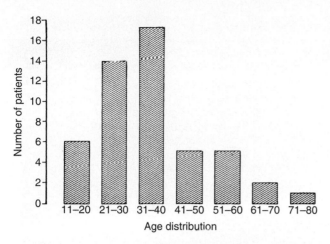

FIG. **5-23** Of the 50 patients with breast abscess, 38 had a subareolar breast abscess and 12 had a peripheral breast abscess. *(Data from Ekland DA, Zeigler MG:* Arch Surg *107:398, 1973.)*

38 had a subareolar abscesses and 12 had a peripheral abscess (Figure 5-23). The age ranges in several series of patients with only subareolar breast abscesses for whom these data were available are combined in Table 5-13. These agree with the age span shown in Figure 5-23 and generally with those previously reported.[28,38,39,44,45] The general impression is that the peak incidence of subareolar abscess occurs in the fourth decade, predominantly in nonlactating premenopausal women.

Investigation. The characteristic features in the history are rapid onset of acute breast pain, tenderness, and swelling of the central subareolar tissue. There is no history of trauma, fibrocystic condition, or cancer. In our experience, a number of our patients who

presented with an acute subareolar breast abscess had a history of antibiotic treatment for breast inflammation that occurred 3 to 4 days after a routine pelvic examination, as previously reported by Leach, Eykyn, and Phillips.[142] At the time they presented for surgery for the acute abscess, which occurred 3 to 4 months later, these patients were found to have gross evidence of duct ectasia, which must have been present but asymptomatic at the time of the pelvic examination.

In subacute cases, symptoms can exist for 1 week, whereas with chronic, poorly drained abscesses treated frequently with antibiotics, symptoms can last for more than 10 years. A medical history of similar problems that were treated either with antibiotics or, if the abscess was well established, with surgical incision and drainage, is often reported. Alternatively, the subareolar abscess drained spontaneously. All acute and subacute symptoms usually resolved with treatment, and this is generally followed by an asymptomatic period, an interval of months to years of apparent resolution followed by recurrence.[28,52] Finally, the patient's smoking habits need to be determined because of the evidence that infectious complications of MDAIDS are associated with heavy smoking (see Figures 5-5 and 5-6).

On physical examination the characteristic features are a florid acute abscess with local tenderness, swelling, erythema, sloughing of skin, and induration or a fluctuation (Figure 5-24). With chronic, recurrent abscesses a draining periarcolar fistula is most often seen (Figure 5-25). On occasion, a purulent nipple discharge is observed.

The diagnosis is made on clinical grounds. In acute subareolar breast abscess, neither mammography, ultrasound, nor FNA cytologic analysis is warranted for diagnostic purposes, although ultrasound can be useful when patients present with early symptoms (Figure 5-26). However, in women older than 40 years

TABLE **5-13** | Age of Patients with Breast Abscess Related to MDAIDS

| INVESTIGATORS | PATIENTS (*n*) | AGE (yr) | | |
		RANGE	MEAN	MEDIAN
Hadfield, 1960[44]	6	27-33	30	—
Abramson, 1969[39]	5	32-38	35	—
Caswell and Maier, 1969[51]	15	25-48	—	—
Habif et al, 1970[28]	146	20-59	36	—
Ekland and Zeigler, 1973[52]	38	14-72	34	—
Leach et al, 1979[53]	9	24-71	35	—
Golinger and O'Neal, 1982[56]	46	13-79	30	—
Watt-Boolsen et al, 1987[22]	34	15-92	—	—
Hartley et al, 1991[46]	13	18-78	—	—
Meguid et al, 1995[19]	24	26-61	—	33

MDAIDS, Mammary duct–associated inflammatory disease sequence.

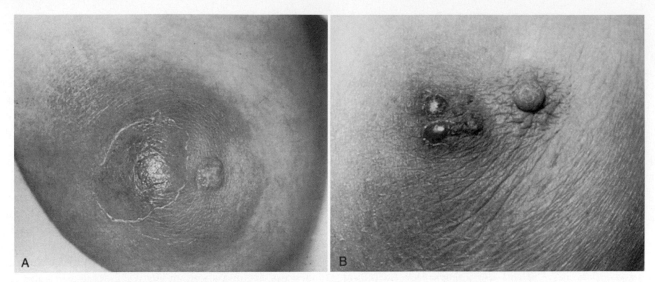

FIG. **5-24 A,** A 38-year-old smoker presented with acute onset of right breast pain. There was no history of symptoms of the mammary duct–associated inflammatory disease sequence (MDAIDS). A red, hot, tender, fluctuant mass was observed. **B,** Another example of a subareolar breast abscess that is about to spontaneously discharge.

of age, these studies are warranted after resolution of the acute process, to rule out unsuspected underlying lesions.

Treatment Plan. The approach to treatment of a primary (nonrecurrent) subareolar breast abscess should include consideration of its stage of development in the pathologic sequence outlined in Figures 5-2 and 5-16.

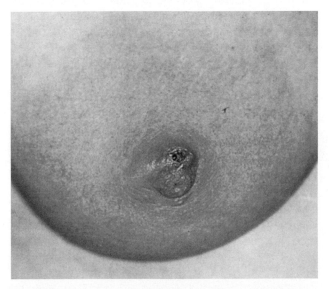

FIG. **5-25** A chronic draining mammary duct fistula in a 32-year-old woman with a history of abscesses. A tender subareolar mass was detected via the finger-and-thumb test. Note invagination of central portion of the nipple.

If a patient presents with an established fistula with induration at the base of the sinus, the entire disease process should be excised, as described next.

Surgical Management. When a patient presents with a primary subareolar breast abscess, treatment should be determined by the degree of inflammation and the stage of abscess development.

Early Abscess. If the abscess is in its early stages (consisting of an indurated mass), a 2-week course of antibiotics consisting of a cephalosporin and metronidazole, each at a dosage of 500 mg by mouth three times a day, is prescribed. Hot packs are recommended for comfort, and a well-fitted bra provides support and further comfort. The patient is scheduled for weekly appointments for follow-up until the process has resolved, and elective excision is planned for 2 to 4 weeks thereafter.

Mature Abscess. If the abscess is fluctuant or has already drained spontaneously, treatment with the patient under general anesthesia consists of making a wide incision to obtain effective drainage and to culture the pus. The patient is then given the two antibiotics for 10 days and monitored weekly to ensure satisfactory resolution with healing. Operative treatment of the abscess and the associated duct under general anesthesia is then planned for 4 to 6 weeks later.

If a patient presents with a recurrent subareolar abscess, the abscess should be incised and drained, as described in the following sections, with antibiotic coverage. After the acute phase has subsided, the major subareolar ducts should be totally excised with a technique similar to that proposed by Urban and

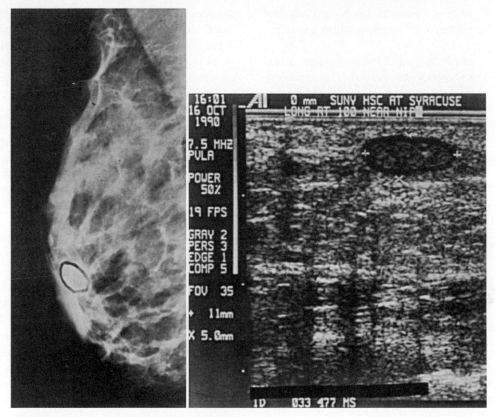

FIG. **5-26** Ultrasound imaging of early subareolar breast abscess.

Hadfield.[44,55] The distal intralobular ducts atrophy, thus dispelling any fear of complications arising during a subsequent pregnancy.

Whereas the conventional treatment for an acute subareolar breast abscess is surgical incision with drainage of the pus—optimally under general anesthesia in the operating room and with perioperative antibiotic coverage for both anaerobes and aerobes—it should be recognized that this is a temporizing measure in the subareolar abscess phase of MDAIDS. Another option, which can be used in the office setting instead of with general anesthesia, is to make the patient comfortable with oral sedation approximately 1 hour before the planned incision and drainage. Then, local analgesia of the incision site is obtained by freezing the skin over the abscess with topical ethyl chloride spray applied from far enough above the abscess to induce skin frosting and freezing. The incision is made through this frozen tissue. Use of conventional local anesthetic agents (e.g., lidocaine) is seldom effective in providing analgesia for the incision because of the low tissue pH in the inflamed skin tissue fluid. It should thus be avoided with an acute inflammatory process. A portion of the anterior abscess wall should be removed for pathologic examination because, although rare, a cancer

could coexist.[52] The abscess may be extensive and multilocular and must be drained completely, but further exploration of the wound and excision of surrounding indurated tissue should be avoided so as not to destroy surrounding breast tissue or disfigure the breast. The pus should be cultured for both aerobic and anaerobic bacteria, and a Gram stain should be performed. Following irrigation of the abscess cavity, a small wick is placed to assist drainage and prevent premature skin closure. Tight packing should be avoided because it deforms the breast. Postoperatively, the two antibiotics should be continued. The healing process may take several weeks and should eventually be followed in 4 to 6 weeks by definitive surgery—major subareolar mammary duct excision (described later in this chapter).

Nonsurgical Management. The advent of percutaneous FNA has introduced nonoperative treatment as a potential alternative, although the criteria for its use have not been defined. The argument given to support needle aspiration of the abscess cavity, coupled with treatment with systemic antibiotics, is that fistulization follows conventional treatment with incision and drainage. This is now a spurious argument, because it is recognized that incision and drainage are temporizing measures for an acute lesion that precede definitive duct surgery, thus avoiding fistulization.

Early reports noted that antibiotic therapy alone for subareolar breast abscesses resulted in complete resolution of only 3% of the infections in 181 breast abscesses because the antibiotics used were effective primarily against aerobes instead of both anaerobes and aerobes.[65,145] The overall success rate of nonsurgical management appears to be less than 50% in two reported series in which the long-term follow-up was inadequate.[128,146] Ignoring the possible role of duct abnormalities in the causation of breast infection leads to (1) inadequate treatment; (2) recurrent infections with periareolar fistulas; (3) mutilating deformities of the breast; and (4) radical breast surgery, including mastectomy.[56] Figure 5-16 summarizes the clinical evaluation and treatment of subareolar breast abscess as it relates to MDAIDS.

PERIAREOLAR MAMMARY DUCT FISTULA AS RELATED TO MDAIDS

A periareolar fistula represents a sequela of treatment failure of the acute subareolar abscess and is the end-stage disease of MDAIDS (Figures 5-1, 5-2, and 5-16). The periareolar mammary duct fistula is an established fistula, a chronically discharging lesion in the region of the areola, usually at the vermilion border (see Figures 5-21 and 5-27) but often at the base of the nipple (see Figure 5-25), which communicates with a centrally situated major subareolar mammary duct (see Figure 5-19). The cause is related to varying degrees of obstruction of a major subareolar mammary duct, secondary to squamous metaplasia of the duct lining. This leads to an accumulation of secretions in acini that becomes infected, forming an acute subareolar abscess. Spontaneous discharge via the shortest and most direct route of least resistance is at the vermilion border. Occasionally, the discharge exits via the nipple. After the sinus has healed, in the vast majority of cases a recurrent abscess appears and discharges once more along the same route, establishing a permanent fistulous tract. Until the underlying cause is removed, repeated episodes of infection are common and seldom self-limiting. This spectrum of MDAIDS and its sequelae is not limited to women but is also occasionally found in men (see Table 5-4).

Clinical Features. The age range (mean and median) of patients who present specifically with periareolar mammary duct fistula, as reported in selected papers in the literature, is summarized in Table 5-14. As expected, this corresponds to the age range of patients presenting with the other features of MDAIDS (i.e., nipple discharge, breast pain, varying degrees of nipple retraction, and acute subareolar abscess). As reported in the literature, the frequency of fistula related to a breast abscess varies from 4% to 20%, depending on whether one considers fistulas subsequent to treatment failure or patients with new fistulas.[36,39] In some reports, more patients presented with fistulas than with breast abscesses.[36,39] The overwhelming data show that most of the tracts studied are lined by granulation tissue.[16] In only a few was squamous metaplasia found.[14] Often,

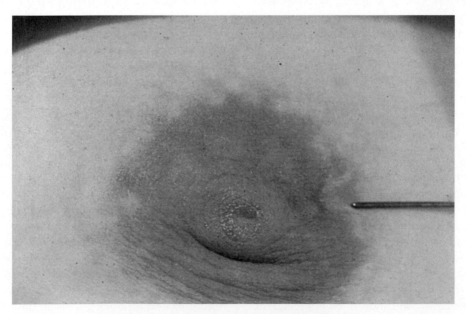

FIG. **5-27** Probe shows opening of chronic sinus at the vermilion border of the areola.

| TABLE **5-14** | Age of Patients Presenting with Periareolar Mammary Duct Fistula |

INVESTIGATORS	FISTULAS (n)	AGE (yr) RANGE	MEAN	MEDIAN	COMMENTS
Zuska et al, 1951[14]	5	29-40	34	—	1 Patient had bilateral large ducts lined by squamous epithelium
Atkins, 1955[48]	35	21-63	34	—	7 bilateral lesions; 19 inverted nipples; 1 carcinoma; nonspecific granulation tissue
Abramson, 1969[39]	14	24-46	35	—	9 patients had previous surgery, 7 with duct ectasia, 2 with squamous metaplasia
Lambert et al, 1986[116]	52	19-63	31	30	1 male; 11 bilateral lesions; 3 patients had more than one fistula on same side
Bundred et al, 1987[49]	46	24-61	—	35	6 recurred after surgery without antibiotic coverage
Mcguid et al, 1995[19]	116	26-61	—	33	All had previous incision and drainage

communication with the underlying subareolar mammary duct can be demonstrated clearly via a lacrimal duct probe.

Investigation. The history should emphasize frequency and time intervals of antecedent acute subareolar abscesses or a subareolar inflammatory mass that had either discharged spontaneously or had been surgically incised and drained. This may also have occurred in the past in the contralateral breast. Other events preceding the fistula, and their time course, need to be ascertained, including nipple discharge, nipple retraction, a history of lactation, and breast biopsies. As stated earlier, inquiry into the patient's smoking habits is essential because of the evidence that periareolar mammary duct fistulas of MDAIDS are associated with heavy smoking (see Figures 5-6 and 5-7).

On physical examination, the site and location of the fistula opening in the involved breast should be noted. Both breasts should be inspected to determine whether the nipples are retracted. Both breasts should be palpated gently and the finger-thumb test performed for subareolar masses (see Figure 5-12, *A*), nipple discharge, or discharge from the fistula of the involved breast. Ipsilateral axillary adenopathy is often present. Mammography and ultrasonography are helpful in defining the nature of a small retroareolar mass (see Figure 5-12, *B*) and detecting signs of prominent subareolar mammary ducts, periductal opacification, and coarse linear and irregular microcalcifications consistent with the radiologic features of MDAIDS.[134,147-150] Intuitively, one would think that a fistulogram would help define the anatomy, but strangely, the literature is lacking in reference to this procedure, although it is generally accepted for gastrointestinal fistulas.

Treatment Plan. Antibiotics—a cephalosporin and metronidazole, each at a dosage of 500 mg by mouth

three times a day for 10 to 14 days—should be given to cover anaerobic and aerobic organisms if there are clinical signs of ongoing, low-grade chronic infection. When the fistula is chronic and well established, the patient should undergo surgery, usually with general anesthesia and continued antibiotic coverage. The fistula tract into the subareolar-retronipple space should be excised, together with the duct (ductectomy) as it emerges through the nipple. The resulting wound is left open and loosely packed or closed primarily, with or without a drain, while further antibiotics are provided. A summary of the clinical evaluation and treatment is shown in Figure 5-16. The surgical techniques are described in the following sections.

General Comments. The term *mammary fistula* was introduced by Atkins in 1955 to describe the fistulas of the subareolar mammary ducts reported by Zuska's group in 1951; they likened it to a fistula in ano.[83,94] It was Walker and Sandison[38] who stressed the association between subareolar abscess and the mammary duct ectasia component of MDAIDS. Other researchers[50,51,59] believe that the fistula originates and remains in the subepidermal glands, because they have failed to identify a communication with a mammary duct, either macroscopically or microscopically. This conservative view does not take into account the concept embodied in the MDAIDS. The fundamental lesion cannot always be determined from the histomorphologic slides because it is destroyed by the repeated acute—and persistent chronic—inflammation that commonly occurs.

Many patients suffer unnecessary pain and discomfort from recurrent sepsis because the diagnosis of a periareolar mammary duct fistula is not suspected. The patient whose breast is depicted in Figure 5-21 was treated with a variety of systemic and topical antimicrobials by her primary care physician for over 3 years

TABLE **5-15**	Treatment Outcome in 31 Surgeries for Periareolar Mammary Duct Fistula			
PROCEDURE	PATIENTS *(n)*	SUCCESSFUL HEALING *(n)*	PROLONGED WOUND DISCHARGE *(n)*	RECURRENT FISTULA *(n)*
Excision and packing	9	8	1	1
Primary closure alone	16	10	6	5
Primary closure with antibiotic coverage	6	6	0	0

From Bundred NJ et al: *Br J Surg* 74:466, 1987.

for "recurrent skin furuncles," during which time her nipple progressively retracted. A high proportion of patients (as many as 60%) have retracted nipples, a known feature of the periductal inflammatory stage of MDAIDS.[49] Although on the basis of the work of Atkins it was initially thought that these are all of congenital origin, in our practice the time relation between retraction and periductal inflammation suggests that it is a consequence of repeated subareolar mammary duct inflammation and, as such, is closely associated with MDAIDS.[48]

Recurrences of mammary fistulas involve other ducts, particularly if only a single ductectomy is performed initially with the fistulectomy. Table 5-15 shows the outcome of surgery for periareolar mammary duct fistula as reported by Bundred and co-workers.[49] For recurrent fistula, we recommend excision of all the major subareolar mammary ducts. In the past, recurrent fistulas and repeated infections have led to mastectomy.[41,44] The most common lesion is consistent with mammary duct ectasia and periductal mastitis,[27,147] although others have also reported granulomatous mastitis.[49]

Operative Techniques

DUCTECTOMY: WHEN ONE DUCT IS INVOLVED

With use of general anesthesia, a radial incision is usually made, starting from the middle of the nipple and encompassing the diseased duct. The incision is extended laterally through the areola and the vermilion border. The nipple is laid open and the duct is isolated and dissected out from its surroundings (Figure 5-28, *A*). The dissection is carried down deep into the middle of the subareolar breast tissue (breast disk), encompassing the enlarged, firm, and inflamed ampulla and the distal duct tissue. The tissue is divided from the remaining breast by electrocoagulation, and the specimen is removed (Figure 5-28, *B*).

Reconstruction. After the diseased portion of the duct is removed, the nipple is carefully reconstructed with No. 4-0 absorbable suture material. The subcutaneous sutures are placed at three critical sites: (1) the circumferential edge of the apex of the nipple

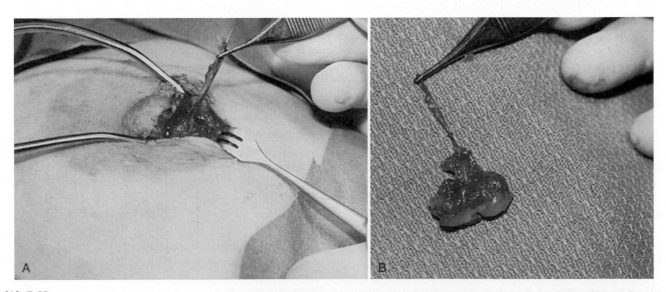

FIG. 5-28 A, A diseased major mammary duct has been dissected out from the nipple/areola complex. **B,** Enlarged, firm, inflamed lactiferous ampulla and distal ductal tissue. *(From Meguid MM et al: Surgery 118:775, 1995.)*

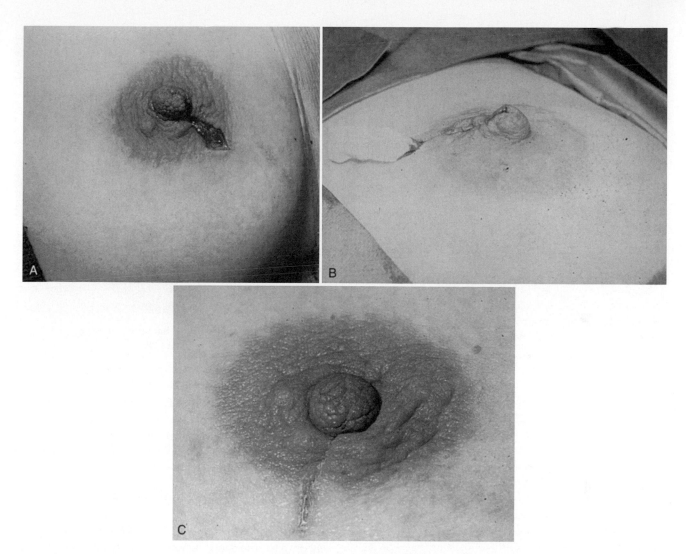

FIG. **5-29** **A** to **C,** Series of surgical steps used to reconstruct nipple/areola complex (see text). *(From Meguid MM et al:* Surgery *118:775, 1995.)*

(Figure 5-29, *A*), (2) the base of the nipple (Figure 5-29, *A*), and (3) the vermilion border of the areola (Figure 5-29, *B*). In patients who present with inverted nipples or a retracted nipple secondary to a previously drained chronic disease site, the nipple is everted and a fourth suture consisting of a purse-string or Z-suture with No. 4-0 Vicryl is placed inside the base of the nipple to prevent it from collapsing. This is done after placement of suture No. 2. Iodoform gauze of appropriate size is placed as a wick into the surgically created defect in the subareolar space and is exteriorized beyond the vermilion border through the lateral aspect of the incision (see Figure 5-29, *B*). The patient is taught to change the wick daily. Antibiotics suitable for coverage against aerobes and anaerobes are selected and prescribed for a course of 10 to 14 days. Figure 5-29, *C,* shows the nipple/areola complex 3 weeks after operation.

RESECTION OF MAJOR MAMMARY DUCTS: WHEN MULTIPLE DUCTS ARE INVOLVED OR FOR RECURRENT SUBAREOLAR ABSCESS

A radial incision can be used similar to that described previously. Alternatively, a circumareolar incision is made below the areola (see Figures 5-14 and 5-30, *A*). Elevation of the nipple from the areolar complex is performed with a knife (Figure 5-30, *B*). The major ducts are separated from the base of the nipple by passing a curved tonsil forceps or hemostat around the nipple base and dividing the ducts with a knife (Figure 5-30, *C*). The nipple base is then carefully cut down to remove all duct tissue (Figure 5-30, *D*). Care is taken to avoid devascularizing the nipple skin. A purse-string or Z-suture of No. 4-0 Vicryl is inserted through the nipple base to hold it everted without causing necrosis. The major subareolar duct system is then dissected out from the middle of the underlying breast

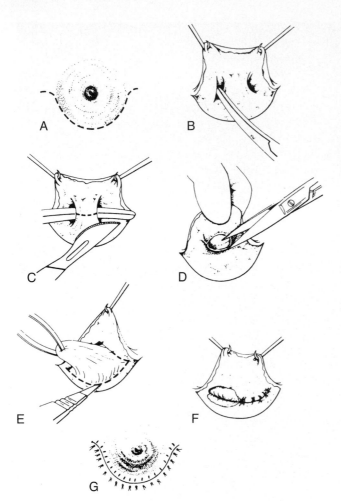

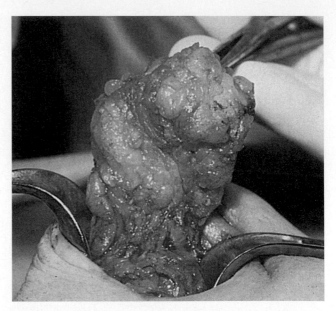

FIG. **5-31** Close-up view of subareolar tissue dissected in a patient following recurrent abscesses.

FIG. **5-30** Technique of subareolar dissection (see text). *(From Hartley MN et al: Br J Surg 78:1187, 1991.)*

tissue (breast disk) (Figures 5-30, *E,* and 5-31). Hemostasis is achieved by electrocoagulation. The wound is irrigated. Primary closure of the subareolar space is performed to obliterate the dead space, and the skin is then closed with fine interrupted suture, absorbable suture with Vicryl, or nonabsorbable suture with fine nylon or prolene, depending on the surgeon's preference (Figure 5-30, *F*). Any dilated ducts are electrocoagulated or ligated individually with No. 5-0 Vicryl. A drain is usually not required in the elective setting. The operation is performed with antibiotic coverage. The areolar skin is sutured in position with subcuticular, interrupted sutures (Figure 5-30, *G*). We prefer to leave the skin open for drainage or to approximate the skin edges with Steri-Strips to obtain the optimal cosmetic result. A firm dressing is placed over the breast. If a drain is used it is removed within 24 hours, and the patient is instructed to wear a well-fitted bra continuously. Patients undergoing surgery should be warned of the potential for recurrent problems and, possibly, loss of nipple sensation. Nipple necrosis is an

uncommon complication of repeated surgery. Reasons for failure of surgery include inadequate removal of major duct tissue, either from the nipple base or from the breast disk itself, and failure to evert the nipple and remove the disease at its base.[1]

CHRONIC SUBAREOLAR BREAST ABSCESS WITH FISTULA

Either a radial or a subareolar incision can be used to encompass the sinus opening and the fistulous tract. The dissection is carried into the substance of the subareolar breast tissue and the tissue is removed en bloc (see Figure 5-30), together with the fistula tract. Injection of the fistula tract with 1% methylene blue before the start of the dissection is often helpful in identifying the corresponding major subareolar duct that connects with the fistula. The wound is irrigated and closed as described earlier. Administration of antibiotics is continued postoperatively.

Peripheral Breast Abscess in Comparison with MDAIDS

A quarter of all abscesses—at any age—are peripheral and present as a pink area in the periphery of the breast. The causes are various. Most common are abscesses related to lactation, folliculitis, and in postmenopausal women, diabetes. In the 3-year series by Petrek[57] of 18 postmenopausal women with breast abscess, half had adult-onset diabetes. These patients often presented without leukocytosis, pain, or accompanying cellulitis.

Gallium-67 citrate in scintigraphy is used to detect latent breast abscesses.

Acute pyogenic abscess of the puerperium is becoming less common, whereas abscesses resulting from the duct ectasia phase of MDAIDS have assumed increasing importance. Nevertheless, acute puerperal breast abscess still causes significant and occasionally serious morbidity. Figure 5-22 shows the distinction between the two types of abscesses. They have different causes, bacteriology, presentations, and treatments. Puerperal abscess is an acute disease of the puerperium, and the pathogen is most often *Staphylococcus aureus*. It remains unclear whether the staphylococci are derived from the skin of the patient or from the mouth of her suckling infant. Perhaps both are sources of infection. The principal cause is blockage of a lactiferous duct or lactiferous ampulla with inspissated secretions and milk, resulting in retention of milk in the peripheral lobules of the breast drained by the blocked duct. This stagnant milk produces breast engorgement and is an excellent bacterial culture medium. The patient usually manifests systemic signs of sepsis, presenting with a fever, tachycardia, and leukocytosis; occasionally, septicemia occurs. Ipsilateral axillary lymphadenopathy is also found.

On physical examination, an exquisitely tender mass is usually present in the peripheral breast tissue. When early cellulitis is found, broad-spectrum antibiotic treatment produces resolution in most instances. If antibiotics are not given or if diagnosis is delayed, an abscess forms unless the blocked duct is rendered patent again by suckling.

Adequate incision and drainage with topical ethyl chloride spray or general anesthesia, with culture of the pus and antibiotic coverage, invariably produce rapid resolution.[151] The incision should be made over the site of maximum tenderness and kept within Langer's lines for optimal cosmesis. The abscess cavity should be explored and all the loculi broken down. In the appropriate age group, a biopsy specimen of the abscess wall is taken to rule out carcinoma. We have favored light packing of the abscess cavity. Although the matter has not been subjected to a randomized controlled clinical trial, others have preferred that the abscess be obliterated by deep mattress sutures and the patient treated with perioperative antibiotics without formal postoperative drainage. This technique has been shown to produce swifter healing with no more complications than formal drainage.[152] Total excision rather than drainage is recommended for smaller lesions. More recently, as discussed earlier, Ferrara and colleagues[146] recommended an attempt at needle aspiration as the primary procedure for selected cases of focal abscess—plus treatment with antibiotics. Antibiotics are continued for 10 days. In approximately 50% of women who develop acute puerperal breast abscess, lactation ceases spontaneously.

For the others, there is no particular reason why breast-feeding should be stopped.

Occasionally unusual pathogens are the cause of abscess. One report described a silent *Mycobacterium chelonei* infection in a young woman who was immunocompromised by large doses of corticosteroids.[153] One of our patients with celiac disease and dermatitis herpetiformis over the legs, arms, and breast, immunosuppressed because of steroid therapy, developed a deep peripheral left breast abscess. This was initially incised and drained and then required treatment with simple mastectomy. Thereafter, she developed a right breast abscess, which was excised and allowed to heal by secondary intention. A case of severe recurrent breast abscess caused by *Corynebacterium minutissimum* resulted from a wound infection after breast biopsy performed through skin that was superficially infected with the same organism.[154] This required four drainage procedures before the infection was finally controlled with intravenous vancomycin and oral erythromycin.

Some cases of mastitis result from exogenous exposure to bacteria. Superficial folliculitis of the breast skin can occur, particularly in the Montgomery glands, and it is commonly caused by gram-positive organisms. This condition is optimally treated by cleansing with soap and water and repeated topical application of Bactroban (mupirocin) three times a day. The condition can also be self-limited and subside spontaneously within 3 or 4 days, although inadvertent use of steroids may cause rapid spread and predispose to invasive disease.[155] Outbreaks of *Pseudomonas aeruginosa* mastitis have been reported from inadequate chlorination of pools and hot tubs.[75] Buchanan and Kominos[156] reported a case of a deep peripheral breast abscess resulting from *P. aeruginosa* in a previously healthy premenopausal woman. The patient showed signs of systemic sepsis, with fever, leukocytosis, and erythema involving the lateral aspect of the breast. The abscess was incised and drained and the wound was left open; Iodophor packs were changed daily. Intravenous tobramycin and ticarcillin were also given, and the patient's condition responded in 2 weeks.

Ekland and Zeigler[52] reported a number of patients with peripheral breast abscess. All were females, ranging in age from 17 to 67 years (mean, 37.4 years). Duration of symptoms varied from 1 day to 4 weeks. Recent trauma was reported by three patients; two had active facial acne, one had a known epidermal cyst at the abscess site, and one had a history of paraffin injections in the affected breast. Insulin-dependent diabetes mellitus occurred in one patient and steroid-treated rheumatoid arthritis in another.

Treatment consisted of incision and drainage or excision. Specimens for bacterial cultures were obtained from 11 patients and were reported to yield no growth in six cultures, coagulase-positive staphylococci in three, coagulase-negative staphylococci in one, and *Proteus* organisms in one. Pathologic examination revealed predominantly acute and chronic inflammation. Other histologic abnormalities noted were epidermal cyst, intraductal papilloma, and cystic duct dilation with apocrine metaplasia in each of three specimens.

Summary

Our concept of the disease process leading to subareolar abscess is based on histomorphologic findings and disease management.[19] On the basis of our work and observations, we postulate an evolutionary process that begins with duct ectasia secondary to hormone imbalance. This mild duct ectasia is aggravated by the development of squamous metaplasia, which leads to duct obstruction and associated stasis of secretion, followed by inflammation. In part, the clinical and morphologic presentation of this disease process reflects the distribution of the aberrations along the duct system—thus the designation *mammary duct–associated inflammatory disease sequence*.

This approach is counter to that recently proposed by Dixon and Bundred and their colleagues, who believe duct ectasia and the inflammatory process are "likely to be totally unrelated."* Their position is based on the observation that, in their patient population, mastitis (1) is associated with an increased number of patients who smoke (whereas duct ectasia is not) and (2) occurs in a younger age group. However, in a prospective study of an equally large patient population, Thomas, Williamson, and Webster[92] did not observe a difference in the percentages of smokers who had mastitis and who had simple ectasia. Although most studies show that mastitis is more common in younger persons, it should be noted that symptomatic duct ectasia does occur in the same age group. The true incidence of simple duct ectasia is unknown because it is likely to be asymptomatic and is observed in women with other mammary diseases. Also lacking in the position taken by Dixon and Bundred and their co-workers is an explanation for a primary infectious etiology as the underlying cause of the mastitis; it appears that the stromal alterations are the same in patients who present with inflammation as in those with simple ectasia.[107]

Our hypothesis takes into consideration (1) the most likely causal factors, (2) the morphologic findings, and (3) the ample clinical experience and documentation that support the necessity for resecting the ducts to manage recurrent subareolar abscess after failed

antibiotic therapy and incision and drainage. The molecular alterations in the duct epithelial cells that result from smoking, vitamin A deficiency, decreased serum prolactin, and inactive estrogen metabolites are still unknown and need to be investigated to enable us to gain a better understanding of the pathogenesis of MDAIDS. Morphologically, as in other organs, cellular alterations must occur before squamous metaplasia is recognizable by light microscopy. For example, there must be changes in the structure and organization of the duct cell microvilli,[89,90] which in some way must affect the function of the epithelium. The necessity to resect the ducts implies that the major distal ducts contribute to persistence of disease; thus, by extension, it can be postulated that the distal duct also has a role during the early stages of evolution of the disease.

Given our current state of knowledge, we view MDAIDS as a disease process related to altered duct epithelial function and structure, the latter evolving into squamous metaplasia. The squamous metaplasia acts as an obstruction, resulting in stasis of secretions, duct ectasia, and accumulation of inflammatory substances such as lipid and keratin. Depending on where along the duct system the obstruction lies and on the kind and degree of altered physiologic events that occur, MDAIDS can be either an asymptomatic entity (symptomatic simple duct ectasia) or an inflammatory process presenting as a subareolar abscess that may evolve into a mammary duct fistula (see Figures 5-1, 5-2, and 5-16).

ACKNOWLEDGMENTS

We thank Jia-Ke Chai, M.D., for retrieving many obscure references; Ms. Deborah Rexine, Mr. George Reynolds, and Mr. Kenneth Peek for photographic service; Patricia Brady, R.N., N.P., Jane D'Antoni, R.N., N.P., for assisting with patient care; and Ms. Darlene Thompson and Ms. Denise Stanton for diligent editorial assistance.

REFERENCES

1. Hughes LE: Non-lactational inflammation and duct ectasia, *Br Med Bull* 47:272, 1991.
2. Payne RL, Strauss AF, Glasser RD: Mastitis obliterans, *Surgery* 14:719, 1943.
3. Bloodgood JC: Clinical picture of dilated ducts beneath the nipple frequently to be palpated as a doughy worm-like mass: the varicocele tumour of the breast, *Surg Gynecol Obstet* 36:486, 1923.
4. Geschickter CF: *Diseases of the breast*, ed 2, Philadelphia, 1948, JB Lippincott.
5. Tice GI, Dockerty MB, Harrington SW: Comedomastitis: a clinical and pathologic study of sata in 172 cases, *Surg Gynecol Obstet* 87:525, 1948.
6. Ingleby H: Normal and pathologic proliferation in the breast with special reference to cystic disease, *Arch Pathol* 33:573, 1942.

*References 18, 26, 29, 30, 49, 58, 109, 134, 148.

7. Deaver JB, McFarland J: *The breast: its anomalies, its diseases and their treatment,* Philadelphia, 1917, Blakiston.
8. Adair FE: Plasma cell mastitis, a lesion simulating mammary carcinoma: a clinical and pathologic study with a report of ten cases, *Arch Surg* 29:735, 1933.
9. Birkett J: *Diseases of the breast and their treatment,* London, 1850, Kangman.
10. Ingier A: Uber obliterienende mastitis, *Virchow's Arch Pathol Anat* 198:338, 1909.
11. Cromar CDL: Correspondence, *BMJ* 1:363, 1921.
12. Foote FW, Stewart FW: Comparative studies of cancerous versus noncancerous breasts, *Ann Surg* 121:197, 1945.
13. Stewart FW: *Tumors of the breast: AFIP fascicle 34,* Washington, DC, 1950, Armed Forces Institute of Pathology.
14. Zuska JJ, Crile G Jr, Ayres WW: Fistulas of lactiferous ducts, *Am J Surg* 81:312, 1951.
15. Haagensen CD: Mammary duct ectasia: a disease that may stimulate carcinoma, *Cancer* 4:749, 1951.
16. Patey DH, Thackray AC: Pathology and treatment of mammary-duct fistula, *Lancet* 2:871, 1958.
17. Ingleby H, Gershon-Cohen J: *Comparative anatomy, pathology and roentgenology of the breast,* Philadelphia, 1960, University of Pennsylvania Press.
18. Dixon JM: Periductal mastitis/duct ectasia, *World J Surg* 13:715, 1989.
19. Meguid MM et al: Pathogenesis-based treatment of recurring subareolar breast abscesses, *Surgery* 118:775, 1995.
20. Bloodgood JC: The pathology of chronic mastitis of the female breast, with special consideration of the blue-domed cyst, *Arch Surg* 3:445, 1921.
21. Kilgore AR, Fleming R: Abscesses of the breast: recurring lesions in the areolar area, *Calif Med* 77:190, 1952.
22. Watt-Boolsen S, Ramussen NR, Blichert-Toft M: Primary periarcolar abscess in the nonlactating breast: risk of recurrence, *Am J Surg* 153:571, 1987.
23. Bonser GM, Dossett JA, Jull JW: *Human and experimental breast cancer,* London, 1961, Pitman Medical.
24. Dossett JA: The normal breast, cystic disease and duct ectasia: a functional and histological study, MD thesis, London, 1959, University of London.
25. Azzopardi JG: *Problems in breast pathology,* London, 1979, WB Saunders.
26. Dixon JM et al: Mammary duct ectasia, *Br J Surg* 70:601, 1983.
27. Toker C: Lactiferous duct fistula, *J Pathol Bacteriol* 84:143, 1962.
28. Habif DV et al: Subareolar abscess associated with squamous metaplasia of lactiferous ducts, *Am J Surg* 119:523, 1970.
29. Bundred NJ et al: The aetiology of periductal mastitis. In Mansel RE (ed): *Recent developments in the study of benign breast disease: proceedings of the 5th International Symposium on Benign Breast Disease,* London, 1993.
30. Dixon JM et al: Smoking in patients with periductal mastitis and duct ectasia. In Mansel RE (ed): *Recent developments in the study of benign breast disease: proceedings of the 5th International Symposium on Benign Breast Disease,* London, 1993.
31. Frantz VK et al: Incidence of chronic cystic disease in so-called "normal breasts": a study based on 225 postmortem examinations, *Cancer* 4:762, 1951.
32. Sandison AT: *An autopsy study of the adult human breast, with special reference to proliferative epithelial changes of importance in the pathology of the breast,* monograph 8, Bethesda, MD, 1962, National Cancer Institute.
33. Sandison AT: Breast changes in fibrocystic disease of the pancreas, *Lancet* 1:691, 1956.
34. Tedeschi LG, Ahari S, Byrne JJ: Involutional mammary duct ectasia and periductal mastitis, *Am J Surg* 106:517, 1963.
35. Davies JD: *Periductal mastitis,* unpublished thesis, London, 1971, University of London.
36. Browning J, Bigrigg A, Taylor I: Symptomatic and incidental mammary duct ectasia, *J R Soc Med* 79:715, 1986.
37. Sandison AT, Walker JC: Inflammatory mastitis, mammary duct ectasia, and mammillary fistula, *Br J Surg* 50:57, 1962/63.
38. Walker JC, Sandison AT: Mammary duct ectasia: a clinical study, *Br J Surg* 51:350, 1964.
39. Abramson DJ: Mammary duct ectasia, mammillary fistula and subareolar sinuses, *Ann Surg* 169:217, 1969.
40. Frischbier HJ, Lohbeck HU: *Fruhdiagnostik des Mammarkarzinomas. Lehrbuch und Atlas,* Stuttgart, 1977, Georg Thieme.
41. Thomas WG et al: The clinical syndrome of mammary duct ectasia, *Br J Surg* 69:423, 1982.
42. Cromar CDL, Dockerty MB: Plasma cell mastitis, *Proc Staff Meet Mayo Clin* 16:775, 1941.
43. Haagensen CD: *Diseases of the breast,* ed 2, Philadelphia, 1971, WB Saunders.
44. Hadfield GJ: Excision of the major duct system for benign disease of the breast, *Br J Surg* 47:472, 1959/60.
45. Hadfield GJ: Further experience of the operation for the excision of the major duct system of the breast, *Br J Surg* 55:530, 1968.
46. Hartley MN, Stewart J, Benson EA: Subareolar dissection for duct ectasia and periareolar sepsis, *Br J Surg* 78:1187, 1991.
47. O'Brien PH, Kreutner A: Another cause of nipple discharge: mammary duct ectasia with periductal mastitis, *Am Surg* 48:577, 1982.
48. Atkins HJB: Mammary fistula, *BMJ* 2:1473, 1955.
49. Bundred NJ et al: Mammillary fistula, *Br J Surg* 74:466, 1987.
50. Caswell HT, Burnett WE: Chronic recurrent breast abscess secondary to inversion of the nipple, *Surg Gynecol Obstet* 102:439, 1956.
51. Caswell HT, Maier WP: Chronic recurrent periareolar abscess secondary to inversion of the nipple, *Surg Gynecol Obstet* 128:597, 1969.
52. Ekland DA, Zeigler MG: Abscess in the nonlactating breast, *Arch Surg* 107:398, 1973.
53. Leach RD et al: Anaerobic subareolar breast abscesses, *Lancet* 1:35, 1979.
54. Urban JA: Excision of the major duct system of the breast, *Cancer* 16:516, 1963.
55. Urban JA, Egeli RA: Non-lactational nipple discharge, *Ca Cancer J Clin* 28:130, 1978.
56. Golinger RC, O'Neal BJ: Mastitis and mammary duct disease, *Arch Surg* 117:1027, 1982.
57. Petrek J: Postmenopausal breast abscess, *South Med J* 75:1198, 1982.
58. Bundred NJ et al: Are the lesions of duct ectasia sterile? *Br J Surg* 72:844, 1985.
59. Maier WP, Berger A, Derrick BM: Periareolar abscess in the nonlactating breast, *Am J Surg* 144:359, 1982.
60. Scholefield JH, Duncan JL, Rogers K: Review of a hospital experience with breast abscesses, *Br J Surg* 74:469, 1987.
61. Guyer PB: The use of ultrasound in benign breast disorders, *World J Surg* 13:692, 1989.

62. MacLeod RM, Lehmyer JR: Studies on the mechanism of the dopamine-mediated inhibition of prolactin secretion, *Endocrinology* 94:1077, 1974.

63. Ransjo U et al: Bacteria in the female breast, *Scand J Plast Reconstr Surg* 19:87, 1985.

64. Thornton JW et al: Studies on the endogenous flora of the human breast, *Ann Plast Surg* 20:39, 1988.

65. Walker AP et al: A prospective study of the microflora of nonpuerperal breast abscess, *Arch Surg* 123:908, 1988.

66. Abul HT et al: Comparison of local and systemic production of interleukin-8 in smoking and non-smoking patients with infectious lung disease, *Med Principles Pract* 5:19, 1996.

67. Michnovicz JJ et al: Increased 2-hydroxylation of oestradiol as a possible mechanism for the antiestrogenic effects of cigarette smoking, *N Engl J Med* 325:1305, 1986.

68. Berta L et al: Smoking effects on the hormonal balance of fertile women, *Hormone Res* 37:45, 1992.

69. Sanchez-Pacheco A, Palomino T, Aranda A: Retinoic acid induces expression of the transcription factor GHF-1/Pit. 1 in pituitary prolactin– and growth hormone–producing cell lines, *Endocrinology* 136:5391, 1995.

70. Berkowitz CD, Inkelish SH: Bloody nipple discharge in infancy, *J Pediatrics* 103:755, 1983.

71. Fenster DL: Bloody nipple discharge, *J Pediatrics* 104:640, 1984.

72. Stringel G, Perelman A, Jimenez C: Infantile mammary duct ectasia: a cause of bloody nipple discharge, *J Pediatr Surg* 21:671, 1986.

73. Kleinberg DL et al: Primate mammary development: effect of hypophysectomy, prolactin inhibition, and growth hormone administration, *J Clin Invest* 75:1943, 1985.

74. Shousha S et al: Mammary duct ectasia and pituitary adenomas, *Am J Surg Pathol* 12:130, 1988.

75. Franks S et al: Prolactin concentration in patients with breast cancer, *BMJ* 4:320, 1994.

76. Kleinberg DL, Noel GL, Frantz AG: Galactorrhea: a study of 235 cases, including 48 with pituitary tumors, *N Engl J Med* 296:589, 1977.

77. Sharp BM, Beyer HS: Rapid desensitization of the acute stimulatory effects of nicotine on rat plasma adrenocorticotropin and prolactin, *J Pharmacol Exp Ther* 238:486, 1986.

78. Massaque J: TGF: beta signal transduction, *Annu Rev Biochem* 67:753, 1998.

79. Patton S, Keenan TW: The milk fat globule membrane, *Biochim Biophys Acta* 415:273, 1975.

80. Gothefors L, Olling S, Winberg J: Breast feeding and biological properties of faecal *E. coli* strains, *Acta Paediatr Scand* 64:807, 1975.

81. Schroten H et al: Inhibition of adhesion of 3-frimbriated Escherichia coli to buccal epithelial cells by human milk fat globule membrane components: a novel aspect of the protective function of mucins in the nonimmunoglobulin fraction, *Infect Immun* 60:2893, 1992.

82. Conney AH: Pharmacological implications of microsomal enzyme induction, *Pharmacol Rev* 19:317, 1967.

83. Barbieri RL, Gochberg J, Ryan KJ: Nicotine, cotinine, and anabasine inhibit aromatase in human trophoblast in vitro, *J Clin Invest* 77:1727, 1986.

84. Mori S: Primary changes in eyes of rats which result from deficiency of fat-soluble A in diet, *JAMA* 79:197, 1922.

85. Darwicke N et al: Retinoid status controls the appearance of reserve cells and keratin expression in mouse cervical epithelium, *Cancer Res* 53:2287, 1993.

86. Ongsakul M, Sirisinha S, Lamb AJ: Impaired blood clearance of bacteria and phagocytic activity in vitamin A–deficient rats, *Proc Soc Exp Biol Med* 178:204, 1985.

87. Chandra RK, Wadhwa M: Nutritional modulation of intestinal mucosal immunity, *Immunol Invest* 18:119, 1989.

88. Spring-Mills E, Elias JJ: Cell surface differences in ducts from cancerous and noncancerous human breasts, *Science* 188:947, 1975.

89. Bradbury E, Mitchell WM: Diseases of the human breast: selective isolation and exposure of epithelia and their correlative surface features and histopathology, *Scan Electron Micros* 3:139, 1978.

90. Biesalki HK et al: Vitamin A and ciliated cells: I. Respiratory epithelia, *Z Ernahungswiss* 25:114, 1986.

91. Schafer P, Furrer C, Mermillod B: An association of cigarette smoking with recurrent subareolar breast abscess, *Int J Epidemiol* 17:810, 1988.

92. Thomas JA, Williamson MER, Webster DJT: The relationship of cigarette smoking to breast disease: the Cardiff experience. In Mansel RE (ed): *Recent developments in the study of benign breast disease: proceedings of the 5th International Symposium on Benign Breast Disease*, London, New York, 1993, Parthenon.

93. Peters EJ et al: Squamous metaplasia of the bronchial mucosa and its relationship to smoking, *Chest* 103:1429, 1993.

94. Wynder EL, Hill P: Nicotine and cotinine in breast fluid, *Cancer Lett* 6:251, 1979.

95. Petrakis NL et al: Mutagenic activity in nipple aspirates of human breast fluid, *Cancer Res* 40:188, 1980.

96. Honjo H et al: Serum estradiol 17-sulfate and lipid peroxides in late pregnancy, *Acta Endocrinol* 126:303, 1992.

97. Ertel A, Eng R, Smith SM: The differential effect of cigarette smoke on the growth of bacteria found in humans, *Chest* 100:628, 1991.

98. Taylor DC et al: An alteration in the host-parasite relationship in subjects with chronic bronchitis prone to recurrent episodes of acute bronchitis, *Immunol Cell Biol* 72:143, 1994.

99. Ohnishi Y et al: Clinical study of anaerobic respiratory infection [in Japanese], *Kansenshogaku Zasshi J Jpn Assoc Infect Dis* 67:336, 1993.

100. Brand KG: Infection of mammary prostheses: a survey and the question of prevention, *Ann Plastic Surg* 30:289, 1993.

100a. Li W et al: Squamous cell carcinoma and mammary abscess formation through squamous metaplasia in Smad[4]/Dpc[4] conditional knockout mice, *Development* 2003 (in press).

101. Cardiff RD et al: The mammary pathology of genetically engineered mice: the consensus reports and recommendations from the Annapolis meeting, *Oncogene* 19:968, 2000.

102. Deng CX, Brodie SG: Knockout mouse models and mammary tumorigenesis, *Semin Cancer Biol* 11:387, 2001.

103. Henninghausen L, Robinson GW: Signaling pathways in mammary gland development, *Dev Cell* 1:467, 2001.

104. Derynck R, Akhurst RJ, Balmain A: TGF beta signaling in tumor suppression and cancer progression, *Nat Genet* 29:117, 2001.

105. Gorska AE et al: Dominant-negative interference of the transforming growth factor beta type II receptor in mammary gland epithelium results in alveolar hyperplasia and differentiation in virgin mice, *Cell Growth Diff* 9:229, 1998.

106. Jhappan C et al: Targeting expression of a transforming growth factor beta 1 transgene to the pregnant mammary

gland inhibits alveolar development and lactation, *Ebo J* 12:1835, 1993.

107. Tedeschi LG, Byrne JJ: A histochemical evaluation of the structure of mammary duct walls, *Surg Gynecol Obstet* 114:559, 1982.

108. Holliday H, Hinton C: Nipple discharge and duct ectasia. In Blamey RW (ed): *Management of breast disease,* London, 1986, Tindall.

109. Bundred NJ et al: Breast abscesses and cigarette smoking, *Br J Surg* 79:58, 1992.

110. The Yorkshire Breast Cancer Group: Symptoms and signs of operable breast cancer, 1976–1981, *Br J Surg* 70:350, 1983.

111. Tedeschi LG, McCarthy PE: Involutional mammary duct ectasia and periductal mastitis in a male, *Hum Pathol* 5:232, 1974.

112. Mansel RE, Morgan WP: Duct ectasia in the male, *Br J Surg* 66:660, 1979.

113. Chan KW, Lau WY: Duct ectasia in the male breast, *Aust NZ J Surg* 54:173, 1984.

114. McClure J, Banerjee SS, Sandilands DGD: Female type cystic hyperplasia in a male breast, *Post Grad Med J* 61:441, 1985.

115. Ashworth MT, Corcoran GD, Haqqani MT: Periductal mastitis and mammary duct ectasia in a male, *Post Grad Med J* 61:621, 1985.

116. Lambert ME, Betts CD, Sellwood RA: Mammillary fistula, *Br J Surg* 73:367, 1986.

117. Tabar L, Dean PB, Pentek Z: Galactography: the diagnostic procedure of choice for nipple discharge, *Radiology* 149:31, 1983.

118. Chaudary MA et al: Nipple discharge: the diagnostic value of testing for occult blood, *Ann Surg* 196:651, 1982.

119. Rimsten A, Skoog V, Stenkvist B: On the significance of nipple discharge in the diagnosis of breast disease, *Acta Chir Scand* 142:513, 1976.

120. Fischermann K et al: Nipple discharge: diagnosis and treatment, *Acta Chir Scand* 135:403, 1969.

121. Donnelly BA: Nipple discharge: its clinical and pathologic significance, *Ann Surg* 131:342, 1950.

122. Kilgore AR, Fleming R, Ramos MM: The incidence of cancer with nipple discharge and the risk of cancer in the presence of papillary disease of the breast, *Surg Gynecol Obstet* 96:649, 1953.

123. Leis HP et al: Nipple discharge, *Int Surg* 58:162, 1973.

124. Funderburk WW, Syphax B: Evaluation of nipple discharge in benign and malignant diseases, *Cancer* 24:1290, 1969.

125. Seltzer MH et al: The significance of age in patients with nipple discharge, *Surg Gynecol Obstet* 131:519, 1970.

126. Ingham HR, Freeman R, Wilson RG: Anaerobic breast abscesses, *Lancet* 1:154, 1979.

127. Wilson WR et al: Anaerobic bacteremia, *Mayo Clin Proc* 47:639, 1972.

128. Rosenthal LJ, Greenfield DS, Lesnick GJ: Breast abscess: management in subareolar and peripheral disease, *NY State J Med* 81:182, 1981.

129. Preece PE: Mastalgia, *Practitioner* 226:1373, 1982.

130. Maddox PR, Mansel RE: Management of breast pain and nodularity, *World J Surg* 13:699, 1989.

131. Preece PE et al: Clinical syndromes of mastalgia, *BMJ* 2:670, 1976.

132. Griffith CDM et al: The breast pain clinic: a rational approach to classification and treatment of breast pain, *Postgrad Med J* 63:547, 1987.

133. Maddox PR et al: Non-cyclical mastalgia: an improved classification and treatment, *Br J Surg* 76:901, 1989.

134. Evans KT, Gravelle IH: Mammography, thermography and ultrasonography in breast disease, London, 1973, Butterworths.

135. Gravelle IH, Lyons K: Radiological evaluation of benign breast disorders, *World J Surg* 13:685, 1989.

136. Hadfield GJ: The pathological lesions underlying discharges from the nipple in women, *Ann R Coll Surg Engl* 44:323, 1969.

137. Pye JK, Mansel RE, Hughes LE: Clinical experience of drug treatments for mastalgia, *Lancet* 2:373, 1985.

138. Rees BI, Gravelle IH, Hughes LE: Nipple retraction in duct ectasia, *Br J Surg* 64:577, 1977.

139. Dixon JM, Lee ECG, Greenall MJ: Treatment of periareolar inflammation associated with periductal mastitis using metronidazole and flucloxacillin: a preliminary report, *Br J Clin Pract* 42:78, 1988.

140. Kleinfeld G: Chronic subareolar breast abscess, *J Fla Med Assoc* 53:21, 1966.

141. Lefrock JL et al: Transient bacteremia associated with sigmoidoscopy, *N Engl J Med* 289:467, 1973.

142. Leach RD, Eykyn SJ, Phillips I: Vaginal manipulation and anaerobic breast abscesses, *BMJ* 282:610, 1981.

143. Brooker BE, Fuller R: The adhesion of coagulase-negative staphylococci to human skin and its relevance to the bacterial flora of milk, *J Appl Bacteriol* 57:325, 1984.

144. Hughes L: Management of recurrent infection following surgery for periductal mastitis, *Br J Clin Pract* 43(suppl 68):81, 1989.

145. Goodman MA, Benson EA: An evaluation of current trends in the management of breast abscesses, *Med J Aust* 1:1034, 1970.

146. Ferrara JJ et al: Nonsurgical management of breast infections in nonlactating women: a word of caution, *Ann Surg* 56:668, 1990.

147. Asch T, Frey C: Radiographic appearance of mammary-duct ectasia with calcification, *N Engl J Med* 266:86, 1962.

148. Dixon JM, Chetty U: The clinical syndrome of mammary duct ectasia, *Br J Surg* 70:57, 1983.

149. Ellerhorst-Ryan JM, Turba EP, Stahl DL: Evaluating benign breast disease, *Nurse Practitioner* 13:13, 1988.

150. Wood CB et al: Ultrasound assessment response to therapy of clinically undetected breast cysts, *Br J Clin Pract* (suppl 68):102, 1989.

151. Benson EA: Management of breast abscesses, *World J Surg* 13:753, 1989.

152. Benson E, Goodman M: Incision with primary suture in the treatment of acute peripheral breast abscess, *Br J Surg* 51:55, 1970.

153. Cua EJ, Oates E: Breast uptake of gallium-67 citrate in disseminated *Mycobacterium chelonae, Clin Nucl Med* 15:705, 1990.

154. Berger SA et al: Recurrent breast abscesses caused by Corynebacterium minutissimum, *J Clin Microbiol* 20:1219, 1984.

155. Bodey GP et al: Infections caused by Pseudomonas aeruginosa, *Rev Infect Dis* 5:279, 1983.

156. Buchanan EB, Kominos SD: Pseudomonas aeruginosa mastitis: a case report, *CMNEEJ* 12:63, 1990.

CHAPTER

6

Gynecomastia

SAMUEL W. BEENKEN
DAVID L. PAGE
KIRBY I. BLAND

Chapter Outline

Gynecomastia is an enlargement of the ductal and stromal tissue of the male breast, which is clinically and histologically different from the neighboring subcutaneous fat. Gynecomastia may be either primary (physiologic) or secondary to an extramammary stimulus. The etiology and natural history of gynecomastia have been redefined in recent years.

Incidence

Wilson and co-workers[1] believed that gynecomastia was so common that they considered it to be part of normal development. Pubertal gynecomastia develops in approximately 60% to 70% of pubertal boys (ages 12 to 15) and is estimated by Schydlower[2] to occur within 1.2 years after an increase in testicular size, the first sign of puberty. Breast enlargement and tenderness, if present, usually regress spontaneously during a 12- to 24-month period. In contrast, prepubertal gynecomastia is extraordinarily rare, with underlying causes that include adrenal carcinoma, testicular tumor, 11β-hydroxylase deficiency, familial gynecomastia, tuberous sclerosis, and sexual precocity.[3]

Nuttall[4] identified gynecomastia in 36% of 306 military reservists and noted a modest increase in prevalence with advancing age. Carlson,[5] in a study of 100 male veterans, noted an overall prevalence of 32% for gynecomastia (30% in 50 inpatients and 34% in 50 outpatients). These results correlate well with those of Ley and colleagues[6] and the autopsy study by Williams,[7] who noted gynecomastia in 40% of 447 aging men. In these clinical series, all male subjects denied breast tenderness or pain, and all had been unaware of breast enlargement or the presence of any palpable breast tissue.

Rubens, Dhont, and Vermeulen[8] considered relative hypogonadism to occur in varying degrees in men beyond age 60 as a consequence of (1) decreased concentrations of total and free serum testosterone, (2) escalations in serum luteinizing hormone (LH), and (3) maintenance of normal serum estradiol. There is evidence that enhanced peripheral aromatization of androgens to estrogens with increasing adiposity contributes to senescent gynecomastia in aging males.

Clinical Presentation

The patient presents with a swelling of the breast, often unilateral, which is commonly tender. The patient may be concerned about the tenderness, the cosmetic appearance, or the possibility of malignancy. Examination reveals a firm disc of retroareolar tissue, which is mobile. There is usually a clear demarcation of the firm breast tissue from softer adjacent fat. The hallmark of gynecomastia is concentricity. If an eccentric mass is found, an alternative diagnosis should be considered and mammography and biopsy performed. To aid in the clinical assessment of gynecomastia, a three-stage classification has been proposed by Simon and colleagues (Table 6-1).[9]

Physiology

Major ductal systems are evident in the normal adult male breast with rare secondary ductal branching. However, with the clinical development of gynecomastia, enlargement of the subareolar portion of the breast is evident as a result of secondary ductal branching and proliferation of fibroblastic stroma. Poulsen[10] presented evidence of a trophic and stimulatory effect of estrogens on mammary epithelial tissue growth, whereas Turkington and Topper[11] demonstrated a less important role for androgens in the inhibition of proliferation. Thus gynecomastia emerges as a result of excess circulating estrogen in the presence of deficient circulating plasma androgen. Defective androgen receptors, as found in testicular insufficiency (feminization) and related syndromes, likewise contribute via the loss of active androgenic influences on ductal breast epithelium. Testosterone, which is synthesized by the testes, and dihydrotestosterone, which is converted from testosterone in the prostate, skin, adipose tissue, and other peripheral sites, are the major active biologic androgens. Testicular secretion of testosterone is primarily regulated by negative feedback inhibition of the pituitary gonadotropin LH. Estradiol is the major biologically active estrogen. In males, most estradiol is synthesized from peripheral conversion of testosterone or androstenedione, a weak androgen secreted by the adrenals.

The loss of inhibitory androgenic influences on breast development, as suggested by MacDonald and associates,[12,13] clarifies the effect of the hypoandrogenic

TABLE **6-1**	Clinical Classification of Gynecomastia
Grade I	Mild breast enlargement without skin redundancy
Grade IIa	Moderate breast enlargement without skin redundancy
Grade IIb	Moderate breast enlargement with skin redundancy
Grade III	Marked breast enlargement with skin redundance and ptosis—simulates a female breast

Modified from Simon BE et al: *Plast Reconstr Surg* 51:48, 1973.

state on the development of gynecomastia. Although the role of prolactin in promoting lactation is evident, its role in gynecomastia is uncertain. Turkington[14] noted normal serum prolactin values in most males with gynecomastia and observed that enlarged breasts do not develop in most subjects with hyperprolactinemia. However, the hyperprolactinemic state may contribute to impotence and gynecomastia through indirect effects on gonadal and possibly adrenal function. Franks and associates[15] confirmed that increased prolactin may lead to alterations in the ratio of circulating estrogens to androgens, thus contributing to an imbalance of sex steroid hormones and, hence, to the emergence of gynecomastia.

Histopathology

The histologic pattern of gynecomastia progresses from an early active phase (florid) to an inactive phase (fibrous), no matter what the cause. Grossly, there is a relatively sharp margin between breast tissue and surrounding subcutaneous fat. The few ductal structures of the male breast enlarge, elongate, and branch along with the encasing connective tissue.[16,17] This combined increase in glandular and stromal elements provides for a regular distribution of each element throughout the enlarged breast. Often, there is an increase in cell number relative to the basement membrane. The loose connective tissue that regularly outlines the ducts as a central feature of gynecomastia is prominent only in the earliest stage of the disease (Figures 6-1 to 6-3). The fibroblasts within this loose tissue are relatively large but lack atypical features and are not clustered, even though they appear more frequently immediately adjacent to the basement membrane of the ducts.

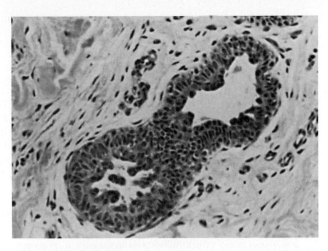

FIG. **6-2** Seen at higher power, the duct (shown in Figure 6-1) demonstrates hyperplastic epithelium. Note the increase in epithelial cell number over the basement membrane.

The epithelial cells are often increased to three or four in height. The cells are primarily cuboidal, without a prominence of basilar or myoepithelial cells. With greater cell numbers, there is a tendency toward a pattern mimicking "tufting," but these small areas, four to five cells in width, are the only foci of cell increase. This very slight hyperplasia, suggesting a papillary pattern, is often enhanced to produce long, narrow papillary proliferations of epithelial cells. These occasionally mimic atypical hyperplastic patterns except that the cells tend to have a regular placement, which differs from the pattern seen in well-developed atypical hyperplasia (Figures 6-2 and 6-4).

The micropapillary pattern is the most common hyperplastic pattern seen with gynecomastia. With a frequent and even distribution throughout the specimen, these micropapillae are benign in appearance.

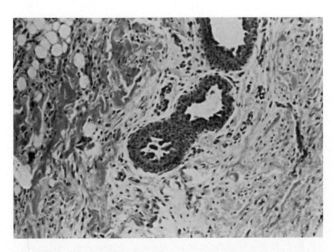

FIG. **6-1** From the florid phase of gynecomastia, a tortuous duct passes through the center of the photograph. A richly vascular, loose connective tissue is present around the duct.

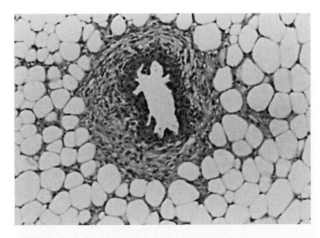

FIG. **6-3** From the florid phase of gynecomastia, this duct has elongated into surrounding fat. Note the cellular, young fibrous tissue ensheathing the duct and insinuating between fat cells.

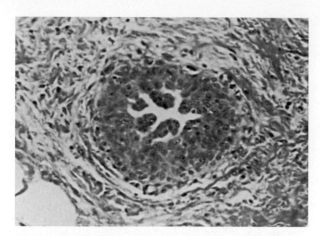

FIG. **6-4** Hyperplasia of epithelial cells is evident in the many layers of cells. The micropapillary fronds that are present centrally are characteristic of the hyperplasia seen in gynecomastia.

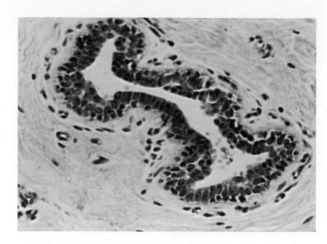

FIG. **6-6** Higher magnification of Figure 6-5 demonstrates compact fibrous tissue applied almost directly on ductal basement membrane. There are fewer capillaries encircling the duct than in the more active earlier stages of gynecomastia.

When present only focally, the pattern resembles that of atypical hyperplasia or even carcinoma in situ. However, the presence of atypical ductal hyperplasia (ADH) in the male breast is not well studied, and its clinical implications are unknown. In fact, these cytologic and histologic forms are only reminiscent of ADH, not diagnostic of that condition. Focal squamous metaplasia also may be found, with islands of squamous metaplastic cells interspersed within the hyperplastic epithelial cells.[18] Foci of apocrine change may be seen but are even less common. The finding of lobular units in the male breast is rare, being reported in 1 in 1000 cases.[19] The formation of lobular units has no known clinical correlate except that it seems to be somewhat more prevalent in florid gynecomastia.

Fibrous gynecomastia describes the later stage of gynecomastia and histologically has a dense collagenous stroma that contains relatively few fibroblasts

(Figures 6-5 to 6-7). This dense collagenous tissue is applied closely to delicate basement membrane regions surrounding sparse epithelial elements in which hyperplasia is usually absent. The loose pattern of periductal stroma that characterizes the florid stage of gynecomastia is lacking. Andersen and co-workers[20] used IHC techniques to show that the majority (89%) of gynecomastia specimens are estrogen receptor (ER) positive. They were unable to demonstrate an association between histopathologic staging of gynecomastia or hormonal parameters and ER status.

Virtually any benign alteration found in the female breast (in particular, fibroadenoma and sclerosing adenosis) may be found in the male breast, although such changes are rare. Differentiating carcinoma of the male breast from gynecomastia may be difficult clinically, but the problem is easily resolved with

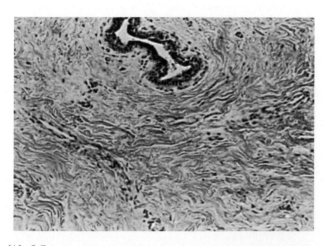

FIG. **6-5** In the late or fibrous stage of gynecomastia, ductal elements are less prominent and a dense collagenous stroma is predominant.

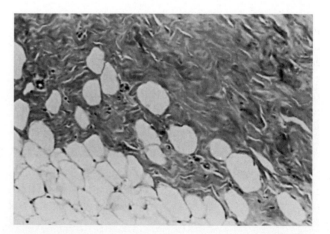

FIG. **6-7** At the interface of mammary connective tissue with subcutaneous fats, there is an intermingling of elements. Note the density of the connective tissue in this case, which is of 6 years' duration.

histologic or cytologic examination. There is significant discrepancy in the literature regarding the association of breast cancer and gynecomastia. Fodor[21] reports an occult focus of cribriform intraductal carcinoma amid gynecomastia identified in a 20-year-old. Ajayi, Osegbe, and Ademiluyi[22] in West Africa found gynecomastia to be present in 22% of cases of male breast cancer. An increased incidence of male breast cancer has been reported in Egypt and Zambia, where gynecomastia is a common finding resulting from hyperestrogenism caused by liver fibrosis and malnutrition. Whether the unusual cases of atypical hyperplasia and carcinoma in the male breast are preceded by gynecomastia is unknown. The carcinomas in situ that are reported to occur in the male breast are most often the solid and comedo types, although complex cribriform patterns are also demonstrated.[23,24]

DNA was analyzed in patients with breast carcinoma, fibroadenoma, and gynecomastia.[25] Specifically, telomeric deletions and *HER2/neu* gene amplification were analyzed. *HER2/neu* amplification was observed in 26.8% of breast carcinoma specimens but not in patients with fibroadenoma or gynecomastia. Significant reductions in telomeric length and concentration were noted in all breast tissue compared with placental control DNA; in addition, no significant differences were noted between carcinoma, fibroadenoma, and gynecomastia.

Physiologic Gynecomastia

Male breast enlargement occurring in the absence of a known or precipitating cause is noted during three phases of life and is regarded as an alteration in steroid hormone physiology rather than a pathologic event.

NEONATAL PERIOD

Palpable enlargement of the male breast in the neonate is normal and is to be distinguished from the rare clinical syndrome of prepubertal gynecomastia. This event occurs from the action of placental estrogens (estradiol, estriol) on neonatal breast parenchyma. Although this breast enlargement usually regresses within a few weeks, Bronstein and Cassorla[26] observed that it may uncommonly persist for prolonged periods.

ADOLESCENCE

Pubertal gynecomastia occurs in approximately two thirds of adolescent males[1] (Figure 6-8). Of 1855 boys of different ages examined at a Boy Scout camp, Nydick and associates[27] noted that 39% had gynecomastia and that 65% of boys aged 14 to 14.5 years were affected. For many of these male patients, the enlarged breasts are grossly asymmetric, tender, and cosmetically and psychologically disturbing. By age 20, only a small

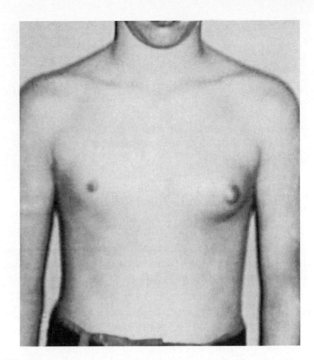

FIG. **6-8** An 11-year-old boy with unilateral (left) gynecomastia at puberty.

number of men have palpable gynecomastia in one or both breasts. Dehner, Hill, and Deschryver[28] found that gynecomastia and juvenile hypertrophy (females) accounted for 36% of the breast diseases seen in patients younger than 20.

The pubertal variant of gynecomastia is explained by a physiologic excess of plasma estradiol relative to the plasma testosterone.[6,29-32] Hemsell and associates[33] observed the production rate of androstenedione to be closely related to body surface area and plasma androstenedione to be the preferred substrate of the extraglandular aromatase system. Therefore, with maximal synthesis of this estrogen precursor during pubertal development and before maximal testosterone secretion by the testes, a relative excess of estrogen is produced and gynecomastia becomes apparent. Sher, Migeon, and Berkovitz[34] found that boys with marked idiopathic breast development had greater body mass than other boys of similar age.

SENESCENCE

The review by Wilson and colleagues[1] suggests that endocrine changes result in breast enlargement, which occurs in virtually all aging men. Others have shown that the prevalence of gynecomastia increases with age and is observed in 32% to 57% of elderly men[4,5,7] (Figure 6-9).

Niewoehner and Nuttall[35] examined 214 hospitalized adult men aged 27 to 92 years for the presence of palpable gynecomastia. The overall prevalence in this series

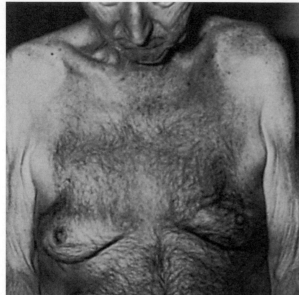

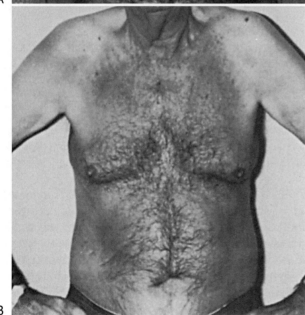

A

B

FIG. **6-9** **A,** Senescent bilateral gynecomastia in an 85-year-old man. The patient had observed a gradual increase in the size of both breasts over the past 4 years. There are no breast masses, and the patient takes no medication. **B,** Senescent bilateral gynecomastia in a 72-year-old man with progressive enlargement of breasts over a 6-year period. The patient has no systemic diseases and takes no medications.

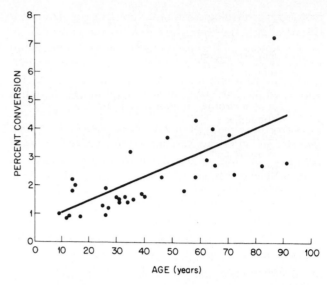

FIG. **6-10** Correlation of the extent of conversion of circulating androstenedione to estrone in men as a function of age. *(From Siiteri PK, MacDonald PC: Role of extraglandular estrogen in human endocrinology. In Greep RO, Astwood EB [eds]: Handbook of physiology, Washington, DC, 1975, American Physiological Society.)*

present in most older men, correlates with the amount of body fat, and does not require clinical evaluation unless symptomatic or of recent onset.

As the plasma testosterone concentration begins to decline at approximately age 70, there is simultaneous elevation of the plasma testosterone-estrogen (sex hormone)–binding globulin (TEBG) such that the level of unbound or free testosterone declines even further. Moreover, there is an associated rise in plasma LH, as suggested by Snyder,[36] with an increase in the rate of conversion of androgens to estrogens in peripheral tissues (Figure 6-10). As the plasma testosterone falls, relative hyperestrinism is evident with the decreasing plasma androgen/estrogen ratio. Siiteri and MacDonald[37] further suggest that the development of obesity increases the rate for peripheral conversion of androgens to estrogens.

Pathophysiologic Mechanisms

A summary of the pathophysiologic mechanisms of gynecomastia is shown in Table 6-2. Most patients have persistent pubertal gynecomastia or breast glandular enlargement from mediations, age-related reduction in testicular function, or idiopathic causes.[38]

ESTROGEN EXCESS STATES

Wilson and colleagues[1] suggest that increased estrogen production (independent of pituitary gonadotropin)

was 65%, being bilateral in all but 11 of these subjects. The prevalence was greatest in the 50- to 69-years group (72%); it was lowest in the 70- to 89-years group (47%) and in the 30- to 49-years group (54%). The authors observed gynecomastia to increase with body mass index (BMI). In particular, more than 80% of those with a BMI of 25 kg/m² or greater had gynecomastia. It was concluded that palpable bilateral gynecomastia is

TABLE 6-2	Pathophysiologic Mechanisms of Gynecomastia

Estrogen excess states
  Gonadal origin
    True hermaphroditism
    Gonadal stroma (nongerminal) neoplasms of the testis
      Leydig's cell (interstitial)
      Sertoli's cell
      Granulosa-theca cell
    Germ cell tumors
      Choriocarcinoma
      Seminoma, teratoma
      Embryonal carcinoma
  Nontesticular tumors
    Skin—nevus
    Adrenocortical neoplasms
    Lung carcinoma
    Malignant mesothelioma
    Hepatocellular carcinoma
  Endocrine disorders
  Diseases of the liver—nonalcoholic and alcoholic cirrhosis
  Nutritional alteration states
Androgen deficiency states
  Senescent causes with aging
  Hypoandrogen states (hypogonadism)
    Primary testicular failure
      Klinefelter's syndrome (XXY)
      Reifenstein's syndrome (XY)
      Rosewater, Gwinup, Hamwi familial gynecomastia (XY)
      Kallmann's syndrome
      Kennedy's disease with associated gynecomastia
      Eunuchoidal males (congenital anorchia)
      Hereditary defects of androgen biosynthesis
      Adrenocorticotropic hormone deficiency
    Secondary testicular failure
      Trauma
      Orchitis
      Cryptorchidism
      Irradiation
      Hydrocele
      Varicocele
      Spermatocele
Drug-related conditions that initiate gynecomastia
Idiopathic mechanisms
  Renal failure
  Nonneoplastic diseases of the lung
  Trauma (chest wall)
  Pituitary adenoma
  Psychologic
  Acquired immunodeficiency syndrome (AIDS) and human immunodeficiency virus (HIV) infection

can be caused by at least three pathophysiologic mechanisms: (1) increased secretion by endocrine organs, including the testes; (2) increased availability of substrate for peripheral conversion to estrogens; and (3) increased aromatase activity within peripheral tissues in the presence of normal substrate levels (Figures 6-11 and 6-12).

Gonadal Origin

True Hermaphroditism. True hermaphroditism occurs when an ovary and a testis or gonad with mixed histologic features of both organs (ovotestis) are present. As indicated by Van Niekerk,[39] four categories are recognized: (1) bilateral, with testicular and ovarian

Normal

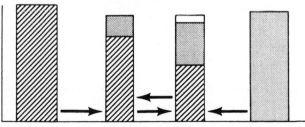

Increased Estrogen Secretion

Increased Substrate Availability

Increased Peripheral Aromatase

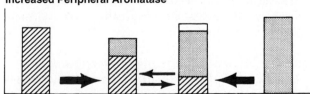

FIG. 6-11 Gynecomastia as the result of increased estrogen formation can arise because of increased estrogen secretion into plasma by the adrenal or the testis, increased availability of substrate for peripheral conversion to estrogen, or an increased rate of aromatization within tissues. (*From Wilson JD, Aiman J, MacDonald PC: The pathogenesis of gynecomastia. In Stollerman GH et al [eds]: Advances in internal medicine, vol 25, St Louis, 1980, Mosby.*)

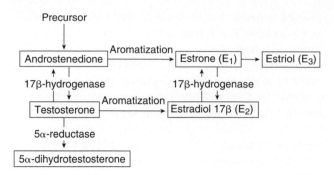

FIG. **6-12** Potential pathways for androgen-estrogen inter-conversion in healthy men. (*Modified from Gordon GG et al: J Clin Endocrinol Metab 40:1018, 1975.*)

tissue (ovotestis) anatomically present on each side; (2) unilateral, in which an ovotestis is evident on one side and an ovary or testis on the contralateral side; (3) lateral, in which a testis is evident on one side and an ovary on the opposite side; and (4) indeterminate, in which the clinical syndrome is expressed but the location and type of gonadal tissue is uncertain.

Significant gynecomastia is evident at puberty in approximately 75% of individuals with true hermaphroditism. Approximately half of these individuals menstruate. For the phenotypic male with true hermaphroditism, menstruation presents as cyclic hematuria. Hormonal activity has been noted by Gallegos and colleagues[40] and Aiman, Hemsell, and MacDonald,[41] who observed gonadal secretion of estradiol in phenotypic men with feminization (gynecomastia and menstruation). Aiman and associates[41] observed excess estradiol secretion relative to androgen production by the ovotestis.

17-Ketosteroid reductase deficiency results in male pseudohermaphroditism with a marked overproduction of androstenedione and estrone and decreased production of testosterone and estradiol. A late-onset form of testicular 17-ketosteroid reductase deficiency can cause gynecomastia and hypogonadism in men.[42] Cavanah and Dons[43] report gynecomastia in a eugonadal adult male secondary to 3β-hydroxysteroid deficiency with an associated alteration in sex hormone ratios.

Gonadal Stromal (Nongerminal) Neoplasms

Leydig's Cell (Interstitial) Tumors of the Testes. Overall, Leydig's cell neoplasms of the testes are relatively uncommon, constituting approximately 2% to 3% of all testicular neoplasms.[44] Such neoplasms are found in children as young as 2 years and in adults as old as 82 years.[33] Leydig's cell tumors account for up to 39% of non–germ cell tumors of the testes and 12% of the testicular neoplasms of children.[45-48]

Camin and colleagues[46] and Turner, Derrick, and Worltmann[49] observed that Leydig's cell tumors of the testes are most often unilateral. Although bilateral neoplasms have been reported, the differential diagnosis of hyperplasia with nodules in each testis from multiple neoplasms may be difficult. These neoplasms are seen in early to middle childhood; Brosman[45] observed the average age for diagnosis to be 4.7 years. Sexual precocity is usually observed in children with these tumors and is accompanied by an increase in muscle mass and stature with advanced bone age in most patients. In children, Leydig's cell tumors are almost uniformly benign. Many believe that therapy should be restricted to unilateral orchiectomy in children.[45,46,50-53] Biopsy of the contralateral testis may be advisable if bilateral enlargement is evident, although bilateral neoplasms occur in only a minority of such patients.

Feminization is less common in the adult, with endocrine signs noted in approximately 30% of these tumors[54]; painful gynecomastia and decreased libido are the most common manifestations. Symptoms may precede the onset of a palpable testicular mass, particularly with Leydig's cell hyperplasia. The diffuseness of the condition explains the delay between onset of symptoms and discovery of the testicular mass.[55]

Malignant behavior of Leydig's cell tumors occurs in approximately 10% of patients, predominantly in adults and older men.[56,57] The carcinomas of interstitial cells may require electron microscopy for certain diagnoses because of poor differentiation at the light microscopic level.[58]

Feminization associated with Leydig's cell tumors is thought to develop after estrogen secretion by these cells.[59] Approximately 25% of the Leydig's cell tumors of adult men secrete predominantly estrogen.[47,48,60,61] For some patients, gynecomastia may be observed despite normal serum estrogen and testosterone levels. In these patients, gynecomastia may occur after in situ conversion of androstenedione to estrone in breast parenchyma, leading to increased local (tissue) estrogen values without elevating serum levels.[62-65] Mellor and McCutchan[66] report the potential occult nature of Leydig's cell tumors first seen with gynecomastia. Gynecomastia associated with Leydig's cell tumors is more often seen when these tumors are benign, especially when 17-ketosteroid values are normal. Malignant Leydig's cell tumors usually demonstrate abnormal estrogen or androgen levels and are associated more frequently with elevated estrogens and 17-ketosteroid levels without gynecomastia.[56,57,67]

Gabrilove and Furukawa[68] performed selective venous sampling of spermatic veins of the testis involved with the Leydig's cell tumor and observed estrogen values to be twentyfold to thirtyfold higher than those in normal subjects. The feminizing effect of excess estradiol is reinforced by the associated hypogonadism. Veldhuis and colleagues[69] and Bercovici and associates[70] observed the inhibitory action of estradiol on testosterone production to occur at two principal sites: the pituitary and the testes. Gabrilove and co-workers[71] observed low-normal LH values for patients with Leydig's cell tumors. For patients with gynecomastia and increased circulating estrogen levels, pituitary suppression of LH release may initiate atrophy of the contralateral testis.[72] Goh and associates[73,74] demonstrated that estrogens inhibit gonadotropin secretion in castrated transsexuals, and Veldhuis and colleagues[69] noted a similar biologic event in patients with feminizing adrenal tumors. A prolonged plasma estradiol response to human chorionic gonadotropin (hCG) is a useful, although nonspecific, adjunct in the diagnosis of Leydig's cell tumors.[75]

Mineur and associates[76] established that estrogen values decrease to normal values soon after tumor removal (orchiectomy). In a study of chronic hyperestrogenism on gonadal function in men who had estrogen-secreting Leydig's cell tumors, these investigators observed men to have low plasma gonadotropin and testosterone levels before unilateral orchiectomy with concurrent increase in estradiol values. Before surgery, spermatogenesis was abnormal in some subjects. Testicular endocrine function and spermatogenesis did not return to normal after surgery. Estradiol values decreased to normal immediately after surgery but returned to upper normal limits in follow-up.[77] Mineur and associates[76] concluded that chronic hyperestrogenism produced hypothalamopituitary inhibition as well as direct steroidogenic blockade at the testicular level.

Other Nongerminal Testicular Neoplasms (Sertoli's Cell and Granulosa-Theca Cell Tumors). The great majority of testicular neoplasms take origin from germ cells. Testicular neoplasms of nongerminal origin having endocrine function, besides the interstitial cell tumor (Leydig's cell), are other tumors of specialized gonadal stroma.[78] This latter group of gonadal stromal lesions, including tumors of Sertoli, granulosa, and theca cell origin,[79] all arise from the primitive gonadal mesenchyme.[47,60,61] Neoplasms of the testes are limited almost entirely to three age groups: infancy, late adolescence/young adulthood, and 50 years or greater.[63] The incidence of testicular tumors in the United States is 2.1 neoplasms per 100,000 males, of which only a small percentage occur in children.[47,80]

The proportion of germinal to nongerminal tumors is greater in children.[47,53] However, 30% of reported Sertoli's cell tumors have been in infants and children younger than 10 years.[57] A calcifying variant of Sertoli's tumor has been described by Waxman and associates.[81]

Gynecomastia has been associated with 26% to 33% of patients with benign Sertoli's cell tumors of the testes, the majority of which rapidly regressed after orchiectomy.[78,82] Fligiel and associates[63] identified five patients with malignant Sertoli's cell tumors with evidence of gynecomastia, two of whom had elevated gonadotropin levels. In most cases there were no elevations of estrogen or testosterone values. Gabrilove and co-workers[57] noted that gynecomastia may reflect an alteration in the estrogen/androgen ratio with or without an increase in the actual estrogen plasma value.

Proppe and Scully[83] note that a variety of Sertoli's cell tumors tend to be bilateral and familial and may be associated with precocious puberty, gynecomastia, and atrial myxomas. Reports by Wilson and associates[84] and Young and associates[85] confirmed multifocal Sertoli's cell tumors associated with the autosomal dominant syndrome of Peutz-Jeghers in young boys. The previous recognition of increased risk of gonadal tumors for females with Peutz-Jeghers syndrome was made by Scully.[86]

Mostofi and Price[61] and Teilum[87,88] suggest that the classification, and consequently the frequency of each cell type, varies according to the degree of cellular differentiation and perceptions of individual observers. Neoplasms of Leydig's and Sertoli's cells make up the bulk of these nongerminal testicular lesions. Thus neoplasms that are composed predominantly of ovarian cellular homologues—theca cell and granulosa cell—are rarely observed in the testes. Some mixed gonadal stromal neoplasms (e.g., Sertoli-Leydig cell tumor) have been described as having undifferentiated gonadal stroma. Early reported cases of the testicular granulosa cell tumor claim a morphologic similarity to the analogous ovarian neoplasm.[89-92] These lesions are of great rarity, with fewer than 10 examples recorded in men aged 20 to 53 years. Only recently has a distinct cystic variant of the granulosa cell tumor of the infant testes been recognized that is morphologically similar to the ovarian juvenile granulosa cell tumor.[93-96]

Sertoli's cell and other gonadal stromal tumors may exhibit malignant behavior after infancy. Rosvoll and Woodard[97] and Kaplan and colleagues[98] report males with distant metastatic disease. No known tumor markers have been identified for the non–Leydig's cell gonadal stromal tumors. α-fetoprotein (AFP) values may be markedly elevated in healthy infants.[99,100] Masterson and colleagues[101] attribute these findings to the production and metabolism of AFP by the infant, which appears to be unrelated to tumor activity. These authors observed elevated values of AFP in only two infants; findings were negative in five other boys, including one with metastatic disease.

Germinal Cell Tumors

Choriocarcinoma, Seminoma, Teratoma, and Embryonal Cell Carcinoma. Precise mechanisms for the pathogenesis of germinal cell testicular neoplasms have not been determined. It has been postulated by Pierce and colleagues[102,103] that any early germ cell has potential for malignant transformation if the factors integrating and controlling its development fail to function. Thus neoplastic transformation of normal germ cells into embryonal carcinoma cells may occur. Neoplasms may be composed solely of the stem embryonal carcinoma cells or may differentiate along somatic and extraembryonic pathways,[102,103] producing teratoma in the former case and trophoblastic tissue (choriocarcinoma) or yolk sac tissue (yolk sac tumor) in the latter.[104] Seminoma may take origin from the totipotential embryonal carcinoma cells.[105,106] This theory of a common origin of germ cell tumors of the testes from embryonal carcinoma cells is supported by the ultrastructural studies of Pierce, Stevens, and Nakane[103] and the experimental production of teratoma from embryonal carcinoma explants by Stevens[107] and Stevens and Hummel.[108] Reports suggest that patients with gynecomastia secondary to elevated estrogen plasma values have increased conversion of dehydroepiandrosterone (DHEA) to estradiol.[63,109-111] Although others[12,112,113] acknowledge that this event occurs with choriocarcinoma, this bioconversion plays a diminutive role in estrogen production for patients with testicular tumors other than choriocarcinoma.[37] Estrogen effects in men with these neoplasms occur secondary to increased aromatization of testosterone and androstenedione into estrogens in peripheral sites because more of the estrogen precursors are synthesized or possibly because of an enhanced activity of aromatizing enzymes.[114] Androstenedione, which has low androgenicity and is readily aromatized to estrone peripherally, may also be produced in increased concentrations by some tumors, with the result of enhanced estrogen production.[37]

Gynecomastia in patients with germ cell tumors correlated with a higher mortality than that in patients without gynecomastia.[110,115] Tseng and colleagues[115] reported a 75% resolution of gynecomastia after orchiectomy and chemotherapy. The persistence of gynecomastia, however, did not indicate residual disease.

Ultrasonographic detection of malignant, nonpalpable germ cell tumors is well documented.[116-119] Such tumors may be small focal lesions within the parenchyma of the testes. Testicular origin is often suggested by feminizing features, including gynecomastia, as well as peripheral lymphadenopathy. Use of testicular ultrasound for detection and localization of these early testicular masses manifested by gynecomastia is essential. Hendry

and associates[120] and Emory and colleagues[121] recommend that any young adult male with unexplained gynecomastia, loss of libido, or impotence have diagnostic testicular ultrasound for evaluation of occult tumors of this organ. Mellor and McCutchan[66] suggest that ultrasound may be insufficiently sensitive to detect the testicular tumor, and they have consequently recommended surgical exploration and biopsy of any suspect testis with associated gynecomastia.

Nagi, Jones, and Belchetz[122] reported a case of gynecomastia associated with a primary mediastinal β-hCG–secreting seminoma. Lemack, Poppas, and Vaughan[123] presented a comprehensive and current review of the urologic causes of gynecomastia

Nontesticular Tumors

Skin—Nevus. The onset of progressive gynecomastia after delivery of a normal fetus with a giant pigmented nevus (3×6.5 cm) has been documented by Leung and colleagues.[124] The removal of this nevus resulted in regression of breast enlargement, suggesting that the association of these two seemingly unrelated problems may be more than coincidental. Nonendocrine tumors (including those of the skin) may result in hormonal imbalance and pathologic signs that are well documented. Salassa, Jowsey, and Arnaud[125] confirmed hypophosphatemic osteomalacia associated with nonendocrine tumors; the removal of these nonendocrine neoplasms resulted in restoration of a normal metabolic state. It is possible that giant pigmented nevi elaborate a mammotrophic substance that is capable of increasing target organ sensitivity to estrogen or may simulate increased conversion of androstenedione or testosterone to estrogen.

In 1970 the review by Fienman and Yakovac[126] included a single case of male prepubertal gynecomastia among 46 patients with neurofibromatosis; since this report, only isolated cases have been documented.[127-134] Etiologic and pathogenetic associations are unproved.

Neoplasms of the Adrenal Cortex. Primary tumors of the adrenal cortex are rare.[135] Although nonfunctional tumors in the adrenal cortex have been reported, the majority of pediatric patients have been initially evaluated for clinical signs of hormonal activity.[136] In a 1966 review by Hayles and colleagues,[137] it was determined that a majority of children had virilization or feminization as a preponderant sign and one third had hyperadrenocorticism. In addition, several symptom complexes that include feminization and hyperaldosteronism have been documented by others.[138-149] Adrenocortical neoplasms have been associated with several congenital anomalies, including astrocytoma, cutaneous lesions, hemihypertrophy, abnormalities of the contralateral adrenal gland, and the Beckwith-Wiedemann syndrome.[150,151]

Ogle[152] reported the first childhood adrenal tumor in 1865. In the 48-year review of surgical experience at Roswell Park Memorial Institute by Didolkar and colleagues,[153] adrenal tumors constituted only 0.04% of all cancer cases. In addition, in a 20-year review of the pediatric population of Manchester, England, Stewart, Morris Jones, and Jolleys[154] found neuroblastoma (a tumor of the adrenal medulla) to be 16 times more frequent than cortical tumors. In the review by Hayles and colleagues,[137] there were 222 cases of functional adrenocortical tumors of childhood. Thus it appears that adrenocortical tumors are rare in the general population and are especially uncommon in the pediatric group. However, there is a bimodal age distribution favoring children and older adults.[155]

Adrenal neoplasms should be suspected in any child with premature or inappropriate signs of progressive virilization or feminization, especially if accompanied by evidence of hyperadrenocorticism or gynecomastia. Feminizing adrenal carcinomas are relatively uncommon.[156] In 1919 Bittorf[157] reported the first estrogen-producing adrenal tumor in an adult male. Since then, a relatively small number of patients have been documented.[142,158,159] In additional patients documented by Gabrilove and associates,[141] an increase in estrogen production with an increased urinary excretion of estrogen was confirmed. Wohltmann, Mathur, and Williamson[160] concluded that the biologic manifestations are a result of alterations in the ratio of estrogen to androgen levels rather than an absolute value of testosterone or estrogen. More recently, Nishiki and colleagues[161] confirmed preoperative elevations of urinary 17-ketosteroids and hydroxycorticosteroids; serum estrogens were dramatically reduced after treatment of the primary adrenal carcinoma.

Feminization with subsequent gynecomastia as a consequence of adrenal adenomas is rare in childhood, with only a few reports in young males.[162] The apparent benignity of physiologic pubertal gynecomastia contrasts with the rare prepubertal gynecomastia that may point to an adrenal or testicular neoplasm. In patients documented by Sultan and associates,[163] the bilateral gynecomastia of an estrogen-producing adrenal adenoma had the unusual appearance of a ballooned areola with prominent venous vascularization. There appears to be overproduction of estrogen by the adrenal adenoma, with consequent persistent adolescent gynecomastia and blockade of pubertal maturation. The gonadal insufficiency in these patients can be related to the negative feedback exerted by estrogens on the hypothalamopituitary axis.[164]

The observations of Latorre and Kenny[132] confirmed that evidence of premature development of secondary sexual characteristics, such as enlarged penis, axillary hair, and pubic hair, may be seen in children with gynecomastia associated with tumors of the adrenal gland or testis.

Desai and Kapadia[165] documented the great infrequency of feminizing adrenocortical adenoma in comparison with the more common feminizing adrenocortical carcinomas of the male. In patients with adrenocortical carcinoma, a diverse pattern of symptoms may become evident during the course of disease, meaning feminization, Cushing's syndrome, and masculinization may predominate at different times in the clinical course.[166] Gabrilove and associates[71,141,142] confirmed that estrogens may be the major functional product, with no evidence of Cushing's syndrome.

Most of the information about the occurrence of neoplasms of the adrenal cortex relates to the time before the introduction of computed tomography,[156] which has replaced other methods of studying the adrenals in situ. This sensitive test may present specific difficulties in the setting of gynecomastia, considering that somewhat enlarged adrenals are relatively common in the older age group. This is not a problem in the pediatric age group, but older persons often have enlarged adrenals, which are perhaps analogous to nodular alteration of the thyroid and have no known physiologic correlate.[155] These incidentally discovered masses have been called *incidentalomas* and should cause no concern in the absence of other indications if they are 3 cm or smaller.

The information of greatest interest with regard to adrenocortical tumors is that those producing feminization in the pediatric age group are not as often malignant as previously thought.[155,167] It is also quite clear that neoplasms producing mixed syndromes in adult males, such as feminization and Cushing's disease, are virtually almost always malignant.[155,168,169] Careful histologic analysis of adrenal tumors is sensitive and specific with regard to indicating the likelihood or unlikelihood of malignant behavior.[170]

Lung Carcinoma. Carcinoma of the lung may initiate an increase in plasma chorionic gonadotropin values with a simultaneous escalation in estrogen secretion.[1,171] Furthermore, it appears that the volume of estrogen-induced breast tissue correlates with estrogen production. Fusco and Rosen[172] were the first to identify gonadotropin in the urine of four male patients who died of bronchogenic carcinoma. In three patients, gonadotropin was also present in tissue samples from the primary lung tumor.

The association of gynecomastia with bronchial carcinoma has previously been reviewed by Camiel, Benninghoff, and Alexander,[173] and with the reports by Fusco and Rosen[172] and Becker and associates,[174] the most plausible explanation is stimulation of the testes, and possibly the adrenals, by chorionic gonadotropin. This physiologic event was previously observed by

Fine, Smith, and Pachter[175] and suggests that gonadotropin stimulation is responsible for the release of estrogens that initiate hyperplasia of the breast. Daily and Marcuse[176] propose that the detection of chorionic gonadotropin may be an aid in the diagnosis of bronchogenic carcinoma. These authors suggest that the appearance of gynecomastia in the adult male should arouse the suspicion of carcinoma of the lung.

The ectopic production of hormones by bronchogenic carcinoma may also initiate lactation, as has been recorded in a single female patient with anaplastic carcinoma of the lung.[177] Behera and associates[178] reported the rare observation of galactorrhea with gynecomastia in a male patient with squamous carcinoma of the lung. This patient was also hypercalcemic, with absence of documented skeletal metastasis. The authors postulate an osteoclast-activating factor or parahormone-like substance secreted by the primary tumor. Furthermore, the abnormal lactation may be secondary to excess secretion of prolactin, as evident in the variance of lactation frequency (2% to approximately 33% of cases) seen in lung cancer.[179,180] For cases in which prolactin values are normal, the intermittent secretion of prolactin or the excessive sensitivity of breast tissue to normal values may initiate clinical gynecomastia.

Malignant Mesothelioma. Okamoto and colleagues[181] describe the only two published cases of hCG-producing malignant pleural mesotheliomas with choriocarcinomatous features. Both patients had bilateral gynecomastia and elevated levels of hCG with tumors that demonstrated α-hCG and β-hCG and human placental lactogen on immunohistochemical staining.

Hepatocellular Carcinoma. Hepatocellular carcinoma may initiate gynecomastia. As confirmed by Kew and associates,[182] feminization in primary liver carcinoma is the consequence of increased aromatase activity in the hepatic neoplasm.

Males develop hepatocellular carcinoma in the cirrhotic liver much more frequently than do females.[183] Furthermore, Andervont[184] determined that in animal models, male castration decreased the incidence of spontaneous hepatocellular carcinoma from 33% to 12%. The administration of testosterone to mice with chemically induced hepatic nodules significantly increased the rate of malignant transformation. Goodall and Butler[185] further determined that control rats fed a diet of aflatoxin B_1 (4 ppm) consistently developed hepatic neoplasms, whereas hypophysectomized animals were resistant to hepatic neoplastic transformation.

Although the mechanism of tumor development remains unknown, gender differences in steroid and drug metabolism is a possibility.[186] A report by Stedman, Moore, and Morgan[187] suggests that primary hepatic neoplasms contain estrogen receptors, as does normal hepatic parenchyma. More recently, Iqbal and colleagues[188] determined that these malignant neoplasms also contain androgen receptors, whereas normal liver parenchyma does not.

Endocrine Disorders (Hyperthyroidism, Hypothyroidism). In 1959 Hall[189] reviewed the English literature for gynecomastia that occurred in association with hyperthyroidism. This author found only 26 cases, and in most instances, gynecomastia appeared during hyperthyroidism and receded after establishment of the euthyroid state. This clinical observation suggests that coexistence of the two diseases is more than coincidental.[190-192] Furthermore, the therapy of the hyperthyroid state has usually resulted in diminution or clinical disappearance of gynecomastia whether the therapy surgery (thyroidectomy),[191,193,194] use of iodine-131 is radioactivity,[192,193,195] or administration of antithyroid medication.[189,190] In rare cases, gynecomastia may not regress after return to the euthyroid state; Larsson, Sundbom, and Astedt[193] documented the need for bilateral mastectomy for gynecomastia that persisted for 6 months after control of the hyperthyroid condition. These authors suggest that the diffuse toxic goiter of Graves' disease is the most common type of hyperthyroidism to occur in association with gynecomastia. Gynecomastia associated with thyroid disease is usually seen clinically with grossly enlarged, tender breasts and, rarely, nipple discharge.[196] In most of the reported cases, gynecomastia is bilateral, and although it may begin unilaterally,[193,194] rarely does it remain unilateral.[197-199] The testes are usually normal in size and consistency, although isolated case reports by Larsson and associates[193] described small testes and others[191,195,197] noted testicular atrophy.

The pathogenesis of gynecomastia with associated thyroid disease remains enigmatic. Nydick and associates[27] observed that size and the occurrence of gynecomastia in clinically euthyroid adolescent boys correlates with the size of the thyroid gland. Furthermore, the mammotrophic effects of thyroid hormone on breast development has been demonstrated by the studies of Weichert and Boyd,[200] who fed thyroid hormones to pregnant rats and noted an earlier and more prominent hypertrophy of breasts than in pregnant controls. Fitzsimons[201] observed a reduction in gynecomastia after administration of exogenous estrogens, making it tempting to identify alterations in endogenous estrogen metabolism as instrumental in the genesis of gynecomastia in the hyperthyroid male. Chopra[202] confirmed that gynecomastia often occurs in men with hyperthyroidism who have high serum free estrogen values and normal free testosterone levels.[203] More recently, Nomura and associates[204] found elevated serum progesterone values in hyperthyroid men, which declined concomitant with serum thyroid hormone levels during antithyroid drug therapy.

The fact that progesterone enhances estrogen stimulation of mammary gland growth[205] strongly intimates that high serum progesterone levels in hyperthyroid men may contribute to the development of this clinical state in conjunction with the imbalance between estrogen and testosterone. Chopra[202] estimates that gynecomastia occurs in approximately 20% to 40% of men with hyperthyroidism. He noted that serum concentrations of total estradiol-17β, total testosterone, and LH are supranormal in these patients. Furthermore, serum concentrations of sex hormone–binding globulin are high in hyperthyroidism. Although serum unbound testosterone is normal, the serum unbound estradiol-17β is above normal in the hyperthyroid male. Furthermore, Chopra suggests that the imbalance in relative concentrations of unbound gonadal steroids is apparently quite favorable to the development of gynecomastia in hyperthyroid states.[202] As a consequence, increased peripheral tissue metabolism of androgens to estrogens seems to be the major factor responsible for the high estradiol-17β value in this state; increased glandular secretion of estradiol-17β may also be important.

Galactorrhea rarely occurs in men; most cases are reported in patients with prolactin-secreting pituitary tumors.[206,207] Kleinberg, Noel, and Frantz[207] and Edwards, Forsyth, and Besser[208] documented hyperprolactinemia and galactorrhea in the presence of hypothyroidism in women. Arnaout and associates[209] reported the occurrence of galactorrhea and gynecomastia in a patient with occult hypothyroidism, both of which resolved after thyroxin replacement therapy. This report is the first to document galactorrhea secondary to hypothyroidism in a male patient. Arnaout suggests that the differential diagnosis of galactorrhea in male patients should include hypothyroidism.[209]

Diseases of the Liver. Although it has been accepted for several decades that the hyperestrogen state is commonly observed in nonalcoholic cirrhosis of the liver, it has only recently been determined that plasma concentrations and urinary excretion of estrogen are both increased. Previous reports confirmed that the peripheral conversion of plasma androgens to estrogens is increased in the cirrhotic state.[210-212]

Kley and associates[213] evaluated estrogen, testosterone, androstenedione, and cortisol values and percentage of binding of these steroids in plasma for normal, young, and old male subjects and in male patients with fatty liver, chronic hepatitis, and cirrhosis of the liver. Alterations of these steroids were most marked in patients with cirrhosis but were also evident

to a lesser degree in patients with fatty metamorphosis of the liver and in normal aging patients. These authors determined a definite increase in estrone, a smaller escalation in estradiol, a decrease in testosterone, and a rise in LH for cirrhosis. Cortisol remained unchanged, whereas ratios of estradiol to testosterone and estrone to testosterone were augmented in patients with cirrhosis and were higher than those in healthy young subjects. These authors suggest that the combination of elevated estrone and estradiol and reduced testosterone, which was strongly bound by increased sex hormone–binding globulin, may be responsible for gynecomastia and hypogonadism in chronic liver diseases. Because patients with hepatic disease and elderly men are observed to have similar alterations of steroid plasma concentrations and the binding of these steroids to plasma proteins, these authors suggest that the etiological mechanism is similar, namely, altered hepatic parenchymal function. In 1985 Kley and colleagues[214] confirmed the absence of gynecomastia in patients with idiopathic hemochromatosis, including those with severe liver disease. The variance in clinical presentation of idiopathic hemochromatosis and alcoholic cirrhosis suggests that the mechanism of hepatic failure is accompanied by different abnormalities in sex hormone metabolism. Kley and associates[214] confirmed the clinical features of hypogonadism and normal estrogen activity in patients with idiopathic hemochromatosis. Conversely, in alcoholic cirrhosis, estradiol and estrone were significantly elevated and sex hormone–binding globulins was increased. In idiopathic hemochromatosis, sex hormone–binding globulin levels were in the same range as for normal men. For idiopathic hemochromatosis, the instantaneous conversion of plasma androstenedione to estrone and estradiol was normal, whereas that of plasma testosterone to plasma estrogen was decreased by about half. The converse was observed in alcoholic cirrhosis: The instantaneous conversion of plasma androstenedione to estrogen was greatly increased, and that of testosterone was within the normal range.

Farthing and associates[215] observed that plasma progesterone values were increased in 72% (36 of 50) of men with liver disease compared with 20 healthy male controls. The plasma progesterone values were significantly higher for men with nonalcoholic cirrhosis and gynecomastia; however, this hormonal relationship was not observed for men with alcoholic fatty change and alcoholic cirrhosis. Although hyperprolactinemia was observed in 14% of males with hepatic disease, it was believed that levels were unrelated to the presence of gynecomastia. The authors suggest that increased circulating values of progesterone and prolactin do not explain the development of gynecomastia in patients with liver disease but that these sex steroids may be a factor acting in concert with other hormones to initiate breast hypertrophy. Furthermore, Johnson[216] and other reviewers concluded that observed increases in estradiol are not great enough to contribute to the feminization seen in cirrhosis. These conclusions are drawn from results of free estradiol estimations that have been equally varied and from the fact that estrone is only a weak estrogen. Kley and coinvestigators[213,214] confirmed the variations in free testosterone and estradiol values in control subjects and for patients with varying stages of hepatic cirrhosis (from well compensated to decompensated with ascites, variceal hemorrhage, gynecomastia, and testicular atrophy). The progressive rise in estradiol was marked, as was the reciprocal fall of free testosterone (Table 6-3). The progressive rise in sex hormone–binding globulins tends to escalate the profound feminizing aspects of alcoholic disease, because testosterone has a significantly higher affinity for sex hormone–binding globulins, thus enhancing the estrogen/testosterone ratio.

Gynecomastia in the Cirrhotic Male. Gynecomastia is observed in approximately 40% of cirrhotic men.[217-223] Total plasma testosterone concentrations were lower than normal as identified by Van Thiel, Lester, and Sherins[224] and by others.[213,214,225-227] Although this relative decrease in testosterone is significant, it is modest and is masked by the far greater fall in the non–protein bound (biologically active) fraction of plasma testosterone.[203,219,225,228] This decrease appears to result from the increased concentration of sex hormone–binding globulin present in cirrhotic males.[229-231] Anderson[232] considers sex hormone–binding globulin the most important plasma protein for determination of the protein binding of plasma testosterone. Biologically, the low plasma testosterone of cirrhotic

men is initiated by a reduction in testosterone synthesis by the testes. Horton and Tait[233] and Gordon and colleagues[210,211] have confirmed with kinetic studies that the atrophic testes of alcoholic cirrhotics contribute approximately one fourth of the normal concentrations of testosterone. Moreover, Gordon and associates[211] suggest that 15% of the testosterone produced in cirrhotic males is derived from peripheral conversion of circulating androstenedione (see Figure 6-11). Green and associates[234] note that unlike biochemical evidence of hypogonadism, the biochemical feminization of the cirrhotic male has not been adequately established. With the advent of sensitive assay methodology to evaluate plasma steroidal concentrations, the measurement of unconjugated plasma estrogens has centered around evaluation of plasma estradiol. In alcoholic cirrhosis, several investigators[219,224,234,235] have noted that the total unconjugated plasma estradiol is normal, mildly elevated,[213,214,236,237] or markedly increased.[212,225,238] Green and associates[234,239] recognized that there is equal disagreement about the role of unbound (biologically active) plasma estradiol in cirrhotic men, with reports of normal, marginally increased, or markedly increased free serum values of this sex steroid.

Temporal Effects of Alcohol Consumption in the Noncirrhotic Male

Short-Term Alcohol Consumption in Noncirrhotic Men. Gordon and associates[210] published a study of short-term (4-week) alcohol consumption with evidence of increased hepatic metabolism and enhanced metabolic clearance rates of testosterone from plasma. Furthermore, the plasma testosterone values declined during the period of the study, as did the protein binding of the plasma testosterone. The authors observed no consistent change in serum LH and interpreted these findings as evidence of direct suppression of hypothalamic-pituitary and testicular function caused by alcohol consumption.

Chronic Alcohol Consumption in the Noncirrhotic Male. The biochemical alterations evident in noncirrhotic chronic alcoholics are somewhat different from those of the short-term alcohol consumers. In the chronic alcohol user, plasma sex hormone–binding globulin was observed to increase markedly, thus reducing the free fraction of plasma testosterone to below normal.[213,214,223,240] Furthermore, there is increasing evidence that many of these patients with fatty livers have augmented plasma gonadotropins[224,241,242] with marginally decreased concentration of free testosterone values.[239]

The hypothesis that explains the aforementioned changes of hypogonadism and overt feminization in men with chronic alcoholic liver disease cannot adequately explain the clinical and biochemical features found in these men. Green and co-workers[234] suggest

TABLE 6-3	Concentrations of Free Testosterone and Free Estradiol in Plasma in Healthy Males (*n* = 8) and in Patients of the Same Age with Alcohol-Induced Cirrhosis of the Liver

	FREE TESTOSTERONE (pg/ml) >	FREE ESTRADIOL (pg/ml) >
Controls	124.7 ± 10.2	0.51 ± 0.06
Group 1	94.9 ± 9.9	0.55 ± 0.03
Group 2	57.8 ± 7.4	0.71 ± 0.05
Group 3	32.0 ± 4.0	1.14 ± 0.15

From Kley HK, Strohmeyer G, Krunkemper HL: *Gastroenterology* 76:235, 1979.
> Values are means ± SEM.
Group 1: Well-preserved liver function. Group 2: Intermediate liver function. Group 3: Decompensated liver disease with ascites, episodes of variceal hemorrhage, gynecomastia, and testicular atrophy.

that the pathogenesis of endocrine changes in the cirrhotic male is multifactorial and includes a combination of decreased hepatic clearance of several estrogenic compounds, an autoimmune-mediated primary testicular defect, and possibly a specific potentiation effect of alcohol consumption. Although all of these explanations are plausible, the precise mechanisms of endocrine, biochemical, and histologic alterations are yet to be confirmed.

Johnson[216] presented data that cast doubt on the hypothesis that chronic liver disease may lead to elevations of estrogen resulting from failure of the liver to metabolize endogenously produced steroids, thereafter initiating low urinary androgen and high urinary estrogen excretion. Johnson[216] reasoned that these hypotheses are dubious because metabolic clearance rates for estradiol and estrone are usually normal in male cirrhotics and the correlation between elevated estrogen values and gynecomastia is poor. Johnson noted the clinical parallels, such as Klinefelter's syndrome (see section discussing Klinefelter's syndrome), in which gynecomastia is also frequent despite normal to marginally increased estrogen values.[243]

Rose and associates[244] presented data to suggest that spironolactone initiates gynecomastia via a blockade of the androgen receptor in the male breast that leads to the unopposed action of estrogen. As a consequence of this metabolic activity, perhaps, gynecomastia in cirrhosis occurs after the treatment of ascites with spironolactone. The biochemical and histopathologic abnormalities induced by the drug are strikingly similar to those of cirrhosis. In this metabolic syndrome, testosterone is decreased, estrogen is increased, and the rate of conversion between the steroids is escalated.

Evidence of hypogonadism is common in men with advanced hepatic disease.[220,245-247] Earlier, investigators explained this observation on the basis of an increased circulating level of estrogen and assumed that a prehepatic accumulation of female sex hormones results in hepatic inactivation or clearance of these hormones.[224] Using the technology of assay systems, investigators showed that plasma estradiol values, and presumably those of other steroidal estrogens, were not elevated in men with hepatic insufficiency.[219,225,226] Total and free plasma levels of testosterone in males with cirrhosis have been uniformly reduced.[217-219,225,226,248] Furthermore, plasma values of LH and follicle-stimulating hormone (FSH) were reported as normal or elevated for subjects in whom they were evaluated.[217-219,225,226] Van Thiel and associates[224] evaluated hypothalamic-pituitary-gonadal function in 40 men with a wide spectrum of alcoholic liver disease in an effort to identify an anatomic location and biochemical mechanism responsible for the observed hypogonadism and feminization. Mean plasma testosterone values were lower ($p < .05$) and associated with severe derangements of hepatic histology. Both FSH and LH concentrations were normal to moderately elevated compared with those of normal men. These authors[224] confirmed that total plasma estradiol values were normal or reduced and that these mean values did not differ from normal. In contradistinction, plasma testosterone was reduced in more than 50% of the men and differed significantly ($p < .01$) from values for normal subjects.

Nutritional Alteration States. Gynecomastia produced by nutritional deprivation has been well documented. Case-control studies of World War II American prisoners of war determined that approximately 15% of males in Japanese prisoner camps developed gynecomastia.[249-251] Approximately one third of the cases of gynecomastia occurred during refeeding after release from prison, and other cases were associated with temporary increases in food supplied during imprisonment. In most of these subjects, gynecomastia was bilateral and disappeared within 5 to 7 months after refeeding. A confounding variable to such studies is the potential for concurrent diseases (e.g., hepatic disease, infectious hepatitis), which may have played a significant role in the development of gynecomastia, because many of these prisoners had fatty infiltration of the liver and spider angiomas. Thus the exact etiologic mechanisms are unclear, and the similarities to primary liver disease are so close that pathogenesis is assumed to be secondary to the gynecomastia of hepatic disease.[249] Bardin[114] and Paulsen[243] suggested that refeeding gynecomastia may be related to a resumption of pituitary gonadotropin secretion after pituitary shutdown that initiates a secondary puberty as a consequence of protein deprivation.

Sattin and associates[252] documented an epidemic of gynecomastia among illegal Haitian entrants of the United States in 1981 and 1982. These authors postulated that refeeding may have been the cause (in view of the probable nutritional deficiencies in the Haitians). Although refeeding gynecomastia has not been reported in other entrant or refugee populations, this may be because the phenomenon is poorly understood and thus was not documented. The transient nature of refeeding gynecomastia, with differences in geographic location, dietary practices, the indigenous population and available medical care, may explain the discrepancies in previous reports.

ANDROGEN DEFICIENCY STATES

The Influence of Aging in Gynecomastia. As noted in the discussion of physiologic gynecomastia, senescent gynecomastia (see Figure 6-9) appears to increase in incidence with advancing age; it was observed by Nuttall[4] in more than half of the men older than age 45. Furthermore, Williams[7] noted that more than 40% of elderly men have true gynecomastia. Plasma testosterone concentration values begin to diminish at approximately 70 years. In addition, there is concurrent elevation in the plasma sex hormone–binding globulin, so the levels of free or unbound testosterone concentrations decline even further. Snyder[36] suggested that the simultaneous increase in plasma LH causes a concurrent increase in the rate of conversion of androgen to estrogen in peripheral tissues (see Figure 6-12). The net result is an effective increase in the relative plasma estradiol values for these elderly men with a synchronous fall in testosterone values resulting from the affinity of this molecule for sex hormone–binding globulin. Overall, relative hyperestrinism is evident with a decrease in the plasma androgen/estrogen ratio. Because senescent gynecomastia develops in the elderly male population, the lesion must be differentiated from carcinoma of the breast. Haagensen[253] suggests that senescent hypertrophy occurs most commonly in men between the ages of 50 and 70 years and that, classically, the hypertrophy takes the form of a tender, 2- to 4-cm discoid tumor beneath the areola. Its tenderness and bilateral occurrence, if present, are considered important physical findings that differentiate hypertrophy from carcinoma. In a great majority of such cases, the lesions are unilateral and the hypertrophy is located centrally beneath the areola with well-defined, smooth, tender margins. In contradistinction, carcinoma of the male breast (Figure 6-13) is poorly defined clinically, with irregular edges and a hard, nontender mass that is fixed to the underlying fascia or skin, possibly with associated retraction of the nipple. The physician who identifies these ominous physical findings must perform a biopsy on suspicious lesions to exclude the presence of carcinoma.

Hypoandrogen States (Hypogonadism)
Primary Testicular Failure
Klinefelter's Syndrome (XXY). The syndrome of 47,XXY karyotype was described more than four decades ago by Klinefelter, Reifenstein, and Albright.[254] The syndrome was first observed in adult phenotypic males with gynecomastia, hypergonadotropic hypogonadism, and azoospermia. Subsequently, the syndrome was found to be associated with the presence of the extra X chromosome. Because the condition was rarely diagnosed until later in life, little was known about the natural history of hypogonadism in young males with the karyotype. The chromosomal pattern XXY is common; Gerald[255] estimated that the syndrome occurs in approximately 1 in 600 live births. When the syndrome is associated with hypergonadotropic hypogonadism and a negative buccal smear, a chromosomal analysis should be done to search for a mosaicism. If the buccal smear is positive, it should have a karyotype confirmation of the extra X chromosome. Tennes and associates[256] noted that in addition to XXY, patients with Klinefelter's syndrome may have multiple X (XXXY) or Y (XXYY) chromosomes or mosaic patterns (e.g., XXY/XY).

Klinefelter's syndrome represents the most common variant of male hypogonadism. Children with the 47,XXY karyotype demonstrate relatively few clinical findings, although there may be an occasional patient who has reduced testicular size or penile length. The clinical picture of gynecomastia, eunuchoidism, and macroorchidism does not usually emerge until well after midpuberty and may never be fully expressed. Testicular biopsy confirms a reduced number of spermatogonia; however, tubular fibrosis and hyalinization of seminiferous tubules are not observed until well after the onset of puberty.[257] Ahmad and associates[258] noted that the testes of adult patients revealed extensive fibrosis and hyalinization and that Leydig's cell volume may be preserved. Biochemical findings confirm reduced levels of serum testosterone with high-normal or enhanced values of serum estradiol.[259] Gabrilove and associates[260] noted that this increased estradiol/testosterone ratio is maintained in elderly patients despite the reduction in testicular function with aging.

Salbenblatt and associates[261] evaluated the serum concentrations of FSH, LH, testosterone, and estradiol at intervals before and during puberty in 40 individuals with Klinefelter's syndrome. Before the appearance of

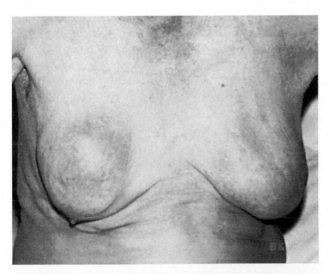

FIG. **6-13** Advanced bilateral gynecomastia in a 70-year-old man. The patient also has a palpable, discrete mass in the right breast confirmed mammographically and on biopsy to be a carcinoma.

secondary sexual changes in these patients, basal serum hormone concentrations and acute responses to stimulation with gonadotropin-releasing hormone and hCG were confirmed to be normal. Although onset of clinical puberty was normal in these patients, serum FSH and estradiol concentrations were significantly elevated. Early pubertal males showed initial testicular growth and normal serum testosterone values. By midpuberty, subjects were uniformly hypergonadotropic and testicular growth had ceased. Serum testosterone concentrations after age 15 remained in the low-normal range, but serum estradiol values were increased, irrespective of the presence or absence of gynecomastia. Drucker and associates[262] distinguished the primary nature of tubular atrophy in myotonic dystrophy and indicated that the testicular lesion differs morphologically and clinically from the seminiferous tubule dysgenesis of Klinefelter's syndrome, with which it often has been confused.

Klinefelter[263] noted that mental deficiency, manic-depressive psychoses, and schizophrenia do not occur more commonly in affected individuals than in control subjects, and most patients work regularly and lead normal lives except for their inability to procreate. There is no treatment for the sterility associated with the syndrome.

Therapy directed toward Klinefelter's syndrome is surgical and medical. Gynecomastia is best treated with excision of the hypertrophic breast tissue and preservation of the nipple/areola complex. This should not be done for cosmetic reasons but because carcinoma of the breast, as confirmed by Cole,[264] is 20 times more frequent in individuals with this condition than in normal men. Jackson and associates[265] suggested that breast carcinoma associated with the syndrome is 66.5 times more frequent than for normal controls. Bilateral carcinoma of the breast has also been reported in affected individuals by Robson, Santiago, and Huang.[266] In the presence of hypogonadism, treatment should include testosterone injections, which appear to be effective in most patients. Klinefelter[263] suggested that testosterone treatment in adolescent patients may abrogate some of the personality traits and abnormalities that emerge in later life.

Reifenstein's Syndrome (XY). In 1947 Reifenstein described hereditary familial hypogonadism with a characteristic phenotype that includes severe hypospadias, incomplete virilization at the time of expected puberty, and azoospermia associated with maturational arrest of spermatogenesis.[267-269] Patients with the syndrome have profound gynecomastia. The family history suggests X-linkage of the phenotype. Endocrinologic studies confirm elevated levels of plasma LH and estradiol, with normal to high values of testosterone.[269] With this endocrine profile, feminization of affected

subjects results from a combination of enhanced estradiol secretion and resistance to androgen action.[270] Schweikert and associates[270] suggested that the endocrine features of Reifenstein's syndrome are the consequence of diminished feedback of testosterone on LH secretion with a subsequent rise in the plasma LH and, consequently, an enhancement in mean secretion of estradiol and testosterone by the testes. These authors also confirmed that plasma levels of free estradiol and free testosterone are elevated even in the presence of elevated sex hormone–binding globulins. These findings further support the concept that the disorder is the result of a resistance to hormone action rather than a defect in androgen physiology.

Rosewater, Gwinup, Hamwi Familial Gynecomastia (XY). In 1965 Rosewater, Gwinup, and Hamwi[271] described a family in which four males had gynecomastia as part of a syndrome previously unreported. In these patients, blood chemistries, including hepatic function tests, were normal, as were urinary 17-ketosteroids and 17-hydroxysteroids. Pituitary gonadotropins and LH were low or absent. Urinary estradiol levels were within normal ranges for males. The patients demonstrated a defect in spermatogenesis. Testicular biopsies confirmed tubular maturation arrest and decreased number of Leydig's cells. Breast tissue biopsy was compatible with estrogenic stimulation despite normal plasma 17-hydroxycorticosteroid and 17-ketosteroids and normal urinary 17-ketosteroids fraction. Estrone and estradiol values were within normal limits. Analysis of the family pedigree suggested that the syndrome resulted as a sex-linked recessive or sex-limited autosomal dominant defect. The authors concluded that familial gynecomastia is a genetic trait associated with a secondary suppression of gonadotropins and that the testes produced an adequate concentration of androgens but were a potential site of increased estrogen production. These patients have a normal XY buccal epithelium chromatin pattern. No enhanced risk of male breast carcinoma appears evident with this syndrome of familial gynecomastia.

More recently, Berkovitz and associates[272] reported a variant of the syndrome for a family in which gynecomastia occurred in five males over two generations. For each affected subject, gynecomastia and male sexual maturation began at an early age. The ratio of plasma concentration of estradiol to 17β-testosterone was elevated in each subject. For three siblings with gynecomastia, the transfer constant for conversion of androstenedione to estrone was 10 times normal. Despite elevation in extraglandular aromatase activity, there was a normal response of the hypothalamic-pituitary axis to provocative stimuli. This report and that of Hemsell and colleagues[33] note the association of gynecomastia with increased extraglandular aromatase activity. The Berkovitz report was the first to document the defect as familial with a probable X-linked (autosomal dominant, sex-limited) mode of inheritance.

Kallmann's Syndrome. Van Dop and colleagues[273] noted that isolated gonadotropin deficiency comprises a heterogeneous group of disorders. The most common variant, Kallmann's syndrome, is a familial deficiency of hypothalamic luteinizing hormone–releasing factor (LHRF) that is transmitted as an autosomal dominant trait with variable penetrance. Described in 1944,[274] this syndrome occurs with a frequency of approximately 1 per 10,000 males and 1 per 50,000 females. A cardinal feature of the syndrome is an impairment or defect of the sense of smell (hyposmia or anosmia)[275] as a consequence of hypoplasia or aplasia of the rhinencephalon. Associated congenital anomalies are multiple and include the kidneys,[276] the skeleton,[277,278] the reproductive system (testes),[278,279] and the nasopharynx with associated cleft palate and congenital deafness.[280] Abnormalities commonly include gynecomastia and obesity.[277]

Patients with the syndrome (genito-olfactory dysplasia) have more associated anomalies than do those patients without an impaired sense of smell. Van Dop and co-authors[273] observed the occurrence of undescended testes in approximately half of their patients, which is not surprising in view of the postulated role of gonadotropins to initiate testicular descent during embryogenesis.[281] The association of cryptorchidism with severe gonadotropin deficiency in the syndrome possibly has predictive value for evaluation of boys with cryptorchidism and hyposmia. In these males, treatment with testosterone is appropriate. However, the therapy for boys who are not clearly hypogonadal may present problems. Patients with delayed puberty and low serum gonadotropin in the absence of intracranial lesions should be examined closely for ocular and skeletal anomalies in addition to the assessment of olfactory function.[273] Replacement testosterone therapy should be initiated at an appropriate age to induce full virilization if the diagnosis of isolated gonadotropin deficiency is established in males with any of these anomalies.

Kennedy's Disease with Associated Gynecomastia. In 1966 Kennedy, Alter, and Foreman[282] described a condition in which patients have muscle cramps, weakness, and atrophy of the limb girdles by age 30 to 40 years. All patients had diffuse fasciculations, especially of the chin and lips, dysarthria, and dysphagia. The clinical course of the disease was slow, and life expectancy was unaffected. On electromyography and muscle biopsy, the condition was confirmed to be frankly neurogenic in origin. This clinical syndrome differs from other spinal muscle atrophies of adulthood and is thought to have an X-linked mode of inheritance.

Guidetti and associates[283] described an X-linked adult-onset neurogenic muscular atrophy that was chiefly proximal, with late involvement of distal musculature and the medulla oblongata. Affected kindred all had gynecomastia, impotence, and essential tremor. Hormonal stimulation tests confirmed borderline low testicular response in the younger of two patients and a pathologic response in older patients. Of the endocrine disturbances, gynecomastia has been cited as one of the signal features of the syndrome since Kennedy's first description. Hausmanowa-Petrusewicz, Barkowsky, and Janczewski[284] and Arbizu and associates[285] established the testicular origin of the deficit. These authors consider gynecomastia, which is not necessarily present, a symptom that occurs secondary to the peripheral transformation of testosterone into estrogen.[286]

Eunuchoidal Males (Congenital Anorchia). Embryonic testicular regression (congenital anorchia) is a disorder, often familial, in which the testes are absent in the phenotypically normal male with the 46,XY karyotype.[287-291] In this example of deficient testosterone production, gynecomastia results despite normal estrogen production rates in adult men. Levitt and colleagues[292] emphasize that the individuals are often considered to have bilateral cryptorchidism at birth; however, plasma testosterone values are undetectable after stimulation with pharmacologically active doses of chorionic gonadotropin. Furthermore, no testes can be identified on abdominal or scrotal exploration. Kirschner, Jacobs, and Fraley[290] confirmed that even when the testes cannot be located anatomically, Leydig's cell remnants may be identified along the urogenital ridge and may secrete diminutive amounts of testosterone. It is estimated that approximately half of subjects who have anorchia develop gynecomastia.

Hereditary Defects of Androgen Biosynthesis. At least five enzymatic defects have been identified to occur in embryogenesis that result in defective androgen biosynthesis with incomplete virilization of the male embryo.[1,269,293-295] The enzymes responsible for these failures in biosynthesis include 20,22-desmolase, 17,20-desmolase, 3β-hydroxysteroid dehydrogenase, 17α-hydroxylase, and 17β-hydroxysteroid dehydrogenase. Each enzyme represents a critical pathway for the conversion of cholesterol to testosterone. In addition, congenital adrenal hyperplasia (see Figure 6-13) may be associated with 20,22-desmolase, 3β-hydroxysteroid dehydrogenase, and 17α-hydroxylase deficiencies. As a consequence of the variability in the blockade of these enzymatic biochemical reactions, affected individuals have a profound escalation in gonadotropin secretion after negative feedback. For individuals with complete or partial deficiencies of 17β-hydroxysteroid dehydrogenase, feminization, which includes gynecomastia, develops at the time of expected puberty in the male.

Gynecomastia is a common occurrence in male patients with 11-β-hydroxylase deficiency; however, it is seldom seen in the 21-β-hydroxylase form of congenital adrenal hyperplasia.[296] Presumably, the gynecomastia results from diminished testosterone biosynthesis in the presence of enhanced or normal estrogenic formation. Furthermore, escalated estrogen biosynthesis may occur from increased availability of androstenedione for conversion to estrogen in peripheral tissues or may secondarily occur from increased estrogen secretion from the testes as a consequence of enhanced gonadotropin secretion.[1]

Adrenocorticotropic Hormone Deficiency. The association between gynecomastia and isolated adrenocorticotropic hormone (ACTH) deficiencies, an uncommon cause of adrenocortical insufficiency,[297] has only rarely been documented.[298,299] Recently, Shimatsu, Suzuki, and Tanaka[300] described a patient with ACTH deficiency who had gynecomastia with elevated estrogens, LH, and prolactin serum values that normalized after replacement therapy with glucocorticoids. Similar cases of isolated deficiency of ACTH associated with gynecomastia have been reported by Uehara and associates[298] and Yoshida and associates.[299] The cause of gynecomastia with ACTH deficiency remains enigmatic. In these subjects, normal values of thyroid hormone, testosterone, and hCG are evident. Low values of androstenedione and urinary 17-ketosteroid were seen in the subjects with high estrogen values. As a consequence of the high estrogen values with normal testosterone levels in the presence of elevated LH concentrations, a decreased testosterone/estrogen ratio is maintained and presumably is the cause of the breast enlargement. High LH values in the presence of normal testosterone suggest that patients have a compensated Leydig's cell insufficiency. However, there is evidence that hyperreactive responses to LH may be related to glucocorticoid deficiency. The high estrogen levels may reflect increased peripheral conversion of estrogens. Furthermore, these augmented values may occur with secretion of testicular estradiol after stimulation by elevated LH. The biochemical role of glucocorticoids in the regulation of estrogen metabolism in men remains to be elucidated.

Secondary Testicular Failure. Gynecomastia is common after testicular failure resulting from trauma, viral orchitis (mumps), or bacterial infections (e.g., tuberculosis, leprosy). These causes of organic failure of the testes for active androgen biosynthesis are extraordinarily rare in the United States. Bilateral testicular atrophy may occur as a consequence of major direct trauma to the penis and testis or from pelvic trauma. The progressive loss of androgen function relates to the deprivation of active testosterone secretion and biosynthesis by the devascularized testes as a result of massive hematoma, direct testicular injury, or both. Mumps represents the most common cause of viral orchitis, although echovirus, lymphocytic choriomeningitis virus, group B arboviruses, and other viruses have been implicated in secondary testicular failure.[301,302] Bjorvatn[303] suggests that viral orchitis occurs as a result of the direct effects of the virus on testicular parenchyma, as evidenced by the mumps virus having been isolated from the testes of affected subjects. This serious complication of mumps occurs in approximately one fourth of men infected with the virus; two thirds have unilateral orchitis. Atrophy appears to result as a direct action of the virus on the seminiferous tubules or to the ischemia of pressure and edema within the tunica albuginea. There is no correlation of the clinical severity of the orchitis and the degree of atrophy of the testes. Atrophy occurs in approximately one third of subjects with viral orchitis and is bilateral in approximately one tenth of infected patients. In a survey of 2000 adult men, Werner[302] observed atrophy to occur in one or both testes in approximately 2%; in half of these patients, the atrophy occurred as a result of mumps.

The use of irradiation and chemotherapy in children treated for malignancies may initiate gonadal failure. Testicular biopsies have shown the absence of spermatogenesis in azoospermic patients.[304,305] Although prepubertal gonads were found to be less sensitive to toxicity,[304,306-308] the testes of boys in early puberty are very sensitive to drug toxicity, as reflected by elevated basal levels of gonadotropins, normal testosterone concentration, and enhanced LH responses to gonadotropin-releasing hormone. Shalet and associates[309] suggested that for children with malignant disease, gonadal damage may occur after the irradiation or chemotherapy that initiates these gonadotropin elevations. Furthermore, irradiation to the hypothalamic-pituitary axis in children with brain tumors may ultimately result in gonadotropin deficiency or hyperprolactinemia, which, in turn, results in gonadal insufficiency. If the testicular damage in prepubertal males is transient, androgen function will return and the chemotherapy- or irradiation-induced gynecomastia will abate.

Testicular failure as a consequence of hydrocele, varicocele, or spermatocele is rare and would be expected to have a higher frequency after trauma in the patient with unilateral cryptorchidism. In such patients, surgical treatment of the hydrocele, varicocele, or spermatocele may be indicated. The testicles should be salvaged if clinically possible, but when orchiectomy is necessary (e.g., major trauma), testosterone replacement with therapeutic doses is indicated.

Wilson and associates[1] pointed out that estrogen and androgen serum concentration dynamics have not been measured in these traumatic, therapeutic, and infectious states. Gynecomastia is also recognized with other causes of testicular failure, including neurologic diseases in which testicular atrophy supervenes,[310,311] postcastration states,[312] and ranulomatous diseases of the testes, especially lepromatous leprosy.[313,314]

Renal Failure. Gynecomastia is common in males in whom uremia develops. Furthermore, data suggest that approximately half of patients undergoing chronic hemodialysis develop gynecomastia.[315-320] Wilson and colleagues[1] noted that the endocrine changes of chronic renal failure are complex and that the relationships of these to the pituitary-testicular axis are only now being elucidated. Holdsworth, Atkins, and de Kretzer[317] observed that plasma LH and FSH values are increased approximately fourfold in men with creatinine clearance rates of 4 ml/min or less. Plasma testosterone concentrations are 30% of normal for these subjects. These authors[317] cite evidence of histologic damage to the testes, with hypospermia and a subnormal response for plasma testosterone secretion after chorionic gonadotropin administration.

Holdsworth and colleagues[317] further state that elevated plasma LH values occur secondary to a reduction in metabolic clearance from the renal failure; a secondary increase in the secretion of LH by the pituitary is evident. Wilson and colleagues[1] explained this sequence of renal failure and gynecomastia as a consequence of increased gonadotropin secretion after the subnormal response of Leydig's cells to gonadotropin stimulation. The biochemical and histologic transformation to gynecomastia remains enigmatic. To date, no studies have confirmed estrogen or androgen alterations that result from chronic renal failure. A plausible hypothesis for the development of gynecomastia is enhanced estradiol secretion by the testes after elevation of the plasma gonadotropins.

DRUG-RELATED GYNECOMASTIA

The development of gynecomastia in the adult male is often recognized as a consequence of drug administration. In contrast to the development of gynecomastia in the pubertal or prepubertal male because of endogenous sex-steroid hormonal production from various organ sites, in the adult a specific inquiry into drug use and a review of past history are essential. Table 6-4 identifies the categories in which exogenous drugs or their metabolic products initiate gynecomastia, including (1) drugs with estrogenic or estrogen-related activity, (2) drugs that inhibit the action and/or synthesis of testosterone, (3) drugs that enhance estrogen synthesis by the testes, and (4) drugs that have idiopathic mechanisms for induction of gynecomastia.

Drugs with Estrogenic or Estrogen-Related Activity. The administration of estrogens or compounds with estrogen-like activity can induce severe gynecomastia in

TABLE 6-4   Drugs Etiologic for Gynecomastia
DRUGS WITH ESTROGENIC OR ESTROGEN-RELATED ACTIVITY
Anabolic steroids (nandrolone, testosterone cypionate)
Clomiphene citrate
Diethylstilbestrol
Digitalis
Estrogens
Heroin
Oral contraceptives
Tamoxifen
Tetrahydrocannabinol (cannabis, marijuana)
DRUGS THAT INHIBIT THE ACTION AND/OR SYNTHESIS OF TESTOSTERONE
Antineoplastic agents
Cimetidine
Cyproterone acetate
D-Penicillamine
Diazepam
Finasteride cyclosporine
Flutamide
Ketoconazole
Medroxyprogesterone acetate
Phenytoin
Spironolactone
DRUGS THAT ENHANCE ESTROGEN SYNTHESIS BY THE TESTES
Gonadotropin hormone–releasing hormone (leuprolide acetate, goserelin acetate)
Human chorionic gonadotropin
DRUGS WITH IDIOPATHIC MECHANISM FOR INDUCTION OF GYNECOMASTIA
Amiodarone
Bumetanide
Busulfan
Calcitonin
Domperidone
Ethionamide
Furosemide
Isoniazid
Methyldopa
Nifedipine
Reserpine
Sulindac
Theophylline
Tricyclic antidepressants
Verapamil

males. The development of breast masses in men with prostate carcinoma is common after therapy with estrogen. Hendrickson and Robertson[321] reported gynecomastia after administration of diethylstilbestrol (DES) for prostate carcinoma. Miller and Ahmann[322] conducted a small clinical trial of low-dose DES to alleviate postcastration menopausal symptoms in prostate cancer patients and noted 75% symptomatic relief, with a 41% incidence of gynecomastia. Brandt, Cohn, and Hilder,[323] reporting on the use of oral contraceptives in hemophilia, identified rapid onset of gynecomastia with estrogen administration. Orentreich and Dur[324] described mammogenesis in transsexuals after administration of oral estrogen. Symmers[325] identified transsexual males who develop metastasizing mammary adenocarcinoma after castration, augmentation mammoplasty, and administration of large doses of estrogen. In contrast, Holleb, Freeman, and Farrow[326] reported in 1968 on a survey of 17,000 patients with cancer of the prostate treated with estrogen by 150 urologists. Only two cases of carcinoma of the breast (incidence, 0.012%) were observed. Holleb and colleagues[326] and Wilson and Hutchinson[327] concluded that it is highly improbable that a causal relationship exists between estrogen administration and breast carcinoma. Only six reported cases of primary breast carcinoma in males with prostate cancer have been reported in the English literature, which further supports this view.[327] Furthermore, prepubertal gynecomastia was described after topical inunction of estrogen-containing ointment,[328] and persistent gynecomastia resulted from scalp inunction of estradiol.[128,329] Beas and colleagues[330] and Landolt and Murset[331] noted the extraordinary sensitivity of men and young boys to dermal ointments that contain estrogens.

Gynecomastia is a common consequence of digitalis administration[332]; Navab, Koss, and LaDue[333] attributed gynecomastia induction from the estrogen-like activity of this cardiac glycoside. Wolfe[334] observed a 10% incidence of gynecomastia in patients who received digitalis preparations for 12 months or longer. Stouffer and associates[335] reported that an increase in total serum estrogens and a decrease of plasma testosterone was evident in patients treated with digoxin. Novak, Kass, and LaDue[336] suggested that the mechanism of initiating gynecomastia by digitalis is the estrogen or estrogen-precursor activity of the drug, similar to the estrogen effect evident in the vaginal mucosa of menopausal women.

Clomiphene citrate has been used to treat ovulatory disturbances in selected infertile women and, more recently, for the treatment of male infertility.[337] The administration of clomiphene has been shown to induce gynecomastia,[338] and gynecomastia has also been induced by withdrawal of the drug.[339]

With the current enthusiasm for use of the anabolic steroids nandrolone and testosterone cypionate, clinics have observed the induction of severe gynecomastia after administration of these injectable steroids. The report by Spano and Ryan[340] admonishes physicians to be aware of the potential deleterious application of tamoxifen to prevent gynecomastia from a similar drug regimen.

Successful application of external radiation to the breast to prevent the estrogen-induced gynecomastia evident with the treatment of prostate cancer has been reported.[341,342] For patients with prostate cancer who are receiving DES, radiation to breast tissue was administered with superficial x-rays, 4-mV cobalt-60, with doses from 1200 to 1500 cGy in three fractions.

Drug abuse in the form of intravenous heroin administration or cannabis (marijuana) smoking may induce gynecomastia as a consequence of depression of plasma androgen levels.[343-346] Olusi[347] reported on the hyperprolactin state induced by cannabis smoking. Although the etiologic mechanism through which marijuana initiates gynecomastia is conjectural, there are structural resemblances between tetrahydrocannabinol (the metabolite of marijuana) and estradiol. Furthermore, tetrahydr cannabinol has been observed to stimulate the development of breast tissue in rats.[344] However, epidemiologic evidence to support an association between cannabis use and gynecomastia was not substantiated by Cates and Pope.[348]

Drugs That Inhibit the Action and/or Synthesis of Testosterone. The mechanisms of drug-induced gynecomastia are less ambiguous with regard to the effects of spironolactone on breast parenchyma in the male. This commonly used diuretic initiates a substantial incidence of gynecomastia when administered at high dosages.[349] Siiteri and MacDonald[37] confirmed that the drug interferes with testosterone biosynthesis. A reduction in the relative concentration of free testosterone is evident because the conversion of androstenedione and testosterone to estrone and estradiol is normal. Bellati and Ideo[350] and Dupont[351] reported the disappearance of spironolactone-induced gynecomastia after treatment with canrenoate potassium. Although gynecomastia is rare after administration of canrenoate potassium or canrenone,[352,353] 30% to 62% of patients taking long-term spironolactone experienced this side effect.[352-355] Rose and associates[244] noted that spironolactone alters the peripheral metabolism of testosterone, with resultant changes in the testosterone/estradiol ratio. These changes appear primarily from significant increases in the metabolic clearance of testosterone and in the rate of peripheral conversion of testosterone into estradiol after spironolactone therapy. Caminos-Torres, Lisa, and Snyder[356] postulated that spironolactone-induced gynecomastia does not occur from alterations in the serum concentrations of testosterone or estradiol. Rather, changes may be related to binding of canrenone to tissue androgen receptors. Therefore it is plausible that the drug has at least two effects on androgen metabolism: inhibition of testosterone biosynthesis and binding of androgen to its receptor, thus effectively reducing the active androgenic effect of testosterone. At low-dose levels, it is possible that gynecomastia is induced by receptor blockade at testosterone-binding sites. Conversely, after high-dose administration, inhibition of testosterone synthesis may initiate gynecomastia.

In 1979 Moerck and Magelund[357] reported a patient with gynecomastia related to abuse of diazepam. Bergman and associates[358] described five patients with gynecomastia related to diazepam use in therapeutic doses. Diazepam-induced gynecomastia associated with other endocrine or hepatic diseases was ruled out by laboratory tests. These patients had elevated serum estradiol concentrations, normal hepatic and thyroid function, and normal serum testosterone values. The discontinuance of diazepam was associated with a fall of the estradiol levels to normal values and clinical improvement in the gynecomastia. These authors postulated that diazepam contributes to gynecomastia through three potential mechanisms: (1) enhanced conversion of testosterone to estradiol, (2) increased sex hormone–binding globulin, and (3) decreased peripheral metabolism or decreased excretion of estrogen.

Although D-penicillamine therapy is associated with a variety of side effects, some occur more commonly in patients with rheumatoid arthritis.[359] Breast gigantism was reported in six women, five of whom suffered from rheumatoid arthritis, after therapy with penicillamine. Reid, Martynoga, and Nuki[360] confirmed this clinical report with evidence of gynecomastia in a man with rheumatoid arthritis who was receiving penicillamine. The infrequent association of breast gigantism with penicillamine use[361-364] confirms that gynecomastia associated with this drug is a rare adverse side effect. The gynecomastia usually disappears promptly after withdrawal of penicillamine and differs from the course observed in patients with breast gigantism. Desai[361] indicated the need for mastectomy and prosthetic surgery in one case and the successful administration of danazol to reverse D-penicillamine–induced breast gigantism in another.[363] It appears that breast gigantism and gynecomastia are initiated by stimulatory effects of D-penicillamine, which inhibits synthesis of testosterone in males and the augmentation of estrogenic activity in females.

Cimetidine is an effective drug for the healing of peptic ulcers and for preventing their recurrence. In vivo animal studies demonstrated that cimetidine can inhibit the binding of dihydrotestosterone to androgen receptors in the prostates of rats and the kidneys of mice.[9,365-368] Thereafter, gynecomastia[369,370] was observed, especially in pathologic hypersecretory states,[371] and was associated with impotence in patients treated with the drug.[372,373] Jensen and associates[374] prospectively evaluated male patients with gastric hypersecretory states and examined the ability of cimetidine to initiate clinically important antiandrogen side effects. These investigators confirmed that impotence, breast tenderness, or gynecomastia developed in exactly half of the patients and that these side effects disappeared when cimetidine was replaced by ranitidine, the newer antagonist of histamine H_2 receptors.[9,367] Moreover, cimetidine has been shown to block testosterone synthesis.[375] These investigators confirmed low plasma testosterone values and elevated plasma gonadotropin concentrations that suggest a primary testicular disorder after administration of cimetidine hydrochloride. These alterations of sexual function improved and plasma testosterone values rose to normal after discontinuance of the drug. Furthermore, readministration of cimetidine resulted in prompt recurrence of sexual problems and low testosterone values. Despite the reversal of gynecomastia after discontinuance of cimetidine and initiation of ranitidine, Tosi and Cagnoli[376] confirmed painful gynecomastia after ranitidine administration. Mignon and associates[372,377] observed divergent effects of cimetidine and ranitidine on androgen receptors, pituitary hormones, and plasma testosterone levels. These data are in accord with the work by Brittain and Daly[378] and Edwards and associates,[379] which suggests minimal effects of ranitidine on these sex hormone parameters. Rodriguez and Jick[380] conducted a large open-cohort study comparing the relative risk of developing gynecomastia among patients receiving cimetidine, ranitidine, misoprostol, or omeprazole versus nonusers. The relative risk of gynecomastia for current users of cimetidine was 7.2; for misoprostol, omeprazole, and ranitidine, 2.0, 0.6, and 1.5, respectively. Adverse endocrine effects have been reported with the use of omeprazole; however, the mechanism of action has not been identified.[381,382] Other drugs, such as cyproterone acetate[383] and flutamide (glutamine),[384] may cause gynecomastia by interfering with the binding of androgens to their receptor proteins. Finasteride, a 5α-reductase inhibitor used in the treatment of benign prostatic hypertrophy, has been implicated in the development of breast tenderness.[385] Jacobs, Klein, and Klehr[386] suggested a possible cumulative effect of cyclosporine and calcium channel blockers that produced gynecomastia in the transplant population.

In attempts to find a technique of medical castration useful as therapy for prostate cancer without the side effects of estrogen or surgical castration, Geller and associates[387] conducted clinical trials with megestrol acetate (Megace), a progestational antiestrogen. Megace was well tolerated by patients and rarely initiated gynecomastia, thromboembolic events, or salt retention, in contrast to the side effects evident with high-dose medroxyprogesterone acetate. Medroxyprogesterone acetate will lower mean plasma testosterone values.[388,389] Meyer and colleagues[390] have shown that the drug is effective in decreasing serum gonadotropin and plasma testosterone concentrations in males.

The oral antifungal ketoconazole has been shown to produce gynecomastia through transit blockade of testosterone synthesis and the adrenal response to corticotropin.[391-393] Therapeutic doses of the drug will suppress serum testosterone concentrations markedly; serum estradiol values are suppressed to a much lesser extent. The percentage of either bound or free androgens and estrogens were not significantly altered. It was postulated by Pont and associates[392,393] that because gynecomastia appears to be the result of an elevated estradiol/testosterone ratio, selective hormonal effects would be demonstrated after use of ketoconazole. Hormonal effects of the drug are generally unrelated to duration of therapy, and occasionally there may be partial reversal of gynecomastia with continual therapy. Side effects appear to be reversible with discontinuance of ketoconazole therapy. Patients receiving the drug should be considered potentially unable to mount an adrenal stress response and may require testosterone supplementation. Because the drug also has a propensity for hepatotoxicity, Moncada and Baranda[394] argue that indications for ketoconazole therapy are not completely established and suggest that it be reserved for cases of chronic deep mycoses in life-threatening situations, or perhaps in recalcitrant superficial mycoses. Trivial diseases should not be treated with this drug because of its potential (and severe) side effects.

The commonly used anticonvulsant phenytoin (Dilantin) may initiate gynecomastia in men with epilepsy. Graybill and Drutz[395] noted resolution of gynecomastia when phenytoin was discontinued and suggested that phenytoin may cause gynecomastia. Several investigators[395-399] have suggested that a reduction in the circulating free testosterone concentrations occurs in patients receiving long-term therapy with various anticonvulsants. These data and the data of Graybill and Drutz[395] are consistent with the hypothesis that phenytoin therapy diminishes free testosterone concentrations, possibly as a result of increasing the concentration of sex hormone–binding globulins with induction of an increased conversion of testosterone to 17β-estradiol. Turkington and Topper[11] indicated that gynecomastia may result from either of these effects or a combination, with a loss of libido and subfertility as a possible side effect of long-term therapy.

Antineoplastic (cytotoxic) drugs are recognized to initiate amenorrhea, disturbances of gonadal estrogen and androgen secretion, oligospermia, and increased plasma concentrations of gonadotropins.[400-404] Gynecomastia has been commonly observed in pubertal males after administration of cytotoxic chemotherapy,[405] but it is considered a rare event in adult men.[406] Trump and Anderson[407] and Trump, Pavy, and Staal[408] described six men with painful gynecomastia after the administration of antineoplastic therapy, with sharp increases in levels of plasma FSH and LH. Plasma testosterone concentrations were within or above normal ranges in most of the subjects evaluated; plasma estradiol concentrations were modestly increased. These authors could not define the precise mechanisms responsible for gynecomastia that occurred after cytotoxic chemotherapy. Damage to germinal epithelium and Leydig's cells, as well as changes in peripheral metabolism of testosterone and estrogen, may be important. Unilateral or bilateral tender gynecomastia may occur in adult men after therapy with cytotoxic drugs.[409-412] Gynecomastia seen in these patients does not necessarily indicate recurrent carcinoma after therapy with single or combination antineoplastic agents. Gynecomastia induction may occur with administration of the chemotherapeutic agents busulfan,[411] vincristine,[412] nitrosoureas,[413] and methotrexate.[414,415]

A Danish study[416] reported a 4% incidence of gynecomastia in patients with Hodgkin's disease; several of the patients with breast enlargement had been treated with alkylating agents. The use of these chemotherapeutic agents in the treatment of lymphoma and various renal disorders is routinely associated with damage to the testicular germ cells and is manifested by elevation of serum FSH and oligospermia or azoospermia.[308,405,417-419] These patients as a group often have reduced serum testosterone, although individual values are usually within normal ranges.[405,420,421] It appears that the testicular toxicity from chemotherapeutic agents could result in impaired androgen production; the resulting increase in the serum estrogen/androgen ratio might then initiate gynecomastia.

Drugs That Enhance Estrogen Synthesis by the Testes. Smith[413] identified an adult patient with acquired gynecomastia who had elevated urinary estrogens, borderline to low FSH and LH, and borderline high serum estradiol. It was thought that the patient potentially had a semiautonomous lesion of the testis that led to an increase of estrogen production, with suppression of LH and FSH causing mild atrophic changes of the contralateral testis. After administration of hCG, there was a 300% increase in urinary estrogens. Morse and co-workers[422] gave a similar dose of hCG (5000 units daily for 4 days) to healthy adult males and measured urinary estrogens on the third and fourth days. These authors confirm that the mean increase in estrogen excretion from baseline to the hCG-stimulated situation was 137%. Lipsett and associates[423] gave a similar dose of hCG per day to males and measured estradiol production rates initially and on the fourth day of hCG administration. The increase in estradiol production averaged 194% (range, 119% to 265%). Therefore it appears that urinary estrogen in these patients is more responsive to hCG than is usually the case among young adult males. These data are compatible with enhanced estrogen synthesis and secretion by the testes or an increased conversion of testosterone to estrogen. In healthy men, the majority of estradiol is thought to be produced by conversion from circulating testosterone.[424,425]

Acquired feminization secondary to testicular neoplasms is seen most often with choriocarcinoma or other germ cell–derived neoplasms that are associated with high values of hCG.[112,243] The hyperestrogen state with associated gynecomastia may be caused by any germ cell–derived neoplasm and can be ruled out based on the low radioimmunoassay values for LH because hCG is measured by the same assay.[426] As noted earlier, Leydig's cell, Sertoli's cell, or gonadal mesenchymal tumors of the testes have been reported to be estrogen-producing. These neoplasms do not produce hCG, but patients commonly have gynecomastia as the most prominent clinical finding. Maddock and Nelson[427] identified severe gynecomastia in adult men after administration of therapeutic doses of hCG. Similar effects can result in the pubertal male and are predictable, because hCG initiates an increase in secretion of estradiol and testosterone by the testes, which was identified by Weinstein and associates.[428]

Clinical practice has witnessed the introduction of potent analogs of gonadotropin hormone–releasing hormone (GnRH), including leuprolide acetate, and goserelin acetate for use in patients with metastatic prostate cancer.[429] A multiinstitutional, randomized, phase III clinical trial[430] compared the efficacy and side effects of bilateral orchiectomy versus a combination of luteinizing hormone–releasing hormone agonist (LHRH-A), goserelin acetate, and flutamide in patients with metastatic prostate cancer. The most common side effects for both treatments included hot flashes and gynecomastia. However, GnRH provides an effective alternative to the exogenous administration of pharmacologic doses of estrogen or surgical castration. The advantage of GnRH over estrogen is primarily related to a decrease in the incidence of cardiovascular toxicity and gynecomastia. The therapeutic potential of GnRH was first suggested by the recognition that pituitary secretion of FSH and LH could be modulated by administration of exogenous GnRH. Clayton and Catt[431] determined that the effects of GnRH depend largely on the dosage and schedule of administration of this hormone. Frequent small doses of GnRH and other agonists mimic physiologic pulsatile secretion and

thereafter activate gonadotropin secretion. Sandow[432] noted the paradoxic effect seen with administration of large doses of GnRH daily or by continuous infusion in causing inhibition of pituitary/gonadal function. Prolonged treatment with GnRH to decrease levels of LH and testosterone to subnormal ranges that reach nadirs after 4 weeks of daily therapy have been noted.[258,433,434] Eisenberger, O'Dwyer, and Friedman[435] suggested that these hormonal changes are consistent with a gradual physiologic selective hypophysectomy and represent the basis for the oncological application of GnRH agonists.

Drugs with Mechanisms for Induction of Gynecomastia. As identified in Table 6-5, a variety of drugs may be etiologic for gynecomastia by inexplicable pathophysiologic mechanisms. Drugs with potential to initiate idiopathic gynecomastia include amiodarone, bumetanide, busulfan, domperidone, ethionamide, furosemide, isoniazid, methyldopa, nifedipine, reserpine, sulindac, theophylline, tricyclic antidepressants, and verapamil.[436] Although mechanisms for drug-induced gynecomastia have not been elucidated for these medications, several authors have attempted to explain the basis of the clinical syndrome without exclusion of concurrent drugs that have the known side effect of gynecomastia. The medical literature does not conclusively exclude other established physiologic causes of gynecomastia in patients using these medications.

Van der Steen, Du Caju, and Van Acker[437] identified gynecomastia in a male infant treated for nausea and vomiting with the investigational antiemetic domperidone. These authors postulated that the gynecomastia and galactorrhea seen in this infant produced a concomitant increase in serum levels of prolactin. Serum thyroid-stimulating hormone and estradiol values were normal for this age group. This clinical syndrome was thought to be the consequence of activation of prolactin secretion by domperidone. A similar physiologic effect was produced after calcium channel blocker therapy with verapamil and nifedipine. Tanner and Bosco[438] identified elevated prolactin values after verapamil treatment. This report is confounding because most of these patients had concomitant therapy with other drugs, although the majority experienced amelioration of symptoms after discontinuation of the calcium channel blocker.

The development of gynecomastia after the use of human growth hormone (hGH) in prepubertal males with growth hormone (GH) deficiency or short stature syndromes has been described.[439] Similarly, elderly men with low circulating levels of insulin-like growth factor-I (IGF-I) treated with hGH to achieve plasma IGF-I levels above 1.0 units/ml demonstrate

TABLE 6-5	Differential Diagnosis of Prepubertal Gynecomastia in Boys*

| CONDITION | SEXUAL MATURATION | CIRCULATING OR URINARY STEROIDS | | | IVP AND RETROPERITONEAL PNEUMOGRAM |
		ESTROGENS	TESTOSTERONE	17-KS AND DHEA	
Idiopathic	Preadolescent	Normal or high	Normal	Normal	Normal
ADRENAL					
Feminizing tumor	Accelerated	Elevated	Normal	Elevated	May be normal or tumor may be seen
Isosexual tumor	Accelerated	Elevated	Normal or elevated	Elevated	
TESTICULAR (Tumor usually palpable)					
Interstitial cell tumor	Accelerated	Elevated	Elevated	Normal	Normal
Choriocarcinoma†	Accelerated	Elevated	Normal	Normal	Normal

From Latorre H, Kenny F: *Am J Dis Child* 126:772, 1973.

17-KS, 17-Ketosteroids; *DHEA*, dehydroepiandrosterone; *IVP*, intravenous pyelogram.

*Exposure to hormonal or nonhormonal drugs that may produce gynecomastia must be ruled out by careful history. Persistent elevation of estrogens or gonadotropins or both indicates need for exploratory laparotomy.

†Not yet reported in prepubertal age. Chorionic gonadotropin levels are elevated.

a substantial frequency of gynecomastia.[440] These side effects can be minimized if levels are maintained in the range of 0.5 to 1.0 units/ml. The mechanism underlying this response to hGH has not been determined, although it may be related to GH receptors or indirectly through the production of IGF.

In most patients with idiopathic gynecomastia related to drug therapy, discontinuance of the suspected drugs led to regression of the gynecomastia. Resolution of drug-induced gynecomastia after discontinuance of the medication has been confirmed for bumetanide,[441,442] sulindac,[436] theophylline,[443] amiodarone,[444] domperidone,[437] and salcatonin (a synthetic calcitonin).[445]

IDIOPATHIC MECHANISMS

Renal Failure. As noted previously, most male patients presenting with gynecomastia have documentable pathophysiologic or drug-related causes to explain this clinical syndrome. For the prepubertal male, idiopathic gynecomastia may be differentiated based on the normal values of estrogen, testosterone, 17-ketosteroids, and DHEA (see Table 6-5). Latorre and Kenny[132] differentiated adrenal and testicular causes of prepubertal gynecomastia in boys who have normal circulating or urinary sex steroids. Male secondary sexual development is accelerated in patients with adrenal or testicular lesions but not in those with idiopathic gynecomastia. Urinary estrogen levels are consistently elevated with adrenal/testicular lesions and may be normal or high in the idiopathic variant. In contrast, 17-ketosteroids and DHEA are elevated in patients with adrenal abnormalities; patients with adrenal or testicular tumors will have elevated serum testosterone values (see Table 6-5).

Although the English literature is replete with inconsistent and confounding reports that lack documentation for the cause of gynecomastia, explanations may be forthcoming in the future after assessment of endocrine and pharmacologic induction mechanisms.

Nonneoplastic Diseases of the Lung. Braude and associates[446] described transient gynecomastia in four of seven patients with cystic fibrosis having associated hypertrophic osteoarthropathy. Thereafter, Russi[447] reported a similar case in a 23-year-old male with cystic fibrosis. The gynecomastia seen with cystic fibrosis is usually transient and associated with severe mastalgia. In most cases, patients were not taking drugs known to cause gynecomastia and had no evidence of liver or testicular disease. Lemen and associates[448] correlated digital clubbing with the severity of lung disease and elevation of the serum prostaglandin $F_{2\alpha}$ and E concentrations in these patients. Russi[447] suggested that the diseased lungs may incompletely metabolize these sex steroids and that an escalation in the estrogenic component of the circulating steroids may be seen.

Trauma (Chest Wall). Although uncommon, unilateral and rarely bilateral gynecomastia may be observed after trauma to the chest wall. Such trauma is most commonly seen after blunt injury, but it also may be noted with penetrating damage of the chest wall. This idiopathic mechanism for gynecomastia may result as a consequence of (1) increased secretion of GnRH; (2) decreased testosterone synthesis and, thus, an androgen-deficiency state; or (3) decreased metabolic clearance of estrogen-like compounds secreted endogenously or administered exogenously. The precise mechanism by which trauma initiates gynecomastia has not been documented.

Central Nervous System–Related Causes

Pituitary Adenoma. Prolactin-secreting macroadenomas (prolactinomas) of the pituitary gland have been associated with gynecomastia, which resolves in response to bromocriptine therapy.[449,450] Adolescent (rare) and adult cases have been reported. Although endocrine deficiencies of varying extent may include gonadotropin deficiencies, gynecomastia may be present in the presence of prolactin oversecretion alone, with resolution after effective therapy.[449]

Psychologic. Endocrine responses to stress and psychologic stimuli have been documented by Rose and colleagues[158] to increase secretion of GH, prolactin, and cortisol with a concomitant decrease in testosterone production. An interaction of the latter two hormones has been proposed. The carefully documented report by Gooren and Daantje[451] correlated the occurrence of gynecomastia with psychologic stress. These authors documented hormonal parameters during episodes of gynecomastia and regression in five men. These data provide evidence that stressful life events associated with increased adrenal secretion and a fall in testosterone production may initiate transitory gynecomastia. The gynecomastia resolved spontaneously (without therapy) when subjects were able to cope successfully with their environment. Thereafter, hormonal functions returned to normal values in all subjects.

Psychologic stress may be an etiologic factor to be considered in gynecomastia. Frantz and Wilson[452] found that in more than 50% of the cases, no underlying endocrine or pathologic cause could be identified. Certainly, one has to consider the mechanism of refeeding gynecomastia (see previous discussion) in individuals who are stressed and have increased consumption of foodstuffs that contain compounds or metabolites with estrogenic or estrogen-like activity. Furthermore, such confounding reports must also exclude concurrent administration of drugs that are known to cause gynecomastia.

Acquired Immunodeficiency Syndrome and Human Immunodeficiency Virus Infection.
Couderc and Clauvel[453] reported the association of transient gynecomastia in two patients with human immunodeficiency virus (HIV) infection. A 36-year-old homosexual intravenous drug abuser had serum antibodies to HIV detected with the enzyme-linked immunosorbent assay (ELISA) technique and Western blot. The patient developed unilateral, then bilateral, painless gynecomastia that resolved spontaneously 6 months after identification of acquired immunodeficiency syndrome (AIDS). Another homosexual patient had generalized lymphadenopathy and bilateral gynecomastia that also resolved spontaneously. Both patients showed transient gynecomastia, with normal plasma values of testosterone, estrone, estradiol, and prolactin. Qazi and associates[454] recently reviewed their experience with gynecomastia accruing in HIV-infected men. They pointed out that gynecomastia in these patients is often a side effect of antiviral therapy.

Assessment of Gynecomastia

Figure 6-14 provides an algorithm for diagnostic approaches to the male patient with unilateral or bilateral breast masses suspicious for gynecomastia.

PATIENT EVALUATION

Unilateral gynecomastia is common in the pubertal male, and most of these young men are asymptomatic. In the older male, prevalence increases with age, as demonstrated by Nuttall.[4] The systematic evaluation of gynecomastia involves a thorough history and physical examination, and in selected cases, it may require laboratory and imaging studies to define the etiologic process.

Pertinent characteristics to elicit while obtaining a history include the duration and timing of breast enlargement, as well as any symptoms—rapid, painful enlargement of recent onset is of more concern than long-standing asymptomatic breast enlargement. Symptoms associated with hypogonadism, including infertility, erectile dysfunction, and decreased libido, are elicited. Systemic diseases associated with hypogonadism and/or gynecomastia are also elicited. A complete medication history and social history, to determine alcohol and drug abuse, is obtained.

Niewoehner and Nuttall[35] described the physical examination of the male breast for gynecomastia. Breast tissue is elevated up and off the chest wall in a pinching fashion for measurement. In the nonobese patient, at least 2 cm of subareolar breast tissue must be present before gynecomastia can be defined. When in doubt about whether the tissue is glandular or adipose, its consistency is compared with that of adipose tissue in the anterior or lateral axillary folds. The examination also determines whether breast enlargement is unilateral or bilateral and whether there is tenderness or nipple discharge. Specific characteristics of the breast enlargement can distinguish between benign and malignant processes. Dominant masses or local areas of firmness, irregularity, asymmetry, eccentricity, ulceration, and immobility, as well as bloody nipple discharge and axillary adenopathy, suggest a malignant process. Examination of the liver, testes, and chest, as well as the gynecomastia itself, is clearly important.

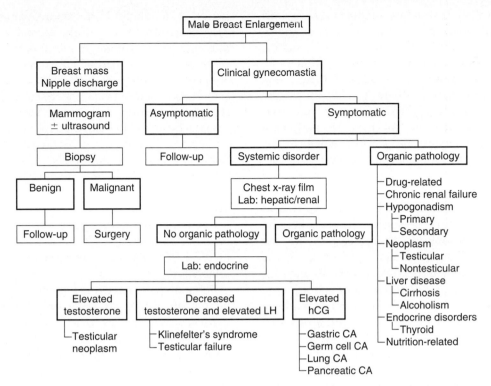

FIG. **6-14** An algorithm for diagnostic approaches to the male patient with unilateral/bilateral breast mass(es) suspicious for gynecomastia. *CA,* Carcinoma; *hCG,* human chorionic gonadotropin. *(Modified from Lucas LM, Kumar KL, Smith DL:* Postgrad Med *82:73, 1987.)*

Investigation. Investigations are confined to liver function tests and a chest radiograph in the older patient, unless there is reason to think that there is an underlying endocrine abnormality, when more sophisticated investigations are indicated. Serum markers for testicular tumors are measured when appropriate, especially in patients with testicular swelling or maldescent.

Biochemical investigations, when warranted, are aimed at establishing an underlying cause. Endocrine investigations include serum estradiol (or estrone), testosterone, LH, sex hormone–binding globulin, hCG, prolactin, and thyroid function tests.[455]

Exclusion of Malignancy. In addition to clinical and endocrinologic studies of male patients with breast disease, fine-needle aspiration (FNA), cytologic examination, and radiology are used to exclude malignant disease in the older patient. This is particularly important in the absence of a well-defined cause, in unilateral disease, and when the palpable mass is eccentric instead of having the usual concentricity. Mammography images gynecomastia well, and its role in the male breast has been reviewed by Dershaw.[456] Gynecomastia appears as a flame-shaped opacity extending into the surrounding fat. Cases of pseudogynecomastia can be readily identified by the absence of breast tissue, and malignancy can often be diagnosed with mammography.[457] Evans and associates[458]

reported that mammography can accurately distinguish between malignant and benign male breast disease. When mammography and clinical examination suggest benign disease, FNA biopsy can be avoided.

FNA Cytology. FNA cytologic examination of the male breast initially was regarded as problematic because the hyperplastic epithelial cells associated with gynecomastia were occasionally erroneously reported as malignant. Now that the cytologic features of gynecomastia are well described, this test can be performed with confidence.

Treatment of Gynecomastia

MEDICAL THERAPY

Most patients with gynecomastia require no therapy other than the correction of an identified cause. If gynecomastia causes sufficient pain or emotional discomfort, specific treatments are available for the enlarged breast tissue. However, gynecomastia has a high rate of spontaneous regression, especially pubertal gynecomastia, in which regression is the anticipated outcome. This makes it difficult to judge the true effectiveness of any medical therapy, unless double-blind randomized studies have been carried out.

Correction of the estrogen/testosterone ratio can lead to resolution of gynecomastia. For disorders of androgen deficiency, Hopwood[459] claimed that testosterone administration would improve (decrease) this ratio, with some regression of the gynecomastia. Conversely, on occasion, testosterone therapy will make the condition worse, especially when there is increased conversion of androgens to estrogens by the peripheral tissues. When the breast diameter is less than 4 cm, the clinician can expect a spontaneous regression; consequently, reassurance of the patient and a period of observation are indicated.

LeRoith, Sobel, and Glick[460] and Plourde, Kulin, and Santner[461] reported varying success in reducing the breast size of gynecomastia after therapy with the antiestrogen clomiphene citrate, which acts at the level of the hypothalamic-pituitary axis to increase gonadotropin secretion. Stephanas and associates[462] reported a 95% success rate with the use of clomiphene citrate to treat pubertal-adolescent gynecomastia. However, the side effects of clomiphene therapy were significant and included adverse gastrointestinal reactions, rashes, and visual impairment. At present, clomiphene citrate is considered investigational in the therapy of gynecomastia and is not approved as a primary drug for the medical management of this disorder.

Ricciardi and Ianniruberto[463] used tamoxifen citrate (Nolvadex) as a treatment for benign breast disorders under the assumption that these lesions have estrogen receptors that may respond to hormonal influences. The authors determined that 71% of patients with symptomatic benign breast disease who were treated with tamoxifen experienced complete regression of symptoms and disappearance of the lesions as assessed with clinical examination and ultrasonography.

Alagaratnam[464] reported 80% complete regression of idiopathic gynecomastia in 61 men treated with 40 mg of tamoxifen daily for 1 to 4 months (median, 2 months). The author noted no long-term side effects of tamoxifen for patients observed through a median follow-up period of 36 months. Furthermore, pain and tenderness disappeared by the end of the second week of therapy, although breast swelling required prolonged therapy to produce complete regression. An inconsistent relationship between duration of therapy and reduction in the size of the gynecomastia and relief of symptoms was reported. Two controlled studies with small numbers of subjects treated with tamoxifen found the medication to be effective therapy for gynecomastia.[465,466] Tamoxifen therapy is reserved exclusively for idiopathic gynecomastia after exhaustive evaluation of endocrine and metabolic profiles and comprehensive radiologic evaluation of potential organ sites that can be etiologic for gynecomastia. Side effects, efficacy, and long-term toxicities associated with the use of tamoxifen in the medical therapy of gynecomastia have not been established.

Pubertal patients treated with dihydrotestosterone heptanoate demonstrate a significant reduction in gynecomastia.[467,468] Decreased serum levels of estradiol, LH, FSH, and free testosterone accompany the clinical improvement.[467] The report by Kuhn and colleagues[469] encourages the use of percutaneous dihydrotestosterone in therapy of idiopathic gynecomastia, but this agent requires prospective clinical trials to establish its efficacy and safety. The synthetic heterocyclic steroid danazol (Danocrine) is the 2,3,isoxazol derivative of 17α-ethyl testosterone. This compound is devoid of estrogenic or progestational activities but possesses well-defined antigonadotropic properties. Prolonged therapy with danazol for women with endometriosis has resulted in atrophy of breasts.[470,471] Greenblatt and colleagues[470] were the first to report improvement in gynecomastia after danazol therapy; beneficial effects have been further described by Buckle.[472] Buckle[473] identified response rates for 77% to 100% of patients with gynecomastia induced by several causes (idiopathic, thyrotoxic, spironolactone, and pubertal); these results are depicted in Table 6-6. Overall, there was marked or moderate improvement in 83% of patients with gynecomastia treated with danazol. Buckle determined

TABLE 6-6   Response of Gynecomastia to Treatment with Danazol

| TYPE OF PATIENTS | NO. OF PATIENTS | REGRESSION OF GYNECOMASTIA | | | |
		MARKED	MODERATE	NIL	MARKED/MODERATE IMPROVEMENT (%)
Adult idiopathic	17	8	5	4	77
Thyrotoxic	1	1			100
Spironolactone-induced	13	9	2	2	85
Pubertal	11	7	3	1	91
TOTAL	42	25	10	7	83

From Buckle R: *Drugs* 19:356, 1980.

that danazol initiated a progressive diminution in plasma concentrations of FSH and LH during the 3- to 16-week duration of therapy, with dose schedules of 300 to 600 mg per day in adults and 200 to 300 mg per day in adolescents. Side effects of danazol therapy relate primarily to the androgenic properties of the compound, which can result in acne and weight gain with fluid retention. Muscle weakness and cramps and spasms occur in a small percentage of patients. Testolactone, an aromatase inhibitor, appears to be effective in the reduction of gynecomastia in an uncontrolled study of pubertal patients.[474]

The management of gynecomastia is governed by two premises. First, most cases are caused by minor hormonal imbalances or by drugs and carry no serious significance. Second, a serious cause is considered in each case, and in the older patient, breast cancer is excluded. In most cases, reassurance that this is a benign, self-limiting condition, which is not premalignant, will suffice. A minority of patients will require treatment either for tenderness or for cosmesis.

RADIOTHERAPY

Prophylactic breast irradiation has been used in the past with some success in the prevention of gynecomastia associated with estrogen use for patients with prostate cancer, but now it is only of historical interest. Waterfall and Glaser[475] noted an 85% incidence of gynecomastia after estrogen therapy in patients not receiving radiation pretreatment, compared with an 11% incidence in those pretreated with radiation. Dosing ranged from 1200 to 1500 cGy and was given in three fractions before or shortly after the initiation of estrogen therapy.[476]

SURGICAL THERAPY

The original surgical approach to gynecomastia was a simple mastectomy. However, the cosmetic results of this procedure were often unacceptable. Surgical treatment now depends on the grade of gynecomastia and the amount of associated adipose tissue. The majority of grade I or IIa cases (see Table 6-1) can be dealt with by subcutaneous mastectomy through a periareolar incision.[477] This, however, can lead to further cosmetic deformity, with a sunken nipple. A small disk of underlying breast tissue can be spared to prevent this abnormality. In cases of grade IIb or III gynecomastia, excess skin is present and requires removal to restore the contour of the breast and prevent nipple ptosis. Various techniques have been designed to improve the cosmetic results in these patients; these techniques include excising an ellipse of the areolar margin or simple mastectomy with free nipple graft. Ward and Khalid[478] recommend a horizontal elliptical incision similar to that used for breast reduction for the removal of excess tissue in grade III gynecomastia.

Liposuction has recently been advocated as a useful adjunct to the excision of breast tissue,[479,480] as well as a primary technique to correct the gynecomastia defect, whether caused by excess fat or parenchymal hypertrophy. Rosenberg[481,482] described a cannula for suction removal of parenchymal tissue of gynecomastia, in addition to the standard 7-mm cannula to remove adipose tissue. Used in conjunction, the technique is successful for gynecomastia associated with excess fat.

TREATMENT OF SECONDARY GYNECOMASTIA

If a cause for the gynecomastia is identified, the gynecomastia will resolve with treatment of the underlying abnormality or withdrawal of the offending drug. If the disease is not amenable to treatment or if continuation of a drug is essential and treatment of gynecomastia is still considered necessary, the plan for treatment of primary gynecomastia can be followed. Three injections of nandrolone 25 mg at 3-week intervals have been recommended for gynecomastia of the elderly, but there is minimal experience with treatment.

REFERENCES

1. Wilson JD, Aiman J, MacDonald PC: The pathogenesis of gynecomastia, *Prog Intern Med* 25:1, 1980.
2. Schydlower M: Breast masses in adolescents, *Am Fam Physician* 25:141, 1982.
3. Haibach H, Rosenholtz MJ: Prepubertal gynecomastia with lobules and acini: a case report and review of the literature, *Am J Clin Pathol* 80:252, 1983.
4. Nuttall FQ: Gynecomastia as a physical finding in normal men, *J Clin Endocrinol Metab* 48:338, 1979.
5. Carlson HE: Gynecomastia, *N Engl J Med* 303:795, 1981.
6. Ley SB et al: Palpable breast tissue versus gynecomastia as a normal physical finding, *Clin Res* 28:24A, 1980 (abstract).
7. Williams MJ: Gynecomastia: its incidence, recognition, and host characterization in 447 autopsy cases, *Am J Med* 34:103, 1963.
8. Rubens R, Dhont M, Vermeulen A: Further studies on Leydig cell function in old age, *J Clin Endocrinol Metab* 39:40, 1974.
9. Brittain RT et al: The outline of the animal pharmacology of ranitidine. In Misiewicz JJ, Wormsley KJ (eds): *The clinical use of ranitidine,* Medicine Publishing Foundation Symposium Series No. 5, Oxford, 1982, Medicine Publishing Foundation.
10. Poulsen HS: Demonstration of hormonal sensitivity in gynaecomastic tissue by thymidine incorporation in vitro, *Acta Pathol Microbiol Scand* 85A:19, 1977.
11. Turkington RW, Topper YJ: Androgen inhibiting of mammary gland differentiation in vitro, *Endocrinology* 80:329, 1967.
12. MacDonald PC et al: Plasma precursors of estrogen. III. Conversion of plasma dehydroisoandrosterone to estrogen in young nonpregnant women, *Gynecol Invest* 7:165, 1976.
13. MacDonald PC et al: Origin of estrogen in normal men and in women with testicular feminization, *J Clin Endocrinol Metab* 49:905, 1979.

14. Turkington RW: Serum prolactin levels in patients with gynecomastia, *J Clin Endocrinol Metab* 34:62, 1972.

15. Franks S et al: Hyperprolactinemia and impotence, *Clin Endocrinol* 8:277, 1978.

16. Karsner HT: Gynecomastia, *Am J Pathol* 22:235, 1946.

17. Nicolis GL, Modlinger RS, Gabrilove JL: A study of the histopathology of human gynecomastia, *J Clin Endocrinol* 32:173, 1971.

18. Gottfried MR: Extensive squamous metaplasia in gynecomastia, *Arch Pathol Lab Med* 110:971, 1986.

19. Bannayan GA, Hajdu SI: Gynecomastia: clinicopathologic study of 351 cases, *Am J Clin Pathol* 57:431, 1972.

20. Andersen J et al: Gynecomastia: immunohistochemical demonstration of estrogen receptors, *Acta Pathol Microbiol Immunol Scand* 95:263, 1987.

21. Fodor PB: Breast cancer in a patient with gynecomastia, *Plast Reconstr Surg* 84:976, 1989.

22. Ajayi DOS, Osegbe DN, Ademiluyi SA: Carcinoma of the male breast in West Africans and a review of world literature, *Cancer* 50:1664, 1982.

23. Johnson RL: The male breast and gynaecomastia. In Page DL, Anderson TJ (eds): *Diagnostic histopathology of the breast*, New York, 1988, Churchill Livingstone.

24. Visfeldt J, Scheike O: Male breast cancer: histologic typing and grading of 187 Danish cases, *Cancer* 32:985, 1973.

25. Odagiri E et al: Reduction of telomeric length and c-erbB-2 gene amplification in human breast cancer, fibroadenoma, and gynecomastia, *Cancer* 73:2978, 1994.

26. Bronstein IP, Cassorla E: Breast enlargement in pediatric practice, *Med Clin North Am* 30:121, 1946.

27. Nydick M et al: Gynecomastia in adolescent boys, *JAMA* 178:449, 1961.

28. Dehner LP, Hill DA, Deschryver K: Pathology of the breast in children, adolescents, and young adults, *Semin Diagn Pathol* 16:235, 1999.

29. Bidlingmaier R, Knorr D: Plasma testosterone and estrogens in pubertal gynecomastia, *Z Kinderheilkd* 115:89, 1973.

30. Dexter CJ: Benign enlargement of the male breast, *N Engl J Med* 254:996, 1956.

31. LaFranchi SH et al: Pubertal gynecomastia and transient elevation of serum estradiol level, *Am J Dis Child* 129:927–931, 1975.

32. Lee PA: The relationship of concentrations of serum hormones to pubertal gynecomastia, *J Pediatr* 86:212, 1975.

33. Hemsell DL et al: Massive extraglandular aromatization of plasma androstenedione resulting in the feminization of a prepubertal boy, *J Clin Invest* 60:455, 1977.

34. Sher ES, Migeon CJ, Berkovitz GD: Evaluation of boys with marked breast development at puberty, *Clin Pediatr* 37:367, 1998.

35. Niewoehner CB, Nuttall FQ: Gynecomastia in a hospitalized male patient, *Am J Med* 77:633, 1984.

36. Snyder PF: Effect of age on the serum LH and FSH responses to gonadotropin-releasing hormone. In Grayhack JT, Wilson JD, Scherbenske MJ (eds): *Benign prostatic hyperplasia*, Washington, DC, 1976, DHEW Publication No. (NIH) 76–1113.

37. Siiteri PK, MacDonald PC: Role of extraglandular estrogen in human endocrinology. In Greep RO, Aswood EB (eds): *Handbook of physiology*, vol 2, part 1, Baltimore, 1973, Waverly Press.

38. Mathur R, Braunstein G: Gynecomastia: pathomechanisms and treatment strategies, *Horm Res* 48:95, 1997.

39. Van Niekerk WA: True hermaphroditism: an analytic view with a report of three new cases, *Am J Obstet Gynecol* 126:890, 1976.

40. Gallegos AJ: Familial true hermaphroditism in three siblings: plasma hormonal profile and in vitro steroid biosynthesis in gonadal structures, *J Clin Endocrinol Metab* 42:653, 1976.

41. Aiman J, Hemsell DL, MacDonald PC: Production and origin of estrogen in two true hermaphrodites, *Am J Obstet Gynecol* 132:401, 1978.

42. Castro-Magana M, Angulo M, Uy J: Male hypogonadism with gynecomastia caused by late-onset deficiency of testicular 17-ketosteroid reductase, *N Engl J Med* 328:1297, 1993.

43. Cavanah SFW, Dons RF: Partial 3b-hydroxysteroid dehydrogenase deficiency presenting as new-onset gynecomastia in a eugonadal adult male, *Metabolism* 42:65, 1993.

44. Castle WN, Richardson JR Jr: Leydig cell tumor and metachronous Leydig cell hyperplasia: a case associated with gynecomastia and elevated urinary estrogens, *J Urol* 136:1307, 1986.

45. Brosman SA: Testicular tumors in prepubertal children, *Urology* 13:581, 1979.

46. Camin AJ et al: Interstitial cell tumor of the testis in a seven-year-old child, *Am J Dis Child* 100:389, 1960.

47. Mostofi FK, Price EB: Tumors of the testis in children. In *Tumors of the male genital system, atlas of tumor pathology*, series 2, fasc 16, Washington, DC, 1973, Armed Forces Institute of Pathology.

48. Symington T, Cameron KM: Endocrine and genetic lesions. In Pugh RCB (ed): *Pathology of testes*, Oxford, 1976, Blackwell.

49. Turner WR, Derrick FC, Worltmann H: Leydig cell tumor in identical twins, *Urology* 7:194, 1976.

50. Blundon KE, Russi S, Bunts RC: Interstitial cell hyperplasia or adenoma, *J Urol* 70:759, 1953.

51. Damjanov I, Katz SM, Jewett MAS: Leydig cell tumors of the testis, *Ann Clin Lab Sci* 9:157, 1979.

52. Davis M et al: Adenome testiculaire à cellules de Leydig chez l'enfant, *Pediatrie* 31:457, 1976.

53. House R, Izant RJ, Persky L: Testicular tumors in children, *Am J Surg* 110:876, 1965.

54. Caldamone AA et al: Leydig cell tumor of the testis, *Urology* 14:39, 1979.

55. Wilson BE, Netzloff ML: Primary testicular abnormalities causing precocious puberty Leydig cell tumor, Leydig cell hyperplasia, and adrenal rest tumor, *Ann Clin Lab Sci* 13:315, 1983.

56. Gabrilove JL: Some recent advances in virilizing and feminizing syndrome and hirsutism, *Mt Sinai J Med* 41:636, 1974.

57. Gabrilove JL et al: Feminizing and nonfeminizing Sertoli cell tumors, *J Urol* 124:757, 1980.

58. Feldman PS et al: Malignant Leydig cell tumor: clinical histologic and electron microscopic features, *Cancer* 49:714, 1982.

59. Shimp WS et al: Leydig cell tumor of the testis with gynecomastia and elevated estrogen levels, *Am J Clin Pathol* 67:562, 1977.

60. Mostofi FK, Price EB: Tumors of the testis. In *Tumors of the male genital system, atlas of tumor pathology*, series 2, part 8, Washington, DC, 1973, Armed Forces Institute of Pathology.

61. Mostofi FK, Price EB: Tumors of specialized gonadal stroma. In *Tumors of the male genital system, atlas of tumor pathology*, fasc. 8, Washington, DC, 1973, Armed Forces Institute of Pathology.

62. Brogard JM, Maurer C, Philippe E: Gyneácomastia et tumeur aá cellules de Leydig, *Press Med* 75:1253, 1967.

63. Fligiel Z, Kaneko M, Leiter E: Bilateral Sertoli cell tumor of the testes with feminizing and masculinizing activity occurring in a child, *Cancer* 38:1853, 1976.

64. Lucas LM, Kumar KL, Smith DL: Gynecomastia: a worrisome problem for the patient, *Postgrad Med* 82:73, 1987.

65. Pierrepoint CG: The metabolism in vitro of dehydroepiandrosterone and hydroepiandrosterone sulphate by Sertoli cell tumours of the testis of two dogs with clinical signs of hyperoestrogenism, *J Endocrinol* 42:99, 1968.

66. Mellor SG, McCutchan JDS: Gynaecomastia and occult Leydig cell tumour of the testis, *Br J Urol* 63:420, 1989.

67. Davis S, DiMartino NA, Schneider G: Malignant interstitial cell carcinoma of the testis: report of two cases with steroid profiles, response to therapy, and review of the literature, *Cancer* 47:425, 1981.

68. Gabrilove JL, Furukawa H: Gynecomastia in association with a complex tumor of the testis secreting chorionic gonadotropin: studies on the testicular venous effluent, *J Urol* 131:348, 1984.

69. Veldhuis JD et al: Pathophysiology of male hypogonadism associated with endogenous hyperestrogenism, *N Engl J Med* 312:1371, 1985.

70. Bercovici JP et al: Leydig call tumor with gynecomastia: further studies—the recovery after unilateral orchiectomy, *J Clin Endocrinol Metab* 61:957, 1985.

71. Gabrilove JL et al: Feminizing interstitial cell tumor of the testis: personal observations and a review of the literature, *Cancer* 35:1184, 1975.

72. Selvaggi FP et al: Interstitial cell tumor of the testis in an adult: two case reports, *J Urol* 109:436, 1973.

73. Goh HH et al: Control of gonadotrophin secretion by steroid hormones in castrated male transsexuals. I. Effects of oestradiol infusion on plasma follicle-stimulating hormone and luteinizing hormone, *Clin Endocrinol* 12:16, 1980.

74. Goh HH, Karim SMM, Ratnam SS: Control of gonadotrophin secretion by steroid hormones in castrated male transsexuals. II. Effects of androgens alone and in combination with oestradiol on the secretions of FSH and LH, *Clin Endocrinol* 15:301, 1981.

75. Kuhn JM et al: hCG test in gynaecomastia: further study, *Clin Endocrinol* 31:581, 1989.

76. Mineur P et al: Feminizing testicular Leydig cell tumor: hormonal profile before and after unilateral orchiectomy, *J Clin Endocrinol Metab* 64:686, 1987.

77. Mikuz G et al: Leydig cell tumor of the testis: morphological and endocrinological investigations in two cases, *Eur Urol* 6:293, 1980.

78. Hopkins GB, Parry HD: Metastasizing Sertoli cell tumor, *Cancer* 23:463, 1969.

79. Mostofi FK: Pathology of germ cell tumors of testis: a progress report, *Cancer* 45:1735, 1980.

80. Mostofi FK: Testicular tumors, *Cancer* 32:1186, 1973.

81. Waxman M et al: Large cell calcifying Sertoli tumor of the testis: light microscopic and ultrastructural study, *Cancer* 54:1574, 1984.

82. Richie JP: Neoplasms of the testis. In Campbell MF, Walsh PC (eds): *Campbell's urology*, vol 2, ed 6, Philadelphia, 1992, WB Saunders.

83. Proppe KH, Scully RE: Large-cell calcifying Sertoli cell tumor of the testis, *Am J Clin Pathol* 74:607, 1980.

84. Wilson DM et al: Testicular tumors with Peutz-Jeghers syndrome, *Cancer* 57:2238, 1986.

85. Young S et al: Feminizing Sertoli cell tumors in boys with Peutz-Jeghers syndrome, *Am J Surg Pathol* 19:50, 1995.

86. Scully RE: Sex cord tumor with annular tubules: a distinctive ovarian tumor of the Peutz-Jeghers syndrome, *Cancer* 25:1107, 1970.

87. Teilum G: Estrogen-producing Sertoli cell tumors of the human testis and ovary, *J Clin Endocrinol* 9:301, 1958.

88. Teilum G: Classification of testicular and ovarian androblastoma and Sertoli cell tumors, *Cancer* 11:769, 1958.

89. Cohen J, Diamond I: Leiontiasis ossea, slipped epiphysis and granulosa cell tumor of the testis with renal disease, *Arch Pathol Lab Med* 56:488, 1953.

90. Laskowski J: Feminizing tumors of the testis: general review with case report of granulosa cell tumor of the testis, *Endokrynol Pol* 3:337, 1952.

91. Marshall FF et al: Sex cord–stromal (gonadal stroma) tumors of the testis: a report of 5 cases, *J Urol* 117:180, 1977.

92. Melicow MM: Classification of tumors of the testis: a clinical and pathological study based on 105 primary and 13 secondary cases in adults and 8 primary and secondary cases in children, *J Urol* 73:547, 1955.

93. Crump WD: Juvenile granulosa cell tumor in an infant, *J Urol* 129:1057, 1983.

94. Lawrence WD, Young RH, Scully RE: Juvenile granulosa cell tumor of the infantile testis, *Am J Surg Pathol* 9:87, 1985.

95. Raju U et al: Congenital testicular juvenile granulosa cell tumor in a neonate with X/XY mosaicism, *Am J Surg Pathol* 10:577, 1986.

96. Young RH, Lawrence DW, Scully RE: Juvenile granulosa cell tumors: another neoplasm associated with abnormal chromosomes and ambiguous genitalia—a report of 3 cases, *Am J Surg Pathol* 9:737, 1985.

97. Rosvoll RV, Woodard JR: Malignant Sertoli cell tumor of the testis, *Cancer* 22:8, 1968.

98. Kaplan GW et al: Gonadal stromal tumors: a report of the prepubertal testicular tumor registry, *J Urol* 136:300, 1986.

99. Mizejewski GJ, Bellisario R, Carter TP: Birth weight and alpha-fetoprotein (AFP) levels in the newborn, *Pediatrics* 73:736, 1984 (letter).

100. Wu JT, Book L, Sudar K: Serum alpha fetoprotein (AFP) levels in normal infants, *Pediatr Res* 15:50, 1981.

101. Masterson JST et al: Neonatal gonadal stromal tumor: limitations of tumor markers. Presented at the Annual Meeting of Section on Urology of the American Academy of Pediatrics, San Francisco, October 1983.

102. Pierce GB Jr: Ultrastructure of human testicular tumors, *Cancer* 19:1963, 1966.

103. Pierce GB Jr, Stevens LC, Nakane PK: Ultrastructural analysis of the early development of teratocarcinomas, *J Natl Cancer Inst* 39:755, 1967.

104. Pearson JC: Endocrinology of testicular neoplasms, *Urology* 17:119, 1981.

105. Dixon FJ, Moore RA: Tumors of the male sex organs. In Dixon FJ, Moore RA (eds): *Atlas of tumor pathology*, Washington, DC, 1952, Armed Forces Institute of Pathology.

106. Friedman NB, Moore RA: Tumors of the testis: a report on 922 cases, *Mil Surg* 99:573, 1946.

107. Stevens LC: Experimental production of testicular teratomas in mice, *Proc Natl Acad Sci USA* 52:661, 1964.

108. Stevens LC, Hummel KP: A description of spontaneous congenital teratomas in strain 129 mice, *J Natl Cancer Inst* 18:719, 1957.

109. Mostofi FK, Thiess EA, Ashley DJB: Tumors of specialized gonadal stroma in human male patients, *Cancer* 12:944, 1959.

110. Stephanas AV et al: Endocrine studies in testicular tumor patients with and without gynecomastia, *Cancer* 41:369, 1978.

111. von Eyben FE: Biochemical markers in advanced testicular tumors, *Cancer* 41:648, 1978.

112. Kirschner MA, Cohen FB, Jespersen D: Estrogen production and its origin in men with gonadotrophin-producing neoplasms, *J Clin Endocrinol Metab* 39:112, 1974.

113. MacDonald PC, Siiteri PK: The in vivo mechanisms of origin of estrogen in subjects with trophoblastic tumors, *Steroids* 8:589, 1966.

114. Bardin CW: Pituitary-testicular axis. In Yen SSC, Jaffe RB (eds): *Reproductive endocrinology*, Philadelphia, 1978, WB Saunders.

115. Tseng A et al: Gynecomastia in testicular cancer patients: prognostic and therapeutic implications, *Cancer* 56:2534, 1985.

116. Glazer HS et al: Sonographic detection of occult testicular neoplasms, *AJR Am J Roentgenol* 138:673, 1982.

117. Leopold GR et al: High-resolution ultrasonography of scrotal pathology, *Radiology* 131:719, 1979.

118. Moudy P, Makhija JS: Ultrasonic demonstration of a nonpalpable testicular tumor, *J Clin Ultrasound* 11:54, 1983.

119. Peterson LJ, Catalona WJ, Koehler RE: Ultrasonic localization of a nonpalpable testis tumor, *J Urol* 122:843, 1979.

120. Hendry WS et al: Ultrasonic detection of occult testicular neoplasms in patients with gynaecomastia, *Br J Radiol* 57:571, 1984.

121. Emory TH et al: Occult testicular interstitial-cell tumor in a patient with gynecomastia: ultrasonic detection, *Radiology* 151:474, 1984.

122. Nagi DK, Jones WG, Belchetz PE: Gynaecomastia caused by a primary mediastinal seminoma, *Clin Endocrinol* 40:545, 1994.

123. Lemack GE, Poppas DP, Vaughan ED: Urologic causes of gynecomastia: approach to diagnosis and management, *Urology* 45:313, 1995.

124. Leung A et al: Resolution of prepubertal male gynecomastia following removal of a giant pigmented nevus, *Ann Plast Surg* 15:167, 1985.

125. Salassa RM, Jowsey J, Arnaud CD: Hypophosphatomic osteomalacia associated with "non-endocrine" tumors, *N Engl J Med* 283:65, 1970.

126. Fienman NL, Yakovac WC: Neurofibromatosis in childhood, *J Pediatr* 76:339, 1970.

127. August GP, Chandra R, Hung W: Prepubertal male gynecomastia, *J Pediatr* 80:259, 1972.

128. Edidin DV, Levitsky LL: Prepubertal gynecomastia associated with estrogen-containing hair cream, *Am J Dis Child* 136:587, 1982.

129. Fontaine G, Lacheretz M, Dupont A: Tumor de la cortico-surrenale avec puberteá preácoce et gynecomastie chez un garcon de 3 ans 1/2, *Ann Pediatr* 17:463, 1970.

130. Hung W, August GP, Glasgow AM: *Pediatric endocrinology*, New York, 1978, Medical Examinations Publishing.

131. Johnstone G: Prepubertal gynecomastia in association with an interstitial tumor of the testes, *Br J Urol* 39:211, 1967.

132. Latorre H, Kenny F: Idiopathic gynecomastia in seven preadolescent boys: elevation of urinary estrogen secretion in two cases, *Am J Dis Child* 126:771, 1973.

133. Marchandise B, Lederer J: Gynecomastia par exces de dihydroepiandrosterone, *Rev Fr Endocrinol Clin* 7:383, 1966.

134. Saenz CA, Bongiovanni AM: An outbreak of premature thelarche in Puerto Rico, *Pediatr Res* 17:171A, 1983 (abstract).

135. Javadpour N, Woltering EA, Brennan MF: Adrenal neoplasms, *Curr Probl Surg* 17:1, 1980.

136. Lee PDK, Winter RJ, Green OC: Virilizing adrenocortical tumors in childhood: eight cases and a review of the literature, *Pediatrics* 76:437, 1985.

137. Hayles AB et al: Hormone-secreting tumors of the adrenal cortex in children, *Pediatrics* 37:19, 1966.

138. Bacon GE, Lowrey GH: Feminizing adrenal tumor in a 6-year-old boy, *J Clin Endocrinol* 25:1403, 1965.

139. Bhettay E, Bonnici F: Pure oestrogen-secreting feminizing adrenocortical adenoma, *Arch Dis Child* 52:241, 1977.

140. Crane MG, Holloaway JE, Winsor WG: Aldosterone-secreting adenoma: report of a case in a juvenile, *Ann Intern Med* 54:280, 1961.

141. Gabrilove JL et al: Feminizing adrenocortical carcinoma in a man, *Cancer* 25:153, 1970.

142. Gabrilove JL et al: Feminizing adrenocortical tumors in the male: a review of 52 cases including a case report, *Medicine* 44:37, 1965.

143. Ganguly A et al: Childhood primary aldosteronism due to an adrenal adenoma: preoperative localization by adrenal vein catheterization, *Pediatrics* 65:605, 1980.

144. Howard CP, Takashashi H, Hayles AB: Feminizing adrenal adenoma in a boy, *Proc Mayo Clin* 52:354, 1977.

145. Kepler EJ, Walters W, Dixon RK: Menstruation in a child aged nineteen months as a result of tumor of the left adrenal cortex: successful surgical treatment, *Proc Mayo Clin* 13:362, 1938.

146. Mosier HD, Goodwin WE: Feminizing adrenal adenoma in a seven-year-old boy, *Pediatrics* 27:1016, 1961.

147. Snaith AH: A case of feminizing adrenal tumor in a girl, *J Clin Endocrinol* 18:318, 1958.

148. Wallach S et al: Adrenocortical carcinoma with gynecomastia: a case report and review of the literature, *J Clin Endocrinol* 17:945, 1957.

149. Wilkins L: A feminizing adrenal tumor causing gynecomastia in a boy of five years contrasted with a virilizing tumor in a five-year-old girl, *J Clin Endocrinol* 8:111, 1948.

150. Beckwith JB: Macroglossia, omphalocele, adrenal cytomegaly, gigantism and hyperplastic visceromegaly, *Birth Defects* 5:188, 1969.

151. Wiedemann HR: Tumours and hemihypertrophy associated with Wiedemann-Beckwith syndrome, *Eur J Pediatr* 141:129, 1983.

152. Ogle JW: Unusually large mass of carcinomatous deposit in one of the suprarenal capsules of a child, *Trans Pathol Soc Lond* 16:250, 1865.

153. Didolkar MS et al: Natural history of adrenal cortical carcinoma: a clinicopathologic study of 42 patients, *Cancer* 47:2153, 1981.

154. Stewart DR, Morris Jones PH, Jolleys A: Carcinoma of the adrenal gland in children, *J Pediatr Surg* 9:59, 1974.

155. Page DL, DeLellis RA, Hough AF Jr: Tumors of the adrenal. In *Atlas of tumor pathology*, second series, fasc 23, Washington, DC, 1985, Armed Forces Institute of Pathology.

156. Wittenberg J: Computed tomography of the body, *N Engl J Med* 309:1224, 1983.

157. Bittorf A: Nebennieren tumor and geschlechtsdrusenausfall beim mann, *Berl Klin Wochenschr* 56:776, 1919.

158. Rose LI et al: Steroidal and gonadotropin evaluation of a patient with feminizing tumor of the adrenal gland: in vivo and in vitro studies, *J Clin Endocrinol Metab* 29:1526, 1969.

159. Lanigan D, Choa RG, Evans J: A feminizing adrenocortical carcinoma presenting with gynaecomastia, *Postgrad Med J* 69:481, 1993.

160. Wohltmann H, Mathur RS, Williamson HO: Sexual precocity in a female infant due to feminizing adrenal carcinoma, *J Clin Endocrinol Metab* 50:186, 1980.

161. Nishiki M et al: Feminizing adrenocortical carcinoma in man, *Jpn J Surg* 10:159, 1980.

162. Leditschke JF, Arden F: Feminizing adrenal adenoma in a five-year-old boy, *Aust Paediatr J* 10:217, 1974.

163. Sultan C et al: Pubertal gynecomastia due to an estrogen-producing adrenal adenoma, *J Pediatr* 95:744, 1979.

164. Landau RL et al: Gynecomastia and retarded sexual development resulting from a long-standing estrogen secreting adrenal tumor, *J Clin Endocrinol* 14:1097, 1954.

165. Desai MB, Kapadia SN: Feminizing adrenocortical tumors in male patients: adenoma versus carcinoma, *J Urol* 139:101, 1988.

166. Bondy PK: Disorders of the adrenal cortex. In Wilson JD, Foster DW (eds): *Williams' textbook of endocrinology*, ed 7, Philadelphia, 1985, WB Saunders.

167. Neblett WW, Frexes-Steed M, Scott HW Jr: Experience with adrenocortical neoplasms in childhood, *Am Surg* 53:117, 1987.

168. Malchoff CD et al: Adrenocorticotropin-independent bilateral macronodular adrenal hyperplasia: an unusual cause of Cushing's syndrome, *J Clin Endocrinol Metab* 68:855, 1989.

169. Thompson NW, Cheung PSY: Diagnosis and treatment of functioning and nonfunctioning adrenocortical neoplasms including incidentalomas, *Surg Clin North Am* 67:423, 1987.

170. Hough AJ Jr: Flow cytometry and adrenal cortical tumors, *J Urol* 134:931, 1985.

171. Smith LG, Lyubsky SL, Carlson HE: Postmenopausal uterine bleeding due to estrogen production by gonadotropin-secreting lung tumors, *Am J Med* 92:327, 1992.

172. Fusco FD, Rosen SW: Gonadotropin-producing anaplastic large-cell carcinomas of the lung, *N Engl J Med* 275:507, 1966.

173. Camiel MR, Benninghoff DL, Alexander LL: Gynecomastia associated with lung cancer, *Dis Chest* 52:445, 1967.

174. Becker KL et al: Endocrine studies in a patient with a gonadotropin-secreting bronchogenic carcinoma, *J Clin Endocrinol Metab* 28:809, 1968.

175. Fine G, Smith RW Jr, Pachter MR: Primary extragenital choriocarcinoma in a male subject: case report and review of literature, *Am J Med* 32:776, 1962.

176. Dailey JE, Marcuse PM: Gonadotropin secreting giant cell carcinoma of the lung, *Cancer* 24:388, 1969.

177. Grillo IA: Endocrine manifestations of pulmonary carcinoma in a Nigerian, *Br J Cancer* 25:266, 1971.

178. Behera D et al: Galactorrhea with gynecomastia in a male with lung cancer, *Indian J Chest Dis Allied Sci* 29:112, 1987.

179. Behera D et al: Circulating hormones in lung cancer, *Indian J Med Res* 79:636, 1984.

180. Gropp C, Havemann K, Scheur A: Ectopic hormones in lung cancer patients at diagnosis and during therapy, *Cancer* 46:347, 1980.

181. Okamoto H et al: Malignant pleural mesothelioma producing human chorionic gonadotropin, *Am J Surg Pathol* 16:969, 1992.

182. Kew MC et al: Mechanism of feminization in primary liver cancer, *N Engl J Med* 296:1084, 1977.

183. Johnson PJ et al: Hepatocellular carcinoma in Great Britain: influence of age, sex, HBsAg status and aetiology of underlying cirrhosis, *Gut* 19:1022, 1978.

184. Andervont HB: Studies on the occurrence of spontaneous hepatomas in mice of strains C_3H and CBA, *J Natl Cancer Inst* 11:581, 1952.

185. Goodall CM, Butler WH: Aflatoxin carcinogenesis: inhibition of liver cancer induction in hypophysectomized rats, *Int J Cancer* 4:422, 1969.

186. Neuberger J et al: Oral contraceptive-associated liver tumours: occurrence of malignancy and difficulties in diagnosis, *Lancet* 1:273, 1980.

187. Stedman KC, Moore GE, Morgan RT: Estrogen receptor proteins in diverse human tumours, *Arch Surg* 115:244, 1980.

188. Iqbal MJ et al: Sex steroid receptor proteins in foetal, adult and malignant human liver tissue, *Br J Cancer* 48:791, 1983.

189. Hall PH: Gynaecomastia. Monographs of the Federal Council of the British Medical Association in Australia, No. 2, 1959.

190. Rosenthal FD, Lees F: Thyrotoxicosis with glucosuria and adrenocortical hyperactivity, *Lancet* 2:340, 1958.

191. Starr P: Gynecomastia during hyperthyroidism, *JAMA* 104:1988, 1935.

192. Stokes JF: Unexpected gynaecomastia, *Lancet* 2:911, 1962.

193. Larsson O, Sundbom CM, Astedt B: Gynaecomastia and diseases of the thyroid, *Acta Endocrinol* 44:133, 1963.

194. Treves N: Gynecomastia, *Cancer* 11:1083, 1958.

195. Hartemann P et al: Gynecomastie et hyperthyroidie: rapport de deux observations, *Ann Med Nancy* 2:1104, 1963.

196. Berson SA, Schreiber SS: Gynecomastia and hyperthyroidism, *J Clin Endocrinol* 13:1126, 1953 (letter).

197. Albright F, cited in Hall PH: Gynaecomastia. Monographs of the Federal Council of the British Medical Association in Australia No. 2, 1959.

198. Becker KL et al: Gynecomastia and hyperthyroidism: an endocrine and histological investigation, *J Clin Endocrinol Metab* 28:277, 1968.

199. Rupp J et al: Hormone excretion in liver disease and in gynecomastia, *J Clin Endocrinol* 11:688, 1951.

200. Weichert CK, Boyd RW: Stimulation of mammary gland development in the pregnant rat under conditions of experimental hyperthyroidism, *Anat Rec* 59:157, 1934.

201. Fitzsimons MP: Gynecomastia in stilbestrol workers, *Br J Ind Med* 1:235, 1944.

202. Chopra IJ: Gonadal steroids and gonadotropins in hyperthyroidism, *Med Clin North Am* 59:1109, 1975.

203. Chopra IJ, Tulchinsky D: Status of estrogen-androgen balance in hyperthyroid men with Graves' disease, *J Clin Endocrinol Metab* 38:269, 1974.

204. Nomura K et al: High serum progesterone in hyperthyroid men with Graves' disease, *J Clin Endocrinol Metab* 66:230, 1988.

205. Freeman CS, Topper YG: Progesterone is not essential to the differentiative potential of mammary epithelium in the male mouse, *Endocrinology* 103:186, 1978.

206. Finn JE, Mount LA: Galactorrhea in males with tumors in the region of the pituitary gland, *J Neurosurg* 35:723, 1971.

207. Kleinberg DL, Noel GL, Frantz AG: Galactorrhea: a study of 235 cases, including 48 with pituitary tumors, *N Engl J Med* 296:589, 1977.

208. Edwards CRW, Forsyth IA, Besser GM: Amenorrhea, galactorrhea, and primary hypothyroidism with high circulating levels of prolactin, *BMJ* 3:462, 1971.

209. Arnaout MA et al: Galactorrhea, gynecomastia, and hypothyroidism in a man, *Ann Intern Med* 106:779, 1987 (letter).

210. Gordon GG et al: Effect of alcohol (ethanol) administration on sex-hormone metabolism in normal men, *N Engl J Med* 295:793, 1976.

211. Gordon GG et al: Conversion of androgens to estrogens in cirrhosis of the liver, *J Clin Endocrinol Metab* 40:1018, 1975.

212. Olivo J et al: Estrogen metabolism in hyperthyroidism and in cirrhosis of the liver, *Steroids* 26:47, 1975.

213. Kley HK et al: Steroid hormones and their binding in plasma of male patients with fatty liver, chronic hepatitis and liver cirrhosis, *Acta Endocrinol* 79:275, 1975.

214. Kley HK et al: Conversion of androgens to estrogens in idiopathic hemochromatosis: comparison with alcoholic liver cirrhosis, *J Clin Endocrinol Metab* 61:1, 1985.

215. Farthing MJG et al: Progesterone, prolactin, and gynaecomastia in men with liver disease, *Gut* 23:276, 1982.

216. Johnson PJ: Sex hormones and the liver, *Clin Sci* 66:369, 1984.

217. Baker HWG et al: A study of the endocrine manifestations of hepatic cirrhosis, *QJM* 45:145, 1976.

218. Baker HWG et al: Endocrine aspects of hepatic cirrhosis, Washington, DC, June 1972, Fourth International Endocrine Congress (abstract).

219. Galvaáo-Teles A et al: Biologically active androgens and oestradiol in men with chronic liver disease, *Lancet* 1:173, 1973.

220. Lloyd CW, Williams RH: Endocrine changes associated with Laennec's cirrhosis of the liver, *Am J Med* 4:315, 1948.

221. Powell LW, Mortimer R, Harris OD: Cirrhosis of the liver: a comparative study of the four major aetiological groups, *Med J Aust* 1:941, 1971.

222. Southern AL et al: Androgen metabolism in cirrhosis of the liver, *Metabolism* 22:695, 1973.

223. Summerskill WHJ et al: Cirrhosis of the liver: a study of alcoholic and nonalcoholic patients in Boston and London, *N Engl J Med* 262:1, 1960.

224. Van Thiel DH, Lester R, Sherins RJ: Hypogonadism in alcoholic liver disease: evidence for a double defect, *Gastroenterology* 67:1188, 1974.

225. Chopra IJ, Tulchinsky D, Greenway FL: Estrogen-androgen imbalance in hepatic cirrhosis: studies in 13 male patients, *Ann Intern Med* 79:198, 1973.

226. Kent JR et al: Plasma testosterone, estradiol and gonadotrophins in hepatic insufficiency, *Gastroenterology* 64:111, 1973.

227. Pincus IJ et al: Hormonal studies in patients with chronic liver disease, *Gastroenterology* 19:735, 1951.

228. Mowat NAG et al: Hypothalamic-pituitary-gonadal function in men with cirrhosis of the liver, *Gut* 17:345, 1976.

229. Rosenbaum W, Christy NP, Kelly WG: Electrophoretic evidence for the presence of an estrogen-binding β-globulin in human plasma, *J Clin Endocrinol Metab* 26:1399, 1966.

230. Rosner W: A simplified method for the quantitative determination of testosterone-estradiol-binding globulin activity in human plasma, *J Clin Endocrinol Metab* 34:983, 1972.

231. Vermeulen A et al: Capacity of the testosterone-binding globulin in human plasma and influence of specific binding of testosterone on its metabolic clearance rate, *J Clin Endocrinol Metab* 29:1470, 1969.

232. Anderson DC: Sex-hormonal-binding globulin, *Clin Endocrinol* 3:69, 1974.

233. Horton R, Tait JF: Androstenedione production and interconversion rates measured in peripheral blood and studies on the possible site of its conversion to testosterone, *J Clin Invest* 45:301, 1966.

234. Green JRB et al: Plasma oestrogens in men with chronic liver disease, *Gut* 17:426, 1976.

235. Geisthövel W, von zur Mühlen A: Studies on the pituitary-testicular axis in patients with chronic hepatic failure, *Acta Endocrinol (Suppl)* 199:256, 1975 (abstract).

236. Korenman SG, Perrin LE, McCallum T: Estradiol in human plasma: demonstration of elevated levels in gynecomastia and in cirrhosis, *J Clin Invest* 48:45a, 1969 (abstract).

237. Pentikäinen PJ et al: Plasma levels and excretion of estrogens in urine in chronic liver disease, *Gastroenterology* 69:20, 1975.

238. Cedard L, Mosse A, Klotz HP: Les oestrogenes plasmatiques dans les gynecomasties et les hepatopathies, *Ann Endocrinol* 31:453, 1970.

239. Green JRB: Mechanism of hypogonadism in cirrhotic males, *Gut* 18:843, 1977.

240. Liegel J et al: Plasma testosterone and sex hormone binding globulin (SHBG) in alcoholic subjects, *Physiologist* 15:198, 1972 (abstract).

241. Van Thiel DH et al: Evidence for an isolated defect in pituitary secretion of LH in chronic alcoholic men, *Gastroenterology* 71:40, 1976.

242. Van Thiel DH, Lester R: Alcoholism: its effect on hypothalamic-pituitary-gonadal function, *Gastroenterology* 71:318, 1976.

243. Paulsen CA: The testes. In Williams RH (ed): *Textbook of endocrinology*, ed 4, Philadelphia, 1968, WB Saunders.

244. Rose LI et al: Pathophysiology of spironolactone-induced gynecomastia, *Ann Intern Med* 87:398, 1977.

245. Barr RW, Som SC: Endocrine abnormalities accompanying hepatic cirrhosis and hepatoma, *J Clin Endocrinol Metab* 17:1017, 1957.

246. Bennett HS, Baggenstoss AH, Butt HR: Testes, breast, and prostate of men who die of cirrhosis of liver, *Am J Clin Pathol* 20:814, 1950.

247. Morrione TG: Effects of estrogens on testes in hepatic insufficiency, *Arch Pathol* 37:39, 1944.

248. Coppage WS, Cooner AE: Testosterone in human plasma, *N Engl J Med* 273:902, 1965.

249. Jacobs EC: Effects of starvation on sex hormones in the male, *J Clin Endocrinol* 8:228, 1948.

250. Klatskin G, Saltin WT, Humm FD: Gynecomastia due to malnutrition, *Am J Med Sci* 213:19, 1947.

251. Zurbiran S, Gomez-Mont F: Endocrine disturbances in chronic human malnutrition, *Vitam Horm* 11:97, 1953.

252. Sattin RW et al: Epidemic of gynecomastia among illegal Haitian entrants, *Public Health Rep* 99:504, 1984.

253. Haagensen CD: Abnormalities of breast growth, secretion and lactation. In Haagensen CD (ed): *Diseases of the breast,* Philadelphia, 1986, WB Saunders.

254. Klinefelter HF, Reifenstein EC, Albright F: Syndrome characterized by gynecomastia, aspermatogenesis without aleydigism, and increased excretion of follicle-stimulating hormone, *J Clin Endocrinol* 2:615, 1942.

255. Gerald PS: Sex chromosome disorders, *N Engl J Med* 294:707, 1976.

256. Tennes K et al: The early childhood development of 17 boys with sex chromosome anomalies: a prospective study, *Pediatrics* 59:574, 1977.

257. Ferguson-Smith MA: The prepubertal testicular lesion in chromatin-positive Klinefelter's syndrome (primary microorchidism) as seen in mentally handicapped children, *Lancet* 1:219, 1959.

258. Ahmad KN et al: Leydig cell volume in chromatin-positive Klinefelter's syndrome, *J Clin Endocrinol Metab* 33:517, 1971.

259. Forti G et al: Klinefelter's syndrome: a study of its hormonal plasma pattern, *J Endocrinol Invest* 2:149, 1978.

260. Gabrilove JL et al: Effect of age on testicular function in patients with Klinefelter's syndrome, *Clin Endocrinol* 11:343, 1979.

261. Salbenblatt JA et al: Pituitary-gonadal function in Klinefelter syndrome before and during puberty, *Pediatr Res* 19:82, 1985.

262. Drucker WD et al: The testis in myotonic muscular dystrophy: a clinical and pathologic study with a comparison with the Klinefelter syndrome, *J Clin Endocrinol Metab* 23:59, 1963.

263. Klinefelter HF: Klinefelter's syndrome: historical background and development, *South Med J* 79:1089, 1986.

264. Cole EW: Klinefelter's syndrome and breast cancer, *Johns Hopkins Med J* 138:105, 1976.

265. Jackson AW et al: Carcinoma of the male breast in association with the Klinefelter syndrome, *BMJ* 1:223, 1965.

266. Robson MC, Santiago Q, Huang TW: Bilateral carcinoma of the breast in a patient with Klinefelter's syndrome, *J Clin Endocrinol* 28:897, 1968.

267. Amrhein JA et al: Partial androgen insensitivity: the Reifenstein syndrome revisited, *N Engl J Med* 297:350, 1977.

268. Reifenstein EC Jr: Hereditary familial hypogonadism, *Proc Am Fed Clin Res* 3:86, 1947.

269. Wilson JD et al: Familial incomplete male pseudohermaphroditism, type 1: evidence for androgen resistance and variable clinical manifestations in a family with the Reifenstein syndrome, *N Engl J Med* 290:1097, 1982.

270. Schweikert H et al: Clinical and endocrinological characterization of two subjects with Reifenstein syndrome associated with qualitative abnormalities of the androgen receptor, *Hormone Res* 25:72, 1987.

271. Rosewater S, Gwinup G, Hamwi GJ: Familial gynecomastia, *Ann Intern Med* 63:377, 1965.

272. Berkovitz GD et al: Familial gynecomastia with increased extraglandular aromatization of plasma carbon 19 steroids, *J Clin Invest* 75:1763, 1985.

273. Van Dop C et al: Isolated gonadotropin deficiency in boys: clinical characteristics and growth, *J Pediatr* 111:684, 1987.

274. Kallmann FJ, Schoenfeld WA, Barrera SE: The genetic aspects of primary eunuchoidism, *Am J Ment Defic* 48:203, 1944.

275. Sparkes RS, Simpson RW, Paulsen CA: Familial hypogonadotropic hypogonadism with anosomia, *Arch Intern Med* 121:534, 1968.

276. Wegenke JD et al: Familial Kallmann syndrome with unilateral renal aplasia, *Clin Genet* 7:368, 1975.

277. Boyar RM et al: Studies of endocrine function in "isolated" gonadotropin deficiency, *J Clin Endocrinol Metab* 36:64, 1973.

278. Lieblich JM et al: Syndrome of anosmia with hypogonadotropic hypogonadism (Kallmann syndrome): clinical and laboratory studies in 23 cases, *Am J Med* 73:506, 1982.

279. Bardin CW et al: Studies of the pituitary–Leydig cell axis in young men with hypogonadotropic hypogonadism and hyposmia: comparison with normal men, prepubertal boys, and hypopituitary patients, *J Clin Invest* 48:2046, 1969.

280. Santen RJ, Paulsen CA: Hypogonadotropic eunuchoidism I. Clinical study of the mode of inheritance, *J Clin Endocrinol Metab* 36:47, 1973.

281. Grumbach MM, Conte FA: Disorders of sex differentiation. In Wilson JB, Foster DW (eds): *Williams' textbook of endocrinology,* ed 7, Philadelphia, 1985, WB Saunders, 1985.

282. Kennedy WR, Alter M, Foreman RT: Hereditary proximal spinal muscular atrophy of late onset, *Neurology* 18:306, 1966.

283. Guidetti D et al: Kennedy disease in an Italian kindred, *Eur Neurol* 25:188, 1986 (abstract).

284. Hausmanowa-Petrusewicz I, Barkowsky J, Janczewski Z: X-linked adult form of spinal muscular atrophy, *J Neurol* 229:175, 1983.

285. Arbizu T et al: A family with adult spinal and bulbar muscular atrophy X-linked inheritance and associated testicular failure, *J Neurol Sci* 59:371, 1983.

286. McFadyen IJ et al: Gonadal-pituitary hormone levels in gynecomastia, *Clin Endocrinol* 13:77, 1980.

287. Edman CD et al: Embryonic testicular regression: a clinical spectrum of XY agonadal individuals, *Obstet Gynecol* 49:209, 1977.

288. Hall JG, Morgan A, Blizzard RM: Familial congenital anorchia, *Birth Defects* 11:115, 1975.

289. Heller CG, Nelson WO, Roth AC: Functional prepubertal castration in males, *J Clin Endocrinol* 3:573, 1943.

290. Kirschner MA, Jacobs JB, Fraley EE: Bilateral anorchia with persistent testosterone production, *N Engl J Med* 289:240, 1970.

291. Kirschner MA, Wider JA, Rose GT: Leydig cell function in men with gonadotrophin producing testicular hormones, *J Clin Endocrin Metab* 30:504, 1970.

292. Levitt SB et al: Endocrine tests in phenotypic children with bilateral impalpable testes can reliably predict "congenital" anarchism, *Urology* 11:11, 1978.

293. Bongiovanni AM: Congenital adrenal hyperplasia and related conditions. In Stanbury JB, Wyngaarden JB, Fredrickson DS (eds): *The metabolic basis of inherited disease,* New York, 1978, McGraw-Hill.

294. Griffin JE, Wilson JD: Hereditary male pseudohermaphroditism, *Clin Obstet Gynecol* 5:457, 1958.

295. Wilson JD, Goldstein JL: Classification of hereditary disorders of sexual development, *Birth Defects (Original Article Series)* 11:1, 1975.

296. Hochberg Z, Even L, Zadik Z: Mineralcorticoids in the mechanism of gynecomastia in adrenal hyperplasia caused by 11β-hydroxylase deficiency, *J Pediatr* 118:258, 1991.

297. Stacpoole PW et al: Isolated ACTH deficiency: a heterogenous disorder, *Medicine* 61:13, 1982.

298. Uehara Y et al: A case of isolated ACTH deficiency associated with gynecomastia, *J Jpn Soc Intern Med* 67:328, 1978 (abstract).

299. Yoshida T et al: Isolated ACTH deficiency accompanied by "primary hypothyroidism" and hyperprolactinemia, *Acta Endocrinol* 104:397, 1983.

300. Shimatsu A, Suzuki Y, Tanaka S: Gynecomastia associated with isolated ACTH deficiency, *J Endocrinol Invest* 10:127, 1987.

301. Riggs S, Sanford JP: Viral orchitis, *N Engl J Med* 266:990, 1962.

302. Werner CA: Mumps orchitis and testicular atrophy, *Ann Intern Med* 32:1066, 1950.

303. Bjorvatn B: Mumps virus recovered from testes by fine-needle aspiration biopsy in cases of mumps orchitis, *Scand J Infect Dis* 5:3, 1973.

304. Pennisi AJ, Grushkin CM, Lieberman E: Gonadal function in children with nephrosis treated with cyclophosphamide, *Am J Dis Child* 129:315, 1975.

305. Penso J et al: Testicular function in prepubertal and pubertal male patients treated with cyclophosphamide for nephrotic syndrome, *J Pediatr* 84:831, 1974.

306. DeGroot GW, Faiman C, Winter JSD: Cyclophosphamide and the prepubertal gonad: a negative report, *J Pediatr* 84:123, 1974.

307. Kirkland RT et al: Gonadotropin responses to luteinizing releasing factor in boys treated with cyclophosphamide for nephrotic syndrome, *J Pediatr* 89:941, 1976.

308. Parra A et al: Plasma gonadotropins and gonadal steroids in children treated with cyclophosphamide, *J Pediatr* 92:117, 1978.

309. Shalet SM et al: Ovarian failure following abdominal irradiation in childhood, *Br J Cancer* 33:655, 1976.

310. Clarke BG, Shapiro S, Monroe RG: Myotonia atrophica with testicular atrophy, *J Clin Endocrinol* 16:1235, 1956.

311. Cooper IS et al: The relation of spinal cord disease to gynecomastia and testicular atrophy, *Proc Staff Meet Mayo Clin* 25:320, 1950.

312. Woodham CWB: Hyperplasia of the male breast, *Lancet* 2:307, 1938.

313. Dass J et al: Androgenic status of lepromatous leprosy patients with gynecomastia, *Int J Lepr* 44:469, 1976.

314. Morley JE et al: Hormonal changes associated with testicular atrophy and gynaecomastia in patients with leprosy, *Clin Endocrinol* 6:299, 1977.

315. Freeman RM, Lawton RL, Fearing MO: Gynecomastia: an endocrinologic complication of hemodialysis, *Ann Intern Med* 69:67, 1968.

316. Gupta D, Burdschu HD: Testosterone and its binding in the plasma of male subjects with chronic renal failure, *Clin Chim Acta* 36:479, 1972.

317. Holdsworth MB, Atkins RC, de Kretzer DM: The pituitary testicular axis in men with chronic renal failure, *N Engl J Med* 296:1245, 1977.

318. Nagel TC et al: Gynecomastia, prolactin, and other peptide hormones in patients undergoing chronic hemodialysis, *J Clin Endocrinol Metab* 36:428, 1973.

319. Sawin CT et al: Blood levels of gonadotropins and gonadal hormones in gynecomastia associated with chronic hemodialysis, *J Clin Endocrinol Metab* 36:988, 1973.

320. Schmitt GW, Shehadeh I, Sawin CT: Transient gynecomastia in chronic renal failure during chronic intermittent hemodialysis, *Ann Intern Med* 69:73, 1968.

321. Hendrickson DA, Robertson WR: Diethylstilbestrol therapy: gynecomastia, *JAMA* 213:468, 1970.

322. Miller JI, Ahmann FR: Treatment of castration-induced menopausal symptoms with low dose diethylstilbestrol in men with advanced prostate cancer, *Urology* 40:499, 1992.

323. Brandt NJ, Cohn J, Hilder M: Controlled trial of oral contraceptives in haemophilia, *Scand J Haematol* 11:225, 1973.

324. Orentreich N, Dur NP: Mammogenesis in transsexuals, *J Invest Dermatol* 63:142, 1974.

325. Symmers WS: Carcinoma of breast in transsexual individuals after surgical and hormonal interference with the primary and secondary sex characteristics, *BMJ* 2:82, 1968.

326. Holleb AI, Freeman HP, Farrow JH: Cancer of the male breast, *NY State J Med* 68:544, 656, 1968.

327. Wilson SE, Hutchinson WB: Breast masses in males with carcinoma of the prostate, *J Surg Oncol* 8:105, 1976.

328. Halperin DS, Sizonenko PC: Prepubertal gynecomastia following topical inunction of estrogen containing ointment, *Helv Paediatr Acta* 38:361, 1983.

329. Gabrilove JL, Luria M: Persistent gynecomastia resulting from scalp inunction of estradiol: a model for persistent gynecomastia, *Arch Dermatol* 114:1672, 1978.

330. Beas F et al: Pseudoprecocious puberty in infants caused by a dermal ointment containing estrogens, *J Pediatr* 75:127, 1969.

331. Landolt R, Murset G: Premature signs of puberty as late sequelae of unintentional estrogen administration, *Schweiz Med Wochenschr* 98:638, 1968.

332. LeWinn EB: Gynecomastia during digitalis therapy: report of eight cases with liver function studies, *N Engl J Med* 248:316, 1953.

333. Navab A, Koss LG, LaDue JS: Estrogen-like activity of digitalis: its effect on the squamous epithelium of the female genital tract, *JAMA* 194:30, 1965.

334. Wolfe CJ: Gynecomastia following digitalis administration, *J Fla Med Assoc* 62:54, 1975.

335. Stouffer SS et al: Digoxin and abnormal serum hormone levels, *JAMA* 225:1643, 1973.

336. Novak A, Kass LF, LaDue JS: Estrogen-like activity of digitalis, *JAMA* 194:142, 1965.

337. Sorbie PJ, Perez-Marrero R: The use of clomiphene citrate in male infertility, *J Urol* 131:425, 1984.

338. Check JH et al: Case report: cystic gynecomastia in a male treated with clomiphene citrate, *Fertil Steril* 30:713, 1978.

339. Lee PA: The occurrence of gynecomastia upon withdrawal of clomiphene citrate treatment for idiopathic oligospermia, *Fertil Steril* 34:285, 1980.

340. Spano F, Ryan WG: Tamoxifen for gynecomastia induced by anabolic steroids? *N Engl J Med* 311:861, 1984.

341. Brown JS, Rubenfeld S: Irradiation in preventing gynecomastia induced by estrogens, *Urology* 3:51, 1974.

342. Foss D et al: Radiotherapeutic prophylaxis of estrogen-induced gynecomastia: a study of late sequelae, *Int J Radiat Oncol Biol Phys* 12:407, 1985.

343. Cicero TJ et al: Function of the male sex organs in heroin and methadone users, *N Engl J Med* 292:822, 1975.

344. Harmon J, Aliapoulios MA: Gynecomastia in marijuana users, *N Engl J Med* 287:936, 1972.

345. Harmon J, Aliapoulios MA: Marijuana induced gynecomastia: clinical and laboratory experience, *Surg Forum* 25:423, 1974.

346. Mendelsohn JH et al: Plasma testosterone levels before, during and after chronic marijuana smoking, *N Engl J Med* 291:1051, 1974.

347. Olusi SO: Hyperprolactinaemia in patients with suspected cannabis-induced gynaecomastia, *Lancet* 1:255, 1980 (letter).

348. Cates W Jr, Pope JN: Gynecomastia and cannabis smoking, *Am J Surg* 134:613, 1977.

349. Marcus R, Korenman SG: Estrogens and the human male, *Annu Rev Med* 27:357, 1976.

350. Bellati G, Ideo G: Gynaecomastia after spironolactone and potassium canrenoate, *Lancet* 1:626, 1986.

351. Dupont A: Disappearance of spironolactone-induced gynecomastia during treatment with potassium canrenoate, *Lancet* 2:731, 1985.

352. Fromantin M: Surveillance clinique et hormonale des traitements prolongeás de l'hypertension arteriele par les anti aldosterones, *Mises Jour Cardiol* 11:95, 1980.

353. Marco J et al: Effets sexuels secondaire de la spironolactone: inteárèt d'une thërapeutique substitutive par la canrenone, *Nouv Presse Med* 7:3668, 1978.

354. Greenblatt DJ, Koch-Weser J: Adverse reactions to spironolactone, *JAMA* 225:40, 1973.

355. Huffman DH et al: Gynecomastia induced in normal males by spironolactone, *Clin Pharmacol Ther* 24:465, 1978.

356. Caminos-Torres R, Lisa MA, Snyder PJ: Gynecomastia and semen abnormalities induced by spironolactone in normal men, *J Clin Endocrinol Metab* 45:255, 1977.

357. Moerck HJ, Magelund G: Gynecomastia and diazepam abuse, *Lancet* 1:1344, 1979.

358. Bergman D et al: Increased oestradiol in diazepam related gynaecomastia, *Lancet* 2:1225, 1981.

359. Lyle WH: Penicillamine, *Clin Rheum Dis* 5:569, 1979.

360. Reid DM, Martynoga AG, Nuki G: Reversible gynaecomastia associated with D-penicillamine in a man with rheumatoid arthritis, *BMJ* 285:1083, 1982.

361. Desai SN: Sudden gigantism of breasts: drug induced? *Br J Plast Surg* 26:371, 1973.

362. Passas C, Weinstein A: Breast gigantism with penicillamine therapy, *Arthritis Rheum* 21:167, 1978.

363. Taylor PJ, Cumming DC, Corenblum B: Successful treatment of D-penicillamine-induced breast gigantism with danazol, *BMJ* 282:362, 1981.

364. Thew DCN, Stewart IM: D-Penicillamine and breast enlargement, *Ann Rheum Dis* 39:200, 1980.

365. Funder JW, Mercer JE: Cimetidine, a histamine H$_2$ receptor antagonist, occupies androgen receptors, *J Clin Endocrinol Metab* 48:189, 1979.

366. Pearce P, Funder JW: Histamine H$_2$ receptor antagonist: radioreceptor assay for antiandrogenic side effects, *Clin Exp Pharmacol Physiol* 7:442, 1980.

367. *The H$_2$-receptor antagonist anthology: worldwide Tagamet experience,* Philadelphia, 1982, Smith, Kline and French International.

368. Winters SJ, Banks JL, Loriaux DL: Cimetidine is an anti-androgen in the rat, *Gastroenterology* 76:504, 1979.

369. Cimetidine Postmarket Surveillance Program, Philadelphia, 1981, Medical Affairs Department, Smith, Kline and French Laboratories.

370. Spence RW, Celestin LR: Gynaecomastia associated with cimetidine, *Gut* 20:154, 1979.

371. Hall WH: Breast changes in males on cimetidine, *N Engl J Med* 295:841, 1976.

372. Mignon M et al: Ranitidine and cimetidine in Zollinger-Ellison syndrome, *Br J Clin Pharmacol* 10:173, 1980.

373. Wolfe MM: Impotence on cimetidine treatment, *N Engl J Med* 300:94, 1979.

374. Jensen RT et al: Cimetidine-induced impotence and breast changes in patients with gastric hypersecretory states, *N Engl J Med* 308:883, 1983.

375. Lardinois CK, Mazzaferri EL: Cimetidine blocks testosterone synthesis, *Arch Intern Med* 145:920, 1985.

376. Tosi S, Cagnoli M: Painful gynaecomastia with ranitidine, *Lancet* 2:160, 1982 (letter).

377. Mignon M, Vallot T, Bonfils S: Gynaecomastia and histamine-2 antagonists, *Lancet* 2:499, 1982.

378. Brittain RT, Daly MJ: A review of the animal pharmacology of ranitidine: a new selective histamine H$_2$ antagonist, *Scand J Gastroenterol* 16(suppl 69):1, 1981.

379. Edwards CRW et al: In vitro studies on the effects of ranitidine on isolated anterior pituitary and adrenal cells, *Scand J Gastroenterol* 16(suppl 69):75, 1981.

380. Rodriguez LAG, Jick H: Risk of gynaecomastia associated with cimetidine, omeprazole, and other antiulcer drugs, *BMJ* 308:503, 1994.

381. Carvajal A, Arias LHM: Gynecomastia and sexual disorders after the administration of omeprazole, *Am J Gastroenterol* 90:1028, 1995 (letter).

382. Lindquist M, Edwards IR: Endocrine adverse effects of omeprazole, *BMJ* 305:451, 1992.

383. Geller J et al: The effect of cyproterone acetate on advanced carcinoma of the prostate, *Surg Gynecol Obstet* 127:748, 1968.

384. Caine M, Perlberg S, Gordon R: The treatment of benign prostatic hypertrophy with flutamide (SCH 13521): a placebo controlled study, *J Urol* 114:564, 1975.

385. Gormley GJ et al: The effect of finasteride in men with benign prostatic hyperplasia, *N Engl J Med* 327:1185, 1992.

386. Jacobs U, Klein B, Klehr HU: Cumulative side effects of cyclosporine and Ca antagonists: hypergalactinemia, mastadenoma, and gynecomastia, *Transplantation Proc* 26:3122, 1994.

387. Geller J et al: Medical castration with megestrol acetate and minidose of diethylstilbestrol, *Urology* 17:27, 1981.

388. Novak E et al: Sebum production and plasma testosterone levels in man after high-dose medroxyprogesterone acetate treatment and androgen administration, *Acta Endocrinol* 95:265, 1980.

389. Novak E, Hendrix JW, Seckman CE: Effects of medroxy-progesterone acetate on some endocrine functions of healthy male volunteers, *Curr Ther Res* 21:320, 1977.

390. Meyer WJ III et al: Pituitary function in adult males receiving medroxyprogesterone acetate, *Fertil Steril* 28:1072, 1977.

391. Nashan D et al: The antimycotic drug terbinafine in contrast to ketoconazole lacks acute effects on the pituitary-testicular function of healthy men: a placebo-controlled double-blind trial, *Acta Endocrinol* 120:677, 1989.

392. Pont A et al: Ketoconazole-induced increase in estradiol-testosterone ratio, *Arch Intern Med* 145:1429, 1985.

393. Pont A et al: High-dose ketoconazole therapy and adrenal and testicular function in humans, *Arch Intern Med* 144:2150, 1984.

394. Moncada B, Baranda L: Ketoconazole and gynecomastia, *J Am Acad Dermatol* 7:557, 1982.

395. Graybill JR, Drutz DJ: Ketoconazole: a major innovation for treatment of fungal disease, *Ann Intern Med* 93:921, 1980.

396. Barragry JM et al: Effects of anticonvulsants on plasma testosterone and sex hormone binding globulin levels, *J Neurol Neurosurg Psychiatr* 41:913, 1978.

397. Dana-Haeri J, Oxley J, Richens A: Reduction of free testosterone by ant epileptic drugs, *BMJ* 284:85, 1982.

398. Rodin E, Subramanian MG, Gilroy J: Investigation of sex hormones in male epileptic patients, *Epilepsia* 25:690, 1984.

399. Toone BK et al: Sex hormones, sexual drive and plasma anticonvulsant levels in male epileptics. In Parsonage M et al (eds): *Advances in epileptology: IVth Epilepsy International Symposium,* New York, 1983, Raven Press.

400. Asbjornsen G et al: Testicular function after combination chemotherapy for Hodgkin's disease, *Scand J Haematol* 16:66, 1976.

401. Chapman RM, Sutcliffe SB, Malpas JS: Cytotoxic-induced ovarian failure in women with Hodgkin's disease, *JAMA* 242:1877, 1979.

402. Chapman RM et al: Cyclical combination chemotherapy and gonadal function, *Lancet* 1:285, 1979.

403. Fossa SD, Klepp O, Aakvaag A: Serum, hormone levels in patients with malignant testicular germ cell tumours without clinical and/or radiological sign of tumour, *Br J Urol* 52:151, 1980.

404. Wang C et al: Effect of combination of chemotherapy on pituitary-gonadal function in patients with lymphoma and leukemia, *Cancer* 45:2030, 1980.

405. Sherins RJ, Olweny CLM, Ziegler JL: Gynaecomastia and gonadal dysfunction in adolescent boys treated with combination chemotherapy for Hodgkin's disease, *N Engl J Med* 299:12, 1978.

406. Schilsky RL et al: Gonadal dysfunction in patients receiving chemotherapy for cancer, *Ann Intern Med* 93:109, 1980.

407. Trump DL, Anderson SA: Painful gynecomastia following cytotoxic therapy for testis cancer: a potentially favorable prognostic sign? *J Clin Oncol* I:416, 1983.

408. Trump DL, Pavy MD, Staal S: Gynecomastia in men following antineoplastic therapy, *Arch Intern Med* 142:511, 1982.

409. Saeter G, Fossa SD, Norman N: Gynecomastia following cytotoxic therapy for testicular cancer, *Br J Urol* 59:348, 1987.

410. Schorer AE, Oken MM, Johnson GJ: Gynecomastia with nitrosourea therapy, *Cancer Treat Rep* 62:574, 1978.

411. Galton DAG, Till M, Wiltshaw W: Busulfan: summary of clinical results, *Ann NY Acad Sci* 68:967, 1957.

412. Smith RH, Barrett O Jr: Gynecomastia associated with vincristine therapy, *Calif Med* 107:347, 1967.

413. Smith SR: Acquired gonadotropin-responsive hyperestrogenism in a male without evidence of neoplasia, *J Clin Endocrinol Metab* 32:77, 1971.

414. Del Paine DW et al: Gynecomastia associated with low dose methotrexate therapy, *Arthritis Rheum* 26:691, 1983.

415. Thomas E, Leroux JL, Blotman F: Gynecomastia in patients with rheumatoid arthritis treated with methotrexate, *J Rheumatol* 21:1777, 1994 (letter).

416. Bichel J: Gynecomastia in Hodgkin's disease, *Dan Med Bull* 4:157, 1957.

417. Glass AR, Berenberg J: Gynecomastia after chemotherapy for lymphoma, *Arch Intern Med* 139:1048, 1979.

418. Guersy P, Lenoir G, Broyer M: Gonadal effects of chlorambucil given to prepubertal and pubertal boys for nephrotic syndrome, *J Pediatr* 92:299, 1978.

419. Van Thiel DH et al: Evidence for a specific seminiferous tubular factor affecting follicle-stimulating hormone secretion in man, *J Clin Invest* 51:1009, 1972.

420. Jacobson RF et al: Leydig cell dysfunction in male patients with Hodgkin's disease receiving chemotherapy, *Clin Res* 26:437A, 1978 (abstract).

421. Large DM et al: Gynaecomastia complicating the treatment of myeloma, *Br J Cancer* 48:69, 1983.

422. Morse WI et al: Urine estrogen responses to human chorionic gonadotropin in young, old and hypogonadal men, *J Clin Endocrinol* 22:678, 1982.

423. Lipsett MB et al: Studies in Leydig cell physiology and pathology: secretion and metabolism of testosterone, *Recent Prog Horm Res* 22:245, 1966.

424. Baird DT et al: Steroid dynamics under steady-state conditions, *Recent Progr Horm Res* 25:628, 1969.

425. Lipsett MB: The testis. In Bondy PK (ed): *Diseases of metabolism,* ed 6, Philadelphia, 1969, WB Saunders.

426. Lipsett MB et al: Metabolism of testosterone and related steroids in metastatic interstitial cell carcinoma of the testis, *J Clin Invest* 45:1700, 1966.

427. Maddock WO, Nelson WO: The effects of chorionic gonadotropin in adult men, *J Clin Endocrinol* 12:985, 1952.

428. Weinstein RL et al: Secretion of unconjugated androgens and estrogens by the normal and abnormal testis before and after human chorionic gonadotropin, *J Clin Invest* 53:1, 1974.

429. Ahmad SR et al: Treatment of advanced prostatic cancer with LHRH analogue 118630: clinical response and hormonal mechanisms, *Lancet* 2:415, 1983.

430. Denis LJ et al: Goserelin acetate and flutamide versus bilateral orchiectomy: a phase III EORTC trial (30853), *Urology* 42:119, 1993.

431. Clayton RN, Catt KJ: Gonadotropin-releasing hormone receptors: characterization, physiological regulation, and relationship to reproductive function, *Endocr Rev* 2:186, 1981.

432. Sandow J: Clinical application of LHRH and its analogues, *Clin Endocrinol* 18:571, 1983.

433. Borgmann V et al: Sustained suppression of testosterone production by the luteinizing hormone-releasing hormone agonist buserelin in patients with advanced prostatic cancer, *Lancet* 1:1097, 1982.

434. Walker KJ et al: Therapeutic potential of the LHRH agonist, ICI 118630 in the treatment of advanced prostatic carcinoma, *Lancet* 2:413, 1983.

435. Eisenberger MA, O'Dwyer PJ, Friedman MA: Gonadotropin hormone-releasing analogues: a new therapeutic approach for prostatic carcinoma, *J Clin Oncol* 4:3:414, 1986.

436. Kapoor A: Reversible gynecomastia associated with sulindac therapy, *JAMA* 250:2884, 1983.

437. Van der Steen M, Du Caju MVL, Van Acker KJ: Gynaecomastia in a male infant given domperidone, *Lancet* 2:884, 1982.

438. Tanner LA, Bosco LA: Gynecomastia associated with calcium channel blocker therapy, *Arch Intern Med* 148:379, 1988.

439. Malozowski S, Stadel BV: Prepubertal gynecomastia during growth hormone therapy, *J Pediatr* 126:659, 1995.

440. Cohn L et al: Carpal tunnel syndrome and gynaecomastia during growth hormone treatment of elderly men with low circulating IGF-1 concentrations, *Clin Endocrinol* 39:417, 1993.

441. Dixon DW, Barwolf-Gohlke C, Gunnar RM: Comparative efficacy and safety of bumetanide and furosemide in long-term treatment of edema due to congestive heart failure, *J Clin Pharmacol* 21:680, 1981.

442. Stone WJ, Bennett WM, Cutler RE: Long-term bumetanide treatment of patients with edema due to renal disease. Cooperative Studies, *J Clin Pharmacol* 21:587, 1981.

443. Dardick KR: Gynecomastia associated with theophylline, *J Fam Pract* 18:141, 1984.

444. Antonelli D, Luboshitzky R: Amiodarone-induced gynecomastia, *N Engl J Med* 315:1553, 1986.

445. Vankrunkelsven PJ, Thijs MM: Salcatonin and gynaecomastia, *Lancet* 344:482, 1994.

446. Braude S et al: Hypertrophic osteoarthropathy in cystic fibrosis, *BMJ* 288:822, 1984.

447. Russi EW: Gynaecomastia in cystic fibrosis, *BMJ* 288:1660, 1984.

448. Lemen RJ et al: Relationship among digital clubbing, disease severity, and serum prostaglandins $F_{2\alpha}$ and E concentrations in cystic fibrosis patients, *Am Rev Respir Dis* 117:639, 1978.

449. Ciccarelli E et al: Long-term therapy of patients with macroprolactinoma using repeatable injectable bromocriptine, *J Clin Endocrinol Metab* 76:484, 1993.

450. Tyson D et al: Prolactin-secreting macroadenomas in adolescents: response to bromocriptine therapy, *Am J Dis Child* 147:1057, 1993.

451. Gooren LJG, Daantje CRE: Psychological stress as a cause of intermittent gynecomastia, *Horm Metabol Res* 18:424, 1986.

452. Frantz AG, Wilson JD: Endocrine disorders of the breast. In Wilson JB, Foster DW (eds): *Williams' textbook of endocrinology,* ed 7, Philadelphia, 1985, WB Saunders.

453. Couderc LJ, Clauvel JP: HIV-infection induced gynecomastia, *Ann Intern Med* 107:257, 1987.

454. Qazi N et al: Diagnosis and management of male breast enlargement in patients with HIV/AIDS, *AIDS Read* 10:703, 2000.

455. Ismail AA, Barth JH: Endocrinology of gynaecomastia, *Ann Clin Biochem* 38:596, 2001.

456. Dershaw DD: Male mammography, *AJR Am J Roentgenol* 146:127, 1986.

457. Dershaw DD et al: Mammographic findings in men with breast cancer, *AJR Am J Roentgenol* 160:267, 1993.

458. Evans GF et al: The diagnostic accuracy of mammography in the evaluation of male breast disease, *Am J Surg* 181:96, 2001.

459. Hopwood NJ: Pathogenesis and management of abnormal puberty, *Spec Top Endocrinol Metab* 7:175, 1985.

460. LeRoith D, Sobel R, Glick SM: The effect of clomiphene citrate on pubertal gynecomastia, *Acta Endocrinol* 95:177, 1980.

461. Plourde PV, Kulin HE, Santner SJ: Clomiphene in the treatment of adolescent gynecomastia, *Am J Dis Child* 137:1080, 1983.

462. Stephanas AV et al: Clomiphene in the treatment of pubertal-adolescent gynecomastia: a preliminary report, *J Pediatr* 90:651, 1977.

463. Ricciardi I, Ianniruberto A: Tamoxifen-induced regression of benign breast lesions, *Obstet Gynecol* 54:80, 1979.

464. Alagaratnam TT: Idiopathic gynecomastia treated with tamoxifen: a preliminary report, *Clin Ther* 9:483, 1987.

465. McDermott MT, Hofeldt FD, Kidd GS: Tamoxifen therapy for painful idiopathic gynecomastia, *South Med J* 83:1283, 1990.

466. Parker LN et al: Treatment of gynecomastia with tamoxifen: a double-blind crossover study, *Metabolism* 35:705, 1986.

467. Eberle AJ, Sparrow JT, Keenan BS: Treatment of persistent pubertal gynecomastia with dihydrotestosterone heptanoate, *J Pediatr* 109:144, 1986.

468. Keenan BS et al: Androgen-stimulated pubertal growth: the effects of testosterone and dihydrotestosterone on growth hormone and insulin-like growth factor I in the treatment of short stature and delayed puberty, *J Clin Endocrinol Metab* 76:996, 1993.

469. Kuhn JM et al: Studies on the treatment of idiopathic gynecomastia with percutaneous dihydrotestosterone, *Clin Endocrinol* 19:513, 1983.

470. Greenblatt RB et al: Clinical studies with an antigonadotrophin—danazol, *Fertil Steril* 22:102, 1971.

471. Sherins RJ et al: Pituitary and testicular function studies. 1. Experience with a new gonadal inhibitor, 17α-pregn-4-en-20-yno (2,3-d) isoxazol-17-01 (danazol), *J Clin Endocrinol Metab* 32:521, 1971.

472. Buckle R: Studies on the treatment of gynaecomastia with danazol (Danol), *J Intern Med Res* 5(suppl 3):114, 1977.

473. Buckle R: Danazol in the treatment of gynaecomastia, *Drugs* 19:356, 1980.

474. Zachmann M et al: Treatment of pubertal gynaecomastia with testolactone, *Acta Endocrinol Suppl* 279:218, 1986.

475. Waterfall NB, Glaser MG: A study of the effects of radiation on prevention of gynaecomastia due to oestrogen therapy, *Clin Oncol* 5:257, 1979.

476. Fass D et al: Radiotherapeutic prophylaxis of estrogen-induced gynecomastia: a study of late sequela, *Int J Radiat Oncol Biol Phys* 12:407, 1986.

477. Webster JP: Mastectomy for gynecomastia through a semicircular intra-areolar incision, *Ann Surg* 124:557, 1946.

478. Ward CM, Khalid K: Surgical treatment of grade III gynaecomastia, *Ann R Coll Surg Engl* 71:226, 1989.

479. Courtiss EH: Reduction mammoplasty by suction alone, *Plast Reconstr Surg* 92:1276, 1993.

480. Samdal F et al: Surgical treatment of gynaecomastia: five years' experience with liposuction, *Scand J Plast Reconstr Hand Surg* 28:123, 1994.

481. Rosenberg GJ: A new cannula for suction removal of parenchymal tissue of gynecomastia, *Plast Reconstr Surg* 94:548, 1994.

482. Rosenberg GJ: Gynecomastia: suction lipectomy as a contemporary solution, *Plast Reconstr Surg* 80:379, 1987.

IV

PATHOLOGY OF BENIGN AND PREMALIGNANT LESIONS OF THE BREAST

CHAPTER

7

Benign, High-Risk, and Premalignant Lesions of the Breast

DAVID L. PAGE

JEAN F. SIMPSON

Chapter Outline

This chapter presents a classification of the incredible variety of noncancerous lesions presenting in the human female breast, largely as they are identified histopathologically with clinical biopsies. This chapter is stratified into categories that have relevance for the prediction of breast cancer risk in broad terms.[1,2]

The magnitude of risk in these various strata are based on the following assumption: Any changes not reliably indicating an increased risk of subsequent breast cancer greater than 50% above that of similar women controlled for age and length of time at follow-up will be accorded *no elevation of risk*. The great majority of lesions are not associated with seeming cellular increase and are designated as *nonproliferative*. These alterations occasion biopsy or present clinical symptoms without an association of increased risk. The other categories with an association or predictability of subsequent breast cancer risk are defined as *proliferative lesions*.

Benign Lesions without Cancer Risk Implications

Benign breast conditions have a diverse array of clinical presentations; the subjective discomfort of mammary pain and clinical signs of lumpiness have little correlation with histologic alterations. Thus the establishment of clear-cut clinicopathologic entities is impossible. *Lumpiness* on physical examination is common to many benign and malignant situations. *Pain* is notorious for its seemingly spontaneous appearance and departure, making careful study of dietary and therapeutic interventions precarious.[3] Rigorous quantitative study in this area is in its infancy.[4,5] A flurry of terms has been used, none of which has a precise meaning.[6] These terms were largely "lumping" or catch-all phrases, most with an emphasis on one or another sign, symptom, or anatomic finding. These terms may be clarified, but not adequately defined, in terms of disease entities or may be completely absolved of controversy. The continued use of such broad terms of convenience as *fibrocystic disease* or *fibrocystic change* (FCD or FCC) and *benign breast disease* (BBD) is not only because they are deeply embedded in clinical parlance. Despite their imprecision, these terms have utility precisely because of their imprecision, familiarity, and wide reference. In surgical pathology or histopathology, these terms had no precise reference and provided no clear understanding of pathogenesis; they essentially denoted that a biopsy had been clinically indicated because microscopic alterations were present. The following discussion highlights anatomic pathology while acknowledging that histopathology is an empty exercise without clinical correlates and predictability. Thus we are highlighting those changes that have clinical implications.

The term *BBD* may be appropriate in some settings, because it refers to a solitary, although intrinsically imprecise, term, avowedly including all elements except carcinoma. However, the use of the analogous term *FCD* has caused problems despite its intent of giving ready clinicopathologic correlation between lumpiness and histologic alterations.[7] The difficulty probably arises from the use of the term *disease* without *benign*, which has reinforced the widely held belief that cancer risk was elevated in this setting.[8] With the introduction of *FCD* in the 1940s, an association with cancer was implied by concurrent associations.[9] It was the intent of many in the recent past to remove the cancer implications of FCD by changing the term to *fibrocystic change* (FCC).[10-12] The need to further define this risk indication has been only partially met through histologic evaluations of breast biopsies (see later discussion and Chapter 23).[13] The link between BBD and FCD is made clear with the understanding that most benign biopsies have been termed *FCD*, and studies of cancer risk have held that the performance of a biopsy constituted BBD with its attendant increased risk of cancer. These broad groupings or associations are referable to the era preceding mammography. It is evident that the introduction of mammography has aided the acceptance of a rigorous reductionist approach in which terms are technique bound (e.g., physical examination, mammogram) and must be individually compared. Thus a large cyst may produce a lump, but is it termed *fibrosis* when cysts are absent or when there is regional variation in fat interposed between breast parenchyma, which might be responsible for a palpable abnormality. These questions often are not resolvable. The net cast by the term *BBD* may be too broad, and the term *FCD* inappropriately implicates the presence of disease. All of these terms are in wide and appropriate use, and we prefer FCC.

The aforementioned view that considers FCCs as an imprecise term of convenience is not held uniformly. Many would consider that placing some confines of definition on this condition supports its acceptance as an entity. Bartow and colleagues[14] have studied different ethnic groups and have evidence that supports the idea of FCCs or FCD as an entity, because these alterations are uncommon in low-risk cancer groups. All of these fibrous and cystic changes increase rapidly in incidence in the 10 or 15 years before menopause.[15,16] Although it may be difficult to draw sharp borders of definition for these changes, it is certain that they occur in more than 50% of the immediately premenopausal population of high-risk North Americans. The presence of cysts without hyperplasia and other changes noted as proliferative breast disease does not identify a higher-risk group of women when compared with others within the same ethnic or geographically defined risk group.[10]

Hyperplastic changes may be more common in breasts that are clinically lumpy, but no formal recent analysis of co-occurrence of these conditions is available. Similarly, reliable mammographic correlates of epithelial hyperplasia are not at hand. Mammograms with increased density have imperfect associations with histologic findings because fibrosis is as common as hyperplasia, although hyperplastic lesions are somewhat more common in dense breasts.[17]

HISTOPATHOLOGY OF BENIGN BREAST DISEASE

Foremost of all the benign histologic changes in the breast are *cysts* and the pink cell *apocrine change* that so commonly accompanies them. Cysts range in size from approximately 1 mm to many centimeters. It is remarkable that cysts are usually unilocular within the breast. The reason for this configuration is thought to be that they arise as lobular lesions in which the individual acini or terminal ductules dilate, untwist, and unfold to enlarge as a cyst (Figure 7-1).[18] Whether other lobular units and duct structures are recruited during enlargement is unknown. The small cysts are often inapparent on gross tissue examination. Whether associated fibrosis may make smaller cysts palpable is unclear but possible. Haagensen noted that clusters of cysts, each 2 to 3 mm in diameter, were palpable and termed them, along with larger examples, *gross cysts*.[19,20] In any case, these correlates of palpability have become less important, particularly when many accept the fact that a biopsy may be appropriate based on clinical or mammographic findings, even if histology demonstrates no determinate abnormality. Understandably, fibrosis is often reported by pathologists in an attempt to explain clinical palpability or mammographic density. The gross appearance of large cysts is often blue, a reflection of the slightly cloudy, brown fluid usually found within. These are accorded the eponymous designation *blue-domed cysts of Bloodgood*, after Joseph Bloodgood, who studied them and their possible cancer association in the first part of the twentieth century.[21]

Many cysts are lined by cells that have characteristic cytologic features of apocrine glands. The cells have many mitochondria *lysosomal* and *secretory* granules that appear pink with eosin staining. The nuclei are also characteristic but less defining in that they are regularly round and often have a prominent round and eosinophilic nucleolus as well. This epithelium is often columnar, with a single protuberance of apical aspect of the cytoplasm appearing as a bleb or snout. Such changes may be prominent in enlarged lobular units and may have minor associations with concurrent atypical lesions.[22,23] Often, the apocrine cells are grouped in tufted or papillary clusters and sometimes produce prominent papillary prolongations from the basement membrane region, which may or may not contain fibrovascular stalks (Figures 7-2 and 7-3). This papillary apocrine change may demonstrate highly complex patterns but is not associated with a significant increased risk of later cancer development unless there is concurrent atypical hyperplasia (see later discussion).[24] Breast cysts, particularly larger ones, may show no evidence of epithelial lining or may have a simple squamous lining with an extremely flattened and undifferentiated epithelialized surface. Several studies have differentiated these two types of cysts, apocrine and simple, indicating that apocrine cysts have a high potassium content and different steroid hormones.[25] A suggestion of a difference in cancer risk between the two kinds of cysts is unproved.[26,27] Apocrine cysts are probably more commonly associated with multiplicity and recurrence than are nonapocrine cysts.[18,28,29] Whether this alteration of mammary epithelium to resemble that of apocrine sweat glands is a true metaplasia seems a point of practical irrelevance. However, many scholars believe that

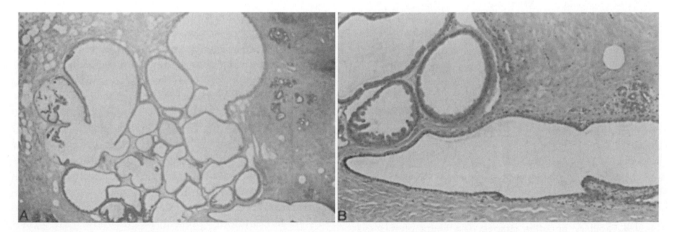

FIG. **7-1** **A,** Apocrine cysts. Acini of this lobular unit have dilated and become distorted. Note entering lobular terminal duct at lower right. Low magnification. (×40.) **B,** Higher power of **A** showing apocrine-like epithelium lining dilated terminal duct and cysts. (×80.)

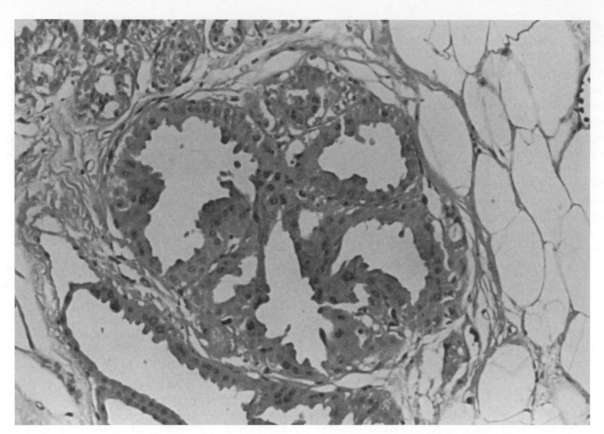

FIG. **7-2** These dilated spaces of a lobular unit show prominent coalescent arches. Note prominent apical blebs, or "snouts." (×225.)

enzymatic profiles and ultrastructural evidence support a true metaplasia.[30] Even so, the frequency of a slight to marked protuberance of cell groups (papillary apocrine change) rather than a smooth, single cell layer is different in the breast compared with the apocrine sweat glands. A protein marker, GCDFP-15, is characteristically present within the cytoplasm and may be a useful marker.[31] Not only is the characteristic apocrine

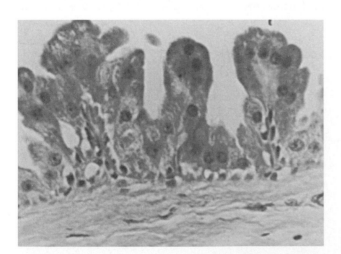

FIG. **7-3** Papillary apocrine change. The lining of this cyst shows complex papillary tufts. Note prominent centrally placed nucleoli. (×320.)

alteration decorated with this marker, but it is also found in other settings with eosinophilic cytoplasm, such as nondistended lobular units and, less often, sclerosing adenosis (SA).

Intensive studies have not indicated that cysts alone are associated with risk, even when larger ones are separately analyzed.[10,32,33] However, recurrent larger cysts may have a cancer risk indication, as presented by Dixon and associates.[34] Cysts are more common in high-risk geographic groups but are not determinants of cancer risk within geographic groups. Dupont and Page[10] demonstrated a very slight elevation of risk for women with a family history of breast cancer and cysts as opposed to women with a family history of breast cancer alone. This is very mild evidence for premalignant indication of cysts, particularly because this interaction was not present with other indicators and remains an isolated observation. Although epithelial hyperplasia (see later discussion), which is related to increased cancer risk, often coexists with cysts,[32] either change may be present without the other in an individual biopsy specimen or entire breast. The apocrine cytoplasmic alteration is also of no proven importance in breast cancer risk. Apocrine change was found by Wellings and Alpers[35] to be more commonly present concurrently with breasts associated with cancer than those without. However, it is not an indicator of breast cancer risk in a predictive fashion. Moreover, when only cases of papillary apocrine change without concurrent patterns of proliferative disease are considered, the risk of later cancer development is not increased over the expected risk level.[24] In summary, neither cysts nor apocrine change significantly elevate cancer risk in an individual woman in the absence of other considerations.[11,12]

Chronic inflammation, edema, and pigment-laden macrophages are often found around cysts. Pigment-laden macrophages are likely the result of cytochromes from dead cells present at some time in the past. Occasionally, some of the pigment material may represent hemosiderin. Although duct ectasia and cysts have some histologic similarities, they are usually easily separable based on the general contour of the lesions and the greater degree of inflammation and/or scarring associated with duct ectasia.[36] Duct ectasia is usually present adjacent to the nipple, although it may extend a distance into the breast.

Epithelial Hyperplasia and Proliferative Breast Disease

The classification of epithelial hyperplasia in the breast espoused here is based on a large follow-up (cohort) epidemiologic study (see Chapter 23) that sought to link epithelial histologic patterns to magnitudes of breast cancer risk.[10] The positive relationship of more extensive and complex examples of hyperplasia with carcinoma is supported in many concurrent and, more important, prospective studies.[18,37-45] Although the categories of histologic alteration can be readily compared with many classification systems that have been proposed, a major consideration marks this approach as different.

Rather than supposing a regular stepwise progression or continuum from no change through carcinoma in situ, this approach proposes an absolute separation between carcinoma in situ and other hyperplastic appearances, using several criteria.[46] Furthermore, it recognizes that small examples of lesions with features of carcinoma in situ may be reproducibly recognized because of their small size or their lack of some of the features of well-developed carcinoma in situ. These less than fully developed examples of carcinoma in situ are recognized by the term *atypical hyperplasia* (AH).[47] This term does not, if it is taken to indicate a moderate increased risk of later carcinoma, include all examples of hyperplasia thought to be generically unusual. On the contrary, the specifically defined AH lesions are recognized by a combination of cytologic, histologic, and extent cues,[48] some of which serve to differentiate them from carcinoma in situ and others to differentiate them from "benign."

DEFINITION AND BACKGROUND

Consistent with its definition elsewhere in the body, epithelial hyperplasia of the breast may be understood to mean an increased number of cells relative to a basement membrane. Thus the increased number of glands without a concomitant increase relative to the basement membrane would not constitute hyperplasia but rather adenosis. Hyperplasia may be considered to represent an increased number of cells above the basement membrane, and because this number is normally two, the presence of three or more cells above the basement membrane constitutes hyperplasia. The discussion that follows is based on the presentations of Wellings, Jensen and Marcum,[18] as well as those of our own group.[10] These are a series of concurrent and prospective studies that seek to reproducibly define subgroups of patients and to demonstrate their relationship or lack of relationship to carcinoma present at the same time[18] or developing in the future in a prospective fashion.[10,47]

In most cases, other terms in general usage may be analogized and compared if the same definitions for atypical hyperplasia are used. The term *papillomatosis*, proposed by Foote and Stewart,[9,49] is still used in North America to indicate the common or usual hyperplasias of moderate and florid degree.

Our approach to the stratification of the hyperplasias is to recognize an atypical lobular type, an apocrine type, and a usual type that includes the remainder of the hyperplastic lesions found in the breast.[50] The three groups recognize patterns regularly found within the breast and do not imply a pathogenetic sequence or a site of origin. The intent of the term *usual* is to denote that these are the common patterns of cytology and cell relationships seen when cell numbers are increased within the basement membrane–bound spaces within the human breast. The usual type or common patterns of hyperplasia have been termed *ductal* in the past largely to contrast them with the lobular series. Because these lesions regularly occur within acini of lobular units, the designation of *ductal* is avoided as an implication for either site of occurrence or site of origin of these cellular populations. Proliferative lesions in true ducts are unusual and are often truly papillary, that is, having branching, fibrous stalks (see later discussion).

The stratification of these hyperplastic lesions of usual type depends largely on quantitative changes. When the alterations begin to approximate patterns seen in carcinoma in situ, these lesions must be differentiated from those termed *atypical ductal hyperplasia* (ADH). Note that the features of the lesser end of the spectrum, between mild and moderate hyperplasia of usual type, depend on quantity and that the differentiation of the larger lesions from ADH depends on qualitative features of intercellular patterns and cytology (see later discussion).[48]

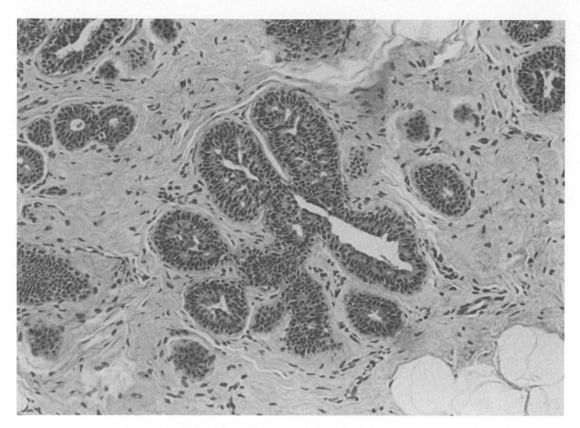

FIG. **7-4** Moderate hyperplasia of the usual type. The ductules are partially filled by a heterogeneous population of cells. Note the normally polarized layer of cells just above the basement membrane. (×175.)

Mild hyperplasia of usual type is characterized by the presence of three or more cells above the basement membrane in a lobular unit or duct and is not associated with any increased cancer risk. Hyperplastic lesions that reach five or more cells above the basement membrane and tend to cross and distend the space in which they occur are called *moderate*. *Florid* is used for more pronounced changes, without any firm definition separating the moderate and the florid categories (Figure 7-4). The reason for this is not to deny that there are quantitatively lesser and greater phenomena; rather, their reliable separation is not accomplished. Moderate and florid hyperplasia of the usual type are found in more than 20% of biopsies. In follow-up studies, the cancer risk between these two groups was found to be similar (see Chapter 23).

Risk categories may be stratified into slight, moderate, and marked, with *slight* indicating a risk of 1.5 to 2 times that of the general population and *marked* indicating about a tenfold increased risk (see Chapter 23). The current status of these assignments of histologic parameters to risk groups is shown in Box 7-1 and has changed little from that presented by a consensus conference that was supported by the American Cancer Society and the College of American Pathologists.[1,2] The clinical significance of usual hyperplasia of moderate and florid degree rests in the positive demonstration of a slight increased risk (1.5 to 2 times) of subsequent invasive carcinoma.

BOX 7-1 Relative Risk for Invasive Breast Carcinoma Based on Histologic Examination of Breast Tissue without Carcinoma*

NO INCREASED RISK (NO PROLIFERATIVE DISEASE)
Apocrine change
Duct ectasia
Mild epithelial hyperplasia of usual type

SLIGHTLY INCREASED RISK (1.5-2 TIMES)
Hyperplasia of usual type, moderate or florid
Sclerosing adenosis,[†] papilloma

MODERATELY INCREASED RISK (4-5 TIMES) (ATYPICAL HYPERPLASIA OR BORDERLINE LESIONS)
Atypical ductal hyperplasia and atypical lobular hyperplasia

HIGH RISK (8-10 TIMES) (CARCINOMA IN SITU)
Lobular carcinoma in situ and ductal carcinoma in situ (noncomedo)

Modified from Hutter RVP et al: *Arch Pathol Lab Med* 110:171, 1986.
*Women in each category are compared with women matched for age who have had no breast biopsy with regard to risk of invasive breast cancer in the ensuing 10 to 20 years. *Note:* These risks are not lifetime risks.
†Jensen and colleagues[51] have shown sclerosing adenosis to be an independent risk factor for subsequent development of invasive breast carcinoma.

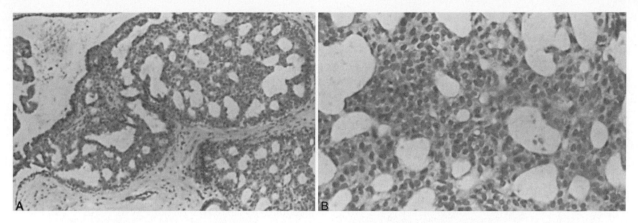

FIG. **7-5 A,** Florid hyperplasia of usual type. Ductules are partially filled with irregular arcade of cells. Note the irregularly shaped secondary lumens. (×150.) **B,** Higher power of **A.** There is mild nuclear variability and irregular placement of cells, features supporting the lack of atypia. (×280.)

A major change in concept since 1985 is the acceptance of SA as an indicator of slightly increased risk.[51]

The positive histologic features of this group (Figures 7-5 to 7-7) are as follows:

1. There is a mild variation of size, placement and shape of cells, and more specifically, nuclei. This feature is of great importance in differentiating these lesions from those of atypical hyperplasia and noncomedo ductal carcinoma in situ. They are most commonly present within lobular units and terminal ducts.

2. The cells often exhibit patterns of swirling or streaming.

3. This change in cellular polarity is associated with a redistribution of a structural protein, fodrin, around the cell membrane.[52] As the epithelial cells proliferate, there is a varied shape of secondary lumens, which are often slitlike and are present between the cells within individual spaces.

4. The secondary lumens, particularly in larger, more cellular lesions, may be present peripherally, immediately above the cells that surmount the basement membrane of the containing space.

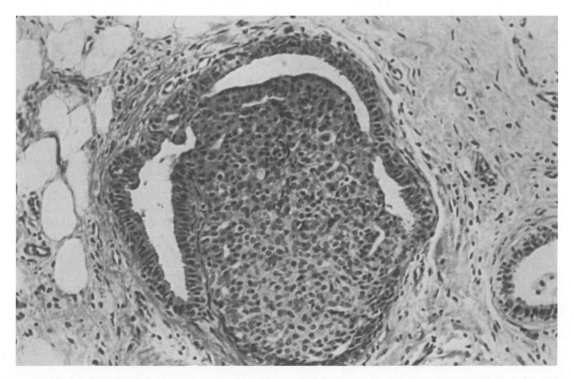

FIG. **7-6** Florid hyperplasia of usual type with solid pattern and peripheral placement of secondary spaces. Nuclei are predominantly heterogeneous. (×350.)

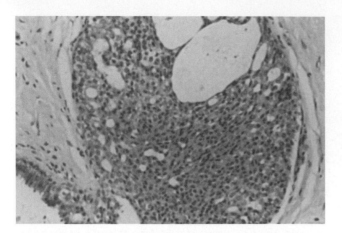

FIG. **7-7** Florid hyperplasia of usual type demonstrating prominent nuclear streaming or swirling. (×200.)

5. The cells appear to be varied, in cytologic appearance and in placement. Thus nuclei are not evenly separated one from the other. This is concomitant to the swirling or streaming change noted earlier.[53,54]

Atypical Hyperplasia

The intent of the term *AH* is to indicate a group of fairly specific histologic patterns that are not generically "atypical" or "unusual" but whose specific criteria have been shown to implicate an increased risk of later breast cancer development (see Box 7-1 and Chapter 23).[47] The link of specific histologic patterns to a moderate magnitude of breast cancer risk depends on the use of defined criteria. This link of AH lesions to risk is the result of a group of studies that sought to restrict the term *AH* to a small number of histologic patterns that have some of the same features as the analogous carcinoma in situ lesions. Many other studies[18,55] have supported the link of epithelial hyperplasia to premalignant states in the breast and have led to the current prospective studies.[42,44,45] Basically, the cases of AH seen by the authors are most analogous to the categories termed level 4 (on a scale of 1 to 5, with 5 equal to carcinoma in situ) by Black and Chabon[55] as well as Wellings, Jensen, and Marcum.[18] Even when diagnostic terms used by hospital pathologists in the 1970s were grouped into analogous categories, a similar but lesser separation of risk groups was accomplished.[37] AH has been shown to be more common in the contralateral breast of women who have breast carcinoma.[56] The atypical hyperplastic lesions have some of the same features as those of carcinomas in situ but either lack a major defining feature of carcinoma in situ or have the features in less developed form.[47,48] The three major defining criteria are cytology, histologic pattern, and lesion extent.[48]

These criteria have also been used by others.[30,57-59] Specific histologic features differentiate each of the AHs from lesser categories, as well as from the analogous carcinoma in situ lesions after which they are named: lobular and ductal carcinoma in situ. Thus the histologic definitions are not viewed as resting within spectra of changes. On the contrary, these histologic categories attempt to accept natural pattern groupings within the complex array of mammary alterations reflected in histologic preparations. However, when no natural grouping is identified, an arbitrary separation is accepted. Arbitrary separation was used to differentiate atypical lobular hyperplasia (ALH) from lobular carcinoma in situ (see later discussion).

Lobular carcinoma in situ (see also Chapter 11) is recognized when there is a well-developed example of filling, distention, and distortion of over half the acini of a lobular unit by a uniform population of characteristic cells. This follows the intent of the original description.[9,49] The analogous AH lesion, ALH, is recognized when fewer than half of the acini in a lobular unit are completely involved, but the appearance is otherwise similar (Figure 7-8).[60]

This arbitrary recognition of ALH and lobular carcinoma in situ in a series of changes from a few cells of appropriate appearance within a lobular unit to extreme examples with uniform cellular populations and extreme distortion and filling of acini imposes a stratification in what is otherwise an undivided continuum. Many pathologists prefer to use one diagnostic term for this range of histologic appearances, for example, *lobular neoplasia*.[61] We espouse this term because it covers both ALH and lobular carcinoma in situ. However, in diagnostic practice, more clinical guidance is given by the use of the separate designations lobular carcinoma in situ and ALH (see Chapter 23 for risk implications).[62]

A specific feature of lobular neoplasia is its tendency to undermine an otherwise normal and certainly different cell population. Because this is the interposition of an abnormal epithelial cell population within another, it has been termed *pagetoid spread* (because of the obvious analogy to Paget's disease of the nipple). Some have used this phenomenon to indicate diagnostic certainty for lobular carcinoma in situ; however, pagetoid spread does occur when the degree of involvement within lobular units reaches only the diagnostic level of ALH. The histologic patterns produced are usually more subtle in ALH,[63] and the solid pattern of ductal involvement in lobular carcinoma in situ is not seen with ALH. This pattern of involvement of ductal spaces outside of lobular units by the cells of lobular neoplasia in the presence of ALH has been termed *ductal involvement in ALH* and has been shown to be associated with a *slightly* higher risk of subsequent breast carcinoma than is found with involvement of the lobular units alone.[64]

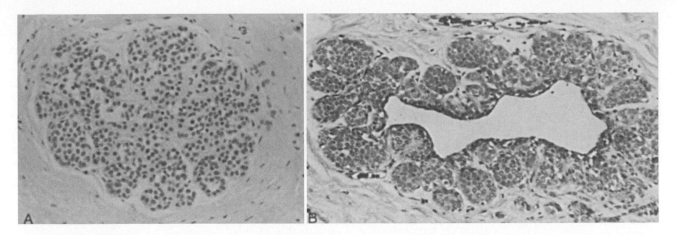

FIG. **7-8 A,** Atypical lobular hyperplasia (ALH). There is a resemblance to lobular carcinoma in situ (LCIS), but less than 50% of the individual acini are uniformly distended. (×180.) **B,** ALH undermining a different luminal cellular population. The same appearance may occur in LCIS; the defining diagnostic features must be present in lobular units to distinguish ALH from LCIS. (×180.) *(From Page DL, Anderson TJ:* Diagnostic histopathology of the breast, *Edinburgh, 1987, Churchill Livingstone.)*

The philosophical underpinnings of the diagnostic term *ADH* are the same as those for ALH. Thus the same features present in the analogous carcinoma in situ lesion are evident, but in a less developed form. Because the criteria of ADH are derived from those of ductal carcinoma in situ, histologic criteria for the latter must be understood. Two major criteria are required for the diagnosis of ductal carcinoma in situ (low grade, non-comedo). First, a uniform population of neoplastic cells must populate the entire basement membrane–bound space. Furthermore, this alteration must involve at least two such spaces (Figures 7-9 and 7-10). An adjunct to assessing the extent of involvement has been put forth by Tavassoli and Norris.[65] They consider lesions smaller than 2 or 3 mm as ADH, with a resulting moderate increase in later cancer development. In addition to extent, an intercellular pattern of rigid arches and even placement of cells must be uniformly present. A helpful secondary criterion is hyperchromatic nuclei, which may not be present in all cases.[48,66] The pattern of comedo ductal carcinoma in situ is not even discussed here because its characteristic extreme nuclear atypia is far beyond the patterns seen in ADH. Without the uniform application of criteria, consistency in diagnosis is unlikely[67]; however, when standardized criteria are applied, concordance is most often ensured.[68]

Some cases of ADH share features with the so-called clinging carcinoma described by Azzopardi.[30] A study from northern Italy indicates a considerable overlap of clinging carcinoma with ADH in histologic patterns and in risk of subsequent cancer development.[40,69,70] The authors do not believe that the diagnosis of clinging carcinoma as a form of ductal carcinoma in situ is appropriate because it obviously indicates a different behavior from that expected of widely accepted forms of ductal carcinoma in situ (see Chapter 11).

Four separate groups[38,42,44,45] have now applied these criteria to large cohorts in long-term follow-up studies, with remarkably similar subsequent risks of cancer development.

Localized Sclerosing Lesions

The classic example of localized sclerosing lesions is *SA*, which has been long accepted as a gross and histologic mimicker of invasive carcinoma. It is in that capacity that it still has its greatest utility as a recognized diagnostic term and histologic pattern in the armamentarium of histopathologists. In its most usual form, SA is present as a microscopic lesion, probably unrecognized in both clinical and gross examination of tissues. SA is diagnosed only when a clearly lobulocentric change gives rise to enlargement and distortion of lobular units with a combination of increased numbers of acinar structures and a coexistent fibrous alteration (Figure 7-11). The normal two-cell population is maintained above the basement membrane in most areas, and the glandular units are regularly deformed. The term was proposed by Ewing[71] and further described by Dawson[72] to clearly separate this increase in glands from lesions involving increased numbers of cells within an enclosure of basement membrane (hyperplasia of usual type, epitheliosis).

Enlarged lobular units that appear otherwise normal, or with slight gland deformity, may not be recognized as SA but may rather be diagnosed using the noncommittal and appropriately descriptive term *adenosis*. There is a favored association of SA with ALH.[51] Diagnostic patterns of ALH are usually present in nonsclerosed lobules elsewhere in the biopsy and are certainly difficult to recognize when present within a

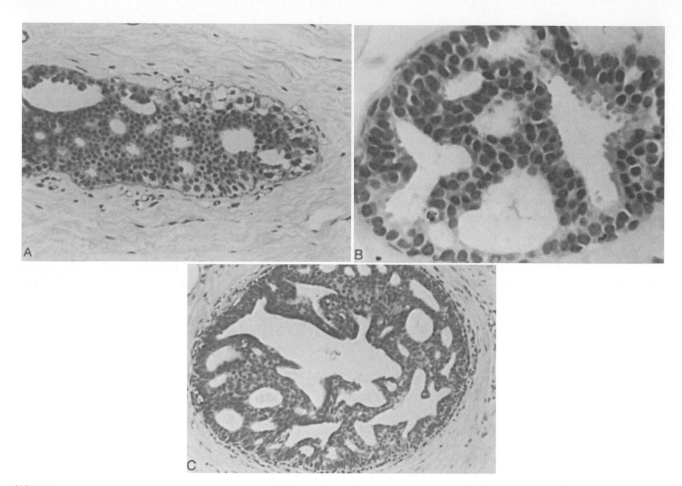

FIG. **7-9** **A,** Atypical ductal hyperplasia (ADH) is evident in this ductule cut longitudinally. Note the regular placement of hyperchromatic nuclei and the regularity of centrally placed secondary lumens. (×190.) **B,** Rigid bar crossing the central portion of the photograph suggests ductal carcinoma in situ (DCIS); however, the cell pattern is not maintained throughout the remainder of the space. Note the polarity of the cells at the lower portion of the space, a finding that indicates ADH rather than DCIS. (×350.) **C,** Although there is some uniformity of some of the intercellular spaces, the cellular prolongations tend to taper and there is a tendency for peripheral placement of secondary spaces. The pattern and cytologic criteria for DCIS are not clearly uniformly met; therefore this is an example of ADH. (×170.) *(From Page DL, Anderson TJ:* Diagnostic histopathology of the breast, *Edinburgh, 1987, Churchill Livingstone.)*

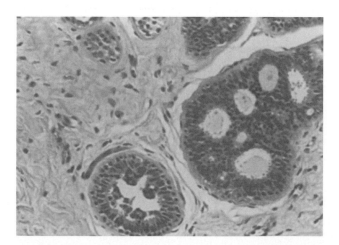

FIG. **7-10** Florid hyperplasia of usual type. Although there are hyperchromatism and regularly spaced secondary spaces, there is not a uniform population of evenly spaced cells; this is not diagnostic of atypical ductal hyperplasia. (×225.)

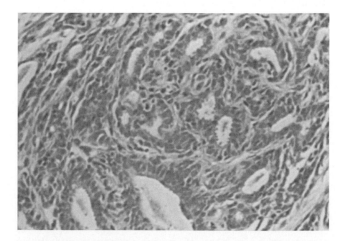

FIG. **7-11** Sclerosing adenosis. Glandular elements are deformed and surrounded by stromal fibrous alteration. Two-cell population (basal or myoepithelial and luminal) is focally inapparent. (×240.)

focus of SA. This may be because of the maintenance of relatively small spaces within readily identifiable lesions of SA (see discussion of ALH). The cytologic features of apocrine change may also be seen in adenosis, so-called apocrine adenosis.[73,74] The enlarged nuclei and prominent nucleoli of apocrine cells, when present in a deformed, sclerotic lesion, can occasionally mimic invasive carcinoma. Some have used the appellation *atypical* to describe this setting.[75] We believe that it is not clearly atypical because it is merely apocrine cytology in an unusual site, not a combination of pattern and cytologic atypia. Although it is unusual, we reserve the designation *atypical* for those histopathologic entities that have a proven risk implication for later cancer development.[10]

A palpable mass may be created by aggregations of microscopic foci of SA (aggregate adenosis). This situation has been termed *adenosis tumor*[20] to indicate that a clinically palpable tumor may be produced. SA also commonly contains foci of microcalcification and, when present in this aggregate form, may be detectable with mammography.

The differential diagnosis of these lesions has often been presented as a series or listing of criteria. These most often seek to differentiate SA from infiltrating tubular carcinoma and its variants. In the formation of these listings, little thought has been given to what is done if, for example, three criteria are consistent and the remaining are not. They must, then, be regarded as guidelines and not as hard-and-fast criteria. Fortunately, most of the time the various criteria are consistent. Such is the variation of the biology of breast disease, or at least the variation of the anatomic expression of breast disease, that occasionally the guidelines will fail or be inconsistent. Usually, careful attention to the fact that SA is lobulocentric will suffice to correctly identify it. It is also true in SA that adjacent tubules tend to take approximately the same or similar shape as their immediate neighbors, although minor variations become marked if one skips to several tubular structures away. Equally true is that occasional ductal structures may be surrounded by a periodic acid–Schiff–positive basement membrane in a benign condition, which tends to be lost in carcinoma. However, many carcinomas have at least an irregular basement membrane and may show immunolocalization of proteins or basement membrane, such as type 4 collagen or laminin.[76,77] Decoration by special stains for myoepithelial markers are also not an absolute indicator of differential diagnosis, largely because these elements are often lost in densely sclerotic foci with glandular atrophy. This is then a helpful but not an absolute criterion. The spaces of a tubular carcinoma tend to be open, occasionally producing an irregular extension of the cluster of cells at one edge, resembling a teardrop. The cells of an infiltrating tubular carcinoma usually are layered singly, and when they are multilayered, the cells appear similar.

A rare condition known as *microglandular adenosis* (MGA), which may also mimic tubular carcinoma, has been well described.[78-81] In this condition, irregular, nonlobulocentric, small glandular spaces are present in increased numbers and appear to dissect and infiltrate through stroma and fat. A clinically palpable mass of several centimeters' diameter may be produced, which may be irregularly demarcated from surrounding tissue. The importance of this rare lesion is its ability to mimic tubular carcinoma. A similar lesion consisting of myoepithelial cells has been described and may show multiple recurrences.[82] MGA complicated by hyperplastic foci has been documented in two patients in whom carcinoma subsequently developed.[80] An additional 13 cases have been described in which infiltrative carcinoma was present in the background of MGA.[83,84] Because of the rarity of this condition, such associations are not certain. Clinical judgment may suggest various options in this setting, but a conservative stance should be emphasized. In other words, in the differential diagnosis between a benign lesion and cancer of little lethality (tubular carcinoma), one should favor benignancy in enigmatic settings.

RADIAL SCAR AND COMPLEX SCLEROSING LESIONS

Radial scar and complex sclerosing lesions have some similarities to SA: Carcinoma may be mimicked either clinically or histologically; it is with mammography that the mimicry of carcinoma by the larger complex sclerosing lesions is complete. Similar lesions were first described by Fenoglio and Lattes[85] as mimickers of carcinoma. Indeed, the advent of mammography has made the formal recognition of these lesions mandatory. The lesions appear spiculated, hence the term *radial scar*. The lesions are not lobulocentric but evidently incorporate several very deformed lobular units within their makeup, having as their probable origin a major stem of the duct system. This is particularly true of very large lesions. These are all characterized by a central scar from which elements radiate. The scar may vary through the full range of histologic appearances of the breast, including cystic dilation and units demonstrating hyperplasia and lobulocentric sclerosis like that of SA. Indeed, evaluation of these dense scars with special immune markers may be made difficult by the disappearance of myoepithelial markers in these epithelial elements within the scars. The microscopic features are determined by the degree of maturation, because it is now realized that the

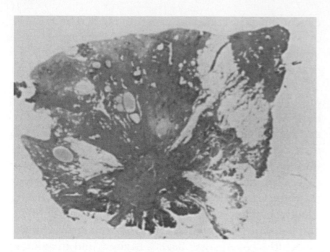

FIG. **7-12** Mature radial scar with sclerotic center showing microcystic peripheral parenchyma. (×5.)

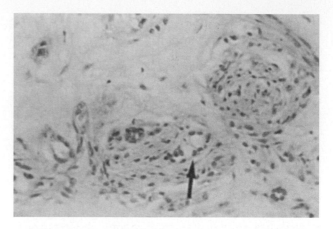

FIG. **7-13** Pseudoinfiltration of glandular elements adjacent to a nerve *(arrow)* from a case of radial scar. The entrapped epithelial elements may closely mimic tubular carcinoma. (×300.)

classic appearance (Figure 7-12) represents the well-developed stage 2. Lesions at an earlier stage show noticeable spindle cells and chronic inflammatory cells around the central parenchymal components, which are less distorted. The association of hyperplasia and cystic and apocrine change becomes more evident as the lesion matures. There is evidence that the presence of these sclerosing lesions may further elevate cancer risk over other histologic risk indicators when they are present together.[86]

The progressive nature of these lesions was studied ultrastructurally by Battersby and Anderson.[87] A feature associated with early lesions was myofibroblasts in close proximity to degenerating parenchymal structures. Mature radial scars showed relatively few, sparsely distributed stromal myofibroblasts. Within the central scar, there are entrapped epithelial elements that have been appropriately characterized as pseudoinvasive (Figure 7-13). Although these are the elements that most commonly mimic carcinoma histologically, atypical hyperplastic lesions may be found within the preformed epithelial spaces in the outer portions of the lesion. The entrapped epithelial units may closely mimic tubular carcinoma, and this differential diagnosis may be difficult. However, it should be recalled that tiny tubular carcinomas pose little threat to life and a conservative posture in the diagnosis of these lesions will benefit more patients.

Anderson and Battersby[88] analyzed the qualitative and quantitative features of more than 100 examples of radial scars from cases with and without cancer. Their frequency is similar in both groups and depends heavily on the diligence of search and the amount of tissue assessed. Bilaterality and multifocality were present in both groups, as was the full range of histologic appearance. No premalignant definition of these lesions was supported.

A variety of terms have been proposed for these lesions. However, it is likely that *radial scar* will maintain dominance. We favor the term *complex sclerosing lesion* for the larger examples in this series. This is because they do tend to have a variety of appearances, and their complexity with regard to mimicry of carcinoma is clearly portrayed by the term *complex*. The term *radial* also is useful to indicate the spiculated nature of the lesions.

Duct Ectasia and Fat Necrosis

DUCT ECTASIA

Duct ectasia is an entity or group of entities that has somewhat unclear confines of definition.[89] Some recognize only dilated ducts, as the term would indicate, as representing this condition. When this approach is taken, the condition is very common but is typically not associated with clinical pain or scarring. The separation of this entity into two large groups affecting different age groups and having different causes is becoming widely recognized.[36]

Most observers reserve the diagnostic term for those conditions in which a clinical presentation includes palpable lumpiness in the region of the breast under the areola. Ducts tend to be involved in a segmental fashion; that is, adjacent ducts extending out into the breast from the nipple are involved. Nipple discharge is a common but not invariable accompaniment of this condition, and undoubtedly the periductal scarring attendant to the later stages of this process is responsible for most cases of benign, acquired nipple inversion.[90] Periductal inflammation is a histologic hallmark of this condition.[30] It is now generally believed that the process begins with such a change and proceeds by destroying the elastic network to ectasia and periductal fibrosis.[91]

Most cases described are found in the perimenopausal age group. There are also younger women who present with inflammation of the ducts in the region of the nipple, which may produce fissures and fistulas with connections from the nipple ducts to the skin at the edges of the areola. The presentation of fistulas in younger women seems to be clearly connected with infection. This so-called periductal mastitis is commonly associated with a history of previous periareolar inflammation.[36] The more classic appearance of duct ectasia in older women may be a more smoldering infection of the larger ducts, and infection as the basis of this condition has been strongly suggested but remains unproved for most cases.[36,92] Very few with duct ectasia have a history of periductal mastitis, suggesting that these two conditions are probably unrelated. There is no association with parity or lactation.[91] As is the case with so many of these benign conditions of the breast, the greatest importance clinically is the mimicry of carcinoma. The plaquelike calcifications that occur within the scarred wall are, of course, visible with mammography (Figure 7-14). Usually, these calcifications can be differentiated from the more irregular punctate calcifications of comedo carcinoma, but this is not always clear. Besides this frequent approximation to the mammographic appearance of comedo ductal carcinoma in situ, the localized scarring of duct ectasia can produce lumps that are fixed within inflamed scar in the breast. These lumps can very closely mimic carcinoma on occasion. One variant of this condition containing many plasma cells has been termed *plasma cell mastitis*. This is probably not a separate condition but rather part of the spectrum of duct ectasia. This is known to be a close mimicker of breast carcinoma of lobular infiltrating type, both grossly and microscopically.

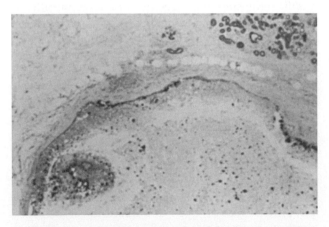

FIG. **7-14** Large duct affected by duct ectasia. There is periductal fibrosis and inflammation. Note calcification in the wall of duct. (×50.)

FAT NECROSIS

Fat necrosis is relatively uncommon but may present in a most dramatic fashion, mimicking a well-developed scirrhous carcinoma or even inflammatory carcinoma. In its late, scarred phase, fat necrosis may not have an identifiable preceding traumatic cause; however, the mammographic appearance in the late stages is characteristic.[93] Most cases seen in the more acute phases, with some inflammatory activity still apparent, are associated with an identifiable recent traumatic event.

The histology of fat necrosis in the breast is no different from its appearance in other organs. The characteristic active chronic inflammatory cells are usually evident, with lymphocytes and histiocytes predominating. In the unusual very acute cases presenting within 1 week after an inciting event, polymorphonuclear leukocytes and free, oily, lipid material may be most apparent, particularly upon needle aspiration. In this stage the clinical features of swelling, redness, and warmth are present.

In the later stage, collagenous scar is the predominant finding, with seemingly granular histiocytes surrounding oil cysts of varying size. These "oil cysts" contain the free lipid material released by lipocyte necrosis.[94]

The greatest clinical importance of fat necrosis is in its mimicry of carcinoma, as noted earlier. There is no known association with carcinoma or carcinoma risk.

Miscellaneous Conditions

GRANULOMATOUS MASTITIS

Granulomatous mastitis should be understood as a descriptive diagnostic term only. Within the broad confines of such a descriptive designation, there are variants of duct ectasia, granulomatous infectious diseases, and idiopathic granulomatous conditions. Idiopathic granulomatous mastitis may be difficult to distinguish from duct ectasia or from infectious granulomatous mastitis. Specific granulomatous infections such as tuberculosis may present in the breast, although this is uncommon.[95,96] Recognition of granulomatous inflammation at the time of frozen section should prompt a search for the etiologic agent through culture. Granulomatous mastitis may be the presenting sign of a systemic disorder such as Wegener's granulomatosis.[97-99] Sarcoidosis is another diagnostic consideration when granulomas are found in the breast.[100,101] The associated features of duct ectasia should be absent in sarcoidosis. The variety of infectious and noninfectious granulomatous mammary conditions are listed by Symmers and McKeown.[102]

Fibroadenoma and Phyllodes Tumor

FIBROADENOMA

Fibroadenomas (FAs) most often have a characteristic clinical presentation with an easily movable mass, seemingly unfixed to surrounding breast tissue. The gross appearance is usually characteristic. The sharp circumscription and smooth interface with surrounding breast tissue, usually producing an elevation of the FA on cut section, is characteristic. The cut surface is white, although one may identify the epithelial elements, if they are numerous, as light-brown areas. The cut surface is shiny and occasionally may seem to present an almost papillary appearance if the clefts lined by epithelium are larger. There may be slight variation from one area to another, with more dense fibrosis in the stroma and, occasionally, calcification. The latter two features are more common in older women.

Although traditionally the risk for subsequent carcinoma in patients with typical FA has not been considered to be higher than that for the general population,[26] one study reported that, overall, FAs were found to be associated with a slight increased relative risk for later cancer.[103] The level of risk varies, depending on the characteristics of the FA itself and the status of the adjacent epithelium. If the adjacent epithelium shows proliferative changes or if the FA is complex, defined as the presence of cysts, SA, epithelial calcifications, or papillary apocrine changes within the FA, the risk is slightly higher than when these changes are absent.[103] Indeed, without these specific features, the women have no increased risk. One of the interesting aspects of this study, also shown by Levi and co-workers,[104] is that the risk identified by FA may not decrease in relative terms in the next 5 or 10 years after identification with biopsy.[103]

Carcinoma arising in FAs is distinctly uncommon. In this setting, lobular carcinoma in situ is the predominant type.[105-107] Risk implications for lobular neoplasia within an FA are not known for certain but probably are no greater than when lobular neoplasia is seen in the usual setting[103]; indeed, a large study indicates that atypical hyperplasia within FAs presents no increased risk of later cancer development.[108] Microscopically, fibrous tissue makes up most of the FA; either the stroma may surround rounded and easily definable ductlike epithelial structures, or the epithelium may be stretched into curvilinear arrangements (Figures 7-15 and 7-16). This latter pattern has been termed *intracanalicular,* and the former pattern has been termed *pericanalicular.* These two terms are still useful as descriptors but are of no practical or prognostic importance and therefore are not used to define supposed subtypes of FA. Smooth muscle is an extremely rare

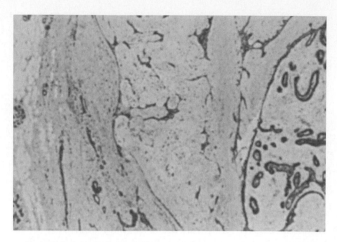

FIG. **7-15** Fibroadenoma showing prominent intracanalicular pattern. (×30.)

component of FAs.[109] The epithelium within an FA may have the same appearance as elsewhere in the breast, including apocrine metaplasia.[30] Rarely, squamous metaplasia is present.[110]

FAs that are allowed to grow after initial detection usually cease to grow when they reach 2 to 3 cm in diameter.[20] Blacks more commonly develop FAs than whites, and they develop them at a younger age as well. FAs in blacks are also more likely to recur.[111] Because FAs are more common in blacks, related lesions are also probably more common in blacks.[112] Infarcts of the breast may occur during pregnancy or lactation with a resultant discrete mass.[113] Approximately 1 of 200 FAs shows infarction.[114,115] Pain and tenderness may occur during pregnancy, and an inflammatory reaction may be accompanied by lymphadenopathy, leading to the clinical impression of carcinoma.

FA may also be regarded as a generic term, referring to any benign, confined tumor of the breast (mass-occupying lesion) that has a mixture of glandular and mesenchymal elements. When it is viewed as a more specific term, special or specific variants of the general pattern are recognized as being separate entities. These include *hamartoma, tubular adenoma, lactating adenoma, adenolipoma, juvenile fibroadenoma,* and *giant adenoma.*

Hamartomas of the breast have received greater attention with the introduction of mammography.[116] The series of Hessler, Schnyder, and Ozzello[117] and Linell and co-workers[118] are important in establishing the notation of hamartomas as first proposed by Arrigoni, Dockerty, and Judd.[119] These are lesions made up of recognizable lobular units, often present at the sharply demarcated margins of these lesions. Fat is rare in FAs, which are also rarely characterized by well-ordered lobular units throughout their substance. Another feature supporting the recognition of hamartomas as separate entities is that their average age of presentation is almost two decades after that for FAs in

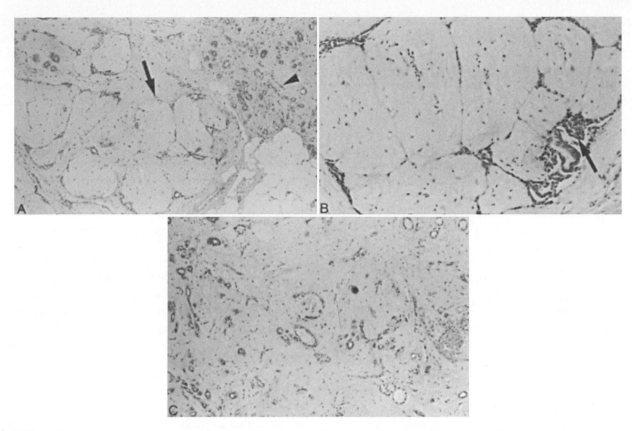

FIG. **7-16 A**, Fibroadenoma with irregular border. Both intracanalicular *(arrow)* and pericanalicular *(arrowhead)* patterns are well demonstrated. (×30.) **B**, Higher power of **A**. Fixation artifact gives appearance of hyperplastic epithelium *(arrow)*. (×125.) **C**, Same case as **A**. Complex epithelial patterns are evident. (×50.)

general. It is the sharp, smooth borders of these lesions and their intermixture with fat that allows mammographic identification in pronounced examples. Duchatelle, Auberger, and Amouroux[120] support the formation of these lesions as more likely to be developmental than neoplastic. A similar lesion is the adenolipoma.[121] These lesions are only one tenth as common as ordinary lipomas.[20]

Other types of FA, perhaps better regarded as variants rather than as separate entities, are lesions tending to occur in women in the younger age range that are characterized by increased cellularity of stroma or epithelium, or both. Duray and colleagues[122] described cellular FAs as being most likely to occur in adolescents and more likely to recur locally as adolescent cellular FA. These lesions bear some resemblance to benign phyllodes tumors of some other classifications. *Juvenile FA* is a diagnostic term based on clinical grounds.[123] Oberman[124] initially suggested the use of the term *juvenile adenofibroma* in a review of breast lesions in juveniles. He believed that 5% to 10% of the adenofibromas that occurred in that age group were notable for rapid growth and large size. Pike and Oberman,[125] further elaborating on juvenile adenofibroma, characterized the lesions by their tendency to occur around the time of

menarche, the common ductal pattern of epithelial hyperplasia, and the defining stromal hypercellularity. Local recurrence was not believed to be a feature of these lesions. Mies and Rosen[126] have also described a series of patients with an average age of 26 years who had an unusual and atypical pattern of epithelial hyperplasia within FAs, which is likely to be misinterpreted as carcinoma in situ. No specific clinical feature was suggested. There is certainly no overlap between the latter series of patients and those described by Duray and co-workers,[122] whereas the cases of Pike and Oberman[125] appear to be somewhere intermediate. The practical utility of these interesting approaches to unusual FAs appears to be that rapidly growing lesions in juveniles are usually benign, often have a densely cellular stroma, and less often have prominent epithelial hyperplasia.

The histologic definitions separating FA from phyllodes tumors are even less well defined than are the definitions of benign versus malignant among the phyllodes tumors (see following discussion). It seems clear that the term *phyllodes tumors* is often applied to most large FAs with any suggestion of hypercellularity. As long as the descriptor *benign* is added to the designation (particularly if the synonymous diagnostic phrase *benign cystosarcoma phyllodes* is used), no harm will come of this usage. Fechner[116] considers up to three mitoses per high-power field as acceptable in FA. Perhaps with the designation of cellular FAs[122] indicating a slightly greater likelihood of local recurrence, the separation of phyllodes tumors from FAs may become more precise. In a carefully reported series of phyllodes tumors, Chua and Thomas[127] recognized 92% as being benign based on the presence of fewer than five mitoses per 10 high-power fields, only mild stromal pleomorphism, and circumscribed tumor margins. An 18% local recurrence rate for these lesions is within the range of 15% cited for FAs alone, further evidence that clinical terminology for these lesions might be considered a matter of personal choice.

There remains the possibility that FAs may evolve into phyllodes tumors, but that occurrence is not well documented; there are lesions with areas of characteristic FA and other areas with leaflike patterns characteristic of phyllodes tumors.[128] Certainly there has been a recent major change from the prior clinical dictum that any determinate mass had to be surgically removed from the breast. Many surgical groups have noted that characteristic 2- to 3-cm FAs could be watched clinically after careful notation, this being most appropriate in patients younger than 25 years and acceptable for those 25 to 30 years, although probably not thereafter.[129,130] Also, needle aspiration with characteristic findings should confirm the fact that such lesions are FAs. The natural history of most FAs supports this approach.[131] A condition that may resemble FA is fibromatosis.[132,133] Fibromatosis is benign histologically and as many as one fourth of these cases may recur after simple excision.[132,133]

Another variant of FA is tubular adenoma. These lesions are uncommon and are recognized as having dominant tubular elements in a circumscribed mass with minimal supporting stroma.[134,135] Grossly tubular adenomas have a fine nodularity.[136] Portions of otherwise characteristic FAs may have the appearance of a tubular adenoma.[137] Uniform tubular structures are seen, and lobular anatomy is usually not evident. Tubular adenomas may have evidence of secretory activity, but when they do not occur in association with pregnancy or lactation, they should not be termed *lactating adenomas.* Lactating adenomas are certainly analogous in some ways to tubular adenomas and may represent a physiologic response of the tubular adenoma to pregnancy.[137] In addition to showing lactational changes, the adenomas presenting in pregnancy have a more evident lobular anatomy than that seen in most tubular adenomas. James, Bridger, and Anthony[138] have supported the notion that the lesions arising in pregnancy, formerly termed *lactating adenomas,* be termed *breast tumor of pregnancy.* This term is proposed because they are distinct from tubular adenomas and should not

be related to lactation (despite histologic changes) because they arise during pregnancy, not during the time of breastfeeding. The microscopic changes seen in the breast tumor of pregnancy are similar to those seen in the normal pregnant breast but are variable in degree and are often out of phase with the normal breast changes resulting from pregnancy.

PHYLLODES TUMOR

The series of mammary tumors known as *phyllodes tumors* continue to pose problems for the physician managing breast disease, largely because of their rarity. Three problems remain incompletely resolved: (1) The confusing terminology of cystosarcoma phyllodes is still in frequent usage; (2) rarity of these lesions has made clear understanding of the borderline between benign and malignant difficult; and (3) there remain a fairly large number of cases, relative to the entire group of lesions, that must continue to be regarded as borderline malignant, presenting obvious problems in patient management, although such "borderline" cases should present a threat of local recurrence only.

First, the replacement of the classic terminology that placed the suffix *sarcoma* on benign and malignant examples of these lesions is a necessary recognition of the evolution of the term *sarcoma.* When first coined by Müller[139] in 1838, the term meant only a fleshy tumor. The general acceptance of the term to mean predicted malignant behavior did not arise until decades later, and we may regard *cystosarcoma* as a vestigial example of the nineteenth century descriptive use of that term.[140]

Second, the rarity of these lesions has led them to be misunderstood. Two differential diagnostic problems are represented by this situation: (1) the separation of the benign phyllodes tumors from some similar, and probably closely related, unusual FA, and (2) the recognition of the truly malignant end of the spectrum of phyllodes tumors.

There is no reliable way to differentiate grossly a giant FA (or the so-called juvenile FA) from a benign phyllodes tumor. Indeed, the tendency to recognize the large size as the dominant characteristic of phyllodes tumor has led to the frequent confusion of these entities. They may be interrelated in any case. A classic gross pattern for a phyllodes tumor includes sharp demarcation from the surrounding normal breast tissue, with the normal tissue obviously compressed. The connective tissue that makes up the greatest bulk of the mass is firm and varies from dense and white to glistening and edematous. Local areas of degeneration lead to cystic and discolored areas. The classic pattern that gave these tumors their name may be evident with smoothly contoured leaflike areas separated from others by narrow, epithelial-lined spaces.[141]

The histologic appearance of phyllodes tumors may be considered the same as that of large FAs unless some

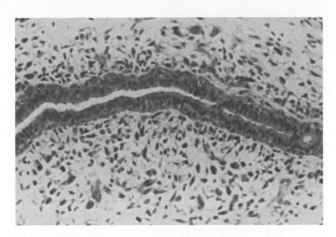

FIG. **7-17** Phyllodes tumor. Hypercellular stroma shows nuclear pleomorphism and atypia. (×300.)

specific guidelines are accepted. Fechner[116] believes that the stroma in phyllodes tumors should have greater cellularity and cell activity but that up to three mitoses per high-power field should be accepted within the definition of FA. Page, Anderson, and Johnson[142] have also accepted that approach and have suggested that the close application of a particularly cellular connective tissue element to the basement membrane region of the epithelial element be the defining factor and that size should have no part in the differential diagnosis of these mixed tumors of the breast (Figure 7-17). The proliferating stroma is usually rich and cellular, regularly deforming the epithelium into extreme examples of the intracanalicular pattern seen in the more common FAs. The classic paper of Norris and Taylor[143] inaugurated the approach to documenting histologic features as rigorously as possible. Later papers have supported counting mitoses and evaluating the margins with care to

determine whether there is an infiltrating focus.[144-146] Evaluated in this way, Chua and Thomas[127] identified five borderline phyllodes tumors, two of which recurred after local excision. A predominantly circumscribed margin, 5 to 10 mitoses per high-power microscopic field, and moderate nuclear pleomorphism were believed to be the defining factors in this group. Thus borderline lesions are unlikely to reveal evidence of truly malignant behavior and may be more likely to recur locally than the usual phyllodes tumor. Special note should be made of the fact that malignant behavior in phyllodes tumors of young women is extremely rare.[147,148] Most malignant phyllodes tumors reported in the literature that have metastasized have had overgrowth of an obvious sarcomatous element (Figure 7-18). This malignant element has often been something other than fibrosarcoma (e.g., liposarcoma, rhabdomyosarcoma). Close examination of the stroma with multiple sections is mandatory. The truly malignant phyllodes tumor may be so only in a portion of the tumor where easily diagnostic foci of sarcoma may be evident. On the other hand, a richly cellular fibrosarcoma-like stroma present in many foci or diffusely throughout the tumor presents the greatest difficulty in differential diagnosis. This difficulty primarily leads to overdiagnosis of malignancy, as evidenced by the 27 patients reported by Blumencranz and Gray,[149] in which 13 of the phyllodes tumors were diagnosed as malignant because of any combination of increased mitotic activity, invasive borders, or marked pleomorphism. In none of the women in this study did recurrences or metastases develop. Similar experience is reported in other series with patients who had well-sampled, benign phyllodes tumors that were successfully treated with careful excision.[150-152] Incomplete excision of phyllodes tumors

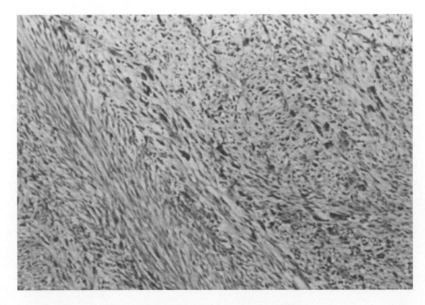

FIG. **7-18** Phyllodes tumor. Low-grade fibrosarcomatous element is evident. (×110.)

has been stressed as a major determinant for local recurrence.[153]

Although it is often stated that histologic criteria are not reliable and that lesions appearing to be benign histopathologically may metastasize, these events are poorly characterized or poorly documented. With the use of a borderline category (tumors that usually do not act in a malignant fashion but may be more likely to recur locally), this unpredictability is no longer completely true. Certainly, even tumors with diffuse features of low-grade fibrosarcoma in the stroma rarely act in a malignant fashion. It is not even clear that such borderline tumors reliably recur locally more often than other benign tumors. However, local recurrence has been reported in up to 59% of cases.[154-156] Other series have found that the approximate 15% local recurrence rate accorded FAs was not reliably different from that of phyllodes tumors. Very important, local recurrences are unlikely to evolve into malignancy if this feature was not present in the primary tumor.[157]

PAPILLOMA

The usual and classic solitary papilloma is a mass lesion of the large ducts most often presenting in the subareolar region. In the periphery, papillary lesions are often multiple and continuous with hyperplastic alterations within lobular units, as shown by Ohuchi and colleagues[158] in three-dimensional reconstruction studies of papillomas. Particularly when they are extensive, these lesions may be associated with atypical hyperplasia and ductal pattern carcinoma in situ within and adjacent to the peripheral papillomas.

There is an important clinical correlate of these papillary lesions—they commonly present with a hemorrhagic discharge that is usually unilateral from the nipple.[30] This is true for the more central and larger lesions but may be also seen in smaller, more peripheral lesions. A careful follow-up of women with a solitary papilloma showed an increased risk of subsequent carcinoma development.[159] It was suggested that accompanying epithelial hyperplasia was responsible for further elevating the increased risk (see Box 7-1). From the Nashville series of patients, a nested case-control study evaluated the risk of carcinoma development after having a papilloma identified with biopsy.[160] A papilloma with or without ordinary patterns of hyperplasia was associated with only a slight increased risk, similar to other features of proliferative breast disease without atypia.[10,160] The presence of atypical hyperplasia (pattern and extent analogous to ADH) within a papilloma increased the risk of subsequent breast cancer development, predominantly near the site of the original papilloma. This single study suggests that women who have papillomas with AH may have a similar or higher cancer risk than others who have patterns of AH within breast parenchyma. Other researchers believe that women with multiple papillomas have an increased risk for subsequent carcinoma development.[20] The co-occurrence of highly atypical hyperplastic lesions (including carcinoma in situ) with these multiple papillomas has been illustrated.[160-162]

Histopathology. Papillomas are truly papillary lesions with a branching fibrovascular core surmounted by epithelium (Figure 7-19). They are most often identified on careful gross examination as lying within dilated ductal sacs. The papillomas may attain several centimeters in size, causing them to appear encysted with the continuity of the duct within which they arose, less apparent than in smaller examples. The texture of papillomas varies from soft to firm with dense sclerotic foci.

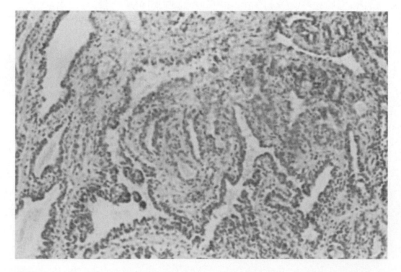

FIG. **7-19** Delicate fibrovascular fronds of papilloma covered by single or double epithelial cell layers. (×280.)

Focal areas of necrosis and hemorrhage are a natural part of the basic elements of papillomas. Infarction may cause compression and distortion of epithelium, producing the appearance of carcinoma.[163] Squamous metaplasia may also be present.[164] The epithelial lining in benign papillomas varies greatly but is usually easily identified as benign (see Figure 7-19). A double cell layer with more rounded cells adjacent to the basement membrane and surmounted by more columnar cells is commonly seen. When the cell numbers are increased beyond that, the same rules for atypia (usually ADH) and carcinoma in situ used for hyperplasia may be applied. Thus there are papillomas with focal atypia that may qualify for atypical hyperplasia (see earlier discussion). When the cell proliferation is uniform and attains the features seen in patterns in ductal carcinoma in situ, noninvasive papillary carcinoma is diagnosed (see Chapter 11).

Other lesions bearing resemblance to papilloma are discussed here for convenience, because they remain a portion of the differential diagnosis of those lesions. These include nipple adenoma (florid papillomatosis of the nipple) and nodular adenosis (ductal adenoma).

Nipple adenoma is a term used to describe a variety of appearances that may present in the nipple or immediately adjacent tissues. Patterns of hyperplasia with pseudoinvasion of dense stroma may be taken to be the basic features of these lesions. They may be misinterpreted clinically as Paget's disease because of irregularities of the surface of the nipple. However, they rarely ulcerate and therefore do not have the moist, red appearance of the eczematous features of Paget's disease. These lesions have localized areas of hyperplasia of slightly varying patterns intermixed with fibrous and cystic changes that may suggest atypia. Nipple adenomas or subareolar papillomatosis usually are diagnosed when they are approximately 1 cm or smaller. Patterns of papilloma are also mimicked. Careful histologic sampling and complete excision are important, because foci of carcinoma have been described in such lesions but apparently are rare.[165,166] These lesions often have nuclear hyperchromatism and a relatively high nuclear cytoplasmic ratio, as well as fibrosis—features that may be worrisome.[167] Complex patterns of epithelial hyperplasia enveloped by fibrosis may lead to the mistaken diagnosis of malignancy. Careful attention to these features avoids overdiagnosis of malignancy.[168]

Nodular adenosis and *ductal adenoma* are similar terms for an important group of lesions presenting varied histology. These lesions are most closely related to papillomas with unusual patterns of sclerosis and adenosis.[169] Because these lesions are characteristically surrounded by dense fibrous tissue within which epithelial cells are pseudoinvasive, they may be overdiagnosed as malignancy by the unwary (Figure 7-20).

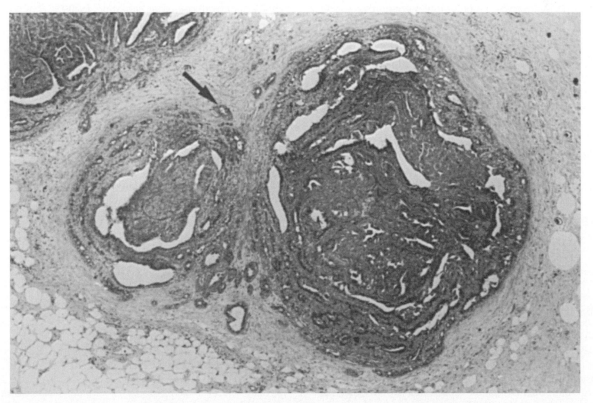

FIG. **7-20** Proliferating glandular epithelium of a "ductal adenoma." Irregularities at the interface between adenotic elements and fibrous capsule simulate invasion *(arrow).* (×70.)

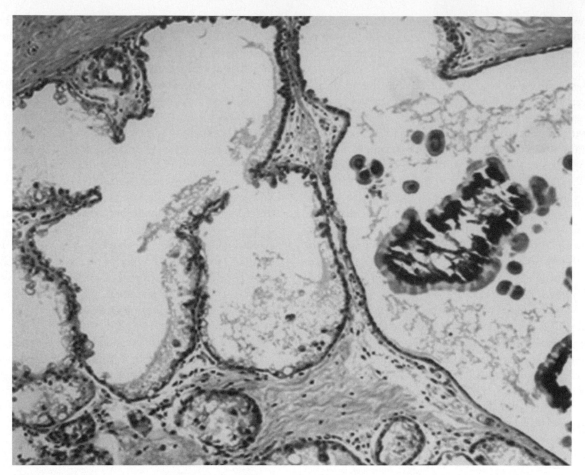

FIG. **7-21** Portion of a dilated lobular unit meriting the term *enlarged lobular unit with columnar alteration.* (×200.)

An increasingly important and benign lesion comes under many different terms and is often found with mammography because of secretory calcifications within. It is a favored site for the appearance of ADH and may be associated with other atypical lesions in the area.[22,23] We prefer the descriptive term *enlarged lobular unit with columnar alteration,* adding whatever other features may be present, such as prominent apocrine or secretory change (Figure 7-21).

REFERENCES

1. Is "fibrocystic disease" of the breast precancerous? *Arch Pathol Lab Med* 110:171, 1986.
2. Fitzgibbons PL, Henson DE, Hutter RV: Benign breast changes and the risk for subsequent breast cancer: an update of the 1985 consensus statement: Cancer Committee of the College of American Pathologists, *Arch Pathol Lab Med* 122:1J053, 1998.
3. Ernster VL et al: Effects of caffeine-free diet on benign breast disease, *Surgery* 91:263, 1982.
4. Kersey P et al: Cyclical mastopathy: an evaluation of methods of assessment, *J Clin Epidemiol* 42:53, 1989.
5. Leinster SJ, Whitehouse GH, Walsh PV: Cyclical mastalgia: clinical and mammographic observations in a screened population, *Br J Surg* 74:220, 1987.
6. Warren JC: The surgeon and the pathologist, *JAMA* 100:1, 1905.
7. Bartow SA et al: Fibrocystic disease: a continuing enigma, *Pathol Annu* 17:93, 1982.
8. Davis HH, Simons M, Davis JB: Cystic disease of the breast: relationship to carcinoma, *Cancer* 17:957, 1964.
9. Foote FW, Stewart FW: Comparative studies of cancerous versus noncancerous breasts. I. Basic morphologic characteristics, *Ann Surg* 121:6, 1945.
10. Dupont WD, Page DL: Risk factors for breast cancer in women with proliferative breast disease, *N Engl J Med* 312:146, 1985.
11. Hutter RV: Goodbye to "fibrocystic disease", *N Engl J Med* 312:179, 1985.
12. Love SM, Gelman RS, Silen W: Sounding board: fibrocystic "disease" of the breast—a nondisease? *N Engl J Med* 307:1010, 1982.
13. Ernster VL: The epidemiology of benign breast disease, *Epidemiol Rev* 3:184, 1981.
14. Bartow SA et al: Prevalence of benign, atypical, and malignant breast lesions in populations at different risk for breast cancer, *Cancer* 60:2751, 1987.
15. Frantz VK et al: Incidence of chronic cystic disease in so-called "normal breasts": a study based on 225 postmortem examinations, *Cancer* 4:762, 1951.
16. Sandison AT: *An autopsy study of the adult human breast: with special reference to proliferative epithelial changes of importance*

in the pathology of the breast, Bethesda, MD, 1962, National Cancer Institute Monograph.

17. Urbanski S et al: The association of histological and radiological indicators of breast cancer risk, *Br J Cancer* 58:474, 1988.

18. Wellings SR, Jensen HM, Marcum RG: An atlas of subgross pathology of the human breast with special reference to possible precancerous lesions, *J Natl Cancer Inst* 55:231, 1975.

19. Haagensen CD: The relationship of gross cystic disease of the breast and carcinoma, *Ann Surg* 185:375, 1977.

20. Haagensen CD (ed): *Diseases of the breast,* ed 3, Philadelphia, 1986, WB Saunders.

21. Bloodgood JC: The pathology of chronic cystic mastitis of the female breast, with special consideration of the blue-domed cyst, *Arch Surg* 3:445, 1921.

22. Shaaban AM et al: Histopathologic types of benign breast lesions and the risk of breast cancer: case-control study, *Am J Surg Pathol* 26:421, 2002.

23. Fraser JL et al: Columnar alteration with prominent apical snouts and secretions: a spectrum of changes frequently present in breast biopsies performed for microcalcifications, *Am J Surg Pathol* 22:1521, 1998.

24. Page DL, Dupont WD, Jensen RA: Papillary apocrine change of the breast associated with atypical hyperplasia and risk of breast cancer, *Cancer Epidemiol Biomarkers Prev* 5:29, 1996.

25. Dixon JM et al: The morphological basis of human breast cyst populations, *Br J Surg* 70:604, 1983.

26. Dixon JM: Cystic disease and fibroadenoma of the breast: natural history and relation to breast cancer risk, *Br Med Bull* 47:258, 1991.

27. Dixon JM, Lumsden AB, Miller WR: The relationship of cyst type to risk factors for breast cancer and the subsequent development of breast cancer in patients with breast cystic disease, *Eur J Cancer Clin Oncol* 21:1047, 1985.

28. Dixon JM, Scott WN, Miller WR: Natural history of cystic disease: importance of cyst type, *Br J Surg* 72:190, 1985.

29. Vilanova JR et al: Early apocrine change in hyperplastic cystic disease, *Histopathology* 7:693, 1983.

30. Azzopardi JG: *Problems in breast pathology,* Philadelphia, 1979, WB Saunders.

31. Mazoujian G et al: Immunohistochemistry of a breast gross cystic disease fluid protein (GCDFP-15): a marker of apocrine epithelium and breast carcinomas with apocrine features, *Am J Pathol* 110:105, 1983.

32. Bundred NJ et al: Is there an increased risk of breast cancer in women who have had a breast cyst aspirated? *Br J Cancer* 64:953, 1991.

33. Page DL, Dupont WD: Are breast cysts a premalignant marker? *Eur J Cancer Clin Oncol* 22:635, 1986.

34. Dixon et al: Risk of breast cancer in women with palpable breast cysts: a prospective study—Edinburgh Breast Group, *Lancet* 353:1742, 1999.

35. Wellings SR, Alpers CE: Apocrine cystic metaplasia: subgross pathology and prevalence in cancer-associated versus random autopsy breasts, *Hum Pathol* 18:381, 1987.

36. Dixon JM et al: Periductal mastitis and duct ectasia: different conditions with different aetiologies, *Br J Surg* 83:820, 1996.

37. Carter CL, Corle DK, Micozzi MS: A prospective study of the development of breast cancer in 16,692 women with benign breast disease, *Am J Epidemiol* 128:467, 1988.

38. Dupont WD et al: Breast cancer risk associated with proliferative breast disease and atypical hyperplasia, *Cancer* 71:1258, 1993.

39. Dupont WD et al: The epidemiologic study of anatomic markers for increased risk of mammary cancer, *Pathol Res Pract* 166:471, 1980.

40. Eusebi V et al: Long-term follow-up of in situ carcinoma of the breast with special emphasis on clinging carcinoma, *Semin Diagn Pathol* 6:165, 1989.

41. Kodlin D et al: Chronic mastopathy and breast cancer: a follow up study, *Cancer* 39:2603, 1977.

42. London SJ, Connolly JL, Schnitt SJ: A prospective study of benign breast disease and risk of breast cancer, *JAMA* 267:941, 1992.

43. Moskowitz M et al: Proliferative disorders of the breast as risk factors for breast cancer in a self-selected screened population: pathologic markers, *Radiology* 134:289, 1980.

44. Palli D et al: Benign breast disease and breast cancer: a case-control study in a cohort in Italy, *Int J Cancer* 47:703, 1991.

45. Marshall LM et al: Risk of breast cancer associated with atypical hyperplasia of lobular and ductal types, *Cancer Epidemiol Biomarkers Prev* 6:297, 1997.

46. Page DL: Cancer risk assessment in benign biopsies, *Hum Pathol* 17:871, 1986.

47. Page DL et al: Atypical hyperplastic lesions of the female breast: a long-term follow-up study, *Cancer* 55:2698, 1985.

48. Page DL, Rogers LW: Combined histologic and cytologic criteria for the diagnosis of mammary atypical ductal hyperplasia, *Hum Pathol* 23:1095, 1992.

49. Foote FW, Stewart FW: Comparative studies of cancerous versus noncancerous breasts. II. Role of so-called chronic cystic mastitis in mammary carcinogenesis; influence of certain hormones on human breast structure, *Ann Surg* 121:197, 1945.

50. Page DL: The woman at high risk for breast cancer: importance of hyperplasia, *Surg Clin North Am* 76:221, 1996.

51. Jensen RA et al: Invasive breast cancer (IBC) risk in women with sclerosing adenosis (SA), *Cancer* 64:1977, 1989.

52. Simpson JF, Page DL: Altered expression of a structural protein (fodrin) within epithelial proliferative disease of the breast, *Am J Pathol* 141:285, 1992.

53. Bocker W et al: An immunohistochemical study of the breast using antibodies to basal and luminal keratins, alpha-smooth muscle actin, vimentin, collagen IV and laminin. Part II: epitheliosis and ductal carcinoma in situ, *Virchows Arch A Pathol Anat Histopathol* 421:323, 1992.

54. Going JJ: Stages on the way to breast cancer, *J Pathol* 199:1, 2003.

55. Black EM, Chabon AB: In-situ carcinoma of the breast, *Pathol Annu* 4:185, 1969.

56. McCarty KS Jr et al: Histopathologic study of subcutaneous mastectomy specimens from patients with carcinoma of the contralateral breast, *Surg Gynecol Obstet* 147:682, 1978.

57. Ackerman LV, Katzenstein AL: The concept of minimal breast cancer and the pathologist's role in the diagnosis of "early carcinoma", *Cancer* 39:2755, 1977.

58. Ashikari R, Huvos AG, Snyde RE: A clinicopathologic study of atypical lesions of the breast, *Cancer* 33:310, 1974.

59. Fisher ER: The pathology of breast cancer as it relates to its evolution, prognosis and treatment, *Clin Oncol* 1:703, 1982.

60. Page DL, Anderson TJ (eds): *Diagnostic histopathology of the breast,* Edinburgh, 1987, Churchill Livingstone.

61. Haagensen CD et al: Lobular neoplasia (so-called lobular carcinoma in situ) of the breast, *Cancer* 42:737, 1978.

62. Page DL et al: Lobular neoplasia of the breast: higher risk for subsequent invasive cancer predicted by more extensive disease, *Hum Pathol* 22:1232, 1991.

63. Fechner RE: Epithelial alterations in the extralobular ducts of breast with lobular carcinoma, *Arch Pathol* 93:164, 1972.

64. Page DL, Dupont WD, Rogers LW: Ductal involvement by cells of atypical lobular hyperplasia in the breast, *Hum Pathol* 19:201, 1988.

65. Tavassoli FA, Norris HJ: A comparison of the results of long-term follow-up for atypical intraductal hyperplasia and intraductal hyperplasia of the breast, *Cancer* 65:518, 1990.

66. Jensen HM: Breast pathology, emphasizing precancerous and cancer-associated lesions. In Bulbrook RD, Taylor DJ (eds): *Commentaries on research in breast disease*, New York, 1981, Liss.

67. Rosai J: Borderline epithelial lesions of the breast, *Am J Surg Pathol* 15:209, 1991.

68. Schnitt SJ et al: Interobserver reproducibility in the diagnosis of ductal proliferative breast lesions using standardized criteria, *Am J Surg Pathol* 16:1133, 1996.

69. Eusebi V et al: Long-term follow-up of in situ carcinoma of the breast, *Semin Diagn Pathol* 11:223, 1994.

70. Bijker N et al: Risk factors for recurrence and metastasis after breast-conserving therapy for ductal carcinoma-in-situ: analysis of European Organization for Research and Treatment of Cancer Trial 10853, *J Clin Oncol* 19:2263, 2001.

71. Ewing J: *Neoplastic disease*, Philadelphia, 1919, WB Saunders.

72. Dawson EK: A histological study of the normal mamma in relation to tumor growth: early development to maturity, *Edinburgh Med J* 41:653, 1934.

73. Eusebi V et al: Adenomyoepithelioma of the breast with a distinctive type of apocrine adenosis, *Histopathology* 11:305, 1987.

74. Simpson JF, Page DL, Dupont WD: Apocrine adenosis: a mimic of mammary carcinoma, *Surg Pathol* 3:289, 1990.

75. Carter DJ, Rosen PP: Atypical apocrine metaplasia in sclerosing lesions of the breast: a study of 51 patients, *Mod Pathol* 4:1, 1991.

76. D'Ardenne AJ: Use of basement membrane markers in tumour diagnosis, *J Clin Pathol* 42:449, 1989.

77. Siegel GP et al: Stages of neoplastic transformation of human breast tissue as monitored by dissolution of basement membrane components: an immunoperoxidase study, *Invasion Metastasis* 1:54, 1981.

78. Clement PB, Azzopardi JG: Microglandular adenosis of the breast: a lesion simulating tubular carcinoma, *Histopathology* 7:169, 1983.

79. McDivitt RW, Stewart FW, Berg JW: *Tumors of the breast*, ed 2, Washington, DC, 1968, Armed Forces Institute of Pathology.

80. Rosen PP: Microglandular adenosis: a benign lesion simulating invasive mammary carcinoma, *Am J Surg Pathol* 7:137, 1983.

81. Tavassoli FA, Norris HJ: Microglandular adenosis of the breast: a clinicopathologic study of 11 cases with ultrastructural observations, *Am J Surg Pathol* 7:731, 1983.

82. Kiaer H et al: Adenomyoepithelial adenosis and low-grade malignant adenomyoepithelioma of the breast, *Virchows Arch A Pathol Anat Histopathol* 405:55, 1984.

83. James BA, Cranor ML, Rosen PP: Carcinoma of the breast arising in microglandular adenosis, *Am J Clin Pathol* 100:507, 1993.

84. Rosenblum MK, Parrazella R, Rosen PP: Is microglandular adenosis a precancerous disease? A study of carcinoma arising therein, *Am J Surg Path* 10:237, 1986.

85. Fenoglio C, Lattes R: Sclerosing papillary proliferations in the female breast, *Cancer* 33:691, 1974.

86. Jacobs TW et al: Radial scars in benign breast-biopsy specimens and the risk of breast cancer, *N Engl J Med* 340:430, 1999.

87. Battersby S, Anderson TJ: Myofibroblast activity of radial scars, *J Pathol* 147:33, 1985.

88. Anderson TJ, Battersby S: Radial scars of benign and malignant breasts: comparative features and significance, *J Pathol* 147:23, 1985.

89. Hughes LE: Non-lactational inflammation and duct ectasia, *Br Med Bull* 47:272, 1991.

90. Rees BI, Gravelle IH, Hughes LE: Nipple retraction in duct ectasia, *Br J Surg* 64:577, 1977.

91. Dixon JM et al: Mammary duct ectasia, *Br J Surg* 70:601, 1983.

92. Bundred NJ, Dixon JM, Lumsden AB: Are the lesions of duct ectasia sterile? *Br J Surg* 72:844, 1985.

93. Orson LW, Cigtay OS: Fat necrosis of the breast: characteristic xeromammographic appearance, *Radiology* 146:35, 1983.

94. Bargum K, Moller NS: Case report: fat necrosis of the breast appearing as oil cysts with fat-fluid levels, *Br J Radiol* 66:718, 1993.

95. Ikard RW, Perkins D: Mammary tuberculosis: a rare modern disease, *South Med J* 70:208, 1977.

96. Wapnir IL et al: Latent mammary tuberculosis: a case report, *Surgery* 98:976, 1985.

97. Deininger HK: Wegener's granulomatosis of the breast, *Radiology* 154:59, 1985.

98. Douglas AC et al: Midline and Wegener's granulomatosis, *Ann N Y Acad Sci* 278:618, 1976.

99. Wilson ME: Wegener's granulomatosis: another cause of breast masses, *Am J Med* 95:116, 1993.

100. Banik S et al: Sarcoidosis of the breast, *J Clin Pathol* 39:446, 1986.

101. Fitzgibbons PL, Simley DF, Kern WH: Sarcoidosis presenting initially as breast mass: report of two cases, *Hum Pathol* 16:851, 1985.

102. Symmers WS, McKeown KC: Tuberculosis of the breast, *BMJ* 289:48, 1984.

103. Dupont WD et al: Long-term risk of breast cancer in women with fibroadenoma, *N Engl J Med* 331:10, 1994.

104. Levi F et al: Incidence of breast cancer in women with fibroadenoma, *Int J Cancer* 57:681, 1994.

105. Diaz NM, Palmer JO, McDivitt RW: Carcinoma arising within fibroadenomas of the breast: a clinicopathologic study of 105 patients, *Am J Clin Pathol* 95:614, 1991.

106. Fondo EY et al: The problem of carcinoma developing in a fibroadenoma: recent experience at Memorial Hospital, *Cancer* 43:563, 1979.

107. Pick PW, Iossifides IA: Occurrence of breast carcinoma within a fibroadenoma: a review, *Arch Pathol Lab Med* 108:590, 1984.

108. Carter BA et al: No elevation in long-term breast carcinoma risk for women with fibroadenomas that contain atypical hyperplasia, *Cancer* 92:30, 2001.

109. Goodman ZD, Taxy JB: Fibroadenomas of the breast with prominent smooth muscle, *Am J Surg Pathol* 5:99, 1981.

110. Salm R: Epidermoid metaplasia in mammary fibroadenoma with formation of keratin cysts, *J Pathol Bacteriol* 74:221, 1957.

111. Organ CH Jr, Organ BC: Fibroadenoma of the female breast: a critical clinical assessment, *J Natl Med Assoc* 75:701, 1983.

112. Kovi J, Chu HB, Leffall LD Jr: Sclerosing lobular hyperplasia manifesting as a palpable mass of the breast in young black women, *Hum Pathol* 15:336, 1984.

113. Hasson J, Pope CH: Mammary infarcts associated with pregnancy presenting as breast tumors, *Surgery* 49:313, 1961.

114. Majmudar B, Rosales-Quintana S: Infarction of breast fibroadenomas during pregnancy, *JAMA* 231:963, 1975.

115. Wilkinson L, Green WO Jr: Infarction of the breast lesion during pregnancy and lactation, *Cancer* 17:1567, 1964.

116. Fechner RE: Fibroadenoma and related lesions. In Page DL, Anderson TJ (eds): *Diagnostic histopathology of the breast*, Edinburgh, 1987, Churchill Livingstone.

117. Hessler C, Schnyder P, Ozzello L: Hamartoma of the breast: diagnostic observation of 16 cases, *Radiology* 126:95, 1979.

118. Linell F et al: Breast hamartomas: an important entity in mammary pathology, *Virchows Arch A Pathol Anat Histol* 383:253, 1979.

119. Arrigoni MG, Dockerty MB, Judd ES: The identification and treatment of mammary hamartoma, *Surg Gynecol Obstet* 133:577, 1971.

120. Duchatelle V, Auberger E, Amouroux J: Hamartomas du sein, *Ann Pathol* 6:335, 1986.

121. Dyreborg U, Starklint H: Adenolipoma mammae, *Acta Radiol Diagn (Stockh)* 16:362, 1975.

122. Duray PH et al: Adolescent cellular fibroadenomas: a clinical and pathologic study, *Lab Invest* 50:17A, 1984.

123. Ashikari R, Farrow JH, O'Hara J: Fibroadenomas in the breast of juveniles, *Surg Gynecol Obstet* 132:259, 1971.

124. Oberman HA: Breast lesions in the adolescent female, *Ann Pathol* 14:175, 1979.

125. Pike AM, Oberman HA: Juvenile (cellular) fibroadenoma: a clinicopathologic study, *Am J Surg Pathol* 9:730, 1985.

126. Mies C, Rosen PP: Juvenile fibroadenoma with atypical epithelial hyperplasia, *Am J Surg Pathol* 11:184, 1987.

127. Chua CL, Thomas A: Cystosarcoma phyllodes tumors, *Surg Gynecol Obstet* 166:302, 1988.

128. Maier WP et al: Cystosarcoma phyllodes mammae, *Oncology* 22:145, 1968.

129. Cant PJ et al: Case for conservative management of selected fibroadenomas of the breast, *Br J Surg* 74:857, 1987.

130. Cant PJ et al: Non-operative management of breast masses diagnosed as fibroadenoma, *Br J Surg* 82:792, 1995.

131. Wilkinson S et al: Fibroadenoma of the breast: a follow-up of conservative management, *Br J Surg* 76:390, 1989.

132. Rosen PP, Ernsberger D: Mammary fibromatosis: a benign spindle-cell tumor with significant risk for local recurrence, *Cancer* 63:1363, 1989.

133. Wargotz ES et al: Fibromatosis of the breast: a clinical and pathological study of 28 cases, *Am J Surg Pathol* 11:38, 1987.

134. Hertel BG, Zaloudek C, Kempson RL: Breast adenomas, *Cancer* 37:2891, 1976.

135. Persaud V, Talerman A, Jordan RP: Pure adenoma of the breast, *Arch Pathol* 86:481, 1968.

136. Moross T, Lang AP, Mahoney L: Tubular adenoma of breast, *Arch Pathol Lab Med* 107:84, 1983.

137. O'Hara MF, Page DL: Adenomas of the breast and ectopic breast under lactational influences, *Hum Pathol* 16:707, 1985.

138. James K, Bridger J, Anthony PP: Breast tumour of pregnancy ("lactating adenoma"), *J Pathol* 156:37, 1988.

139. Müller J: *Uber den Feinern Bau und die Formen der Krankhaften Geschwulste*, Berlin, 1838, G Reimer.

140. Hough AJ, Page DL: Prospectives on cartilaginous tumors: nomenclature, nosology, and neologism, *Hum Pathol* 20:927, 1989.

141. Blichert-Toft M et al: Clinical course of cytosarcoma phyllodes related to histologic appearance, *Surg Gynecol Obstet* 140:929, 1975.

142. Page DL, Anderson TJ, Johnson RL: Sarcomas of the breast. In Page DL, Anderson TJ (eds): *Diagnostic histopathology of the breast*, Edinburgh, 1987, Churchill Livingstone.

143. Norris HJ, Taylor HB: Relationship of histologic features to behavior of cystosarcoma phyllodes: analysis of 94 cases, *Cancer* 22:22, 1967.

144. Hart WR, Bauer R, Oberman H: Cystosarcoma phyllodes: a clinicopathologic study of twenty-six hypercellular periductal stromal tumors of the breast, *Am Clin Pathol* 70:211, 1978.

145. Murad TM et al: Histopathological and clinical correlations of cystosarcoma phyllodes, *Arch Path Lab Med* 112:752, 1988.

146. Pietruszka M, Barnes L: Cystosarcoma phyllodes: a clinicopathologic analysis of forty-two cases, *Cancer* 41:1974, 1978.

147. Briggs RM, Walters M, Rosenthal D: Cystosarcoma phyllodes in adolescent female patients, *Am J Surg* 146:712, 1983.

148. Leveque J et al: Malignant cystosarcomas phyllodes of the breast in adolescent females, *Eur J Obstet Gynecol Reprod Biol* 54:197, 1994.

149. Blumencranz PW, Gray GF: Cystosarcoma phyllodes: clinical and pathological study, *N Y State J Med* 78:623, 1978.

150. Chaney AW et al: Primary treatment of cystosarcoma phyllodes of the breast, *Cancer* 89:1502, 2000.

151. Meneses A et al: Prognostic factors on 45 cases of phyllodes tumors, *J Exp Clin Cancer Res* 19:69, 2000.

152. Reinfuss M et al: The treatment and prognosis of patients with phyllodes tumor of the breast: an analysis of 170 cases, *Cancer* 77:910, 1996.

153. Moffat C et al: Phyllodes tumour of the breast: a clinicopathological review of thirty-two cases, *Histopathology* 27:205, 1995.

154. Hajdu SI, Espinosa MH, Robbins GF: Recurrent cystosarcoma phyllodes: a clinicopathologic study of 32 cases, *Cancer* 38:1402, 1976.

155. Lindquist KD et al: Recurrent and metastatic cystosarcoma phyllodes, *Am J Surg* 144:341, 1982.

156. West TL, Weiland JH, Clagett OT: Cystosarcoma phyllodes, *Ann Surg* 173:520, 1971.

157. Martin RG, Gallager HS: Sarcomas of the breast. In Gallager HG et al (eds): *The breast*, St Louis, 1978, Mosby.

158. Ohuchi N et al: Origin and extension of intraductal papillomas of the breast: a three-dimensional reconstruction study, *Breast Cancer Res Treat* 4:117, 1984.

159. Carter D: Intraductal papillary tumors of the breast: a study of 78 cases, *Cancer* 39:1689, 1977.

160. Page DL et al: Subsequent breast carcinoma risk after biopsy with atypia in a breast papilloma, *Cancer* 78:258, 1996.

161. Ohuchi N, Rikiya A, Kasai M: Possible cancerous change of intraductal papillomas of the breast: a 3D reconstruction study of 25 cases, *Cancer* 54:605, 1984.

162. Haagensen CD et al (eds): *Breast carcinoma risk and detection,* Philadelphia, 1981, WB Saunders.
163. Flint A, Oberman HA: Infarction and squamous metaplasia of intraductal papilloma: a benign breast lesion that may simulate carcinoma, *Hum Pathol* 15:764, 1984.
164. Reddick RL, Jennette JC, Askin FB: Squamous metaplasia of the breast, *Am J Clin Pathol* 84:530, 1985.
165. Gudjonsdottir A, Hagerstrand I, Ostberg G: Adenoma of the nipple with carcinomatous development, *Acta Pathol Microbiol Scand [A]* 79:676, 1971.
166. Rosen PP, Caicco JA: Florid papillomatosis of the nipple: a study of 51 patients, including nine with mammary carcinoma, *Am J Surg Pathol* 10:84, 1986.
167. Oberman HA: Benign breast lesions confused with carcinomas. In McDivitt RW et al (eds): *The breast,* Baltimore, 1984, Williams & Wilkins.
168. Perzin KH, Lattes R: Papillary adenoma of the nipple (florid papillomatosis, adenoma, adenomatosis): a clinicopathology study, *Cancer* 54:605, 1984.
169. Azzopardi JG, Salm R: Ductal adenoma of the breast: a lesion which can mimic carcinoma, *J Pathol* 144:11, 1984.

8

Congenital and Acquired Disturbances of Breast Development and Growth

KIRBY I. BLAND

LYNN J. ROMRELL

Chapter Outline

Development of the Breast

The mammary glands, or breasts, are considered highly modified sudoriferous glands. Basically, the glands develop as ingrowths from the ectoderm, which form the ducts and alveoli. The supporting vascularized connective tissue is derived from mesenchyme. At about the fifth or sixth week of development, two ventral bands of somewhat thickened ectoderm, called the *mammary ridges* (or *milk lines*), are present in the embryo (Figure 8-1). In many mammals, paired mammary glands develop along these ridges, which extend from the base of the forelimb (future axilla) to the region of the hindlimb (inguinal region). The ridges are not prominent in the human embryo and disappear shortly after their formation, except for a small portion that persists in the pectoral region, where a single pair of glands usually develops. Accessory nipples (polythelia) or accessory mammary glands (polymastia) may occur along the original mammary ridges or milk lines (Figure 8-2) if the structure fails to undergo its normal regression.

Each gland develops as the ingrowth of the ectoderm forms a primary bud of tissue in the underlying mesenchyme (Figure 8-3, *A*). Each primary bud gives rise to 15 to 20 secondary buds, or outgrowths (Figure 8-3, *B*). During the fetal period, epithelial cords develop from the secondary buds and extend into the surrounding connective tissue. By the end of prenatal life, lumens have developed in the outgrowths, forming the lactiferous ducts and their branches (Figure 8-3, *C*). At birth, the lactiferous ducts open into a shallow epithelial

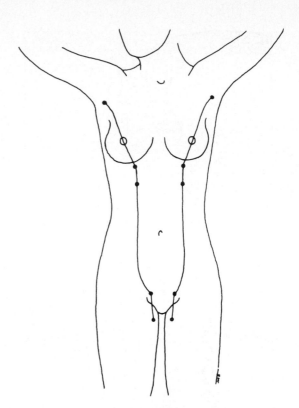

FIG. **8-2** Mammary milk line. After development of the milk bud in the pectoral area of ectodermal thickening, the "milk streak" extends from the axilla to the inguinal areas. At week 9 of intrauterine development, atrophy of the bud has occurred except for the presence of the supernumerary nipples or breast.

depression, known as the *mammary pit*. The pit becomes elevated and transformed into the nipple shortly after birth as a result of proliferation of the mesenchyme underlying the presumptive nipple and areola (Figure 8-3, *D*). Failure of the elevation of the pit to occur results in a congenital malformation known as *inverted nipple*.

In newborn infants of both sexes, the breasts often show a transient enlargement and may produce some secretion, often called *witch's milk*. These transitory changes occur in response to maternal hormones that cross the placenta during fetal development. At birth, the breasts appear similar in both sexes, demonstrating the presence of only the main lactiferous ducts. The glands remain underdeveloped until puberty, when in the female the breasts enlarge rapidly in response to estrogen and progesterone secretion by the ovaries. The hormonal stimulation causes proliferation of the glandular tissue as well as fat and other connective tissue elements associated with the breast. The glandular tissue remains incompletely developed until pregnancy occurs. At this time, the intralobular ducts undergo rapid development and form buds that become alveoli.

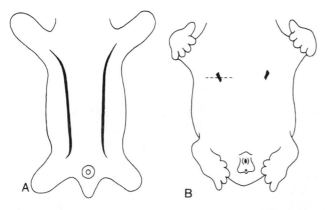

FIG. **8-1** The mammary ridges and their regression. **A,** Ventral view of an embryo at the beginning of the fifth week of development (about 28 days), showing the mammary ridges that extend from the forelimb to the hindlimb. **B,** A similar view of the ventral embryo at the end of the sixth week, showing the remains of the ridges located in the pectoral region.

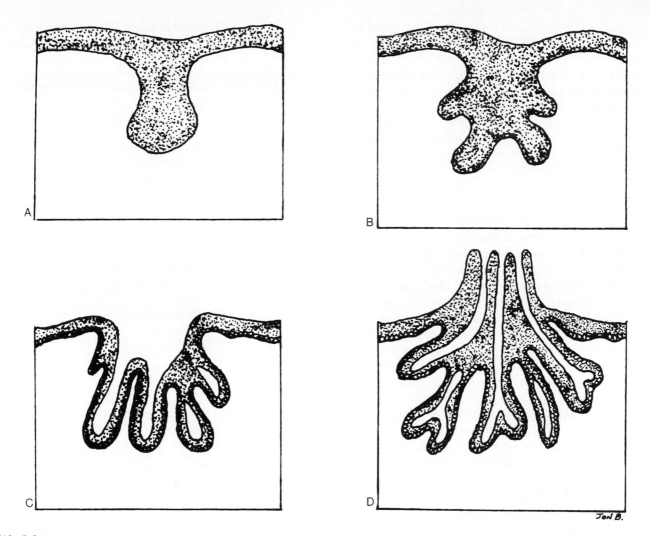

FIG. **8-3** Sections through evolutionary development and growth of the mammary bud. **A** to **C,** Similar sections showing the developing gland at successive stages between the twelfth week and birth. The mammary pit develops, and major lactiferous ducts are present at the end of gestation. **D,** A similar section showing the elevation of the mammary pit by proliferation of the underlying connective tissue forming the nipple soon after birth.

Russo and Russo[1-3] have shown that the risk of developing breast cancer is heavily influenced by endocrinologic and reproductive influences, especially those created during pregnancy. The risk of breast cancer has long been known to show inverse relationship with early parity (for review, see Russo and colleagues[4]). The risk of breast cancer increases with the age at which a woman bears her first child. This protection appears to be inversely related to the length of time between menarche and the first pregnancy, as evidenced by the increased risk of cancer if the length of this interval is more than 14 years. Pregnancy has to occur before age 30 to have a protective effect on breast cancer risk. Women who become pregnant after age 30 have a risk above that of nulliparous women. Multiparity does confer additional protection; however, the protective effect is primarily limited to the first birth and persists at all subsequent ages. The mechanism responsible for early first-term pregnancy protection remains largely unknown. Evidence suggests that the differentiation of the mammary gland that is induced by full-term pregnancy inhibits carcinogenic initiation. Studies summarized by Russo and colleagues[4] suggest that the breast of late parous and nulliparous women exhibit characteristics of undifferentiated breast cells that are predisposed to undergo neoplastic differentiation.

The role of genes in both normal development and neoplastic changes in the breast is of major interest. Lewis[5] has recently reviewed the growing literature on the genetic determinants that establish and maintain the integrity of the mammary cells. Recently, there has been a great deal of interest in families of regulatory genes, called *homeobox genes*. These genes encode for proteins that recognize and bind to specific DNA sequences of other genes that control the sequential development of structures and organs. Recent studies of gene expression strongly suggest that homeobox genes may function in the development of the mammary gland and may play a role in the development of breast cancer.

Amastia

The congenital absence of one or both breasts (amastia) is a rare clinical anomaly.[6] The first recorded reference to amastia is found in "The Song of Solomon" in the Bible (8:viii): "We have a little sister, and she hath no breast: What shall we do for our sister in the day when she shall be spoken for?" Froriep first described true absence of the breast in 1839.[7] The association of bilateral amastia with other congenital anomalies was described in 1882 by Gilly,[8] who described a 30-year-old woman who presented with absence of the ulna and the ulnar aspect of the right hand. Approximately 50 case reports of amastia were recorded by Deaver and McFarland[9] in their treatise of the breast in 1917. Reports in the literature before the 1960s rarely gave details of amastia or its less severe manifestations.[10] There have been only a few reports of bilateral amastia, defined as complete absence of both breasts and nipples. An extensive review of the literature by Trier[11] documented 43 cases for which data were available. Three presentations were observed: (1) bilateral absence of breasts with congenital ectodermal defects (7 cases), (2) unilateral absence of the breasts (20 cases), and (3) bilateral absence of the breast (16 cases) with variable associated anomalies (Table 8-1).

Subsequently, Tawil and Najjar[12] reported an additional case of congenital bilateral absence of breasts and nipples in a 12-year-old Arab girl with abnormal ears, macrostomia, and chronic glomerulonephritis. Previously, Goldenring and Crelin[13] described a mother and daughter with similar phenotypes. More recently, Nelson and Cooper[14] documented a family in which the father and two of three daughters were found to have bilateral absence or hypoplasia of the nipples or breast tissue with associated minor defects. The mode of inheritance of this combination of defects is autosomal dominant.[15]

Unilateral absence of the breast (Figure 8-4) is more common than bilateral amastia, and such subjects are most commonly female. This rare physical defect occurs as a result of complete failure of the development of the mammary ridge at about the sixth week in utero. Most often, abnormalities are not associated with bilateral absence of nipple and breast tissue. However, Trier[11] has observed amastia in association with cleft

TABLE 8-1	Congenital Anomalies Associated with Bilateral Absence of the Nipples and Breast Tissues
NO. OF PATIENTS	**REPORTED ANOMALIES**
1	Atrophy of the right pectoral muscle; absence of the ulna and ulnar side of the hand
1	Absence of finger on the right hand; deformity of the right foot
1	Bilateral lobster-claw deformity of the hands and feet; cleft palate
2	Sparse axillary and pubic hair; saddle nose; hypertelorism; high-arched palate
1	Short status; short, small nose; broad nasal root; protrusion of the external ear; high-arched palate
10	No anomalies

From Trier WC: *Plast Reconstr Surg* 36:431, 1965.

palate; hypertelorism and saddle nose; and anomalies of the pectoral muscle, ulna, hand, foot, palate, ears, genitourinary tract, and habitus. Occasionally, several members of a family have been affected. At least four reports[11,13,16,17] document the transmission of this anomaly with pedigree penetrance consistent with dominant inheritance.

Triolo and associates[18] observed a case of athelia and amastia in a 28-year-old woman with associated severe dental alterations, nail dystrophies, and irregular cutaneous hyperpigmentation but normal sweating. The diagnosis was hidrotic ectodermal dysplasia, an autosomal dominant hereditary disease. The syndrome was present in the father and two brothers of the patient. The patient also had urinary incontinence due to sphincter urethrae agenesis.

Rich and associates[19] described a case of ureteral triplication as a component of an autosomal dominant syndrome consisting of bilateral amastia, pectus excavatum, umbilical hernia, patent ductus arteriosus, dysmorphic low-set ears, ptosis, epicanthic folds with an antimongoloid slant of the eyes, ocular hypertelorism, high-arched palate, flat broad nasal bridge, tapered digits, cubitus valgus, and syndactyly. Nelson and Cooper[14] have also reported the autosomal dominant transmission of breast hypoplasia or absence of the nipples in association with webbing of the fingers. Rich and colleagues[19] are the only investigators to report genetically transmitted ureteral triplication, either alone or in association with bilateral amastia.

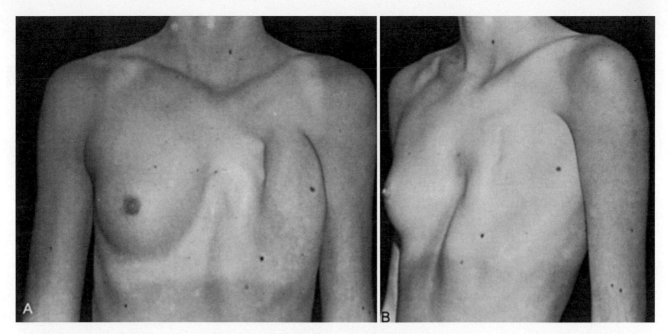

FIG. **8-4 A** and **B,** Unilateral amastia in 20-year-old woman with concomitant chest wall deformity of ipsilateral ribs 3 to 6 and cartilage. In contrast to those with Poland's syndrome, this patient has accessory musculature of the shoulder, including pectoralis major and minor, latissimus dorsi, and serratus anterior muscles. *(Courtesy Dr. John McCraw, Norfolk, VA.)*

Unilateral Congenital Defects of the Breast with Associated Defects of the Chest Wall, Ipsilateral Musculature, Subcutaneous Tissues, and Brachysyndactyly (Poland's Syndrome)

In 1841, Alfred Poland[20] published in *Guy's Hospital Report* the description of a patient who presented with absence of musculature (pectoralis major and minor) of the shoulder girdle and malformations of the ipsilateral upper limb. In this original report of unilateral congenital absence of the pectoralis major and minor muscles, there was associated absence of the external oblique and partial absence of the serratus anterior. Thereafter, numerous authors[21] have reported similar findings, with the additional observation of hypoplasia or complete absence of the breast or nipple, costal cartilage and rib defects (ribs 2, 3, and 4 or ribs 3, 4, and 5), hypoplasia of subcutaneous tissues of the chest wall, and brachysyndactyly. This constellation of clinical findings, whether all or partially present, is currently termed *Poland's syndrome.* Clinical manifestations of this disorder are extremely variable, and rarely can all features be recognized in a single individual.[22-24] Fabian and Fischer[25] reported an unusual case of Poland's syndrome in a newborn infant. There was extension of the

liver through the chest defect and absence of a whole arm rather than hypoplasia and brachysyndactyly.

Poland's syndrome is invariably unilateral, with a higher incidence in female than in male patients. When the chest wall defect (ribs, cartilage, or both) is evident, there is usually a deep concavity on expiration and lung herniation with inspiration (Figure 8-5). The right side is more commonly affected than the left.[26] The most common defect, breast hypoplasia, is readily recognized, and the rudimentary breast tissue is usually higher on the involved side and medially displaced from its normal anatomic position.

Although the cause is unclear, this syndrome is seldom familial. Leukemia has been associated with the syndrome, as have other rare congenital anomalies. Similar defects have been noted with exposure to drugs, such as thalidomide.

Treatment of patients with Poland's syndrome varies with the number of anomalies and their physical expression. With the presentation of one or two typical characteristics of Poland's syndrome, patients usually complain only about their appearance. These patients are not functionally embarrassed by their lack of anterior chest wall muscle mass or the small size of their breast. Only in extreme cases, as with total absence of the costal cartilage or segments of the anterior ribs, are patients physically impaired and emotionally disturbed by their deformity. Surgical procedures to correct the deformities of the chest wall have been documented[24]

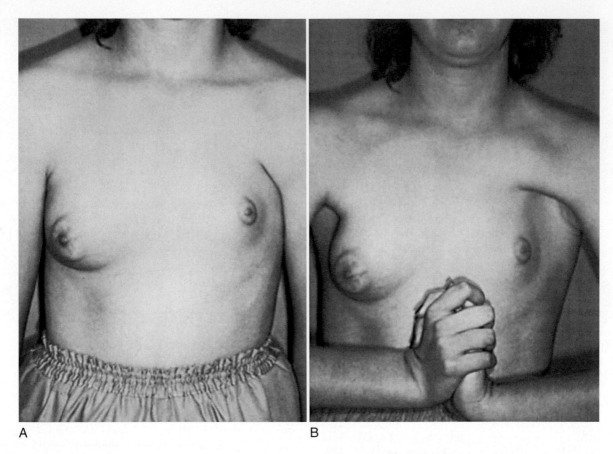

A   B

FIG. **8-5** Poland's syndrome. A 15-year-old girl with Poland's syndrome of left breast. **A,** With shoulder girdle musculature actively contracted. **B,** There is accentuation of the left hypoplastic breast. There is absence of the sternal head of the pectoralis major although the clavicular head is present. *(Courtesy Dr. Hollis H. Caffee, Division of Plastic and Reconstructive Surgery, University of Florida College of Medicine, Gainesville, FL.)*

and include (1) subperiosteal grafts from adjacent ribs with free flaps of latissimus dorsi or external oblique,[27] (2) autologous split-rib grafts,[28] (3) split-rib grafts with periosteum that has been detached posteriorly and rotated from the anterior aspect of the defective rib to the sternum,[29] (4) heterologous bone grafts,[30] (5) metallic mesh implants followed by rib grafts from the opposite chest wall,[31] and (6) customized silicon breast and chest wall prostheses to reconstruct both structures in difficult cases.[32] Ravitch[33] popularized the use of split-rib grafts from the opposite chest wall that are placed across the defect and reinforced with Teflon felt. The technique described by Amoroso and Angelats[34] uses autologous tissue of the latissimus dorsi myocutaneous flap to augment the hypoplastic breast and to contour the anterior chest wall while simultaneously augmenting the involved hypoplastic breast. This procedure, initially attempted by Asp and Sulamaa[27] of Finland, was unsuccessful using a free latissimus dorsi flap. Thus the procedure was abandoned because transplanted muscle atrophied as a result of the omission of the neurovascular pedicle from the

transplant, emphasizing the value of preservation of the pedicle when employing this technique. In 1950, Campbell[35] described the use of a latissimus dorsi muscle flap transferred through the axilla for anterior chest wall reconstruction with preservation of the neurovascular bundle. He, too, abandoned this technique because the flap was associated with a cutaneous component or applied over a breast prosthesis unsuccessfully.

Schneider, Hill, and Brown[36] emphasized the value of a single-stage reconstruction. The high success rate and the reliability of this technique, which uses the latissimus dorsi myocutaneous flap, represents remarkable advance over the aforementioned methods. The cosmetic and functional results of this technique appear superior to those obtained with standard multiple-stage procedures.

Computed tomography (CT) provides useful information in planning reconstructive surgery in patients with Poland's syndrome.[37] Hurwitz, Stofman, and Curtin[38] have recently suggested the use of a three-dimensional CT scan as an adjunct for planning chest wall and breast reconstruction in Poland's syndrome. Follow-up with three-dimensional MRI reformation was used to demonstrate the results of the implant reconstruction. The authors suggest that these imaging techniques can be used to accurately portray the three-dimensional tissue deficit and assist in the selection of muscle transposition flaps and reconstructive technique.

At least two reports confirm a variant of Poland's syndrome associated with large melanotic spots. Because breasts and melanocytes both originate from the ectoderm, abnormalities of breast hypoplasia and hyperpigmentation probably develop from within this germinal layer. Moore and Schosser[39] reported on Becker's melanosis associated with hypoplasia of the breast and pectoralis major muscle. Zubowicz and Bostwick[40] also confirmed two patients with areas of diffuse hyperpigmentation overlying a unilaterally hypoplastic breast. Treatment was directed at reconstructing the breast mound and symmetrically sizing the two areolae. Patients often do not request treatment of the pigmented abnormalities, and standard methods used in the therapy of hyperpigmentation often yield unsatisfactory results. Such hyperpigmented areas appear to have no neoplastic risk.

Iatrogenic Factors That Initiate Breast Hypoplasia

Failure of complete development of the vestigial male or female breast may occur as a consequence of developmental hypomastia (Figure 8-6) or may be initiated by therapeutic manipulation or injury of the mammary anlage in infancy or in the prepubertal interval. Rudimentary breast tissue in the male or female infant lies beneath the primitive nipple/areola complex at approximately the fourth intercostal space. Thus *trauma, incisions, abscess, infectious lesions,* or *radiation therapy* to the breast bud in the infantile or prepubertal era can initiate maldevelopment with hypoplasia of the vestigial breast. The surgeon must be especially aware of the necessity and technique of any incision for drainage of lesions of the areolar complex or masses within the breast bud to avoid subsequent maldevelopment. Furthermore, unilateral development of breast tissue in the adolescent female may represent nonisometric growth of breast tissue in precocious or early pubertal states. With this presentation, cautious observation of the contralateral breast is in order. The surgeon should not perform a biopsy on the rudimentary breast structure or the nipple/areola complex using incisional or excisional techniques. The risk of neoplastic lesions is infinitesimally small in this younger age group, whereas the travesty of irreversible damage to

the breast bud with subsequent hypoplasia of the breast or amastia is a distinct possibility. The bilaterally symmetric nipple/areola and breast complexes overlie the fourth intercostal space of the infant. In the fully developed breasts of the sexually mature female, the complex may extend to the seventh and eighth intercostal spaces. Thus excisional biopsies of any chest wall lesions that are initiated before full maturation of the mammae must be approached cautiously.

Cherup, Siewers, and Futrell[41] documented breast and pectoral muscle maldevelopment after *anterolateral* and *posterolateral thoracotomies* in children. Incisions placed through the third and fourth intercostal spaces for repair of congenital heart lesions were evaluated in 28 patients by these authors. In this series, standard anterolateral thoracotomies resulted in a high frequency of breast or pectoral muscular maldevelopment. Using measurements of volumes of the breast and pectoral muscles with plaster molds and linear dimensions of each chest side, the authors concluded that 60% of patients with these incisions had greater than a 20% difference in volume between the two sides. To avoid these maldevelopment syndromes, when the anterolateral or posterolateral thoracotomy must be used, it should be started anteriorly in the seventh or eighth interspace, below the level to which the breast will extend by adulthood, and the incision should be carried no higher than the sixth interspace to avoid the extension of the breast to the axilla. Furthermore, the pectoralis muscles should not be divided but elevated superiorly as a unit from the inferior edge and retracted to avoid subsequent injury to this organ as well. This technique avoids injury to the neurovascular pedicles of the pectoralis muscles and the breast bud itself.

In 1959 Moss[42] reported that in the prepubertal interval, when the human breast consists mainly of an expanding ductular system, 1500 to 2000 rad of radiation delivered through a single portal over an 8-day period will initiate striking maldevelopment of this organ. Furthermore, 3000 to 4000 rad administered over 30 days not only permanently arrests growth of glandular epithelium but also concomitantly produces severe fibrosis and hypoplasia of the breast. Following 3000 rad, the result was essentially complete loss of lobules and shrinkage of ductules of breast tissue. Williams and Cunningham,[17] in evaluating the histologic changes of irradiated breasts of women, state that irradiated areas show intense obliterative endarteritis and, in the end stages, marked fragmentation of elastic tissue.

Underwood and Gaul[43] documented severe breast hypoplasia as a consequence of *radium therapy implants* for a cavernous hemangioma in the region of the left breast of an infant. Subsequently, the contralateral breast matured normally, whereas the ipsilateral

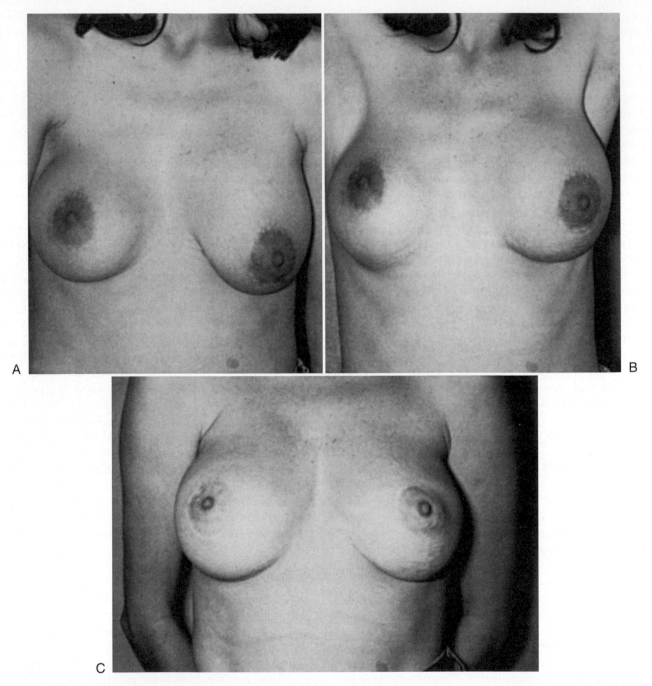

FIG. **8-6 A,** Developmental hypomastia of right breast in a 27-year-old woman. **B,** Elevation of arms confirms presence of pectoralis major and shoulder girdle musculature on side of hypomastia. **C,** Final cosmetic appearance of breasts following augmentation mammaplasty of right breast and reduction mammaplasty with mastopexy of left breast. *(Courtesy Dr. Hal G. Bingham, Division of Plastic and Reconstructive Surgery, University of Florida, College of Medicine, Gainesville, FL.)*

involved breast failed to develop. Similar reports of hypoplasia have been recorded by Mathews,[44] who used radium needles applied to the surface of the hemangioma, close to the nipple, when the patient was in her infancy. The report by Weidman, Zimany, and Kopf[45] addresses the necessity of observation of breast hemangiomas and the cautious application of

radiotherapy in the treatment of hemangiomas or other lesions of the breast with ionizing radiation. Furthermore, contemporary approaches to the therapy of intrathoracic or chest wall neoplasms dictate modification of irradiation portals that traverse the nipple/areola complex or the breast bud in infantile or prepubertal patients.

Premature Thelarche

The term *premature thelarche* refers to isolated breast development in the *absence* of additional signs of sexual maturation.[46, 47] This clinical presentation is represented by precocious development (Figure 8-7) with out other signs of puberty in girls younger than 8 years. Wilkins, Blizzard, and Migeon[48] postulate that an increased sensitivity of breast tissue to low circulating levels of estrogens (estrone, estradiol) secreted during early childhood is the cause of this premature breast development. Several authors have suggested normal or slightly increased plasma estradiol and basal gonadotropin (luteinizing hormone [LH] and follicle-stimulating hormone [FSH]) levels with the presentation.[49] Conflicting results with regard to gonadotropin responsiveness by synthetic gonadotropin-releasing hormone (luteinizing hormone–releasing hormone [LHRH]) have been observed. In premature thelarche, the basal LH and FSH concentrations have been reported as normal or slightly elevated.[50,51] In a series of 15 patients reported by Caufriez and co-workers,[52] all patients with premature thelarche had normal basal LH and FSH levels for

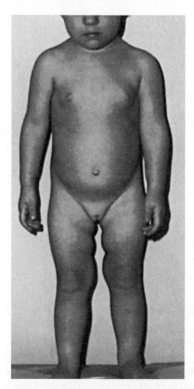

FIG. **8-7** Premature thelarche in a 19-month-old girl with isolated breast development in the absence of additional signs of sexual maturation. *(Courtesy Dr. Arlan L. Rosenbloom, Department of Pediatrics, University of Florida College of Medicine, Gainesville, FL.)*

their age and normal responses to LHRH. The observations of these investigators are in agreement with those of Reiter and colleagues[53] and Tenore and co-workers.[54] These reports suggest that patients with premature thelarche have normal regulation of the hypothalamic-pituitary-gonadal axis.

Caufriez and co-workers[52] confirmed a normal prolactin secretion in basal conditions and in response to thyrotropin-releasing hormone (TRH) for girls with premature thelarche. Prolactin does not convincingly appear to have a role in the genesis of isolated breast development in prepubertal girls. The endocrinologic relationship of this clinical presentation has been further investigated by Pasquino and associates[55] in nine young girls with premature thelarche who were compared with nine healthy girls and six girls with true precocious puberty. The gonadotropin stimulation test with LHRH was used. Girls with premature thelarche were observed to have LH responses that resemble those of normal girls, and FSH responses were similar to those of patients with precocious puberty. This study suggests that in premature thelarche there is partial activation of the diencephalic-hypophyseal-gonadal axis, which affects FSH alone. The authors conclude that premature thelarche should be considered as one of the disorders that results from altered sensitivity of the hypothalamic receptors that regulate sexual maturation. From a practical point of view, this study emphasizes the utility of the gonadotropin stimulation test with LHRH in girls with premature breast development as a test to distinguish between *premature thelarche* and true *precocious puberty*.

Data from Ilicki and co-workers[56] in the long-term follow-up of 68 girls with premature thelarche confirmed that 85% of patients with the disorder had onset before the age of 2 years. In 30.8%, this clinical finding was recognized at birth; in 44%, there was a regression after $3^{3}/_{12} \pm 2^{8}/_{12}$ years (standard deviation). In this study, basal levels of plasma FSH and response to LHRH were significantly higher ($p\ 11 < .001$) than in prepubertal controls. Of 52 patients, 27 evaluated had increased plasma estradiol, and in 27 of 40 patients tested, urocystograms or vaginal smears confirmed estrogenization. Basal levels of LH and responses to LHRH were prepubertal. In this study, girls with premature thelarche were significantly taller than normal controls of the same age ($p < .001$). These investigators suggest that premature thelarche is an incomplete form of precocious sexual development, probably occurring secondary to a derangement in the maturation of the hypothalamic-pituitary-gonadal axis that results in a higher-than-normal secretion of FSH. The authors conclude that the end result appears to be a defect in the peripheral sensitivity to the sexual hormones.

In follow-up of the natural history and endocrine findings of premature thelarche, a longitudinal study from the Institute of Paediatrics, University of Rome, Italy, was completed by Pasquino and associates.[57] This study of 40 girls with premature thelarche confirmed that when the disorder occurred before the age of 2 years, it usually regressed completely, thus representing an isolated and transient phenomenon. However, when this disorder occurred *after* 2 years of age, it persisted more frequently and may represent the first sign of sexual development, generally leading to early simple puberty. These observations were confirmed by Mills and colleagues,[51] who likewise conducted longitudinal studies of the natural history of the disorder by contacting 46 patients with previously diagnosed cases. These authors observed palpable breast tissue that persisted for 3 to 5 years in 57% of the subjects. Only 11% reported that their breast tissue had continued to enlarge. Patients in whom breast tissue had been present at birth and had persisted were significantly more likely to have progressive enlargement. Comparison of these patients with matched-control subjects showed no relationship between premature thelarche and maternal obstetrical problems, exposure to medications, diet, or prenatal infections. Furthermore, girls with premature thelarche were no more likely than control subjects to have other medical or sexual problems develop during the interval of follow-up.

Escobar, Rivarola, and Bergadaá[58] evaluated the plasma concentration of extradiol-17β in premature thelarche and in varying types of sexual precocity. All patients with idiopathic precocious puberty had elevated plasma estradiol concentrations for their ages that showed wide variations. No correlation between the grade of sexual development and the level of estradiol was observed. The plasma estradiol concentrations confirmed good correlation with clinical signs of estrogenic effects in prepubertal and adolescent normal girls (Figure 8-8). Of their 10 patients with premature thelarche, 7 had prepubertal levels of estradiol. Girls with higher estradiol levels were 7 years older and had urocystograms with moderate estrogenic activity. The findings in these younger girls confirmed the hypothesis that premature thelarche specifically resulted from higher sensitivity of breast tissue to prepubertal estrogen levels, because other estrogen target tissues did not show this stimulatory effect.

Tenore and associates[54] used multivariate analysis (chronologic age, FSH, LH, and bone age/chronologic age ratio) to predict the evolution of premature thelarche to central precocious puberty. In a study of 32 girls with premature thelarche, they reported that all subjects with isolated premature thelarche could be sharply distinguished from those who progressed to precocious puberty. In a related long-term study,

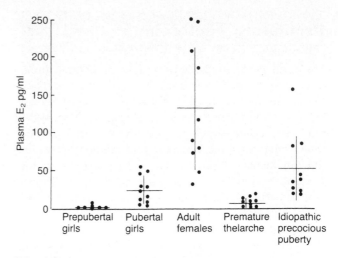

FIG. **8-8** Estradiol-17β plasma values in normal females, premature thelarche, and idiopathic precocious puberty. Mean values are indicated by horizontal lines and standard deviations by vertical lines. *(From Escobar ME et al: Acta Endocrinol 81:351, 1976.)*

Pasquino and colleagues[59] retrospectively examined 100 girls with premature thelarche to evaluate whether girls with premature thelarche progress to central precocious puberty. Fourteen of the patients with characteristic premature thelarche progressed during follow-up to precocious or early central precocious puberty. The chronologic age of the 14 girls in this group was 5.1 (standard deviation of 2.0) years at the onset of premature thelarche and 7.8 (standard deviation of 0.6) years after progression to central precocious puberty. No clinical or hormonal characteristics could be established that separated the 14 girls who progressed to precocious puberty from the 86 girls who did not. The authors conclude that premature thelarche is not always a self-limited condition and that it may sometimes accelerate the timing of puberty. Rosenfield[60] warns that although premature pubarche, premature thelarche, and precocious puberty are usually simply normal phenomena occurring at an early age, they may sometimes be harbingers of reproductive endocrine disturbances in adulthood. Consequently, girls with these complaints should be followed to ascertain that pubertal reproductive function is eventually normal.

Juvenile (Adolescent, Virginal) Hypertrophy of the Female Breast

Juvenile, or adolescent, hypertrophy of the breast is a commonly observed occurrence in the young adolescent female following a normal puberty. This clinical presentation denotes the adolescent breast that does not cease its rapid pubertal growth and continues to enlarge even into mature years. Most patients with juvenile

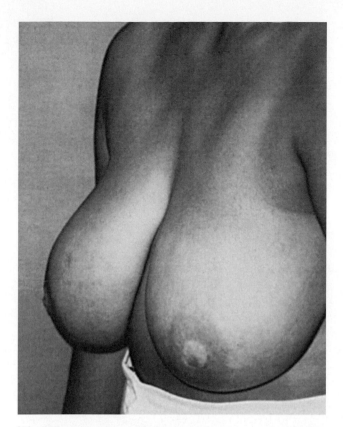

FIG. 8-9 Bilateral juvenile hypertrophy in a 17-year-old nulliparous Hispanic girl. The patient presented with mastodynia related to her large breast size. She was not taking any medications known to induce breast gigantism. Therapy consisted of reduction mammaplasty. *(Courtesy Dr. Hollis H. Caffee, Division of Plastic and Reconstructive Surgery, University of Florida College of Medicine, Gainesville, FL.)*

hypertrophy of the breast have symmetric, *bilateral* involvement (Figure 8-9), although *unilateral* juvenile hypertrophy has been described.[61] There have been a few reported cases of massive breast hypertrophy during pregnancy,[62-64] in which rapid enlargement is evident soon after conception, with predominant growth occurring during the second trimester.

Several conditions may initiate breast asymmetry, including maldevelopment, neoplasms, incisional or excisional biopsies, trauma, and radiotherapy.[65] As noted earlier, developmental abnormalities account for most of these lesions. Mayl, Vasconez, and Jurkiewicz[66] suggested that juvenile hypertrophy, also referred to as *macromastia*, may occur secondary to a primary defect of the breast or an endocrinologic disorder.[67] The general tenet has been that an augmented plasma level of estrone or estradiol may induce hypertrophy of the mamma. However, the measurement of various mammotropic hormones as etiologic for the disorder has not yielded precise clinical correlates with breast enlargement. Nonetheless, substantial *decreases* in plasma *progesterone* levels have been documented for

juvenile hypertrophy in the presence of *normal* plasma *estrogen* and *growth hormone* values. These substantial decreases of progesterone in the hormonal milieu may be causing the abnormality. One could also postulate that target organ tissues (ductal epithelium, collagen and stroma of the adolescent female breast) may have estrogen receptors that are highly responsive to minimal concentrations of the mammotropic steroid hormones (e.g., estrogens, progesterone) that regulate breast growth and development.[68]

Sperling and Gold[69] and Mayl and associates[66] have recommended the use of the antiestrogen drugs dydrogesterone (Gynorest) and medroxyprogesterone acetate (Provera) in the treatment of virginal hypertrophy. Ryan and Pernoll[70] were successful in preventing regrowth of breast parenchyma following reduction mammaplasty in several patients with adolescent hypertrophy by using the drug dydrogesterone. However, a subsequent follow-up report by these investigators suggested its ineffectiveness. Thereafter, partial success for prevention of regrowth was achieved with tamoxifen citrate (Nolvadex). Treatment with tamoxifen may be of value after reduction mammaplasty (subcutaneous mastectomy) in patients with strongly positive estrogen receptor profiles in the removed breast tissue. Using an escalating dose of 10 to 40 mg of tamoxifen citrate per day, these authors were able to achieve reduction of breast bulk with the drug. Theoretically, with the use of this compound, estrogen receptors can be converted to a negative profile status. The infrequent use of tamoxifen in the treatment of juvenile hypertrophy of the breast suggests that a prospective controlled clinical trial may be of value to determine its efficacy for this condition.

The most commonly applied technique for the treatment of adolescent (juvenile) hypertrophy continues to be the *subcutaneous mastectomy* described by Furnas[71] as a reduction mammaplasty. However, the technique, as reported by Cardoso de Castro[72] does not represent a panacea for this disorder. Modifications of the subcutaneous mastectomy have subsequently been described by Courtiss and Goldwyn,[73] who used an inferior pedicle technique as an alternative to free nipple and areola grafting for severe *macromastia* or *extreme ptosis*. For recurrent adolescent hypertrophy following previously successful reduction mammaplasty, the *total glandular mastectomy* with *subpectoral augmentation* may be considered. This aggressive technique, as previously described by Bland and co-workers,[74] should only rarely be necessary in the premenopausal female (Figure 8-10). The success of this more radical approach depends on the extirpation from the chest wall of all breast tissue that has estrogen hypersensitivity and, thus, the potential for regrowth.

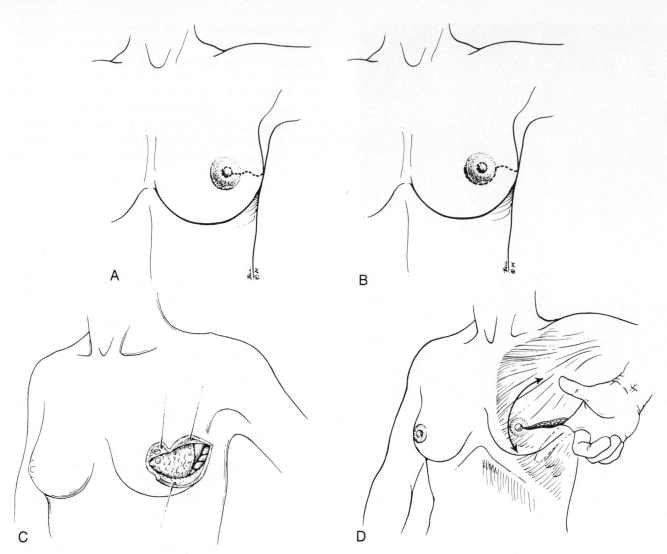

A

B

C

D

FIG. **8-10** Technique for one-stage mastectomy with immediate reconstruction. **A,** Circumferential nipple incision extended transareolarly and in "lazy S" pattern over lateral portion of breast. Nipple and ductal system remain with breast specimen. **B,** When preexisting paraareolar scar is present, or inferior skin envelope must be reduced, circumareolar incision is used. Nipple is circumscribed as in **A. C,** Flap elevation via circumareolar incision with development of skin thickness and extent of dissection identical to modified radical mastectomy technique. **D,** Entering submuscular plane via muscle-splitting incision of serratus anterior at fifth rib level, serratus anterior muscle origins are avulsed from their ribs to beyond sixth rib, and blunt dissection of subpectoralis major plane is continued superiorly to clavicle and medially to sternum. *(From Bland KI et al: Arch Surg 121:221, 1986.)*

Drug Induction of Gigantism

Drug-related induction of *breast gigantism* has previously been described. This disorder may occur in the adolescent or in the fully mature adult breast (Figure 8-11). D-Penicillamine as an etiologic factor in breast enlargement is poorly understood but is a well-recognized cause of sudden gigantism. Desai[75] postulates an effect on sex hormone–binding globulin by D-penicillamine to increase the amount of circulating free estrogen. Taylor, Cumming, and Corenblum[76] suggest that it is likely that D-penicillamine produces a local effect on the

breast, because patients do not show changes in menstrual function while receiving the drug or during the time of maximal breast growth. These authors confirm the effect of danazol (17-α-pregna-2, 4-dien-20-ynol(2,3-d) isoxazol-17β-0; Danocrine) to act by interfering with the sensitivity of the breast parenchymal estrogen receptor, thereby diminishing growth.[77] These studies confirmed both diminution in breast size during the first courses of danazol administration and that these reductions occurred simultaneously with a reduction in plasma circulating estradiol concentrations. Furthermore, the cessation of danazol administration with an increase in breast volume

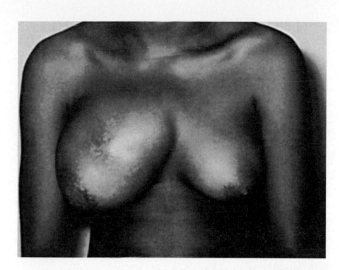

FIG. **8-11** Gigantism of drug induction. An 18-year-old black woman with painful unilateral gigantism of the right breast following treatment with D-penicillamine.

indicated that a reduction in breast size was not simply a coincidental spontaneous remission. This clinical trial did not determine whether the breast shrinkage that resulted with the drug was produced by a reduction in circulating estrogen concentrations or by a local effect. The blocking of estrogen receptors by danazol may mimic the postmenopausal condition and has been successfully applied by Buckle[78] for the treatment of gynecomastia in males.

Breast Hypertrophy with Pregnancy (Gigantomastia)

Massive hypertrophy of the breast with pregnancy is a rare condition of unknown cause. It is often referred to as *gigantomastia of pregnancy*.[79] The first recorded report of this condition was made by Palmuth in 1648.[80] In the exhaustive review of 55 cases in the world literature by Moss,[63] 33 patients with this condition had previously been reported by Deaver and McFarland in 1917.[9] These reviews reveal that this condition may affect women of all races during the childbearing years. The disorder is less common than juvenile (virginal) hypertrophy of the breast, which classically progresses independent of pregnancy and occurs usually between the ages of 11 and 19 years. In distinction, gigantomastia of pregnancy usually occurs during the first few months of pregnancy and may progress to necrosis, incapacity, and possibly death.[63]

The typical history is that of a healthy pregnant woman who observed gradual bilateral massive enlargement of her breasts within the first few months of pregnancy. The breasts may enlarge to several times their normal weight and size to become grotesque, huge, and incapacitating. The skin and parenchyma become firm, edematous, and tense and may have prominent subcutaneous veins with a diffuse peau d'orange appearance. As a consequence of rapid breast enlargement and skin pressure, insufficient vascularity of the skin may initiate ulceration, necrosis, infection, or hemorrhage.

In the immediate postpartum period, the hypertrophied breasts recede to approximately their previous volume. When the woman delivers, the breasts regress in size but almost always hypertrophy again with succeeding pregnancies. Most authors agree that this condition is hormonal in etiology, but its precise mechanism is unclear. Whether there is an overproduction of mammotropic hormone from the pituitary or an enhanced sensitivity of breast parenchyma to the hormones of pregnancy (e.g., estriol, estradiol, human chorionic gonadotropin [hCG], progestins) has not been established. Parham[81] determined that estrogen and testosterone were of no value in the treatment of gigantism of pregnancy; however, norethindrone may be of value.[82] Hydrocortisone therapy has been attempted without success by Nolan[64]; testosterone has been used with divided results. Moss[63] used fluoxymesterone without results, whereas diuretics were successfully used, with moderate temporary effect.

Luchsinger[62] was one of the first to suggest that this condition may occur as a consequence of specific individual reactivity of the breast to hormonal stimuli. This author questioned whether in addition to possible hormonal dysfunction, estrogenic placental hormones were sufficiently metabolized in the presence of insufficient liver function. Lewison and colleagues[83] postulated that gigantism of pregnancy may be related to the depression of all steroid hormones and decreased liver function as measured by the salicylate conjugation test. These investigators advocated the use of the progestational agent norethindrone to reduce breast size; however, it was used with mestranol and had to be discontinued when thrombophlebitis occurred. Although liver dysfunction and the inability to metabolize estrogenic hormones have been postulated to be a possible cause for the disorder, it must be noted that many normal pregnancies are accompanied by severe liver failure without the development of gigantomastia.

In most instances, gigantomastia is self-limiting and does not progress to pyogenic abscesses, skin ulcerations, necrosis, or systemic illness. For most patients, breast size will spontaneously regress to its approximate nonpregnant configuration. The patient should be advised of proper brassiere support, good skin hygiene, and adequate nutrition. On occasion, diuretics are of value. Operative intervention may be necessary to relieve severe pain, massive infection, necrosis, slough, and ulceration or hemorrhage if delivery is not imminent. After delivery, the patient should be advised that gigantism will almost certainly recur with subsequent pregnancies, and *reduction mammaplasty* may be considered.

See Scott-Conner and Shorr[84] for a review of the diag-nosis and management of breast problems during pregnancy and lactation. See Howard and Gusterson[85] for a review of the histology of the normal physiologic states of the human breast, including prenatal, prepubertal, and pubertal development; adult resting gland; pregnancy; lactation; and postinvolution.

Symmastia: Medial Confluence of the Breast

Symmastia (Greek, *syn*, meaning "together" and *mastos*, meaning "breast") is the contemporary terminology for medial confluence of the breast. This rare clinical anomaly represents a webbing across the midline in breasts that are usually symmetric (Figure 8-12). More common, however, is the presternal blending (confluence) of the breast tissue that is associated with macromastia. These conditions are most often recognized in individuals who seek reduction mammaplasty.[86]

Like many anomalies of ectodermal origin, a broad spectrum of defects may be observed with this congenital lesion. Cases may range from an empty skin web to those with an apparent confluence of major portions of symmetric breast tissue within the midline. The common denominator is the need for resection of presternal skin to varying degrees. Spence, Feldman, and Ryan[86] recommend correction of the web defect using three methods. (1) The first method is elevation of an *inferiorly based triangular skin flap* that is advanced superiorly in an inverted Y-V manner following division of excessive medial soft tissue. Thereafter, the divided medial soft tissue is sutured superiorly to the medial pectoralis fascia to create a brassiere-band sling effect. (2) These authors have also used *a superiorly based medial flap* that contains both skin and soft tissue. Excess skin and soft tissue were excised, and the remaining flap was tailored to fit into a V-shaped defect in the inferior incision. (3) A third option suggested by the authors consists of the vertical division and superior rotation of the excess subcutaneous tissue flaps with elevation of a *superiorly based skin flap* inserted into a V-shaped defect in the inferior incision. The use of *liposuction* as an integral part of a surgical correction of symmastia has been reported by Schonegg and associates.[87] Regarding the use of liposuction, McKissock[88] predicts that the same limitations will apply to the breast as advocates of liposuction have professed exist elsewhere in the body. Thus the amount of skin involved in the web medially, and its resiliency, will determine the applicability of liposuction techniques for this anomaly.

Supernumerary Nipples (Polythelia)

Velanovich[89] has recently reviewed the embryology, clinical presentation, diagnosis, treatment, and clinical significance of supernumerary nipples, supernumerary breasts, and ectopic breast tissue. Important considerations concerning these common anomalies include the following:

1. Supernumerary nipples, supernumerary breasts, and ectopic breast tissue most commonly develop along the milk lines.

2. Whereas polythelia is evident at birth, supernumerary and ectopic breast tissue is evident only after hormonal stimulation that occurs at puberty or during pregnancy.

3. Ectopic breast tissue is subject to the same pathologic changes that occur in normally positioned breasts.

4. Axillary ectopic breast tissue may be confused with other malignant and benign lesions occurring in the area.

5. Polythelia may indicate associated conditions, most notably urologic malformations or urogenital malignancies.

The presence of supernumerary or accessory nipples (Figure 8-13) is a relatively common, minor congenital anomaly that occurs in both sexes, with an estimated frequency of 1 in 100 to 1 in 500 persons.[90] Meáhes[91,92] and Meáhes and associates[93] reported the frequency of supernumerary nipples as 0.22% in a white European population, which is significantly lower than the incidence of 1.63% found by Rahbar[94] in black American neonates. This represents a 7.4-fold increase for the anomaly in blacks. In the newborn Jewish population reported by Mimouni and associates,[95] the higher incidence of 2.5% for polythelia was observed. This high frequency of supernumerary nipples could possibly be related to ethnic differences but, as acknowledged by some authors, may be related to a systematic technique for examination of the newborn.

Polythelia should be searched for in the routine physical examination of every newborn, and the presence of the condition should be reported to the

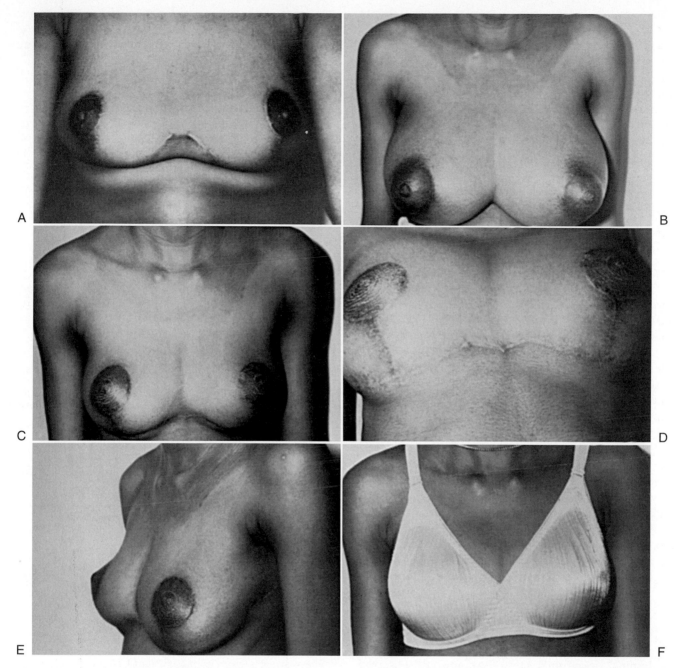

FIG. **8-12** Symmastia. **A,** A 24-year-old woman following reduction mammaplasty with persistent central breast web of symmastia. Cosmetic congenital defect was corrected with inserted Y-V advancement flap. **B,** A 19-year-old woman with large, painful breasts and prominent central webbing reportedly present since the beginning of breast development. **C** to **F,** Postoperative appearance of breasts after correction of symmastia with reduction mammaplasty using the inferior pedicle technique. *(From Spence RJ et al: Plast Reconstruct Surg 73:2, 1984.)*

parents. This is important for the following reasons, as reported by Mimouni and co-workers[95]:

1. Supernumerary breasts in females may respond to fluctuations in hormones in a physiologic manner such that pubertal enlargement, premenstrual swelling, tenderness, and lactation during pregnancy and parturition may occur.

2. Patients with polythelia may be subject to the same spectrum of pathologic diseases observed in

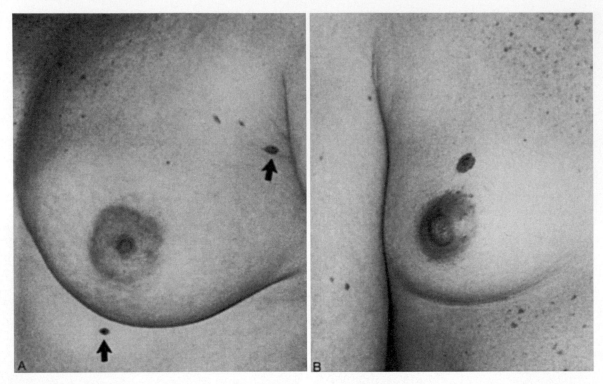

F I G. **8-13** Supernumerary nipple. **A,** A 38-year-old woman with supernumerary nipples above (in axilla) and below the normal left breast in the mammary milk line. **B,** Supernumerary nipple and areolar complex (rudimentary) in upper right breast of a 22-year-old woman. Excisional biopsy was the preferred treatment.

normal breasts (e.g., neoplasms, fibroadenomas, papillary adenomas, cysts, or carcinomas).[96-99]

3. The supernumerary nipples may be associated with other congenital diseases such as vertebral anomalies,[100,101] cardiac arrhythmias, or renal anomalies.[96,102-106]

Table 8-2 summarizes the associated abnormal conditions that may occur with polythelia.

Moore and Schosser[39] observed that supernumerary nipples usually develop just below the normal breast in the white population, with less common occurrence in abdominal or inguinal sites.[107] Abramson[108] observed bilateral supernumerary nipples in approximately half

of patients with polythelia. In the ectopic sites, polythelia takes origin from the extra mammary buds that are present along the ventral embryonic mammary ridges (see Figure 8-3, *A*). Only a minority of persons with this clinical anomaly have more than two extra nipples.[39]

Although various malformations have been associated with polythelia (see Table 8-2), attention has been drawn to the high incidence of *renal anomalies* and *malignancies in children* with supernumerary nipples.[109] The association between supernumerary nipples and occult anomalies of the urogenital system has been reported in at least two non-U.S. pediatric populations. These studies from Hungary[42] and Israel[110] report that 23% and 40%, respectively, of children with polythelia

TABLE **8-2**	Polythelia and Associated Conditions	
URINARY TRACT ABNORMALITIES	**CARDIAC ABNORMALITIES**	**MISCELLANEOUS ABNORMALITIES**
Renal agenesis	Cardiac conduction	Pyloric stenosis
Renal cell	disturbances, especially	Epilepsy
carcinoma	left bundle branch block	Ear abnormalities
Obstructive disease	Hypertension	Arthrogryposis
Supernumerary	Congenital heart	multiplex congenita
kidney(s)	anomalies	

From Pellegrini JR, Wagner RF Jr: *Am Fam Physician* 28:129, 1983.

had obstructive renal abnormalities or duplications of the excretory system. Studies in Hungarian children show no link between polythelia and renal anomalies. Jojart and Seres[111] found 504 supernumerary nipples in healthy newborns, infants, schoolchildren, and pediatric ward and clinic patients. The prevalence of supernumerary nipples was 4.29% among newborns and 5.86% among schoolchildren. Ultrasound was used to examine 496 of the children with supernumerary nipples and 410 acutely ill patients who served as controls. Another control group consisted of 1957 newborns infants routinely screened with ultrasound. The prevalence of renal anomalies was 3.74% in children with supernumerary nipples and 3.17% in the control group; 2.86% in newborns with supernumerary nipples and 1.89% in control newborns. The differences were not significant.

In embryogenesis, polythelia occurs during the third month of gestation, when the embryonic mammary ridge fails to regress normally—an event coincident with the development of the urogenital and other organ systems. Therefore it is not surprising that various congenital anomalies, particularly of the genitourinary tract, appear to occur excessively with polythelia. The studies by Goedert and colleagues[112,113] and Meáhes and co-workers[93] suggest that polythelia is also associated with cancers of the testis and kidney. *Familial occurrence* has been reported by the authors, including the association of polythelia with renal cancer and in three families, the combination of urogenital anomalies, germ cell tumors, and renal cancer.[101,114]

Goedert and associates[113] evaluated 299 medical students, of whom 8 (2.7%) had polythelia. This frequency of the anomaly yielded an estimated relative risk of testicular cancer for men with polythelia of 4.5 (95% confidence interval, 1.6 to 12.4). In the first Health and Nutrition Examination Survey (HANES) dermatologic examination, polythelia was observed in 108 (0.5%) of the total series of 20,749 persons and in 27 (0.4%) of the 7004 white males. Using the HANES white males as controls, these authors estimate the relative risk of testicular cancer associated with polythelia to be 31.8 (95% confidence interval, 13.9 to 72.6). Obviously, the estimated magnitude for risk of testicular cancer in men with polythelia is expected to vary according to the nature of the comparison group and the methods for determination of the disorder. The prevalence of polythelia of 2.5% as reported by Mimouni and colleagues[95] suggests that this rate closely resembles the 2.7% prevalence evident in the medical student population determined by Goedert and associates.[113] Thus an intensive evaluation and search for the anomaly would expectantly change the frequency when compared with the HANES dermatologic examination. Overall, it would appear that the estimated 4.5-fold relative risk

of testicular cancer in men with polythelia is a more accurate determination than the relative risk of 31.8 based on the HANES survey. Although the association between the disorder and testicular cancer is statistically highly significant, the estimated incidence of testicular cancer in men with polythelia appears to be fewer than five cases per 10,000 per year. Despite this low frequency of testicular carcinoma, the association with renal anomalies must be sought. It was also suggested that children with polythelia, especially male children, should be evaluated to exclude urinary tract anomalies. For these children, kidney ultrasonography is indicated. Radiologic examinations of the urogenital tract are indicated in every patient in whom a pathologic condition in this organ system is suspected. As noted earlier, Rahbar[94] acknowledged the high frequency of accessory nipples in black Americans to be almost 7.4-fold greater than in white Europeans. However, the association of the wide range of anomalies reported in whites with polythelia has thus far not been experienced in black Americans.

Only a few cases of bilateral *intraareolar polythelia* have been recorded. Multiplicity of nipples is not uncommon, and they are bilateral in approximately half of patients so affected. As many as 10 nipples have been recorded in a single patient.[115] Atypical locations[116] have been noted secondary to the displaced embryonal primordium. Intraareolar polythelia represents a nipple/areola unit within the mammary ridge such that a dichotomy of the vestigial breast and nipple/areola complex exists.

The presence of supernumerary nipples may necessitate operative therapy in instances in which discharge, tumor, or cyst formation is evident. Simple excision elliptically placed in lines of cleavage or skin folds is preferred to achieve maximum cosmesis. Primary closure is usually possible and allows the surgeon to achieve a superior cosmetic result.

Supernumerary Breast (Polymastia)

Although congenital supernumerary nipples or breasts may occur in any size or configuration along the mammary milk line, the most common site to observe the abnormally placed mamillae is a line extending from the nipple to the symphysis pubis. As noted earlier, the supernumerary nipple anomaly may be easily overlooked in young infants, in whom these ectopic lesions often appear only as a small spot with a diameter of 2 to 3 mm. Clearly, the importance of recognition of this anomaly is the potential need for investigation of other associated anomalies. In contradistinction, polymastia results when the embryonic mammary ridge (see Figure 8-1, *A*) fails to undergo normal regression (see Figure 8-1, *B*). Causal factors are as yet unknown.

A familial occurrence of the polymastia anomaly has been observed.[76,117] DeGrouchy and Turleau[118] document the association of polymastia with *congenital cytogenetic syndromes,* especially those involved with chromosomes 3 and 8. The prevalence of polymastia was 0.1% in the Collaborative Perinatal Project reported by Chung and Myrianthopoulos,[119] although Orti and Oazi[117] suggest a frequency approaching 1%. In a longitudinal survey of minor congenital defects, Meáhes[91,92] and Meáhes and associates[93] observed that supernumerary breasts were present in 0.2% of children; 8 of the 20 affected children in the study also had *major renal anomalies.* Furthermore, other congenital anomalies, notably *Turner's syndrome* (ovarian agenesis and dysgenesis with chromosomal karyotypes of 45,X, but mosaic patterns [45,X/46,XX or 45,X/46,XX/47, XXX] are seen) and *Fleischer's syndrome* (lateral displacement of the nipples to the midclavicular lines with bilateral renal hypoplasia[120]), may have polymastia as a component of the syndrome (Figure 8-14).

Goeminne[121] documented that renal anomalies often occur together with an abnormal number or location of nipples. Previous reports suggest an association between renal adenocarcinoma and renal malformations,[109,122] and half of the patients with polymastia and kidney cancer in the study by Goedert and co-workers[112] had duplicate renal arteries. The aforementioned reports suggest the association between polymastia, renal anomalies, and renal adenocarcinoma. The observations of

Cohen and associates[90] and Fraumeni[123] of renal cancer in young patients with polymastia are consistent with the earlier onset of several hereditary neoplasms.[124]

Accessory (Ectopic) Axillary Breast Tissue

Ectopic axillary breast tissue is a relatively uncommon occurrence but is a relatively common variant of supernumerary breast tissue.[125] In the human embryo, the mammary ridge first becomes apparent in the 7- to 8-mm-long embryo and atrophies before birth. It is the persistence of mammalian tissue along the milk line that results in ectopically displaced or accessory breast tissue (see Figures 8-1 and 8-2). This congenital anomaly is commonly bilateral and is often unaccompanied by the areola or the nipple (Figure 8-15). Greer[126] noted the presence of accessory axillary breast tissue to be apparent only at or after puberty, with the most rapid growth observed during pregnancy. Another study[127] classified accessory axillary breast tissue into eight categories as follows: (1) the presence of a complete breast with mammary gland tissue and the nipple/areola complex, (2) the presence of gland tissue and nipple, (3) gland tissue and areola, (4) solitary gland tissue, (5) nipple/areola with fat replacement of the mammary gland tissue (*pseudomamma*), (6) the nipple alone (*polythelia*), (7) the areola alone (*polythelia areolaris*), and (8) the presence of a small patch of hair-bearing tissue (*polythelia pilosa*). Clearly, polythelia represents the most common variant of supernumerary breast components and occurs predominantly between the breast and the umbilicus.[126] However, glandular tissue compatible with complete or variable components of breast parenchyma can occur within the mammary ridge at sites between the axilla and the groin. Jeffcoate[128] suggests that axillary breast tissue may represent true ectopic tissue not contiguous with the breast but more commonly represents an enlargement of the axillary tail of Spence. Thus, to determine the presence or absence of accessory axillary breast tissue, one must distinguish between an enlargement of the axillary tail and ectopically displaced mammary tissues of the milk line. The occurrence of ectopic breast tissue outside the axilla is exceedingly rare. Dworak and associates[129] and Reck and colleagues[130] are the first to report a hamartoma of ectopic breast tissue in the inguinal region. The finding, confirmed with histopathologic examination, occurred in a 50-year-old woman suspected of having a chronic incarcerated hernia.

The discovery of accessory axillary breast tissue usually occurs during the first pregnancy as a consequence of the secondary changes initiated with

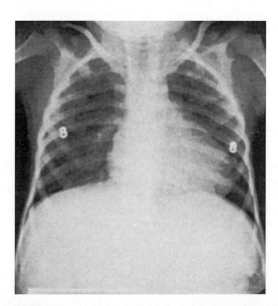

FIG. **8-14** Fleischer's syndrome. Posteroanterior chest roentgenogram of a 5-year-old with bilateral renal hypoplasia. Although the clavicles are not horizontal, the lateral displacement of the nipples (designated by the lead markers 8) is apparent. *(From Fleischer DS: J Pediatr 69:806, 1966.)*

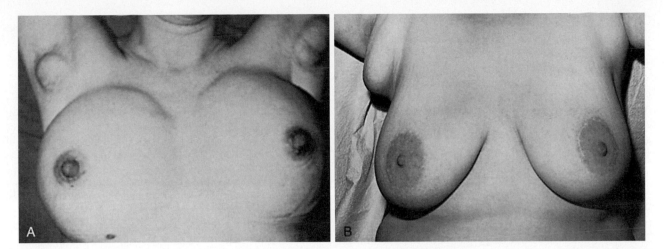

FIG. **8-15 A** and **B,** Supernumerary breasts presenting as accessory (ectopic) breast tissue bilaterally in the axilla. **A,** Right supernumerary inframammary nipple presenting in the mammary milk line. *(A, from Greer KE:* Arch Dermatol *109:88, 1974. Copyright 1974, American Medical Association. **B,** courtesy Dr. Michael M. Meguid, SUNY Health Sciences Center, Syracuse, NY.)*

hormonal stimulation by ovarian estradiol and placental estriol. The symptomatic axillary breast tissue becomes painfully enlarged and, on rare occasion, may develop galactoceles with milk secretion via contiguous skin pores.[131] Although these anomalies may not become evident until the first pregnancy, once the lesions are recognized, they continue to recur with subsequent pregnancies and may undergo cyclical changes during menstruation. DeCholnoky[116] noted pathologic findings in 26 cases of axillary breast tissue that included normal breast tissue (9), cystic disease (10), fibroadenoma (3), mastitis (4), and atypical ductal hyperplasia (1) or carcinoma (2). Bilateral fibroadenomata have been reported in supernumerary breasts of the vulva.[132] Often, the clinician will identify the lesion as excess axillary fat, although lymphadenitis, lymphoma, metastatic carcinoma, and hidradenitis suppurativa are common misdiagnoses. After identification of the hormonal dependency with pregnancy or menstruation, the clinician can often establish the diagnosis, especially if a history of lactation during the puerperium is confirmed.

Management consists of reassuring the patient of its common benignity and its embryologic origin. However, accessory axillary tissue may be misdiagnosed as the symptomatic alterations inherent with pathologic changes of breast tissue (e.g., carcinoma and the benign breast tissue spectrum). Treatment of symptomatic accessory breast tissue during the puerperium and pregnancy involves conservative management for most clinical presentations. The presence of dense, nodular masses suggestive of malignant transformation necessitates aggressive

approaches to rule out carcinoma.[133] As this hormonally dependent accessory breast tissue rapidly regresses when lactation ceases, the patient can be reassured but should be admonished that enlargement and painful, lactating, accessory tissue may recur with subsequent pregnancy. Elliptically placed incisions in skin folds of the axilla allow complete dissection and removal of the breast tissue beneath the skin and over the underlying fascia. The cosmetically oriented resections of the accessory tissue are usually curative, although the lesion may recur if excision is incomplete.

In a 1995 case presentation and review of the literature regarding carcinoma of ectopic breast tissue, Evans and Guyton[134] reported that of a total of 90 cases of carcinoma of ectopic breast tissue, 64 occurred in the axilla. The combined survival beyond the 4-year posttreatment period was 9.4%. No survival advantage was found for radical or modified radical mastectomy over local excision combined with axillary dissection or radiation. They found that the correct preoperative diagnosis was rarely made, and they suggest that improved prognosis requires diagnostic suspicion and early biopsy of suspicious ectopic masses that occur along the embryonic milk lines. In related studies, fine-needle biopsy has been found to be useful in the diagnosis and management of ectopic breast tissue.[115,135,136]

ACKNOWLEDGMENTS

The authors gratefully acknowledge the technical assistance and photographs supplied by Dr. Arlan L. Rosenbloom, Department of Pediatrics, and Drs. Hal G. Bingham and H. Hollis Caffee, Division of Plastic Surgery, University of Florida.

REFERENCES

1. Russo J, Russo IH: Development of the human mammary gland. In Neville MC, Daniel CW (eds): *The mammary gland development, regulation, and function,* New York, 1987, Plenum Press.
2. Russo J, Russo IH: Biological and molecular bases of mammary carcinogenesis, *Lab Invest* 57:112, 1987.
3. Russo J, Russo IH: Mammary gland neoplasia in long-term rodent studies, *Environ Health Perspect* 104:938, 1996.
4. Russo J et al: Cancer risk related to mammary gland structure and development, *Microsc Res Tech* 52:204, 2001.
5. Lewis MT: Homeobox genes in mammary gland development and neoplasia, *Breast Cancer Res* 2:158, 2000.
6. Hubert C: Etude sur l'amastic, thesis, Paris, 1907, A Michalon.
7. Froriep L: Beobachtung eines Falles von Mangel der Brustdruse, *Notizen aus dem Gebiete der Natur and Heilkunst* 1:9, 1839.
8. Gilly E: Absence complete de mamelles chez une femme mère: atrophie de membre supéárieur droit, *Courrier Med* 32:27, 1882.
9. Deaver JB, McFarland J: *The breast: anomalies, diseases and treatment,* Philadelphia, 1917, P Blakiston's & Sons.
10. Weinberg W: Zur vererbung des zwergwuchses, *Arch Rass Ges Biol* 9:710, 1912.
11. Trier WC: Complete breast absence: case report and review of the literature, *Plast Reconstr Surg* 36:431, 1965.
12. Tawil HM, Najjar SS: Congenital absence of the breasts, *J Pediatr* 73:751, 1968.
13. Goldenring J, Crelin ES: Mother and daughter with bilateral congenital amastia, *Yale J Biol Med* 33:466, 1961.
14. Nelson MM, Cooper CK: Congenital defects of the breast: an autosomal dominant trait, *S Afr Med J* 61:434, 1982.
15. Wilson MG, Hall EB, Ebbin AJ: Dominant inheritance of absence of the breast, *Humangenetik* 15:268, 1972.
16. Fraser FC: *Dominant inheritance of absent nipples and breasts. Novanta anni delle leggi mendeliane,* Roma, 1956, Istituto Gregorio Mendel.
17. Williams IG, Cunningham GJ: Histological changes in irradiated cancer of the breast, *Br J Radiol* 24:123, 1951.
18. Triolo O et al: Familial ectodermal dysplasia with agenesis of the breasts and the external urethral sphincter: description of a case, *Minerva Ginecol* 45:139, 1993.
19. Rich MA et al: Autosomal dominant transmission of ureteral triplication and bilateral amastia, *J Urol* 137:102, 1987.
20. Poland A: Deficiency of the pectoral muscles, *Guys Hosp Rep* 6:191, 1841.
21. Pers M: Aplasias of the anterior thoracic wall, the pectoral muscles, and the breast, *Scand J Plast Reconstr Surg* 2:125, 1968.
22. Mace JW et al: Poland's syndrome: report of seven cases and review of the literature, *Clin Pediatr* 11:98, 1972.
23. Martin LW, Helmsworth JA: The management of congenital deformities of the sternum, *JAMA* 179:82, 1962.
24. Urschel HC et al: Poland's syndrome: improved surgical management, *Ann Thorac Surg* 37:204, 1984.
25. Fabian MC, Fischer JD: A variant of Poland's syndrome, *Can J Surg* 37:67, 1994.
26. David TJ: Nature and etiology of the Poland anomaly, *N Engl J Med* 287:487, 1972.
27. Asp K, Sulamaa M: On rare congenital deformities of the thoracic wall, *Acta Chir Scand* 118:392, 1959.
28. Ravitch MM: Operative treatment of congenital deformities of the chest, *Am J Surg* 101:588, 1961.
29. Ravitch MM: *Congenital deformities of the chest wall and their operative correction,* Philadelphia, 1977, WB Saunders.
30. Heeker WC, Daum R: Chirurgisches vorgchen bei kongenitalen brustwanddefekten, *Chirurg* 11:482, 1964.
31. Fevre M, Hannouche D: Les breáches thoraciques par aplasie ou par anomalies costales, *Ann Chir Infant* 9:153, 1968.
32. Hochberg J et al: Complex reconstruction of the chest wall and breast utilizing a customized silicone implant, *Ann Plast Surg* 32:524, 1994.
33. Ravitch MM: Disorders of the sternum and the thoracic wall. In Sabiston DC Jr, Spencer FC (eds): *Gibbon's surgery of the chest,* ed 3, Philadelphia, 1976, WB Saunders.
34. Amoroso PJ, Angelats J: Latissimus dorsi myocutaneous flap in Poland syndrome, *Ann Plast Surg* 6:287, 1981.
35. Campbell DA: Reconstruction of the anterior thoracic wall, *J Thorac Surg* 19:456, 1950.
36. Schneider WJ, Hill HL Jr, Brown RG: Latissimus dorsi myocutaneous flap for breast reconstruction, *Br J Plast Surg* 30:277, 1977.
37. Bainbridge LC, Wright AR, Kanthan R: Computed tomography in the preoperative assessment of Poland's syndrome, *Br J Plast Surg* 44:604, 1991.
38. Hurwitz DJ, Stofman G, Curtin H: Three-dimensional imaging of Poland's syndrome, *Plast Reconstr Surg* 94:719, 1994.
39. Moore JA, Schosser RH: Becker's melanosis and hypoplasia of the breast and pectoralis major muscle, *Pediatr Dermatol* 3:34, 1985.
40. Zubowicz V, Bostwick J III: Congenital unilateral hypoplasia of the female breast associated with a large melanotic spot: report of two cases, *Ann Plast Surg* 12:204, 1984.
41. Cherup LL, Siewers RD, Futrell JW: Breast and pectoral muscle maldevelopment after anterolateral and posterolateral thoracotomies in children, *Ann Thorac Surg* 41:492, 1986.
42. Moss TW: *Therapeutic radiology,* St Louis, 1959, Mosby.
43. Underwood GB, Gaul LB: Disfiguring sequelae from radium therapy: results of treatment of a birthmark adjacent to the breast of a female infant, *Arch Dermatol* 57:918, 1948.
44. Mathews DN: Treatment of hemangiomata, *Br J Plast Surg* 6:83, 1953.
45. Weidman AI, Zimany A, Kopf AW: Underdevelopment of the human breast after radiotherapy, *Arch Dermatol* 93:708, 1966.
46. Job JC et al: Le deáveloppement preámatureá isoleá des seins chez les fillettes, *Arch Fr Peádiatr* 32:39, 1975.
47. Nelson KG: Premature thelarche in children born prematurely, *J Pediatr* 103:756, 1983.
48. Wilkins L, Blizzard RM, Migeon CJ: *The diagnosis and treatment of endocrine disorders in childhood and adolescence,* ed 3, Springfield, IL, 1965, Charles C Thomas.
49. Guyda HF et al: Determination of serum luteinizing hormone (SLII) by radioimmunoassay in disorders of adolescent sexual development, *Pediatr Res* 3:538, 1969.
50. Kenny FM et al: Radioimmunoassayable serum LH and FSH in girls with sexual precocity, premature thelarche and adrenarche, *J Clin Endocrinol Metab* 29:1272, 1969.
51. Mills JL et al: Premature thelarche, *Am J Dis Child* 135:743, 1981.
52. Caufriez A et al: Gonadotropins and prolactin pituitary reserve in premature thelarche, *J Pediatr* 91:751, 1977.

53. Reiter EO et al: Responsivity of pituitary gonadotrophins to luteinizing hormone–releasing factor in idiopathic precocious puberty, precocious thelarche, precocious adrenarche, and in patients treated with medroxyprogesterone acetate, *Pediatr Res* 9:111, 1975.

54. Tenore A et al: Prognostic signs in the evolution of premature thelarche by discriminant analysis, *J Endocrinol Invest* 14:375, 1991.

55. Pasquino AM et al: Hypothalamic-pituitary-gonadotrophic function in girls with premature thelarche, *Arch Dis Child* 55:941, 1980.

56. Ilicki A et al: Premature thelarche: natural history and sex hormone secretion in 68 girls, *Acta Paediatr Scand* 73:756, 1984.

57. Pasquino AM et al: Premature thelarche: a follow up study of 40 girls: natural history and endocrine findings, *Arch Dis Child* 60:1180, 1985.

58. Escobar ME, Rivarola MA, Bergadaá C: Plasma concentration of oestradiol-17β in premature thelarche and in different types of sexual precocity, *Acta Endocrinol* 81:351, 1976.

59. Pasquino AM et al: Progression of premature thelarche to central precocious puberty, *J Pediatr* 126:11, 1995.

60. Rosenfield RL: Normal and almost normal precocious variations in pubertal development premature pubarche and premature thelarche revisited, *Horm Res* 41(suppl 2):7, 1994.

61. Lorino CO, Finn M: Unilateral juvenile hypertrophy of the breast, *Br J Radiol* 60:193, 1987.

62. Luchsinger J: Bilateral mammary hypertrophy during pregnancy, *Rev Obstet Ginecol Venez* 20:707, 1960.

63. Moss WM: Gigantomastia with pregnancy: a case report with review of the literature, *Arch Surg* 96:27, 1968.

64. Nolan JJ: Gigantomastia: report of a case, *Obstet Gynecol* 19:526, 1962.

65. Martin JA: Treatment of cystic hygromas, *Tex State J Med* 50:217, 1954.

66. Mayl N, Vasconez LO, Jurkiewicz MJ: Treatment of macromastia in the actively enlarging breast, *Plast Reconstr Surg* 54:6, 1974.

67. Li Z et al: Congenital hypertrichosis universalis associated with gingival hyperplasia and macromastia, *Chin Med J* 99:916, 1986.

68. Bland KI, Copeland EM III: Breast disease: physiologic considerations. In Miller T, Rowlands B (eds): *The physiological basis of modern surgical care*, St Louis, 1988, Mosby.

69. Sperling RL, Gold JJ: Use of an anti-estrogen after a reduction mammaplasty to prevent recurrence of virginal hypertrophy of breasts: case report, *Plast Reconstr Surg* 52:439, 1973.

70. Ryan RF, Pernoll ML: Virginal hypertrophy, *Plast Reconstr Surg* 75:737, 1985.

71. Furnas DW: Subcutaneous mastectomy for juvenile hypertrophy of the breast: report of a case, *Br J Plast Surg* 35:367, 1982.

72. De Castro CC: Subcutaneous mastectomy for gigantomastia in an adolescent girl: case report, *Plast Reconstr Surg* 59:575, 1977.

73. Courtiss EH, Goldwym RM: Reduction mammaplasty by the inferior pedicle technique: an alternative to free nipple and areola grafting for severe macromastia or extreme ptosis, *Plast Reconstr Surg* 59:500, 1977.

74. Bland KI: One-stage simple mastectomy with immediate reconstruction for high-risk patients: an improved technique: the biologic basis for ductal-glandular mastectomy, *Arch Surg* 121:221, 1986.

75. Desai SN: Sudden gigantism of the breasts: drug induced? *Br J Plast Surg* 26:371, 1973.

76. Taylor PJ, Cumming DC, Corenblum B: Successful treatment of D-penicillamine–induced breast gigantism with danazol, *BMJ* 282:362, 1981.

77. Guillebaud J et al: Endocrine effects of danazol in menstruating women, *J Int Med Res* 5(suppl 3):57, 1977.

78. Buckle R: Studies on the treatment of gynecomastia with danazol (Danol), *J Int Med Res* 5(suppl 3):114, 1977.

79. Blaydes RM, Kinnebrew CA: Massive breast hyperplasia complicating pregnancy, *Obstet Gynecol* 12:601, 1958.

80. Palmuth P: *Observationem medicarum centuriae tres poshumae*, Braunschweig, Cent ii, 1648, OBS.

81. Parham KJ: Gigantomastia: report of a case, *Obstet Gynecol* 18:375, 1961.

82. Jessing A: Excessive mammary hypertrophy in pregnancy treated with androgenic hormones, *Nord Med* 63:237, 1960.

83. Lewison EF et al: Gigantomastia complicating pregnancy, *Surg Gynecol Obstet* 110:215, 1960.

84. Scott-Conner CE, Schorr SJ: The diagnosis and management of breast problems during pregnancy and lactation, *Am J Surg* 170:401, 1995.

85. Howard BA, Gusterson BA: Human breast development, *J Mammary Gland Biol Neoplasia* 5:119, 2000.

86. Spence RJ, Feldman JJ, Ryan JJ: Symmastia: the problem of medial confluence of the breasts, *Plast Reconstr Surg* 73:261, 1984.

87. Schonegg WD et al: Reduction-plasty of the breast in symmastia, *Geburtshilfe Frauenheilkd* 51:853, 1991.

88. McKissock PK: Discussion of symmastia: the problem of medial confluence of the breast, *Plast Reconstr Surg* 73:267, 1984.

89. Velanovich V: Ectopic breast tissue, supernumerary breasts, and supernumerary nipples, *South Med J* 88:903, 1995.

90. Cohen AJ et al: Hereditary renal-cell carcinoma associated with a chromosomal translocation, *N Engl J Med* 301:592, 1979.

91. Mehes K: Association of supernumerary nipples with other anomalies, *J Pediatr* 94:274, 1979.

92. Mehes K: Association of supernumerary nipples with other anomalies, *J Pediatr* 102:161, 1983.

93. Mehes K et al: Supernumerary nipples and urologic malignancies, *Cancer Genet Cytogenet* 24:185, 1987.

94. Rahbar F: Clinical significance of supernumerary nipples in black neonates, *Clin Pediatr* 21:46, 1982.

95. Mimouni F et al: Occurrence of supernumerary nipples in newborns, *Am J Dis Child* 137:952, 1983.

96. Kumar S, Cederbaum AI, Pletka PG: Renal cell carcinoma in polycystic kidneys: case report and review of literature, *J Urol* 124:708, 1980.

97. Mate K: Association of polythelia and aberrant ventricular conduction, *Orv Hetil* 117:1863, 1976.

98. Mate K et al: Polythelia associated with disturbances of cardiac conduction, *Cor Vasa* 21:112, 1979.

99. Miller G, Bernir I: Adenomatose erosive du mamelon, *Can J Surg* 8:261, 1965.

100. Carella A et al: Case report on supernumerary breast associated with multiple vertebral malformations, *Acta Neurol* 26:136, 1971.

101. Cellini A, Offidani A: Familial supernumerary nipples and breasts, *Dermatology* 185:56, 1992.

102. Brightmore TG: Cystic lesion of a dorsal supernumerary breast in a male, *Proc R Soc Med* 64:662, 1971.

103. Kenney RD, Flippo JL, Black EB: Supernumerary nipples and renal anomalies in neonates, *Am J Dis Child* 141:987, 1987.

104. Lau FT, Henline RB: Ureteral anomalies: report of a case manifesting three ureters on one side with one ending blindly in an aplastic kidney and a bifid pelvis with a single ureter on the other side, *JAMA* 96:587, 1931.

105. McFarland WL, Wallace S, Johnson DE: Renal carcinoma and polycystic disease, *J Urol* 107:530, 1972.

106. Ng RC, Suki WN: Renal cell carcinoma occurring in a polycystic kidney of a transplant recipient, *J Urol* 124:710, 1980.

107. Camisa C: Accessory breast on the posterior thigh of a man, *J Am Acad Dermatol* 3:467, 1980.

108. Abramson DJ: Bilateral intra-areolar polythelia, *Arch Surg* 110:1255, 1975.

109. Blackard CE, Mellinger GT: Cancer in a horseshoe kidney: a report of two cases, *Arch Surg* 97:616, 1968.

110. Varsano IB et al: Urinary tract abnormalities in children with supernumerary nipples, *Pediatrics* 73:103, 1984.

111. Jojart G, Seres E: Supernumerary nipples and renal anomalies, *Int Urol Nephrol* 26:141, 1994.

112. Goedert JJ, McKeen EA, Fraumeni JF Jr: Polymastia and renal adenocarcinoma, *Ann Intern Med* 95:182, 1981.

113. Goedert JJ et al: Polythelia and testicular cancer, *Ann Intern Med* 101:646, 1984.

114. Tollerud DJ et al: Familial testicular cancer and urogenital developmental anomalies, *Cancer* 55:1849, 1985.

115. Das DK et al: Fine needle aspiration cytologic diagnosis of axillary accessory breast tissue, including its physiologic changes and pathologic lesions, *Acta Cytol* 38:130, 1994.

116. DeCholnoky T: Accessory breast tissue in the axilla, *NY State J Med* 51:2245, 1951.

117. Orti E, Qazi QH: Polymastia. In Bergsma D (ed): *Birth defects compendium*, New York, 1979, Alan R Liss.

118. DeGrouchy J, Turleau C: *Clinical atlas of human chromosomes*, New York, 1977, John Wiley & Sons.

119. Chung CS, Myrianthopoulos NC: Factors affecting risks of congenital malformations. I. Analysis of epidemiologic factors in congenital malformations. Report from the Collaborative Perinatal Project, *Birth Defects Orig Artic Ser* 11:1, 1975.

120. Fleisher DS: Lateral displacement of the nipples, a sign of bilateral renal hypoplasia, *J Pediatr* 69:806, 1966.

121. Goeminne L: Synopsis of mammo-renal syndromes, *Humangenetik* 14:170, 1972.

122. Lorbek W: Ein Fall von Ureter trifidus, *Wien Med Wochenschr* 102:222, 1952.

123. Fraumeni JF Jr: Clinical patterns of familial cancer. In Mulvihill JJ, Miller RW, Fraumeni JF, Jr (eds): *Genetics of human cancer*, New York, 1977, Raven Press.

124. Mulvihill JJ: Genetic repertory of human neoplasia. In Mulvihill JJ, Miller RW, Fraumeni JF Jr (eds): *Genetics of human cancer*, New York, 1977, Raven Press.

125. John C: Uber akzessorische Milchdrüsenaand Warzen, insbesondere über milchdrüsemähnliche Bildungen in der Achselhoêe, *Arch Gynakol* 126:689, 1925.

126. Greer KE: Accessory axillary breast tissue, *Arch Dermatol* 109:88, 1974.

127. Brightmore T: Bilateral double nipples, *Br J Surg* 59:55, 1972.

128. Jeffcoate TN: *Principles of gynecology*, London, 1967, Butterworth.

129. Dworak O et al: Hamartoma of an ectopic breast arising in the inguinal region, *Histopathology* 24:169, 1994.

130. Reck T et al: Hamartoma of aberrant breast tissue in the inguinal region, *Chirurg* 66:923, 1995.

131. Raux JP: Lactation from axillary tail of breast, *BMJ* 1:28, 1955.

132. Hassim AM: Bilateral fibroadenoma in supernumerary breasts of the vulva, *J Obstet Gynaecol Br Commonw* 76:275, 1969.

133. Guerry RL, Pratt-Thomas HR: Carcinoma of supernumerary breast of vulva with bilateral mammary cancer, *Cancer* 38:2570, 1976.

134. Evans DM, Guyton DP: Carcinoma of the axillary breast, *J Surg Oncol* 59:190, 1995.

135. Vargas J et al: Fine needle aspiration diagnosis of carcinoma arising in an ectopic breast: a case report, *Acta Cytol* 39:941, 1995.

136. Velanovich V: Fine needle aspiration cytology in the diagnosis and management of ectopic breast tissue, *Am Surg* 61:277, 1995

V

CLINICAL ASPECTS OF BENIGN DISEASE

Evaluation and Treatment of Benign Breast Disorders

SAMUEL W. BEENKEN

KIRBY I. BLAND

The term *benign breast disorder* (BBD) can be defined as any nonmalignant breast condition and encompasses a wide range of clinical and pathologic disorders. Although BBD is not life threatening, clinicians require an in-depth understanding of its significance so that clear explanations can be given to affected patients, appropriate treatment can be instituted, and unnecessary long-term follow-up can be avoided.

In the 1950s, several studies demonstrated that the histologic changes of fibrocystic disease were widely distributed in patients who were not symptomatic and who had not demonstrated overt disease. From studies of both surgical and autopsy specimens, a spectrum of changes between normal histology and disease was demonstrated.[1] Epithelial hyperplasia was shown to be very common at menopause and could regress without treatment. In 1961, Obermand and French wrote, "Adenofibroma, fibrocystic disease and intraductal papilloma do not appear to represent distinct entities, but rather form a spectrum of conditions having their basis in an abnormality between hormonal stimulus to the breast and stromal and epithelial response."[2] Unfortunately, since then, *fibrocystic disease* and related terms have too often been used as blanket terms to describe symptoms, rationalize the need for breast biopsy, and explain biopsy results. This has led to confusion regarding the true nature of fibrocystic disease and its relationship to breast cancer. Autopsy studies have shown that most of the benign breast changes previously considered as disease are so common that they can be regarded as normal. An autopsy study of 200 breasts from 100 postmenopausal patients (mean age, 62 years) without clinical breast disease showed changes of "fibrocystic condition" in 54% of cases, while 46% were histologically free of this condition.[3] Hyperplasia with severe atypia was seen in only 3% of cases.

The goals of this chapter are (1) to provide an overview of BBD that will define the place that the more common conditions occupy in the overall spectrum of breast disease, (2) to provide some insight into current thinking regarding the pathogenesis of BBD and its relation to histologic changes of breast development and involution, and (3) to describe accepted treatments for common BBD conditions.

Breast Development, Cyclical Change, and Involution

The most significant feature during perimenarchal development of the breast is the addition of lobular structures to a rudimentary duct system. The lobules develop primarily between 15 and 25 years of age. Early lobules are gradually replaced by more mature and less active lobules during the menstrual cycle and especially during pregnancy. The luteal phase of the menstrual cycle is also associated with enhanced acinar sprouting from the ductules. A distinctive element of the lobule is its highly specialized connective tissue and the close interaction between epithelium and connective tissue, which are separated only by a basement membrane. Both the epithelial and stromal elements of lobules are under hormonal control, and there is evidence that the two work in tandem.

The details of the interaction of hormones and growth factors on epithelium, myoepithelium, basement membrane, and stroma are now being elucidated. As the mechanisms underlying these relationships become more clearly defined, it is apparent that interference with these relationships is responsible for many BBD conditions. The changes occurring with each menstrual cycle demonstrate a peak of mitosis in the late cycle followed by apoptosis.[4] These changes provide a continuing opportunity for alterations to occur. Over time, these alterations can produce marked differences in the structure and appearance of various areas of a breast on a purely random basis. A microscopic section of healthy breast from a patient who has no breast complaints or overt clinical disease can display a wide spectrum of histologic variation. Often one can see well-developed lobules, poorly developed lobules, dilated ducts and normal ducts, lobule-deficient fibrous tissue, and fatty tissue. These appearances provide for the "fibrosis" and "adenosis" described in biopsies taken from patients with nodular breasts. It has not always been appreciated that the same changes may be evident without any clinical complaint or finding.

Involutional changes in the breast are apparent by 35 years of age and often earlier, so cyclical change and involution can run in tandem for up to 20 years. Involution particularly affects the lobules where loose, hormone-responsive intralobular connective tissue is replaced by more dense interlobular fibrous tissue. By the time menopause is reached, involution is extensive, with only a few ducts remaining and very few lobular structures. As might be expected, minor aberrations of this process are common. Epithelial involution of the lobule is dependent on the continuing presence of surrounding specialized stroma. If the stroma disappears early, the epithelial acini remain and can form microcysts. Microcysts proceed to macroscopic cyst formation when a pressure disparity exists between secretion and drainage, as can occur with obstruction of the draining ductule. Microcyst formation is common in healthy breasts, as demonstrated by Parks.[1] In the process of cystic lobular involution, microcysts can appear even though specialized stroma is still present. Presumably, this arises from minor obstruction to the duct secondary to kinking or compression from fibrous tissue, or perhaps from vigorous secretion by still active epithelial tissue.

Aberrations of Normal Development and Involution

The aberrations of normal development and involution (ANDI) classification of BBD provides an overall framework for benign conditions of the breast that encompasses both pathogenesis and the degree of abnormality.[5] It is a bidirectional framework based on the fact that most BBD arise from normal physiologic processes (Table 9-1). The horizontal component defines BBD along a spectrum from normal to mild abnormality ("disorder") to severe abnormality ("disease"). The vertical component defines the pathogenesis of the condition. Together, the two provide a comprehensive framework into which can be fitted most BBD conditions. The basic principles underlying the ANDI classification are presented in Table 9-2.

The concept that BBD results from ANDI was first published in 1987. Since then, a great deal of information relating both to physiology and to pathology has provided support to those elements of the concept that were originally speculative. The ANDI classification was accepted and recommended by an international multidisciplinary working group in 1992.[6] Mastalgia provides an example of horizontal assessment. The clinical significance of mastalgia is quantified in the Cardiff Mastalgia Clinic through classification and assessment of the impact of mastalgia on patients' lives by visual linear analogue scales and breast pain charts.[7] It has been found that two thirds of a population of working women experience mastalgia. A majority of mastalgia cases evaluated are considered "normal," some are sufficiently troublesome to warrant attention and are regarded as a "disorder," but only a minority are sufficiently severe to be a major interference in the patient's life and are regarded as "disease."

DISORDERS OF DEVELOPMENT

Fibroadenoma. Fibroadenomas, which arise from lobules, are seen predominantly in women age 15 to 25. Parks showed that hyperplastic lobules are histologically identical to fibroadenomas and can be found in virtually all breast tissues.[1] All the cellular elements of fibroadenomas are normal on conventional and electron microscopy, and the epithelium and myoepithelium maintain a normal relationship.[8] Molecular biology studies show that fibroadenomas are polyclonal in keeping with hyperplasia, whereas phyllodes tumors are monoclonal in keeping with a neoplastic condition. Fibroadenomas usually grow to 1 or 2 cm in diameter and then remain constant. They show hormonal dependence similar to that of normal lobules. In particular, they lactate during pregnancy and involute to be replaced by hyaline connective tissue in the perimenopausal period. A fibroadenoma will occasionally grow to a size of 3 cm, but growth beyond 5 cm is very uncommon in Western populations and is regarded as disease (giant fibroadenoma). Similarly, multiple fibroadenomas (more than five lesions in one breast) are very uncommon in Western populations and are considered a disease. Fibroadenoma fits well into the ANDI classification: Small fibroadenomas are normal, clinical fibroadenomas (1 to 3 cm) are a disorder of the normal process, and giant and multiple fibroadenomas fit in the disease end of the spectrum.

Adolescent Hypertrophy. Adolescent hypertrophy is associated with gross stromal hyperplasia at the time of breast development. The cause is unknown, but there is

TABLE 9-1 ANDI Classification of Benign Breast Disease

	NORMAL→	DISORDER→	DISEASE
Early reproductive years (age 15-25)	Lobular development Stromal development	Fibroadenoma Adolescent hypertrophy	Giant fibroadenoma Gigantomastia
	Nipple eversion	Nipple inversion	Subareolar abscess/mammary duct fistula
Mature reproductive years (age 25-40)	Cyclical changes of menstruation	Cyclical mastalgia Nodularity	Incapacitating mastalgia
	Epithelial hyperplasia of pregnancy	Bloody nipple discharge	
Involution (age 35-55)	Lobular involution	Macrocysts Sclerosing lesions	
	Duct involution/dilation/sclerosis	Duct ectasia Nipple retraction	Periductal mastitis/abscess
	Epithelial turnover	Epithelial hyperplasia	Epithelial hyperplasia with atypia

TABLE 9-2	Principles Underlying the ANDI Classification

- Most BBDs are related to the normal processes of reproductive life.
- There is a spectrum of conditions that range from normal to "disorder" and occasionally to "disease."
- The ANDI classification embraces all aspects of the breast condition: symptoms, signs, histology, and physiology.

BBDs, Benign breast disorders.

a hormonal basis to the condition. The spectrum from a small breast through massive hyperplasia fits the horizontal element of the ANDI concept: An excessively large breast is a disorder, whereas gigantomastia is at the disease end of the spectrum.

DISORDERS OF CYCLICAL CHANGE

Mastalgia and Nodularity. Some discomfort and nodularity are so commonly associated with premenstrual enlargement and postmenstrual involution of the breast that they are regarded as normal. *Cyclical pronounced mastalgia* and *severe painful nodularity* are terms used to differentiate distressing symptoms from the more common physiologic discomfort and lumpiness. Painful nodularity that persists for more than 1 week of the menstrual cycle is considered a disorder. An underlying physiologic abnormality is excess prolactin release from the pituitary following stimulation of the hypothalamic-pituitary axis.[9]

DISORDERS OF INVOLUTION

Cyst Formation. Over a many-year period of cyclic changes, the integrated involution of stroma and epithelium is not always seen and disorders of the process are common. The exact mechanism of involution is not well understood, but it appears that involution of a lobular epithelium is dependent on the specialized stroma around it.[10] If the stroma involutes too quickly, the epithelial acini remain and can form microcysts, which are precursors for macrocyst formation. The frequent occurrence of macrocysts and the fact that they are often multiple and subclinical suggest that macrocysts are a disorder, not a disease requiring specific treatment. The fact that macrocysts can be either apocrine or nonapocrine in nature is poorly understood, but evidence suggests that they both develop along a common pathway.[10,11]

Sclerosing Adenosis. Sclerosing adenosis can be considered a disorder of either the proliferative or the involutional phase of the breast cycle (or both) because of histologic changes that are both proliferative and involutional in nature. Considering the complex interrelationship of the stromal fibrosis and epithelial regression that occur during involution, along with the concomitant cyclical change of ductal sprouting, it is not surprising that the characteristic distortion of epithelial acini by fibrous tissue seen in sclerosing adenosis is occasionally present.

Duct Ectasia and Periductal Mastitis. Another major group of BBD is that associated with duct ectasia and periductal mastitis. The pathogenesis of duct ectasia is obscure. Haagensen regarded duct ectasia (dilated ducts) as a primary event, which subsequently led to stagnation of secretions, epithelial ulceration, and leakage of duct secretions (containing chemically irritant fatty acids) into periductal tissue.[12] This sequence produced a local inflammatory process with periductal fibrosis and subsequent fibrous contraction and nipple retraction.

An alternative theory states that periductal mastitis is the primary process, which leads to weakening of the muscular layer of the ducts and secondary dilation. It is likely that both processes occur. Together, they explain the wide spectrum of clinical behavior seen in this condition: nipple discharge, nipple retraction, inflammatory masses, and abscesses. Both duct dilation and duct sclerosis represent disorders of involution. Periductal fibrosis can occur in the absence of duct ectasia or inflammation and probably represents part of the normal involutional process.[13] Duct ectasia is so common in the postmenopausal breast that it is considered part of the normal aging process.

Epithelial Hyperplasia. Parks showed that lobular and intraductal papillary hyperplasia is common in the premenopausal period and tends to regress spontaneously after menopause.[1] It is regarded as a disorder of normal involution. In an autopsy study, Kramer and Rush[14] found that 59% of women older than age 70 exhibited some degree of epithelial hyperplasia. Sloss, Bennett, and Clagett[15] concluded from another autopsy study, "the mere presence of blunt duct adenosis, apocrine epithelium and intraductal epithelial hyperplasia in the breast of women is insufficient to warrant such changes being called disease." However, studies by Page and colleagues[16] and Wellings, Jensen, and Marcum[17] have shown that the other end of the spectrum—atypical lobular hyperplasia and atypical ductal hyperplasia, particularly as seen in the terminal ductal lobular unit (TDLU)—is commonly associated with malignancy. There is insufficient evidence to determine whether these conditions present a continuous spectrum.

OTHER BENIGN BREAST DISORDERS

Nipple Inversion. Nipple inversion is a disorder of the development of the terminal ducts, preventing the normal protrusion of ducts and areola.

Mammary Duct Fistula. Nipple inversion predisposes to terminal duct obstruction, leading to recurrent subareolar abscess and mammary duct fistula—the usual form of periductal mastitis seen in younger women. Extraneous factors include smoking and oronipple contact.

Epithelial Hyperplasia of Pregnancy. Marked hyperplasia of the duct epithelium occurs in pregnancy. The papillary projections sometimes give rise to bilateral bloody nipple discharge.

Benign Duct Papilloma. Benign duct papilloma is a common condition that occurs during the years of cyclical activity. It shows minimal if any malignant potential and is regarded as a disorder of cyclical epithelial activity.

Pathology of Benign Breast Disorders

Of paramount importance for the optimal management of BBD is the histologic differentiation between benign, atypical, and malignant changes.[18,19] The histologic evaluation of a biopsy specimen also helps determine the subsequent risk of developing cancer. This information, together with the surgeon's knowledge of other risk factors, determines the frequency of follow-up and future mammography as well as the necessity of additional biopsies. Determining the clinical significance of the spectrum of histologic changes in BBD is a difficult problem that has been compounded by a lack of consistent nomenclature. This problem was addressed by Page and co-workers, whose work led to the development of a classification system that was subsequently adopted by the American College of Pathologists.[16,18-22] This system emphasizes the uselessness of the term *fibrocystic disease* and provides a practical classification of BBD histology that is clinically relevant. The classification system developed by Page separates the various types of BBD into three clinically relevant groups: nonproliferative lesions, proliferative lesions without atypia, and proliferative lesions with atypia (Table 9-3). This classification eliminates potentially confusing terminology and incorporates histologic criteria that are associated with an increased risk for the development of breast cancer.[23] The histologic features of the breast biopsy specimen, together with the surgeon's knowledge of the family history, establishes the relative risk for cancer. These data, combined with mammographic and physical examination findings, determine the management strategy and follow-up for the patient. This system is outlined in Table 9-3.

TABLE 9-3	Pathologic Classification System of Benign Breast Disorders

NONPROLIFERATIVE LESIONS OF THE BREAST
- Cysts and apocrine metaplasia
- Duct ectasia
- Mild ductal epithelial hyperplasia
- Calcifications
- Fibroadenoma and related lesions

PROLIFERATIVE BREAST DISORDERS WITHOUT ATYPIA
- Sclerosing adenosis
- Radial and complexing sclerosing lesions
- Florid ductal epithelial hyperplasia
- Intraductal papillomas

ATYPICAL PROLIFERATIVE LESIONS
- Atypical lobular hyperplasia (ALH)
- Atypical ductal hyperplasia (ADH)

Modified from Consensus Meeting: *Arch Pathol Lab Med* 110:171, 1986; and Dupont WD, Page DL: *N Engl J Med* 312:146, 1985.

NONPROLIFERATIVE LESIONS OF THE BREAST

Nonproliferative lesions of the breast account for approximately 70% of benign lesions and carry no increased risk of cancer.[16,17] Cysts and apocrine metaplasia, duct ectasia, mild ductal epithelial hyperplasia, calcifications, fibroadenomas, and related lesions are included in this category.

Cysts and Apocrine Metaplasia. Cysts are defined by the presence of fluid-filled epithelialized spaces.[24,25] Cysts in the breast vary greatly in size and number and can be microscopic or macroscopic. These lesions are almost always multifocal and bilateral and are almost never malignant.[26-29] Cysts originate from the terminal duct lobular unit (TDLU) or from an obstructed ectatic duct. The typical macroscopic cyst is round, appears bluish (blue-domed cyst), and usually contains dark fluid ranging in color from green-gray to brown. The epithelium of the cyst is often flattened, and apocrine metaplasia of the epithelium lining the wall of the cyst is occasionally seen (Table 9-4). The stroma surrounding these cysts is generally fibrotic and is often infiltrated with lymphocytes, plasma cells, and histiocytes.

Duct Ectasia. Duct ectasia involves the large and intermediate ductules of the breast.[10] It is most often recognized by the presence of palpable dilated ducts filled with desquamated ductal epithelium and proteinaceous secretions. Duct ectasia is common, being present in nearly half of women older than 60 years.[30] Periductal inflammation is a distinguishing histologic characteristic in this condition. The clinical significance

TABLE **9-4**	Epithelial Hyperplasia of the Breast

APOCRINE TYPE
- Apocrine metaplasia (most commonly seen in the lining of cysts)

DUCTAL TYPE
- Sclerosing adenosis
- Mild ductal hyperplasia
- Moderate ductal hyperplasia
- Florid ductal hyperplasia
- Atypical ductal hyperplasia (ADH)

LOBULAR TYPE
- Atypical lobular hyperplasia (ALH)
- Ductal involvement of cells of ALH

Modified from Consensus Meeting: *Arch Pathol Lab Med* 110:171, 1986; and Dupont WD, Page DL: *N Engl J Med* 312:146, 1985.

TABLE **9-5** Risk for Development of Invasive Carcinoma	
LESION	**RELATIVE RISK**
Nonproliferative lesions of the breast	No increased risk
Sclerosing adenosis	No increased risk
Intraductal papilloma	No increased risk
Florid hyperplasia	1.5- to 2-fold
Atypical lobular hyperplasia	4-fold
Atypical ductal hyperplasia	4-fold
Ductal involvement by cells of atypical ductal hyperplasia	7-fold
Lobular carcinoma in situ	10-fold
Ductal carcinoma in situ	10-fold

Data from Dupont WD, Page DL: *N Engl J Med* 312:146, 1985; and Page DL et al: *J Natl Cancer Inst* 61:1055, 1978.

of severe duct ectasia lies in its mimicry of invasive ductal carcinoma, but there is no demonstrated relationship to cancer risk.[31,32]

Mild Ductal Epithelial Hyperplasia. The fundamental feature of epithelial hyperplasia is an increased number of cells relative to what is normally observed along the basement membrane.[16] Normally, two cell layers are evident. The presence of three or more cell layers along the basement membrane is pathognomonic of hyperplasia of the duct epithelium.[16,33] Epithelial hyperplasia does not include conditions in which glandular (stromal) cells are increased in number relative to the basement membrane, a condition known as *adenosis*.[34]

The diagnosis of epithelial hyperplasia of ductal tissue is often made by exclusion. It represents any epithelial hyperplasia that lacks lobular, apocrine, or atypical features. Mild and moderate epithelial hyperplasia are recognized primarily to distinguish them from the more marked changes of florid epithelial hyperplasia, which carries an increased risk of breast cancer[16,20] (see Tables 9-4 and 9-5). A breast biopsy specimen showing mild hyperplasia does not imply any clinically significant risk of cancer.

Calcifications. Calcifications are common in the ductal, lobular, and stromal tissues of the breast. They can be macroscopic or microscopic and can be seen in blood vessels or lobules, free in the stroma, or associated with epithelium. Diffuse microcalcifications are commonly seen in sclerosing adenosis.[33,34]

Fibroadenoma and Related Lesions. Fibroadenomas are benign tumors composed of fibrous and epithelial elements.[35] The gross appearance of a fibroadenoma is usually diagnostic. It is a sharply circumscribed spherical mass that can be unilobular or multilobular. The cut surface is white or yellow, and on gross examination a fibroadenoma is pseudoencapsulated and sharply delineated from the surrounding breast tissue.[33] Microscopically, fibroadenomas have both an epithelial and a stromal component. The histologic pattern depends on which of these components is predominant. In general, the epithelial component consists of well-defined gland-like and ductlike spaces with varying degrees of epithelial hyperplasia. The stromal component consists of connective tissue with variable collagen content and rarely mature adipose tissue or smooth muscle.[10,36] Autopsy studies demonstrate that fibroadenomas are present in approximately 10% of women.[37] Although the peak incidence occurs between the second and third decades of life, fibroadenomas are occasionally seen in the elderly. In elderly patients, fibroadenomas can become dense as a result of calcification and the lack of epithelial elements. Fibroadenomas have a doubling time of approximately 1 year and generally cease growing once they reach 3 cm in diameter. The tumors are usually painless, are spherical, have smooth margins, and are mobile within the breast.

Adenomas of the breast are well-circumscribed tumors composed of benign epithelial elements with sparse stroma.[33,38] The sparse stroma is the histologic feature that differentiates adenomas from fibroadenomas, in which the stroma is abundant. Adenomas can be divided into tubular adenomas and lactating adenomas.[35] Tubular adenomas present in young women as well-defined, freely mobile tumors that clinically resemble fibroadenomas. Lactating adenomas present during pregnancy or during the postpartum period. On microscopic examination, they have lobulated borders and are composed of glands lined by cuboidal cells that possess secretory activity identical to that normally observed in breast tissue during pregnancy and lactation.

Hamartomas are discrete breast tumors, which are commonly 2 to 4 cm in diameter, firm, and sharply circumscribed.[35,39] Microscopically, numerous lobules are present that can coalesce to form a homogeneous mass. Hamartomas and fibroadenomas share the feature of gross circumscription and the presence of lobules. The lobules in hamartomas are a major component of the tumor, whereas the stroma of a fibroadenoma is usually more cellular than the stroma of a hamartoma. Hamartomas have areas of fat replacement, which is a rare observation in fibroadenomas.

Adenolipomas consist of sharply circumscribed nodules of fatty tissue that have normal lobules and ducts interspersed.[40] Microscopically, the fat is normal and the lobules and ducts are fairly evenly distributed throughout the tumor. Most of the lobules are not associated with fibrous stroma.

PROLIFERATIVE BREAST DISORDERS WITHOUT ATYPIA

Proliferative breast disorders without atypia include sclerosing adenosis, intraductal papillomas, and florid ductal epithelial hyperplasia.[41] There is an increased risk of invasive breast cancer (approximately 1.5 to 2 times normal) when the breast specimen demonstrates florid ductal epithelial hyperplasia (see Table 9-5).

Sclerosing Adenosis. Sclerosing adenosis is a proliferation of glandular and stromal elements resulting in an enlargement and distortion of lobular units.[34,42] Microscopically, the condition is characterized by an increased number of acinar structures and by fibrosis of the lobular stroma while the normal two-cell population along the enveloping basement membrane is maintained. Sclerosing adenosis commonly occurs in the context of multiple microscopic cysts but occasionally presents as a palpable mass.[43] Diffuse microcalcifications are commonly seen in sclerosing adenosis. The significant clinical aspect of sclerosing adenosis is its mimicry of cancer.[44]

Sclerosing adenosis can be confused with cancer on physical examination, by mammography, and at gross pathologic examination. The borders of the lesion are irregular. Maintenance of the lobular architecture as determined by low-power evaluation under the light microscope allows sclerosing adenosis to be identified as a benign lesion. Sclerosing adenosis is confined for the most part to the childbearing and perimenopausal years. It has no proven premalignant implications. Excisional biopsy and histologic study of these lesions is often necessary to exclude the diagnosis of cancer.

Radial Scars and Complex Sclerosing Lesions. Radial scars and complex sclerosing lesions of the breast are characterized by central sclerosis and varying degrees of epithelial proliferation, apocrine metaplasia,

and papilloma formation.[45] The term *radial scar* is reserved for smaller lesions (up to 1 cm in diameter), whereas *complex sclerosing lesion* is used for larger masses. Radial scars originate at the point of terminal duct branching.[46] With the naked eye, the appearance is often unremarkable, but with magnification the characteristic histologic changes radiate from a central white area of fibrosis, which contains elastic elements. Complex sclerosing lesions closely resemble radial scars but on a larger scale. All of the histologic features of a radial scar are seen in these larger lesions, but the involved elements show a greater disturbance of structure with papilloma formation, apocrine metaplasia, and occasionally sclerosing adenosis.[47]

Florid Ductal Epithelial Hyperplasia. Florid hyperplasia is found in more than 20% of biopsy samples and thus is the most common proliferative lesion of the breast.[16] This entity is characterized by an increase in cell number within the ducts. Florid hyperplasia consists of a proliferation of cells that occupy at least 70% of the duct lumen and often distend the involved spaces. Architecturally, epithelial hyperplasia is either solid or papillary and is characterized by intracellular spaces that are irregular, slitlike, and variably shaped.

Intraductal Papillomas. Solitary intraductal papillomas are tumors of the major lactiferous ducts and are most commonly observed in premenopausal women.[33,48] A common presenting symptom is nipple discharge, which may be serous or bloody. Intraductal papillomas are generally smaller than 0.5 cm in diameter but may be as large as 4 or 5 cm.[49] Grossly, these lesions are pinkish tan, friable, and usually attached to the wall of the involved duct by a stalk. Microscopically, these lesions are composed of multiple branching papillae with a central fibrous vascular core that is lined by a layer of epithelial cells. Variable amounts of fibrosis are present between the epithelial elements. It is often difficult to differentiate between benign papilloma and papillary cancer on frozen section.[50] Moreover, there has been considerable debate regarding the malignant potential of papillomas. In any case, it is rare for these lesions to undergo malignant transformation, and their presence does not appear to increase a woman's overall risk of developing breast cancer.

Multiple intraductal papillomas tend to occur in younger patients and are less frequently associated with nipple discharge than are solitary intraductal papillomas.[33] Multiple intraductal papillomas are often peripheral, tend to be bilateral, and most important, appear to be susceptible to malignant transformation. In Haagensen's series of 39 patients with multiple papillomas, simultaneous cancer was observed in 38%.[51]

ATYPICAL PROLIFERATIVE LESIONS

Atypical proliferative lesions include both ductal and lobular lesions. These lesions have some, but not all, of the features of carcinoma in situ. At times, even the most experienced pathologists disagree as to whether a given lesion is atypical hyperplasia or carcinoma in situ.

Atypical Lobular Hyperplasia. Atypical lobular hyperplasia fulfills some, but not all, of the criteria of lobular carcinoma in situ.* The cytology of atypical lobular hyperplasia is usually quite bland, with round, lightly stained eosinophilic cytoplasm. The uniformity and roundness of the cell population is pathognomonic of atypical lobular hyperplasia. The lobular unit is less than half filled with these cells, and no significant distortion of the lobular unit is present.[16] If any lobular unit fulfills the criteria for lobular carcinoma in situ, this diagnosis overrides the presence of atypical lobular hyperplasia from a prognostic and therapeutic perspective. Cells of atypical lobular hyperplasia can involve the ducts and present histologic features identical to those of lobular carcinoma in situ.[54,55] In 1978, the spectrum of disease ranging from atypical lobular hyperplasia to lobular carcinoma in situ was termed *lobular neoplasia* by Haagensen and associates.[56] The risk of subsequent invasive cancer in women with atypical lobular hyperplasia is four times that of women who did not have this diagnosis.[19-21] (see Table 9-5) This risk is approximately tenfold in women with lobular carcinoma in situ. The incidence of atypical lobular hyperplasia present in benign biopsies is slightly greater than 1%, with the great majority of cases occurring in the perimenopausal period. As with atypical ductal hyperplasia, there appears to be an increased incidence in patients with a strong family history of breast cancer. Women with atypical lobular hyperplasia and a family history of breast cancer in a first-degree relative have a risk of invasive cancer that is twice that of the patient who presents with atypical lobular hyperplasia alone.[20]

Atypical Ductal Hyperplasia. Atypical ductal hyperplasia is diagnosed when atypia is present and either the cytologic or architectural criteria for ductal carcinoma in situ (DCIS) is absent. Page and co-workers[19] have emphasized that each of the following criteria must be met for a diagnosis of DCIS: (1) a uniform population of cells, (2) smooth geometric spaces between cells or micropapillary formation with uniform cellular placement, and (3) hyperchromatic nuclei. Atypical ductal hyperplasia has some, but not all, of these features. The natural history of atypical ductal hyperplasia suggests an intermediate risk (approximately fourfold) for the development of invasive cancer[19] (see Table 9-5). Women with atypical ductal hyperplasia who were followed for 15 years after breast biopsy alone developed invasive breast cancer about four times as frequently as women in the general population.[19,21] This relative risk translates into an absolute risk that 10% of women with atypical ductal hyperplasia will develop invasive carcinoma over a 10- to 15-year period following biopsy.

Clinical Features of Benign Breast Disorders

A useful classification system for BBD was described by Love and colleagues[33] and Love, Gelman, and Silen[57] and is based on symptoms and physical findings. Six general categories were identified (Table 9-6): physiologic swelling and tenderness, nodularity, mastalgia, dominant masses, nipple discharge, and breast infection.

PHYSIOLOGIC SWELLING AND TENDERNESS

Many women experience premenstrual tenderness, which is often associated with mild breast swelling. These changes are physiologic and generally limited to the reproductive years because they are hormonally regulated. Cyclical alterations in breast structure, contour,

TABLE 9-6 Classification of Benign Breast Disease Based on Clinical Features

Physiologic swelling and tenderness

Nodularity

Mastalgia (breast pain)

Dominant lumps
- Gross cysts
- Galactoceles
- Fibroadenoma

Nipple discharge
- Galactorrhea
- Abnormal nipple discharge

Breast infections
- Intrinsic mastitis
  - Postpartum engorgement
  - Lactational mastitis
  - Lactational breast abscess
- Chronic recurrent subareolar abscess
- Acute mastitis associated with macrocystic breasts
- Extrinsic infections

Modified from Love SM et al: *N Engl J Med* 307:1010, 1982; and Love SM et al: *Benign breast disorders*, Philadelphia, 1987, JB Lippincott.

*References 16, 18, 19, 21, 52, 53.

and size result from variations in plasma concentrations of gonadotrophic and ovarian hormones.[58] Before the onset of menses, the mammary lobules, stroma, and ducts become engorged. The connective stroma and ductal epithelial cells begin to increase in size and number by the second week of the cycle.[58] With the onset of menses, the epithelial cells lining the ducts desquamate.

NODULARITY

A cyclical pattern of diffuse lumpiness or nodularity is common and represents the responsiveness of breast parenchyma and stroma to circulating estrogenic and progestational hormones.[5,59] The nodularity can be finely granular or grossly lumpy, and it can involve the entire breast or a specific region. Patey coined the term *pseudolump* to describe a dominant area of lumpiness that coalesces into the surrounding breast tissue.[60,61]

MASTALGIA

Mastalgia (pain in the breast) is both common and of concern to the patient, as evidenced by the large number of women who present to their surgeons with such complaints.[62] These individuals are generally seeking reassurance that they do not have cancer or another serious breast disorder. The surgeon rules out this possibility with a careful history and physical examination and a mammogram. With such patients, an explanation of the hormonal nature of the breast pain is helpful in alleviating anxiety and often no other treatment is necessary.

DOMINANT MASSES

A dominant mass in the breast must be investigated to rule out cancer. Dominant masses that are benign include macroscopic cysts, galactoceles, and fibroadenomas.[10] As a general rule, discrete masses are aspirated with a needle to determine whether they are cystic or solid. If the lesion is cystic, the wall collapses with needle aspiration and the cyst is no longer palpable. If the lesion is solid, further evaluation to rule out cancer is mandatory.

NIPPLE DISCHARGE

Nipple discharge can be classified as galactorrhea or abnormal nipple discharge.[33,63] Galactorrhea is the spontaneous discharge of milklike fluid as a result of stimulation of the breast secondary to elevated prolactin secretion from the pituitary. Prolactin levels can be elevated in patients who use oral contraceptives, in patients with thyroid disease, and as a result of a functional pituitary adenoma. Appropriate management includes thyroid tests and determination of the serum prolactin level. Abnormal nipple discharge can be bloody or nonbloody. Takeda and colleagues noted that the presence of red blood cells or clusters of more

than 30 ductal cells is suggestive of malignancy.[64] The most common causes of bloody discharge from the nipple are intraductal papilloma, duct ectasia, and cancer.

BREAST INFECTIONS

Excluding the postpartum period, infections of the female breast are rare. They are classified as intrinsic (secondary to abnormalities in breast architecture or function) or extrinsic (secondary to an infection in an adjacent organ or structure that involves the breast) infections of the breast.[63] Intrinsic mastitis includes postpartum engorgement, lactational mastitis, and lactational breast abscess. Chronic recurrent subareolar abscesses occur primarily in women in the reproductive years and have a high incidence of squamous metaplasia of the involved ducts. Antibiotics are generally not of therapeutic benefit in this setting, and resolution of the infection depends on excision of the chronically involved site. Acute mastitis associated with gross cysts is observed in the patient with macrocystic breasts who develops a localized area of redness, pain, edema, and fever. Because this entity mimics inflammatory cancer, the involved lesion is often aspirated or sampled by incisional biopsy for culture and histology. Extrinsic infections develop secondary to an infectious process within the thoracic cavity or in the skin overlying the breast.

Treatment of Benign Breast Disease[7]

Most BBD can be regarded as minor aberrations of normality and hence do not demand specific treatment. This being the case, any active management of these conditions is based on considerations such as an accurate diagnosis, the patient's concern, and interference with quality of life.

CYSTS OF THE BREAST

Because needle aspiration of breast masses can produce artifacts that make mammographic assessment more difficult, many radiologists prefer to image ill-defined breast masses before aspiration. In practice, the first investigation of easily palpable masses in the breast is often the insertion of a needle. When this approach is practiced, cysts will often be diagnosed when the patient is first seen. A 21-gauge needle with a syringe of appropriate size (10 or 20 ml) is placed directly into the mass, which is fixed by two fingers of the opposite hand. The volume of a typical cyst is 5 to 10 ml but it can be 75 ml or more. If the mass proves to be solid, a cytologic specimen is obtained. If the fluid is not bloodstained, the cyst is aspirated to dryness, the needle removed, and the fluid discarded. Cytologic examination of cyst fluid is not useful or cost effective unless the fluid is bloodstained. Many have advocated cytologic examination of all cyst fluid, but it is now recognized to be unnecessary.[61,65-67] After aspiration, the breast is carefully palpated to exclude a residual mass. If one exists, another needle biopsy is performed under ultrasound guidance for cytologic examination (and to exclude a persistent cyst) before excisional biopsy.

If the fluid is bloodstained, 1 to 2 ml only of fluid is taken for cytologic examination. The mass is then imaged with ultrasound, and any solid area in the cyst is biopsied. The presence of blood is usually obvious, but in cysts with dark fluid, examining for blood using microscopy or via a chemical occult blood test can eliminate any doubt. Blood must be regarded as synonymous with tumor (usually benign, but sometimes malignant). To summarize, there are two cardinal rules for safe cyst aspiration, and these must always be observed: (1) The mass must disappear completely after aspiration. If it does not, it must be approached like any other persistent mass with mammography, repeat needle biopsy and open biopsy as indicated. (2) The fluid must not be bloodstained. If it is, ultrasound and cytologic examination as outlined previously will be helpful but open biopsy is recommended, even if all other assessments are negative.

FIBROADENOMA AND RELATED TUMORS

In the past, removal of all fibroadenomas has been advocated irrespective of age or other considerations. Yet most fibroadenomas are self-limiting, and many go undiagnosed. In practice, solitary fibroadenomas in young women are often removed to alleviate patient concern. However, it is reasonable to take a more conservative approach. The safety of conservation has been assessed in a prospective study[68] in which the criteria for conservation were age younger than 40 years and a clinical diagnosis confirmed by cytologic examination and ultrasound (and mammography if older than 35 years). Ninety percent of patients opted for conservation and were monitored regularly. Excision was advised if the volume of the tumor increased by 20%, as occurred in 9% of the patients. Patients were discharged after 2 years if the tumor remained static or regressed. No tumor under observation proved to be a cancer. The authors suggest that core needle biopsy can further increase the safety of this conservative approach. No cancers were missed or subsequently developed in another smaller series of patients who were younger than 30 years.[69] In this series, 53 of the 85 fibroadenomas originally treated conservatively came to excision and none were found to be malignant.

Transformation of a fibroadenoma to a phyllodes tumor is an extremely rare occurrence, but it is desirable to identify such a tumor within a conservative management policy. Noguchi and colleagues[70] demonstrated that it is impossible to identify a phyllodes tumor on the basis of age, tumor size, multiplicity, or conventional histology, but they were able to do so by clonal analysis. They claimed that the technique was reliably performed on fine-needle aspiration specimens. This may become a practical procedure in the future, at least in those fibroadenomas that show progression on ultrasound monitoring.

SCLEROSING ADENOSIS, RADIAL SCAR, AND COMPLEX SCLEROSING LESIONS

The diagnostic workup for radial scars, complex sclerosing lesions, and sclerosing adenosis is similar: stereoscopic or open biopsy depending on (1) the facilities and experience available and (2) the perceived risk of malignancy from the radiologic appearance. It is widely accepted that it is impossible to differentiate these lesions with certainty from cancer by mammographic features. Frouge and colleagues[71] reported the pathologic findings in 40 radial scars diagnosed by mammography: 20 were radial scars, 12 were cancers, and 8 were cancers (7 tubular) associated with a radial scar. On review of the antecedent mammograms, it was impossible to differentiate the three groups based on the size and shape of the spicule, the size of the central core, or associated calcifications. Local excision is adequate management for benign lesions.

THE DUCT ECTASIA/PERIDUCTAL MASTITIS COMPLEX

Mildly painful and tender masses behind the areola are observed initially with the likelihood that they will resolve spontaneously. More painful masses are explored with a 21-gauge needle, and any fluid aspirated is submitted for cytologic examination and culture using a transport medium appropriate for the detection of anaerobic organisms. If pus is not present, patients are started on a combination of metronidazole and dicloxacillin while awaiting the results of culture. Antibiotics are then continued on the basis of sensitivity tests. Many early cases respond satisfactorily, especially in the short term. When there is more than a minimum amount of pus, one proceeds to surgical drainage with continuing antibiotic cover. Once a large amount of pus has formed, repeated aspiration is unlikely to lead to resolution and can result in destruction of breast tissue and skin with a less satisfactory cosmetic result. Duct excision is the recommended option in this setting. Antibiotic therapy is particularly useful in recurrent inflammation after formal duct excision. A prolonged course—at least 2 weeks and repeated once if necessary—is tried before resorting to further surgery. Table 9-7 presents indications for surgery for patients with duct ectasia or periductal mastitis.

TABLE **9-7** Duct Ectasia and Periductal Mastitis: Indications for Surgery

Nipple discharge

Correction of nipple inversion

Diagnosis of retroareolar mass

Subareolar abscess

Recurrent abscess with fistula

Nipple Discharge. Nonbloody nipple discharge, typically from several ducts and sometimes bilateral, is a benign condition with no increased cancer risk. It is not normally an indication for surgical treatment. Investigation and treatment is not necessary except in those rare cases in which the discharge is so profuse as to require wearing a breast pad to avoid social embarrassment. In this situation, one excludes a prolactinoma and then offers the patient the operation of total duct excision, which is bilateral when necessary. When bloody nipple discharge is present, there is a significant risk of cancer or hyperplastic lesions, especially when the patient is older than age 40. In this setting, the operation of total duct excision has some advantages over more conservative procedures. In particular, it provides a good histologic specimen and relieves the patient's anxiety.

Correction of Nipple Inversion. Patients are more likely to request correction of congenital nipple inversion than retraction due to duct ectasia occurring later in life, but some patients do request correction of retraction for the latter condition. Although the results are usually satisfactory, patients seeking correction for cosmetic reasons should be aware of the possibility of nipple necrosis, interference with sensation, inability to breastfeed and the possibility that postoperative fibrosis will lead to late recurrent inversion. Because the condition results from shortening of the ducts, a complete division of the subareolar ducts is the only procedure that can correct it permanently. The surgeon should not encourage operative correction for cosmetic reasons alone. When patients have duct excision or division carried out for complications of periductal mastitis, the resulting correction of nipple inversion is an appreciated side effect. Such patients may then ask for operative correction of the contralateral inverted nipple. Accumulation of debris in an inverted nipple can be malodorous and provides another indication for correction.

Diagnosis of a Retroareolar Mass. The tender acute retroareolar mass of periductal mastitis often resolves spontaneously, so surgery is delayed if aspiration biopsy is suggestive of this diagnosis. When a mass persists for several weeks, one can treat it by performing a simple excisional biopsy, even if dilated ducts filled

with proteinaceous material are encountered. When an abscess is encountered during surgery, the surgeon can either undertake simple drainage with a view to further surgery should the problem recur or proceed immediately to total duct excision under appropriate antibiotic cover. The first course is favored in young women, whereas the latter course is favored in older women who are past the childbearing period.

Subareolar Abscess. A subareolar abscess is confirmed with needle aspiration, which also provides a specimen for cytologic examination and bacterial culture. An established abscess is best treated with open drainage. Unlike a puerperal abscess, the abscess is usually unilocular and often associated with a single duct system. Therefore it is desirable to confine the process to a single segment and drainage is conservative. Preoperative ultrasound will accurately show the extent of the abscess.

Most patients with anaerobic bacteria will develop recurrent infection and/or a fistula. Therefore it is advisable to proceed to a definitive procedure (fistulectomy or duct excision) after 6 to 8 weeks in most cases. The resulting wound can be managed satisfactorily by permitting healing by secondary intention or by primary closure under antibiotic cover.[72] If the patient prefers a more conservative approach, aspiration under antibiotic cover is a reasonable alternative and has been advocated by Dixon.[73] In this setting, aspiration is facilitated by ultrasound guidance. Repeated aspirations are often necessary, and 40% of cases involving anaerobic bacteria recur after a short follow-up period. Scholefield, Duncan, and Rogers,[74] reporting on a

TABLE **9-8** Treatment of Recurrent Subareolar Sepsis

SUITABLE FOR FISTULECTOMY	SUITABLE FOR TOTAL DUCT EXCISION
Small abscess–localized to one segment	Large abscess–affecting >50% of areolar circumference
Recurrence always at the same site	Recurrence involving a different segment
Mild or no nipple inversion	Gross nipple inversion
Patient unconcerned about nipple inversion	Patient requests correction of nipple inversion
Younger patient	Older patient
No discharge from other ducts	Purulent discharge from other ducts between episodes
	Recurrence after fistulectomy

TABLE 9-9	Causes of Recurrent Duct Ectasia/Periductal Mastitis
Persisting abscess cavity	
Persistent proximal ducts	
Persistent distal ducts	
Persisting or recurrent nipple inversion	
Early pregnancy	
Contralateral disease	
Factitial disease	

10-year follow-up, found that 90% of patients with anaerobic infections had recurrent infections.

Recurrent Abscess with Fistula. When a patient has a recurrent abscess with fistula, the surgeon must make the difficult decision as to whether the condition is best treated with fistulectomy or major duct excision. Some of the factors bearing on this decision are presented in Table 9-8. When a localized periareolar abscess recurs at the same point and a fistula is clearly present, the operation of choice is fistulectomy. It is a simple procedure with minimal complications and a high degree of success. If it fails (Table 9-9), total duct excision can still be performed. When subareolar sepsis is diffuse rather than localized to one segment or when more than one fistula opening is present, total duct excision is the procedure of choice. The former situation is likely to be seen in young women with squamous metaplasia of a single duct, whereas the latter is likely to be seen in an older woman with multiple ectatic ducts. However, age is not a reliable guide, and fistula excision is considered the best initial procedure for localized lesions irrespective of age. One exception is when there is marked nipple inversion and the patient wishes to have this corrected. These circumstances tip the balance toward total duct excision, particularly if the patient will not be breast-feeding in the future.

REFERENCES

1. Parks AG: The microanatomy of the breast, *Ann Roy Coll Surgeons Engl* 25:295, 1959.
2. Oberman HA, French AJ: Chronic fibrocystic disease of the breast, *Surg Gynecol Obstet* 112:647, 1961.
3. Sarnelli R, Squartini F: Fibrocystic condition and 'at risk' lesions in asymptomatic breasts: a morphologic study of postmenopausal women, *Clin Exp Obstet Gynecol* 18:271, 1991.
4. Vorherr H: *The breast: morphology, physiology and lactation,* New York, 1974, Academic Press.
5. Hughes LE, Mansel RE, Webster DJTW: Aberrations of normal development and involution (ANDI): a new perspective on pathogenesis and nomenclature of benign breast disorders, *Lancet* 2:1316, 1987.
6. Hughes LE, Smallwood J, Dixon JM: Nomenclature of benign breast disorders: report of a working party on the rationalisation of concepts and terminology of benign breast conditions, *Breast* 1:15, 1992.
7. LE Hughes, RE Mansel, DJT Webster (eds): *Benign disorders and diseases of the breast concepts and clinical management,* ed 2, Philadelphia, 2000, WB Saunders.
8. Archer F, Omar N: The fine structure of fibroadenoma of the human breast, *J Pathol* 99:113, 1969.
9. Kumar S et al: Prediction of response to endocrine therapy in pronounced cyclical mastalgia, using dynamic tests of prolactin release, *Clin Endocrinol* 23:699, 1985.
10. Azzopardi JG: *Problems in breast pathology,* Philadelphia, 1979, WB Saunders.
11. Miller WR et al: Classification of human breast cysts according to electrolyte and androgen conjugate composition, *Clin Oncol* 9:227, 1983.
12. Page DL, Anderson TJ: Miscellaneous, non-neoplastic conditions. In *Diagnostic histopathology of the breast,* Edinburgh, 1987, Churchill Livingstone.
13. Elston CW, Ellis IO (eds): *The breast,* ed 3, vol 13, *Symmer's Systematic Pathology,* Edinburgh, 1998, Churchill Livingstone.
14. Kramer WM, Rush BF: Mammary duct proliferation in the elderly: a histological study, *Cancer* 31:130, 1973.
15. Sloss PT, Bennett WA, Clagett OT: Incidence in normal breasts of features associated with chronic cystic mastitis, *Am J Pathol* 33:1181, 1957.
16. Page DL et al: Relationship between component parts of fibrocystic disease complex and breast cancer, *J Nat Cancer Inst* 61:1055, 1978.
17. Wellings SR, Jensen HM, Marcum RG: An atlas of subgross pathology of the human breast with reference to possible precancerous lesions, *J Nat Cancer Inst* 55:231, 1975.
18. Page DL: Cancer risk assessment in benign biopsies, *Hum Pathol* 17:871, 1986.
19. Page DL et al: Atypical hyperplastic lesions of the female breast: a long-term follow-up study, *Cancer* 55:2698, 1985.
20. Dupont WD, Page DL: Risk factors for breast cancer in women with proliferative breast disease, *N Engl J Med* 312:146, 1985.
21. Page DL, Dupont WD, Rogers LW: Breast cancer risk of lobular-based hyperplasia after biopsy: "ductal" pattern lesions, *Cancer Detect Prevent* 9:441, 1986.
22. Consensus Meeting: Is "fibrocystic disease" of the breast precancerous? *Arch Pathol Lab Med* 110:171, 1986.
23. Hutchinson WB et al: Risk of breast cancer in women with benign breast disease, *J Natl Cancer Inst* 65:13, 1980.
24. Hughes LE, Mansel RE, Webster DJT: Cysts of the breast. In *Benign disorders and diseases of the breast: concepts and clinical management,* London, 1989, Bailliere Tindall.
25. Page DL, Anderson TJ: Cysts and apocrine change. In *Diagnostic histopathology of the breast,* New York, 1987, Churchill Livingstone.
26. Harrington E, Lesnick G: The association between gross cysts of the breast and breast cancer, *Breast* 7:13, 1981.
27. Herrman JB: Mammary cancer subsequent to aspiration of cysts in the breast, *Ann Surg* 173:40, 1971.
28. Kodlin D et al: Chronic cystic mastopathy and breast cancer: a follow-up study, *Cancer* 39:2603, 1977.
29. Page DL, Dupont WD: Are breast cysts a premalignant marker? *Eur J Cancer Clin Oncol* 22:635, 1986.
30. Frantz VK et al: Incidence of chronic cystic disease in so-called "normal breasts," a study based on 225 postmortem examinations, *Cancer* 4:762, 1951.

31. Haagensen CD: Mammary-duct ectasia: a disease that may stimulate carcinoma, *Cancer* 4:749, 1951.

32. Page DL, Anderson TJ: Miscellaneous non-neoplastic conditions. In *Diagnostic histopathology of the breast*, New York, 1987, Churchill Livingstone.

33. Love SM et al: *Benign breast disorders*, Philadelphia, 1987, JB Lippincott.

34. Page DL, Anderson TJ: Adenosis. In *Diagnostic histopathology of the breast*, New York, 1987, Churchill Livingstone.

35. Fechner RE: Fibroadenoma and related lesions. In Page DL, Anderson TJ (eds): *Diagnostic histopathology of the breast*, New York, 1987, Churchill Livingstone.

36. Goodman ZD, Taxy JB: Fibroadenomas of the breast with prominent smooth muscle, *Am J Surg Pathol* 5:99, 1981.

37. Hughes LE, Mansel RE, Webster DJT: Fibroadenoma and related tumors. In *Benign disorders and diseases of the breast: concepts and clinical management*, London, 1989, Bailliere Tindall.

38. Moross T, Land AP, Mahoney L: Tubular adenoma of breast, *Arch Pathol Lab Med* 107:84, 1983.

39. Arrigoni MG, Dockerty MB, Judd ES: The identification and treatment of mammary hamartoma, *Surg Gynecol Obstet* 133:577, 1971.

40. Spalding JE: Adenolipoma and lipoma of the breast, *Guy's Hosp Rep* 94:80, 1945.

41. Azzopardi JG: Benign and malignant proliferative epithelial lesions of the breast: a review, *Eur J Cancer Clin Oncol* 19:1717, 1983.

42. Hughes LE, Mansel RE, Webster DJT: Sclerosing adenosis. In *Benign disorders and diseases of the breast: concepts and clinical management*, London, 1989, Bailliere Tindall.

43. Greenblatt RB, Nazhat C, Ben-Nun I: The treatment of benign breast disease with danazol, *Fertil Steril* 34:242, 1980.

44. MacErlean DP, Nathan BE: Calcification in sclerosing adenosis simulating malignant breast calcification, *Br J Radiol* 45:944, 1972.

45. Page DL, Anderson TJ: Radial scars and complex sclerosing lesions. In *Diagnostic histopathology of the breast*, New York, 1987, Churchill Livingstone.

46. Anderson JA, Battersby S: Radial scars of benign and malignant breast: comparative features and significance, *J Pathol* 147:23, 1985.

47. Andersen JA, Gram JB: Radial scar in the female breast: a long term follow-up study of 32 cases, *Cancer* 53:2557, 1984.

48. Page DL, Anderson TJ: Papilloma and related lesions. In *Diagnostic histopathology of the breast*, New York, 1987, Churchill Livingstone.

49. Carter D: Intraductal papillary tumors of the breast: a study of 78 cases, *Cancer* 39:1689, 1977.

50. Hughes LE, Mansel RE, Webster DJT: Operations. In *Benign disorders and diseases of the breast: concepts and clinical management*, London, 1989, Bailliere Tindall.

51. Haagensen CD: *Diseases of the breast*, ed 3, Philadelphia, 1986, WB Saunders.

52. Ashikari R et al: A clinicopathological study of atypical lesions of the breast, *Cancer* 33:310, 1974.

53. Black MM et al: Association of atypical characteristics of benign breast lesions with subsequent risk of breast cancer, *Cancer* 29:338, 1972.

54. Page DL, Dupont WD, Rogers LW: Ductal involvement by cells of atypical lobular hyperplasia in the breast, *Hum Pathol* 19:201, 1988.

55. Rosen PP et al: Lobular carcinoma in situ of the breast: detailed analysis of 99 patients with average follow-up of 24 years, *Am J Surg Pathol* 2:225, 1978.

56. Haagensen CD et al: Lobular neoplasia (so-called lobular carcinoma in situ) of the breast, *Cancer* 42:737, 1978.

57. Love SM, Gelman RS, Silen WS: Fibrocystic "disease" of the breast: a non-disease, *N Engl J Med* 307:1010, 1982.

58. Hughes LE, Mansel RE, Webster DJT: Breast anatomy and physiology. In *Benign disorders and diseases of the breast: concepts and clinical management*, London, 1989, Bailliere Tindall.

59. Bland KI, Copeland EM: Breast disease: physiologic considerations in normal benign and malignant states. In Miller T, Rowlands B (eds): *The physiologic basis of modern surgical care*, St Louis, 1988, Mosby.

60. Patey DH: Two common non-malignant conditions of the breast, *BMJ* 1:96, 1949.

61. Patey DH, Nurck AW: Natural history of cystic disease of breast treated conservatively, *BMJ* 1:15, 1953.

62. Hughes LE, Mansel RE, Webster DJT: Breast pain and nodularity. In *Benign disorders and diseases of the breast: concepts and clinical management*, London, 1989, Bailliere Tindall.

63. Hughes LE, Mansel RE, Webster DJT: Nipple discharge. In *Benign disorders and diseases of the breast: concepts and clinical management*, London, 1989, Bailliere Tindall.

64. Takeda T et al: Cytologic studies of nipple discharges, *Acta Cytol* 26:35, 1982.

65. Tong D: The treatment of solitary cysts in the breast: a new technique, *Br J Surg* 56:885, 1969.

66. Forrest APM, Kirkpatrick JR, Roberts MM: Needle aspiration of breast cysts, *BMJ* 3:30, 1975.

67. Cowen PN, Benson EA: Cytological study of fluid from benign breast cysts, *Br J Surg* 66:209, 1979.

68. Dixon JM et al: Assessment of the acceptability of conservative management of fibroadenoma of the breast, *Br J Surg* 83:264, 1996.

69. Dent DM, Cant PJ: Fibroadenoma, *World J Surg* 13:706, 1989.

70. Noguchi S et al: Progression of fibroadenoma to phyllodes tumor demonstrated by clonal analysis, *Cancer* 76:1779, 1995.

71. Frouge C et al: Mammographic lesions suggestive of radial scars: microscopic findings in 40 cases, *Radiology* 195:623, 1995.

72. Bundred NJ, Webster DJT, Mansel RE: Management of mamillary fistula, *J Roy Coll Surgeons Edinburgh* 36:381, 1991.

73. Dixon JM: Outpatient treatment of non-lactational breast abscesses, *Br J Surg* 79:56, 1992.

74. Scholefield JM, Duncan JL, Rogers K: Review of hospital experience of breast abscess, *Br J Surg* 74:469, 1987.

CHAPTER

10

Etiology and Management of Breast Pain

V. SUZANNE KLIMBERG

RONDA S. HENRY-TILLMAN

Chapter Outline

Although mastalgia is one of the most commonly reported symptoms in women with breast complaints at dedicated breast clinics or general practice,[1] it is still underreported and poorly characterized. In a 1985 survey nearly 66% of women reported having breast pain, of which 21% of cases were reported to be severe.[2] However, only half of women with breast pain had consulted a family physician,[2] and in another study, only 5% were referred to a dedicated breast clinic.[3] Because of the increasing awareness of breast cancer and the possibility that mastalgia may indicate disease, more women than ever are seeking help for breast pain. At present, most physicians are ill trained for the treatment of mastalgia, which usually balances management of relatively minor complaints with the side effects of treatment. More than 90% of patients with cyclic mastalgia and 64% of patients with noncyclic mastalgia can obtain relief by using a combination of nonprescription and prescription drugs.[4]

Assessment of Mastalgia

CLINICAL ASSESSMENT

The degree, severity, and relationship of breast pain to the menstrual cycle are best assessed with the use of a daily breast pain chart that uses a visual analog scale. This chart should be kept during at least two menstrual cycles. Breast pain that is mild (<3 on visual analog scale) and that lasts fewer than 5 days before a menstrual cycle is considered normal. The extent to which mastalgia disrupts the patient's normal lifestyle in terms of sleep, work, and sex provides a useful assessment of severity. For more severe pain, a thorough history that includes diet, methylxanthine intake, use of new medications (especially hormones and promethazines), and a history of recent stress should be recorded. Possible sites of referred pain, such as cervical radiculopathy, myocardial ischemia, lung disease, hiatal hernia, and cholelithiasis, should be excluded. The keystone to the management of mild mastalgia is reassurance; this is successful in 80% to 85% of patients.[2] Patients are reassured that they do not have breast cancer only after clinical examination and mammography are performed and reveal no malignancy. Ultrasonography and fine-needle aspiration may be used, when indicated, to further reassure the patient. Cancer must be considered seriously as a diagnosis in any patient who has well-localized and persistent breast pain. In a series of 240 patients with operable breast cancer seen during a 4-year period at the Cardiff Mastalgia Clinic, 15% had breast pain as one of their presenting symptoms and 7% had mastalgia alone.[5] After clinical assessment excludes overt disease, subsequent neoplasia is rare (0.5%).[6] Although a study of 5319

patients by Leinster and colleagues showed there was a higher incidence of "high-risk" mammographic patterns according to the Wolfe classification in premenopausal women with cyclic mastalgia that correlated with the severity, duration, and need for treatment,[7] no study to date has reported an increased risk of breast cancer with cyclic mastalgia. Initial evaluation should exclude breast pain from localized benign lesions of the breast that require needle aspiration or surgical therapy, such as painful cysts, fibroadenomas, subareolar duct ectasia, lipomas, and fibrocystic changes.[8]

Classification. Classification of mastalgia provides a baseline measurement of pain and severity, dividing symptoms into the categories of cyclic mastalgia, noncyclic mastalgia, and chest wall pain.[8] This distinction is important because presentation, occurrence of spontaneous remission, and likelihood of a response to treatment differs for these three conditions; a useful response is obtained in 92% of patients with cyclic mastalgia, 64% of those with noncyclic mastalgia,[4] and 97% of those with chest wall pain.[9]

Cyclic mastalgia accounts for approximately 67% of cases and usually is first seen during the third decade of life as dull, burning, or aching pain.[9] However, one breast is usually involved to a greater extent than the other, and the pain may be sharp and shooting, with radiation to the axilla or arm because of glandular entrapment of the intercostobrachial nerve. Cyclic mastalgia usually starts in the upper outer quadrant of the breast 5 days or more before the menstrual cycle, although pain can persist throughout the cycle and may be accompanied by premenstrual exacerbation. Exacerbation of symptoms just before menopause is common, and resolution of symptoms at menopause is predictable; spontaneous resolution before menopause occurs in about 22% of patients.

Noncyclic mastalgia peaks during the fourth decade of life and tends to occur much less frequently (26% of patients).[9] The duration of noncyclic mastalgia tends to be shorter, with spontaneous resolution occurring in nearly 50% of patients.[10] In contrast to cyclic mastalgia, noncyclic mastalgia is almost always unilateral. Exacerbations of pain occur for no apparent reason and are difficult to treat.

Mastalgia from other origins includes costochondritis,[11] lateral extramammary pain syndrome,[12] cervical radiculopathy,[13] or other nonbreast causes. Chest wall pain from these etiologies is almost always felt either on the lateral chest wall or at the costochondral junction.[12] Musculoskeletal pain may be improved with analgesics or local injection of steroid or anesthetic.[9] If it is more generalized, nonsteroidal antiinflammatory drugs are the treatment of choice.[14] Neurogenic pain is much more difficult to diagnose and treat. If pain of neurogenic origin is suspected, an empirical trial of amitriptyline or carbamazepine may be beneficial for diagnosis and treatment. Musculoskeletal pain accounts for only 7% of cases seen at a dedicated mastalgia clinic.[9]

Pathophysiology of Mastalgia

NOMENCLATURE

The term *fibrocystic disease*, of which mastalgia is the most common symptom, is not helpful because it fails to delineate the full spectrum of disease. With no consistent relationship between histology and symptoms, Love and co-workers have classified fibrocystic changes as a nondisease.[15] The greatest source of confusion in the evaluation of fibrocystic conditions has been evaluation of symptoms or histologic appearance in isolation, without reference to the normal breast morphology and the changes that occur throughout reproductive life. Postmortem studies of "normal" breast specimens indicate that fibrocystic changes occur in 50% to 100% of individuals.[16-18] In 1987 Hughes and colleagues introduced the concept of aberrations of normal development and involution (ANDI) to classify benign breast disorders, such as mastalgia, into those arising secondary to abnormalities of breast development, cyclic changes, or involution rather than as disease.[19]

PATHOGENESIS AND ETIOLOGY

Epithelial and stromal activity, as well as regression, constantly occur within the breast. Fibrosis, adenosis, and lymphoid infiltration, commonly used to characterize mastalgia, cannot be correlated with clinical episodes.[19] Watt-Boolsen and colleagues found no histologic differences between women with cyclic and noncyclic mastalgia and asymptomatic patients.[20] Jorgensen and Watt-Boolsen reported fibrocystic changes in 100% of 41 women with breast pain who underwent breast biopsy.[21] Although a higher incidence of fibrocystic change was seen in this cohort than in asymptomatic controls, the total incidence of breast abnormalities did not differ between groups. Attempts to demonstrate edema as the main cause of cyclic pain and nodularity have been unsuccessful. Cysts that commonly occur with ANDI and mastalgia are secondary to changes of involution, periductal inflammation, and fibrosis, which may narrow the ducts distally and cause proximal dilation.[19] Although the involution process is not well understood, it seems to depend on the continuing presence of the surrounding stroma. Disappearance of this stroma is patchy; if it occurs too early, there may be localized cystic enlargement of the remaining acini.[22] Although enlarged cysts can be painful and aspiration helpful, aspiration itself does not relieve generalized mastalgia.

There has never been any correlation between benign fibrocystic changes of the breast or chronic mastalgia and breast cancer. However, Page and colleagues (and others) have demonstrated that atypical hyperplasia, either ductal or lobular, is clearly associated with an increased risk of malignancy.[23]

ENDOCRINE INFLUENCES

The natural history of mastalgia is clearly linked to the reproductive cycle, with onset at the age of menarche, monthly cycling, and cessation of symptoms at menopause. Gateley and colleagues reported, in a prospective study of reproductive factors associated with mastalgia, that women with cyclic mastalgia were more likely to be premenopausal, to be nulliparous, or to have been at a young age when they had their first child.[4] However, theories of the exact hormonal events, including progesterone deficiency,[24] excess estrogen,[25] changes in progestin/estrogen ratio,[26] differences in receptor sensitivity,[27] disparate follicle-stimulating hormone (FSH) and luteinizing hormone (LH) secretion,[28] low androgen levels,[29] and high prolactin (PRL) levels,[30] have been difficult to prove or have not abated with hormone therapy.

Under normal circumstances, PRL exerts structural growth and secretory differentiation, enteromammary immune system development, and initiation and maintenance of milk secretion.[31] PRL secretion is episodic and shows circadian rhythm, with clustering of more intense episodes after midnight. In addition, PRL secretion has menstrual and seasonal variations.[32] These variations may, to some extent, account for the discrepancies in available reports.[30] Mastalgia may be related to an upward shift in the circadian PRL profile, a possible downward shift in menstrual profiles, and loss of seasonal variations.[32,33] Patients with mastalgia also show a heightened PRL secretion in response to thyrotropin-releasing hormone (TRH) and antidopaminergic drugs[28,33] (Figure 10-1). In addition, stress can cause a rise in PRL response.[34]

Disturbances in the pituitary–ovarian steroid axis have long been associated with breast pain (see Figure 10-1). However, numerous studies have not shown differences in estrogen and progesterone between asymptomatic controls and mastalgia patients[35-44] (Table 10-1). Available reports have measured estrogen over various time courses, from single midluteal phase samples to daily for an entire cycle. Clearly, circadian, menstrual, seasonal, or episodic changes could have been overlooked. More important, normal breast function is a balance between estrogen and progesterone, which is a part of the neuroendocrine control exerted by the hypothalamic-pituitary-gonadal axis (see Figure 10-1). The theory of an inadequate luteal phase defect has never been confirmed. Three studies[35-37] (see Table 10-1)

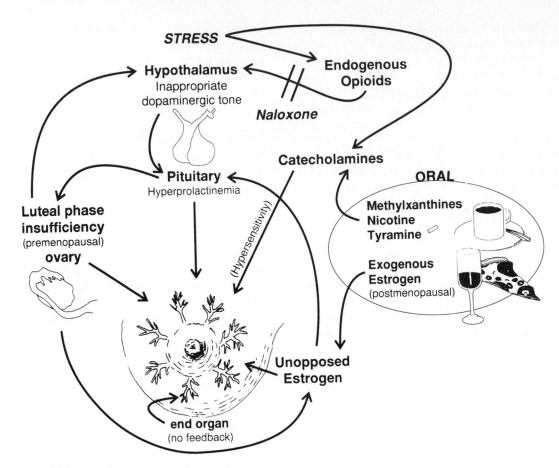

FIG. **10-1** Suggested theories of causation of breast pain.

demonstrated a significant decrease in luteal phase progesterone in women with mastalgia versus pain-free controls; however, four other comparable studies have not confirmed these results.[39,40,42,43] Nevertheless, an estrogen-proges terone imbalance could affect PRL secretion. An impairment of the normal ability to counteract estrogen-induced PRL release by increasing the central dopaminergic tone has been suggested as a cause of mastalgia.[45] Administration of naloxone has been shown to decrease PRL response to stress[46] (see Figure 10-1).

NONENDOCRINE INFLUENCES

Serum studies in animals demonstrate that caffeine intake can increase PRL,[47] insulin,[48] and corticosterone[49]

| TABLE 10-1 | Estrogen and Progesterone Levels in Women with Mastalgia |

REFERENCE	NO. OF PATIENTS	METHOD	ESTROGEN*	PROGESTERONE*
Ayers and Gidwani[35]	25	1 LS	NS	↓, $p < .05$
Sitruk-Ware et al.[36]	66	3 LS	NS	↓, $p < .0005$
Sitruk-Ware et al.[37]	109	1 LS	NS	↓, $p < .001$
Walsh et al.[38]	82	3 LS	NS	NP
Walsh et al.[39]	115	3 LS	NP	NS
England et al.[40]	19	Daily	NS	NS
Golinger et al.[41]	7	Weekly	NS	NP
Kumar et al.[42]	17	1 LS	NS	NS
Kumar et al.[43]	8	Salivary levels qd	NP	NS
Watt-Boolsen et al.[44]	20	Days 7, 16, 20, 24	NS	NP

LS, Luteal sample(s); NP, not performed; NS, not significant.
*Pain level in patients with mastalgia compared with asymptomatic controls.

and can decrease thyroid-stimulating hormone (TSH), free triiodothyronine (T_3), and thyroxine (T_4).[47] Minton and associates[50,51] originally hypothesized that methylxanthines, either by inhibiting phosphodiesterase and breakdown of cyclic adenosine monophosphate (cAMP) or by increasing catecholamine release, increase cAMP, leading to cellular proliferation in the breast[52] (see Figure 10-1). Tissue from patients with breast disease showed unchanged phosphodiesterase activity but appeared to have increased adenylate cyclase levels and increased responsiveness to the biochemical-stimulating effects of methylxanthines.[50,51] Caffeine itself has no direct effect on cAMP, but catecholamines can increase cAMP. Studies in Minton's laboratory have shown increased release of circulating catecholamines in response to caffeine consumption[53] (see Figure 10-1). Indeed, studies from Minton and colleagues have shown "catecholamine supersensitivity" in patients with ANDI. In symptomatic patients ($n = 21$), there were significantly higher levels of β-adrenergic receptors than in asymptomatic controls ($n = 13$).[54] Basal receptors and stimulation of receptors, with isoprenaline or epinephrine, were higher in the symptomatic group. The increased activity and sensitivity of the β-adrenergic–adenylate cyclase system in symptomatic patients suggest a genetic predisposition for ANDI that is stimulated by the biochemical or hormonal effects of methylxanthines. Moreover, Butler and colleagues have been able to categorize patients genetically into fast and slow acetylators based on their caffeine metabolism.[55] Like the methylxanthines, a common biochemical effect of nicotine, tyramine, and physical and emotional stress is enhancement of catecholamine release and an increase of circulating catecholamines[54] (see Figure 10-1). Arsiriy showed that women with mastalgia and ANDI had significantly higher levels of urinary catecholamines than did asymptomatic controls.[56] Studies have shown increased serum epinephrine and norepinephrine and decreased baseline dopamine levels in patients with cyclic as well as noncyclic mastalgia.[54] The increase or stimulation of adenylate cyclase activity in breast tissue appears to be an important step for triggering the intracellular cAMP-mediated events leading to symptomatic ANDI.[54] Randomized studies on smoking, tyramine, or stress reduction have not been performed.

The theory that fat increases endogenous hormone levels, and thus breast pain, has led to dietary fat-restriction studies.[57] In these studies women with breast pain show lower levels of plasma essential fatty acid gamma-linolenic acid (GLA) than do asymptomatic controls. It has been hypothesized that essential fatty acid deficiencies may affect the functioning of the cell membrane receptors of the breast by producing a supersensitive state.[58,59] High levels of saturated fats inhibit the rate-limiting delta-6 desaturation step between linoleic acid and GLA. Catecholamines, diabetes, glucocorticoids, viral infections, and high cholesterol levels likewise limit this step.[58,59] Both with estrogen and progesterone receptors, a supersensitive state can be produced with a higher ratio of saturated to unsaturated fatty acids. Administration of essential fatty acids in the form of evening primrose oil (9% GLA) bypasses the delta-6 desaturation step, leading to a gradual reduction in the proportions of the saturated fatty acids[58] and diminishing the abnormal sensitivity of the breast tissue. Likewise, Ghent and colleagues have theorized that the absence of dietary iodine may also render terminal intralobular duct epithelium more sensitive to estrogen stimulation.[60]

Management of Mastalgia

As might be anticipated, there is a long list of suggested modalities for the treatment of an entity that is ubiquitous, whose cause is unknown, and whose relationship to fibrocystic breast disease and cancer is poorly understood. Breast pain may resolve spontaneously, and 19% of patients have marked responses to placebo therapy. Therefore double-blind, placebo-controlled trials are required to prove the effectiveness of drugs in the treatment of mastalgia.[61] GLA, bromocriptine, danazol, luteinizing hormone–releasing hormone (LHRH) agonists, molecular iodine, and tamoxifen have all been shown by such trials to be of use in the treatment of breast pain. The safety and efficacy of these therapies, as well as less proven therapies, are discussed in the next section (Table 10-2).

NUTRITIONAL THERAPY

Nutritional factors have been less well documented than other modalities in the cause and treatment of breast pain. Although they are the least expensive and least prone to side effects, dietary changes are often the most difficult to institute in the noncompliant patient.

Methylxanthines. Chemicals classified as methylxanthines include caffeine, theophylline, and theobromine. These substances are found in coffee, tea, chocolate, and cola beverages, as well as in many respiratory medications and stimulants. Minton and colleagues reported complete disappearance of all palpable nodules, pain, tenderness, and nipple discharge 1 to 6 months after eliminating methylxanthines from the diet of 13 of 20 women (65%).[62] In a subsequent clinical trial involving 87 women, complete resolution was seen in 82.5%, with significant improvement in 15% of women abstaining from methylxanthines.[51] Resumption of methylxanthines was associated with recurrence of symptoms in this cohort. These data are supported by nonrandomized

TABLE **10-2** | Effectiveness of Preferred Drug Treatments for Mastalgia

| DRUG | MASTALGIA | | | SIDE EFFECTS |
	CYCLICAL	NONCYCLICAL	COMBINED	
Methylxanthines[54]	—	—	78%	None
↓ Dietary fat[73]	90%	73%	83%	None
EPO[4]	58%	38%	—	2%-4%
Molecular iodine[60]	—	—	65%	11%
Danazol*[86]	70%	31%	—	50%
Gestrinone[92]	—	—	55%	None
LHRH agonist[96]	—	—	81%	All
Thyroid replacement[98,99]	—	—	73%	None
Analgesics[107]	—	—	97%	3%
Combination†[4]	92%	64%	—	—

*Low-dose regimen demonstrated a 55% complete response rate without side effects.
†Combination of danazol, bromocriptine, and EPO.

studies, including retrospective data from 90 pairs of twins[63] in which the twin with breast pain was found to be more likely to consume more coffee than the unaffected twin. Ernster and colleagues randomized 82 of 158 women to abstain from methylxanthine and 76 women to no dietary instruction.[64] Differences in clinically palpable breast findings were significantly less in the caffeine-abstaining group, but absolute changes were minor. Bullough and colleagues studied daily methylxanthine ingestion from drug and dietary sources by means of questionnaires from a sample of 102 women.[65] Fibrocystic breast disease assessed with mammography and breast pain were found to be positively correlated with both caffeine and total methylxanthine ingestion.

Minton reported evaluation of 315 patients with ANDI for a mean of 3 years (range, 1 to 11 years).[54] Each patient was asked to abstain from methylxanthines and nicotine and examined at 8-week intervals. During the course of the study, 254 of the 315 patients completely abstained from caffeine intake; 78% of the 254 patients improved, 6% became worse, and 15% remained the same. Seventy-two patients who had stopped all caffeine consumption resumed consumption at a later date; 85% of these went from better to worse. Forty-one patients stopped intake of methylxanthines and nicotine, with 85% achieving a positive response. Other case-controlled studies, however, have not confirmed these clinical findings.[66-69] A study of an age- and race-matched cohort of approximately 3000 women who were a part of the Breast Cancer Detection Demonstration Project demonstrated no association between methylxanthine consumption and breast tenderness in women with fibrocystic disease or in controls.[70] Consumption of chocolate-containing foods and candies or caffeine-containing medication was not recorded. In a single-blind clinical trial of 56 women randomized to a control

(no dietary restrictions), a placebo (cholesterol-free diet), and an experimental group (caffeine-free diet) for 4 months, Allen and Froberg showed that caffeine restriction did not lessen breast pain or tenderness.[71]

Another factor is the significant difference in the length of withdrawal of caffeine seen between positive and negative studies. Minton's work has been criticized for lack of controls and blinding as well as the general instability of findings in patients with mastalgia.[72] An unflawed, large-scale, prospective, long-term study, either to prove or disprove the value of methylxanthine withdrawal, that would count methylxanthines from all sources and use reliable dependent variables to assess pain has yet to be performed. Until then, clinicians may want to suggest a methylxanthine-restricted diet, especially in light of its no cost, no side effect status and the other unwanted health consequences of caffeine.

Dietary Fat. As with breast cancer, mastalgia is less common in the East and in Eskimos, whose diets are notably lower in fat. Reduction of dietary fat intake (to <15% of total calories for 6 months) significantly improves cyclic breast tenderness and swelling.[57] In one study Sharma and colleagues demonstrated significant elevations in high-density lipoprotein cholesterol (HDL-C) and the ratio of HDL-C to low-density lipoproteins, and a decrease in the total cholesterol to HDL-C between 32 cyclic and 25 noncyclic mastalgia patients.[73] Response to a low-fat dietary regimen was significant only in the cyclic mastalgia group, suggesting that cyclic mastalgia may be from cyclic aberrations in lipid metabolism and that dietary management may need to be pursued. A good or partial response was seen in 19 of 21 of the cyclic and 11 of 15 of the noncyclic patients. It is unclear what would lead to such a lipid profile abnormality, whether it is excessive intake or a genetic predisposition. Nevertheless, dietary manipulation of this kind is difficult to achieve, is difficult to monitor, and requires a high degree of compliance.[74]

Evening Primrose Oil

Gamma-Linolenic Acid. Studies have shown that women with severe cyclic mastalgia have abnormal blood levels of some essential fatty acids,[75] which have been implicated in the control of PRL secretion and steroid hormone/receptor alterations.[27] Clinical experience with evening primrose oil (EPO) produces a 58% response rate with cyclic mastalgia and a 38% response rate with noncyclic mastalgia.[4] The side effects of EPO are far less than those of danazol, making it a more attractive first-line treatment.[76] Symptoms of pain and nodularity were significantly improved with EPO (3 g/day) in a placebo-controlled trial after 4 months, and treatment was associated with an elevation of essential fatty acids toward normal levels.[77] In a double-blind crossover trial,[4] 44 women with severe cyclic (36%) and noncyclic mastalgia (8%) were randomized to active or placebo arms. A clinically useful response was noted in 16 of 38 (42%) patients completing 2 months of therapy and in 9 of 18 (50%) patients completing 4 months of therapy. Of 324 patients receiving therapy for cyclic mastalgia at the Cardiff Mastalgia Clinic, initial treatment with EPO was given to 85 patients, and a clinically useful response was seen in 58%. In patients in whom initial treatment with either bromocriptine or danazol failed, EPO as a second-line therapeutic agent had a clinically useful response in 12 of 29 (41%). In 24 patients in whom two previous therapies failed, EPO had a response in 8 (33%). Treatment of noncyclic mastalgia with EPO produced a clinically useful therapeutic response in 38% of patients as a first-line treatment, in 33% as a second-line treatment, and in 30% as a third-line therapy. Adverse effects in the form of mild gastrointestinal symptoms were seen in less than 2% of patients receiving EPO.[5]

Unless the severity of symptoms requires a rapid response, and in view of the low incidence of adverse events, EPO (3 g/day) should be considered a first-line treatment in the fertile patient or in patients requiring repeated courses of treatment because of recurrent pain.

Iodine. The exact influence of iodine on breast tissue is not understood. In contrast to iodides, which are thyrotrophic, Eskin and colleagues demonstrated that iodine is involved primarily in extrathyroidal activities, particularly in the breast.[78] Ghent and colleagues theorized that the absence of iodine may render the epithelium of the terminal intralobular ducts more sensitive to estrogen stimulation and proceeded to perform three studies.[60] In an uncontrolled study with sodium-bound iodide (313 volunteers for 2 years) and protein-bound iodide (588 volunteers for 5 years), subjects had 70% and 40% clinical improvement, respectively. The rate of side effects was high. In a prospective controlled crossover study, 145 patients in whom treatment with protein-bound iodide failed were given molecular iodine (0.08 mg/kg) and compared with 108 volunteers treated initially with molecular iodine. Objective improvement was noted in 74% of the patients in the crossover series and in 72% of those receiving molecular iodine as first-line therapy. The third part of the study was a controlled double-blind study in which 23 patients received molecular iodine (0.07 to 0.09 mg/kg) and 33 patients received placebo. In the treatment group, 65% had subjective and objective improvement. In the control group, 33% had subjective placebo effect and 3% had objective deterioration. Molecular iodine was found to be nonthyrotropic, without side effects, and beneficial for breast pain. No further studies have been published, and a source of molecular iodine is difficult to find.

ENDOCRINE THERAPY

Although it is difficult to prove, hormonal factors clearly play a role in the cause of cyclic mastalgia. This is evidenced by the fact that the condition manifests itself primarily during the ovulatory years, with symptoms that fluctuate during the course of the menstrual cycle, intensifying premenstrually and subsiding with menses.[79]

Androgens

Testosterone. One of the earliest effective hormonal treatments for mastalgia was testosterone injections. Its use has been limited by its adverse side effects. However, results from a recently conducted placebo-controlled trial using 40 mg twice daily of the undecenoate oral form of testosterone demonstrated a reduction in mastalgia pain scores of 50%, with acceptable tolerance.[80]

Danazol. Danazol is an attenuated androgen and is the 2,3-isoxazol derivative of 17α-ethinyl testosterone (ethisterone). Danazol competitively inhibits estrogen and progesterone receptors in the breast, hypothalamus, and pituitary[81]; inhibits multiple enzymes of ovarian steroidogenesis[82]; inhibits the midcycle surge of LH in premenopausal women[83]; and reduces gonadotrophin levels in postmenopausal women.[83] The precise mechanism of danazol in reducing breast pain is unknown. It is the only medication approved by the U.S. Food and Drug Administration (FDA) for the treatment of mastalgia.

In initial studies a double-blind crossover trial comparing two dosages of danazol (200 versus 400 mg/day) in 21 patients with mastalgia was performed and demonstrated significant decreases in pain and nodularity at both dosages. Onset of response and side effects were higher with the higher dosage. Of the participants, 30% had amenorrhea and weight gain.[84] There was significant reduction in mean pain scores and mammographic density using danazol in a randomized trial with daily treatments of 200 or 400 mg of danazol for 6 months.[85] Patients relapsed more quickly (9.2 versus 12.2 months) and to a greater extent (67% versus 52%) in women taking 200 versus 400 mg of danazol. Pye and colleagues treated 120 women in a nonrandomized fashion daily with 200 mg of danazol and found that 70% of patients with cyclic mastalgia and 31% of those with noncyclic mastalgia obtained a useful response.[86] Side effects were seen in 22% and were severe in 6%, with menstrual irregularity in up to 50% of patients. This compared with a 47% response rate with bromocriptine, a 44% response rate with EPO, and a 19% response rate with placebo. Because side effects of danazol are dose related, Harrison and colleagues[87] and Sutton and O'Malley[88] developed low-dose regimens. Patients responding to a dosage of 200 mg/day of danazol after 2 months were given a dosage of 100 mg/day for 2 months and then 100 mg every other day[87] or 100 mg daily only during the second half of the menstrual cycle. If previous reductions were well tolerated,[88] the danazol was discontinued. Symptoms were controlled without side effects at a total average monthly dose of 700 mg. Of 20 women, 13 (65%) of whom had experienced previous side effects, none reported side effects while taking this low dosage. Some relief of pain was seen in all women, with a complete response maintained in 55%. Other side effects that have been reported include muscle cramps, acne, oily hair, hot flashes, nervousness, hirsutism, voice change, fluid retention, increased libido, depression, headaches, and dyspareunia, which usually resolved after discontinuation of the treatment. Danazol is contraindicated in women with a history of thromboembolic disease. For women of childbearing age, adequate nonhormonal contraception is essential.

Gateley and colleagues recently reported a series of 126 patients with refractory mastalgia who had failed to respond to various first-line therapies.[89] The response rate of those with cyclic mastalgia treated with danazol was 57% as a second-line therapy and 25% as a third-line therapy. Equivalent figures for noncyclic mastalgia were 24% and 21%, respectively. Danazol was confirmed to be the most effective therapy, regardless of the treatment sequence.

Recommendations for the administration of danazol are 100 mg twice daily for 2 months while the patient keeps a breast pain record. If no response or an incomplete response is obtained, the dosage may be increased to 200 mg twice daily. If there is still no response, another drug should be tried. Therapy should not continue longer than 6 months (because side effects may develop) and should be tapered, as described by Harrison and associates[87] and Sutton and O'Malley.[88]

Gestrinone. Gestrinone is an androgen derivative of 19-nortestosterone. As such, its mode of action and side effects are similar to those of danazol. However, side effects result less frequently with the reduced dosage required for treatment (5 mg versus 1400 to 4200 mg per week). With its androgenic, antiestrogenic, and antiprogestagenic properties, gestrinone may inhibit the midcycle gonadotrophin surge and act directly on the pituitary gland, in the ovary, directly at the estrogen receptor of the mammary gland.[90]

In a multicenter trial evaluating the safety and efficacy of gestrinone,[91] 105 patients were randomized to receive gestrinone or placebo 2.5 mg twice weekly for 3 months. Of patients treated with gestrinone, 55% had a clinically favorable response, with a placebo effect of 25%. Complete resolution of symptoms with gestrinone occurred in 22% of patients. The major side effect is contraception, although this has been disputed and barrier protection is now suggested. Further trials with gestrinone are warranted.

Others

Luteinizing Hormone–Releasing Hormone Agonist. The mechanisms of LHRH analogs are thought to be their antigonadotrophic action and direct inhibition of ovarian steroidogenesis, which almost completely induce ovarian ablation, resulting in extremely low levels of the ovarian hormones estradiol, progesterone, androgens, and PRL.[92] The initial report of clinical use of LHRH analogs was in a small trial using nafarelin, a nasal spray that demonstrated effective relief of mastalgia in 50% of the patients.[93] However, the number of patients evaluated was small (32 patients receiving treatment and 8 receiving placebo), the efficacy of the drug delivered nasally is not ideal, the method of assessment was heterogenous, and side effects were high. Case reports[94] using 1 mg/day of LHRH analog subcutaneously for 3 months and then 0.5 mg/day for 2 months show response in patients with resistant mastalgia. In a nonrandomized trial Monosonego and colleagues[95] gave intramuscular LHRH agonist (3.75 mg as a monthly depot) to 66 patients during a 3- to 6-month period. A complete response was observed in 44% of the patients treated with an LHRH agonist alone, and a partial response was seen in 45%. Monthly injections of an LHRH analog resulted in an overall response rate of more than 81% in patients with both cyclic and noncyclic mastalgia. Side effects, which included hot flashes, myasthenia, depression, vaginal atrophy, decreased libido, visual disorders, and hypertension, were experienced by most participants but reportedly were not severe enough to require cessation of therapy.[96] Significantly, treatment with an LHRH agonist induced remarkable loss of trabecular bone.[97] For this reason, only short courses of LHRH analogs should be administered and only for acute and severe cases of mastalgia.

Thyroid Hormone. Data from in vitro studies have suggested that thyroid hormones may antagonize the effects of estrogen at the pituitary receptor levels of lactotrophs, such as TRH, although there is no conclusive support for this.[33] Relative estrogen dominance is suggested as a cause for the increase in PRL responsiveness to TRH in patients with mastalgia.

Kumar and colleagues[33] found a generalized abnormality of hypothalamic-pituitary axis in 17 patients with cyclic mastalgia compared with 11 controls by using a combined TRH and gonadotrophin-releasing hormone test. The release of PRL, LH, and FSH was significantly greater in patients with cyclic mastalgia than in controls; estrogen and progesterone levels were normal. Carlson and co-workers showed a 50% response rate to thyroid hormone replacement in 16 of 18 patients with mastodynia who had elevated TRH-induced PRL responses; 13 of the patients had endemic goiter.[98] In 17 patients with mastalgia, Estes demonstrated that in patients given 0.1-mg doses of levothyroxine for 2 months, 47% obtained complete relief and 26% obtained partial relief without side effects.[99] A large, randomized, placebo-controlled trial of levothyroxine is needed before any recommendation is made for its use as a standard treatment.

NONENDOCRINE THERAPY

Bromocriptine. Results of recent studies point toward a PRL secretory hypersensitivity for estradiol in patients with cyclic mastalgia (see Figure 10-1). Watt-Boolsen and colleagues[44] studied 20 women with cyclic mastalgia and compared them with 10 women who were asymptomatic. Basal serum PRL levels were significantly elevated, although within the normal range, in the mastalgia group versus controls. Cole and colleagues[30] have demonstrated that PRL is involved in the regulation of water and electrolyte balance in the nonlactating breast. An increase in serum PRL levels could possibly cause an influx of water and electrolytes in the breast, thus increasing tension and causing pain. Further support for this theory comes from Blichert-Toft and colleagues' observation that the breast becomes smaller, softer, and less tender during PRL-suppressive therapy.[100] However, PRL is probably not the only factor. In women with true hyperprolactinemia, levels of mammotrophic hormones are entirely different because ovarian steroid levels are suppressed. Bromocriptine is an ergot alkaloid that acts as a dopaminergic agonist on the hypothalamic-pituitary axis. One result of this action is suppression of PRL secretion.

Mansel and colleagues[101] reported a double-blind crossover study using bromocriptine in a group of patients with mastalgia. Lowered PRL levels associated with a significant clinical response were seen in patients

with cyclic breast pain but not in those with noncyclic breast pain. In a double-blind controlled trial of danazol and bromocriptine, Hinton and associates[102] reported a clinical response with bromocriptine in two thirds of patients with cyclic pain but no response in patients with noncyclic pain. In contrast, Pye and colleagues[103] reported a minimal response rate of 20% with bromocriptine in patients with noncyclic mastalgia versus 47% in those with cyclic mastalgia. Clearly, bromocriptine is not as effective as danazol; in one report 17% of the patients were unable to continue with treatment because of side effects, which included nausea, vomiting, constipation, dizziness, fatigue, and headaches. The European Multi-Center Trial of bromocriptine in cyclic mastalgia[104] confirmed the efficacy of bromocriptine. Side effects occurred in 45% of patients and were severe enough to warrant discontinuation of therapy in 11%. Side effects were reduced by an incremental buildup of doses over 2 weeks. However, recent reports of serious side effects of bromocriptine prescribed for lactation cessation, including seizures (63), strokes (31), and deaths (9), have resulted in its removal from the indication list of the FDA.[105] Bromocriptine has not been approved by the FDA for use in treating mastalgia. Despite its apparent effectiveness, because of the seriousness and frequency of the reported side effects, we do not recommend bromocriptine for use in mastalgia. A multicenter, double-blind, randomized study is underway in Europe to study a new, highly selective, potent, and long-lasting dopamine agonist, cabergoline. Initially used in lactation cessation, it appears to be better tolerated than bromocriptine and has the added advantage of only twice-weekly administration.[104]

Analgesics. In a retrospective questionnaire survey of 71 patients, a negligible response was seen to conium cream, phytolacca cream, metronidazole, aspirin, cyproterone acetate, and ibuprofen cream.[106] Recently, a prospective but nonrandomized trial administering nimesulide, an oral analgesic, was reported. All but 2 of 60 patients had a clinically useful response (97%) after 2 weeks of therapy. Of 60 patients, 28 (47%) had complete resolution of their symptoms. Two patients could not take the analgesic because of complaints of gastritis.[107] A prospective randomized trial of oral analgesics has not been reported.

Abstention from Medications. Onset of breast pain with the recent prescription of any medication should be suspect. This is particularly so with estrogen replacement therapy (ERT), and withdrawal of such can produce dramatic results.[108] Tenderness caused by ERT can be circumvented with initial low-dose therapy and dosage escalation or with short "drug holidays" when patients become symptomatic.

MASTALGIA REFRACTORY TO DRUG THERAPY

Tamoxifen. Tamoxifen is an estrogen agonist-antagonist commonly used in the treatment of breast cancer. It is thought to competitively inhibit the action of estradiol on the mammary gland. In 1985 Cupceancu[109] first reported a noncontrolled prospective study of tamoxifen given for 10 to 20 days of the menstrual cycle at a dosage of 20 mg/day for up to six cycles; breast pain disappeared in 71% of patients, and symptoms were ameliorated in 27%. Controlled trials at dosages of 10 and 20 mg/day produced greater than 50% reduction in mean pain scores in 90% of patients with cyclic mastalgia and in 56% of those with noncyclic mastalgia.[110,111] The higher dosage was no more effective, but side effects were more prominent. In a double-blind, controlled, crossover trial of tamoxifen (20 mg/day) given during a 3-month period, pain relief was seen in 75% of patients receiving tamoxifen and in 22% of those receiving placebo. Major side effects included hot flashes (26%) and vaginal discharge (16%). In an effort to reduce side effects while maintaining efficacy, the tamoxifen dosage was lowered to 10 mg/day for 3 to 6 months. Side effects were seen in approximately 65% of patients taking 20 mg and in 20% of those taking 10 mg.[111] European investigators have been evaluating tamoxifen for the treatment of patients with mastalgia for several years. Possible links between tamoxifen use and endometrial carcinoma have relegated its use only for patients in whom symptoms are severe and in whom all standard therapies have failed.[112] It should be reserved for patients in whom standard first-line therapies have failed and then used only under close supervision and for a limited time.

Psychiatric Approaches. Lack of treatment for patients with mastalgia stems from the prevailing belief, as first proclaimed by Sir Astley Cooper, that all unexplained breast pain is a psychosomatic complaint seen in the neurotic female, not a real physiologic entity.[113] Indeed, in states of acute emotional stress, PRL is released and may form a physiologic basis for mastalgia (see Figure 10-1). A study by Preece and colleagues found no difference between patients with cyclic and noncyclic mastalgia and those with varicose veins. However, a small subgroup of patients (5.4%) with treatment-resistant mastalgia had characteristics that were similar to those of a psychiatric patient group.[114] Jenkins and colleagues[115] hypothesized that patients with severe or resistant mastalgia are likely to exhibit psychiatric problems. To investigate this hypothesis, researchers had 25 patients with severe mastalgia complete a psychiatric evaluation using the Composite International Diagnostic Interview (CIDI) and a general health questionnaire. Based on the CIDI examination, 17 had current anxiety, 5 had panic disorders, 7 had somatization disorders, and 16 had current major depressive disorders. Jenkins suggests that in patients in whom "standard pharmacologic interventions" for mastalgia fail, evaluation by a psychiatrist and a trial of tricyclic antidepressants may be indicated.

Surgical Approaches. Surgery, such as a subcutaneous mastectomy or excisional breast biopsy for mastodynia, should be a tool of last resort. It should be offered only at the behest of the patient and then only after significant counseling. In general, surgical excision of localized trigger spots is unsuccessful 20% of the time and runs the risk of replacing a painful area with a painful scar.[116]

Ineffective Treatments

Diuretics. Diuretics have never been tested in a double-blind, placebo-controlled trial. However, Preece and colleagues demonstrated that premenstrual fluid retention in patients with mastalgia is no different than in symptom-free controls, limiting the rationale for the use of diuretics.[117]

Progesterones. Studies by Maddox and colleagues (and others) with a randomized, controlled, double-blind, crossover design with 20 mg of medroxyprogesterone acetate during the luteal phase showed no benefit for the patient with mastalgia.[118]

Vitamins. Abrams[119] reported a favorable response to vitamin E in an uncontrolled trial nearly 30 years ago. In a small, prospective, double-blind, crossover study of the efficacy of vitamin E or placebo, 10 of 12 patients receiving 300 IU/day and 22 of 26 patients receiving 600 IU/day showed improvement after 4 weeks of taking vitamin E. Serum levels of dehydroepiandrosterone (DHEA), but not estrogen or progesterone, were significantly higher in the responders to the drug before and normalized after administration of vitamin E. Meyer and associates[120] randomized 105 women into a double-blind, placebo-controlled, crossover trial with vitamin E (600 IU/day) for 3 months. Although 37% reported improvement while taking vitamin E, versus 19% reporting improvement with placebo, this was not statistically significant. Double-blind, placebo-controlled trials by London and co-workers[121] (128 patients receiving 150, 300, and 600 IU vitamin E for 2 months) and Ernster and colleagues[122] (73 patients receiving 600 IU for 2 months) reported no benefits from vitamin E.

Supplementation with vitamins B_1 and B_6[123,124] is thought to be of no benefit. A recent report by McFayden and colleagues[106] retrospectively reviewed treatment of 289 patients with pyridoxine (100 mg/day) for 3 months; 49% had a beneficial response, with only 2% reporting side effects. However, a double-blind controlled trial in 42 patients showed no benefit.

Vitamin A was first used for mastodynia by Brocq and colleagues in 1956 at a daily dose of 50,000 IU for 2 months, which led to significant reductions of pain.[125] In a small, nonrandomized trial in patients with symptomatic breast pain, 9 of 12 patients had marked pain reduction after 3 months of therapy with daily doses of 150,000 IU of vitamin A (all-*trans* retinal).[126] These results were associated with toxic effects often severe enough to stop or interrupt treatment. Santamaria and Bianchi-Santamaria developed a protocol of daily doses of 20 mg of beta-carotene interrupted with 300,000 IU of retinol acetate starting 7 days before each menstrual period and continuing for 7 days for each cycle.[127] Twenty-five patients with cyclic mastalgia were treated with this regimen for 6 months. Two patients had a complete response, and the remaining patients had a modest partial response. No side effects were reported. This regimen was not effective for noncyclic mastalgia. Controlled trials have failed to demonstrate a role for vitamins in the treatment of breast pain.

Mastalgia Management Summary (Figure 10-2)

1. As with any workup of a problem, a *thorough history* is vital. A history of a serous or bloody nipple discharge, nodularity, infection, or inflammation in addition to diffuse, pinpoint, or cyclic breast pain signifies an abnormality and should be treated accordingly. Other factors to be evaluated through the history include diet, medication use, pregnancy status, menses, exercise, and recent trauma.

2. *Physical examination* determines the presence of a breast mass, skin changes (peau d'orange or dimpling), nipple retraction, crusting or discharge (single duct versus multiple ducts, unilateral versus bilateral, spontaneous versus pressure at a single site to elicit discharge), or axillary or supraclavicular lymphadenopathy.

3. *Mammography* is indicated in women age 40 or older with or without a specific abnormality on history or physical examination. Ultrasound is a useful adjunct to determine whether a palpable abnormality is cystic or solid. If nipple discharge is present, it should be tested for blood. A milky discharge from multiple ducts may be the result of a persistently elevated PRL level and may require an endocrine evaluation.

4. Any abnormality, whether it be a palpable mass, bloody nipple discharge, or mammographic concern, should be followed with a *biopsy*. Seven percent of patients with breast cancers have breast pain alone as the first symptom.

5. A critical history will *classify* patients into categories of cyclic mastalgia (67%), noncyclic mastalgia (26%), or chest wall pain (7%). Documentation of the pain with charts may help clarify the type of pain. In general, cyclic breast pain is much more responsive to available therapies than is noncyclic mastalgia. Identification of chest wall pain is important because this type of pain may respond to local anesthesia and analgesics. Classification of pain into mild to

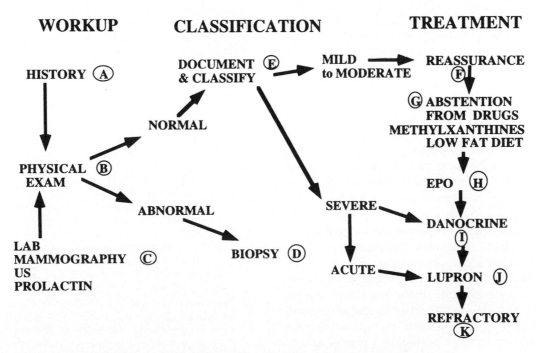

FIG. **10-2** Algorithm for the management of mastalgia. *EPO*$_2$—Evening primrose oil; *US*, ultrasound.

moderate versus severe and acute will help the physician decide on more or less aggressive therapies.

6. *Reassurance* that the patient does not have breast cancer may be all that is needed. In the Cardiff Mastalgia Clinic, 80% to 90% of patients needed no further therapy. Reassurance must be based on a negative history and negative physical and radiographic examinations.

7. *Abstention from certain medications* (e.g., cimetidine, β-blockers, theophyllines) may be helpful. Methylxanthines are also found in coffee, tea, chocolate, and many carbonated drinks. Whether abstention from methylxanthines is helpful is debated. A large randomized study that controls for all sources of methylxanthine has not been completed. In light of the abundance of available decaffeinated drinks and the negative health consequences of caffeine, many physicians recommend abstinence from methylxanthines. Minton supports avoidance of substances containing high amounts of tyramine (e.g., high-fat foods, wine) and nicotine,[53,54] although randomized studies have not been performed.

8. *EPO* is a mixture of essential fatty acids and 9% GLA. Randomized studies of 3 g/day of EPO (270 g/day of GLA) have demonstrated a 44% response rate with cyclic pain and a 27% response rate with noncyclic pain. Although EPO is slow in onset (about 2 months), it has virtually no side effects and costs about $30 per month. EPO is probably the first-line drug for mastalgia, as reported in many surveys.

9. *Danazol* is an attenuated androgen. At dosages starting at 100 mg twice daily and escalating to 200 mg twice daily, response rates are excellent—70% for cyclic pain and 31% for noncyclic pain. Side effects include hirsutism and menstrual irregularities. Danazol treatment costs approximately $70 to $80 per month.

10. An *LHRH antagonist (leuprolide acetate)* is used in acute severe cases of mastalgia. In such cases the response rate is approximately 80%. Use is limited to severe cases because more than three doses of leuprolide acetate can have detrimental effects on bone mass. The cost is also prohibitive—$223 for a single dose of 3.75 mg (given as a monthly depot).

11. *Refractory cases* should be examined for evidence of other pathologic conditions. Occasionally, patients respond to antidepressants. Only in rare cases should tamoxifen be prescribed, and then for only a limited time because of the published reports of increased incidence of uterine cancer and thrombophlebitis. Surgery for mastalgia is to be discouraged and runs the risk of trading a painful area of the breast for a painful scar.

REFERENCES

1. Nichols S, Water WE, Wheeler MJ: Management of female breast disease by Southampton general practitioner, *BMJ* 281:1450, 1980.
2. Maddox PR, Mansel RE: Management of breast pain and nodularity, *World J Surg* 13:699, 1989.
3. Wisbey JR et al: Natural history of breast pain, *Lancet* 2:672, 1983.
4. Gateley CA et al: Drug treatments for mastalgia: 17 year experience in the Cardiff Mastalgia Clinic, *J R Soc Med* 85:12, 1992.
5. Preece PE et al: The importance of mastalgia in operable breast cancer, *BMJ* 248:1299, 1982.
6. Jenkins PL et al: Psychiatric illness in patients with severe treatment-resistant mastalgia, *Gen Hosp Psychiatry* 15:55, 1993.
7. Leinster SJ, Whitehouse GH, Walsh PV: Cyclical mastalgia: clinical and mammographic observations in a screen population, *Br J Surg* 74:220, 1987.
8. Preece PE et al: Clinical syndromes of mastalgia, *Lancet* 2:670, 1976.
9. Maddox PR et al: Non-cyclical mastalgia: improved classification and treatment, *Br J Surg* 76:901, 1989.
10. Harrison BJ, Maddox PR, Mansel RE: Maintenance therapy of cyclical mastalgia using low-dose danazol, *J R Coll Surg Edinb* 34:79, 1989.
11. Gateley CA, Mansel RE: Management of painful nodular breast, *BMJ* 47:284, 1991.
12. Abramson DJ: Lateral extra mammary pain syndrome, *Breast* 6:2, 1980.
13. LaBan MM, Meerschaert JR, Taylor RS: Breast pain: symptom of cervical radiculopathy, *Arch Phys Med Rehabil* 60:315, 1979.
14. Galea MH, Blomey RW: Non-cyclical breast pain: 1 year audit of improved classifications. In Mansel RE (ed): *Recent developments in the study of benign breast disease*, Carnforth, England, 1992, Parthenon.
15. Love SM, Gelman RS, Silen W: Fibrocystic "disease" of the breast: a nondisease, *N Engl J Med* 307:1010, 1982.
16. Foote F, Stewart F: Comparative studies of cancerous versus noncancerous breasts, *Ann Surg* 121:6, 1945.
17. Davis H, Simons M, Davis J: Cystic disease of the breast: relationship to cancer, *Cancer* 17:957, 1964.
18. Rush BF, Kramer WM: Proliferative histologic changes and occult carcinoma in the breast of the aging female, *Surg Gynecol Obstet* 117:425, 1962.
19. Hughes LE, Mansel RE, Webster JT: Aberrations of normal development and involution (ANDI): a new perspective on pathogenesis and nomenclature of benign breast disorders, *Lancet* 2:1316, 1987.
20. Watt-Boolsen S, Emus H, Junge J: Fibrocystic disease and mastalgia, *Dan Med Bull* 29:252, 1982.
21. Jorgensen J, Watt-Boolsen S: Cyclical mastalgia and breast pathology, *Acta Chir Scand* 151:319, 1985.
22. Davids JD: Inflammatory change to ducts in mammary dysplasia: a cause of duct obliteration, *J Pathol* 117:47, 1975.
23. Page DI et al: Relationship between component parts of fibrocystic disease complex and breast cancer, *J Natl Cancer Inst* 61:1055, 1978.
24. Mauvais-Jarvis P et al: Luteal insufficiency: a common pathophysiologic factor in the development of benign and malignant breast disease. In Bulbrook RD, Taylor DJ (eds): *Commentaries on research in breast disease*, New York, 1979, Alan R Liss.

25. Fechner RE: Benign breast disease in women on estrogen therapy, *Cancer* 29:566, 1970.

26. Sitruk-Ware AR et al: Inadequate corpus luteum function in women with benign breast diseases, *J Clin Endocrin Metab* 44:771, 1977.

27. Horrobin DF, Manku MS: Clinical biochemistry of essential fatty acids. In Horrobin DF (ed): *Omega-6 essential fatty acids: pathophysiology and roles in clinical medicine,* New York, 1990, Wiley-Liss.

28. Kumar S et al: Altered responses of prolactin, luteinizing hormone and follicle stimulating hormone secretion to thyrotrophin releasing hormone/gonadotrophin releasing hormone stimulation in cyclical mastalgia, *Br J Surg* 71:870, 1984.

29. Brennan MJ et al: Urinary and plasma androgens in benign breast disease, *Lancet* 1:1076, 1973.

30. Cole EM et al: Serum prolactin concentrations in benign breast disease throughout the menstrual cycle, *Eur J Cancer* 13:597, 1977.

31. Robyn C: Endocrinological aspects of breast physiology. In Angeli A, Bradlow HL, Dogliotti L (eds): *Endocrinology of cystic breast disease,* New York, 1983, Raven.

32. Parker DC, Rossman LG, Vanderlaan ER: Sleep-related nychthemeral and briefly episodic variations in human plasma prolactin concentrations, *J Clin Endocrinol Metab* 36:119, 1973.

33. Kumar S, Mansel RE, Hughes LE: Prolactin response to thyrotrophin-stimulating hormone stimulation in dopaminergic inhibition in benign breast disease, *Cancer* 53:1311, 1984.

34. Dogliotti L et al: Experimental and clinical evidences for a role of prolactin in human breast cancer and the possible usefulness of combining hypoprolatinemic drugs with standard hormonal treatments. In Baulier EE, Jacobell S, McGuire WL (eds): *Endocrinology and malignancy,* Carnforth, England, 1986, Parthenon.

35. Ayers J, Gidwani G: The "luteal breast" and hormonal and sonographic investigation of benign breast disease in patients with cyclic mastalgia, *Fertil Steril* 408:779, 1983.

36. Sitruk-Ware R, Sterkers N, Mauvais-Jarvis P: Benign breast disease: hormonal investigation, *Obstet Gynecol* 53:457, 1979.

37. Sitruk-Ware L et al: Inadequate corpus-luteal function in women with benign breast disease, *Clin Endocrinol Metab* 44:771, 1977.

38. Walsh P et al: Serum oestradiol-17b and prolactin concentrations during the luteal phase in women with benign breast disease, *Eur J Cancer Clin Oncol* 20:1345, 1984.

39. Walsh P et al: Serum progesterone concentration during the luteal phase in women with benign breast disease, *Eur J Cancer Clin Oncol* 20:1339, 1984.

40. England P et al: Sex hormones in breast disease, *Br J Surg* 62:806, 1975.

41. Golinger R et al: Hormones and the pathophysiology of fibrocystic mastopathy: elevated luteinizing hormone levels, *Surgery* 84:212, 1978.

42. Kumar S et al: Altered response of prolactin, luteinizing hormone and follicle stimulating hormone secretion to thyrotrophin releasing hormone/gonadotrophin releasing hormone stimulation in cyclical mastalgia, *Br J Surg* 71:870, 1984.

43. Kumar S et al: Daily salivary progesterone levels in cyclical mastalgia patients and their controls, *Br J Surg* 73:260, 1986.

44. Watt-Boolsen S, Andersen A, Blichert-Toft M: Serum prolactin and oestradiol levels in women with cyclical mastalgia, *Horm Metab Res* 13:700, 1981.

45. Angeli A, Fagiuolo R, Berruti A: Abnormalities of prolactin secretion in patients with fibrocystic disease. In Dogliotti L, Mansel RE (eds): *Fibrocystic breast disease,* Aulendorf, France, 1986, Editio Cantor.

46. Pontiroli AE et al: Effects of naloxone on prolactin, luteinizing hormone and cortisol responses to surgical stress in humans, *J Clin Endocrinol Metab* 55:378, 1982.

47. Spindel E et al: Effects of caffeine on anterior pituitary and thyroid hormones in the rat, *J Pharmacol Exp Ther* 214:58, 1980.

48. Schlosber AJ et al: Acute effects of caffeine injection on neutral amino acids and brain monoamine levels, *Life Sci* 29:173, 1981.

49. Krantz JC, Carr JC (eds): *The pharmacologic principles of medical practice,* Baltimore, 1969, Williams & Wilkins.

50. Minton JP et al: Response of fibrocystic disease to caffeine withdrawal and correlation of cyclic nucleotides with breast disease, *Am J Obstet Gynecol* 135:157, 1979.

51. Minton JP et al: Clinical and biochemical studies on methylxanthine-related fibrocystic disease, *Surgery* 90:299, 1981.

52. Bar H: Epinephrine and prostaglandin-sensitive adenyl cyclase in mammary gland, *Biochem Biophys Acta* 321:397, 1973.

53. Minton JP: Dietary factors in benign breast disease, *Cancer Bull* 40:44, 1988.

54. Minton JP, Abou-Issa H: Nonendocrine theories of etiology of benign breast disease, *World J Surg* 13:680, 1989.

55. Butler M et al: Determination of CYP1A2 and acetylator phenotypes in several human populations by analysis of caffeine urinary metabolites, *Pharmacogenetics* 2:116, 1992.

56. Arsiriy SA: Urine catecholamine content in patients with malignant and benign breast neoplasms, *Vopr Onkol* 15:50, 1969.

57. Boyd NF et al: Effect of a low fat high-carbohydrate diet on symptoms of cyclical mastopathy, *Lancet* 2:128, 1988.

58. Horrobin DF, Manku MS: Clinical biochemistry of essential fatty acids. In Horrobin DF (ed): Omega-6 essential fatty acids: pathophysiology and roles in clinical medicine, New York, 1990, Wiley-Liss.

59. Horrobin DF: The effects of gamma-linolenic acid on breast pain and diabetic neuropathy: possible non-eicosanoid mechanisms, *Prostaglandins Leukot Essent Fatty Acids* 48:101, 1993.

60. Ghent WR et al: Iodine replacement in fibro-cystic disease of the breast, *Can J Surg* 36:453, 1993.

61. Hinton CP et al: Double blind controlled trial of danazol and bromocriptine in the management of severe cyclical breast pain, *Br J Surg* 40:326, 1986.

62. Minton JP et al: Caffeine, cyclic nucleotides and breast disease, *Surgery* 86:105, 1979.

63. Odenheimer DJ et al: Risk factors for benign breast disease: a case controlled study of discordant twin, *Am J Epidemiol* 120:585, 1984.

64. Ernster VL et al: Effects of caffeine-free diet on benign breast disease: a randomized trial, *Surgery* 91:263, 1982.

65. Bullough B, Hindei-Alexander M, Fetou HS: Methylxanthine and fibrocystic breast disease: a study of correlations, *Nurse Pract* 15:36, 1990.

66. Lubin F et al: A case-control study of caffeine and methylxanthines in benign breast disease, *JAMA* 253:2388, 1985.

67. Lawson D, Jick H, Rothman K: Coffee and tea consumption and breast disease, *Surgery* 90:801, 1981.

68. Marshall J, Graham S, Swanson M: Caffeine consumption and benign breast disease: a case control comparison, *Am J Public Health* 72:610, 1982.

69. Boyle CA et al: Caffeine consumption of fibrocystic disease: a case control epidemiologic study, *J Natl Cancer Inst* 72:1015, 1984.

70. Schaierer C, Brinton LA, Hoover RN: Methylxanthines in benign breast disease, *Am J Epidemiol* 124:603, 1986.

71. Allen SS, Froberg DG: The effect of decreased caffeine consumption on benign proliferative disease: a randomized clinical trial, *Surgery* 101:720, 1987.

72. Heyden S, Muhlbaier LH: Prospective study of fibrocystic breast disease and caffeine consumption, *Surgery* 96:479, 1984.

73. Sharma AK et al: Cyclical mastalgia: is it a manifestation of aberration in lipid metabolism? *Indian J Physiol Pharm* 38:267, 1994.

74. Vobecky J et al: Nutritional profile of women with fibrocystic disease, *Natl J Epidemiol* 22:989, 1993.

75. Gateley CA et al: Plasma fatty acid profiles in benign breast disorders, *Br J Surg* 79:407, 1992.

76. Gateley CA et al: Evening primrose oil (Efamol), a safe treatment option for breast disease, *Breast Cancer Res Treat* 101:720, 1989.

77. Mansel RE, Pye JK, Hughes LE: Effects of essential fatty acids on cyclical mastalgia and non-cyclical breast disorder. In Horrobin DF (ed): *Omega-6 essential fatty acids: pathophysiology and roles in clinical medicine,* New York, 1990, Wiley-Liss.

78. Eskin BA et al: Etiology of mammary gland pathophysiology induced by iodine deficiency. In Medeiros-Neto G, Gaitan E (eds): *Frontiers in thyroidology,* vol 2, Proceedings of the Ninth International Thyroid Congress, 1985, Sao Paolo, Brazil, New York, 1986, Plenum.

79. Andrews WC: Hormonal management of fibrocystic disease, *J Reprod Med (Suppl)* 35:87, 1990.

80. Laidlaw I et al: The Manchester Restandol trial. In Mansel RE (ed): *Recent developments in the study of benign breast disease,* Carnforth, England, 1992, Parthenon.

81. Chambers GC, Asch RH, Pauerstein CJ: Danazol binding and translocation of steroid receptors, *Am J Obstet Gynecol* 136:426, 1980.

82. Barbier RS et al: Danazol inhibits steroidogenesis, *Fertil Steril* 22:102, 1971.

83. Greenblatt RB et al: Clinical studies with the antigonadotrophin danazol, *Fertil Steril* 22:102, 1971.

84. Hinton CP et al: Double blind controlled trial of danazol and bromocriptine in the management of severe cyclical breast pain, *Br J Surg* 40:326, 1986.

85. Tobiasson T et al: Danazol treatment of severely symptomatic fibrocystic breast disease and long-term-follow-up: the Hjorring Project, *Acta Obstet Gynecol Scand* 123(suppl):159, 1984.

86. Pye JK, Mansel RE, Hughes LE: Clinical experience of drug treatments for mastalgia, *Lancet* 2:373, 1985.

87. Harrison BJ, Maddox PR, Mansel RE: Maintenance therapy of cyclical mastalgia using low-dose danazol, *J R Coll Surg Edinb* 34:79, 1989.

88. Sutton GLJ, O'Malley UP: Treatment of cyclical mastalgia with low dose short-term danazol, *Br J Clin Pract* 40:68, 1986.

89. Gateley CA, Maddox PR, Mansel RE: Mastalgia refractory to drug treatment, *Br J Surg* 77:1110, 1990.

90. Snyder BW, Beecham GD, Winneker RC: Studies on the mechanism of action of danazol and gestrinone, *Fertil Steril* 51:705, 1989.

91. Peters F: Multicentre study of gestrinone in cyclical breast pain, *Lancet* 339:205, 1991.

92. Clayton RN: Gonadotrophin releasing hormone: from physiology to pharmacology, *Clin Endocrinol* 26:231, 1987.

93. Roberts JV: Experience in the use of nafarelin for treatment of benign breast disease, *Br J Clin Pract (Suppl)* 68:37, 1989.

94. Richardson MR, Njemanze J: Management of severe fibrocystic disease of the breast with leuprolide acetate, *Fertil Steril* 54:942, 1990.

95. Monosonego J et al: Fibrocystic disease of the breast in premenopausal women: histohormonal correlation and response to luteinizing hormone releasing hormone analogue treatment, *Am J Obstet Gynecol* 164:1181, 1991.

96. Hamed H et al: LHRH analogue for treatment of recurrent and refractory mastalgia, *Ann R Coll Surg Engl* 72:221, 1990.

97. Dawood MY, Lewis V, Ramos J: Cortical and trabecular bone mineral content in women with endometriosis: effective gonadotrophin releasing hormone agonist and danazol, *Fertil Steril* 52:21, 1989.

98. Carlson HE et al: Effect of thyroid hormones on prolactin response to thyrotrophin releasing hormone in normal persons and euthyroid goiterous patients, *J Clin Endocrinol Metab* 47:275, 1978.

99. Estes NC: Mastodynia due to fibrocystic disease controlled with thyroid hormone, *Am J Surg* 142:764, 1981.

100. Blichert-Toft M, Henriksen OB, Mygind T: Treatment of mastalgia with bromocriptine: a double-blind crossover study, *BMJ* 1:237, 1979.

101. Mansel RE, Preece PE, Hughes LE: Double-blind trial of prolactin inhibitor bromocriptine in painful benign breast disease, *Br J Surg* 65:274, 1978.

102. Hinton CP et al: A double-blind controlled trial of danazol and bromocriptine in the management of severe cyclical breast pain, *Br J Surg* 40:326, 1986.

103. Pye JK, Mansel RE, Hughes LE: Clinical experience of drug treatments for mastalgia, *Lancet* 2:373, 1985.

104. Mansel RE, Dogliotti L: A European multi-center trial of bromocyptine in cyclical mastalgia, *Lancet* 335:192, 1990.

105. Arrowsmith-Lowe T: Bromocriptine indications withdrawn, *FDA Med Bull* 24:2, 1994.

106. McFayden IJ et al: Cyclical breast pain: some observations and the difficulties in treatment, *Br J Clin Pract* 46:161, 1992.

107. Gabrielli G et al: Nimesulide in the treatment of mastalgia, *Drugs* 46(suppl 1):137, 1993.

108. Maddox PR: Management of mastalgia in the UK, *Horm Res* 32(suppl 1):21, 1989.

109. Cupceancu B: Short-term tamoxifen treatment in benign breast diseases, *Endocrinologie* 23:169, 1985.

110. Fentimen IS et al: Double-blind controlled trial of tamoxifen therapy for mastalgia, *Lancet* 1:287, 1986.

111. Fentimen IS et al: Studies of tamoxifen in women with mastalgia, *Br J Clin Pract* 43(suppl 68):34, 1989.

112. van Leeuwen FE et al: Risk of endometrial cancer after tamoxifen treatment with breast cancer, *Lancet* 343:448, 1994.

113. Cooper A: *Illustration of the diseases of the breast,* London, 1829, Longman, Rees, Orme, Brown and Green.

114. Preece PE, Mansel RE, Hughes LE: Mastalgia: psycho-neurosis or organic disease? *BMJ* 1:29, 1978.

115. Jenkins PI et al: Psychiatric illness in patients with severe treatment-resistant mastalgia, *Gen Hosp Psychiatry* 15:55, 1993.

116. Hinton CP: Breast pain. In Blamey RW (ed): *Complications and management of breast disease,* London, 1986, Bailliere & Tindall.

117. Preece PE et al: Mastalgia and total body water, *BMJ* 4:498, 1975.

118. Maddox PR et al: A randomized controlled trial of medroxyprogesterone acetate in mastalgia, *Ann Coll Surg Engl* 72:71, 1990.

119. Abrams AA: Use of vitamin E in chronic cystic mastitis, *N Engl J Med* 272:1080, 1965.

120. Meyer EC et al: Vitamin E in benign breast disease, *Surgery* 107:549, 1990.

121. London RS et al: Mammary dysplasia: a double-blind study, *Obstet Gynecol* 65:104, 1985.

122. Ernster VL et al: Vitamin E in benign breast disease: a double-blind randomized clinical trial, *Surgery* 97:490, 1985.

123. Pye JK, Mansel RE, Hughes LE: Clinical experience of drug treatments for mastalgia, *Lancet* 2:373, 1985.

124. Smallwood J, Ah-Kye D, Taylor I: Vitamin B6 in the treatment of premenstrual mastalgia, *Br J Clin Pract* 40:532, 1986.

125. Brocq P, Stora C, Bernheim L: De l'emploi de la vitamin A dans le traitement des mastoses, *Ann Endocrinol (Paris)* 17:193, 1956.

126. Band PR et al: Treatment of benign breast disease with vitamin A, *Prev Med* 13:549, 1984.

127. Santamaria L, Bianchi-Santamaria A: Cancer chemoprevention by supplemental carotenoids and synergism with retinol in mastodynia treatment, *Med Oncol* 7:153, 1990.

VI

PATHOLOGY OF MALIGNANT LESIONS

CHAPTER

11

In Situ Carcinomas of the Breast: Ductal Carcinoma In Situ, Paget's Disease, Lobular Carcinoma In Situ

DAVID L. PAGE
MICHAEL D. LAGIOS
ROY A. JENSEN

Chapter Outline

The widespread adoption of mammographic screening as an integral component of women's health has driven dramatic changes in the incidence, diagnosis, classification, nature, and treatment of breast disease in the last two decades. These changes have been particularly profound concerning in situ carcinoma of the breast, as reflected in the explosive increase in the publication of studies of this disease relating to the definition, diagnostic criteria, and both short- and long-term risks associated with specific histologic variants or types of in situ carcinoma.

In situ carcinomas of the breast were first recognized in the early twentieth century and were identified morphologically as cells cytologically similar to those of invasive carcinomas but confined to duct structures. These lesions were usually found adjacent to areas of invasive carcinoma. The definitions were arbitrary, and opportunities to study the behavior of an in situ carcinoma independent of an invasive component, or after a surgical procedure less than that of mastectomy, were rare.[1-3] A number of studies relying on the review of archival slide material demonstrated basic differences between distinct histologic patterns of in situ carcinomas and led to the concept of risk markers (e.g., lobular carcinoma in situ [LCIS], atypias with increased cancer risk implications; see Chapter 7 and the discussion of LCIS later), which identified subsequent risk essentially equally distributed to either breast, and committed lesions (e.g., ductal carcinoma in situ [DCIS]), which identify risks largely confined to the ipsilateral breast and usually the same quadrant.[4,5] The two pivotal studies of DCIS, which followed the women for 10 to 30 years, were similar and identified small, noncomedo-type DCIS lesions undiagnosed at time of initial biopsy.[6] The studies of Wellings and Jensen[7] focused attention on the terminal ductal-lobular units (TDLUs)

as a common anatomic site for the development of hyperplastic changes of both the ductal and the lobular type as well as corresponding neoplastic lesions. The terms *DCIS* and *LCIS* were once meant to signify separate anatomic origins—one in ducts, the other in lobules—but this concept is now accepted as an anachronism. Unfortunately, the myth of distinct lobular and ductal origins for breast neoplasms continues to persist despite our understanding of neoplastic development in the breast. Currently, the term *ductal* refers to patterns of abnormal epithelial cell proliferation associated with a prominent involvement of true ducts in the carcinoma in situ (CIS) category and a high risk of local recurrence without adequate local treatment. Thus DCIS is essentially a diagnosis of exclusion, including in its broad sweep any lesion deemed CIS that does not exhibit the cytologic features of lobular neoplasia cells.[8-10] The distinction is important, however, because distribution of lesions in the breast as well as between breasts is one of the major differences between the ductal and lobular patterns of CIS. The few studies devoted to bilaterality of DCIS report fewer later cancers in the contralateral breast than is seen after diagnosis of an invasive carcinoma[11,12]—a very different association from lobular disease (Table 11-1).

Ductal Carcinoma In Situ

DCIS comprises a heterogeneous group of noninvasive neoplastic proliferations with diverse morphologies and risks of subsequent recurrence and invasive transformation (Figures 11-1 to 11-17). DCIS probably arises predominantly in the TDLU but often extends out to involve extralobular ducts. As compared with LCIS, DCIS is generally more variable histologically

TABLE 11-1   Comparative Features of Ductal (DCIS) and Lobular Carcinoma In Situ (LCIS)

	DCIS	LCIS
Average age	Late 50s	Late 40s
Menopausal status	70% postmenopausal	70% premenopausal
Clinical signs	Breast mass, Paget's disease, nipple discharge	None
Mammographic signs	Microcalcification	None
Risk of subsequent carcinoma	30%-50% at 10-18 yr	23%-30% at 15-20 yr
Site of subsequent invasive carcinoma:		
Same breast	99%	50%-60%
Other breast	1%	40%-50%

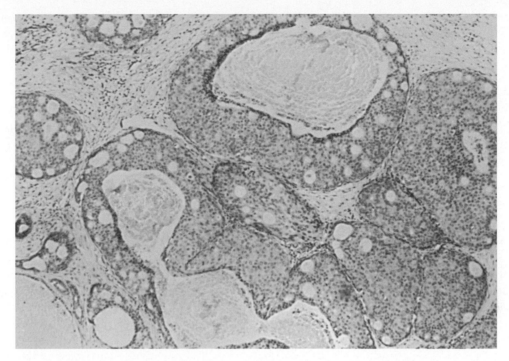

FIG. **11-1** This low-power view of a common form of DCIS shows solid cellular masses distending basement membrane–bound spaces. Within these cellular masses are sharply defined, rounded secondary lumens. There are central areas of necrosis, and evident distention and distortion of the involved spaces. (×75.)

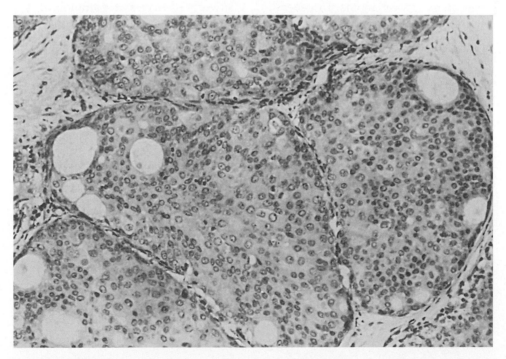

FIG. **11-2** This high-power view of Figure 11-1 demonstrates that the nuclei are of low grade, being similar one to another and without demonstrated irregularity. The presence of necrosis and low-grade nuclei is indicative of a condition intermediate between well-developed comedo carcinoma and the usual ductal noncomedo carcinoma in situ. (×200.)

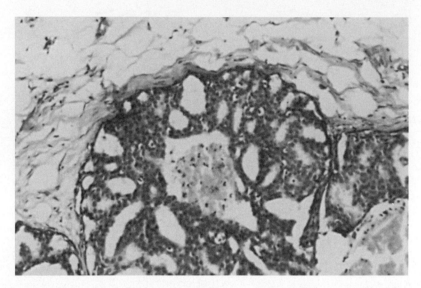

FIG. **11-3** This example of ductal carcinoma in situ is characterized by sinuous, interconnecting strands of hyperchromatic cells. Note few necrotic cells centrally. (×100.)

and cytologically, with larger and more pleomorphic nuclei and a tendency to form microacini, cribriform spaces or papillary structures. In some cases, the periphery of these lesions may include patterns overlapping with atypical hyperplasia.[13] There has been a lack of concordance between different pathologists in determining whether small lesions should be considered atypical hyperplasia or in situ carcinoma. In general,

lesions that involve only a few membrane-bound spaces and that measure less than 2 to 3 mm in greatest dimension should be regarded as hyperplastic lesions (with or without atypia) and not in situ carcinoma. There is a greater degree of concordance in larger lesions.[14] Even the diagnosis of difficult, smaller, borderline lesions will approach concordance between observers if pathologists agree on criteria[15]

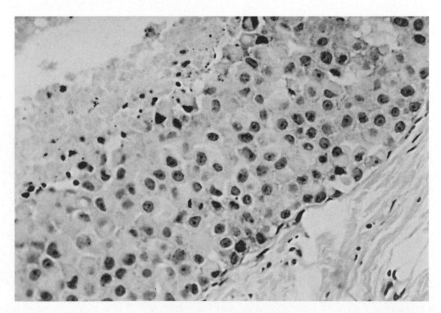

FIG. **11-4** This example of intermediate-grade ductal carcinoma in situ (DCIS) presents highly atypical nuclei but not the most advanced, bizarre, and varied cytologic patterns often seen in comedo DCIS. Although one might debate whether these represented intermediate-grade nuclei, the limited luminal necrosis (here at upper left and elsewhere in this case) indicated an intermediate-grade designation. (×350.)

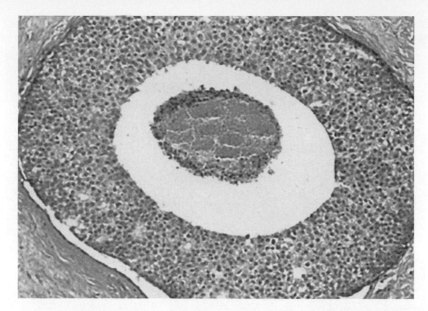

FIG. **11-5** In this example of intermediate-grade ductal carcinoma in situ, the presence of necroses helps define the category. Low- to intermediate-grade nuclei are present. (×200.) *(From Anderson TJ, Page DL: Risk assessment in breast cancer. In Anthony PP, MacSween RNM, Lowe DG [eds]: Recent advances in histopathology, vol 17, Edinburgh, 1997, Churchill Livingstone.)*

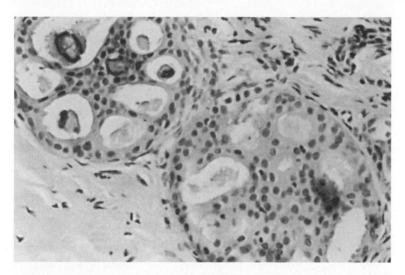

FIG. **11-6** Rigid arches of a cribriform pattern variant of ductal carcinoma in situ. Note: Calcified material in central spaces is not indicative of cellular necrosis. (×225.)

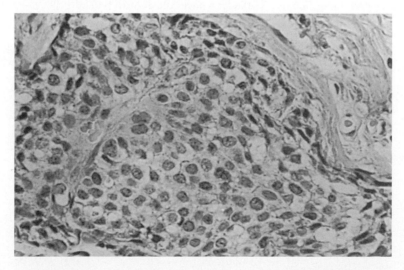

FIG. **11-7** An example of a solid pattern variant of ductal carcinoma in situ. There are no evident intercellular spaces, and the slightly irregular placement of cells and sharply defined intercellular contours are not consistent with the lobular pattern of carcinoma in situ. (×450.)

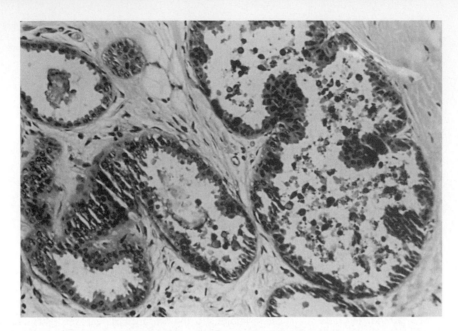

FIG. **11-8** Micropapillary carcinoma in situ with necrosis. Although some cells have lighter cytoplasm, the nuclear pattern is similar throughout. (×400.)

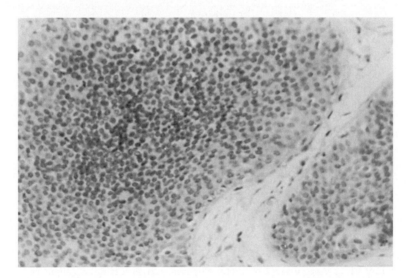

FIG. **11-9** This solid variant of atypical ductal hyperplasia (ADH) is diagnostically very similar to solid ductal carcinoma in situ. The more vesicular nuclei in the second population of cells render a diagnosis of ADH. (×150.)

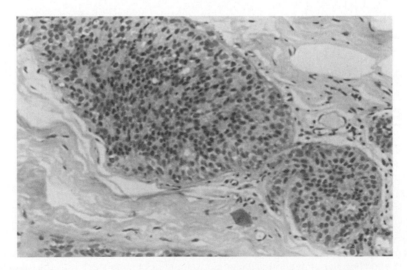

FIG. **11-10** The microglandular or "endocrine" pattern of solid ductal carcinoma in situ. (×150.)

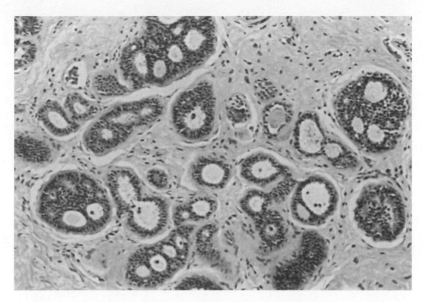

FIG. **11-11** Low-power photograph demonstrating the full extent of the evidence supporting a diagnosis of atypical ductal hyperplasia. Note that there are only three or four spaces in which a central population of uniform cells may be seen. In the others, only narrow bars cross from one side to the other. Thus there are pattern and cell population features of ductal carcinoma in situ. However, in the three largest spaces involved, there are cells adjacent to the basement membrane that appear different; thus a diagnosis of atypical ductal hyperplasia rather than ductal carcinoma in situ is made. (×75.)

(see Table 11-4). Occasionally, it may be difficult to distinguish histologically between DCIS and LCIS, with some forms of DCIS characterized by small uniform cells with a solid growth pattern simulating LCIS. Rare in situ neoplastic proliferations are indeterminate; in such cases, they are presumed to have the prognostic implications of both diagnoses (i.e., local evolution to invasion for DCIS and increased general risk in each

breast for LCIS).[9] It has been proposed that E-cadherin stains are useful in such overlap cases,[16,17] but it should be pointed out that no long-term follow-up study has examined the implications of E-cadherin staining or absence thereof for regional breast cancer risk. It has been our approach to diagnose such cases as CIS, mixed pattern, and to indicate that a regional risk for local recurrence should be assumed.

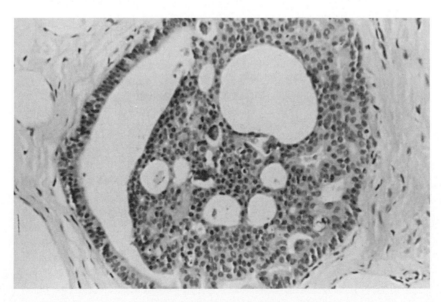

FIG. **11-12** Photomicrograph exhibiting a detail of the polarization of luminal cells near the basement membrane that are quite different from the evenly placed and "suspicious" cells present in the central proliferation. This is atypical ductal hyperplasia. (×200.)

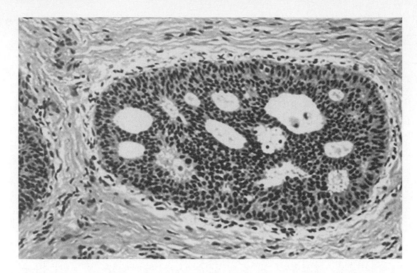

FIG. **11-13** This central cribriform pattern of similar cells with outer cells normally polarized (above basement membrane) is probably the most common pattern of atypical ductal hyperplasia. (×150.) *(From Anderson TJ, Page DL: Risk assessment in breast cancer. In Anthony PP, MacSween RNM, Lowe DG [eds]: Recent advances in histopathology, vol 17, Edinburgh, 1997, Churchill Livingstone.)*

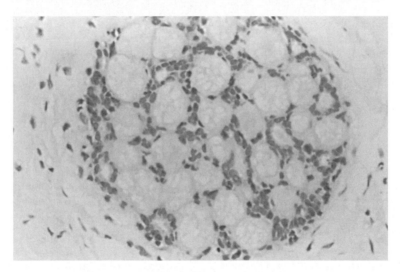

FIG. **11-14** Collagenous spherulosis, a pattern sometimes confused with atypical ductal hyperplasia or ductal carcinoma in situ.[79] Note that the spaces are defined by a secreted material that may be seen faintly. The spaces are surrounded by a sparse population of cells that everywhere is tapered or thinned in its extent. Such a pattern is not recognized as atypical. (×150.)

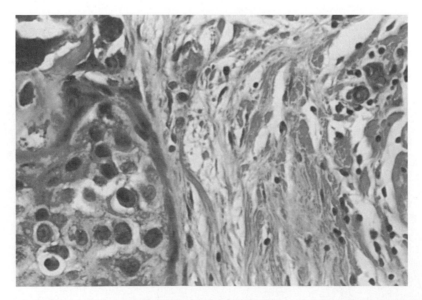

FIG. **11-15** High-power view of ductal comedo carcinoma in situ demonstrating necrosis in the upper left-hand corner. Note also that the stroma is altered about this area, which occurs frequently in this type of carcinoma in situ. (×700.)

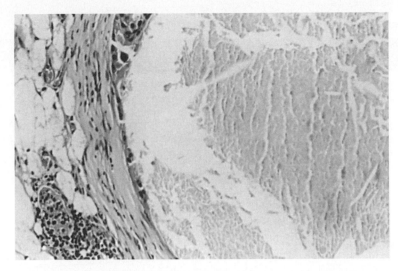

FIG. **11-16** Occasionally cellular necrosis in comedo carcinoma in situ is so extensive that very few atypical cells remain. Indeed, the necrosis may appear to extend to the basement membrane. (×125.)

Terminology is an important consideration here, and as noted earlier, there are distinct clinical implications for the terms *lobular* and *ductal*. Although the inherited terms have a historical legacy that may carry other significance, they have the impelling merit of familiarity. It is for us to develop more specific criteria for subtypes and to accept that it is the criteria linked to clinical end point analysis that will guide clinical practice.[14] One significant problem is the wonderfully earthy word *comedo*. It refers to the lowly comedones of common experience from our teen years, an unfailing image of the gross appearance of these lesions. When used by Bloodgood,[18] he coined the term *comedo-adenoma* because when treated with mastectomy in the Halstedian era it was associated with long-term survival. For Bloodgood, the alternative to carcinoma was adenoma, a lesion capable of cure when adequately excised. The term *comedo* remains descriptive and is now somewhat confusingly used to indicate both a type of DCIS with a coagulation-type necrosis and frequent nuclear debris, as well as merely the evidence of necrosis alone (comedo necrosis). Now, most students of DCIS use *comedo* as a modifier for DCIS, signifying high-grade lesions that exhibit necrosis.

A major transition in our thinking regarding DCIS was the idea that perhaps not all DCIS cases were the same and the different histologic appearances of DCIS might in fact have important clinical implications. Translating this concept into practical terms, it was suggested that if comedo-type DCIS did have a more menacing clinical import, then one should err on the side of including any questionable case within this

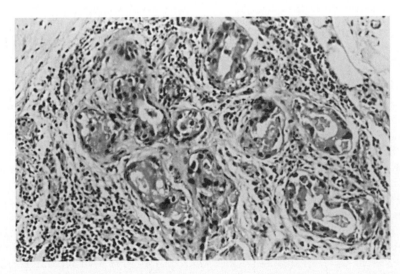

FIG. **11-17** Characteristic of more advanced and comedo carcinoma–type examples of ductal carcinoma in situ is the spread of highly atypical cells into lobular units. Here this phenomenon of so-called cancerization of lobules is demonstrated. (×200.)

| TABLE 11-2 | DCIS Classifications Based on Nuclear Grade and Necrosis |

	NECROSIS	NUCLEAR GRADE		
		I	II	III
Lagios et al[19]	+ -	Low	Intermediate	High
Silverstein et al[33]	- -		Group 2 Group 1	Group 3
Solin et al[35]	+ -		Noncomedo	Comedo

Modified from Lagios MD: *Breast J* 1:67, 1995.
High, Intermediate, Low = High, intermediate, and low nuclear grade, respectively.

category.[9] Thus in 1989 the critically important concept of further stratification was introduced[19] as a part of the inception of the modern era of understanding of DCIS (see Chapter 48). Because minor amounts of necrosis may be seen in the common hyperplasias without features of atypia, specific guidelines are necessary to make appropriate stratifications. Thus inclusion of an intermediate-grade category has been adopted by the majority of DCIS classifications put forth since the early 1990s (see later and Table 11-2) to recognize examples with minimal necrosis and a moderate degree of nuclear pleomorphism.

Conventionally, DCIS has been classified on the basis of architectural features such as comedo, cribriform, papillary, solid, and micropapillary.[20,21] Although comedo-type DCIS includes advanced nuclear abnormalities within the neoplastic proliferation as part of the definition, the diagnosis of other patterns of DCIS were based on architecture alone. These patterns were accepted to be overlapping when DCIS was considered one entity and not held to have separate clinical or biologic implications.[21,22] The first indication that distinguishing among comedo, noncomedo, and micropapillary subtypes,[23] as well as separation by grade,[19] may have clinical utility inaugurated the modern era of DCIS in 1989.

The increasing use of breast-conserving therapy (BCT) in the treatment of mammographically detected DCIS has permitted studies on factors that predict local recurrences and invasive events in the remaining breast after excisional biopsy. Before a large number of small mammographically detected DCIS cases were found with screening, mastectomy was the only acceptable treatment for DCIS, and it remains a standard treatment for larger examples today (see also Chapter 48).[24,25]

Three prognostic factors have been shown to be important in local control of DCIS after attempts at BCT.[26] These are (1) the extent (size) of disease in the breast (and its corollary, the residuum after an attempt

at excision), (2) the status of margins (also reflecting residual disease in the breast), and (3) the grade of the DCIS (and possibly pure subtype, particularly micropapillary). The most significant of these factors appears to be margin status, followed by histologic grade.[27-31] High nuclear grade and necrosis together define forms of DCIS at much higher risk of local recurrence and invasive transformation. The grade of a DCIS is largely independent of the conventional pattern classification. For example, lesions of high nuclear grade can exhibit any architectural pattern (although lack of precise patterns is most common).[19,32] However, as recognized in the classification system of Holland and associates[32] (see Table 11-4), ordered intercellular relationships are most common in lesions of low nuclear grade. There is a growing consensus that classifications based on nuclear grade and necrosis can identify the majority of patients with DCIS who are at risk for short-term local recurrence and invasive transformation after excision[19,33-36] with or without irradiation. Most of these short-term recurrences are associated with DCIS exhibiting high (3/3 or grade III) nuclear grade morphology and significant coagulative necrosis. Such lesions would be conventionally classified as comedo DCIS. Studies using conventional classification schemes have shown that most short-term failures are associated with comedo-type DCIS.[36-39] It should be recalled that the term *comedo-type DCIS* is not synonymous with high nuclear grade when it is used to indicate necrosis only. Some lesions exhibiting comedo-type necrosis and a solid growth pattern are composed of intermediate-grade and, in rare cases, borderline low-grade nuclei (see Figures 11-1 to 11-10).

Information regarding the potential for recurrence of low-grade (noncomedo-type) DCIS after biopsy or BCT resides in a small number of published studies. It is clear that in the short term (5 to 10 years), few local recurrences or invasive transformations occur; however, a recent update of the only study of low-grade DCIS present at biopsy (without planned excision[5]) and with extended follow-up[6] noted a substantial delayed recurrence rate of invasive lesions (i.e., approximately 37% at 25 years of follow-up). Although the sample is small, it is significant that recurrences were in the same quadrant and, in some women, in the site of the prior biopsy—a biology identical to that of higher-grade DCIS and a risk that does not diminish after menopause. This biology should be contrasted with that of marker lesions (e.g., atypical ductal hyperplasia [ADH],[14] atypical lobular hyperplasia [ALH]), which do not predict the side of involvement and in which risk diminishes postmenopausally (at least for ALH and LCIS).[40-42]

There are several published classifications of DCIS,[43] many of which use nuclear grade and necrosis as the major distinguishing features in a general classification applying to most cases of specific subtypes. The separations achieved by these classifications are different and in part may affect the interpretation of outcome results (Table 11-3). DCIS characterized by nuclear morphology (high grade III) (e.g., advanced atypia) and necrosis is uniformly classified as high grade.[13,19,33-35,37,44] The European Organisation for Research and Treatment of Cancer (EORTC) classification,[32] although it does not use conventional nuclear grade or necrosis as major discriminates, would also regard this as a high grade or, in their terminology, a poorly differentiated DCIS. Fisher and colleagues[45] summarized the pathology analysis from the National Surgical Adjuvant Breast and Bowel Project (NSABP) studies on DCIS and noted that DCIS with grade III nuclei and DCIS that exhibited larger areas of necrosis (greater than one third of ducts involved) had a higher local recurrence rate. The authors reported these results separately, not analyzing the risk associated with the two features in concert. Despite the differences in classification,[46] it would appear that high-grade DCIS can be recognized uniformly; all investigators have shown that high-grade subtype so defined has the highest risk of local recurrence and invasive transformation.

The recognition that necrosis and high nuclear grade usually cluster together[47] may foster agreement between observers by using limited necrosis as a way of defining an intermediate grade category.[19,44,48] The separate classifications are less consistent with regard to the remainder of the heterogeneous noncomedo-type group (see Table 11-2). DCIS with grade III nuclei but without necrosis, an uncommon situation, is classified as high grade by Silverstein and coworkers,[33] but "noncomedo" (a lower grade) by Solin and associates.[35] Lagios and colleagues[19] and Silverstein and co-workers[33] use nuclear grade to separate the remaining DCIS groups; however, Lagios and co-workers classify low-grade DCIS as grade I nuclei without necrosis and intermediate-grade DCIS as grade II with or without necrosis. Silverstein and colleagues[33] separate DCIS with nuclear grades I and II on the basis of necrosis. Group I (low grade) may exhibit grade I or II nuclei but no necrosis, whereas DCIS with grade I or II nuclei but with any necrosis is classified as intermediate (group II). Solin and associates[35] regard all DCIS without grade III nuclei and necrosis as noncomedo-type DCIS. Despite these differences in classification, all investigators have shown a substantially diminished local recurrence rate for DCIS that is not characterized by grade III nuclei and necrosis. Moreover, in those studies in which DCIS is divided into three groups, as opposed to the dichotomous comedo/noncomedo structure, there is a recognizable intermediate group (intermediate grade, group II, intermediately differentiated) that exhibits a morphology and a risk intermediate between low-grade and high-grade DCIS.

Summary of DCIS Classification

Although nuclear grade and necrosis would appear to define most of the risk associated with DCIS, certain architectural patterns appear to carry significance independent of nuclear grade. DCIS with almost pure micropapillary architectural features, for example, is

TABLE 11-3　Subclassification of Ductal Carcinoma In Situ (DCIS) of the Breast (The Common Presentation)

HISTOLOGY	DETERMINING FEATURES		FINAL DCIS GRADE
	NUCLEAR GRADE	NECROSIS	
Comedo	High	Extensive	High
Intermediate*	Intermediate	Focal or absent	Intermediate
Noncomedo†	Low	Absent	Low

*Often a mixture of noncomedo patterns.
†Solid, cribriform, papillary, or focal micropapillary.

strongly associated with extensive disease, that is, seemingly separate foci in different quadrants.[23,37] This growth pattern makes adequate excision extremely difficult. In some cases, mammographic and histopathologic evidence of disease is present in all four quadrants. As a result, most clinical studies that define DCIS with micropapillary features and low nuclear grade were based on excisions without adequate margins.

Conventional classification of DCIS covers perhaps 85% of what is recognized as noninvasive ductal carcinoma. A number of less common subtypes remains to be fully defined morphologically and with regard to risk. Proliferations with apocrine features, bridging the spectrum from minimal atypia to frank DCIS, were the subject of a proposed classification by O'Malley and associates.[49] Because of the difficulty of applying traditional rules regarding cellular atypia and architecture to apocrine lesions, this schema proposed that definitive diagnoses of low-grade apocrine DCIS be limited to cases measuring at least 8 mm in size. In addition, a borderline category was proposed for lesions measuring 4 to 8 mm, with the suggestion that these lesions had the relative risk implications of at least ADH. Confirmation of the utility of this approach awaits long-term follow-up analysis.

Another contender for special-type status is the so-called endocrine type of DCIS,[50,51] which presents a particularly low-grade pattern of disease. Similarly, a possible special type characterized by hypersecretory features is discussed later. In all of these less common special types of DCIS, a major limitation is the lack of precise confines of histologic definition that specifically and reproducibly describes the entire spectrum of changes with a linkage to clinical implications corroborated by long-term follow-up studies. In this background of uncertainty it is our philosophy to apply the traditional rules to the extent possible and to not overdiagnose CIS without firm evidence.

We anticipate additional efforts in this and other areas in the future, and present our system here (Lagios, revised from 1989)[19,48] (see Tables 11-2 and 11-3[44]). Also, several DCIS classifications are presented in Table 11-4, providing a basis on which to understand the slightly

TABLE **11-4**	Classification Schema for Ductal Carcinoma In Situ*

1. *Differentiation,* mainly based on nuclear morphology and cell polarization[32]
2. *Nuclear grade and necrosis*[33]
3. *Intersection of nuclear grade and extent of necrosis* similar to Silverstein, but with separate identification of special types[44]

*It is evident that the classification scheme should promote consistency.

varied approaches. The major differences between our approach and most of the other proposals is that we use the intersection of two variables—necrosis and nuclear grade—to foster agreement. It is common to debate between adjacent nuclear grades, viz, 1 or 2, and 2 or 3. The extensiveness of the necrosis is to be used to aid in the resolution of these issues. In a test set, agreement was fostered by this approach.[44] The second feature of our suggested schema is to separate some special types of DCIS because they present patterns not readily allowing grading. In the special case of pure (not intermixed with solid or cribriform) micropapillary DCIS, we believe that the usual extensiveness of disease is independent of the nuclear grade. Note that separating special types from the majority of cases is precisely what we do with invasive disease (see Chapter 12).

Extent of Disease

Clinical concern with the evaluation of size or extent of the area of the breast occupied by DCIS was an early focus during the development of BCT for this disease. By using a serial subgross sectioning technique correlated with specimen radiography, developed by Egan and associates,[52,53] a clear association was shown between the likelihood of invasive growth and the extent of disease.[22] Egan's technique permitted correlative studies of radiographic images and pathologic mapping of areas of involvement by DCIS in mastectomy specimens. The initial concern was whether occult invasion might exist in the breast separate from an adequately excised focus of DCIS. This was shown not to be the case. DCIS cases measuring 25 mm or less, completely excised by the standards of the day, were not associated with occult areas of invasion in those cases that subsequently went to mastectomy. Silverstein[54] demonstrated a similar correlation between the extent of disease and the likelihood of invasion, as did Patchefsky and colleagues.[23] What was not clearly described at the time was that the invasive focus always occurred within the area occupied by DCIS and that the area occupied by DCIS had a segmental distribution, as clearly noted subsequently.[55,56] Using the same serial subgross technique but applying it to radial segments of the breast, which more closely approximate the true anatomy of the ductal system (see Chapter 13), Holland and colleagues[56] were able to define more clearly the relationships of DCIS to mammographic microcalcification and to the remaining breast. They identified different distribution patterns among DCIS of different subtypes. High-grade DCIS (poorly differentiated) was more closely defined by the extent of mammographic microcalcifications; therefore its extent could be estimated with more certainty preoperatively. It was also associated with fewer discontinuities or "skip areas" in its distribution. In contrast, DCIS of lower grades (intermediate and well differentiated) were poorly associated with microcalcification and often exhibited a discontinuous distribution. However, Faverly and colleagues[55] note that 85% of low-grade (well-differentiated) DCIS would be excised with a 10-mm margin. Despite the greater likelihood of residual disease, lower grades of DCIS have a much lower frequency of local recurrence after attempts at BCT, at least in the first 10 years of follow-up.[31,39]

Extensiveness, Multicentricity, and Multifocality

The literature on the multicentricity and multifocality of DCIS remains confusing because of the different definitions, methods of tissue processing, and sampling techniques used, as well as differences in the perspective of the investigators. Two groups of investigators, both of which used Egan's serial subgross technique of examination, exemplify useful approaches to resolving this problem. The focus of Lagios and co-workers was on the question of residual disease after segmental mastectomy (or lumpectomy), a new and radical direction for American surgeons at the time. They defined as multicentric any focus lying beyond 5 cm of the border of the resection. In most cases, this feature defined involvement in another quadrant. Holland and co-workers[56] and Faverly and colleagues[55] (although clearly concerned about the success of a surgical resection) were focused more on the distribution of the disease. Multicentric DCIS, by very definition, required a 4-cm zone of uninvolved breast tissue between the primary and any potential multicentric site. Discontinuous foci of DCIS within 4 cm were defined as multifocal. Holland and co-workers noted that only 5% of cases of DCIS were multicentric using this definition. To what extent these data reflect the large size of DCIS in their patient population remains unknown. However, Faverly and colleagues reported that 63% of the cases of DCIS studied at mastectomy had an extent greater than 5 cm (50 mm), whereas Lagios and co-workers,[22] in a similar mastectomy series, noted that 52% were 25 mm or less and 25% were 50 mm or more. We believe that the most prudent approach is to clearly describe the extent and distribution of disease within the breast in unequivocal terms that cannot be misinterpreted.

Distribution

The considerations of the extent of DCIS are discussed primarily in Chapter 13. Basically, in the field of breast surgery, we are moving rapidly toward a wide acceptance of the peculiar segmental anatomy of the breast. The lobes are not precisely placed or sized, rather they are now viewed as subtending regions drained by major ducts and are overlapping (see Chapter 13). DCIS may indeed have as its hallmark the spread through the large duct system. The lobes are not precisely demarcated anatomically, but the major spread in any given case of DCIS appears to be in the same lobe toward and away from the nipple and in adjacent lobes as well. This clinical situation may be varied in that a major lesion deep within the breast may involve many lobular units, and then a single duct may seem to ascend toward the nipple with few other lobular elements involved, as demonstrated by Ohtake and colleagues[57] and also illustrated by the three-dimensional reconstruction studies of Moffat and Going.[58]

Mammographic Correlations

The distribution of DCIS within the breast, its association with microcalcification, the types of microcalcification, and the likelihood that DCIS may exhibit an extensive growth pattern with a substantial risk of residual disease after attempts at excision is also correlated with grade and subtype. High-grade DCIS with comedo necrosis exhibits a greater extent, is often segmental[56,58,59] (see Chapter 13) and contiguous in distribution, is more closely associated with microcalcifications, and is less likely to show an intermittent or discontinuous distribution in the breast.[55,60] In contrast, DCIS of intermediate and low grades is less likely to exhibit a contiguous growth pattern, especially on mammography, even if its distribution can be understood to lie within a segmental duct system. DCIS of these lower grades is more likely to exhibit discontinuous but regional growth and to show less association with microcalcification, although many cases are continuous on three-dimensional reconstruction studies. From a clinical and mammographic point of view, high-grade comedo-type DCIS is more likely to be adequately excised, given its association with microcalcification and contiguous growth pattern; nonetheless, it is associated with the greatest risk of local recurrence and invasive transformation. An important study of the growth pattern of DCIS in time has come from the group in Nottingham.[61] Rates of change and direction of change in mammographic calcifications was correlated with DCIS histology. Growth rates increased with increasing nuclear grade of DCIS, and the DCIS growth rate was greatest along an axis toward and away from the nipple. The latter finding demonstrated preferential growth of DCIS along the radiating anatomy of the ducts from the nipple to the end of the breast disk.

There may be a special form of DCIS that demonstrates discontinuous spread histologically within ducts[62] and that is associated with recurrence despite performance of an extensive quadrantectomy. Low-grade DCIS is more likely to be inadequately excised unless margins are carefully assessed with means other than mammography for residual disease in the same quadrant, but nonetheless it is associated with a lower risk of subsequent recurrence and invasive transformation.

Margin Status

Assessment of resection margins has been a major focus in BCT in the United States since the increasing use of that surgical procedure in the mid-1970s. The most common method of margin assessment is based on the use of India ink or some other permanent dye or pigment and selective sampling. This method works well for invasive carcinomas in which a likely area of involved margins can be estimated with palpation in most cases and confirmed with a few appropriate sections. The method is still practicable but more difficult in DCIS, in which the lesion is generally nonpalpable, is grossly invisible, and may not be uniformly associated with microcalcification. In these circumstances, margins must be examined completely rather than sampled. This often substantially increases the number of tissue samples or cassettes (blocks) prepared; however, neither the margin involvement nor occult microinvasion can be excluded without complete tissue processing. Differences in the kind of tissue processing used can contribute significantly to outcome results in BCT in DCIS.[10,63] This is a major limitation of large multicenter clinical trials in which the patients may be randomized but the pathologists and their technique for processing the specimen are not.

Considering that careful and precise assessment of margin status is likely the most critical variable in determining the recurrence rate for DCIS (if the lesion has been completely removed, further therapy should not make a difference), it is little wonder that carefully designed single-institution studies with consistent and rigorous pathologic assessment of the specimens have proved so useful. Ideally, breast specimens should be oriented by the surgeon in reference to the nipple and axilla and processed such that the extent of the lesion and its proximity to margins in all three dimensions can be determined. Multicolor inking protocols considerably facilitate analysis, along with uniform sectioning of the specimen at 2- to 3-mm intervals. In addition, we advocate specimen radiography before and after sectioning to foster lesion identification and the focused submission of blocks on larger specimens. However, the histologic appearance of the lesion should *never* be compromised by compression of the specimen for radiography.

The definitions of an adequate margin initially used by several investigators[19,22,64] were, in retrospect, not adequate for cases of DCIS that exhibited a discontinuous distribution. At that time (about 1990), 1 mm was a standard acceptable margin, whereas the NSABP advocated that anything short of transection of an involved duct was adequate.[45,65] The work of Holland and co-workers[56,66] and Silverstein and colleagues[64] subsequently documented that a 1-mm margin was inadequate. In analyzing the results of initial attempts at excision biopsy, Silverstein and associates noted that 45% of cases of DCIS that were thought to be adequately excised had residual disease, either at reexcision or on mastectomy, and that, all other factors being equal, the distance of the free margin was directly related to local recurrence-free survival.[30] However, even using a definition of 1 mm as an adequate margin achieves a better local recurrence-free survival than did the NSABP-B-17 criterion of nontransection (e.g., 16% of local recurrence at 124 months' mean follow-up[27] versus 22% local recurrence rate at 43 months' mean follow-up).[65] At present, a 5-mm minimum free margin, as assessed with ocular micrometry in the fixed and sectioned material, is often recommended. Although a 10-mm margin may be more desirable, it may be impractical, even for small lesions in large breasts. It is likely that narrower margins are adequate for lower-grade lesions. It is anticipated that the use of larger free margins would reduce the local recurrence of DCIS following BCT. This factor has already been demonstrated by the studies of Veronesi and colleagues[67] and Veronesi and Zurrida[68] and by personal communication with Veronesi in 1989, whose local recurrence rates after quadrectomy for DCIS and without the aid of radiation are only 7% at 8 years of follow-up. These findings are consistent with those of Schnitt and associates[26] and Schnitt, Harris, and Smith.[69]

Receptor Proteins, Oncogenes, Tumor-Suppressor Genes, and Ploidy

A rapidly expanding literature since 1987 describes the presence and distribution of specific oncogenes, receptor proteins, and measures of ploidy and proliferative activity in DCIS. Initially, there was an expectation that such investigations would be able to identify DCIS subgroups that are at increased risk for invasive transformation or local recurrence after BCT, particularly among patients at highest risk. In part, these expectations were met, but largely by demonstrating a correlation between specific oncogenes or gene products and DCIS subtypes recognized with conventional morphologic analysis as being a high risk for recurrence (i.e., high-grade [poorly differentiated], comedo-type DCIS, or both).

The clearest association between an oncogene and a DCIS subtype is seen with *HER2/neu* oncogene and its *erbB2* product, which is largely restricted to DCIS subtypes characterized by large cell type and higher nuclear grade.[70-75] Bartkova and colleagues[76] have shown that among those cases of DCIS that are of mixed subtypes, *HER2/neu* expression is seen only in the large cell component, and this factor is dramatically evident in cases in which the mixed cell population occurs within single ductules (Figure 11-18).

DePotter and associates[71] demonstrated a significant association between *HER2/neu*-positive large cell–type DCIS and the extent of disease in the breast, which was independent of mitotic index, and hypothesized that *HER2/neu/erbB2* has a role in motility of in situ carcinomas within the ductal epithelium. Gupta and co-workers[77] have shown that E-cadherin expression is associated with the apparent degree of differentiation or orderliness. The cadherins are related to lateral complex integrity, polarity, and probably cell-cell communication.

p53, largely studied with immunoperoxidase techniques in noninvasive lesions, is also correlated with high nuclear grade subtypes.[5,70,75,78] O'Malley and colleagues,[49] among others, noted that p53 protein overexpression was largely limited to high-grade, comedo-type DCIS. Immunohistochemical studies have shown overexpression in some cases in which *p53* mutations were not detected by sequencing in the most highly conserved portion of the gene. Poller and co-workers[78] concluded that there was no relationship between *p53* and *HER2/neu* status but nonetheless noted that almost all cases of *p53*-positive DCIS were large cell: 35.8% of large cell DCIS and only 4.1% of small cell DCIS were *p53* positive. Others have documented similar relationships between high-grade DCIS, *HER2/neu*, and *p53*.[32,70,74,79]

Estrogen receptor (ER) and progesterone receptor (PR) protein expression, as demonstrated with immunohistochemistry, shows consistent, but not absolute, correlation with DCIS subtypes.[80] Bobrow and co-workers[70] noted an association between cytonuclear differentiation and PR status. DCIS with "poor" cytonuclear differentiation, as opposed to "good" differentiation, tended to lack demonstrable PR. Similarly, Poller and associates[81] noted ER expression to be related to noncomedo architecture, negative *HER2/neu* status, small cell size, and surprisingly higher S-phase fraction on flow cytometry. Wilbur and Barrows[80] noted a similar trend between grade (i.e., cytonuclear differentiation) and receptor status. They noted that 75% of ER-negative DCIS exhibited nuclear grade III morphology (high grade), whereas only 14% of ER-positive DCIS were nuclear grade III. Leal and colleagues[72] and Zafrani and co-workers[75] noted no relationship between DCIS subtype and receptor status. These studies suggest that there is a weak association between high nuclear grade

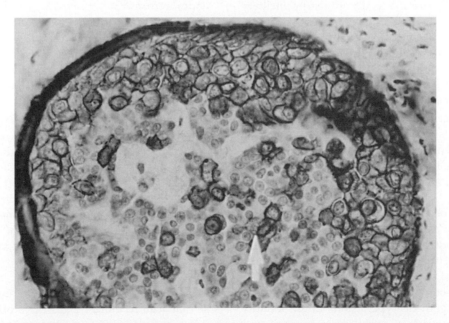

FIG. **11-18** Immunocytochemical stain for *erbB2* with strong membrane staining of large cells in a higher-grade DCIS. Note the presence of a negative, small cell population. (×200.)

and negative receptor status similar to that noted in many high-grade invasive carcinomas.

Despite the fact that some investigators used two-tiered classification and others used three-tiered classifications, agreement between the studies has been substantial. DCIS subtypes characterized by large cell type and high nuclear grade tend to be *HER2/neu* positive, are more likely *p53* positive[49] and ER negative,[80] are aneuploid, and are more likely to exhibit a higher S-phase fraction or other measurement of proliferation. They are also more likely to exhibit significant comedo-type necrosis, periductal stromal desmoplasia, and a diffuse increase in microvessel density.[34,82,83] In contrast, DCIS of small cell size, and of intermediate or low nuclear grade, or of noncomedo-type architecture tend to be *erbB2* and *p53* negative and diploid and, in most studies, exhibit a lower S-phase fraction and a tendency toward positive receptor status.[84] They also tend to lack significant necrosis and stromal reaction.

Despite concerted efforts using immunohistochemical demonstration of oncogenes and determination of ploidy and S-phase fraction with flow and image cytometry, identification of a subset of morphologically defined high-grade DCIS at even greater risk of invasive transformation remains elusive. Somewhat surprisingly, cyclin D expression was found to be similar and high in all grades of DCIS, with low levels in most ADH lesions.[85] In contrast, most genetic and molecular analyses have shown that the low-grade DCIS lesions are more similar to ADH than they are to high grade DCIS lesions. The cyclins D, especially cyclin D1, control important transitional events in the cell cycle, especially entrance into DNA synthesis. Morphologic grading achieves as much separation as do numerous ancillary tests. Susnik and associates,[86] using a classification based on nuclear texture features quantified with high-resolution image cytometry, were able to identify 100% of high-grade comedo-type DCIS concurrently associated with invasion and 80% of noncomedo-type lesions associated with invasion. The study design was necessarily retrospective, but the results are suggestive. If further validated, automated quantitative analysis of nuclear texture features in DCIS may be able to identify patients at different levels of risk. However, prospective studies are needed to certify the prospective utility of these approaches.

Simpson and associates[87] compared NM23 expression in in situ carcinoma associated with an invasive component with those not associated concurrently with an invasive component and found there was a higher expression of NM23 in comedo-type DCIS unassociated with an invasive component, suggesting that NM23 expression within comedo-type lesions might identify lesions with a lesser risk of evolution to invasion and metastatic capacity. Goldstein and Murphy[88] evaluated

nuclear grade in a three-scale system and found grades of invasive and in situ components to agree most of the time.

Special Types of DCIS with Special Implications

HYPERSECRETORY DUCTAL CARCINOMA IN SITU

Hypersecretory changes in the breast represent a type of cellular presentation and cytoplasmic differentiation. Although they are poorly understood at present, these histologic elements coexisting with atypia appear to be associated with special features in the distribution and perhaps evolution of in situ disease toward malignancy. These lesions tend not to produce a lump within the breast and often have benign-appearing, lobular-type calcifications because it is the central secretion that calcifies. Often the mammogram produces patterns that outline the lobules in an area of the breast. The presentation of the disease is commonly regional but does not have the uniformity of continuity seen in most forms of DCIS.

This entity was first described by Rosen and Scott in 1984.[89] The original paper and the follow-up presentation by the same group in 1988[90] emphasized the cystic dilation of the spaces involved and allowed for a category of atypia without the designation of DCIS. The association with the development of clinically evident malignancy in most of these cases was inapparent or unproved.[91] Often these cases present striking patterns of hugely enlarged nuclei abutting into the lumen, as seen in hypersecretory changes in the endometrium.[92,93]

Our approach to these extremely difficult cases is to recognize atypicality in a biopsy and recommend careful continued mammographic surveillance. Unfortunately, calcifications may be present in clearly benign secretory alterations in the same region, representing a challenge for mammographic follow-up.[60]

However, there are a certain number of cases in which the diagnosis of DCIS is mandatory, and this diagnostic plateau is reached definitively when true ducts are involved. The recognition of DCIS status is particularly evident when patterns of micropapillary DCIS are reached.[94] It is indeed this favorite association with micropapillary DCIS that may be one of the more interesting elements in this complex of newly recognized diseases.[95] It is because of the regional presentation of this disease that we have occasionally suggested segmentectomy or quadrantectomy, although again the regionality of this disease appears to be not as precise as that seen in more typical cases of DCIS. It is clearly different from ALH (see Chapter 7) and does not often coexist with ALH.

PAGET'S DISEASE OF THE NIPPLE

Paget's disease of the breast has been recognized as a specific clinical entity for more than 100 years, but it does not inherently imply any extension of the disease process beyond the nipple.[96] Thus the diversity of disease from within the breast after presentation of Paget's disease of the nipple is what needs to be emphasized, and Paget's disease of the breast should no longer be viewed as a type of breast cancer; rather, it is a presentation of breast cancer. After complete evaluation of the presentation, the disease may be local or extensive in the breast.[97,98]

The classic and still relevant presentation is with an eczematous area of the nipple. This feature may be subtle or evolve to an obviously eroded, weeping lesion. The underlying process is population of the epidermis of the nipple surface with a scattering of neoplastic breast epithelial cells. Often, but not uniformly, these cells are identical with a DCIS lesion in the underlying ducts.[99,100] In advanced cases the process may extend from the nipple to the areola and even to adjacent skin. The terms *pagetoid change* and *pagetoid features* are used for the interspersion of one cell type within another anywhere within the ducts and lobules of the breast. Immunohistochemical stains for *erbB2* (see Figure 11-18) are useful in demonstrating these cells and are often helpful in the differential diagnosis, because *erbB2* expression is common to virtually all examples of Paget's disease of the nipple.[71,101]

Paget's disease is usually associated with extensive DCIS within the breast.[102] In the early mammographic era, Paget's disease of the nipple was associated with invasive carcinoma and DCIS in 50% of cases. The practical importance with regard to accepting conservation, when possible, is that at present about 10% of cases are associated with disease confined to the immediate area of the nipple and are amenable to excision of the nipple/areola complex for cure.[103,104]

ENCYSTED, NONINVASIVE PAPILLARY CARCINOMA

Encysted, noninvasive papillary carcinoma contain patterns otherwise diagnostic for DCIS and have been a valuable recent addition to the diagnostic armamentarium of neoplastic breast disease. These lesions are essentially anatomically confined and probably represent DCIS arising in and overtaking the residual aspects of an intraductal papilloma. The DCIS component usually is low grade, but it can be intermediate. The clinical importance of these lesions was clarified by Carter, Orr, and Merino,[105] who introduced the concept of an encysted lesion and produced a clear conclusion: In the absence of adjacent DCIS in neighboring ducts, local excision of these lesions is curative.[106,107] This valuable study has not been improved on. It is consistent with all the information we have at present about the importance of the extensiveness of regional DCIS with regard to the likelihood of local recurrence. It is widely recognized that a pattern of these lesions has very tall cells similar to those seen in villous adenoma of the colon with enlarged hyperchromatic nuclei. These nuclei are present without an increased cell number above fibrovascular stalks. We might consider such lesions as an encysted, noninvasive lesion in this category (Figure 11-19).

It should be noted that the cutoff point between papillomas with atypia (analogous to ADH), encysted or otherwise, from the nonencysted and encysted papillary

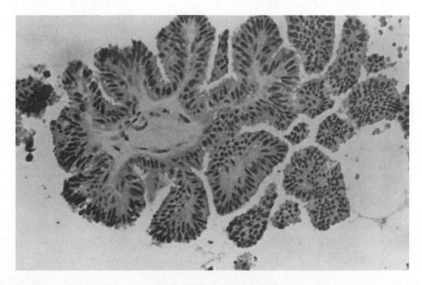

FIG. **11-19** The presence of tall and hyperchromatic cells surmounting these papillary fronds supports the possibility of a diagnosis of encysted papillary carcinoma. Usually the epithelium is much more atypical and closely mimics that found in other ductal carcinoma in situ patterns. (×125.)

carcinoma lesions is unclear. Reports by Raju and Vertes[108] and Page and colleagues[109] have stated that some degrees of atypia similar to that of ADH present within papillomas may increase the likelihood of later cancer occurrence, but the two studies are in disagreement. There is an indication from the study by Page and co-workers[109] that well-developed atypical hyperplasia within papillomas of any size indicates increased likelihood of local occurrence of carcinoma, or at least regional occurrence of carcinoma after local excision for biopsy alone. There is no certainty at this time that wider excision after such a finding is necessary. However, we suggest careful mammographic surveillance of the area until this situation is better determined. When an encysted papillary lesion is partially, but not completely, involved by patterns of low-grade DCIS, we diagnose partial involvement and pay close attention to the possibility of regional local occurrence of DCIS similar to the lesions that are fully involved.

SUMMARY

Comedo or high-grade DCIS lesions are at high risk for evolution to invasion and metastatic capacity, and it is clear that extensive high-grade, comedo lesions are not easily cured and that recurrences are common even after radiation therapy.[30,64] In contrast, small examples of noncomedo DCIS are nonobligate precursor lesions, and only 25% to 30% of them eventuate in invasive carcinomas if left untreated. They may be regarded as increased-risk lesions because their relative risk of later invasive cancer development is about 10 times that of the general population. There is strong evidence that DCIS of small size and low histologic grade is easily cured with local excision without radiation therapy. This is certainly true of lesions that are smaller than 1 cm in largest diameter. Thus the best estimate of the size of a DCIS lesion should be stated even for core biopsy specimens to help facilitate clinical management. The greatest extent of a lesion is assessed most easily with careful pathologic-mammographic correlation, which is mandatory in most instances. Precisely which concurrence of histologic grade, size, and margin clearance is to be the determinant of therapeutic decision making is an area under investigation currently. However, it should be understood that local recurrence in the setting of a low-grade lesion is unlikely to be a life-threatening event and that a woman's desire for breast conservation with a willingness to accept the possibility of local recurrence may be as important with regard to therapeutic decision making as any other consideration. In contrast, local recurrence in the setting of a high-grade DCIS lesion is much more likely to be associated with invasion, high-grade histology, and distant metastases.[36,110] Thus careful pathologic assessment of DCIS lesions that includes histologic pattern, grade, size, and margin status is essential for optimal clinical management and should be considered essential components of any breast biopsy report for DCIS.

Lobular Carcinoma In Situ

Epithelial proliferative lesions (noninvasive or in situ) of the human breast termed *lobular* were inaugurated by

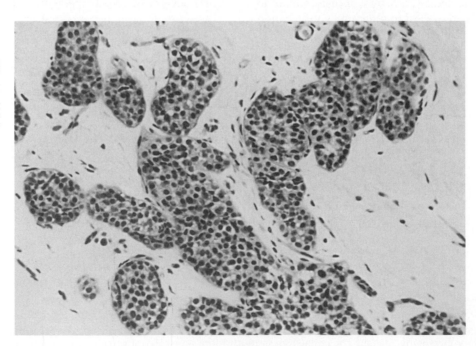

FIG. **11-20** An example of lobular carcinoma in situ showing complete distention and filling of the majority of spaces in this area by characteristic population of cells. (×200.)

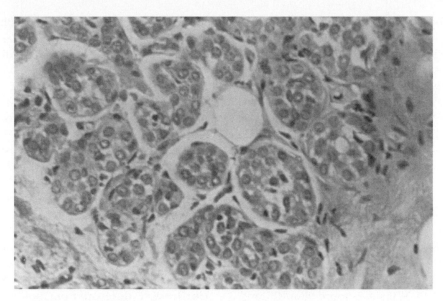

FIG. **11-21** Portion of a lobular unit demonstrating some distention and little filling of the involved acini. This is atypical lobular hyperplasia. (×300.)

the introduction of the term *LCIS* in 1941 by Foote and Stewart.[111] Critical to the definition and concept was the distinctive caricature of lobular units produced by the diagnostic clustering of three major criteria: distention, distortion, and filling by a population of characteristic cells (Figures 11-20 to 11-22). Also important to the definition, in all probability, was that more than 60% of invasive cancers presenting with single filing of cancer cells with similar cytology have such in situ lesions present in the same breast. Through the 1970s and 1980s, an important general acceptance of LCIS as an elevated cancer risk marker was established (see Table 11-1).[21,112] The two important papers of 1978 agreed that

there was no difference in risk between well-developed and less-well-developed histologic examples.[113,114] However, the first papers from Memorial Hospital in New York stated that lesser examples were not included.[42,112] Clearly, the later papers[113,114] did include minor histologic examples with little distortion of lobular units. Studies of a large Nashville cohort of benign breast biopsies did separate lesser examples and found lesser risk for these lesions,[42] as have two more recent reports by Bodian, Perzin, and Lattes[115] and Fisher and colleagues.[116]

Bodian, Perzin, and Lattes[115] apparently seek to continue to call the full range of changes termed *LCIS*

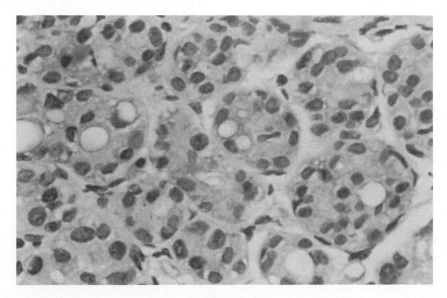

FIG. **11-22** The vacuoles or globules in the cytoplasm are characteristic of lobular neoplasia. Note that some of the cells have the appearance of signet ring cells. (×400.)

and *ALH* lobular neoplasia (LN) and further hold that LCIS is essentially identical to their LN. Others have different terminology and have used *ALH* to refer to histologically less-well-developed examples in the broad range of cytologically similar images; this approach is useful, because ALH is associated with a lower risk of cancer.[41,42] Of importance, Bodian, Perzin, and Lattes[115] and another paper from the NSABP[116] have divided the LN spectrum into well-developed examples and less-well-developed ones on a numeric basis. Considering that the study by Fisher and associates[116] is based on cases originally diagnosed by study pathologists as DCIS, it is evidently a biased series. Both recent studies found a lower risk for less-well-developed examples, whether it is called *ALH* or *LN numbers 1 and 2* as opposed to LN 3. In the review of Bodian, Perzin, and Lattes,[115] the incidence of LN in a group of 2134 biopsies is more than 10% and indicates that it is a highly selected series. It is clear that what many call *ALH* includes most of the cases within the broad range of cases in LN. Indeed, using our restricted criteria for LCIS, we found an incidence of only 0.5% of LCIS in an unselected series of just over 10,000 biopsies.[42] We continue to use the term *LN* as applying to a wide range of changes from maximal to minimal, *LCIS* to refer to maximal changes, and *ALH* to refer to the rest. Besides supporting the belief that less extensive histologic disease has less cancer risk, Bodian, Perzin, and Lattes[115] also support the finding of the Nashville series[42] that LN identified in a patient older than 55 years has less clinical importance.

Another difference among series is that the occurrence of noninvasive carcinoma of ductal type is sometimes considered a positive end point,[113,115] despite increasing the positive end point of cancer development; others have included only invasive carcinoma, and the magnitude of cancer risk is still smaller than in other studies. We have discussed this element as likely to be due to including lesser examples of histologic changes such as minimal changes that we found did not meaningfully or statistically increase the risk of subsequent carcinoma.[42]

Many foster the notion that protection should be an absolute concept; that is, there are no options referred to other than surveillance and bilateral mastectomy. Review of the experience with LCIS at Memorial Hospital in New York strongly supports the idea that removal of breast tissue (single mastectomy) does reduce the risk,[117] although nothing can provide absolute protection. Thus unilateral mastectomy provides some reduction in later cancer risk but is not a popular treatment choice.

Bodian, Perzin, and Lattes do not indicate that ductal involvement by LN incurs a greater risk. However, using the criteria of Page and associates,[42] ductal involvement is common in rigorously applied criteria

for LCIS and identified a somewhat increased risk when present in cases with ALH in lobular units.[118]

Thus ALH, LCIS, and LN continue to signify an increased risk of later cancer development in either breast, and other useful interactive associations remain to be evaluated fully. Although the usual and common examples of LN are clearly multifocal with sparing of scattered lobular units, there is a suggestion that the risk of later cancer favors the breast that had ALH on biopsy,[119,120] with about 65% of later cancer occurring in the breast homolateral to the biopsy with ALH. Whatever the terminology, it is clear that lesser examples of histologic involvement (ALH) are associated with lower risk than more classic and more extensive examples recognized as fully developed LCIS, and most findings in this series are best regarded as ALH.[119-121] The LNs, with LCIS as the fully developed example, are clearly very different from the pattern of DCIS (see Table 11-1), although rare examples of local proliferation share features of each and may be best regarded as exemplifying each lesion for patient care purposes.

A current concern is the importance of finding ALH and/or LCIS in core needle biopsies. There is a full range of opinions with regard to the possible need for further excision, with little apparent agreement.[122-126] It is likely that extent of disease is important here and that several lobular units showing only standard ALH should not necessitate formal excision without other indications.

Summary

LN should probably not be termed *LCIS* as a generic indication of the full range of histologic changes from trivial to maximal and classic. LN indicates risk elevation for later cancer throughout the breast tissues and is usefully stratified by the extent of histologic disease and age. Considerations of margins do not apply for this admittedly multicentric condition.

Understanding DCIS of the breast has been a consistent challenge because of changing presentations of DCIS and changing concepts and therapeutic options. It is impossible to understand DCIS without a historical background. This is because the diseases so named in the premammographic era were uniformly of palpable and usually high-grade type. There were only a small number of cases recognized incidentally to the indications for the biopsy procedure (i.e., palpable lump) and another few cases presenting because of bloody nipple discharge. As with most other aspects of breast disease, mammography has changed all of this and demanded that we alter our insights and practical approach. Most important, we must now understand DCIS that includes a broad range of conditions—it has become a generic term including specific categories within its confines of definition. Fortunately, it is relatively easy to include within this broad group the smaller lesions that now predominate and that are usually of lower grade. Recognition of stratification of this group of diseases is the fundamentally important conceptual change from the past and has become broadly accepted in the last decade of the twentieth century.[6,29,48]

The growing evidence that smaller lesions of DCIS can be locally excised with successful results (see Chapter 48) has demanded that we develop careful stratification and speciation of the broad range of lesions included under the broad term of *DCIS*. Planned wide excision to negative margins for smaller lesions is being widely practiced. Ernster and co-workers[24] documented that 30% of the cases of DCIS treated in 1992 in the United States were treated with local excision without radiation therapy. Size or extent of the DCIS, histologic grade, and margin status are the determinants of local recurrence after excision in the conserved breast.

Some special subtypes of DCIS will be separated out, but basically there is now a fundamental understanding that low-grade lesions by any name that are less than approximately 2 cm in size (greatest extent) can be adequately treated with careful wide excision. Also, larger (certainly those >3 cm in greatest extent) and high-grade lesions can be treated successfully with mastectomy and are probably not adequately treated by other means, although special radiotherapeutic approaches in some of these cases may prove to be successful (see other relevant chapters on radiotherapy and Chapter 48).

The terms and concepts developed over the last 10 years seem to be serving us nicely for most presentations of DCIS in high- and low-risk categories, with precise categorizations within the intermediate, and special-type categories to await further study. However, the diverse patterns of the nonclassic cases and the fact that they make up only 10% to 20% of all uses of DCIS may mean that the precise definition of the borders in heterogenous lesions may not be possible. This will remain an exciting and somewhat controversial area for some time; however, looking at the optimistic side, there is an incredibly broad range of agreement of the concepts and approaches championed in the literature of the late 1990s. Precisely structured questions of therapeutic efficacy are ideally tested in a multicenter trial with prospective design and performance. Such trials constructed to answer which women may be treated for smaller examples of DCIS with surgery alone will not be completed until the first years of the twenty-first century. However, many surgeons are following the leads of the few carefully constructed single-center studies, such as those reviewed here.

REFERENCES

1. Dean L, Geschickter CF: Comedo carcinoma of the breast, *Arch Surg* 36:225, 1938.
2. Geschickter CF: *Diseases of the breast,* Philadelphia, 1993, JB Lippincott.
3. Gillis DA, Dockerty MB, Clagett OT: Preinvasive intraductal carcinoma of the breast, *Surg Gynecol Obstet* 110:555, 1960.
4. Betsill WL, Jr et al: Intraductal carcinoma: long-term follow-up after treatment by biopsy alone, *JAMA* 239:1863, 1978.
5. Page DL et al: Intraductal carcinoma of the breast: follow-up after biopsy only, *Cancer* 49:751, 1982.
6. Page DL et al: Continued local recurrence of carcinoma 15–25 years after a diagnosis of low grade ductal carcinoma in situ of the breast treated by biopsy only, *Cancer* 76:1197, 1995.
7. Wellings SR, Jensen HM: On the origin and progression of ductal carcinoma in the human breast, *J Natl Cancer Inst* 50:1111, 1973.
8. Page DL, Anderson TJ: How should we categorize breast cancer? *Breast* 2:217, 1993.
9. Page DL, Anderson TJ, Rogers LW: Carcinoma in situ (CIS). In Page DL, Anderson TJ (eds): *Diagnostic histopathology of the breast,* Edinburgh, 1987, Churchill Livingstone.
10. Page DL, Lagios MD: Pathology and clinical evolution of ductal carcinoma in situ (DCIS) of the breast, *Cancer Lett* 86:1, 1994.
11. Habel LA et al: Risk of contralateral breast cancer among women with carcinoma in situ of the breast, *Ann Surg* 225:69, 1997.
12. Webber BL et al: Risk of subsequent contralateral breast carcinoma in a population of patients with in-situ breast carcinoma, *Cancer* 47:2928, 1981.
13. Lennington WJ et al: Ductal carcinoma in situ of the breast: heterogeneity of individual lesions, *Cancer* 73:118, 1994.
14. Page DL, Rogers LW: Combined histologic and cytologic criteria for the diagnosis of mammary atypical ductal hyperplasia, *Hum Pathol* 23:1095, 1992.
15. Schnitt SJ et al: Interobserver reproducibility in the diagnosis of ductal proliferative breast lesions using standardized criteria, *Am J Surg Pathol* 16:1133, 1992.
16. Acs G et al: Differential expression of E-cadherin in lobular and ductal neoplasms of the breast and its biologic and diagnostic implications, *Am J Clin Pathol* 115:85, 2001.
17. Jacobs TW et al: Carcinomas in situ of the breast with indeterminate features: role of E-cadherin staining in categorization, *Am J Surg Pathol* 25:229, 2001.
18. Bloodgood JC: Comedo carcinoma (or comedo-adenoma) of the female breast, *Am J Cancer* 22:842, 1934.
19. Lagios MD et al: Mammographically detected duct carcinoma in situ, *Cancer* 63:619, 1989.
20. Azzopardi JG: *Problems in breast pathology,* Philadelphia, 1979, WB Saunders.
21. McDivitt RW, Stewart FW, Berg JW: *Tumors of the breast,* Washington, DC, 1968, Armed Forces Institute of Pathology.
22. Lagios MD et al: Duct carcinoma in situ: relationship of extent of noninvasive disease to the frequency of occult invasion, multicentricity, lymph node metastases, and short-term treatment failures, *Cancer* 50:1309, 1982.
23. Patchefsky AS et al: Heterogeneity of intraductal carcinoma of the breast, *Cancer* 63:731, 1989.
24. Ernster VL et al: Incidence of and treatment for ductal carcinoma in situ of the breast, *JAMA* 275:913, 1996.

25. Winchester DP et al: Treatment trends for ductal carcinoma in situ of the breast, *Ann Surg Oncol* 2:207, 1995.

26. Schnitt SJ et al: The relationship between microscopic margins of resection and the risk of local recurrence in patients with breast cancer treated with breast-conserving surgery and radiation therapy, *Cancer* 74:1746, 1994.

27. Lagios MD: Ductal carcinoma in situ: controversies in diagnosis, biology and treatment, *Breast J* 1:67, 1995.

28. Silverstein MJ et al: Ten-year results comparing mastectomy to excision and radiation therapy for ductal carcinoma in situ of the breast, *Eur J Cancer* 9:1425, 1995.

29. Silverstein MJ et al: A prognostic index for ductal carcinoma in situ of the breast, *Cancer* 77:2267, 1996.

30. Silverstein MJ et al: The influence of margin width on local control of ductal carcinoma in situ of the breast, *N Engl J Med* 340:1455, 1999.

31. Chan KC et al: Extent of excision margin width required in breast conserving surgery for ductal carcinoma in situ, *Cancer* 91:9, 2001.

32. Holland R et al: Ductal carcinoma in situ, a proposal for a new classification, *Semin Diagn Pathol* 11:167, 1994.

33. Silverstein MJ et al: Prognostic classification of breast ductal carcinoma-in-situ, *Lancet* 345:1154, 1995.

34. Sneige N et al: Ductal carcinoma in situ treated with lumpectomy and irradiation: histopathological analysis of 49 specimens with emphasis on risk factors and long term results, *Hum Pathol* 26:642, 1995.

35. Solin LJ et al: Ductal carcinoma in situ (intraductal carcinoma) of the breast treated with breast-conserving surgery and definitive irradiation: correlation of pathologic parameters with outcome of treatment, *Cancer* 71:2532, 1993.

36. Bijker N et al: Risk factors for recurrence and metastasis after breast-conserving therapy for ductal carcinoma-in-situ: analysis of European Organisation for Research and Treatment of Cancer Trial 10853, *J Clin Oncol* 19:2263, 2001.

37. Bellamy CO et al: Noninvasive ductal carcinoma of the breast: the relevance of histologic categorization, *Hum Pathol* 24:16, 1993.

38. Bornstein BA et al: Results of treating ductal carcinoma in situ of the breast with conservative surgery and radiation therapy, *Cancer* 67:7, 1991.

39. Schwartz GF et al: Subclinical ductal carcinoma in situ of the breast: treatment by local excision and surveillance alone, *Cancer* 70:2468, 1992.

40. London SJ et al: A prospective study of benign breast disease and risk of breast cancer, *JAMA* 267:941, 1992.

41. Page DL et al: Atypical hyperplastic lesions of the female breast: a long-follow-up study, *Cancer* 55:2698, 1985.

42. Page DL et al: Lobular neoplasia of the breast: higher risk for subsequent invasive cancer predicted by more extensive disease, *Hum Pathol* 22:1232, 1991.

43. Douglas-Jones AG et al: A critical appraisal of six modern classifications of ductal carcinoma in situ of the breast (DCIS): correlation with grade of associated invasive carcinoma, *Histopathology* 29:397, 1996.

44. Scott MA et al: Ductal carcinoma in situ of the breast: reproducibility of histological subtype analysis, *Hum Pathol* 28:967, 1997.

45. Fisher ER et al: Pathologic findings from the National Surgical Adjuvant Breast Project (NSABP) protocol B-17: intraductal carcinoma (ductal carcinoma in situ), *Cancer* 75:1310, 1995.

46. Douglas-Jones AG et al: A critical appraisal of six modern classifications of ductal carcinoma in situ of the breast (DCIS): correlation with grade of associated invasive carcinoma, *Histopathology* 29:397, 1996.

47. Harrison M et al: Comparison of cytomorphological and architectural heterogeneity in mammographically detected ductal carcinoma in situ, *Histopathology* 28:445, 1996.

48. Lagios MD: Duct carcinoma in situ: pathology and treatment, *Surg Clin North Am* 70:853, 1990.

49. O'Malley FP et al: Ductal carcinoma in situ of the breast with apocrine cytology: definition of a borderline category, *Hum Pathol* 25:164, 1994.

50. Ashworth MT, Haqqani MT: Endocrine variant of ductal carcinoma in situ of breast: ultrastructural and light microscopical study, *J Clin Pathol* 39:1355, 1986.

51. Tsang WY, Chan JK: Endocrine ductal carcinoma in situ (E-DCIS) of the breast: a form of low-grade DCIS with distinctive clinicopathologic and biologic characteristics, *Am J Surg Pathol* 20:921, 1996.

52. Egan RL: Multicentric breast carcinomas: clinical-radiographic pathologic whole organ studies and 10-year survival, *Cancer* 49:1123, 1982.

53. Egan RL, Ellis JR, Powell RW: Team approach to the study of disease of the breast, *Cancer* 71:847, 1971.

54. Silverstein MJ: Intraductal breast carcinoma: two decades of progress? *Am J Clin Pathol* 14:534, 1991.

55. Faverly DR et al: Three dimensional imaging of mammary ductal carcinoma in situ: clinical implications, *Semin Diagn Pathol* 11:193, 1994.

56. Holland R et al: Extent, distribution, and mammographic/histological correlations of breast ductal carcinoma in situ, *Lancet* 335:519, 1990.

57. Ohtake T et al: Intraductal extension of primary invasive breast carcinoma treated by breast-conservative surgery: computer graphic three-dimensional reconstruction of the mammary duct–lobular systems, *Cancer* 76:32, 1995.

58. Moffat DF, Going JJ: Three dimensional anatomy of complete duct systems in human breast: pathological and developmental implications, *J Clin Pathol* 49:48, 1996.

59. Johnson JE et al: Recurrent mammary carcinoma after local excision: a segmental problem, *Cancer* 75:1612, 1995.

60. Liberman L et al: Mammographic features of local recurrence in women who have undergone breast-conserving therapy for ductal carcinoma in situ, *Am J Roentgenol* 168:489, 1997.

61. Thomson JZ et al: Growth pattern of ductal carcinoma in situ (DCIS): a retrospective analysis based on mammographic findings, *Br J Cancer* 85:225, 2001.

62. Ohuchi N, Furuta A, Mori S: Management of ductal carcinoma in situ with nipple discharge: intraductal spreading of carcinoma is an unfavorable pathologic factor for breast-conserving surgery, *Cancer* 74:1294, 1994.

63. Page DL, Lagios MD: Pathologic analysis of the National Surgical Adjuvant Breast Project (NSABP) B-17 trial: unanswered questions remaining unanswered considering current concepts of ductal carcinoma in situ, *Cancer* 75:1219, 1995.

64. Silverstein MJ et al: Intraductal carcinoma of the breast (208 cases): clinical factors influencing treatment choice, *Cancer* 66:102, 1990.

65. Fisher B et al: Lumpectomy compared with lumpectomy and radiation therapy for the treatment of intraductal breast cancer, *N Engl J Med* 328:1581, 1993.

66. Holland R et al: The presence of an extensive intraductal component following a limited excision correlates with prominent residual disease in the remainder of the breast, *J Clin Oncol* 8:113, 1990.

67. Veronesi U et al: Local recurrences and distant metastases after conservative breast cancer treatments: partly independent events, *J Natl Cancer Inst* 87:19, 1995.

68. Veronesi U, Zurrida S: Breast cancer surgery: a century after Halsted, *J Cancer Res Clin Oncol* 122:74, 1996.

69. Schnitt SJ, Harris JR, Smith BL: Developing a prognostic index for ductal carcinoma in situ of the breast: are we there yet? *Cancer* 77:2189, 1996.

70. Bobrow LG et al: The classification of ductal carcinoma in situ and its association with biological markers, *Semin Diagn Pathol* 11:199, 1994.

71. DePotter CR et al: Neu overexpression correlates with extent of disease in large cell ductal carcinoma in situ of the breast, *Hum Pathol* 26:601, 1995.

72. Leal CB et al: Ductal carcinoma in situ of the breast: histologic categorization and its relationship to ploidy and immunohistochemical expression of hormone receptors, p53, and c-erb B-2 protein, *Cancer* 75:2123, 1995.

73. Simpson JF, Page DL: Pathology of preinvasive and excellent-prognosis breast cancer, *Curr Opin Oncol* 7:501, 1995.

74. Steeg PS et al: Molecular analysis of premalignant and carcinoma in situ lesions of the human breast, *Am J Pathol* 149:733, 1996.

75. Zafrani B et al: Mammographically-detected ductal in situ carcinoma of the breast analyzed with a new classification: a study of 127 cases: correlation with estrogen and progesterone receptors, p53 and c-erB-2 proteins, and proliferative activity, *Semin Diagn Pathol* 11:199, 1994.

76. Bartkova J et al: Immunohistochemical demonstration of c-erbB-2 protein in mammary ductal carcinoma in situ, *Hum Pathol* 21:1164, 1990.

77. Gupta SK et al: E-cadherin (E-cad) expression in duct carcinoma in situ (DCIS) of the breast, *Virchows Arch* 430:23, 1997.

78. Poller DN et al: p53 protein expression in mammary ductal carcinoma in situ: relationship to immunohistochemical expression of estrogen receptor and c-erbB-2 protein, *Hum Pathol* 24:463, 1993.

79. Barnes DM et al: Overexpression of the c-erb B-2 oncoprotein: why does this occur more frequently in ductal carcinoma in situ than in invasive mammary carcinoma and is this of prognostic significance? *Eur J Cancer* 28:644, 1992.

80. Wilbur DC, Barrows GH: Estrogen and progesterone receptor and c-erbB-2 oncoprotein analysis in pure in situ breast carcinoma: an immunohistochemical study, *Mod Pathol* 6:114, 1993.

81. Poller DN et al: Oestrogen receptor expression in ductal carcinoma in situ of the breast: relationship to flow cytometric analysis of DNA and expression of the c-erbB-2 oncoprotein, *Br J Cancer* 68:156, 1993.

82. Guidi AJ et al: Microvessel density and distribution in ductal carcinoma in situ of the breast, *J Natl Cancer Inst* 86:614, 1994.

83. Sasano H et al: Expression of p53 in human esophageal carcinoma: an immunohistochemical study with correlation to proliferating cell nuclear antigen expression, *Hum Pathol* 23:1238, 1992.

84. Zafrani B et al: Conservative treatment of early breast cancer: prognostic value of the ductal in situ component and other pathological variables on local control and survival: long-term results, *Eur J Cancer Clin Oncol* 25:1645, 1989.

85. Weinstat-Saslow D et al: Overexpression of cyclin D mRNA distinguishes invasive and in situ breast carcinomas from nonmalignant lesions, *Nat Med* 1:1257, 1995.

86. Susnik B et al: Differences in quantitative nuclear features between ductal carcinoma in situ (DCIS) with and without accompanying invasive carcinoma in the surrounding breast, *Anal Cell Pathol* 8:39, 1995.

87. Simpson JF et al: Heterogeneous expression of nm23 gene product in noninvasive breast carcinoma, *Cancer* 73:2352, 1994.

88. Goldstein NS, Murphy T: Intraductal carcinoma associated with invasive carcinoma of the breast: a comparison of the two lesions with implications for intraductal carcinoma classification systems, *Am J Clin Pathol* 106:312, 1996.

89. Rosen PP, Scott M: Cystic hypersecretory duct carcinoma of the breast, *Am J Surg Pathol* 8:31, 1984.

90. Guerry P, Erlandson RA, Rosen PP: Cystic hypersecretory hyperplasia and cystic hypersecretory duct carcinoma of the breast: pathology, therapy, and follow-up of 39 patients, *Cancer* 61:1611, 1988.

91. Jensen RA, Page DL: Cystic hypersecretory carcinoma: what's in a name? *Arch Pathol Lab Med* 112:1176, 1988.

92. Arias-Stella J: Atypical endometrial changes associated with the presence of chorionic tissue, *Arch Pathol* 58:112, 1954.

93. Arias-Stella J: Atypical endometrial changes produced by chorionic tissue, *Hum Pathol* 3:450, 1972.

94. Anderson TJ, Page DL: Risk assessment in breast cancer. In Anthony PP, MacSween RN, Lowe DG (eds): *Recent advances in histopathology,* vol 17, Edinburgh, 1997, Churchill Livingstone.

95. Page DL, Kasami M, Jensen RA: Hypersecretory hyperplasia with atypia in breast biopsies, *Pathol Case Rev* 1:36, 1996.

96. Fechner RE: One century of mammary carcinoma in situ: what have we learned? *Am J Clin Pathol* 100:654, 1993.

97. Bulens P et al: Breast conserving treatment of Paget's disease, *Radiother Oncol* 17:305, 1990.

98. Salvadori B, Fariselli G, Saccozzi R: Analysis of 100 cases of Paget's disease of the breast, *Tumori* 62:529, 1976.

99. Chaudary MA et al: Paget's disease of the nipple: a ten year review including clinical, pathological, and immunohistochemical findings, *Breast Cancer Res Treat* 8:139, 1986.

100. Dixon AR et al: Paget's disease of the nipple, *Br J Surg* 78:722, 1991.

101. Ramachandra S et al: Immunohistochemical distribution of c-erbB-2 in in situ breast carcinoma: a detailed morphological analysis, *J Pathol* 161:7, 1990.

102. Page DL, Steel CM, Dixon JM: ABC of breast diseases: carcinoma in situ and patients at high risk of breast cancer, *BMJ* 310:39, 1995.

103. Lagios MD et al: Paget's disease of the nipple: alternative management in cases without or with minimal extent of underlying breast carcinoma, *Cancer* 54:545, 1984.

104. Bijker N et al: Breast-conserving therapy for Paget disease of the nipple: a prospective European Organization for Research and Treatment of Cancer study of 61 patients, *Cancer* 91:472, 2001.

105. Carter D, Orr SL, Merino MJ: Intracystic papillary carcinoma of the breast: after mastectomy, radiotherapy or excisional biopsy alone, *Cancer* 52:14, 1983.

106. Corkill ME et al: Fine-needle aspiration cytology and flow cytometry of intracystic papillary carcinoma of breast, *Am J Clin Pathol* 94:673, 1990.

107. Estabrook A et al: Mammographic features of intracystic papillary lesions, *Surg Gynecol Obstet* 170:113, 1990.

108. Raju U, Vertes D: Breast papillomas with atypical ductal hyperplasia: a clinicopathologic study, *Hum Pathol* 27:1231, 1996.

109. Page DL et al: Subsequent breast carcinoma risk after biopsy with atypia in a breast papilloma, *Cancer* 78:258, 1996.

110. Bijker N et al: Histological type and marker expression of the primary tumour compared with its local recurrence after breast-conserving therapy for ductal carcinoma in situ, *Br J Cancer* 84:539, 2001.

111. Foote FW, Stewart FW: Lobular carcinoma in situ, *Am J Pathol* 17:491, 1941.

112. McDivitt RW et al: In situ lobular carcinoma: a prospective follow-up study indicating cumulative patient risks, *JAMA* 201:96, 1967.

113. Haagensen CD et al: Lobular neoplasia (so-called lobular carcinoma in situ) of the breast, *Cancer* 42:737, 1978.

114. Rosen PP et al: Lobular carcinoma in situ of the breast: detailed analysis of 99 patients with average follow-up of 24 years, *Am J Surg Pathol* 2:225, 1978.

115. Bodian CA, Perzin KH, Lattes R: Lobular neoplasia: long term risk of breast cancer in relation to other factors, *Cancer* 78:1024, 1996.

116. Fisher ER et al: Pathologic findings from the National Surgical Adjuvant Breast Project (NSABP) protocol B-17: five-year observations concerning lobular carcinoma in situ, *Cancer* 78:1403, 1996.

117. Rosen PP et al: Lobular carcinoma in situ of the breast: preliminary results of treatment by ipsilateral mastectomy and contralateral breast biopsy, *Cancer* 47:813, 1981.

118. Page DL, Dupont WD, Rogers LW: Ductal involvement by cells of atypical lobular hyperplasia in the breast: a long-term follow-up study of cancer risk, *Hum Pathol* 19:201, 1988.

119. Page DL et al: Atypical hyperplastic lesions of the female breast: a long-term follow-up study, *Cancer* 55:2698, 1985.

120. Marshall LM et al: Risk of breast cancer associated with atypical hyperplasia of lobular and ductal types, *Cancer Epidemiol Biomarkers Prev* 6:297, 1997.

121. Fitzgibbons PL: Atypical lobular hyperplasia of the breast: a study of pathologists' responses in the College of American Pathologists Performance Improvement Program in Surgical Pathology, *Arch Pathol Lab Med* 124:463, 2000.

122. Berg WA, Mrose HE, Ioffe OB: Atypical lobular hyperplasia or lobular carcinoma in situ at core-needle breast biopsy, *Radiology* 218:503, 2001.

123. Jacobs TW, Connolly JL, Schnitt SJ: Nonmalignant lesions in breast core needle biopsies: to excise or not to excise? *Am J Surg Pathol* 26:1095, 2002.

124. Liberman L et al: Lobular carcinoma in situ at percutaneous breast biopsy: surgical biopsy findings, *AJR Am J Roentgenol* 173:291, 1999.

125. Renshaw AA et al: Lobular neoplasia in breast core needle biopsy specimens is not associated with an increased risk of ductal carcinoma in situ or invasive carcinoma, *Am J Clin Pathol* 117:797, 2002.

126. Shin SJ, Rosen PP: Excisional biopsy should be performed if lobular carcinoma in situ is seen on needle core biopsy, *Arch Pathol Lab Med* 126:697, 2002.

CHAPTER

12

Malignant Neoplasia of the Breast: Infiltrating Carcinomas

JEAN F. SIMPSON

EDWARD J. WILKINSON

Chapter Outline

Understanding the histopathologic features of breast cancer has been recognized anew as a necessary element for appropriate management of breast carcinoma.[1-3] Standard staging procedures recognize the extremes of the prognostic spectrum, and many therapeutic decisions are based on the tumor, node, metastasis (TNM) system; however, additional prognostic information is available through careful, focused histopathologic examination. The use of chemotherapy in an adjuvant setting has raised the question of whether such therapy will be beneficial—either because the patient already has an excellent prognosis or because the prognosis is so poor that high-dose chemotherapy is indicated. This chapter reviews the histopathology of invasive breast carcinoma, emphasizing the proven and potential settings in which it provides prognostic information.

There have been two general approaches to prognostication via histopathologic analysis. The first categorizes carcinomas based on specific features, recognizing the so-called special-type carcinomas. The second approach evaluates individual characteristics of the carcinoma, such as nuclear pleomorphism or gland formation (grading). Recognizing the special-type carcinomas makes it possible to identify a group of patients with an extremely good prognosis, often approaching or equaling that of the general population. In contrast, a subset of patients who have a very poor prognosis can be identified (representing about 25% of invasive breast carcinomas) with careful histologic grading. We endorse both of these approaches to histopathologic analysis for most cases, as described in the following sections.

Histologic Types of Invasive Carcinoma

Much of the terminology of breast lesions is divided into *lobular* and *ductal,* based principally on historical perspectives. Early classifications of breast carcinomas used the term *lobular* for tumors commonly associated with lobular carcinoma in situ. Because ducts were the other source of epithelium within the breast, lesions that did not have a lobular pattern were referred to as *ductal.* In fact, most breast lesions, both benign and malignant, originate in the terminal duct lobular unit (TDLU),[4] but the terms *lobular* and *ductal* continue to be used because they are so deeply ingrained in clinical parlance. Because fewer than 10% of invasive carcinomas are of the lobular type, the term *ductal* has no specific meaning.

We support the histologic classification that recognizes special types of mammary carcinoma defined in terms of specific histologic criteria (Table 12-1). In general, these special types are associated with less malignant potential than ordinary carcinomas that lack these special features. Terminology varies, but in general the frequency of these special types in different series is comparable. The special-type carcinomas make up about 20% to 30% of all invasive carcinomas (this figure is higher for carcinomas detected in screening programs), the remainder being invasive *ductal* or *no special type (NST)* carcinomas.[11-14] Fisher and colleagues[15] have termed these latter carcinomas *not otherwise specified;* however, we prefer the designation *NST,* to be consistent with the special-type terminology and to serve as a reminder to look for the features of special type in every case.[6] To qualify as a special-type carcinoma, at least 90% of the tumor should contain the defining histologic features; if the features are present in 75% to 90% of the tumor (variant), the prognosis is often better than that for a carcinoma that contains no special features.[9,16] The variant patterns are less powerful indicators of prognosis than their pure counterparts, however. Obviously, it is essential to sample the carcinoma thoroughly, paying attention to the possibility of heterogeneity. Although we stress the precise histopathologic criteria that qualify a carcinoma as a special type, an analysis of outcome from the Surveillance, Epidemiology, and End Results (SEER) programs shows that even without central slide review, an improved survival is seen with these special types of carcinoma.[17]

TABLE **12-1**   Incidence (%) of Special-Type Carcinomas in Different Series

SERIES	LOBULAR	TUBULAR	MEDULLARY	MUCINOUS	TOTAL
Rosen[5]	10	1	10	2	23
Fisher et al[6]	5	1	6	2	14
Fu et al[7]	11	7	15	2	35
Wallgren et al[8]	14	7	6	0	27
Page et al[9]	10	7*	5	2	24
Ellis et al[10]	16	3*	3	1	23
Anderson et al[11] (screen-detected)	7	10	0	0.5	22

*Includes tubular and invasive cribriform carcinoma.

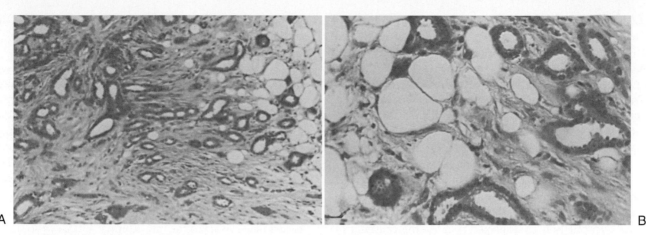

FIG. **12-1** Tubular carcinoma. **A,** Haphazardly arranged angular glands infiltrate stroma and fat. (×100.) **B,** Note the low nuclear grade and absence of mitotic activity. (×250.)

TUBULAR CARCINOMA

Probably the most important special type is *tubular carcinoma*[18-20] because distant metastatic potential is highly unlikely when this tumor is present in pure form.[21,22] The diagnosis is made when characteristic angulated tubules, composed of cells with *low-grade* nuclei, comprise at least 90% of the carcinoma (Figure 12-1). These neoplastic tubules are haphazardly arranged and are often found infiltrating between existing benign structures. Low-grade ductal carcinoma in situ and atypical ductal hyperplasia are common findings.[9] Tubular carcinoma has also been termed *well-differentiated carcinoma*, but this designation lacks precision, because carcinomas of no special type can also be well differentiated.

The prognosis for tubular carcinoma depends on the purity of the histologic pattern.[18,21,23] In the classic series of 54 cases reported by Cooper, Patchefsky, and Krall,[18] all 12 patients whose carcinoma was composed purely of the characteristic low-grade, angulated tubules survived 15 years, regardless of tumor size.

In screening programs, tubular carcinoma represents 9% of detected carcinomas,[11,13] whereas in mammographic series, this special type of carcinoma is responsible for as many as 27% of detected carcinomas.[14] Mammographic features include a spiculated mass, with or without associated microcalcifications, or, less commonly, asymmetric density and architectural distortion with associated calcifications.[24] Diagnostic features of tubular carcinoma seen in fine-needle aspiration specimens have been described.[25]

Tubular carcinoma represents only about 3% to 5% of all invasive carcinomas; thus their significance may be lost when cases are grouped and analyzed only by stage. The importance of tubular carcinoma lies with therapeutic decisions for *individual* patients. Tubular carcinoma has the biologic correlates of a low-grade cancer (estrogen receptor [ER] positive, diploid, low S phase, no expression of *c-erbB-2* or epidermal growth factor receptor) and is more likely to occur in older patients. The survival of patients with tubular carcinoma is generally similar to that of the general population, and systemic adjuvant therapy may be avoided in these patients.[26] A review of surgical therapy states that for cases of pure tubular carcinoma with an adequate negative margin, mastectomy, radiation, or even axillary lymph node dissection may be unnecessary.[27,28]

INVASIVE CRIBRIFORM CARCINOMA

Closely related, histologically and biologically, to tubular carcinoma is *invasive cribriform carcinoma (ICC)*.[29,30] Histopathologically, these carcinomas infiltrate the stroma as islands of cells that have the same appearance as cribriform-type ductal carcinoma in situ (Figure 12-2). Differentiating cribriform in situ from ICC may be difficult because of distortion and scarring.

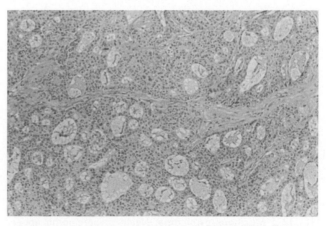

FIG. **12-2** Invasive cribriform carcinoma. Islands of low-grade cribriform structures infiltrate the stroma.

If tumor nests can be demonstrated within fat, beyond the confines of lobular units, the distinction is less difficult. Without this feature, irregular clustering of cellular islands signifies an invasive process. Another helpful feature is that the invasive islands in ICC are usually evenly spaced and often of uniform size.[9] About one fourth of cases have intermixed areas of tubular carcinoma. Because both tubular carcinoma and ICC have equally excellent prognoses, this feature has no bearing on an otherwise excellent prognosis.

In studies of *pure* tubular carcinoma[18] and ICC,[29,30] the presence of one or two positive low axillary lymph nodes did not adversely affect survival. The importance of pattern purity is emphasized because the presence of carcinoma that does not conform to special-type criteria increases the likelihood not only of nodal involvement but also of shorter survival.[18,21,29,30]

MUCINOUS CARCINOMA

Mucinous (colloid) carcinoma, when present in its pure form, is also associated with an excellent prognosis. Its defining histologic characteristic is extracellular pools of mucin in which low-grade tumor aggregates appear to be suspended (Figure 12-3). As with tubular carcinoma, the importance of pure patterns is essential to ensure an excellent prognosis (90% 10-year survival)[31] in the absence of adjuvant chemotherapy.[26] Other studies confirm that the excellent prognosis of mucinous carcinoma is confined to pure examples of this special type of breast carcinoma.[32-37]

Pure and mixed mucinous carcinomas also have different mammographic appearances. Whereas pure mucinous carcinoma has a circumscribed, lobular contour on mammograms (corresponding histologically to pools of extracellular mucin), mixed carcinomas have an ill-defined, irregular mammographic contour. This lack of circumscription corresponds histologically to the interface between invasive carcinoma and the often-fibrotic stroma.[38]

INFILTRATING LOBULAR CARCINOMA

Infiltrating lobular carcinoma (ILC) has important clinical correlates, but there has been disagreement about prognostic implications. The different histologic definitions of this entity, whose incidence ranges from 1% to 20%, reflect this disagreement.[39,40] The two defining features of ILC are cytology and pattern of infiltration. The classic ILC is composed of small cells with cytologic features identical to those of lobular carcinoma in situ: regular, round, bland nuclei and cytoplasm with occasional intracytoplasmic lumina.[41,42] Morphometric analysis of the nuclei in classic ILC shows small nuclear volume, adding a quantitative measure to the cytologic criteria.[43] These cells infiltrate in single-file, frequently encircling existing structures (so-called targetoid pattern). When these two features are found in combination, the classic (or pure) pattern of ILC is diagnosed (Figure 12-4). It is this form of ILC that is most often associated with lobular carcinoma in situ. Variant patterns have been described in which either the cytologic features or infiltrative pattern is present.[9,44-48] These include the solid, alveolar, mixed, and pleomorphic variants of ILC.

Part of the controversy surrounding the prognostic implications of ILC relates to the inconsistent application of histologic definition. Whereas some require at least 80%[44,49] of the carcinoma to have the appropriate ILC features, others have accepted as little as 5% as defining of ILC.[50] Studies that have shown an improved prognosis associated with ILC limit this prediction to the classic form of the disease.[44,49,51,52] The prognosis is intermediate (70% to 80% 5-year survival), falling between the excellent prognosis of tubular and related carcinomas and the often poor prognosis of carcinomas

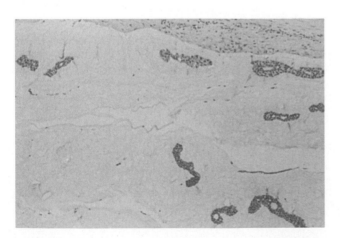

FIG. **12-3** Mucinous carcinoma. Nests of carcinoma appear suspended in extracellular mucin. Note the characteristic sharply circumscribed edge.

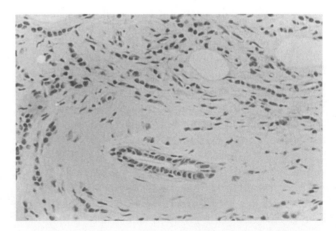

FIG. **12-4** Infiltrating lobular carcinoma, classic type. The carcinoma has bland nuclear features and infiltrates in a single-file pattern.

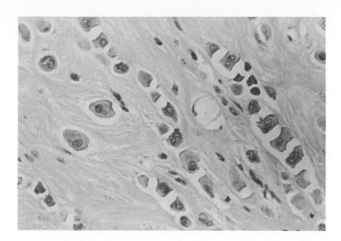

FIG. **12-5** Infiltrating lobular carcinoma, pleomorphic variant. Despite the single-file growth pattern, the nuclei show marked pleomorphism.

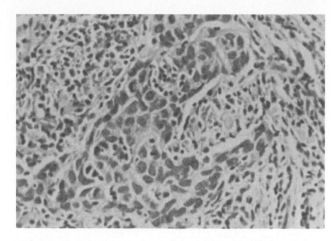

FIG. **12-6** Medullary carcinoma, showing the defining growth pattern of irregular, often interconnecting, islands of neoplastic cells surrounded by a dense, lymphocytic infiltrate.

of no special type.[9] The importance of low-grade cytologic examination in diagnosing classic ILC is emphasized by two studies of so-called pleomorphic lobular carcinoma (PLC). Although the pattern of infiltration (single-file growth pattern) is similar to that of classic ILC, cytologic features are too pleomorphic for that diagnosis (Figure 12-5), and in both series, PLC was associated with aggressive behavior.[45,48] The solid variant of ILC also appears to have a poor prognosis.[53] A molecular correlate of the dyshesive growth pattern that defines ILC has been described in mutations in the cell adhesion molecule E-cadherin.[54]

ILC is notorious for presenting diagnostic difficulties, clinically and radiographically. Although ILC is often associated with a discrete mass, a large proportion of these lesions are difficult to detect because of their insidious growth pattern. When compared with cancers of no special type but of similar size, patients with ILC have a better survival.[55]

ILC is often multifocal and bilateral, especially the pleomorphic variant.[56] These features have little bearing on outcome, either overall survival[56] or disease-free survival after conservative therapy.[52,57]

MEDULLARY CARCINOMA

Medullary carcinoma has characteristic mammographic, clinical, and pathologic correlates. Medullary carcinoma is a common phenotype of hereditary breast cancer and is found in women who are at risk for cancer because of mutations in the tumor-suppressor gene *BRCA1*.[58] This genetic characteristic is in large part attributable to the young age of the patients.[59]

The distinctive smooth, pushing border of medullary carcinoma is reflected mammographically as a sharply circumscribed mass. Grossly, medullary carcinoma has a uniform, soft consistency. The essential histologic features include islands of tumor cells having irregular

borders, without sharp edges, that are often connected (syncytial growth pattern; Figure 12-6). These islands do not invade the adjacent breast tissue; instead they appear to push against it, resulting in a smooth interface with the adjacent normal breast tissue.[9] Unlike the special-type carcinomas discussed earlier, medullary carcinoma is characterized by nuclei that have pronounced anaplastic features. The nuclei are large and pleomorphic, with clumped chromatin, frequent nucleoli, and readily identifiable mitotic figures. The other required histologic feature is a prominent infiltrate of lymphocytes and plasma cells in the loose connective tissue between the cellular islands. Multifactorial analysis has shown that high mitotic count, pushing tumor margins, and a lymphocytic infiltrate are independently associated with *BRCA1* mutations.[60] Unlike medullary carcinoma in other organs, medullary carcinoma of the breast is rarely associated with microsatellite instability.[61]

The special prognostic features of medullary carcinoma have received considerable attention. The need for adhering to careful histologic guidelines is evident, because currently this entity is overdiagnosed,[62] despite the availability of specific histopathologic criteria.[63] When these histologic guidelines are followed, node-negative medullary carcinoma predicts a good prognosis; otherwise, the predictive utility is not clear.[64,65] A better prognosis for the so-called medullary variant, or atypical medullary carcinoma, is not predicted beyond what would be expected for an ordinary intermediate-grade carcinoma of no special type.[65]

INVASIVE MAMMARY CARCINOMAS OF NO SPECIAL TYPE

Approximately three fourths of invasive breast carcinomas do not have histopathologic features that would

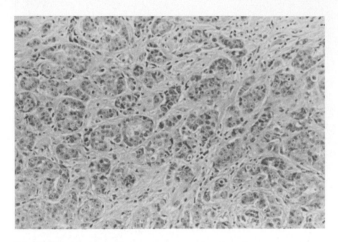

FIG. **12-7** Small, tight clusters of malignant cells are seen in this infiltrating mammary carcinoma of no special type.

allow their inclusion into the aforementioned categories. These have been referred to as *ductal* because they do not have the lobular pattern described previously. Regardless of this common usage, these carcinomas have not been proved to arise in ducts, and in practice, they are diagnosed through exclusion because they do not fit into any of the special-type categories. For these reasons, we support the designation *no special type* (NST) carcinomas, which is equivalent to the descriptor used by Fisher's group, *ductal without special features* or *otherwise not specified type*.[6]

No specific histopathologic features are consistently associated with *infiltrating mammary carcinoma NST.* These NST carcinomas are characterized by a variety of patterns, from solid to small tightly cohesive nests to single-cell infiltrative patterns (Figures 12-7 and 12-8). Gland formation may be present, and often a mixture of these patterns is found in an individual carcinoma. Moreover, any of the patterns described for special-type carcinomas can be found focally.

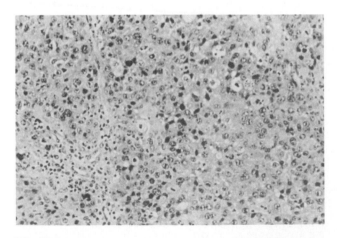

FIG. **12-8** Solid growth pattern of invasive mammary carcinoma of no special type.

These infiltrating NST carcinomas have the worst prognosis. Unlike the special-type carcinomas, limited prognostic information is obtained from the histologic patterns, because these are quite variable. Instead, prognosis is largely based on tumor stage.[66]

Despite the availability of well-defined histologic criteria for the different types of mammary carcinoma, the terminology used by surgical pathologists to report breast cancers is often inconsistent, as shown by the report from the SEER program of the National Cancer Institute. This update listed more than 20 histologic types of invasive carcinomas based on pathology reports.[67] Despite the lack of consistency in reporting, the 5-year survival for the special-type carcinomas was nevertheless better than that for those of NST.[67]

UNUSUAL TYPES OF INVASIVE CARCINOMA

The preceding discussion of types of invasive carcinomas includes those commonly encountered. There are several types of carcinomas that are only occasionally encountered, representing in total less than 2% of all breast carcinomas.[9] Despite their rarity, specific diagnostic terms should be used in pathology reporting because of inherent clinical correlates.[9]

Secretory carcinoma is usually small and well circumscribed. The characteristic histologic feature is the presence of abundant intracellular and extracellular clear areas that contain secretions. Most examples are associated with discontinuous fibrous tissue that is often prominent within the lesion. The secretory material stains with periodic acid–Schiff stain and other mucosubstance stains.

Originally described in juveniles, secretory carcinoma can also affect older women.[68] Features that ensure an excellent prognosis include young age, tumor diameter less than 2 cm, and no stromal invasion at the periphery of the lesion.[9,69,70]

Whereas squamous metaplasia may be a feature of NST carcinomas, *squamous cell carcinoma* as a pure pattern of breast carcinoma is distinctly unusual. Often cystic, squamous cell carcinoma of the breast may also assume a solid pattern with keratinization. The prognosis of squamous cell carcinoma of the breast is probably the same as that for ordinary intermediate-to high-grade carcinoma NST.[71] The importance in its recognition lies with better understanding in the event of later metastases.[9]

Rarely, breast carcinoma displays the same pattern as well-accepted *salivary gland tumors.* The most important salivary gland type of tumor in the breast is *adenoid cystic carcinoma* because of potential confusion in prognosis. In the salivary gland proper, this tumor is infiltrative and, despite a long clinical course, may be lethal. In contrast, adenoid cystic carcinoma of the breast is associated with an excellent prognosis, and death from distant metastases is not recorded.[72-74] The histologic, cytologic, and immunohistochemical features of this unusual breast tumor have been presented.[72,73,75] Adenoid cystic carcinoma regularly lacks ER and shows increased cellular proliferation[76,77]; however, these features do not negate the excellent prognosis associated with adenoid cystic carcinoma. The lack of ER likely reflects derivation from an ER myoepithelial cells, rather than lack of differentiation. *Mucoepidermoid carcinoma* of the breast has the same histopathologic features as the salivary gland counterpart. The salient features—mucin production and squamous differentiation—can, however, be a nonspecific feature of mammary carcinoma NST. The identification of mucoepidermoid carcinoma is probably important only when it is a low-grade tumor.[78,79] Case reports of high-grade mucoepidermoid carcinoma have demonstrated an aggressive course.[80,81] The histogenesis of this unusual neoplasm has been studied ultrastructurally,[82] immunohistochemically,[82,83] and biochemically.[83]

The term *metaplastic carcinoma* encompasses a group of tumors that show both epithelial and mesenchymal features. The mesenchymal component may show squamous, spindled, cartilaginous, or osseous differentiation. With ultrastructural and immunohistochemical analysis, the sarcomatoid areas have been demonstrated to be of epithelial origin.[84,85] Despite the unusual appearance of these heterogeneous tumors,[86,87] the prognosis is similar to that for stage-matched invasive mammary carcinomas NST.[84,88] A subset of metaplastic carcinoma has been recognized as having distinct clinicopathologic correlates.[89] Tumors with growth patterns resembling fibromatosis were found to be associated with local but not distant recurrence. This is important because such lesions were previously classified with other metaplastic carcinomas.

Prognosis of Invasive Breast Carcinoma

Predicting outcome for patients with breast carcinoma, especially those whose carcinoma is confined to the breast, is of critical importance. Enormous efforts have been expended to identify predictors of prognosis. Evaluating which of these factors gives significant *independent* information is difficult because available studies have differences in the end points being evaluated, patient groups, length of follow-up, and treatments, as well as inconsistent inclusion of known prognostic factors to test for independent significance in the final analysis.[2,90,91]

The College of American Pathologists (CAP) Cancer Committee continues to address the clinical relevance of prognostic markers for solid tumors.[1,92] Previous CAP conferences have classified prognostic factors into three general categories based on their clinical utility and results of clinical investigation.[1]

The most recent CAP conference refined these classifications as follows: The clinically important category included factors that are well supported by the literature and are in general use in patient management, including TNM staging information, histologic tumor type, histologic grade, mitotic figure count, and hormone receptor status.[92]

TUMOR STAGE

Tumor stage is the most useful means for predicting survival. The TNM staging system, the mainstay for prognostication for breast cancer, considers three variables[90]: diameter of the primary tumor (T), lymph node metastasis (N), and distant metastasis (M). The primary tumor is categorized as T_1 if 2 cm or smaller in diameter, T_2 if greater than 2 but not greater than 5 cm, and T_3 if larger than 5 cm. The size of the primary tumor and the status of axillary lymph nodes are independent and additive in predicting survival.[66] Both parameters reflect the tumor's ability to spread distantly.[66,93]

As important as the tumor size is, it is important to distinguish the invasive component in establishing the T stage, because the in situ component does not have metastatic capacity.[94,95] Staging is especially useful at the extremes of the scale. Clearly, the prognosis associated with a small carcinoma (1 cm) that does not involve axillary lymph nodes is so good that adjunctive measures are unlikely to have any impact.[96,97] On the other hand, most would agree that patients with 3-cm carcinomas should receive adjuvant therapy. However, *pure special type carcinomas,* such as tubular and mucinous carcinomas, have an excellent long-term prognosis, even if they attain this size.[16] The challenge for surgical pathologists is to consistently apply the specific histologic criteria that would allow their recognition, thus ensuring good prognosis.

There have been some recent changes in the TNM staging system[98] that address status of lymph nodes. These changes are especially timely considering the current emphasis placed on sentinel lymph node examination. A category of pN_{1mi} is created for micrometastasis (>0.2 mm and ≤2 mm). The category of pN_0 is subcategorized to address the identification of isolated tumor cells (ITC) detected with ancillary methods, such as immunohistochemical or molecular methods, but verified on routine hematoxylin and eosin (H&E) stained slides.[98] Other changes include the classification of metastases to the infraclavicular lymph nodes (now N_3) and the supraclavicular lymph nodes (now N_3 rather than M_1).

The status of axillary lymph nodes continues to be essential in the staging and prognostication of breast cancer, especially in small tumors. Sentinel lymph node biopsy is an increasingly accepted staging procedure. However, with this procedure comes the opportunity to detect occult disease, the significance of which is still under investigation. The sixth edition of the American Joint Commission for Cancer (AJCC) staging manual allows for the separate reporting of these foci, with clarification of the method of detection. This approach should allow the separate analysis of the impact that occult metastatic cells may have on a patient's outcome. A careful review of this topic has been presented.[99] CAP has recommended that immunohistochemical evidence of metastases to lymph nodes unsupported by documentation with routine H&E stains not be regarded as evidence of regional metastases.[92]

HISTOLOGIC GRADING

Although the prognosis for small or special-type carcinomas is favorable, prognostication for the remainder of patients, especially those with negative lymph nodes, is uncertain. *Histologic grading* of breast carcinomas may help stratify this group of patients. Unfortunately, careful grading of breast carcinoma has not been carried out consistently, despite the requirement for grading other malignancies.

Grading systems may be based on architectural or cytologic features. We endorse the grading system of Scarff, Bloom, and Richardson (SBR), as modified by Elston and Ellis.[100] The most recent CAP consensus conference endorses this system,[92] as well as the sixth edition of the AJCC *Cancer Staging Manual*. Also known as the *combined histologic grade*, this system is a composite of degrees of glandular formation, nuclear pleomorphism, and mitotic activity. Each of these parameters is assigned a numerical score based on specific criteria (Table 12-2). The scores from each category are then summed:

3 (lowest score possible), 4, or 5—equivalent to grade 1
6 or 7—equivalent to grade 2
8 or 9—equivalent to grade 3

The grader who uses this system is required to evaluate each parameter, with the result that interobserver agreement is fostered.

Although the SBR system has been used for many years, modification and extensive application to more than 2000 cases of primary operable breast cancer by Elston and Ellis[100] have clarified criteria, strengthening predictive power and reproducibility. Elston and Ellis have shown a highly significant correlation between grade and both relapse-free and overall survival. The distribution of cases within the three grades is also interesting: 19% were grade 1; 34%, grade 2; and 47%, grade 3. This contrasts with other grading schemes that place approximately two thirds of cases into the poorly differentiated category, thus reducing predictive power.[15] Others have shown that grading is predictive of outcome,[101] being second only to lymph node involvement as an independent prognostic factor.[102] Histologic grade of small carcinomas is especially important in prognostication.[103] In general, the special-type carcinomas have low nuclear grade, as determined both histologically and with cell cycle analysis.[104]

Although in North America histologic grading of breast carcinoma has not been accepted as widely as in Europe, there is a recent trend toward increased use of histologic grading.[105] The reproducibility of histologic grading using the combined histologic grading system has been demonstrated.[106,107]

The Nottingham Prognostic Index (NPI), a prognostic index, incorporates tumor size, lymph node status, and the combined histologic grade with independent prediction of outcome, including small (<1 cm) tumors.[101,108]

PROLIFERATIVE ACTIVITY

An assessment of proliferative activity is an important factor in breast cancer prognosis, although it has not been as widely verified as the parameters described previously. Cellular proliferation may be assessed in several ways, most practically through quantification of mitotic figures. The latter method is endorsed by the most recent CAP consensus conference.[92] As a component of the combined histologic grade, a high mitotic rate is the strongest indicator of a poor prognosis,[109] for both node-negative[110] and node-positive breast cancer.[111] By itself, the mitotic count has been shown to be a powerful predictor of recurrence and survival.[112,113]

| TABLE 12-2 | Combined Histologic Grading System (modified from Elston[100]) |

% TUBULE FORMATION	NUCLEAR PLEOMORPHISM	MITOTIC ACTIVITY*
>75% = 1	Mild = 1	<10 per 10 hpf = 1
10%-75% = 2	Moderate = 2	10-19 per 10 hpf = 2
<10% = 3	Marked = 3	>20 per 10 hpf = 3

*Based on high-power field (hpf) area of 0.274 mm^2.

Proliferation is commonly analyzed through flow cytometric analysis of DNA, from which the percentage of cells in S phase may be calculated. Correlation is also seen between an elevated S-phase fraction and high histologic grade. Although an elevated S-phase fraction appears to be an important predictor of poor disease-free and overall survival, in multivariate analysis the prognostic power of S phase may lose its independent significance if histologic grade is included in the analysis.[114] Standardization of methods and the establishment of meaningful divisions of S phase continue to be investigated.[115]

Disadvantages of flow cytometric analysis relate to the requirement for tissue beyond that necessary for the histopathologic diagnosis and the inability to be sure which cells are being analyzed. These drawbacks are not unique to flow cytometry but relate to any process that requires a tissue homogenate. Another approach for assessing growth fraction is immunohistochemical analysis for nuclear antigens associated with cell proliferation. The most widely studied of these is the Ki-67 antigen, which is present in all phases of the cell cycle except G_0. Expression of Ki-67 correlates with other measures of cell proliferation (thymidine labeling,[116] mitotic count,[117] and S-phase fraction[118]) and is an independent prognostic indicator when present in high levels.[119]

Immunohistochemical methods of determining cell proliferation are attractive because they circumvent the disadvantages described for flow cytometry. The proliferation antigen Ki-67 is easily detected by using antibody MIB1 and antigen retrieval techniques, which allow assessment of routinely processed tissue.[120] Reactivity of this antibody correlates with mitotic activity and tumor grade[121] and, compared with other markers of proliferation, may have the greatest predictive value.[122,123] Along with lymph node status, tumor size, and grade, MIB1 reactivity is an independent prognostic indicator.[121]

ESTROGEN RECEPTOR

The immunohistochemical determination of ER in paraffin-embedded tissue yields results that closely parallel biochemical determinations. These tissue section analyses are advantageous for the following reasons: (1) The same tissue that is used for making the diagnosis is used for the ER analysis; thus tissue is conserved. This is especially important with smaller cancers. (2) The presence of ER is detected in the context of histopathology. Thus the physician is ensured that the positive signal detected is emanating from carcinoma instead of benign epithelium. The biochemical assay is based on a tissue homogenate, so it is impossible to know which cells are responsible for a positive signal. This is also an issue if carcinoma in situ is assayed biochemically,

rather than the invasive component. (3) Greater sensitivity is achievable with the immunohistochemical assay. If a carcinoma is not very cellular or if there are many contaminating stromal or inflammatory cells, a resulting dilutional effect may be encountered in the biochemical assay. In contrast, positive cells, even if very rare, are easily recognized immunohistochemically.

Several studies have shown the benefits of immunohistochemical analysis for ER.[124,125] Although the clinical predictive power of the biochemical method has been well established,[126] the immunohistochemical method for determining ER status is superior in predicting response to adjuvant endocrine therapy[127] and adoption of the immunohistochemical method of ER determination has been supported.[128]

ADDITIONAL ELEMENTS OCCASIONALLY HELPFUL IN PROGNOSTICATION

The prognostic significance of *vascular invasion* has not been completely straightforward. In general, *lymphatics* are the vessels most often involved in breast carcinoma, although blood vessels sometimes contain carcinoma. Misinterpreting carcinoma in soft tissue spaces or intraductal carcinoma as tumor in lymphatic spaces is often responsible for the overdiagnosis of lymphatic invasion. These mistakes may be avoided if the physician requires the presence of tumor cell emboli in a space lined by endothelial cells to make the histologic determination of vascular invasion (Figure 12-9).

Studies that have adhered to this criterion for vascular space involvement have found that peritumoral lymphatic invasion portends a worse prognosis. This has been found in lymph node–positive cases[129] and in node-negative cases.[130,131] Moreover, for primary carcinomas that are smaller than 2 cm in greatest diameter, lymphatic involvement was an independent predictor of the presence of axillary lymph node metastasis.[132]

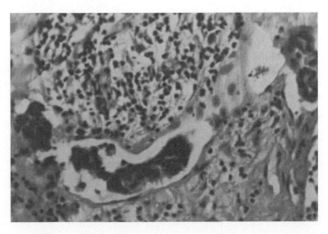

FIG. **12-9** Lymphovascular invasion. Carcinoma cells are present within an endothelial-lined vascular space.

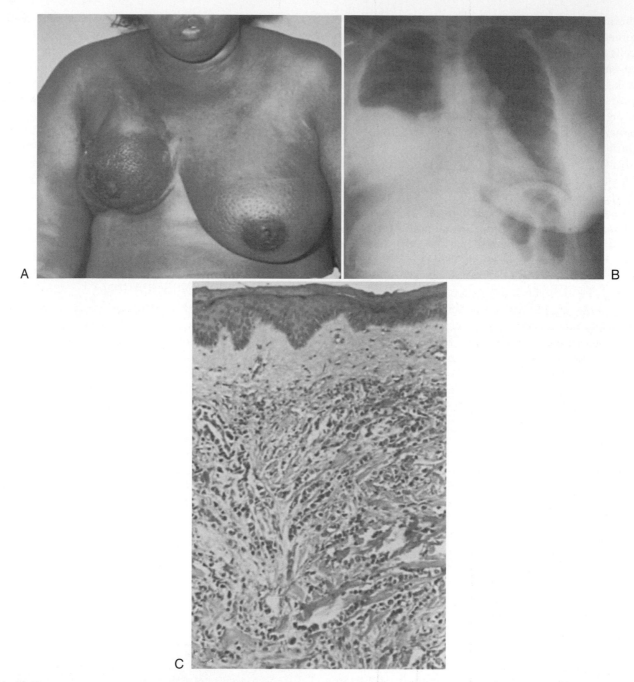

FIG. **12-10 A,** Clinical presentation of bilateral inflammatory breast carcinoma in a 38-year-old woman. The right breast is fixed to the chest wall with ipsilateral extremity lymphedema. The left breast demonstrates the skin changes of peau d'orange, characteristic of inflammatory carcinoma. **B,** Posteroanterior chest radiograph of same patient at clinical presentation with large right pleural effusion and associated hilar adenopathy. **C,** Inflammatory carcinoma, showing characteristic dermal lymphatic involvement.

Carcinoma involving the lymphatic spaces of the dermis often results in the distinctive clinical entity *inflammatory breast carcinoma*. This diagnosis is made when a breast containing carcinoma is red, edematous, and warm. Dermal lymphatic invasion can be demonstrated in most patients so affected (Figure 12-10). The presence of one feature and not the other (clinical signs versus histologic demonstration of dermal lymphatic invasion) has resulted in some controversy about outcome. It is rare for patients with inflammatory carcinoma to survive 5 years, although a multimodality approach—multiagent chemotherapy, surgery, and irradiation—may improve survival.[133]

In summary, prognostication based on tumor stage, histologic recognition of special types of carcinomas, and careful histologic grading are proven predictive factors, and surgical pathology reporting is incomplete without them. Likewise, studies of new prognostic factors should include these proven factors in the final analysis of independent significance.[134]

REFERENCES

1. Henson DE et al: College of American Pathologists Conference XXVI on clinical relevance of prognostic markers in solid tumors: summary, *Arch Pathol Lab Med* 119:1109, 1995.
2. Page DL: Prognosis and breast cancer: recognition of lethal and favorable prognostic types, *Am J Surg Pathol* 15:334, 1991.
3. Reynolds T: Breast cancer prognostic factors: the search goes on, *J Natl Cancer Inst* 86:480, 1994.
4. Wellings SR, Jensen HM, Marcum RG: An atlas of subgross pathology of the human breast with special reference to possible precancerous lesions, *J Natl Cancer Inst* 55:231, 1975.
5. Rosen PP: The pathologic classification of human mammary carcinoma: past, present, and future, *Ann Clin Lab Sci* 9:144, 1979.
6. Fisher B, Redmond C, Fisher ER, and participating NSABP investigators: The contribution of recent NSABP clinical trials of primary breast cancer therapy to aid understand of tumor biology: an overview of findings, *Cancer* 46:1009, 1980.
7. Fu Y et al: The relationship of breast cancer morphology and estrogen receptor protein status, *Progr Surg Pathol* 51:1, 1981.
8. Wallgren A, Silverward S, Eklund G: Prognostic factors in mammary carcinoma, *Acta Radiol* 5:1, 1976.
9. Page DL, Anderson TJ, Sakamoto G: Infiltrating carcinoma: major histological types. In Page DL, Anderson TJ (eds): *Diagnostic histopathology of the breast*, Edinburgh, 1987, Churchill Livingstone.
10. Ellis IO et al: Pathologic prognostic factors in breast cancer. II. Histologic type. Relationship with survival in a large study with long term follow-up, *Histopathology* 20:479, 1992.
11. Anderson TJ et al: Comparative pathology of breast cancer in a randomised trial of screening, *Br J Cancer* 64:108, 1991.
12. Anderson TJ et al: Comparative pathology of prevalent and incident cancers detected by breast screening, *Lancet* 519, 1986.
13. Patchefsky AS et al: The pathology of breast cancer detected by mass population screening, *Cancer* 40:1659, 1977.
14. Rajakariar R, Walker RA: Pathological and biological features of mammographically detected invasive breast carcinomas, *Br J Cancer* 71:150, 1995.
15. Fisher ER, Sass R, Fisher B, and participating NSABP investigators: Pathologic findings from the National Surgical Adjuvant Project for breast cancer (protocol no. 4). Discriminates for tenth year treatment failure, *Cancer* 53:712, 1984.
16. Dixon JM et al: Long term survivors after breast cancer, *Br J Surg* 72:445, 1985.
17. Gamel JW et al: The impact of stage and histology on the long-term clinical course of 163,808 patients with breast carcinoma, *Cancer* 77:1459, 1996.
18. Cooper HS, Patchefsky AS, Krall RA: Tubular carcinoma of the breast, *Cancer* 42:2334, 1978.
19. McDivitt RW, Boyce W, Gersell D: Tubular carcinoma of the breast: clinical and pathological observations concerning 135 cases, *Am J Surg Pathol* 6:401, 1982.
20. Parl FF, Richardson LD: The histological and biological spectrum of tubular carcinoma of the breast, *Hum Pathol* 14:694, 1983.
21. Winchester DJ et al: Tubular carcinoma of the breast: predicting axillary nodal metastases and recurrence, *Ann Surg* 223:342, 1996.
22. Anderson TJ et al: Pathology characteristics that optimize outcome prediction of a breast screening trial, *Br J Cancer* 83:487, 2000.
23. Stalsberg H, Hartmann WH: The delimitation of tubular carcinoma of the breast, *Hum Pathol* 31:601, 2000.
24. Elson BC et al: Tubular carcinoma of the breast: mode of presentation, mammographic appearance, and frequency of nodal metastases, *AJR Am J Roentgenol* 161:1173, 1993.
25. Dawson AE, Logan-Young W, Mulford DK: Aspiration cytology of tubular carcinoma: diagnostic features with mammographic correlation, *Am J Clin Pathol* 101:488, 1994.
26. Diab SG et al: Tumor characteristics and clinical outcome of tubular and mucinous carcinomas, *J Clin Oncol* 17:1442, 1999.
27. Baker RR: Unusual lesions and their management, *Surg Clin North Am* 70:963, 1990.
28. Mailbenco DC et al: Axillary lymph node metastases associated with small invasive breast carcinomas, *Cancer* 85:1530, 1999.
29. Page DL et al: Invasive cribriform carcinoma of the breast, *Histopathology* 7:525, 1983.
30. Venable JG, Schwartz AM, Silverberg SG: Infiltrating cribriform carcinoma of the breast: a distinctive clinicopathologic entity, *Hum Pathol* 21:333, 1990.
31. Komari K et al: Mucinous carcinoma of the breast in Japan: a prognostic analysis based on morphologic features, *Cancer* 61:989, 1988.
32. Andre S et al: Mucinous carcinoma of the breast: a pathologic study of 82 cases, *J Surg Oncol* 58:162, 1995.
33. Clayton F: Pure mucinous carcinomas of the breast: morphologic features and prognostic correlates, *Hum Pathol* 17:34, 1986.
34. Rasmussen BB, Rose C, Christensen IB: Prognostic factors in primary mucinous breast carcinoma, *Am J Clin Pathol* 87:155, 1987.
35. Fentiman IS et al: Mucoid breast carcinomas: histology and prognosis, *Br J Cancer* 75:1061, 1997.
36. Northridge ME et al: The importance of histologic type on breast cancer survival, *J Clin Epidemiol* 50:283, 1997.
37. Avisar E et al: Pure mucinous carcinoma of the breast: a clinicopathologic correlation study, *Ann Surg Oncol* 5:447, 1998.
38. Wilson TE et al: Pure and mixed mucinous carcinoma of the breast: pathologic basis for differences in mammographic appearance, *AJR Am J Roentgenol* 165:285, 1995.
39. Haagensen CD (ed): *Disease of the breast*, ed 2, Philadelphia, 1971, WB Saunders.
40. Donegan WL, Perez-Mesa CM: Lobular carcinoma—an indication for elective biopsy of the second breast, *Ann Surg* 176:178, 1972.
41. Battifora H: Intracytoplasmic lumina in breast carcinoma: a helpful histopathologic feature, *Arch Pathol* 99:614, 1975.
42. Quincy C et al: Intracytoplasmic lumina: a useful diagnostic feature of adenocarcinomas, *Histopathology* 19:83, 1991.
43. Ladekarl M, Sorensen FB: Prognostic, quantitative histopathologic variables in lobular carcinoma of the breast, *Cancer* 72:2602, 1993.
44. Dixon JM et al: Infiltrating lobular carcinoma of the breast, *Histopathology* 6:149, 1982.
45. Eusebi V, Magalhaes F, Azzopardi JG: Pleomorphic lobular carcinoma of the breast: an aggressive tumor showing apocrine differentiation, *Hum Pathol* 23:655, 1992.

46. Fechner RE: Histologic variants of infiltrating lobular carcinoma of the breast, *Hum Pathol* 6:373, 1975.

47. Martinez V, Azzopardi JG: Invasive lobular carcinoma of the breast: incidence and variants, *Histopathology* 3:47, 1979.

48. Weidner N, Semple JP: Pleomorphic variant of invasive lobular carcinoma of the breast, *Hum Pathol* 23:1167, 1992.

49. DiCostanzo D et al: Prognosis in infiltrating lobular carcinoma: an analysis of "classical" and variant tumors, *Am J Surg Pathol* 14:12, 1990.

50. Wheeler JE, Enterline HT: Lobular carcinoma of the breast in situ and infiltrating, *Pathol Annu* 2:161, 1976.

51. Haagensen CD et al: Lobular neoplasia (so-called lobular carcinoma in situ) of the breast, *Cancer* 42:737, 1978.

52. Silverstein MJ et al: Infiltrating lobular carcinoma: is it different from infiltrating duct carcinoma? *Cancer* 73:1673, 1994.

53. du Toit RS et al: Invasive lobular carcinomas of the breast: the prognosis of histopathological subtypes, *Br J Cancer* 60:605, 1989.

54. Berx G et al: E-cadherin is inactivated in a majority of invasion human lobular breast cancers by truncation mutations throughout its extracellular domain, *Oncogene* 13:1919, 1996.

55. Toikkanen S, Pylkkanen L, Joensuu H: Invasive lobular carcinoma of the breast has better short- and long-term survival than invasive ductal carcinoma, *Br J Cancer* 76:1234, 1997.

56. Dixon JM et al: Infiltrating lobular carcinoma of the breast: an evaluation of the incidence and consequence of bilateral disease, *Br J Surg* 70:513, 1983.

57. Schnitt SJ et al: Influence of infiltrating lobular histology on local tumor control in breast cancer patients treated with conservative surgery and radiotherapy, *Cancer* 64:448, 1989.

58. Eisinger F et al: Mutations at *BRCA1*: the medullary breast carcinoma revisited, *Cancer Res* 58:1588, 1998.

59. Marcus JN et al: Hereditary breast cancer: pathobiology, prognosis, and *BRCA1* and *BRCA2* gene linkage, *Cancer* 77:697, 1996.

60. Lakhani SR: The pathology of familial breast cancer: morphologic aspects, *Breast Cancer Res* 1:31, 1991.

61. Lee SC et al: Microsatellite instability is frequently in medullary breast cancer, *Am J Clin Pathol* 115:823, 2001.

62. Rubens JR et al: Medullary carcinoma of the breast: over-diagnosis of a prognostically favorable neoplasm, *Arch Surg* 125:601, 1990.

63. Ridolphi RL et al: Medullary carcinoma of the breast: a clinical pathological study with 10 year follow-up, *Cancer* 40:1365, 1977.

64. Pedersen L et al: Medullary carcinoma of the breast: prevalence and prognostic importance of classical risk factors in breast cancer, *Eur J Cancer* 31A:2289, 1995.

65. Rapin V et al: Medullary breast carcinoma: a reevaluation of 95 cases of breast cancer with inflammatory stroma, *Cancer* 61:2503, 1988.

66. Carter CL, Allen C, Henson DE: Relation of tumor size, lymph node status, and survival in 24,740 breast cancer cases, *Cancer* 63:181, 1989.

67. Berg JW, Hutter RVP: Breast cancer, *Cancer* 75:257, 1995.

68. Oberman HA: Secretory carcinoma of the breast in adults, *Am J Surg Pathol* 4:465, 1980.

69. Akhtar M et al: Secretory carcinoma of the breast in adults: light and electron microscopic study of three cases with review of the literature, *Cancer* 51:2245, 1983.

70. Tavassoli FA, Norris HJ: Secretory carcinoma of the breast, *Cancer* 45:2404, 1980.

71. Azzopardi JG: *Problems in breast pathology*, Philadelphia, 1979, Saunders.

72. Lamovec J et al: Adenoid cystic carcinoma of the breast: a histologic, cytologic, and immunohistochemical study, *Semin Diag Pathol* 6:153, 1989.

73. Pastolero G et al: Proliferative activity and p53 expression in adenoid cystic carcinoma of the breast, *Mod Pathol* 9:215, 1996.

74. Peters GM, Wolff M: Adenoid cystic carcinoma of the breast: report of 11 new cases, review of the literature and discussion of biological behavior, *Cancer* 52:680, 1982.

75. Kasami M et al: Maintenance of polarity and a dual cell population in adenoid cystic carcinoma of the breast: an immunohistochemical study, *Histopathology* 32:232, 1998.

76. Trendell-Smtih NJ, Peston D, Shousha S: Adenoid cystic carcinoma of the breast: a tumor commonly devoid of estrogen receptors and related proteins, *Histopathology* 35:241, 1999.

77. Kleer CG, Oberman HA: Adenoid cystic carcinoma of the breast: value of histologic grading and proliferative activity, *Am J Surg Pathol* 22:569, 1998.

78. Fisher ER et al: Mucoepidermoid and squamous cell carcinomas of the breast with reference to squamous metaplasia and giant cell tumors, *Am J Surg Pathol* 7:15, 1983.

79. Patchefsky AS et al: Low-grade mucoepidermoid carcinoma of the breast, *Arch Path Lab Med* 103:196, 1979.

80. Hastrup N, Sehested M: High-grade mucoepidermoid carcinoma of the breast, *Histopathology* 9:887, 1985.

81. Kovi J, Duong HD, Leffall LDJ: High-grade mucoepidermoid carcinoma of the breast, *Arch Pathol Lab Med* 105:612, 1981.

82. Hanna W, Kahn HJ: Ultrastructural and immunohistochemical characteristics of mucoepidermoid carcinoma of the breast, *Hum Pathol* 16:941, 1985.

83. Luchtrath H, Moll R: Mucoepidermoid mammary carcinoma: immunohistochemical and biochemical analyses of intermediate filaments, *Virchows Archiv A Pathol Anat* 416:105, 1989.

84. Gersell D, Katzenstein AL: Spindle cell carcinoma of the breast: a clinicopathologic and ultrastructural study, *Hum Pathol* 12:550, 1981.

85. Santeusanio G et al: Metaplastic breast carcinoma with epithelial phenotype of pseudosarcomatous components, *Arch Pathol Lab Med* 112:82, 1988.

86. Wargotz ES, Deos PH, Norris HJ: Metaplastic carcinomas of the breast. II. Spindle cell carcinoma, *Hum Pathol* 20:732, 1989.

87. Wargotz ES, Norris HJ: Metaplastic carcinomas of the breast. V. Metaplastic carcinoma with osteoclastic giant cells, *Hum Pathol* 21:1142, 1990.

88. Bauer TW et al: Spindle cell carcinoma of the breast: four cases and review of the literature, *Hum Pathol* 15:147, 1984.

89. Gobbi H et al: Metaplastic breast tumors with a dominant fibromatosis-like phenotype have a high rate of local recurrence, *Cancer* 85:2170, 1999.

90. Burke H, Henson DE: Criteria for prognostic factors and for an enhanced prognostic system, *Cancer* 72:3131, 1993.

91. McGuire WL: Breast cancer prognostic factors: evaluation guidelines, *J Natl Cancer Inst* 83:154, 1991 (editorial).

92. Fitzgibbons PL et al: Prognostic factors in breast cancer: College of American Pathologists consensus statement 1999, *Arch Pathol Lab Med* 124:966, 2000.

93. Veronesi U et al: Local recurrences and distant metastases after conservative breast cancer treatments: partly independent events, *J Natl Cancer Inst* 87:19, 1995.

94. Abner AL et al: Correlation of tumor size and axillary lymph node involvement with prognosis in patients with T1 breast carcinoma, *Cancer* 83:2502, 1998.

95. Fentiman IH et al: Prognosis of patients with breast cancers up to 1 cm in diameter, *Eur J Cancer* 32:417, 1996.

96. McGuire WL, Clark GM: Prognostic factors and treatment decision in axillary-node negative breast cancer, *N Engl J Med* 326:1756, 1992.

97. Osborne CK: Prognostic factors for breast cancer: have they met their promise? *J Clin Oncol* 10:679, 1992.

98. Greene FL et al (eds): *AJCC cancer staging manual,* ed 6, New York, 2002, Springer-Verlag.

99. Weaver DL et al: Pathologic analysis of sentinel and non-sentinel lymph nodes in breast carcinoma: a multicenter study, *Cancer* 88:1099, 2000.

100. Elston CW, Ellis IO: Pathological prognostic factors in breast cancer. I. The value of histologic grade in breast cancer: experience from a large study with long-term follow-up, *Histopathology* 19:403, 1991.

101. Arnesson LG et al: Histopathology grading in small breast cancers <10 mm: results from an area with mammography screening, *Breast Cancer Res Treat* 44:39, 1997.

102. Contesso G et al: The importance of histologic grade in long-term prognosis of breast cancer: a study of 1,010 patients, uniformly treated at the Institut Gustave-Roussy, *J Clin Oncol* 5:1378, 1987.

103. Joensuu H, Pylkkanen L, Toikkanen S: Late mortality from pT1N0M0 breast carcinoma, *Cancer* 85:2183, 1999.

104. Bergers E et al: Prognostic implications of different cell cycle analysis models of flow cytometric DNA histograms of 1,301 breast cancer patients: results from the Multicenter Morphometric Mammary Carcinoma Project (MMMCP), *Int J Cancer* 74:260, 1997.

105. Henson EE et al: Relationship among outcome, stage of disease, and histologic grade for 22,616 cases of breast cancer: the basis for a prognostic index, *Cancer* 68:2142, 1991.

106. Dalton LW, Page DL, Dupont WD: Histological grading of breast cancer: a reproducibility study, *Cancer* 73:2765, 1994.

107. Frierson HFJ et al: Interobserver reproducibility of the Nottingham modification of the Bloom and Richardson histologic grading scheme for infiltrating ductal carcinoma, *Am J Clin Pathol* 103:195, 1995.

108. Kollias J et al: The prognosis of small primary breast cancers, *Eur J Cancer* 35:908, 1999.

109. Parl F, Dupont WD: A retrospective cohort study of histologic risk factors in breast cancer patients, *Cancer* 50:2410, 1982.

110. Page DL et al: Prediction of node-negative breast cancer outcome by histologic grading and S-phase analysis by flow cytometry: an Eastern Cooperative Oncology Group Study (2192), *Am J Clin Oncol* 24:10, 2001.

111. Simpson JF et al: Prognostic value of histologic grade and proliferative activity in axillary node-positive breast cancer: results from the Eastern Cooperative Oncology Group companion study, EST 4189, *J Clin Oncol* 18:2059, 2000.

112. Clayton F: Pathologic correlates of survival in 378 lymph node negative infiltrating ductal breast carcinomas: mitotic count is the best single predictor, *Cancer* 68:1309, 1991.

113. Van Diest PJ, Baak JPA: The morphometric prognostic index is the strongest prognosticator in premenopausal lymph node-negative and lymph node-positive breast cancer patients, *Hum Pathol* 22:326, 1990.

114. O'Reilly SM et al: Node-negative breast cancer: prognostic subgroups defined by tumor size and flow cytometry, *J Clin Oncol* 8:2040, 1990.

115. Hedley DW et al: Consensus review of the clinical utility of DNA cytometry in carcinoma of the breast, *Cytometry* 14:482, 1993.

116. Kamel OW et al: Thymidine labeling index and Ki-67 growth fractions in lesions of the breast, *Am J Pathol* 134:107, 1989.

117. Isola J et al: Evaluation of cell proliferation in breast carcinoma: comparison of Ki-67 immunohistochemical study, DNA flow cytometric analysis, and mitotic count, *Cancer* 65:1180, 1990.

118. Dettmar P et al: Prognostic impact of proliferation-associated factors MIB-1 (Ki-67) and S phase in node negative breast cancer, *Br J Cancer* 75:1525, 1997.

119. Wintzer H-O et al: Ki-67 immunostaining in human breast tumors and its relationship to prognosis, *Cancer* 67:421, 1991.

120. Cattoretti G et al: Monoclonal antibodies against recombinant parts of the Ki-67 antigen (MIB 1 and MIB 3) detect proliferating cells in microwave-processed formalin-fixed paraffin sections, *J Pathol* 168:357, 1992.

121. Pinder SE et al: Assessment of the new proliferation marker MIB1 in breast carcinoma using image analysis: association with other prognostic factors and survival, *Br J Cancer* 71:146, 1995.

122. Keshgegian AA, Cnaan A: Proliferation markers in breast carcinoma: mitotic figure count, S-phase fraction, proliferation cell nuclear antigen, Ki-67, and MIB-1, *Am J Clin Pathol* 104:42, 1995.

123. Clahsen PC et al: The utility of mitotic index, oestrogen receptor and Ki-67 measurements in the creation of novel prognostic indices for node-negative breast cancer, *Eur J Surg Oncol* 25:356, 1999.

124. Allred DC et al: Immunocytochemical analysis of estrogen receptors in human breast carcinomas: evaluation of 130 cases and a review of the literature regarding concordance with the biochemical assay and clinical relevance, *Arch Surg* 125:107, 1990.

125. Pertschuk LP et al: Estrogen receptor immunocytochemistry in paraffin embedded tissues with ER1D5 predicts breast cancer endocrine response more accurately than H222Sp gamma in frozen sections or cytosol-based ligand-binding assays, *Cancer* 77:2514, 1996.

126. Allred DC: Should immunohistochemical examination replace biochemical hormone receptor assays in breast cancer? *Am J Clin Pathol* 99:1, 1993.

127. Harvey JM et al: Estrogen receptor status by immunohistochemistry is superior to the ligand-binding assay for predicting response to adjuvant endocrine therapy in breast cancer, *J Clin Oncol* 17:1474, 1999.

128. Taylor CR: Paraffin section immunocytochemistry for estrogen receptor: the time has come, *Cancer* 77:2419, 1996.

129. Davis BW et al, and the Ludwig Breast Cancer Study Group: Prognostic significance of peritumoral vessel invasion in clinical trials of adjuvant therapy for breast cancer with axillary lymph node metastasis, *Hum Pathol* 16:1212, 1985.

130. Clemente CG et al: Peritumoral lymphatic invasion in patients with node-negative mammary duct carcinoma, *Cancer* 69:1396, 1992.
131. De Mascarel I et al: Obvious peritumoral emboli: an elusive prognostic factor reappraised: multivariate analysis of 1320 node-negative breast cancers, *Eur J Cancer* 34:58, 1998.
132. Chadha M et al: Predictors of axillary lymph node metastases in patients with T1 breast cancer: a multivariate analysis, *Cancer* 73:350, 1994.
133. Perez CA et al: Management of locally advanced carcinoma of the breast. II. Inflammatory carcinoma, *Cancer* 74:466, 1994.
134. Page DL: Special types of invasive breast cancer, with clinical implications, *Am J Surg Pathol* 27:832, 2003.

13

Extent and Multicentricity of In Situ and Invasive Carcinoma

MARY EDGERTON

JOYCE E. JOHNSON

PHILIP L. DUTT

DAVID L. PAGE

The terms *multicentricity* and *multifocality* have been used for decades to indicate seeming or real multiplicity of cancer within an individual breast. The terms have no intrinsically different meaning but have recently been interpreted as follows: *Multicentricity* indicates multiple but independent sites of origin, usually in a separate duct system or relatively remote from one another; *multifocality* indicates multiple foci of the same tumor, relatively close to each other, usually in the same quadrant. Multicentricity has been considered an important factor when planning breast-conserving surgery. However, many cases that would have previously been deemed multicentric in the past are now recognized as multiple lesions within a breast segment that result from spread of intraductal carcinoma within the three-dimensional duct system. Although multicentricity is important in planning surgical therapy, its true prevalence is much less than originally estimated. Indeed, extent of disease, in situ or invasive, is a concept that has essentially replaced that of multifocality and multicentricity, particularly in the planning of surgical therapy. Bilaterality, the occurrence of carcinoma in the contralateral breast is excluded by definition and is discussed separately in Chapters 74 and 76. Also excluded is concurrence of breast carcinoma and sarcoma, which is reviewed in Chapters 12 and 14. Multicentricity associated with lobular carcinoma in situ (LCIS) is discussed separately in Chapter 11. The studies of intraductal carcinoma referenced in this chapter largely apply to ductal carcinoma in situ (DCIS) only, either by exclusion of LCIS or because of the greater proportion of cases with DCIS included in the studies.

The prevalence of true multicentricity is difficult to estimate from the literature. In 1957, Qualheim and Gall[1] published one of the first studies to distinguish between cancerous foci in the vicinity of a primary mass and those that might be regarded as distant. The standard definition of multicentricity applied in studies published by Fisher and colleagues as part of the National Surgical Adjuvant Breast Project (NSABP) required that the second cancer be present in a separate quadrant from the dominant mass.[2,3] These studies produced a conservative estimate of separate cancer sites, in part because cases in which the dominant mass was present in the tail of the breast or beneath the nipple were excluded from analysis. In 1985, Holland and associates[4] published a study of multiple foci of tumor using distance from the primary mass to predict recurrence, thereby bypassing the issue of defining multicentricity.

Since then, the criteria for the definitions of hyperplasia, atypical hyperplasia, in situ carcinoma, and multicentricity itself have evolved. In 1994, Faverly, with Holland and associates,[5] applied three-dimensional imaging to study the distribution of intraductal carcinoma as constrained by the anatomy of the breast duct system. Since then, Ohtake and associates[6,7] and Mai and colleagues[8] have used computer-generated reconstructions of the mammary duct system in three dimensions to study the pattern of distribution of intraductal and invasive carcinoma in relation to the duct systems. They discovered that apparent multicentricity is often the result of intraductal spread of tumor. This finding has highlighted the inherent problem of formulating a useful definition of multicentricity based on distance or quadrants.

Other studies have added the elements of time and biology (natural history) by observing the evolution (or lack of it) of clinical disease in the living breast after partial mastectomy. The results of breast-conserving surgery show that recurrent disease most often occurs locally, within the spatial constraint that the geometry of the duct system places upon the spread of in situ carcinoma. Simply put, more than 90% of local recurrences of breast carcinoma in the many women treated with breast-conserving surgery are in the immediate vicinity of the primary tumor.[9] This implies that the extensiveness of in situ carcinoma within a duct system and margin status are the more relevant issues for predicting outcome in most cases.[4,10]

Definition and Anatomy

A perfect definition of multicentricity referable to all settings is essentially impractical because of the difficulties inherent in visualizing the three-dimensional microanatomy of the breast. Distinguishing independently originating breast carcinomas from multiple foci of invasion resulting from intramammary spread of carcinoma along ducts is difficult. Therefore *multicentricity* as a descriptor is necessarily arbitrary and becomes a function of the method used for detection. Consider here the anatomy of the breast.

The breast is a branching (racemose) gland with 15 to 20 collecting (lactiferous) ducts exiting at the nipple. Each of these ductal systems or lobes subserves hundreds of lobular units, which are collections of acinar elements.[11] In a three-dimensional reconstruction based on one patient, Ohtake and colleagues[7] noted that only 2 of the duct systems actually communicated with one another, and the remaining 14 were anatomically independent. Although the ductal systems are not grossly definable anatomic units separated by septa, only immediately adjacent radiating ductal systems overlap (Figure 13-1), with limited opportunity for communication.[11] Quadrants represent an attempt to divide the breast into independent duct systems; however, the boundaries are drawn arbitrarily, and true duct systems may overlap into an adjacent quadrant at the periphery.

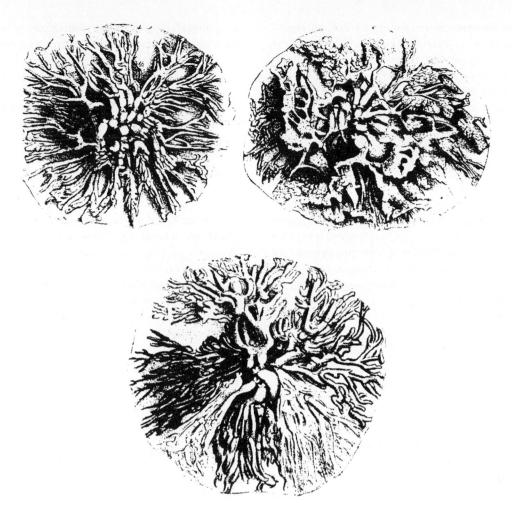

FIG. **13-1** Lobar, radiating anatomy of the ductal system of the breast. *(From Cooper A:* The anatomy and diseases of the breast, *Philadelphia, 1845, Lea and Banchard, plate VI.)*

Given this anatomy, apparent multicentricity resulting from spread along a single duct system would be expected to appear in a radial distribution from nipple to periphery. This radial distribution, combined with the irregular branching system of duct systems that exists in three dimensions, explains the fact that a single intraductal breast cancer may appear as separate foci in the two-dimensional slides routinely used for diagnosis. Mai and colleagues,[8] who performed computer-assisted three-dimensional reconstruction of intraductal and invasive mammary carcinoma (lobular carcinoma was excluded) from 30 mastectomy specimens, found that intraductal carcinoma presented with a radial distribution corresponding to the geometry of each duct system. They also noted that multiple foci of invasive carcinoma were connected by intervening intraductal carcinoma within a single duct system. Ohtake and colleagues[6] have taken the viewpoint that multicentricity requires demonstration of histologic noncontinuity of intraductal tumor through the mammary ductal tree. Of note, there are no cases of lobular carcinoma in their series. As stringent as this requirement appears, even it may allow

an overestimate of true multicentricity. Both Mai and associates[8] and Faverly and colleagues[5] report that discontinuities of intraductal tumor, detected at a subgross level, within a single mammary duct tree are not uncommon. Recent studies indicate that the phenomenon of "pagetoid spread" of intraductal carcinoma[12] may lead to apparent discontinuities in intraductal tumor that originate from the same "index" carcinoma.

Studies using molecular biology to differentiate independent sources for multicentric carcinoma (discussed later) also support the concept of a single index case that spreads through the duct system.[13-15] As such, the true definition of multicentric should require demonstration of independent molecular events that result in the local occurrence of carcinoma in independent duct systems. This definition would require three-dimensional reconstruction of the duct systems along with molecular profiling studies, procedures that are not a part of routine processing of breast specimens. Therefore *multicentricity* is likely to remain arbitrarily defined. Extent of disease is more amenable to measurement in routine pathologic examination of specimens. Given that the prevalence of true multicentricity is overestimated, extent of disease (discussed in more detail later) may be more relevant in the majority of cases when planning breast-conserving surgical therapy.

Historical Review

Cheatle and Cutler[16] first defined multicentricity as two lesions separated by normal breast tissue. Since then, most authors have adhered to the *quadrant rule*, which defines multicentric lesions as second tumors lying in a different quadrant from that in which the primary or dominant lesion is located. Some authors regard the subareolar region as a fifth mammary region, separate from the four quadrants. Others place subareolar lesions in the most closely associated quadrant.

In addition to the quadrant rule, some authors have used a *distance rule*, with specific distances applied ranging from 5 to 2 cm. It should be noted that Lagios[17] uses the 5-cm distance rule because such a distance generally places a second lesion in a different quadrant. European guidelines define the criteria for multicentricity as the presence of two or more distinct tumor foci either at a distance of at least 4 cm and/or present in different quadrants.[18]

All of these definitions have shortcomings. Egan and McSweeney[19] offered a possible solution to the problem by using multiple criteria: (1) wide separation of foci grossly, radiographically, and microscopically; (2) a pattern of multiple areas scattered throughout much of the breast; or (3) sharp delineation of different histologic types. Holland and associates,[4] in their early work, cleverly avoided the problems of both the rule of quadrants and the arbitrary distance definitions of multicentricity by measuring the distance from the secondary foci to the dominant lesion and graphing the frequencies at which invasive and noninvasive foci were located at various distances from the edge of the dominant lesion. Their approach has important therapeutic implications regarding how generous the margins around tumors should be in lumpectomy specimens.

On balance, it should be remembered that the quadrants rule has been the most commonly used definition. The following cases demonstrate the difficulties encountered with identifying multicentric breast carcinoma based on information obtained from standard pathology procedures. The lesion that attracted attention clinically or mammographically and led to diagnostic procedures will be called the *primary* or *dominant lesion*, and other malignant lesions will be called *secondary lesions*. Pathology reports in which multiple simultaneous lesions are grossly identifiable and separately measurable should emphasize the largest lesion.[20]

Case 1. A 46-year-old woman underwent a modified radical right mastectomy for a 2 × 1.7 × 1.3 cm mass in the lower inner quadrant. Histologically, this was an infiltrating mammary carcinoma of predominantly lobular type with an extensive intraductal component (EIC) (Figure 13-2). Sampling of the upper inner quadrant revealed a separate 0.7 × 0.5 × 0.5 cm focus of infiltrative lobular carcinoma with extensive LCIS (Figure 13-3).

Case 2. An 87-year-old woman had two clinically apparent masses in her left breast. The decision to perform mastectomy was based on a diagnosis of carcinoma made on material obtained with fine-needle aspiration of a mass in the upper inner quadrant. The left

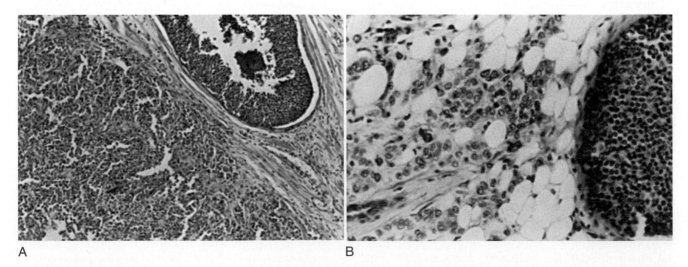

A   B

FIG. **13-2 A** and **B,** Extension of prominent intraductal component (right in both pictures) beyond border of invasive lobular carcinoma (left) in lower inner quadrant mass of Case 1. (**A,** ×60; **B,** ×200.)

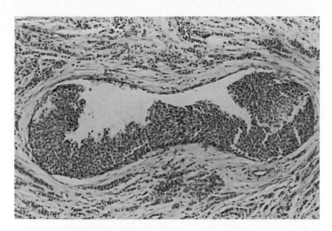

FIG. **13-3** Separate upper inner quadrant lesion from Case 1 contains infiltrating lobular carcinoma with extensive in situ lobular component involving the duct in the center of picture. (×180.)

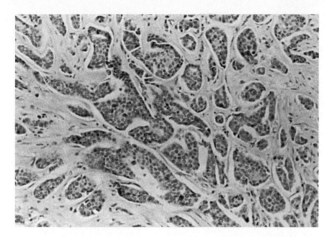

FIG. **13-4** Infiltrating mammary carcinoma of no specific type (invasive ductal carcinoma) found in larger mass in the upper inner quadrant in Case 2. (×250.)

mastectomy specimen contained an $8 \times 5 \times 4$ cm mass in the upper inner quadrant that histologically was invasive mammary carcinoma of no special type (Figure 13-4). The upper outer quadrant contained a separate, smaller $3.5 \times 3 \times 2.5$ cm mass with a similar histological appearance (Figure 13-5). Biopsy of a lesion in the right breast at the time of mastectomy revealed DCIS (Figure 13-6).

Case 3. A 47-year-old woman underwent mastectomy. The mastectomy specimen contained invasive mammary carcinoma of no specific type (Figure 13-7). Elsewhere in the most remote sites were extensive areas of invasive carcinoma with mucinous features (Figure 13-8).

Case 4. A mammogram revealed three lesions in a single quadrant in a 43-year-old woman (Figure 13-9). All three were invasive carcinomas with EICs. As is often the case, each invasive focus appeared histologically similar. Tissue sampled between each of the lesions demonstrated in situ carcinoma only. This case demonstrates the important association of DCIS with the occurrence of multiple carcinomas within one breast.

Case 5. A 30-year-old woman had a palpable mass in the left upper outer quadrant, a few centimeters from the nipple. A biopsy revealed a 15-mm intermediate-grade carcinoma of no special type, with intratumoral and adjacent extensive DCIS of solid, cribriform, and focal comedo types. A quadrantectomy contained two additional foci of invasive carcinoma of similar histology, 8 mm and 6 mm in size (Figure 13-10), in addition to a 1-mm focus of residual carcinoma in the wall of the biopsy cavity. Tissue taken from between each of the three invasive foci showed high-grade (comedo) carcinoma in situ.

Prevalence

The exact prevalence of multicentricity is uncertain. Using either the quadrant rule or a minimum distance rule, the reported prevalence has ranged from 4% to 75%.[21,22] This variation is attributable to many variables, the most obvious of which are (1) a lack of consistency in the definition of multicentricity and (2) the method of examining specimens. In the 20 specimens examined in three dimensions by Ohtake and collaborators,[6] there were no occurrences of multiple carcinoma foci, either invasive or in situ, without intervening intraductal carcinoma. In the three cases of patients each with multiple breast carcinomas that were examined for clonality by Noguchi and colleagues,[14] there were also no cases in the carcinomas could be attributed to independent molecular events.

In any series studying multicentricity, one should be aware of the method used to examine the breast. The most thorough methods involve three-dimensional imaging of the breast and/or molecular techniques. This would require examination of breast tissue using a combination of radiographs, a dissecting microscope, and microscopic examination of whole tissue sections from breasts that have been frozen and serially sectioned at 2- to 5-mm intervals[6-8,17,21] and/or using molecular techniques to evaluate for clonality.[13-15]

IN SITU LESIONS

The reported prevalence of multicentricity has varied, depending on whether the primary lesion is an in situ or an invasive lesion and on the histologic type of the primary lesion. The risk of multicentricity associated

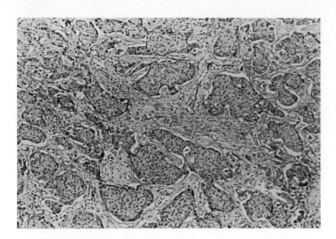

FIG. **13-5** Similar histologic features were present in the smaller upper outer quadrant lesion in Case 2. (×180.)

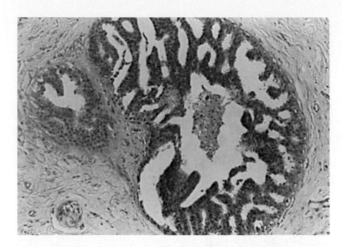

FIG. **13-6** This ductal carcinoma in situ was found simultaneously in the breast contralateral to the one containing the lesion in Figures 13-4 and 13-5. (×200.)

with LCIS is discussed in Chapter 11 and is not repeated here.

DCIS is rarely present without some connection in three dimensions if one considers DCIS with apparent gaps and confined to a single ductal system as connected. As such, it is more likely to be multifocal disease rather than multicentric disease. The frequency with which DCIS has been reported as multicentric has ranged from 0% to 78%.[23-28] The difficulty in assessing true multicentricity (i.e., arising from independent index tumors in separate duct systems) and the variability in pathology procedures to detect multicentricity can explain the broad range in estimates of its prevalence. Faverly and co-workers[5] examined 60 mastectomy specimens in the most detailed study of DCIS to date using three-dimensional reconstruction of the site, extent, and growth pattern of tumor foci. Only one of these had what they

defined as a multicentric occurrence of DCIS (i.e., a separate focus of DCIS present with at least 4 cm of uninvolved glandular structures between it and the primary focus).

Faverly and co-workers[5] determined that 50% of cases of DCIS in their series demonstrated gaps, of which 83% were smaller than 1 cm. Mai and colleagues[8] found that 21% of their 28 cases of invasive carcinoma with associated DCIS also exhibited skip areas in the DCIS. These results were obtained with subgross level imaging. Faverly's group predicted that breast-conserving surgery with an intraductal-free margin of 1 cm should eradicate approximately 90% of DCIS. Interestingly, the three-dimensional reconstruction of duct systems performed by Ohtake and colleagues[7] suggests that removal of a single duct system is adequate therapy in nearly

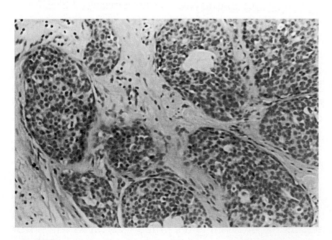

FIG. **13-7** Invasive mammary carcinoma of no specific type described in Case 3. (×200.)

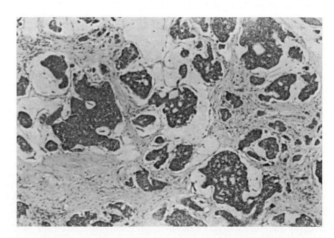

FIG. **13-8** Mucinous carcinoma present elsewhere in the breast of the patient described in Case 3. (×75.)

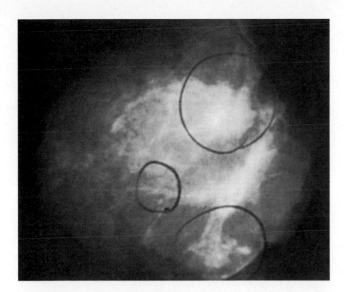

FIG. **13-9** Mammogram described in Case 4 showing three radiographic lesions within the circles. Each contained invasive carcinomas of similar histologic pattern with extensive intraductal components. Note that all three are linked by connective tissue strands that histologically contained ductal carcinoma in situ. *(Courtesy L. Ming Hang, M.D., Escondido, CA.)*

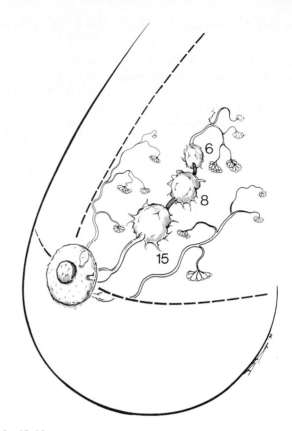

FIG. **13-10** Lateral aspect of left breast in Case 5. Three histologically similar foci of invasive carcinoma of no special type were present in the upper outer quadrant, with intervening in situ carcinoma *(dark hatching)*. The numbers indicate the size of the invasive foci in millimeters.

90% of cases, based on the number of anastomoses connecting otherwise independent duct systems in their reconstruction. This prediction has been borne out in studies by Silverstein and co-workers,[10] who published a study of recurrences as a function of margin. They concluded that breast-conserving surgery with a 1-cm tumor-free margin for DCIS was successful in patients more than 98% of the time.

INVASIVE LESIONS

Although invasive mammary carcinoma of no specific type (invasive ductal carcinoma) is the most common type of invasive mammary carcinoma, it is fortunately associated with one of the lowest rates of multicentricity. Gump and colleagues[29] found that it was the least likely to be multicentric, with a 19% rate of multicentricity, compared with a rate of 27% for all types. The rate of multicentricity increases when other factors are present. For example, the rate of multicentricity associated with minimally invasive ductal carcinoma is apparently greater than that associated with usual invasive ductal carcinoma.[30] This may not be related to the small size of the invasive component per se but rather to its regular presence in cases of extensive DCIS. The rate of multicentricity is increased approximately twofold when infiltrating ductal carcinoma is associated with LCIS.[31]

Infiltrating lobular carcinoma is associated with elevated rates of multicentricity.[31] Fisher and associates[2] showed that invasive lobular carcinoma was more frequently associated with invasive secondary lesions but not with noninvasive secondary lesions. Some authors have pointed out that most of the secondary lesions lie near the primary and probably represent recurrence or spread of the original invasive lobular carcinoma rather than true multicentricity.[32]

Ascertaining accurate rates of multicentricity for special types of invasive mammary carcinoma is difficult because of small sample sizes. Lagios, Rose, and Margolin[33] reported that 56% of tubular carcinomas were multicentric. In a study of minimal invasive carcinoma (lesions ≤10 mm in diameter), 59% of small tubular carcinomas were multicentric.[21] Although other studies have shown lower rates of multicentricity,[34] tubular carcinoma probably has an increased rate of multicentricity compared with the average for all cancers.

In studies with both large[31] and small[35] numbers of examples, medullary carcinoma has been shown to have one of the lowest rates of multicentricity. It is difficult to draw conclusions about the rate of multicentricity associated with colloid or mucinous carcinoma because of the small numbers of cases studied.[21,35]

COMBINED INVASIVE AND IN SITU CARCINOMA

Several authors have noted that multicentricity is more likely if invasive carcinoma coexists with a significant amount of intraductal carcinoma.[2,22,36] Middleton and colleagues[22] have recently studied a series of 32 patients diagnosed with multicentric invasive carcinoma who underwent a mastectomy. Only one patient did not exhibit essentially identical histology across the multiple foci of tumor. Twenty-four of the patients had invasive mammary carcinoma of no special type (invasive ductal carcinoma). Of these, 20 had DCIS that was associated with at least one of the foci of invasion. There were eight cases of infiltrating lobular carcinoma, only four of which were associated with LCIS. The remaining patient with LCIS had mixed DCIS and LCIS, with two foci of invasive mammary carcinoma (ductal). The nipple was involved in 10 of the patients. Spread of intraductal tumor into separate duct systems via communication at the nipple may explain an apparent association with multicentricity.

Mai and co-workers[8] performed three-dimensional reconstructions from 30 mastectomy specimens with invasive mammary carcinoma (ductal). Infiltrating lobular carcinoma was excluded from the study. Of the 30 cases, 28 had coexistent DCIS. Only 1 of the 28 cases with combined invasive and in situ carcinoma had multiple invasive tumor foci, each present in a separate quadrant. These three foci had similar histology, and there was extensive DCIS at the nipple associated with invasion. This finding again supports the argument that multicentricity, defined as multiple independent carcinogenesis events, is not as common as previously thought and suggests that the nipple may be associated with apparent multicentricity because of local duct convergence.

Biologic Studies. Evaluation of multicentric tumors using subcellular and molecular technologies has expanded current understanding of the true biologic nature of multicentric tumors and may allow more precise definitions of *multicentric* and *extensive*. Two different hypotheses, excluding intramammary metastases, have been introduced to explain the etiology of multicentric disease. One of these suggests that the multiple sites develop by intraductal spread, which may appear discontinuous at the subgross level, from an "index" case. The other hypothesis supports the concept of a genetic alteration that occurs during development and distributes extensively or locally in the breast depending on the stage of development at which it occurs. This first hit predisposes the affected region, and a second, localized genetic event results in carcinoma.[37] If the latter hypothesis is correct, there will be a combination of shared and distinct molecular events that define the separate foci of carcinoma.

Noguchi and associates,[14] in a study of 30 patients with invasive mammary carcinoma (ductal), demonstrated that clonality within a tumor could be established by measuring the restriction fragment length polymorphism (RFLP) of the tumor using the X-linked phosphoglycerate kinase gene (*PGK*). They then evaluated individual foci of invasive mammary carcinoma (ductal) in each of three women with three, three, and four separate ipsilateral lesions. They found that the separate foci exhibited the identical RFLP for each patient, strong evidence that seemingly independent foci of cancer are likely to be related.

A study applying cytogenetic analysis[15] to multicentric tumors ("macroscopically distinct," 5 to 15 mm apart) also supports the hypothesis of intraductal spread of tumor as the major mechanism for apparent multifocality. However, the presence of cytogenetically unrelated clones within a single focus suggests that breast cancer may in fact be polyclonal. Thus diverging molecular evolution of a single focus may make it difficult to differentiate between independent "index" cases and evolution of tumor that has spread from a single "index" case. In fact, molecular evolution may in part explain histologic heterogeneity in DCIS within independent duct systems.

Fujii and colleagues[13] studied invasive tumors for allelic losses at seven different chromosomal loci and compared the alterations in these tumors with those present in DCIS within the same breast. A high degree of concordance of specific losses between the in situ and invasive lesions supports the concept of multifocal rather than truly multicentric carcinoma. A variable degree of heterogeneity in allelic losses at one or more loci in 8 of the 20 cases examined is again attributed to some degree of clonal divergence in the evolution of breast cancer.

Early protein-based immunocytochemical techniques,[38] certainly the least reliable of these methodologies, generated conflicting results in a study of 24 cases of "separate" tumors. More recently a study of morphology combined with immunohistochemistry for estrogen receptor, progesterone receptor, *HER2/neu*, and *Ki-67* in 32 patients who had undergone modified radical mastectomy supported the hypothesis that multicentric mammary carcinoma results from intraductal spread.[22] As noted earlier, all but one (97%) of the patients in that study had identical histology in the separate tumor foci.

ASSOCIATED FACTORS

Numerous authors have proposed various factors to be associated with increased risk of multicentricity, defined by occurrence in multiple quadrants or within a minimum distance. The problem with interpreting these studies is the inherently arbitrary definition of multicentricity in standard pathology reports. As described earlier, many of the lesions called *multicentric* are likely multifocal manifestations of DCIS or multiple foci of invasion with intervening intraductal carcinoma. The presence of a lesion in the nipple or subareolar area is perhaps the most clearly and consistently demonstrated risk factor for multicentricity.[2,22,35,39,40] Mai and co-workers[8] discovered that DCIS exhibited a pyramidal shape, "fanning out" from the nipple to the posterior of the breast. As described earlier, it is possible that the convergence of the duct systems at the nipple explains the seemingly increased multicentricity in the subareolar tissue.

Studies looking for a relationship between multicentricity and tumor size,* patient age,[2,31,42,44] family history,[35,42] or nodal status[2,31,42-47] have generated mixed results. Lagios, Westdahl, and Rose[21] found an association of multicentricity with tubular carcinoma. Among other factors studied and shown to have no relationship with an increased rate of multicentricity are estrogen receptor status, height, weight, parity,[31] specific breast or quadrant involved, amount of necrosis,[2] nuclear grade, expression of the adhesion molecule CD44v6,[48] preexisting or concurrent benign breast disease,[2,44] and bilaterality.[44]

Clinical Follow-Up Studies. The primary relevance of multicentric disease is essentially for patients who desire or undergo breast-conserving therapy. Middleton and co-workers,[22] who studied multicentricity in patients who had undergone mastectomies, found no difference in disease-free survival for women with apparently multicentric versus unicentric invasive carcinoma. In their study, 75% of the cases were invasive mammary carcinoma and 25% had infiltrating lobular carcinoma. The authors were unable to determine whether the equivalence in survival rates was due to the type of treatment the women received.

The recent studies described earlier in this chapter with extensive three-dimensional reconstruction suggest that multicentricity of carcinoma, either DCIS or an invasive (not lobular) carcinoma associated with DCIS, defined as independent sources of tumor located in separate duct systems, is actually an unlikely event, whereas multifocality of either invasive or in situ carcinoma is not uncommon. Given the near-complete independence of the ductal systems, breast-conserving surgery may be adequate therapy when disease is localized and, if based on a segmental anatomy, may also be adequate when extensive or multifocal DCIS is present. The latter may also present with multiple foci of invasive carcinoma, but these will originate within the same duct system nearly 90% of the time.

*References 2, 4, 17, 21, 29, 31, 35, 41-44.

As such, the phenomenon of extensive intraductal carcinoma with multifocal invasive or in situ tumor is the more commonly encountered issue than true multicentricity when planning surgical therapy for a patient with breast carcinoma. The collaborative study between medical schools at Nijmegen and Harvard represents the one of the early comprehensive studies to address an EIC as a clinically relevant factor in the study of breast carcinoma.[20] The definition of an EIC for this study was similar to that in a previous study by Schnitt and associates[49] and consisted of two criteria: (1) DCIS was present prominently (≥25%) within the infiltrating tumor, and (2) DCIS was present clearly extending beyond the infiltrating margin of the tumor. Mastectomy specimens from 214 patients were studied with a three-dimensional reconstructive techniques; the study design was predicated on a practical clinical question: Can the findings in an excisional biopsy predict residual tumor within the remaining breast? Excisional biopsies with extensive in situ carcinoma were in fact far more likely (74% versus 42%) to be associated with residual carcinoma, primarily in situ disease, in the mastectomy specimen. The EIC-positive patients were also more likely to have additional foci of invasive carcinoma within the breast at the time of mastectomy. However, this difference was small and reached statistical significance only within the immediate vicinity of the primary tumor (within 2 cm of the margin of the primary tumor). The major difference, then, between the EIC-positive and EIC-negative tumors was in the extent of the in situ disease of ductal type within the remainder of the breast (Figure 13-11).[4] Intralymphatic channel tumor involvement was not different between the two tumor types.

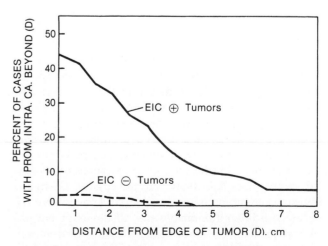

FIG. **13-11** Frequency distribution of prominent intraductal carcinoma at various distances from the edge of the primary tumor. *(From Holland R et al: J Clin Oncol 8:113, 1990.)*

The Holland study on the predictive capability of EIC produced results compatible with other studies on this phenomenon[49-51] and has been confirmed in studies from Amsterdam[52,53] and London.[54] Other earlier studies did not support the predictive usefulness of EIC with regard to local treatment failure. This disparity may be explained by the fact that one of these studies used a large resection[55] and the other required histologic documentation of tumor-free margins.[56]

The more recent studies with three-dimensional reconstruction by Ohtake and co-workers[7] and Mai and co-workers,[8] described earlier in this chapter, also support the concept of extensive intraductal carcinoma as an important factor in determining the effectiveness of breast-conserving therapy. However, this does not necessarily imply that breast-conserving therapy will not be successful. Mai and co-workers attribute the success of segmental resection in treating breast carcinoma to the high prevalence of DCIS restricted to a single duct system. They go even further and suggest that failures using segmental resection for small carcinomas may in part be related to the pyramidal shape of the distribution of the DCIS. Supportive of this hypothesis is a small study of mastectomy specimens obtained following local failure after lumpectomy, which found that recurrences were located in the same quadrant as the primary lesion and were present radial to the initial tumor (either closer to the nipple or toward the axilla).[57] Mai and co-workers also suggested involvement of the nipple and the lack of recognition of an EIC associated with a small, palpable invasive lesion as possible causes for failures in segmental resections.

Other approaches to local therapy may abrogate the negative effect of clinically occult multicentricity on the rate of local recurrence,[9,58-60] even in the setting of a subareolar lesion.[61]

Summary

We have seen the concept of multicentricity evolve from merely an observed phenomenon to a more specific model-based definition using a three-dimensional reconstruction of the breast mammary tree and molecular profiles of the tumor. Observed multicentricity in cases of invasive mammary carcinoma has been strongly associated with involvement of the nipple and the presence of an EIC. Discovery of a focus of invasive carcinoma more than 4 cm from the edge of a definable invasive carcinoma is uncommon, and the rate of this occurrence is approximately that of development of a second primary in the opposite breast. Multicentricity and bilaterality have sometimes been considered related in some respects. Considering that true multicentricity occurs as a result of independent molecular events, one would expect the rates of multicentricity and bilaterality to be similar. The published rates and circumstances of multiple occurrence of ipsilateral and contralateral breast carcinoma are in fact quite different. Most "secondary" lesions in the ipsilateral breast, therefore, likely represent (multifocal) evolution from intraductal extension of the primary lesion. This model is supported by recent imaging and molecular studies of seemingly multicentric tumors,[5-8,14,15] with confirmation in the clinical finding that more than 90% of recurrences after local removal of a carcinoma from a breast are found in the same segment as the original carcinoma[57] (see Chapters 19, 45, 63, 67, and 79).

Difficulties in defining the relationships of multiple tumors should not obscure the recognition that it is important only insofar as it has predictive value for treatment success or failure. True multicentricity, defined as independent index sources of tumor, is difficult to estimate and occurs much less often than has been published. Therefore it may be appropriate to consider extensive intraductal carcinoma, the likely cause of most published instances of multicentric disease, as the more important factor in prognosticating success of treatment.

It is unclear at this juncture whether magnetic resonance imaging (MRI) will play a role in the planning of surgery for women suspected of having multicentric or extensive intraductal carcinoma. To date, MRI is most successful in assessing breast lesions within well-defined groups of women at high risk for breast cancer. It has been demonstrated to be more sensitive but less specific than mammography for the diagnosis of "multicentricity" and for extensive intraductal disease.[62]

REFERENCES

1. Qualheim RE, Gall EA: Breast carcinoma with multiple sites of origin, *Cancer* 10:460, 1957.
2. Fisher ER et al: Pathologic findings from the National Surgical Adjuvant Breast Project (Protocol No. 4). I. Observations concerning the multicentricity of mammary cancer, *Cancer* 35:247, 1975.
3. Fisher ER et al: Pathologic findings from the National Surgical Adjuvant Breast Project (Protocol No. 6). I. Intraductal carcinoma (DCIS), *Cancer* 57:197, 1986.
4. Holland R et al: Histologic multifocality of Tis, T1-2 breast carcinomas: implications for clinical trials of breast-conserving surgery, *Cancer* 56:979, 1985.
5. Faverly DR et al: Three dimensional imaging of mammary duct carcinoma in situ: clinical implications, *Semin Diagn Pathol* 11:193, 1994.
6. Ohtake T et al: Intraductal extension of primary invasive breast carcinoma treated by breast-conservative surgery: computer graphic three dimensional reconstruction of the mammary duct-lobular system, *Cancer* 76:32, 1995.
7. Ohtake T et al: Computer-assisted complete three dimensional reconstruction of the mammary ductal-lobular

systems: implications of ductal anastomoses for breast-conserving surgery, *Cancer* 91:2263, 2001.

8. Mai KT et al: Pattern of distribution of intraductal and infiltrating ductal carcinoma: a three dimensional study using serial coronal giant sections of the breast, *Hum Pathol* 31:464, 2000.

9. Harris EE, Solin LJ: The diagnosis and treatment of ductal carcinoma in situ of the breast, *Breast J* 6:78, 2000.

10. Silverstein MJ et al: The influence of margin width on local control of ductal carcinoma in situ of the breast, *N Engl J Med* 340:1455, 1999.

11. Moffat DF, Going JJ: Three dimensional anatomy of complete duct systems in human breast: pathological and developmental implications, *J Clin Pathol* 49:48, 1996.

12. Mannes KD et al: Pagetoid spread in ductal carcinoma in situ: characterization and computer simulation. Abstract 164. United States and Canadian Academy of Pathology 91st Annual Meeting, Chicago, Feb 23-Mar 1, 2002.

13. Fujii H et al: Genetic divergence in the clonal evolution of breast cancer, *Cancer Res* 56:1493, 1996.

14. Noguchi S et al: Discrimination between multicentric and multifocal carcinomas of the breast through clonal analysis, *Cancer* 74:872, 1994.

15. Teixeira MR et al: Cytogenetic analysis of multifocal breast carcinomas: detection of karyotypically unrelated clones as well as clonal similarities between tumour foci, *Br J Cancer* 70:922, 1994.

16. Cheatle GL, Cutler M: *Tumors of the breast: their pathology, symptoms, diagnosis and treatment*, Philadelphia, 1931, JB Lippincott.

17. Lagios MD: Multicentricity of breast carcinoma demonstrated by routine correlated serial subgross and radiographic examination, *Cancer* 40:1726, 1977.

18. European Commission: *European guidelines for quality assurance in mammography screening*, ed 2, Luxembourg, 1996, Office for Official Publications of the European Communities. II-C-15-II-16.

19. Egan RL, McSweeney MB: Multicentric breast carcinoma, *Recent Results Cancer Res* 90:28, 1984.

20. Holland R et al: The presence of an extensive intraductal component (EIC) following a limited excision correlates with prominent residual disease in the remainder of the breast, *J Clin Oncol* 8:113, 1990.

21. Lagios MD, Westdahl PR, Rose MR: The concept and implications of multicentricity in breast carcinoma, *Pathol Annu* 16:83, 1981.

22. Middleton LP et al: Multicentric mammary carcinoma, *Cancer* 94:1910, 2002.

23. Patchefsky AS et al: Heterogeneity of intraductal carcinoma of the breast, *Cancer* 63:731,1989.

24. Simpson T, Thirlby RC, Dail DH: Surgical treatment of ductal carcinoma in situ of the breast: 10- to 20-year follow-up, *Arch Surg* 127:468, 1992.

25. Ashikari R, Hajdu SI, Robbins GF: Intraductal carcinoma of the breast, *Cancer* 28:1182, 1971.

26. Alpers CE, Wellings SR: The prevalence of carcinoma in situ in normal and cancer associated breasts, *Hum Pathol* 16:796, 1985.

27. Posner MC, Wolmark N: Noninvasive breast carcinoma, *Breast Cancer Res Treat* 21:15, 1992.

28. Ringberg A et al: Bilateral and multifocal breast carcinoma: a clinical and autopsy study with special emphasis on carcinoma in situ, *Eur J Surg Oncol* 17:20, 1991.

29. Gump FE et al: The extent and distribution of cancer in breasts with palpable primary tumors, *Ann Surg* 204:384, 1986.

30. Schwartz GF et al: Multicentricity of non-palpable breast cancer, *Cancer* 45:2913, 1980.

31. Lesser ML, Rosen PP, Kinne DW: Multicentricity and bilaterality in invasive breast carcinoma, *Surgery* 91:234, 1982.

32. Schnitt SJ et al: Influence of infiltrating lobular histology on local tumor control in breast cancer patients treated with conservative surgery and radiotherapy, *Cancer* 64:448, 1989.

33. Lagios MD, Rose MR, Margolin FR: Tubular carcinoma of the breast: association with multicentricity, bilaterally, and family history of mammary carcinoma, *Am J Clin Pathol* 73:25, 1980.

34. McDivitt RW, Boyce W, Gersell D: Tubular carcinoma of the breast: clinical and pathological observations concerning 135 cases, *Am J Surg Pathol* 6:401, 1982.

35. Rosen PP et al: "Residual" mammary carcinoma following simulated partial mastectomy, *Cancer* 35:739, 1975.

36. Arbutina DR et al: Multifocality in the earliest detectable breast cancers, *Arch Surg* 127:421, 1992.

37. Sharpe CR: A developmental hypothesis to explain the multicentricity of breast cancer, *CMAJ* 159:55, 1998.

38. Dawson PJ, Baekey PA, Clark RA: Mechanisms of multifocal breast cancer: an immunocytochemical study, *Hum Pathol* 26:965, 1995.

39. Andersen JA, Pallesen RM: Spread to the nipple and areola in carcinoma of the breast, *Ann Surg* 189:367, 1979.

40. Luttges J, Kalbfleisch H, Prinz P: Nipple involvement and multicentricity in breast cancer: a study on whole organ sections, *J Cancer Res Clin Oncol* 113:481, 1987.

41. Morgenstern L, Kaufman PA, Friedman NB: The case against tylectomy for carcinoma of the breast, *Am J Surg* 130:251, 1975.

42. Sarnelli R, Squartini F: Multicentricity in breast cancer: a submacroscopic study, *Pathol Annu* 21:143, 1986.

43. Squartini F, Sarnelli R: Structure, functional changes, and proliferative pathology of the human mammary lobule in cancerous breasts, *J Natl Cancer Inst* 67:33, 1975.

44. Westman-Naeser S et al: Multifocal breast carcinoma, *Am J Surg* 142:255, 1981.

45. De Laurentiis M et al: A predictive index of axillary nodal involvement in operable breast cancer, *Br J Cancer* 73:1241, 1996.

46. Ariso R et al: What modifies the relation between tumour size and lymph node metastases in T1 breast carcinomas? *J Clin Pathol* 53:846, 2000.

47. Chua B et al: Frequency and predictors of axillary lymph node metastases in invasive breast cancer, *ANZ J Surg* 71:723, 2001.

48. Ruibal A et al: Expression of the adhesion molecule CD44v6 in infiltrating ductal carcinomas of the breast is associated with hormone dependence: our experience with 168 cases, *Rev Esp Med Nucl* 19:350, 2000.

49. Schnitt SJ et al: Pathologic predictors of early local recurrence in stage I and II breast cancer treated by primary radiation therapy, *Cancer* 53:1049, 1984.

50. Harris JR et al: Clinical-pathologic study of early breast cancer treated by primary radiation therapy, *J Clin Oncol* 1:184, 1983.

51. Schnitt SJ, Connolly JL, Khettry U: Pathologic findings on reexcision of the primary site in breast cancer patients considered for treatment by primary radiation therapy, *Cancer* 59:675, 1987.

52. Bartelink JH et al: The impact of tumor size and histology on local control after breast-conserving therapy, *Radiother Oncol* 11:279, 1988.
53. Voogd AC et al: Differences in risk factors for local and distant recurrence after breast-conserving therapy or mastectomy for stage I and II breast cancer: pooled results of two large European randomized trials, *J Clin Oncol* 19:1688, 2001.
54. Lindley R, Bulman A, Parsons P: Histologic features predictive of an increased risk of early local recurrence after treatment of breast cancer by local tumor excision and radical radiotherapy, *Surgery* 105:13, 1989.
55. van Limbergen E et al: Tumor excision and radiotherapy as primary treatment of breast cancer: analysis of patient and treatment parameters and local control, *Radiother Oncol* 8:1, 1987.
56. Fisher B et al: Eight-year results of a randomized clinical trial comparing total mastectomy and lumpectomy with or without irradiation in the treatment of breast cancer, *N Engl J Med* 320:822, 1989.
57. Johnson JE et al: Recurrent mammary carcinoma after local excision: a segmental problem, *Cancer* 75:1612, 1995.
58. Veronesi U et al: Breast conservation is a safe method in patients with small cancer of the breast: long term results of three randomised trials on 1,973 patients, *Eur J Cancer* 31A:1574, 1995.
59. Weng EY et al: Outcomes and factors impacting local recurrence of ductal carcinoma in situ, *Cancer* 88:1643, 2000.
60. Skinner KA, Silverstein MJ: The management of ductal carcinoma in situ of the breast, *Endocr Relat Cancer* 8:33, 2001.
61. Haffty BG et al: Subareolar breast cancer: long-term results with conservative surgery and radiation therapy, *Int J Radiat Oncol Biol Phys* 33:53, 1995.
62. Kinkel K, Vlastos G: MR Imaging: breast cancer staging and screening, *Semin Surg Oncol* 20:187, 2001.

14

Mammary Sarcoma and Lymphoma

CAROLYN MIES

Sarcoma

The term *sarcoma* (from the Greek *sarkoma*, meaning "fleshy growth") denotes nonepithelial tumors. In the past, it was assumed that because "soft tissue" has its principal embryologic origin in mesoderm, sarcomas arise from primitive mesenchymal cells. The pathogenesis of most sarcomas is, of course, unknown; modern classification systems categorize these tumors according to the adult tissue they most resemble— muscle, bone, cartilage, vascular endothelium, and so forth—and not to the putative tissue or cell of origin.[1] Malignant lymphoma—"lymphosarcoma" in the past— is a hematologic system malignancy and is no longer included in the soft tissue sarcoma group.

Soft tissue sarcomas are rare, constituting less than 1% of all human cancers.[1] These tumors tend to arise unifocally and spread along a path of least resistance, generally respecting anatomic boundaries. Sarcomas usually grow as expansile masses that compress surrounding normal tissues; grossly, they often appear well circumscribed, even encapsulated. This circumscription belies the insidious peripheral infiltration that becomes apparent on microscopic examination. Sarcomas have a propensity to metastasize by the bloodstream, usually to lung and bone. Except for particular subtypes, regional lymph node involvement is uncommon and may be prognostically equivalent to metastatic disease.[2]

The American Joint Committee for Cancer Staging developed the TNMG staging system for soft tissue sarcomas that incorporates *t*umor size, lymph *n*ode status, the presence of *m*etastasis and the type and *g*rade of sarcoma.[2] This staging system, summarized in Table 14-1, is applicable to soft tissue sarcomas at all sites and can be used as a general guide to prognosis and therapy.[1]

Mammary Sarcoma

GENERAL ASPECTS

Soft tissue sarcomas are rare, but mammary sarcomas are rarer still, accounting for less than 1% of all breast cancers.[3] They occur in both women and men and are histologically identical to comparable soft tissue tumors at other anatomic sites; by definition, they lack a neoplastic epithelial component.[4-6] Some subtypes— phyllodes tumor, de novo angiosarcoma, and fibromatosis—have distinctive clinicopathologic features that differ significantly from the larger group of mammary sarcoma. Although not a true mammary neoplasm, Stewart-Treves syndrome (angiosarcoma of the skin and soft tissue arising in the setting of postmastectomy lymphedema) is conventionally included

in this group because of its relationship to the treatment of breast carcinoma.

Sarcomas of the breast are a heterogeneous group of tumors, not a single entity.[5,7] This diverse group of neoplasms includes fibrosarcoma-malignant fibrous histiocytoma, fibromatosis (desmoid tumor or low-grade fibrosarcoma), liposarcoma, leiomyosarcoma, rhabdomyosarcoma, malignant schwannoma, osteogenic sarcoma, and chondrosarcoma. All share some common clinical and pathologic features. *Stromal sarcoma* is a term coined more than 30 years ago that has been dropped from the lexicon because it obscures the diversity of this group of neoplasms.[4]

A clear picture of the morphologic and clinical spectrum of each specific subtype of mammary sarcoma has been slow to emerge. There are several reasons for this, not the least of which is that these mammary tumors are rare. Second, the histologic classification of sarcoma has changed considerably during the last few decades. Certain tumor types, such as fibrosarcoma-malignant fibrous histiocytoma, were not recognized as specific entities until relatively recently. Third, discriminating true sarcomas from metaplastic mammary carcinoma, the most important differential diagnosis, was more difficult without modern pathologic techniques. In the 1960s and 1970s, electron microscopy was used to distinguish epithelial from mesenchymal neoplasms. Now, paraffin tissue immunohistochemistry (IHC) is a widely available and cost-effective diagnostic tool that quickly and reliably solves the problem in cases in which the morphology is ambiguous or the diagnostic tissue sample is small (e.g., a core biopsy).

Survival data from past studies of mammary sarcoma are difficult to interpret because of these confounding factors. We also are only beginning to learn about the efficacy of breast-conserving surgery for sarcoma; until the relatively recent past, most patients were treated with mastectomy.

CLINICAL FEATURES

The typical patient with mammary sarcoma is a woman with a painless breast mass.[7,8] When Barnes and Pietruszka[7] reviewed the premammography era literature of "stromal sarcoma," they found the mean age at the time of presentation was 52 years and the median tumor size was 5.3 cm. In older series, more than half the patients describe being aware of their tumors for more than 6 months and seek medical attention because of sudden rapid growth of the mass.[7,9] Bilateral tumors occur in all sarcoma subtypes but are exceptional.

GENERAL PATHOLOGIC FEATURES

Mammary sarcomas are neoplastic proliferations of spindle-shaped cells that grow as expansile masses. In some cases a gross impression of sharp circumscription

TABLE 14-1 | AJCC 2002 TNMG Staging of Soft Tissue Sarcomas

PRIMARY TUMOR (T)

T_1	Tumor <5 cm
T_{1a}	Superficial tumor
T_{1b}	Deep tumor
T_2	Tumor ≥5 cm
T_{2a}	Superficial tumor
T_{2b}	Deep tumor

REGIONAL LYMPH NODES (N)

N_X	Regional nodes cannot be assessed
N_0	No regional lymph node metastasis
N_1	Regional lymph node metastasis

DISTANT METASTASIS (M)

M_X	Distant metastasis cannot be assessed
M_0	No distant metastasis
M_1	Distant metastasis

HISTOLOGIC GRADE (G)

G_X	Grade cannot be assessed
G_1	Well differentiated
G_2	Moderately differentiated
G_3	Poorly differentiated
G_4	Poorly differentiated or undifferentiated

STAGE GROUPING

Stage I	$T_{1a}, T_{1b}, T_{2a}, T_{2b}$	N_0	M_0	G_{1-2}
Stage II	T_{1a}, T_{1b}, T_{2a}	N_0	M_0	G_{3-4}
Stage III	T_{2b}	N_0	M_0	G_{3-4}
Stage IV	Any T	N_1	M_0	Any G
	Any T	N_0	M_1	Any G

Modified from AJCC cancer staging manual, ed 6, New York, 2002, Springer-Verlag.

is paralleled by a rounded, pushing microscopic margin and the tumor seems to "shell out." In others, the advancing edge of the tumor is infiltrative even where it appears grossly well defined. In the latter instance, tumor cells invade fat and tend to grow between the glandular structures of the breast, separating individual acini and expanding the intralobular space; this growth pattern is particularly prominent in mammary angiosarcoma. Neoplastic glands or epithlium are, by definition, never seen in mammary sarcoma.

Mammary sarcomas are graded in the same way as their soft tissue counterparts on the basis of cellular and nuclear pleomorphism and mitotic index; as a practical matter, division into a two-tier low- and high-grade system correlates with outcome and influences some aspects of treatment.[10,11]

The most important pathologic differential diagnosis of mammary sarcoma is metaplastic carcinoma (i.e., invasive ductal carcinoma with spindle cell metaplasia). This entity can mimic sarcoma but is, in fact, an epithelial neoplasm with a completely different prognosis, rate of lymph node metastasis, and treatment. Carcinoma is excluded through ample sampling of the tumor to identify intraductal carcinoma or usual patterns of invasive ductal cancer. Where this fails in an excised tumor or cannot be done because of the small size of the biopsy, IHC staining for cytokeratin and other epithelial markers, which are positive in metaplastic carcinoma, can almost always solve this problem. Because nearly all spindle cell neoplasms stain for vimentin and both metaplastic carcinoma and sarcoma may stain for S-100 protein and actin, none of these are useful in this context.

The second differential diagnosis in this setting is metastatic melanoma, which can have an amelanotic spindle cell morphology and is one of the commonest metastatic tumors found in the breast.[12,13] If there is a known history of melanoma with prior biopsy slides for comparison or if the cells are pigmented, the diagnosis may be straightforward. If not, adding a melanocyte marker to the IHC panel will solve the problem.

DIAGNOSING AND TREATING MAMMARY SARCOMA

Today, fine-needle aspiration (FNA) or core biopsy is often the first step in diagnosing a mammary tumor. Because infiltrating carcinoma is, by far, the most common mass-forming malignancy in the breast, a diagnosis of sarcoma is often unexpected. An FNA that yields atypical or frankly malignant spindle cells mandates a tissue biopsy to make the crucial distinction between metaplastic carcinoma and sarcoma. Large (>2 cm) tumors can be sampled with a core or incisional biopsy; a complete excisional biopsy is recommended for small tumors.

IHC for cytokeratins has a key role in ruling out carcinoma in a core biopsy. If this can be accomplished unambiguously, the surgical options appropriate for carcinoma can be discussed with the patient and a definitive procedure planned. If core biopsy results show spotty or equivocal staining, then incisional biopsy is the prudent course before definitive surgery; some sarcomas have an occasional cytokeratin-positive cell.[1]

The best primary treatment for mammary sarcoma is wide excision with a rim of normal breast tissue. A total mastectomy may be required if the tumor is very large. Local recurrence is best correlated with incomplete excision; therefore the basic principles of sarcoma surgery should not be compromised. Axillary dissection is not indicated unless clinical assessment suggests the lymph nodes are likely to contain metastatic disease. As a nearly universal rule, metastatic mammary sarcoma appears in the lungs or bones, not in axillary lymph nodes.[8] A metastatic spindle cell neoplasm in axillary nodes should be considered carcinoma until proved otherwise.

The usefulness of adjuvant radiotherapy and chemotherapy for sarcomas with high-risk features is unclear and difficult to assess in such uncommon tumors.

Fibrosarcoma-Malignant Fibrous Histiocytoma

Most of the reported cases of primary mammary fibrosarcoma have appeared in general reviews of mammary sarcoma.[5,7,14-16] Similarly, reports describing primary mammary malignant fibrous histiocytoma (MFH) as a specific entity are very uncommon.[17-20]

In the breast, there is considerable morphologic overlap between fibrosarcoma and MFH, leading Weiss and colleagues to consider them as two closely related members of the same family of fibroblastic tumors, which makes sense.[11,21] By definition, mammary fibrosarcoma-MFH arises in the parenchyma, not in the skin or chest wall fascia; postradiation examples in skin and chest wall are not considered primary in the breast.[21-23]

Fibrosarcomas are composed of neoplastic cells with ultrastructural features of fibroblasts and myofibroblasts; in addition, histiocyte differentiation is seen in the MFH pattern.[1,21] The interface with normal breast may be either sharp or infiltrative. The spindle-shaped tumor cells have little cytoplasm and gather in sweeping fascicles. In the well-developed fibrosarcoma pattern, the tumor cells grow—like the woven fabric—in a herringbone pattern. At the MFH end of the spectrum, the cells grow as small fascicular bundles of spindle-shaped cells that form a pinwheel or storiform pattern around small vessels (Figure 14-1). The tumor cells produce variable amounts of collagen. Larger, more rounded fibroblasts, irregularly shaped histiocytes, and multinucleated tumor giant cells are other cellular constituents in the MFH pattern. Mitotic figures are common and can have an abnormal configuration in poorly differentiated tumors.

In the largest series of cases, it was shown that mammary fibrosarcoma-MFH could be categorized as low or high grade based on cytologic atypia and mitotic index.[11] Low-grade tumors may recur locally but do not metastasize or kill. They have the more uniformly fascicular growth pattern of usual fibrosarcoma, little to moderate cytologic atypia, and 5 or fewer mitoses per

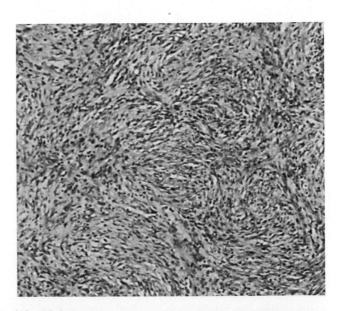

FIG. **14-1** Fibrosarcoma—malignant fibrous histiocytoma. Short fascicles of tumor cells arranged in a storiform pattern. (H&E, ×100.)

10 high-power field (hpf), most 2 or fewer per 10 hpf. Vascular and nerve invasion are not seen and the tumor border is usually circumscribed. In this study, 16 patients had low-grade tumors, 13 treated with wide local excision and 2 with mastectomy; none had axillary dissections. After a median of 8 years follow-up, 10 had local recurrences but none developed metastatic disease. Recurrences occurred in the first 5 years of follow-up.[11]

In contrast, high-grade fibrosarcoma-MFH may both recur locally and metastasize. They exhibit moderate to marked cellular atypia and have numerous mitoses. The storiform MFH pattern is more common among the high-grade tumors and typically infiltrates normal breast at the periphery by entrapping benign mammary structures. Of 16 patients with high-grade fibrosarcoma-MFH in this study, 7 were treated with wide local excision, 2 with simple mastectomy, and 7 with modified radical mastectomy. In the latter group, no lymph node metastases were found. After a median of 7 years follow-up, five (31%) had died of their malignancy and two (12%) were living with it. Bone and lung metastases developed in four (25%) cases. Almost all the high-grade tumors destined to recur did so within 2 years, regardless of type of surgery.[11]

Pathologic diagnosis of mammary fibrosarcoma-MFH is based on the overall morphology of the tumor and the exclusion of metaplastic carcinoma; there are no specific IHC markers for fibrosarcoma-MFH.[19]

Fibromatosis (Desmoid Tumor)

Fibromatosis is a fascinating proliferative lesion that exhibits uncontrolled local growth and a tendency to recur—especially if incompletely excised—but lacks metastatic potential. Modern molecular biology techniques have demonstrated that extraabdominal fibromatosis is monoclonal (i.e., derived from a single progenitor cell, a feature of neoplasia, but not reactive processes).[24] Despite this, there is antecedent trauma in some cases.

Mammary fibromatosis (MF) (desmoid tumor) has become better recognized as a distinct clinicopathologic entity in recent years. In the past, cases were probably grouped with mammary fibrosarcoma, which it resembles histologically. Like fibromatosis at other anatomic sites, it behaves like a low-grade neoplasm that is locally invasive but does not metastasize; it should be distinguished from frank fibrosarcoma.[25-27] MF occurs over a wide age range in both women and men,[28] can be bilateral, and is clinically most significant because its clinical presentation can mimic carcinoma.[26,27,29-34] Like other extraabdominal fibromatoses, MF has occurred after trauma and in association with augmentation and reconstructive mammaplasty.[26,35-37] Axillary

fibromatosis, in one instance, followed mastectomy for mammary carcinoma.[38]

It has long been suspected that MF is related to adenomatous polyposis coli (APC) and its variant, Gardner's syndrome (GS). Three cases of MF in patients with APC/GS have been described, one bilateral.[31,39,40] Molecular biology has now demonstrated a connection at the DNA level. Somatic mutations in either the APC or β-catenin genes were demonstrated in 79% (26/33) of MFs, 25 sporadic and 1 in a patient with known APC/GS. There was evidence for biallelic (germline and somatic) inactivation of the APC gene in four MFs, one from the APC/GS patient, as would be predicted, and in three without polyposis.[39]

PATHOLOGIC FEATURES

MF averages 2 to 3 cm in diameter. Its gross appearance depends on the configuration of the tumor itself and the composition of the breast. In contrast to other types of sarcoma, MF is firm but often poorly circumscribed with an ill-defined margin. The tumor can blend in so well that it can be difficult to grossly distinguish from normal breast tissue, making it difficult to excise completely (Figure 14-2).

Mammary fibromatosis resembles fibrosarcoma in that it is composed of infiltrating sweeping fascicles of spindle-shaped cells with features of fibroblasts and myofibroblasts (Figure 14-2, *B*).[32,33,41] It differs in having low cellularity, inconspicuous mitotic activity, and focally abundant intercellular collagen that, in some cases, is deposited in keloidlike aggregates. Necrosis, hemorrhage, cytologic atypia, and aberrant mitoses are features of frank fibrosarcoma, not fibromatosis.[26,27] IHC stains—except to rule out metaplastic carcinoma—have no role in diagnosis.

Mammary fibromatosis has a local recurrence rate after excision of 21% to 27%.[26,27,30] The only pathologic feature that correlates with recurrence is a positive resection margin.[26,27,30] It appears that MF does not express estrogen and progesterone receptors, indicating that tamoxifen has no role in controlling local disease.[42,43] Because it does not metastasize, the prognosis of patients with this mammary soft tissue tumor is excellent.

Liposarcoma

Despite being one of the more common soft tissue tumors at other anatomic sites, primary mammary liposarcoma is rare. Most reports, which date back to 1883, are single cases; Austin and Dupree (1986) reported the only series of cases, discussed later in this chapter.[45,46] Mammary liposarcoma can arise as a de novo neoplasm or, just as often, as a malignant component in a phyllodes tumor.[45-51] There is a wide age spectrum and, as is true

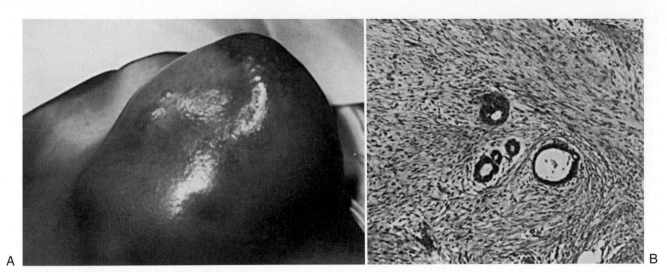

A   B

FIG. **14-2 A,** The right breast is replaced by fibromatosis (desmoid tumor) in an 18-year-old gravid black female. Because this poorly circumscribed neoplasm infiltrated the pectoralis major muscle, a Halsted radical mastectomy was performed. **B,** Mammary fibromatosis. Sweeping fascicles of fibroblasts envelop an atrophic mammary lobule. (H&E, ×100.)

for other types of mammary sarcoma, most patients with liposarcoma are women.[46,52] Bilaterality is rare.[49,53]

One reported case of liposarcoma had coexistent infiltrating ductal carcinoma,[54] and bilateral invasive ductal carcinoma followed excision in another.[55] A few of the first patients described had lymph node metastasis, unusual behavior for liposarcoma at any site.[1,56] It is possible that these tumors were metaplastic carcinoma with liposarcomatous differentiation, not primary liposarcoma. In any event, axillary node dissections in most subsequent reported cases all yielded negative results.[46]

PATHOLOGIC FEATURES

Early reports of mammary liposarcoma describe bulky, multifocal tumors, often involving the entire breast.[57] Liposarcomas unassociated with phyllodes tumor resemble other primary mammary sarcomas except that they tend to be larger—on average, 8 cm.[46] The well-differentiated, myxoid, pleomorphic, and round cell patterns seen at other sites also occur in the breast.[1,46,58] Electron microscopy, no longer used to diagnose mammary liposarcoma, shows ultrastructural features similar to those of liposarcoma at other sites.[59,60]

Liposarcoma diagnosis is based on the overall morphologic pattern and the identification of lipoblasts, vacuolated lipid-containing immature adipose cells that are the sine qua non of liposarcoma. Large tumors should be amply sampled to look for ductal carcinoma and underlying phyllodes tumor. There is no specific IHC stain for liposarcoma, but IHC should be used to rule out metaplastic carcinoma in tumors with undifferentiated spindle cell areas.

Correlating the pathologic features of mammary liposarcoma with outcome is difficult because of this tumor's rarity. In the only published series, Austin and Dupree[46] culled 20 cases from the Armed Forces Institute of Pathology (AFIP) consultation files (1949 to 1981). The series included de novo liposarcoma and liposarcoma in phyllodes tumor. Most patients had been treated with mastectomy; 35% had local excisions. Of 20 patients, for whom follow-up information was available 17 (85%) were cured. Association with phyllodes tumor was a key prognostic feature. One patient with pure mammary liposarcoma treated with mastectomy had a local recurrence; 3 of 13 (23%) developed distant metastases within 1 year of diagnosis. In contrast, one patient with liposarcoma in a phyllodes tumor treated with local excision had a local recurrence; none developed metastatic sarcoma. The two men in the series remained disease free after having radical mastectomy for large tumors, 12 and 19 cm, respectively.[46] Optimal treatment is complete surgical excision with tumor-free margins; axillary node dissection is unnecessary.[46]

Leiomyosarcoma and Rhabdomyosarcoma

Primary mammary leiomyosarcoma and rhabdomyosarcoma are rare; fewer than 40 cases have been described. Mammary *leiomyosarcoma* occurs most often in women and in the occasional man.[61] There is a wide age range, but most patients are 40 to 60 years old. Most tumors arise in the parenchyma proper,[62-73] but some are in the nipple/areola complex.[61,74-76] In one man, leiomyosarcoma developed in ectopic areola.[77] An unusual case of mesocolic leiomyosarcoma metastatic to the breast serves to remind that we should always consider metastasis when we encounter tumor types unexpected in the breast.[78]

Typically, leiomyosarcoma presents as a firm, painless, enlarging mass, most in the 4 to 6 cm range, although larger examples are reported. Mammography and ultrasound show a circumscribed, lobulated mass that suggests a diagnosis of phyllodes tumor.[65,70,71] Gross pathologic findings parallel this image; leiomyosarcoma is characteristically firm, circumscribed, and grows with an expansile, pushing border.[65]

Leiomyosarcoma in the breast, as at other sites, grows as sweeping interlacing fascicles of spindle-shaped cells with abundant cytoplasm, blunt-ended nuclei and, often, small perinuclear vacuoles. Fascicles of cells intersect at right angles in the best-differentiated examples. Multinucleated and bizarre giant cells can be seen, and mitotic activity varies from sparse to abundant.[62,65,67]

Electron microscopy of mammary leiomyosarcoma shows features of smooth muscle differentiation.[1,61-63,67] In the diagnostic realm, IHC stains are used to rule out metaplastic carcinoma and to identify the protein markers specific for smooth muscle differentiation— desmin and/or muscle-specific actin.*

The prognosis of mammary leiomyosarcoma is fairly good, but quirky. Among 16 cases published between 1974 and 2003 with at least 1-year follow-up, 2 (12.5%) suffered local and distant recurrence, the latter occurring 16 and 20 years after initial treatment.[64,75] Four (16%) others had only breast recurrence following local excision. Although the interval to recurrence in one patient was 2 years, it ranged from 3 to 6 years in the others.[62,63,68] This tendency to late recurrence is unusual; in general, primary mammary sarcomas and malignant phyllodes tumors recur within 2 years of treatment, if at all.

Primary mammary *rhabdomyosarcoma* is exceedingly rare in adults,[79-81] children, and adolescents.[82] In the latter groups, rhabdomyosarcoma is the most common metastatic tumor in the breast.[83-86] This may be because rhabdomyosarcoma is one of the most common childhood malignancies, but it also seems that breast is a preferential site of metastasis in adolescent girls.[84] Metastatic rhabdomyosarcoma can also occur in adults.[87]

Mammary rhabdomyosarcoma presents as a rapidly enlarging, bulky, firm mass in the 7 to 12 cm range.[79-81] Microscopy shows a high-grade spindle cell tumor with rhabdomyoblasts at different stages of development, often containing cytoplasmic cross striations, the sine qua non of diagnosis.[80] Because the few published cases

---

*References 62, 63, 65, 67, 69, 70.

of primary rhabdomyosarcoma lack follow-up, prognosis is unknown.[79-81] In contrast, rhabdomyosarcoma metastatic to the breast is almost always accompanied by metastases at other sites and is fatal.

Malignant Schwannoma

It was difficult to accurately diagnose malignant schwannoma (also termed *malignant peripheral nerve sheath tumor*) of the breast before the IHC era because the histomorphology is not that distinctive. There have been a few case reports[88-90] of malignant schwannoma, in addition to one small series of mammary nerve sheath tumors from the AFIP that included three cases.[68] From this report, we learn that the tumors were solitary, rubbery masses, 0.5 cm, 2.7 cm, and 3.2 cm, respectively. One occurred in a woman with von Recklinghausen's disease and was associated with a neurofibroma. All three tumors had infiltrative borders, were very cellular, and had numerous mitotic figures, many with aberrant configurations. IHC showed tumor cells to contain S-100 protein in one of two tumors that could be tested; stains for cytokeratins and smooth muscle actin were negative in both. One patient was treated with mastectomy; the other two had local excision. There were no recurrences during follow-up of 1.5 to 3 years.[68]

Osteogenic Sarcoma and Chondrosarcoma

True mammary osteogenic sarcoma and chondrosarcoma show bone and cartilage formation, respectively, by malignant-appearing stromal cells; by definition, there is no epithelial component.[91] Because bone and cartilage formation are common in metaplastic carcinoma, it is essential to look at any bone- or cartilage-forming breast tumor for signs of carcinoma in numerous sections and with IHC stains.[91-94] Similarly, an underlying phyllodes tumor should be excluded.[3,94-97] When one carefully examines the pathologic descriptions and photomicrographs, it becomes apparent that there are many published cases of primary osteogenic sarcoma and chondrosarcoma that are not what they seem.[98-103]

Before the 1998 AFIP series of 50 cases,[104] there were fewer than 10 reasonably well-characterized examples of true de novo mammary *osteosarcoma*, all in women.[91,92,94,105-107] Silver and Tavassoli[104] studied 50 examples of mammary osteosarcoma without associated phyllodes tumor, one in a man. The tumors, 1.4 to 13.0 cm (mean, 4.6 cm), appeared radiographically circumscribed and lobulated, leading to a clinical diagnosis of fibroadenoma in one third of patients.

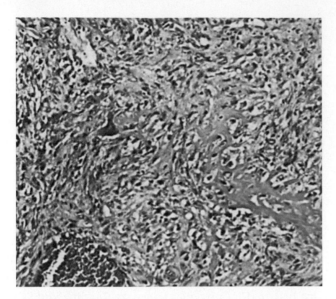

FIG. **14-3** Osteogenic sarcoma. Osteoid formed by malignant cells is seen on the right. (H&E, ×160.)

Microscopically, most tumors were infiltrative, and 18% had tiny satellite nodules. Malignant stroma ranged from minimally atypical spindle cells to large highly pleomorphic forms but always formed osteoid or mineralized bone in at least some portion of the tumor (Figure 14-3). IHC stains for keratins and other markers were feasible in 32 cases and ruled out metaplastic carcinoma. All resected lymph nodes were sarcoma free.[104]

Clinical follow-up for 39 of the 50 patients (78%) showed a poor prognosis, although these referred cases may have been biased toward bad outcome: Sections of metastatic sarcoma were submitted for 11 of the 50 patients at the time of pathologic consultation. Locally recurrent (11) and/or metastatic (16) disease developed in 23 (59%). Local recurrence was strongly correlated with a positive margin in patients who had local excisions. Local and distant recurrence occurred quickly, within 1 and 3 years of primary treatment, respectively. At present, 16 of the 39 (41%) have died from disease and another 7 are alive with disease, leading to a 10-year estimated survival of 32%.[104] Interestingly, osteosarcoma arising in a phyllodes tumor has a 40% mortality rate, with metastasis appearing in a year in the fatal cases.[98-103,108]

Examples of genuine *chondrosarcoma* of the breast are exceedingly rare.[94,109-112] Mammary chondrosarcoma, like cartilaginous tumors at other sites, tends to form a multinodular, bosselated, firm mass with visible foci of calcification. Well-differentiated tumors resemble normal hyaline cartilage; poorly differentiated examples have less cartilage formation, more cytologic atypia, and many mitoses.[109] Cartilage-forming cells are positive for S-100 protein but lack epithelial markers.[110,111] Getting a clear picture of prognosis for this very rare tumor is difficult, if not impossible.

Mammary Angiosarcoma

Angiosarcoma of the breast accounts for less than 10% of primary mammary sarcomas but is striking for its aggressive clinical behavior; high-grade examples are among the deadliest of breast cancers. In addition to case reports, there are four published series of cases comprising 108 patients.[113-116] The most recent review of the Memorial Sloan Kettering Cancer Center experience[116] has 63 patients, including 38 from two prior studies.[117,118] Mammary angiosarcoma is largely a tumor of women: There are only four reported cases in men, not all convincing.[114,115,119-121] The age range is wide (from age 14 to people in their nineties), but the mean is about 40 years.[113-115] Interestingly, a variety of other illnesses—invasive ductal carcinoma, phyllodes tumor, Hodgkin's disease, lymphoma, Kasabach-Merritt syndrome, and different thyroid disorders—occur in women with angiosarcoma.[114,115,122,123]

Although the occurrence of mammary angiosarcoma during pregnancy[124,125] has led some to suggest that these tumors are hormonally influenced, this may simply reflect that they tend to occur during childbearing years.[115,126] Biochemical hormone receptor assays were positive for estrogen and progesterone receptors in two tumors tested,[126] but I am not aware of any studies using the more reliable IHC stains.

Mammary angiosarcoma usually causes a rapidly growing painless mass, sometimes with violaceous or bluish discoloration of the overlying skin (Figure 14-4, *A*).[127] Mammography usually shows a dominant mass that, in a few, is focally calcified. There are no mammographic abnormalities in one third of patients.[127] Magnetic resonance imaging (MRI) in two cases showed an enhancing lesion and detected unsuspected contralateral angiosarcoma, probably metastatic, in one.[127,128] Because this tumor characteristically extends past the grossly observed margin,[115,116,129,130] making wide excision difficult, MRI may prove useful in determining the extent of disease before surgery.

PATHOLOGIC FEATURES

Most angiosarcomas are soft hemorrhagic masses with an ill-defined margin, but a few appear only as a thickened or indurated area in the breast.[114,115,117] Some resected tumors have a honeycomb cut surface, obvious dilated vascular channels, or pools of blood. Average size is 4 to 6 cm (range, 1.5 to 11.0 cm) and is not prognostically significant.[115-117]

Mammary angiosarcoma, as the name implies, is a malignancy of blood vessel cells. These tumors are classified (graded) according to a three-tiered system that correlates with prognosis.[113,115,117] Type I (well-differentiated) tumors grow as well-formed,

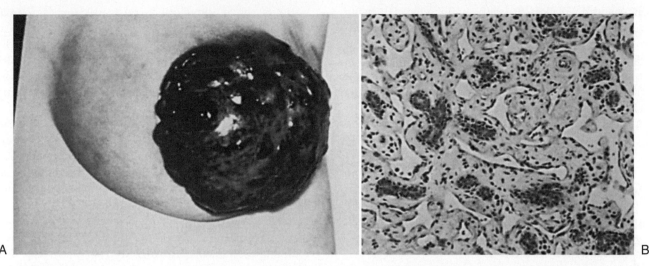

FIG. **14-4 A,** Massive angiosarcoma with extension through nipple/areola complex. Despite its large size (15 cm), this low-grade, well-differentiated lesion was not fixed to the pectoralis major muscle. The patient was managed with total mastectomy and split-thickness skin graft of the large defect. *(Courtesy Dr. Condict Moore, Department of Surgery, University of Louisville.)* **B,** Type I, well-differentiated angiosarcoma. Irregularly shaped, dilated vascular structures infiltrating a mammary lobule. (H&E, ×200.)

interanastomosing vascular channels that subtly infiltrate mammary lobules and acini (Figure 14-4, *B*). Neoplastic endothelial cells are flat, slightly hyperchromatic, and only mildly disordered; mitoses are few or absent.[113,115,117] This pattern is seen at the peripheral margin of virtually all mammary angiosarcomas; where they exist, the less differentiated components are more central.[115,117] Because of this, small biopsies may underestimate grade.

Type II (moderately differentiated) tumors are similar but show increased cellularity with endothelial tufting, mitotic activity, and the occasional solid focus.[117] Type III (poorly differentiated) angiosarcoma contains areas of solid spindle cell growth and prominent mitotic activity; nuclear abnormalities, necrosis, and hemorrhage are the rule. Coexistent type I and II foci, nearly always present, are clues to diagnosis in the least differentiated tumors.[117]

Factor VIII–related antigen, CD31, and CD34 are robust markers of endothelial differentiation, both benign and malignant.[131,132] Positive IHC stain in an undifferentiated malignant spindle cell tumor can confirm a suspected diagnosis of angiosarcoma (e.g., in a small biopsy).[132,133]

PROGNOSIS

The prognosis of patients with angiosarcoma correlates best with tumor type (grade). Patients with type I and II lesions fare significantly better, with 5-year disease-free survival rates of 76% and 70%, respectively, versus only 15% for type III tumors.[115,117] Similar results were obtained in a smaller study of 15 patients.[113] The overall 5-year disease-free survival rate is approximately 30%; the average survival of those who die is 2 to 4 years.[114,115,117]

Complete surgical excision, which may necessitate total mastectomy, is the mainstay of treatment; routine axillary node dissection is not indicated. Adjuvant chemotherapy and irradiation are administered in many cases, but their efficacy remains unproved.[115,134-138]

Postmasectomy Angiosarcoma (Stewart-Treves Syndrome)

In 1948, Stewart and Treves reported the first six cases of cutaneous/soft tissue angiosarcoma (lymphangiosarcoma) occurring in the setting of chronic postmastectomy lymphedema.[139] More than 200 similar cases have been reported, nearly all in patients treated for mammary carcinoma. In earlier decades, this complication occurred in 0.45% of patients surviving at least 5 years after radical mastectomy.[140] The incidence of lymphedema after radical mastectomy is 15% to 25%, but only 5.5% after modified radical mastectomy.[141] The prevalence of STS will probably decrease because of modern breast-conserving surgery, sentinel node biopsy with fewer axillary dissections, and improved surgical and radiation techniques.

The pathogenesis of STS is unclear. It has been speculated for years that chronic lymphedema disrupts the local immune system in the affected limb, making it an immunologically vulnerable site.[139,142-146] The essential features of the syndrome are onset of cutaneous or subcutaneous angiosarcoma an average of 10 years (range, 6 to 24) after mastectomy, complicated by severe long-standing upper extremity lymphedema.[139] In the past, many STS patients also had postmastectomy axillary irradiation that further compromised lymphatic drainage and contributed to lymphedema. Angiosarcoma can complicate chronic lymphedema at other anatomic sites caused by benign conditions such as filariasis infection and congenital disorders.[147-151]

Postmastectomy angiosarcoma occurs in the background of diffuse induration and pitting edema that characterizes long-standing lymphatic obstruction. It commonly begins as one or more innocuous-looking, painless bruises on the ipsilateral upper arm, shoulder, or chest, followed by multiple small dark red-blue papules and dermal nodules. These may become confluent or ulcerate and spontaneously heal, only to reappear after a brief interval.[139,152]

The microscopic appearance of postmastectomy angiosarcoma is identical to that of usual angiosarcoma, except for the associated diffuse proliferation of lymphatic channels (lymphangiomatosis) that characterizes chronic lymphedema and may constitute a premalignant change.[149,150] It is conventional for the pathologist to grade STS angiosarcomas, but tumor grade does not correlate with outcome.

Angiosarcoma occurring in STS exhibits differentiation features characteristic of endothelium. Ultrastructural studies have demonstrated features of both lymphatic- and blood vessel–type endothelium in the same tumor.[153-155] Factor VIII–related antigen, CD31, and CD34 are reliable markers of vascular differentiation in these tumors.[153,154,156]

Superficial skin biopsy of a suspicious cutaneous lesion in the postmastectomy setting may be misleading or difficult to interpret. As in de novo mammary angiosarcoma, the well-differentiated component of these tumors can appear so orderly that it is mistaken for benign. On the other hand, poorly differentiated components can raise the differential diagnosis of recurrent mammary carcinoma, melanoma, or other types of sarcoma.[150,156] An adequate biopsy is essential.

The prognosis for patients with postmastectomy angiosarcoma is poor. The 5-year survival rate is now 29%,[157] an improvement over the 9% in earlier series.[151,158,159] Interscapulothoracic amputation is the primary treatment of choice; the role of adjuvant chemotherapy and radiation is still being defined.[159,160]

Angiosarcoma after Breast-Conserving Treatment for Carcinoma

Breast-conserving surgery followed by adjuvant radiation is now a standard treatment for infiltrating mammary carcinoma, and it is no surprise that some

patients have developed postradiation sarcoma. Numerous case reports[161-171] that began appearing in 1987, and some later surveys, have delineated the complete clinicopathologic syndrome.[172,173] A population-based series from the Netherlands estimates the incidence of angiosarcoma after breast-conserving surgery and radiation to be 0.16%.[173]

Postradiation mammary angiosarcoma is different from postmastectomy cutaneous angiosarcoma occurring in chronic upper extremity lymphedema (STS), although there are two reported cases in which breast lymphedema-complicating radiation preceded angiosarcoma.[161,174] Although other subtypes of sarcoma can be seen in this context, the majority are angiosarcomas. Most cases are unilateral; there are two reports of bilateral angiosarcoma occurring after breast-conserving treatment for metachronous bilateral ductal carcinoma, suggesting there may be a genetic susceptibility to this complication.[164,175]

Postradiation mammary angiosarcoma involves only the skin in about half the cases, the skin and breast in 40% of cases, and only the breast in 10%.[174] Clinical features resemble those of de novo mammary angiosarcoma and develop an average of 6 years (range, 3 to 10 years) after partial mastectomy and irradiation.[172,173] The only difference is that the changes are superimposed on the cutaneous changes that may follow irradiation; angiosarcoma can mimic late-radiation dermatitis.[176,177] Atypical and benign vascular lesions also occur in irradiated skin in this setting.[162]

The histomorphology is identical to that of usual mammary and cutaneous angiosarcoma except that higher-grade tumors are more prevalent.[162] Prognosis is poor, no better than for grade-matched, usual angiosarcoma.[157,172,173] Mastectomy with tumor-free margins is the first line of treatment, and there has been some recent success with postmastectomy hyperfractionated radiotherapy.[178]

Phyllodes Tumor

Phyllodes tumor (PT, cystosarcoma phyllodes) accounts for 0.5% to 1.0% of all breast tumors and only 2.5% of fibroepithelial tumors; fibroadenoma is much more common.[179] PT differs from fibroadenoma in having a very small, but definite, potential to recur locally and/or metastasize. Determining which PTs are most likely to do this is a continuing challenge. Despite its rarity relative to carcinoma, PT is the most common mammary sarcoma.

Investigators are using modern molecular biology techniques to try to answer fundamental questions about fibroadenoma and PT. Microdissection has been used to specifically select stromal cells from these neoplasms, to isolate the DNA, and to determine clonality. The first studies showed that the stromal cells of fibroadenoma can be either polyclonal or monoclonal, whereas those of PT are always monoclonal (i.e., derived from a single progenitor cell; epithelial cells in these fibroepithelial tumors are polyclonal).[180,181] These findings, which support the concept that the neoplastic component of PT is the stroma, have been recently challenged by others who suggest that there are DNA aberrations in both the stromal and epithelial components of PT.[182] Further studies are needed to resolve this issue and to understand the pathogenesis of these biphasic tumors.

Muller[183] coined the term *cystosarcoma phyllodes* in 1838 for what appeared to be, literally, a large, cystic, fleshy (Greek: *sarkoma*), leafy tumor of the breast that usually behaved in a benign fashion, despite its often-harrowing clinical appearance. Since the first description, more than 62 different synonyms have been used to encapsulate this neoplasm's many puzzling features.[184]

Early epidemiology studies suggested that PT is more common in black women, but later studies showed that this was a result of sampling bias related to practice location. The first population-based cancer registry analysis of PT showed that, in Los Angeles County, the average annual age-adjusted incidence rate of malignant PT is 2.1 per million women and that Latina whites and Asian women have a significantly higher rate than do other racial-ethnic groups.[185]

PT occurs predominantly in women, although there have been a few PTs involving breast,[186-190] prostate,[191] and seminal vesicles[192] in adult men. It also occurs rarely in ectopic breast in axilla[193] and vulva.[194] PT has a broad age range, but the average is 45 years, about 10 to 15 years higher than the average for fibroadenoma. This neoplasm occurs uncommonly in adolescents[195,196] and can be fatal in this group.[197,198]

There are some bilateral examples, but PT usually occurs as a solitary, unilateral breast tumor.[199] In the premammography era, a palpable mass or diffuse mammary enlargement was the uniform presentation; now, 20% of cases are detected as nonpalpable masses on screening mammograms.[200] Approximately 20% to 30% of patients give a history of sudden, rapid growth in a stable breast mass.[201] Tumor size has a wide range, but the average is 4 to 5 cm.[202,203] PT is typically firm, painless, and nonfixed unless the tumor has grown very large and has ulcerated the overlying skin. This distressing feature, rarely seen today, does not imply metastatic behavior.[204-206] Although PT has some distinctive imaging features, there is a great deal of overlap among fibroadenoma, benign PT, and malignant PT.[200,207,208] A biopsy is required for diagnosis.

PATHOLOGIC FEATURES

Although some of the large, bulky examples of PT have the gross characteristics Muller described in his original

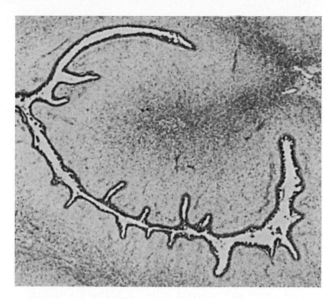

FIG. **14-5** Histologically benign phyllodes tumor. (H&E, ×40.)

report, many more grow as rubbery or firm solid masses without a conspicuous cystic component. PT grossly appears well delineated from the surrounding breast, but the microscopic picture does not always bear this out.[209] Degeneration and hemorrhage are seen in some PTs but are more often a manifestation of infarction than of malignancy.[203,209]

PT, like fibroadenoma, has a biphasic microscopic pattern with both a stromal and epithelial component (Figure 14-5). Current evidence favors that PT is a neoplasm of mammary stroma; the accompanying epithelial expansion is an intrinsic part of the overall histologic picture but is benign and secondary.[139,140] Only malignant spindle cells are found in metastatic PT.[212] The stroma of the usual PT has a fibrous or myxoid appearance, and the cells have features of fibroblasts and myofibroblasts.[211,213-216] Lipomatous, chondroid, or osseous differentiation occurs in some cases and can affect imaging findings.[108,200,217-222]

The ductal epithelial component of PT can become hyperplastic or undergo apocrine or squamous metaplasia; the degree of hyperplasia often parallels the stromal cell density. In situ carcinoma can coincidentally involve the epithelium in PT, which is not surprising given how prevalent breast cancer is in the United States.[223-227]

PROGNOSTIC PATHOLOGIC FEATURES

Many investigators have studied PT in an effort to identify histologic factors that correlate with outcome.* PT is currently subclassified on the basis of a constellation of histologic findings that correlate with local and distant recurrence; no single factor is predictive.[203,233]

---

*References 15, 158, 179, 201-203, 206, 209, 228-234.

Key histologic features of PT are as follows:

- Character of the interface between tumor and normal breast
- Proportion of neoplastic stroma relative to epithelial structures
- Mitotic index (MI), the number of mitoses/10 hpf
- Cytologic anaplasia

Benign PT nearly always has a circumscribed, pushing border; a balanced, homogeneous ratio of stroma to epithelial structures; and a low MI of 0 to 4/10 hpf. *Borderline* or *low-grade malignant* PT commonly has a partially or completely infiltrative border, a denser stroma, and a higher MI of 5 to 9/10 hpf.[203,233] *Malignant* PT (Figure 14-6) has an infiltrative border, densely packed anaplastic stromal cells, an MI of 10/10 hpf or greater, and a feature called *stromal overgrowth* that describes the dominant growth of neoplastic spindle cells relative to the epithelial component.[203,233] Stromal overgrowth exists when the spindle cell component entirely fills a low-power (40×) microscopic field, focally obliterating the characteristic fibroepithelial pattern recognized as PT.[15,201,203,229,234]

Barth[235] recently published an elegant review and meta-analysis of studies that correlate histologic features with outcome in PT. He combined the results of five series that used the Pietruszka and Barnes[233] criteria previously discussed and found that 0/78, 0/26, and 12/42 (29%) of patients with benign, borderline, and malignant PT, respectively, developed metastasis and died.[235] The combined results of three larger series using slightly different criteria showed that metastatic disease developed in 2% (3/138), 9% (5/57),

and 23% (24/105) of patients with benign, borderline, and malignant PT, respectively. In summary, most PTs are in the benign and borderline categories.[235] Histologic criteria, particularly those of Pietruszka and Barnes,[233] clearly identify a large subgroup of patients with minimal to no chance of distant metastasis.[235] Patient age, tumor size, and extent of surgery do not affect survival.

What about in-breast recurrence after breast-conserving therapy? *Local excision* (LE, removal of tumor with little or no margin) and *wide local excision* (WLE, excision with at least 1 to 2 cm of normal tissue around the tumor) are two options. Barth[235] combined the results of 20 comparable studies and found that the risk of in-breast recurrence of PT after LE was 21%, 46%, and 65% for benign, borderline, and malignant tumors, respectively. With WLE, local recurrence drops to 8%, 29%, and 36%, respectively, suggesting that excision with a negative margin is better breast-conserving treatment for PT (data from 13 studies).[205,235,236]

Several retrospective studies of PT have analyzed DNA ploidy and synthetic phase fraction with automated flow cytometry using cells isolated from archived paraffin-embedded blocks of tumor. The results have been conflicting, with most showing no correlation of DNA indices with clinical outcome.[228,230,237,238] A few studies suggest that DNA aneuploidy signifies a more guarded prognosis.[239-241] At this point, there is no proven role for DNA flow cytometry in managing this tumor.

Some early reports suggested that PT recurs locally in more malignant form,[242] but this is an inconsistent finding. That some primary tumors are inadequately sectioned and "undergraded" is a more plausible explanation for this phenomenon. PTs that are destined to recur will usually do so within 2 years of primary diagnosis. Local recurrence does not signal inevitable

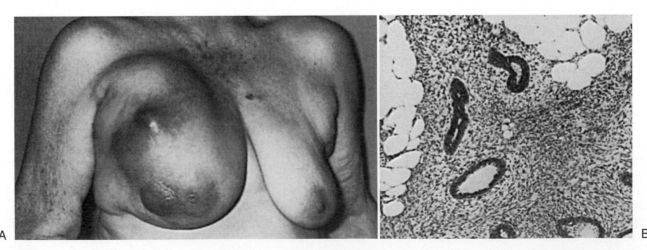

A   B

F I G. **14-6**   **A,** Malignant phyllodes tumor in a 68-year-old woman. The breast is totally replaced with a bulky, fleshy tumor that gives it a "teardrop" contour. Treatment included a total mastectomy with 3-cm margins and skin graft of the chest wall defect. **B,** Histologically malignant phyllodes tumor. Malignant cells infiltrate the surrounding mammary fat at the tumor periphery. (H&E, ×100.)

metastatic disease. Many breast recurrences can be successfully reexcised, and most patients with local recurrence do not develop metastatic disease.[231,243] Metastases always resemble the spindle cell component of the primary tumor; the benign epithelial component of PT is not malignant and does not metastasize.[212,244]

DIAGNOSIS AND TREATMENT

FNA biopsy of a PT may yield cells with features suggesting a fibroepithelial neoplasm, but it is insufficient to distinguish between some fibroadenomas and PTs.[245,246] In most cases a core biopsy can go one step further to identify usual fibroadenoma. A more challenging problem for the pathologist is to distinguish histologically benign or borderline PT from cellular fibroadenoma. This is not always possible with a small tissue sample. In adults, it is prudent to excise fibroepithelial tumors 4.0 cm or larger, enlarging masses, and those of any size where an infiltrative border is seen on the core biopsy.

Primary treatment is currently WLE. Because PT rarely spreads to lymph nodes, there is no role for routine axillary dissection.[243,244,247] PTs contain both estrogen and progesterone receptors, especially the latter.[248-250] There is currently no diagnostic or therapeutic role for hormone receptor analysis in PT.

Metastatic PT can involve any anatomic site, but it travels most commonly to lung, bone, skin, and central nervous system.[44,244,251-254] Metastatic PT is not easily treated; the role of chemotherapy with agents such as ifosfamide is currently under investigation.[252]

Mammary Lymphoma

Primary breast lymphoma is extremely rare; among patients with localized extranodal non-Hodgkin's lymphoma, only 2% have mammary lesions.[255-257] There appear to be two distinct clinicopathologic variants of mammary lymphoma. One type occurs in young women, is often bilateral, and exhibits the histologic features of a Burkitt-type lymphoma. The second, more common, disease pattern is seen in older women and is usually B-cell type.[258] This latter group includes a few mammary lymphomas with features seen in the so-called mucosa-associated lymphoid tissue (MALT) lymphomas that occur in the gastrointestinal tract and salivary glands.[258-261] Rare instances of breast involvement by Hodgkin's lymphoma have also been described.[262-265]

CLINICAL FEATURES

Most mammary lymphomas are seen first as a painless mass that tends to be larger at diagnosis than usual ductal carcinoma; the average size is 4 cm. There are no imaging features that distinguish mammary lymphoma from carcinoma.[266] The mean age at diagnosis is 60 years. In contrast to carcinoma, there is a right breast predominance; the ipsilateral axillary nodes often are involved as well.[263,267] Bilateral breast involvement, which may occur metachronously, is seen in about 10% of patients.[3]

PATHOLOGIC FEATURES

Histologically, mammary lymphoma resembles lymphoma at other anatomic sites. Characteristically, a uniform population of malignant lymphoid cells densely infiltrate the mammary lobules, effacing the normal parenchymal architecture. Diffuse large cell type is, by far, the most common histologic subtype, as is true for most extranodal lymphomas.[268,269] Large cell lymphoma can sometimes be mistaken for carcinoma,[269] but an appropriate index of suspicion and IHC staining for epithelial and lymphocyte markers can easily resolve this problem.[3] Most primary mammary lymphomas are B-cell subtype.[258,261,269] The few T-cell lymphomas appear to have an aggressive clinical course.[269,270]

TREATMENT

Total mastectomy and axillary node sampling are advocated for large, bulky primary lymphomas of the breast. However, some regionally localized tumors can be successfully treated with breast-conserving surgery and radiation.[271] Recurrent local disease and accessible regional nodal disease can be managed with radiotherapy. Chemotherapy using current regimens for non-Hodgkin's lymphoma is used for systemic or multiregional disease. Prognosis is favorable, with 5-year survival rates of 74% and a 10-year survival rate of 51%.[268]

ACKNOWLEDGMENT

Dr. John M. Daly co-authored Mesenchymal Infiltrating Tumors, the first iteration of this chapter in the first edition of *The Breast* and provided the clinical photographs.

REFERENCES

1. Enzinger FM, Weiss SW: *Soft tissue tumors*, ed 3, St Louis, 1995, Mosby.
2. Greene FL et al (eds): *AJCC cancer staging manual*, ed 6, New York, 2002, Springer-Verlag.
3. Rosen PP, Oberman HA: Tumors of the mammary gland, *Atlas of Tumor Pathology, Third Series*, Washington, DC, 1993, Armed Forces Institute of Pathology.
4. Berg JW et al: Stromal sarcomas of the breast: a unified approach to connective tissue sarcomas other than cystosarcoma phyllodes, *Cancer* 13:418, 1962.

5. Callery CD, Rosen PP, Kinne DW: Sarcoma of the breast: a study of 32 patients with reappraisal of classification and therapy, *Ann Surg* 201:527, 1985.

6. Norris HJ, Taylor HB: Sarcomas and related mesenchymal tumors of the breast, *Cancer* 22:22, 1968.

7. Barnes L, Pietruszka M: Sarcomas of the breast: a clinicopathological analysis of 10 cases, *Cancer* 40:1577, 1977.

8. Pitts WC et al: Carcinomas with metaplasia and sarcomas of the breast, *Am J Clin Pathol* 95:623, 1991.

9. Terrier PH et al: Primary breast sarcoma: a review of 33 cases with immunohistochemistry and prognostic factors, *Breast Cancer Res Treat* 13:39, 1989.

10. Fraker D: Personal communication, 2003.

11. Jones MW et al: Fibrosarcoma-malignant fibrous histiocytoma of the breast: a clinicopathological study of 32 cases, *Am J Surg Pathol* 16:667, 1992.

12. Cangiarella J et al: Malignant melanoma metastatic to the breast, *Cancer (Cancer Cytopathol)* 84:160, 1988.

13. Sneige N et al: Fine-needle aspiration cytology of metastatic neoplasms in the breast, *Am J Clin Pathol* 92:27, 1989.

14. Botham RJ, McDonald JR, Clagett OT: Sarcoma of the mammary gland, *Surg Gynecol Obstet* 197:55, 1958.

15. Oberman HA: Sarcomas of the breast, *Cancer* 18:1233, 1965.

16. Pollard SG et al: Breast sarcoma: a clinicopathologic review of 25 cases, *Cancer* 66:941, 1990.

17. Langham MR et al: Malignant fibrous histiocytoma of the breast: a case report and review of the literature, *Cancer* 54:558, 1984.

18. Ostyn C, Spector I, Bremner CG: Malignant fibrous histiocytoma of the breast, *S Afr Med J* 71:665, 1987.

19. Remer S, Tartter PI, Schwartz IS: Malignant fibrous histiocytoma of the breast: a case report and review of the literature, *Breast Dis* 1:37, 1987.

20. van Niekerk JLM et al: Malignant fibrous histiocytoma of the breast with axillary lymph node involvement, *J Surg Oncol* 34:32, 1987.

21. Vera-Sempere F, Llombart-Bosch A: Malignant fibrohistiocytoma (MFH) of the breast: primary and postirradiation variants—an ultrastructural study, *Pathol Res Pract* 178:289, 1984.

22. Hardy, TJ et al: Postirradiation sarcoma (malignant fibrous histiocytoma) of axilla, *Cancer* 42:118, 1978.

23. Tsuneyoshi M, Enjoji M: Postirradiation sarcoma (malignant fibrous histiocytoma) following breast carcinoma: an ultrastructural study of a case, *Cancer* 45:1419, 1979.

24. Lucas DR et al: Desmoid tumor is a clonal cellular proliferation: PCR amplification of HUMARA for analysis of patterns of X-chromosome inactivation, *Lab Invest* 74:10A, 1996.

25. Ali M et al: Fibromatosis of the breast, *Am J Surg Pathol* 12:501, 1979.

26. Rosen PP, Ernsberger D: Mammary fibromatosis: a benign spindle cell tumor with significant risk for local recurrence, *Cancer* 63:1363, 1989.

27. Wargotz ES et al: Fibromatosis of the breast: a clinical and pathological study of 28 cases, *Am J Surg Pathol* 11:38, 1987.

28. Burrell HC, Sibbering DM, Wilson ARM: Case report: fibromatosis of the breast in a male patient, *Br J Radiol* 68:1128, 1995.

29. Cederlund C-G et al: Fibromatosis of the breast mimicking carcinoma at mammography, *Br J Radiol* 57:98, 1984.

30. Gump FE, Steinchein MJ, Wolff M: Fibromatosis of the breast, *Surg Gynecol Obstet* 153:57, 1981.

31. Haggitt RC, Booth JL: Bilateral fibromatosis of the breast in Gardner's syndrome, *Cancer* 25:161, 1970.

32. Hanna WM, Jambrosid J, Fish E: Aggressive fibromatosis of the breast, *Arch Pathol Lab Med* 109:260, 1985.

33. Leal SM et al: Fibromatosis of the breast mimicking infiltrating carcinoma on mammography, *Breast Dis* 1:277, 1989.

34. Ormandi K et al: Extra-abdominal desmoid mimicking malignant male breast tumor, *Eur Radiol* 9:1120, 1999.

35. Dale PS et al: Desmoid tumor occurring after reconstruction mammaplasty for breast carcinoma, *Ann Plast Surg* 35:515, 1995.

36. Jewett ST, Mead JH: Extra-abdominal desmoid arising from a capsule around a silicone breast implant, *Plast Reconstr Surg* 63:577, 1979.

37. Schuh ME, Radford DM: Desmoid tumor of the breast following augmentation mammaplasty, *Plastic Reconstr Surg* 93:603, 1994.

38. Pretorius ES, Hruban RH, Fishman EK: Recurrent fibromatosis in a patient with breast carcinoma, *Invest Radiol* 30:381, 1995.

39. Abraham SC et al: Fibromatosis of the breast and mutations involving the APC/beta-catenin pathway, *Hum Pathol* 33:39, 2002.

40. Simpson RD, Harrison EG, May CW: Mesenteric fibromatosis in familial polyposis: a variant of Gardner's syndrome, *Cancer* 17:526, 1964.

41. Feiner H, Kaye GI: Ultrastructural evidence of myofibroblasts in circumscribed fibromatosis, *Arch Pathol Lab Med* 100:265, 1976.

42. Rasbridge SA, Gillert CE, Millis RR: Oestrogen and progesterone receptor expression in mammary fibromatosis, *J Clin Pathol* 46:349, 1994.

43. Reis-Filho JS et al: Primary fibromatosis of the breast in a patient with multiple desmoid tumors—report of a case with evaluation of estrogen and progesterone receptors, *Pathol Res Pract* 197:775, 2001.

44. Reference deleted in proofs.

45. Stout AP, Bernanke M: Liposarcoma of the female mammary gland, *Surg Gynecol Oncol* 83:216, 1946.

46. Austin RM, Dupree WB: Liposarcoma of the breast: a clinicopathological study of 20 cases, *Hum Pathol* 17:906, 1986.

47. Breckenridge RL: Liposarcoma of the breast: report of a case, *Am J Clin Pathol* 24:954, 1954.

48. Homes RS, Leis HP: Liposarcoma of the female breast: Review of the literature and report of a case, *J Am Geriatr Soc* 10:455, 1962.

49. Hummer CD, Burkart TJ: Liposarcoma of the breast: a case of bilateral involvement, *Am J Surg* 113:558, 1967.

50. Jackson AV: Metastasising liposarcoma of the breast arising in a fibroadenoma, *J Pathol Bacteriol* 83:582, 1962.

51. Kristensen PB, Kryger H: Liposarcoma of the breast: a case report, *Acta Chir Scand* 144:193, 1978.

52. Neal MP: Malignant tumors of the male breast, *Arch Surg* 27:427, 1933.

53. Vivian JB et al: Bilateral liposarcoma of the breast, *Aust NZ J Surg* 63:658, 1993.

54. McGregor JK: Liposarcoma of the breast: case report and review of literature, *Can Med Assoc J* 82:781, 1960.

55. Titius BR, Gohring U-J, Scharl A: Bilateral mammary carcinoma following myxoid liposarcoma of the breast, *Pathologe* 16:230, 1995.

56. Tedeschi CG: Mammary lipoma, *Arch Pathol* 46:386, 1942.

57. Lifvendahl RA: Liposarcoma of the mammary gland, *Surg Gynecol Oncol* 50:81, 1930.

58. Menon M, Velthoven PCM: Liposarcoma of the breast: a case report, *Arch Pathol* 98:370, 1974.

59. Kanemoto K, Nakamura T, Matsuyama A: Liposarcoma of the breast: review of the literature and report of a case, *Jpn J Surg* 11:381, 1981.

60. Rasmussen J, Jensen H: Liposarcoma of the breast: case report and review of the literature, *Virchows Arch A Pathol Anat Histol* 385:117, 1979.

61. Hernandez FJ: Leiomyosarcoma of male breast originating in the nipple, *Am J Surg Pathol* 3:299, 1978.

62. Arista-Nasr J et al: Primary recurrent leiomyosarcoma of the breast, *Am J Clin Pathol* 92:500, 1989.

63. Boscaino A et al: Smooth muscle tumors of the breast: clinicopathologic features of two cases, *Tumori* 80:241, 1994.

64. Chen KTK, Kuo TT, Hoffman KD: Leiomyosarcoma of the breast: a case of long survival and late hepatic metastasis, *Cancer* 47:1883, 1981.

65. Falconieri G et al: Leiomyosarcoma of the female breast: report of two new cases and a review of the literature, *Am J Clin Pathol* 108:19, 1997.

66. Gobardhan AB: Primary leiomyosarcoma of the breast, *Neth J Surg* 36:116, 1984.

67. Gonzalez-Palacios F: Leiomyosarcoma of the female breast, *Am J Clin Pathol* 109:650, 1998.

68. Jones MW et al: Smooth muscle and nerve sheath tumors of the breast: a clinicopathologic study of 45 cases, *Int J Surg Pathol* 2:85, 1994.

69. Kusama R, Fujimori M, Hama Y: Stromal sarcoma of the breast with leiomyosarcomatous pattern, *Pathol Int* 52:534, 2002.

70. Markaki S et al: Leiomyosarcoma of the breast: a clinico-pathologic and immunohistochemical study, *Eur J Obstet Gynecol* 106:233, 2003.

71. Szekely, E et al: Leiomyosarcoma of the female breast, *Pathol Oncol Res* 7:151, 2001.

72. Waterworth PD et al: Primary leiomyosarcoma of the breast, *Br J Surg* 79:169, 1992.

73. Yamashina M: Primary leiomyosarcoma in the breast, *Jpn J Clin Oncol* 17:71, 1987.

74. Lonsdale RN, Widdison A: Leiomyosarcoma of the nipple, *Histopathology* 20:537, 1992.

75. Nielsen BB: Leiomyosarcoma of the breast with late dissemination, *Virchows Arch (Pathol Anat)* 403:241, 1984.

76. Pardo-Mindan J, Garcia-Julian G, Altuna ME: Leiomyosarcoma of the breast: report of a case, *Am J Clin Pathol* 62:477, 1974.

77. Alessi E, Sala F: Leiomyosarcoma in ectopic areola, *Am J Dermatopathol* 14:165, 1992.

78. Taillibert S et al: A mesocolic leiomyosarcoma metastatic to breast: case report and review of the literature, *Anticancer Research* 20:4867, 2000.

79. Evans RW: Rhabdomyosarcoma of breast, *J Clin Pathol* 6:140, 1953.

80. Kyriazis AP, Kyriazis AA: Primary rhabdomyosarcoma of the female breast: report of a case and review of the literature, *Arch Pathol Lab Med* 122:747, 1998.

81. Woodard BH et al: Rhabdomyosarcoma of the breast, *Arch Pathol Lab Med* 104:445, 1980.

82. Herrera LJ, Lugo-Vicente H: Primary embryonal rhabdomyosarcoma of the breast in an adolescent female: a case report, *J Pediatr Surg* 33:1582, 1998.

83. Garcia CJ et al: Breast US in children and adolescents, *RadioGraphics* 20:1605, 2000.

84. Persic M, Roberts JT: Alveolar rhabdomyosarcoma metastatic to the breast: long-term survivor, *Clin Oncol (R Coll Radiol)* 11:417, 1999.

85. Rogers DA et al: Breast malignancy in children, *J Pediatr Surg* 29:48, 1994.

86. Vergier B et al: Metastases to the breast: differential diagnosis from primary breast carcinoma, *J Surg Oncol* 48:112, 1991.

87. Hanna NN, O'Donnell K, Wolfe GR: Alveolar soft part sarcoma metastatic to the breast, *J Surg Oncol* 61:159, 1996.

88. Berrada R et al: Malignant schwannoma of the breast: a case report, *J Gynecol Obstet Biol Reprod* (Paris) 27:441, 1998.

89. Catania S et al: Malignant schwannoma of the breast, *Eur J Surg Oncol* 18:80, 1992.

90. Hauser H et al: Malignant schwannoma of the breast, *Langenbecks Arch Chir* 380:350, 1995.

91. Muffarij AA, Feiner HD: Breast sarcoma with giant cells and osteoid: a case report and review of the literature, *Am J Surg Pathol* 11:225, 1987.

92. Going JJ, Lumsden AB, Anderson TJ: A classical osteogenic sarcoma of the breast: Histology, immunohistochemistry, and ultrastructure, *Histopathology* 10:631, 1986.

93. Remadi S, Doussis-Anagnostopoul I, Gee WM: Primary osteosarcoma of the breast, *Pathol Res Pract* 191:471, 1995.

94. Smith BH, Taylor HB: The occurrence of bone and cartilage in mammary tumors, *Am J Clin Pathol* 51:610, 1969.

95. Gonzalez-Licea A, Yardley JH, Hartmann WH: Malignant tumor of the breast with bone formation: studies by light and electron microscopy, *Cancer* 20:1234, 1967.

96. Spagnolo DV, Shilkin KB: Breast neoplasms containing bone and cartilage, *Virchows Arch (Pathol Anat)* 400:287, 1983.

97. Wester JG, Finlay-Jones LR: Osteogenic sarcoma of the breast, *Trop Geogr Med* 12:222, 1960.

98. Anani PA, Baumann RP: Osteosarcoma of the breast, *Virchows Arch A (Path Anat)* 357:213, 1972.

99. Chan CW, Alagaratnam TT: A bony tumour of the breast, *Aust NZ J Surg* 52:79, 1982.

100. Jernstrom P, Lindberg AL, Meland ON: Osteogenic sarcoma of the mammary gland, *Am J Clin Pathol* 40:521, 1963.

101. Kaiser U et al: Primary osteosarcoma of the breast: case report and review of the literature, *Acta Oncol* 33:74, 1994.

102. Rottino A, Howley CP: Osteoid sarcoma of the breast: a complication of fibroadenoma, *Arch Pathol* 40:44, 1945.

103. Watt AC, Haggar AM, Krasiccky GA: Extraosseous osteogenic sarcoma of the breast: Mammographic and pathologic findings, *Radiology* 150:34, 1984.

104. Silver SA, Tavassoli FA: Primary osteogenic sarcoma of the breast: a clinicopathologic analysis of 50 cases, *Am J Surg Pathol* 22:925, 1998.

105. Benediktsdottir K et al: Osteogenic sarcoma of the breast: report of a case, *Acta Pathol Microbiol Scand* (Section A) 88:161, 1980.

106. Mertens HM, Langnickel D, Staedtler F: Primary osteogenic sarcoma of the breast, *Acta Cytol* 26:512, 1982.

107. Savage AP, Sagor GR, Dovey P: Osteosarcoma of the breast: a case report with an unusual diagnostic feature, *Clin Oncol* 10:295, 1984.

108. Silver SA, Tavassoli FA: Osteosarcomatous differentiation in phyllodes tumor, *Am J Surg Pathol* 23:815, 1999.

109. Beltaos E, Banerjee TK: Chondrosarcoma of the breast: report of two cases, *Am J Clin Pathol* 71:345, 1979.

110. Guymar S et al: Breast chondrosarcoma: a case report and review, *Ann Pathol* 21:168, 2001.

111. Ladefoged C, Nielsen BB: Primary chondrosarcoma of the breast: a case report and review of the literature, *Breast* 10:26, 1984.

112. Llombart-Bosch A, Peydro A: Malignant mixed osteogenic tumours of the breast: an ultrastructural study of two cases, *Virchows Arch A Pathol Anat Histol* 366:1, 1975.

113. Merino MJ, Carter D, Berman M: Angiosarcoma of the breast, *Am J Surg Pathol* 7:53, 1983.

114. Rainwater LM et al: Angiosarcoma of the breast, *Arch Surg* 121:669, 1986.

115. Rosen PP, Kimmel M, Ernsberger D: Mammary angiosarcoma: the prognostic significance of tumor differentiation, *Cancer* 62:2145, 1988.

116. Steingaszner LC, Enzinger FM, Taylor HB: Hemangiosarcoma of the breast, *Cancer* 18:352, 1965.

117. Donnell RM et al: Angiosarcoma and other vascular tumors of the breast, *Am J Surg Pathol* 7:53, 1981.

118. McClanahan BJ, Hogg L: Angiosarcoma of the breast, *Cancer* 7:586, 1954.

119. Manssouri H et al: A rare case of angiosarcoma of the breast in a man: case report, *Eur J Gynaecol Oncol* 21:603, 2000.

120. Procter DSC: Angioma of a male breast with malignant characteristics, *S Afr Med J* 32:407, 1958.

121. Yadov RVS et al: Angiosarcoma of the male breast, *Int J Surg* 61:463, 1976.

122. Mazzocchi A et al: Kasabach-Merritt syndrome associated to angiosarcoma of the breast, *Tumori* 79:137, 1993.

123. Ryan JF, Kealy WF: Concomitant angiosarcoma and carcinoma of the breast: a case report, *Histopathol* 9:893, 1985.

124. Batchelor GB: Haemangioblastoma of the breast associated with pregnancy, *Br J Surg* 46:647, 1958.

125. Enticknap JB: Angioblastoma of the breast complicating pregnancy, *BMJ* 2:51, 1946.

126. Brentani MM, Pacheco MM, Oshima CTF: Steroid receptors in breast angiosarcoma, *Cancer* 51:2105, 1983.

127. Liberman L et al: Angiosarcoma of the breast, *Radiology* 183:649, 1992.

128. Marchant LK et al: Bilateral angiosarcoma of the breast on MR imaging, *AJR Am J Roentgenol* 169:1009, 1997.

129. Chen KTK, Kirkegaard DD, Bocian JJ: Angiosarcoma of the breast, *Cancer* 46:368, 1980.

130. Gulesserian HP, Lawton RL: Angiosarcoma of the breast, *Cancer* 24:1021, 1969.

131. De Young BR et al: CD31: An immunospecific marker for endothelial differentiation in human neoplasms, *Appl Immunohistochem* 1:97, 1993.

132. Sirgi KE, Wick MR, Swanson PE: B72.3 and CD34 immunoreactivity in malignant epithelioid soft tissue tumors: Adjuncts in the recognition of endothelial neoplasms, *Am J Surg Pathol* 17:179, 1993.

133. Burgdorf WHC, Mukai K, Rosai J: Immunohistochemical identification of factor VIII related antigen in endothelial cells of cutaneous lesions of alleged vascular structure, *Am J Clin Pathol* 75:167, 1981.

134. Antman KH et al: Multimodality therapy in the management of angiosarcoma of the breast, *Cancer* 50:2000, 1982.

135. Britt L et al: Angiosarcoma of the breast: initial misdiagnosis is still common, *Arch Surg* 130:221, 1995.

136. Bundred NJ, O'Reilly K, Smart JG: Long-term survival following bilateral breast angiosarcoma, *Eur J Surg Oncol* 15:263, 1989.

137. Myerowitz RL, Pietruszka M, Barnes EL: Primary angiosarcoma of the breast, *JAMA* 239:403, 1978.

138. Rosner D: Angiosarcoma of the breast: long-term survival following adjuvant chemotherapy, *J Surg Oncol* 39:90, 1988.

139. Stewart FW, Treves N: Lymphangiosarcoma in postmastectomy lymphedema: a report of six cases in elephantiasis chirurgica, *Cancer* 1:64, 1948.

140. McConnell AH, Haslam P: Angiosarcoma in postmastectomy lymphedema: a report of five cases and a review of the literature, *Br J Surg* 46:322, 1959.

141. Golematis BC et al: Lymphedema of the upper limb after surgery for breast cancer, *Am J Surg* 129:286, 1975.

142. d'Amore ESG et al: Primary malignant lymphoma arising in postmastectomy lymphedema: Another facet of the Stewart-Treves syndrome, *Am J Surg Pathol* 14:456, 1990.

143. Ruocco V, Schwartz RA, Ruocco E: Lymphedema: an immunologically vulnerable site for development of neoplasms, *J Am Acad Dermatol* 47:124, 2002.

144. Schreiber H, Barry FM, Russell WC: Stewart-Treves syndrome: a lethal complication of postmastectomy lymphedema and regional immune deficiency, *Arch Surg* 114:82, 1979.

145. Stark RB, Dwyer EM, DeForest M: Effect of surgical ablation of regional lymph nodes on survival of skin homografts, *Ann NY Acad Sci* 87:140, 1960.

146. Waxman M et al: Malignant lymphoma of the skin associated with postmastectomy lymphedema, *Arch Pathol Lab Med* 108:206, 1984.

147. Case records of the MGH: *N Engl J Med* 328:1337, 1993.

148. Merrick TA, Erlandson RA, Hajdu SI: Lymphangiosarcoma of a congenitally lymphedematous arm, *Arch Pathol* 91:365, 1971.

149. Muller R, Hajdu SI, Brennan MF: Lymphangiosarcoma associated with chronic filarial lymphedema, *Cancer* 59:179, 1987.

150. Sordillo PP et al: Lymphangiosarcoma, *Cancer* 48:1674, 1981.

151. Woodward AH, Ivins JC, Soule EA: Lymphangiosarcoma arising in chronically lymphedematous extremities, *Cancer* 30:562, 1972.

152. Eby CS, Brennan MJ, Fine G: Lymphangiosarcoma: a lethal complication of chronic lymphedema. Report of two cases and review of the literature, *Arch Surg* 94:223, 1967.

153. Capo V et al: Angiosarcoma arising in lymphedematous extremities: immunostaining of factor VIII-related antigen and ultrastructural features, *Hum Pathol* 16:144, 1985.

154. Kindblom L-G, Stenman G, Angervall L: Morphological and cytogenetic studies of angiosarcoma in Stewart-Treves syndrome, *Virchows Arch A (Pathol Anat)* 419:439, 1991.

155. Tomita K et al: Lymphangiosarcoma in postmastectomy lymphedema (Stewart-Treves syndrome): ultrastructural and immunohistologic characteristics, *J Surg Oncol* 38:275, 1988.

156. Miettinen M, Lehto V-P, Virtanen I: Postmastectomy angiosarcoma (Stewart-Treves syndrome): light microscopic, immunohistological, and ultrastructural characteristics of two cases, *Am J Surg Pathol* 7:329, 1983.

157. Brady MS et al: Post-treatment sarcoma in breast cancer patients, *Ann Surg Oncol* 1:66, 1994.

158. Hines JR, Murad TM, Beal JM: Prognostic indicators in cystosarcoma phylloides, *Am J Surg* 153:276, 1987.

159. Stewart NJ et al: Lymphangiosarcoma following mastectomy, *Clin Orthop Rel Res* 320:135, 1995.

160. Yap B-S et al: Chemotherapy for postmastectomy lymphangiosarcoma, *Cancer* 47:853, 1981.

161. Benda JA, Al-Jurf AS, Benson AB: Angiosarcoma of the breast following segmental mastectomy complicated by lymphedema, *Am J Clin Pathol* 87:651, 1987.

162. Fineberg S, Rosen PP: Cutaneous angiosarcoma and atypical vascular lesions of the skin and breast after radiation therapy for breast carcinoma, *Am J Clin Pathol* 102:757, 1994.

163. Givens SS et al: Angiosarcoma arising in an irradiated breast: a case report and review of the literature, *Cancer* 64:2214, 1989.

164. Joshi MG, Crosson AW, Tahan SR: Paget's disease of the nipple and angiosarcoma of the breast following excision and radiation therapy for carcinoma of the breast, *Mod Pathol* 8:1, 1995.

165. Provencio M, Bonilla F, Espana P: Breast angiosarcoma after radiation therapy, *Acta Oncol* 34:969, 1995.

166. Rubin E, Maddox WA, Mazur MT: Cutaneous angiosarcoma of the breast 7 years after lumpectomy and radiation therapy, *Radiology* 174:258, 1990.

167. Shaikh NA et al: Postirradiation angiosarcoma of the breast: a case report, *Eur J Surg Oncol* 14:449, 1988.

168. Stokkel MPM, Peterse HL: Angiosarcoma of the breast after lumpectomy and radiation therapy for adenocarcinoma, *Cancer* 69:2965, 1992.

169. Weber B: Three cases of breast angiosarcomas after breast-conserving treatment for carcinoma, *Radiother Oncol* 37:250, 1995.

170. Wijnmaalen A et al: Angiosarcoma of the breast following lumpectomy, axillary lymph node dissection, and radiotherapy for primary breast cancer: three case reports and a review of the literature, *Int J Radiat Oncol Biol Phys* 26:135, 1993.

171. Zucali R et al: Soft tissue sarcoma of the breast after conservative surgery and irradiation for early mammary cancer, *Radiother Oncol* 30:271, 1994.

172. Marchal C et al: Nine breast angiosarcomas after conservative treatment for breast carcinoma: a survey from French comprehensive cancer centers, *Int J Radiation Oncology Biol Phys* 44:113, 1999.

173. Strobbe LJA et al: Angiosarcoma of the breast after conservation therapy for invasive cancer, the incidence and outcome: an unforeseen sequela, *Breast Cancer Res Treat* 47:101, 1998.

174. Majeski J, Austin RM, Fitzgerald RH: Cutaneous angiosarcoma in an irradiated breast after breast conservation therapy for cancer: association with chronic breast lymphedema, *J Surg Oncol* 74:208, 2000.

175. de Bree E et al: Bilateral angiosarcoma of the breast after conservative treatment of bilateral invasive carcinoma: genetic predisposition? *EJSO* 28:392, 2002.

176. Deutsch M, Rosenstein MM: Angiosarcoma of the breast mimicking radiation dermatitis arising after lumpectomy and breast irradiation: a case report, *Am J Clin Oncol* 21:608, 1998.

177. Hildebrandt G et al: Cutaneous breast angiosarcoma after conserving treatment of breast cancer, *Eur J Dermatol* 11:580, 2001.

178. Feigenberg SJ et al: Angiosarcoma after breast-conserving therapy: experience with hyperfractionated radiotherapy, *Int J Radiat Oncol Biol Phys* 52:620, 2002.

179. Lester J, Stout AP: Cystosarcoma phyllodes, *Cancer* 7:335, 1954.

180. Noguchi S et al: Clonal analysis of fibroadenoma and phyllodes tumor of the breast, *Cancer Res* 53:4071, 1993.

181. Noguchi S et al: Progression of fibroadenoma to phyllodes tumor demonstrated by clonal analysis, *Cancer* 76:1779, 1995.

182. Sawyer EJ et al: Molecular analysis of phyllodes tumors reveals distinct changes in the epithelial and stroma components, *Am J Pathol* 156:1093, 2000.

183. Muller J: Uber den feinern Ban und die Formen der Krankafter Geschwulste, Lfg. I. Berlin, Reimer, 54, 1838.

184. Fiks A: Cystosarcoma phyllodes of the mammary gland—Muller's tumor: for the 180th birthday of Johannes Muller, *Virchows Arch (Pathol Anat)* 392:1, 1981.

185. Bernstein L, Deapen D, Ross RK: The descriptive epidemiology of malignant cystosarcoma phyllodes tumors of the breast, *Cancer* 71:3020, 1993.

186. Bartoli C, Zurrida SM, Clemente C: Phyllodes tumor in a male patient with bilateral gynaecomastia induced by oestrogen therapy for prostatic carcinoma, *Eur J Surg Oncol* 17:215, 1991.

187. Kahan Z et al: Recurrent phyllodes tumor in a man, *Pathol Res Pract* 193:653, 1997.

188. Nielsen VT, Andreasen C: Phyllodes tumour of the male breast, *Histopathology* 11:761, 1987.

189. Pantoja E, Llobet RE, Lopez E: Gigantic cystosarcoma phyllodes in a man with gynecomastia, *Arch Surg* 111:611, 1976.

190. Reingold IM, Ascher GS: Cystosarcoma phyllodes in a man with gynecomastia, *Am J Clin Pathol* 53:852, 1970.

191. Halling AC, Farrow GM, Bostwick DG: Prostatic phyllodes tumor: a report of six cases, *Am J Clin Pathol* 100:320, 1993.

192. Fain JS et al: Cystosarcoma phyllodes of the seminal vesicle, *Cancer* 71:2055, 1993.

193. Saleh HA, Klein LH: Cystosarcoma phyllodes arising synchronously in right breast and bilateral axillary ectopic breast tissue, *Arch Pathol Lab Med* 114:624, 1990.

194. Tbakhi A et al: Recurring phyllodes tumor in aberrant breast tissue of the vulva, *Am J Surg Pathol* 17:946, 1993.

195. Amerson JR: Cystosarcoma phyllodes in adolescent females: a report of seven patients, *Ann Surg* 171:849, 1970.

196. Mollitt DL, Golladay ES, Jimenez JF: Cystosarcoma phylloides in the adolescent female, *J Pediatr Surg* 22:907, 1987.

197. Hoover CH, Trestioreau A, Ketcham AS: Metastatic cystosarcoma phyllodes in an adolescent girl, an unusually malignant tumor, *Ann Surg* 181:279, 1975.

198. Turalba CIC, El-Mahdi AM, Ladaga L: Fatal metastatic cystosarcoma phyllodes in an adolescent female: case report and review of treatment approaches, *J Surg Oncol* 33:176, 1986.

199. Blumencranz PW, Gray GF: Cystosarcoma phyllodes: a clinical and pathological study, *NY State J Med* 78:623, 1978.

200. Liberman L et al: Benign and malignant phyllodes tumors: mammographic and sonographic findings, *Radiology* 198:121, 1996.

201. Hawkins RE et al: The clinical and histologic criteria that predict metastases from cystosarcoma phyllodes, *Cancer* 69:141, 1992.

202. Hart WR, Bauer RC, Oberman HA: Cystosarcoma phyllodes: a clinicopathologic study of 26 hypercellular periductal stromal tumors of the breast, *Am J Clin Pathol* 70:21, 1978.

203. Norris HJ, Taylor HB: Relationship of histologic features to behavior of cystosarcoma phyllodes: analysis of 94 cases, *Cancer* 20:2090, 1967.

204. Gogas JG: Cystosarcoma phyllodes: a clinicopathological analysis of 14 cases, *Int Surg* 64:77, 1979.

205. Schmidt B et al: Cystosarcoma phyllodes, *Isr J Med Sci* 17:895, 1981.

206. Treves N, Sunderland DA: Cystosarcoma of the breast: a malignant and a benign tumor: clinicopathological study of 75 cases, *Cancer* 4:1286, 1951.

207. Cole-Beuglet C et al: Ultrasound, x-ray mammography, and histopathology of cystosarcoma phylloides, *Radiology* 146:481, 1983.

208. Farria DM et al: Benign phyllodes tumor of the breast: MR imaging features, *AJR Am J Roentgenol* 167:187, 1996.

209. McDivitt RW, Urban JA, Farrow JH: Cystosarcoma phyllodes, *Johns Hopkins Med J* 120:33, 1967.

210. Reference deleted in proofs.

211. Reddick RL et al: Stromal proliferation of the breast: an ultrastructural and immunohistochemical evaluation of cystosarcoma phyllodes, juvenile fibroadenoma, and fibroadenoma, *Hum Pathol* 18:45, 1987.

212. Lindquist KD et al: Recurrent and metastatic cystosarcoma phyllodes, *Am J Surg* 144:341, 1982.

213. Aranda FI, Laforga JB, Lopez JI: Phyllodes tumor of the breast: an immunohistochemical study of 28 cases with special attention to the role of myofibroblasts, *Pathol Res Pract* 190:474, 1994.

214. Auger M, Hanna W, Kahn HJ: Cystosarcoma phylloides of the breast and its mimics: an immunohistochemical and ultrastructural study, *Arch Pathol Lab Med* 113:1231, 1989.

215. Fernandez BB, Hernandez KJ, Spindler W: Metastatic cystosarcoma phyllodes: a light and electron microscopic study, *Cancer* 37:1737, 1976.

216. Harris M, Khan MK: Phyllodes tumour and stromal sarcoma of the breast: an ultrastructural comparison, *Histopathology* 8:315, 1984.

217. Barnes L, Pietruszka M: Rhabdomyosarcoma arising within a cystosarcoma phyllodes: case report and review of the literature, *Am J Surg Pathol* 2:423, 1978.

218. DeLuca LA, Traiman P, Bacchi CE: An unusual case of malignant cystosarcoma phyllodes of the breast, *Gynecol Oncol* 24:91, 1986.

219. Kay S: Light and electron microscopic studies of a malignant cystosarcoma phyllodes featuring stromal cartilage and bone, *Am J Clin Pathol* 53:852, 1970.

220. Oberman HA, Nosanchuk JS, Finger JE: Periductal stromal tumors of the breast with adipose metaplasia, *Arch Surg* 98:384, 1969.

221. Quizilbash AH: Cystosarcoma phyllodes with liposarcomatous stroma, *Am J Clin Pathol* 65:321, 1976.

222. Rosen PP, Romain K, Liberman L: Mammary cystosarcoma with mature adipose stromal differentiation (lipophyllodes tumor) arising in a lipomatous hamartoma, *Arch Pathol Lab Med* 118:91, 1994.

223. Christensen L, Nielsen M, Madsen PM: Cystosarcoma phyllodes: a review of 19 cases with emphasis on the occurrence of associated breast carcinoma, *Acta Path Microbiol Immunol Scand* (Section A) 94:35, 1986.

224. Grove A, Kristensen LD: Intraductal carcinoma within a phyllodes tumor of the breast: a case report, *Tumori* 72:187, 1986.

225. Ishida T, Izuo M, Kawai T: Breast carcinoma arising in cystosarcoma phyllodes: report of a case with a review of the literature, *Jpn J Clin Oncol* 14:99, 1984.

226. Knudsen PJT, Ostergaard J: Cystosarcoma phylloides with lobular and ductal carcinoma in situ, *Arch Pathol Lab Med* 111:873, 1987.

227. Seemayer TA, Tremblay G, Shibata H: The unique association of mammary stromal sarcoma with intraductal carcinoma, *Cancer* 36:599, 1975.

228. Grimes MM: Cystosarcoma phyllodes of the breast: histologic features, flow cytometric analysis, and clinical correlations, *Mod Pathol* 5:232, 1992.

229. Hart J et al: Practical aspects in the diagnosis and management of cystosarcoma phyllodes, *Arch Surg* 123:1079, 1988.

230. Keelan PA et al: Phyllodes tumor: clinicopathologic review of 60 patients and flow cytometric analysis in 30 patients, *Hum Pathol* 23:1048, 1992.

231. Moffat CJC et al: Phyllodes tumours of the breast: a clinicopathological review of 32 cases, *Histopathology* 27:205, 1995.

232. Oberman HA: Cystosarcoma phyllodes: a clinicopathologic study of hypercellular periductal stromal neoplasms of breast, *Cancer* 18:697, 1965.

233. Pietruszka M, Barnes L: Cystosarcoma phyllodes: a clinicopathologic analysis of 42 cases, *Cancer* 41:1974, 1978.

234. Ward RM, Evans HL: Cystosarcoma phyllodes: a clinicopathologic study of 26 cases, *Cancer* 58:2282, 1986.

235. Barth RJ: Histologic features predict local recurrence after breast-conserving therapy of phyllodes tumor, *Breast Cancer Res Treat* 57:291, 1999.

236. Blichert-Toft M et al: Clinical course of cystosarcoma phyllodes related to histologic appearance, *Surg Gynecol Obstet* 140:929, 1975.

237. Layfield LJ et al: Relation between DNA ploidy and the clinical behavior of phyllodes tumors, *Cancer* 64:1486, 1989.

238. Palko MJ et al: Flow cytometric S fraction as a predictor of clinical outcome in cystosarcoma phyllodes, *Arch Pathol Lab Med* 114:949, 1990.

239. El-Naggar A et al: DNA content and proliferative activity of cystosarcoma phyllodes of the breast, *Am J Clin Pathol* 93:480, 1990.

240. Mies C, Rosen PP, Daly J: DNA analysis of cystosarcoma phyllodes, *Lab Invest* 64:13A, 1991.

241. Murad TM et al: Histopathological and clinical correlations of cystosarcoma phyllodes, *Arch Pathol Lab Med* 112:752, 1988.

242. Hajdu SI, Espinosa MH, Robbins GF: Recurrent cystosarcoma phyllodes: a clinicopathologic study of 32 cases, *Cancer* 38:1402, 1976.

243. Salvadori B et al: Surgical treatment of phyllodes tumors of the breast, *Cancer* 63:2532, 1989.

244. Kessinger A et al: Metastatic cystosarcoma phyllodes: a case report and review of the literature, *J Surg Oncol* 4:131, 1972.

245. Simi U et al: Fine-needle aspiration cytopathology of phyllodes tumor: Differential diagnosis with fibroadenoma, *Acta Cytol* 32:63, 1988.

246. Stawicki ME, Hsiu J-G: Malignant cystosarcoma phyllodes: a case report with cytologic presentation, *Acta Cytol* 23:61, 1979.

247. Mincowitz S et al: Cystosarcoma phyllodes: a unique case with multiple unilateral lesions and ipsilateral axillary metastases, *J Pathol* 96:514, 1968.

248. Kesterson GHN et al: Cystosarcoma phyllodes: a steroid receptor and ultrastructure analysis, *Ann Surg* 190:640, 1979.

249. Palshof T et al: Estradiol binding protein in cystosarcoma phyllodes of the breast, *Eur J Cancer* 16:591, 1980.

250. Rao BR, Meyer JS, Fry CG: Most cystosarcomas phyllodes and fibrosarcomas have progesterone receptor but lack estrogen receptor: stromal localization of progesterone receptor, *Cancer* 47:2016, 1981.

251. Grimes MM, Lattes R, Jaretzki A: Cystosarcoma phyllodes: report of an unusual case with death due to intraneural extension to the central nervous system, *Cancer* 56:1691, 1985.

252. Hawkins RE et al: Ifosfamide is an active drug for chemotherapy of metastatic cystosarcoma phyllodes, *Cancer* 69:2271, 1992.

253. Hlavin ML et al: Central nervous system complications of cystosarcoma phyllodes, *Cancer* 72:126, 1993.

254. Rhodes RH et al: Metastatic cystosarcoma phyllodes: a report of two cases presenting with neurological symptoms, *Cancer* 41:1179, 1978.

255. Fischer M, Chideckel N: Primary lymphoma of the breast, *Breast* 10:7, 1984.

256. Smith MR, Brustein S, Straus DJ: Localized non-Hodgkin's lymphoma of the breast, *Cancer* 59:351, 1987.

257. Wiseman C, Liao K: Primary lymphoma of the breast, *Cancer* 29:1705, 1972.

258. Bobrow LG et al: Breast lymphomas: a clinicopathologic review, *Hum Pathol* 24:274, 1993.

259. Aozasa K et al: Malignant lymphoma of the breast: immunologic type and association with lymphocytic mastopathy, *Am J Clin Pathol* 97:699, 1992.

260. Lamovec J, Jancar J: Primary malignant lymphoma of the breast: lymphoma of the mucosa-associated lymphoid tissue, *Cancer* 60:3033, 1987.

261. Pelstring RJ et al: Diversity of organ site involvement among malignant lymphomas of mucosa-associated tissues, *Am J Clin Pathol* 96:738, 1991.

262. Blaustein JC, Lewkow L: Recurrent "syncytial variant" of Hodgkin's disease: an immunohistologic diagnosis, *Hum Pathol* 18:746, 1987.

263. Dixon JM et al: Primary lymphoma of the breast, *Br J Surg* 74:214, 1987.

264. Graeme-Cook F, O'Briain DS, Daly PA: Unusual breast masses: the sequential development of mammary tuberculosis and Hodgkin's disease in a young woman, *Cancer* 61:1457, 1988.

265. Meis J, Butler JJ, Osborne BM: Hodgkin's disease involving the breast and chest wall, *Cancer* 57:1859, 1986.

266. Liberman L et al: Non-Hodgkin lymphoma of the breast: imaging characteristics and correlation with histopathologic findings, *Radiology* 192:157, 1994.

267. DeCosse J et al: Primary lymphosarcoma of the breast: a review of 14 cases, *Cancer* 15:1264, 1962.

268. Brustein S et al: Malignant lymphoma of the breast: a study of 53 patients, *Ann Surg* 205:144, 1987.

269. Lin Y, Govindan R, Hess JL: Malignant hematopoietic breast tumors, *Am J Clin Pathol* 107:177, 1997.

270. Aguilera NSI et al: T-cell lymphoma presenting in the breast: a histologic, immunophenotypic, and molecular genetic study of four cases, *Mod Pathol* 13:599, 2000.

271. DeBlasio D et al: Definitive Irradiation for localized non-Hodgkin's lymphoma of the breast, *Int J Radiat Oncol Biol Phys* 17:843, 1989.

CHAPTER

15

Epithelial Neoplasms and Dermatologic Disorders

FRANKLIN P. FLOWERS
JOY KUNISHIGE
DIANE MULLINS

Chapter Outline

The skin of the breast, similar to other truncal skin, consists of keratinizing stratified squamous epithelium overlying a relatively thick dermis. Adnexal structures, primarily hair follicles and eccrine glands, blood vessels, lymphatics, and cutaneous nerves, reside within the dermis. The subcutaneous fatty tissue that envelops the mammary ducts and glands proliferates, as a result of hormonal influences, especially at puberty and during pregnancy. The highly specialized skin of the nipple has a papillomatous surface and numerous openings for lactiferous ducts, sebaceous glands, and apocrine glands. Areolar skin is similar but may have a few vellus or terminal hairs and clusters of large sebaceous glands (the tubercles of Montgomery). These units also contain lactation ductlike foci that produce milklike substances.[1,2]

Numerous dermal disorders, including congenital anomalies, benign and malignant neoplasms, and manifestations of localized and systemic dermatoses, may involve the skin of the breast. This chapter discusses conditions that are unique to the skin of the breast or that have an unusual or modified appearance compared with a similar lesion elsewhere on the body. Additional information may be found in standard textbooks on dermatology.

Congenital Hypoplasia and Developmental Anomalies

Bilateral hypoplasia of the breast may occur in Turner's (XO) syndrome. *Hypomastia,* defined as breast size of 200 ml or less in an adult female, may occur in otherwise healthy women or in association with mitral valve prolapse.[3] *Acquired hypoplasia* is associated with wasting diseases such as human immunodeficiency virus (HIV) infection, anorexia nervosa, and tuberculosis. *Unilateral hypoplasia* has been described in the Poland anomaly—unilateral absence of the sternocostal portion of the pectoralis major muscle, ipsilateral syndactyly, absence of axillary hair, and abnormal fingerprint patterns.[4] Unilateral hypoplasia has been described in association with large, irregularly shaped melanotic macules that cover the hypoplastic breast and wrap laterally onto the back. Basilar hyperpigmentation of melanocytes without significant melanocytic hyperplasia is seen on histologic examination.[5] *Morphea* (localized scleroderma) of the chest wall in a prepubertal child may lead to deformity and hypoplasia of the breast in later years.[6]

Becker's nevus is a hamartoma of pigmented epidermis, terminal hairs, and erector pili muscles usually found on the chest, shoulder, upper back, or upper arm. It is an androgen-dependent lesion that typically appears in males in the second and third decades but

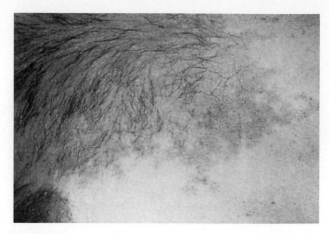

F I G. **15-1** Becker's nevus: large pigmented macule with irregular borders and numerous coarse terminal hairs on the lateral chest wall.

occasionally affects females. Rarely, this benign pigmented lesion, which is often mistaken clinically for a giant pigmented hairy melanocytic nevus, is associated with abnormalities of the underlying musculoskeletal system, including spina bifida, scoliosis, localized lipoatrophy, and hypoplasia of the pectoralis muscle (Figure 15-1).[7-10]

Rudimentary (absent or maldeveloped) nipples may be present as an isolated congenital defect or as a component of the *SEN* (scalp, ears, nipple) *syndrome.*[11-13] This disorder is inherited in an autosomal dominant fashion. Cutaneous manifestations include aplasia cutis congenita of the scalp, protuberant cupped or folded external ears, and sparse axillary hair. The malformed nipple appears as a small dimple without pigmentation or recognizable structure; the breast may also fail to develop.

Polythelia (supernumerary nipples) or *polymastia* (supernumerary breasts) develops along embryonic lines that stretch from the axillas to the inner thighs. Notably, vulvar lesions that previously were termed *supernumerary nipples* actually represent adenomas of vulvar apocrine—or mammary-like glands; the so-called milk lines do not cross the vulva. Most supernumerary breast tissue takes the form of insignificant, gently raised, pigmented papules. Histologically, these accessory structures may consist of nipple, areola, or glandular tissue in any combination. Hyperplasia, adenomas, and rarely carcinomas can involve these tissues, as they do the breast proper.

In a study from Japan, small *benign adnexal polyps* of the areola were reported to involve 4% of neonates. These small (1-mm), firm, pink papules contain hair follicles, eccrine glands, and vestigial sebaceous glands. Most wither rapidly and fall off shortly after birth.[14]

The rare familial syndrome of *hereditary acrolabial telangiectasia* consists of an extensive network of superficial, thin-walled vessels and variable proliferation of vessels in the deeper soft tissues. These superficial vessels impart a bluish hue to the lips, areolas, nipples, and nail beds, which may be mistaken for cyanosis at birth. Varicose veins and migraine headaches may develop in adulthood. No serious vascular or coagulative sequelae have been reported in these persons.[15]

Inflammatory Dermatoses

The most common inflammatory disorders of the skin of the breast fall into the group of papulosquamous and eczematous diseases (Table 15-1). The lesions appear as discrete, oval, or irregular-shaped patches with overlying fine to coarse scale and surrounding erythema. Inflammatory disorders of the nipple, subcutaneous tissue, and vasculature are also discussed here.

Seborrheic dermatitis is marked clinically by its characteristic distribution in the scalp, eyebrows, eyelid margins, cheeks, nasolabial folds and paranasal areas, external ear canals, beard, and presternal area. Although generally a dry, powdery scale, when there is extensive presternal or inframammary involvement, the lesions may have coarser scales on an erythematous base with

TABLE **15-1**	Differential Diagnosis of Common Scaly Disorders of the Skin of the Breast

INFLAMMATORY DERMATOSES

Seborrheic dermatitis

Psoriasis

Pityriasis rosea

Chronic contact dermatitis

Discoid lupus erythematosus

Darier's disease

Nummular eczema

Nipple eczema

Jogger's nipples

INFECTIONS

Erythrasma

Tinea corporis

Tinea versicolor

NEOPLASMS

Lichen planus–like keratosis

Actinic keratosis

Superficial basal cell carcinoma

Bowen's disease

Paget's disease

Mycosis fungoides

follicular pustules. The clinical course is chronic, with remissions and exacerbations. Low-potency topical steroids are the treatment of choice. Topical antifungal treatment (ketoconazole [Nizoral]) has also been successful; the yeast *Pityrosporum ovales* is believed to play a role.[16] Differential diagnosis includes psoriasis, tinea corporis, tinea versicolor, erythrasma, and contact dermatitis. *Psoriasis* is differentiated by characteristic lesions on the elbows, knees, and other extensor body surfaces. Psoriasis, especially when it involves the areola or nipple, may be difficult to distinguish clinically from Bowen's disease (squamous cell carcinoma in situ). A biopsy readily distinguishes the two entities. The expanding oval lesions of *tinea corporis* and *tinea versicolor* have a peripheral collarette of scale and more haphazard distribution, and fungal hyphae may be identified on KOH preparation in the office or in biopsy specimens.

Erythrasma is a superficial cutaneous bacterial infection caused by the organism *Corynebacterium minutissimum*. Although usually intertriginous, disciform erythrasma presents as a well-demarcated, oval, reddish brown patch with fine scaling. Both clinical forms may be diagnosed by the characteristic coral-red fluorescence under Wood's light. Treatment consists of oral or topical erythromycin.[17]

Contact dermatitis most often results from a nickel allergy, and the lesions appear under bra straps and hooks in the shape of the offending metal part. Other common causes of contact dermatitis are topical medications, perfumes, latex, and airborne allergens. A careful history of environmental exposures and the use of patch tests usually identify the offending agent. Histologic examination of a biopsy specimen shows a spongiotic dermatitis with eosinophils; changes resulting from chronic rubbing (lichen simplex chronicus) may also be present if the exposure is of long standing.

Other papulosquamous disorders to consider include *pityriasis rosea*, with its oval, finely scaling, salmon-colored patches, and *lupus erythematosus*.

Darier's disease (keratosis follicularis) is an uncommon, autosomal dominant papulosquamous disorder with a seborrheic dermatitis–like distribution. The affected skin develops firm, discrete, 2- to 3-mm, red to brown spiny papules that make the skin look dirty and that may coalesce to form large plaques (Figure 15-2). The disease can be exacerbated by heat, high humidity, exposure to ultraviolet or ionizing radiation, or trauma. Secondary bacterial or fungal infection is common. This disorder has a characteristic, although not pathognomonic, histologic appearance. Individual keratinocytes in the suprabasal layer dissociate from their adjacent keratinocytes because of loss of intercellular bridges (acantholysis). These acantholytic cells undergo premature keratinization (dyskeratosis) and are shed as

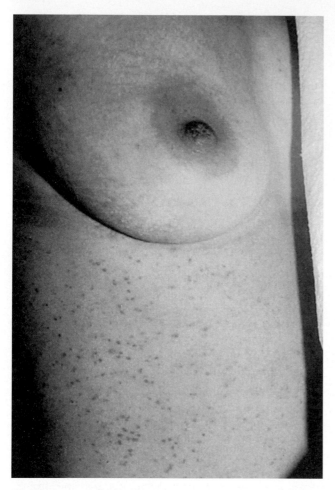

FIG. **15-2** Darier's disease (keratosis follicularis): discrete, red to brown spiny papules on the trunk.

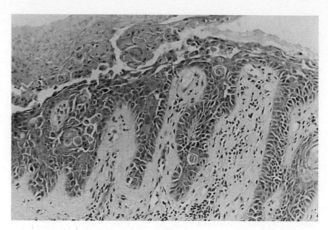

FIG. **15-3** Darier's disease. A thick, compact stratum corneum overlies an acantholytic process within the epidermis. Individual dyskeratotic and acantholytic cells are present within the stratum spinosum, and rounded dyskeratotic cells with shrunken nuclei (corps ronds) and flattened, oat-shaped dyskeratotic cells are seen in the superficial layer of the epidermis immediately beneath the stratum corneum.

shrunken, round, or flattened cells (corp ronds and grains; Figure 15-3). Oral synthetic retinoids may be used to control the primary lesions, although the disease recurs when retinoids are discontinued. Case reports suggest topical 5-fluorouracil and adapalene 0.1% gel are successful and more easily tolerated alternatives.[18,19] Avoiding or minimizing exposure to exacerbating factors is a mainstay of therapy. Appropriate topical or oral antibiotics may be used to combat documented secondary infections. *Grover's disease*, or *transient acantholytic dermatosis*, exhibits a nearly identical histologic picture but is characterized clinically by an eruption of itchy papules and macules on the upper chest and back of adults. There is no familial predisposition, and the disease is self-limited.

Several inflammatory diseases involve the nipple and areola and can mimic a malignant process. *Nummular eczema* presents as single or multiple erythematous, slightly raised plaques with fine to moderate scale, slight oozing, and pruritus. Involvement of the nipple (nipple eczema) may mimic Paget's disease or Bowen's disease. Involvement localized to a mastectomy scar may raise suspicion of breast carcinoma recurrence. A punch biopsy specimen of eczema shows spongiotic dermatitis with variable features of chronicity and rules out malignancy. Nummular eczema may be difficult to distinguish from chronic allergic contact dermatitis; patch testing may identify an offending allergen. *Jogger's nipples* refers to a specific pattern of nipple irritation caused by chronic friction from loose-fitting clothing.[20] Finally, the human mite *Sarcoptes scabiei* can infest the nipple, areola, and inframammary creases and present with extreme pruritus and excoriation. Scrapings mixed on a slide with a drop of oil then coverslipped reveal the organism's eggs and feces. Topical scabicides usually eradicate the mite.

Three forms of *radiation dermatitis* can involve the skin of the breast. The first and most common type is erythema with fine scale that develops during the course of radiotherapy. This is uncomfortable but self-limited and generally can be managed with soothing topical treatments. Months to years later, scarring, atrophy, telangiectasia, and scaling may overlie old radiation portals. This form of radiodermatitis is rare but chronic and may progress to tissue necrosis, ulceration, and de novo cutaneous malignancies (usually squamous cell carcinoma or basal cell carcinoma). Finally, patients who have previously received radiation therapy may develop *radiation recall dermatitis* when exposed to subsequent chemotherapy agents: A painful, erythematous macular papular rash erupts over the previous radiation port site.[21-25] *Vitiligo* has also been reported following radiotherapy.[26] Vascular lesions developing in radiation fields are discussed in the section on neoplasms.

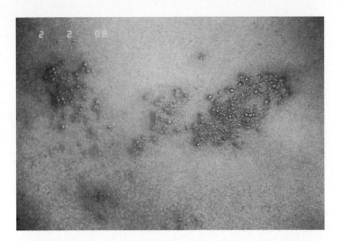

FIG. **15-4** Herpes zoster (shingles): clear fluid-filled grouped vesicles on an erythematous base following a thoracic dermatome.

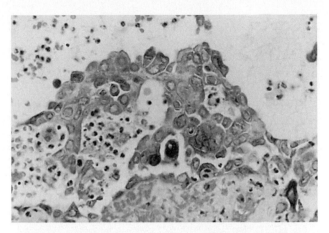

FIG. **15-6** Herpes zoster: viral cytopathic effect. Multinucleated giant keratinocytes within the epidermis and within a hair follicle, and focal leukocytoclastic vasculitis affecting the superficial capillary plexus.

Primary blistering or bullous cutaneous eruptions of the breast are relatively uncommon. Of these, the most common is *herpes zoster (shingles)*, which manifests as severe stinging, burning pain in a dermatomal distribution, followed within a few days by a papulovesicular eruption with small, grouped vesicles on an erythematous base (Figure 15-4). Constitutional symptoms such as fever, headache, and malaise may precede or accompany a severe outbreak. Postherpetic neuralgia persists in as many as 15% of patients. Tzanck smear shows multinucleate keratinocytes with nuclear molding. A biopsy usually is not necessary but shows characteristic viral cytopathologic features of ballooning and reticular degeneration of keratinocytes, multinucleate keratinocytes with ground-glass nuclei and nuclear molding, and leukocytoclastic vasculitis in the underlying small dermal capillaries (Figures 15-5 and 15-6). Prompt administration of antiviral drugs (e.g., famciclovir) leads to resolution of the primary lesion, with a marked decrease in the incidence, severity, and duration

of postherpetic neuralgia. Topical capsaicin may also be used to control the pain of postherpetic neuralgia. Rarely, *cutaneous herpes simplex* with axillary adenopathy infects the nipple of a mother who is breastfeeding a baby with herpetic gingivostomatitis. Viral cultures of mother and baby establish the diagnosis.[27]

Improper or prolonged breastfeeding may result in exquisitely painful, small (1- to 3-mm), translucent vesicles or sore, cracked, fissured nipples. Viral and bacterial cultures are negative. Soothing topical treatments applied immediately after nursing and gently washed off before the next feeding may be helpful.

Panniculitis (inflammation of the subcutaneous tissue) may be encountered in the breast. *Silicone granulomas* appear as painful, irregularly shaped lumps or plaques in patients who have received injections of free silicone or whose silicone implants have ruptured. Microscopic examination of this tissue shows a characteristic "Swiss cheese" granulomatous inflammatory pattern where the silicone has dissolved out of multinucleate giant cells and extracellular areas during histologic processing. *Factitial panniculitis* arises from repetitive self-harm. Possible presentations may mimic virtually any dermatosis and include excoriation, ulceration, puncture wounds and embedded foreign bodies, eczema, vesiculobullous lesions, and nipple discharge. Factitial disease should be considered when an unusual pattern or presentation is not consistent with established clinicopathologic entities or when the patient exhibits an unusual or strange affect or response to the problem. Careful clinical evaluation with mammography and biopsy, if necessary, should be taken to rule out primary organic disease of the breast. Psychiatric evaluation should be recommended.

Scleroderma appears as a firm, indurated, white plaque with a central depression and faintly violaceous

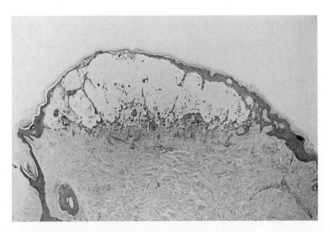

FIG. **15-5** Herpes zoster: a tense, fluid-filled blister containing a few inflammatory cells and degenerated keratinocytes.

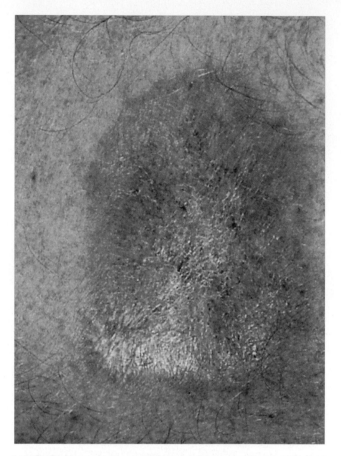

FIG. **15-7** Scleroderma (morphea): well-demarcated patch with central pallor and atrophy and a peripheral violaceous rim.

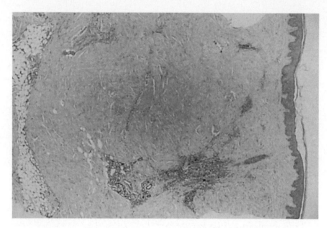

FIG. **15-8** Scleroderma (morphea). Punch biopsy shows dense dermal collagen with sclerosis of the collagen at the dermal-subcutaneous tissue interface and a superficial and deep perivascular and periadnexal lymphoplasmacytic inflammatory infiltrate.

borders (Figure 15-7). This may be the only lesion (localized scleroderma, linear scleroderma, or morphea) or may be associated with systemic sclerosis or the CREST syndrome (calcinosis cutis, Raynaud's phenomenon, esophageal involvement, sclerodactyly, and telangiectasia). The differential diagnosis includes scar, sclerotic carcinoma, sclerodermoid graft-versus-host disease, and dermatomyofibroma.[28,29] Biopsy shows thickened sclerotic collagen, particularly at the interface of the reticular dermis and the subcutaneous tissue with a sparse to mild lymphoplasmacytic inflammatory infiltrate (Figure 15-8). Therapy consists of potent topical steroids or steroids under occlusion, but although progression of the lesion may be inhibited, the plaque generally does not resolve.

Coumarin necrosis occurs in patients with inborn or acquired abnormalities of the coagulation cascade, particularly deficiencies of protein C or protein S. These patients develop seemingly paradoxical intravascular coagulation with initiation of warfarin anticoagulant therapy, owing to depletion of vitamin K–dependent antithrombosis factors. The intravascular thrombi form preferentially in relatively cool, fatty areas of the body such as breasts, buttocks, and abdominal panniculus

and are exquisitely painful. Widespread ischemic tissue necrosis is the usual outcome. Prevention through prior anticoagulation with heparin before initiation of warfarin therapy is recommended.[30] Similar pyoderma gangrenosum–like ulcerative lesions have been reported in patients with *lupus anticoagulant* syndrome.[31]

Mondor's disease is a superficial thrombophlebitis of the thoracoepigastric, lateral thoracic, or superior epigastric vein. The usual presentation is a tender, firm, linear cord. Affected patients are usually in the third to fifth decade, and women outnumber men 3 to 1. Most cases are idiopathic; a few can be related to trauma, surgery, illness, or another skin condition near the involved vessel.[32] One historic case of breast carcinoma presenting as Mondor's disease has been reported; inflammatory breast carcinoma should always be considered.[33] Treatment is symptomatic, and most cases resolve in several weeks.

Cutaneous Neoplasms

Like inflammatory dermatoses, most neoplasms of the skin of the breast occur elsewhere on the integument also, and it is beyond the scope of this chapter to describe all of them. The following discussion has been limited to lesions that are of special interest because of their presentation, implications, or differential diagnosis.

BENIGN EPITHELIAL NEOPLASMS

The most common epithelial neoplasm of the breast is *seborrheic keratosis*. The lesions are unattractive, warty, waxy papules and small plaques that sit on the surface of the skin. Their color generally ranges from tan to brown to shades of gray, but shades of red may also be seen. Bleeding and crusting are common, particularly in lesions that the patient manipulates or that are constantly irritated by clothing. A patient may have only a few or a hundred or more keratoses, which develop synchronously or metachronously. The *sign of Leser-Trelat* is the sudden appearance of numerous seborrheic keratoses in a patient with an internal malignancy and is related to high levels of circulating epidermal growth factor, presumably produced by the tumor. Although many histologic variants of seborrheic keratoses have been described, all exhibit hyperkeratosis, papillomatosis, acanthosis, horn cysts, and variable inflammation. Treatment consists of ablation of bothersome lesions.

Lichen planus–like keratoses, also called *benign lichenoid keratoses*, are solitary (rarely multiple) 5- to 20-mm, bright red, violaceous, or brown plaques on the chest and upper back. Clinically, they can mimic lentigo and other pigmented lesions, superficial basal cell carcinoma, or squamous cell carcinoma in situ. The histologic features are virtually identical to those of lichen planus with hyperkeratosis, hypergranulosis, acanthosis, and a dense bandlike lymphocytic inflammatory infiltrate at the base of the lesion; site and clinical presentation distinguish these two disorders.

Adnexal tumors of pilosebaceous origin that occur on the breast are usually cystic and include the epidermoid cyst (formerly called *cyst of follicular infundibulum, epidermal inclusion cyst*, or *sebaceous cyst*), *trichilemmal cyst (pilar cyst), pilomatrixoma, eruptive vellus hair cyst*, and *steatocystoma. Eruptive vellus hair cysts* are asymptomatic 1- to 2-mm follicular papules that appear suddenly late in childhood or in early adulthood and have an autosomal dominant inheritance pattern (Figure 15-9). Histologic examination reveals a cyst lined by stratified, squamous keratinizing epithelium filled with laminated keratin debris and one to many small, vellus hairs. Rupture with accompanying granulomatous

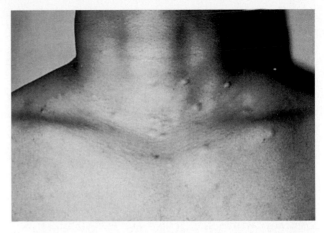

FIG. **15-10** Steatocystoma multiplex: numerous soft, yellow papules on the anterior chest and neck.

inflammation is common. Some hypothesize that eruptive vellus hair cysts and steatocystomas are variants of one disorder.[34] *Steatocystomas* are small, solitary (steatocystoma simplex) or multiple (steatocystoma multiplex), 1- to 5-mm yellowish papules containing a creamy or oily fluid. Steatocystoma multiplex is inherited in an autosomal dominant fashion (Figure 15-10). These cysts are lined by thin, stratified squamous epithelium with a prominent homogeneous, eosinophilic, folded cuticle, mimicking a sebaceous duct. Flattened sebaceous lobules may be seen in contiguity with the epithelial lining (Figure 15-11). The cysts usually appear empty, because the oily substance within them is dissolved during processing. Adnexal tumors can be excised. Successful eradication of multiple eruptive hair cysts with erbium: YAG laser has been reported.[35]

Eccrine tumors that have been reported to occur on the breast include *eccrine poromas* (a tumor of the intraepithelial portion of the eccrine duct), *hidradenomas* (a tumor of the straight portion of the eccrine duct), and

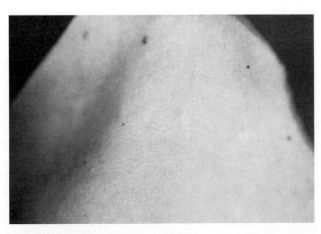

FIG. **15-9** Vellus hair cysts: small, 1- to 2-mm flesh-colored papules on the shoulder and upper chest.

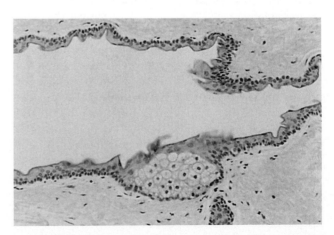

FIG. **15-11** Steatocystoma: cyst lined by thin, stratified squamous epithelium with a hyaline cuticle. Note the sebaceous lobule in the wall.

spiradenomas (a tumor of the deep coiled gland). Eccrine poromas appear clinically as solitary, pedunculated, red or flesh-colored lesions that are often mistaken for pyogenic granulomas. Histologic examination shows a proliferation of broad, anastomosing bands of small, cuboidal cells beneath a flattened epidermis. Within these broad bands of epithelium are small, often slitlike, duct spaces. The absence of peripheral palisading is an important distinguishing feature from basal cell carcinoma. The intervening stroma is edematous and richly vascular.

Hidradenomas are solitary intradermal tumors, 0.5 to 2.0 cm in diameter, with intact overlying skin. Microscopically, within the dermis are well-circumscribed, sometimes encapsulated, lobules of polygonal and cuboidal cells in which are embedded simple tubular ducts. The polygonal cells have round nuclei with basophilic cytoplasm and indistinct cell borders. The cuboidal cells have clear or pale cytoplasm; when clear cells are numerous, the tumor may be termed *clear cell hidradenoma*. Reduplicated basement membrane material, appearing as homogeneous, dull, eosinophilic masses, is often present within or surrounding the tumor. Mitoses may be present and, unless atypical in appearance, should not be taken as a sign of malignancy.

Spiradenomas present as solitary, markedly tender, deep dermal or subcutaneous masses. Microscopic examination reveals deeply basophilic, sharply demarcated lobules of small cuboidal cells within the dermis and subcutaneous tissue. Two types of epithelial cells are present. One cell type consists of cells with relatively large, centrally placed clear nuclei and scant cytoplasm that forms ductular structures. The second cell type— smaller, with small, dark nuclei and wispy basophilic cytoplasm—is found primarily at the periphery of the lobules. As in hidradenomas, abundant hyaline-like, reduplicated basement material may be found. Simple but complete excision of eccrine tumors is the appropriate management.

Erosive adenomatosis or papillary adenoma of the nipple presents most often in a perimenopausal woman with crusting or oozing of one nipple. Clinically the lesion mimics Paget's disease or nipple eczema. The affected nipple appears eroded or ulcerated, and a serous discharge is common; a subareolar mass may be present. On histologic examination, two patterns of growth are evident. The first pattern associated with erosive lesions is adenomatous: A proliferation of round, oval, or irregularly shaped ducts are embedded in a fibrovascular or hyalinized stroma (Figure 15-12). The ducts are lined by cuboidal to columnar epithelium with an outer myoepithelial layer. The second pattern associated with a mass effect is papillomatous: Papillary proliferations of columnar epithelial and cuboidal myoepithelial cells fill and distend the ducts. In both patterns, the overlying

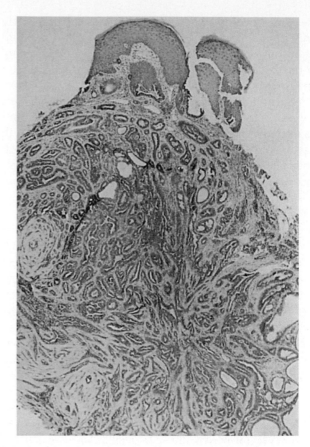

FIG. **15-12** Papillary adenoma: a lobular tumor without discrete borders showing numerous tubular glands, some with luminal papillary projections.

or adjacent epithelium is acanthotic and numerous plasma cells may be seen in the stroma. Important differences from breast carcinoma include absence of (1) significant cytoatypia and (2) atypical mitotic figures. Cribriform intraductal patterns are not seen, and myoepithelial cells are present. This lesion is benign, and simple resection is adequate.

MALIGNANT EPITHELIAL NEOPLASMS

Paget's disease of the breast is an important lesion to recognize, because more than 90% of women with Paget's disease have underlying breast carcinoma, often in situ only (see Chapter 11). The nipple, areola, or adjacent skin exhibits persistent eczematoid dermatitis with scaling, oozing, and crusting. A bloody, sometimes purulent, discharge from the nipple is commonly present. Microscopic examination of involved skin shows Paget's cells scattered singly or in small groups throughout all layers of the epithelium. These cells are larger than the adjacent keratinocytes and have a large nucleus with a crisp nuclear membrane, one or two prominent nucleoli, and abundant clear or pale eosinophilic to amphophilic cytoplasm. Flattened basal cells may be identified between the groups of Paget's

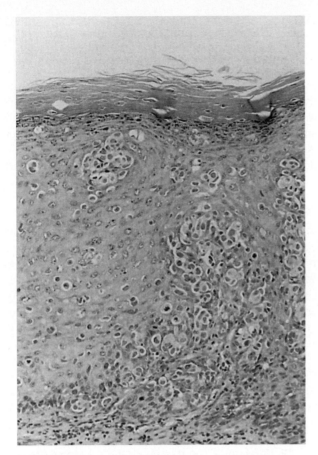

FIG. **15-13** Paget's disease: single and nested epithelioid cells with voluminous, pale cytoplasm in the stratum spinosum, stratum granulosum, and stratum corneum.

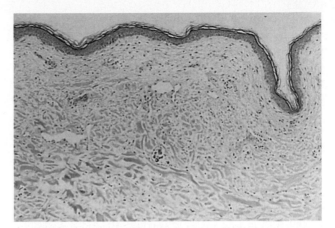

FIG. **15-14** Inflammatory carcinoma (metastatic breast carcinoma): dilated vascular channels, a few of which contain single and clustered malignant cells.

cells and the basement membrane of the epithelium, a histologic feature that distinguishes Paget's disease from melanoma (Figure 15-13). The usual staining properties for these cells are outlined in Table 15-2. Contrary to extramammary Paget's disease, only 40% of mammary Paget's cells contain demonstrable mucin.[36] Cytokeratin-7 and other low-molecular-weight cytokeratins may stain related benign cells in the epidermis of the nipple and are not diagnostic in and of themselves of mammary Paget's disease.[37] Monoclonal cytokeratin preparations and electron microscopic findings support

TABLE **15-2**   Immunoreactivity of Paget's Disease, Bowen's Disease, and Melanoma

	PAGET'S DISEASE	BOWEN'S DISEASE	MELANOMA
S-100	−	−	+
Epithelial membrane antigen	+	−	−
Carcinoembryonic antigen	±	−	−
Cytokeratin	+	+	−

lactiferous duct epithelium as the origin for Paget's cells.[38,39] Any nonhealing, eczematous lesion of the nipple should be regarded as "suspect" for Paget's disease, and a biopsy should be performed and the patient followed accordingly. Exfoliative cytologic examination is a noninvasive screening alternative; however, a negative finding does not exclude Paget's disease.[40-42]

Metastases of breast carcinoma to the skin are not uncommon. Four clinical patterns are observed: *inflammatory carcinoma, telangiectatic carcinoma, nodular carcinoma,* and *carcinoma en cuirasse.* One or more types may be present in the same patient. *Inflammatory carcinoma* appears as red, warm, slightly indurated skin with well-demarcated borders. Dermal and subcutaneous lymphatics contain numerous tumor emboli that are similar in appearance to the primary carcinoma (Figures 15-14 and 15-15). Vascular congestion and tissue edema accompany the lymphatic blockage. *Telangiectatic*

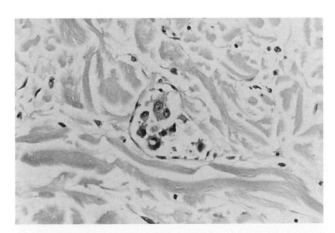

FIG. **15-15** Inflammatory carcinoma (metastatic breast carcinoma): poorly differentiated metastatic breast carcinoma in a vascular space. Finding these cells may require a careful search through multiple levels of tissue.

carcinoma presents as numerous purple plaques and hemorrhagic vesicles that resemble hemangiomas. Congested, dilated capillaries and lymphatics in the superficial dermis are permeated with tumor. *Nodular carcinoma* consists of large and small nodules of tumor within the dermis surrounded by fibrosis. This is the type of metastatic carcinoma most often found in mastectomy scars. Patients with *carcinoma encuirasse,* or *scirrhous carcinoma,* develop woody, indurated plaques that on histologic examination consist of small, easily overlooked hyperchromatic tumor cells embedded in abundant, dense, fibrotic stroma.

Basal cell carcinoma is the most common malignancy in whites and is more prevalent than all other malignancies combined. Fortunately, this tumor usually remains confined to the skin and metastases rarely occur, although local recurrence can be a problem. Basal cell carcinoma arises most frequently on sun-damaged skin but occurs on protected skin also. The most common type of basal cell carcinoma is the noduloulcerative variant, which presents as a pearly nodule with overlying and adjacent telangiectasia. Ulceration may be present. Histologically, the tumor consists of nests of small, basaloid epithelial cells in continuity with the overlying epithelium. Peripheral palisading (the picket fence–like arrangement of the cells at the rim of the nests) distinguishes basal cell carcinoma from appendageal tumors. Two variants are of special interest in this anatomic site: superficial multifocal basal cell carcinoma and fibroepithelioma of Pinkus. *Superficial multifocal basal cell carcinoma* presents clinically as a sharply marginated erythematous patch or plaque with slight scale (Figure 15-16). Histologic examination shows widely spaced nests of basaloid cells budding off the base of the overlying epithelium and surrounded by a loose, myxomatous inflamed stroma. Spontaneous regression,

which is common, leaves a nonspecific superficial scar, and the lesion may be missed on a small punch biopsy. Levels through the submitted tissue or repeat biopsy may be necessary to establish the diagnosis. *Fibroepithelioma of Pinkus* is a pink or tan, sessile nodule that on histologic examination shows thin, anastomosing strands of basaloid cells embedded in abundant stroma. Careful searching reveals foci of peripheral palisading. This tumor is thought to be a basal cell carcinoma that proliferates along the framework provided by preexisting benign eccrine ducts.

Squamous cell carcinomas arise on skin damaged by long-term sun exposure or, rarely, by therapeutic irradiation. Generally, scaly, rough intraepithelial proliferations of atypical keratinocytes called *actinic keratoses* precede the development of invasive carcinoma. *Squamous cell carcinoma* in situ, also called *Bowen's disease,* clinically appears as a velvety red patch that is sharply demarcated from the adjacent skin. The risk of developing invasive carcinoma from Bowen's disease is estimated at 5%.[43]

MELANOCYTIC NEOPLASMS

Pigmented lesions of the breast are common; the average white adult has 40 to 100 benign melanocytic nevi scattered over all body surfaces, including the breast. These lesions range from simple lentigos (basilar hyperpigmentation of keratinocytes with little or no increase in melanocytes) to junctional, compound, and intradermal melanocytic nevi. Nevi are generally smaller than 0.5 cm, oval to round, tan to brown, evenly pigmented, macular or papular lesions with relatively smooth borders; congenital nevi may be larger, darker, and slightly asymmetrical. Pigmented lesions that change, grow, ulcerate, itch, bleed, show significant color variation, or develop border irregularities should be excised to rule out melanoma. *Primary melanoma* of the skin of the breast accounts for 1.8% to 5% of melanomas.[44,45] A properly performed excisional biopsy that includes a narrow rim of clinically normal skin and completely removes the melanocytic lesion is necessary for accurate histologic evaluation and diagnosis. Wood's lamp enhances the pigmentary variation between normal and involved skin and may help delineate the borders of suspect lesions. For lesions larger than 2.0 cm or when total excision poses problems with closure (e.g., in the nipple or areola), an incisional biopsy can be performed from the thickest or darkest portion of the lesion. The initial evaluation of a patient with a suspected melanoma includes a personal history, family history, and appropriate physical examination that includes a whole-body skin examination and palpation of the regional lymph nodes. The focus of this evaluation is to identify risk factors, signs, or symptoms of metastases, atypical moles, and additional melanomas.[46]

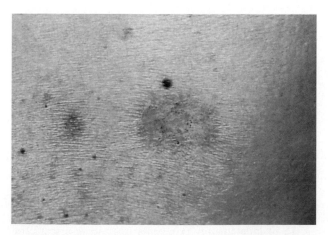

FIG. **15-16** Superficial multifocal basal cell carcinoma: sharply marginated plaque with slight scaling and areas of altered pigmentation (caused by tumor regression and scarring).

Standard therapy for melanoma is surgical excision. For melanoma in situ, excision of the lesion or biopsy site with a 0.5-cm border of clinically normal skin and a layer of the subcutaneous tissue is sufficient. The surgical margin should be histologically free of tumor. Elective (i.e., prophylactic) regional lymph node dissection is not indicated for patients with thin melanomas. Removal and microscopic examination of the sentinel lymph node identified by dye or lymphoscintigraphy for micrometastatic melanoma has emerged as an important management tool for intermediate-thickness (1.00- to 4.00-mm) melanomas. Extensive diagnostic studies (e.g., computed tomography, magnetic resonance imaging, scintigraphy) are not indicated and should not be performed when staging asymptomatic patients[44]; however, origin of the melanoma from the skin of the breast is an independent but significant negative prognostic factor.[47] An exception is primary melanomas of the nipple and areola, which are exceedingly rare and overall have a better prognosis and lower incidence of metastasis than other melanomas of the breast.[48] Other negative prognostic factors include measured thickness of the melanoma from the granular layer of the epidermis to the deepest tumor cell greater than 1.5 mm, ulceration, angioinvasion, neural invasion, and male sex. Obviously, regional or distant lymphadenopathy or symptoms suggesting distant organ metastases are grave prognostic indicators.

The most common subtype of melanoma that arises on the breast is the superficial spreading type. Clinically, the lesions are large, asymmetrical plaques of variable color (from white—indicating areas of regression—to black, brown, blue, or red). Nodules within the plaque indicate areas of dermal invasion (Figure 15-17). Histologic evaluation shows a proliferation of atypical, single and nested melanocytes within the epidermis, often exhibiting pagetoid upward spread. Individual melanocytes are large, with dusty

to chunky pigmentation and large, prominent nucleoli. In situ melanomas are confined to the epidermis and skin appendages. Invasive melanomas invade into the dermis and provoke a variable inflammatory host response. Depth of invasion is generally reported both by Clark's level, which reflects the functional level of invasion, and Breslow's thickness, which is the depth of invasion as measured by a calibrated ocular micrometer (Tables 15-3 and 15-4). Tumor staging in the sixth edition of the *American Joint Committee on Cancer Manual* has major new approaches.[48a] Any invasive melanoma 1 mm or smaller in thickness is tumor stage I. Without ulceration, such thin melanomas are stage T_{1a} if also only level II or III. Stage T_{1b} lesions have ulceration and/or are level IV.

Approximately 25% of melanomas arise in preexisting melanocytic nevi. Attempts to identify which patients are at risk for malignant transformation have led to recognition of the familial melanoma syndromes. These patients have family or personal histories of melanoma and often have large, atypical nevi by both clinical and histologic criteria.[49-53]

CONNECTIVE TISSUE NEOPLASMS

Cherry angiomas are extremely common, red to violaceous papules measuring a few millimeters in diameter that appear on the trunk and proximal extremities of adults. Histologic examination shows a cluster of dilated thin-walled vessels in the superficial dermis. *Angiokeratomas,* similar vascular lesions that extend up

TABLE **15-3**	Clark's Level for Melanomas
LEVEL	**CRITERION**
I	Is confined to the epithelium
II	Invades into the papillary dermis
III	Expands and fills the papillary dermis
IV	Invades into the reticular dermis
V	Invades into the subcutaneous tissue

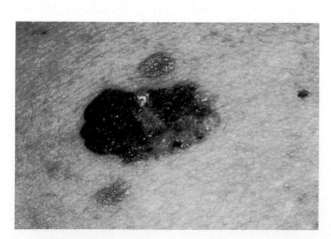

FIG. **15-17** Malignant melanoma, superficial spreading type. Histologic depth 0.35 mm.

TABLE **15-4**	Recommended Surgical Excision Margins	
BRESLOW THICKNESS	**EXCISION MARGINS**	**APPROXIMATE 5-YEAR SURVIVAL**
In situ	2-5 mm	95%-100%
<1 mm	1 cm	95%-100%
1-2 mm	1-2 cm	80%-96%
2-4 mm	2-3 cm (2 cm preferred)	60%-75%
>4 mm	2-3 cm	50%

Modified from Roberts DL et al: *Br J Dermatol* 146:7, 2002.

into the squamous epithelium, may be markers for Fabry's disease (α-galactosidase deficiency) and should prompt a search for clusters of angiokeratomas around the navel and on the genitals, corneal opacities, and symptoms of anhidrosis or hypohydrosis.[54] Enzyme assays establish the diagnosis. *Sinusoidal hemangioma*, a variant of cavernous hemangioma,[55] and *progressive lymphangioma*, a rare benign proliferation of lymph channels,[56,57] have both been reported to involve the breast. *Angiosarcoma* of the skin of the breast has been reported after radiation therapy for carcinoma of the breast.[58-61] Although very rare, incidence should increase with the widespread use of breast conservation therapy.[23]

Piloleiomyomas are benign proliferations of erector pili muscles—the smooth muscle attached to hair follicles that produces "goosebumps." Piloleiomyomas are often exquisitely painful and respond to light touch, stroking, or chilling with painful contraction. Bilateral smooth muscle tumors arising in the areola and nipple have been reported.[62] Calcium channel blockers have been used to control activation of these muscles when excision is not feasible. Piloleiomyomas are also a feature of Becker's nevus but in this setting are not painful.

Dermatomyofibroma (fibrohistiocytic tumor[28,29]) and *granular cell tumor* (a tumor of neural origin) are both rare and benign. Simple excision is curative.

The occurrence of myxomas, spotty pigmentation, endocrine overactivity, and schwannomas define *Carney's complex*, a multisystem connective tissue tumor syndrome inherited in an autosomal dominant fashion. Typical sites for the myxomas include nipples, eyelids, and the external ear canal. Histologic examination of these rare tumors shows a hypocellular tumor with stellate fibroblasts embedded in an abundant gelatinous blue-gray matrix.[63] The identification of a myxoma on biopsy of a mass lesion of the nipple should prompt a search for skin stigmata and metabolic abnormalities.

Cutaneous lymphoid infiltrates, both pseudolymphomas and lymphomas, may involve the skin of the breast. *Rosai-Dorfman disease* (sinus histiocytosis with massive lymphadenopathy), an uncommon benign lymphoproliferative disorder, was reported masquerading as a clinically malignant left breast mass in a male patient.[64] A *cutaneous lymphocytoma* associated with Lyme disease manifested as a nodule in the areola of a child and resolved after treatment with ceftriaxone.[65] *Mycosis fungoides*, a form of cutaneous T-cell lymphoma, appears initially as brownish red patches with fine scale and delicate wrinkling on the skin of the trunk, particularly intertriginous areas such as inframammary folds and axillae. Careful clinical evaluation of the patient and ancillary studies, including biopsy tissue submitted for routine processing and for molecular and genetic analysis, allow accurate categorization of most lymphoproliferative disorders.

REFERENCES

1. Smith DM Jr, Peters TG, Donegan WL: Montgomery's areolar tubercle: a light microscopic study, *Arch Pathol Lab Med* 106:60, 1982.
2. Watkins F, Giacomantonio M, Salibury S: Nipple discharge and breast lump related to Montgomery's tubercles in adolescent females, *J Pediatr Surg* 23:718, 1988.
3. Rosenberg CA, Derman C, Grabb WC: Hypomastia and mitral valve prolapse: evidence of a linked embryologic and mesenchymal dysplasia, *N Engl J Med* 309:1230, 1983.
4. David TJ: Nature and etiology of the Poland anomaly, *N Engl J Med* 287:487, 1972.
5. Zubowicz V, Bostwick J: Congenital unilateral hypoplasia of the female breast associated with a large melanotic spot: report of two cases, *Ann Plast Surg* 12:204, 1984.
6. Treiber ES, Goldberg NS, Levy H: Breast deformity produced by morphea in a young girl, *Cutis* 54:267, 1994.
7. Glinick SE et al: Becker's melanosis: associated abnormalities, *J Am Acad Dermatol* 9:509, 1983.
8. Happle R: Epidermal nevus syndromes, *Semin Dermatol* 14:111, 1995.
9. Moore JA, Schosser RH: Becker's melanosis and hypoplasia of the breast and pectoralis major muscle, *Pediatr Dermatol* 3:34, 1985.
10. Van Gerwen HJ et al: Becker's nevus with localized lipoatrophy and ipsilateral breast hypoplasia, *Br J Dermatol* 129:213, 1993.
11. Edwards MJ et al: Scalp-ear-nipple syndrome: additional manifestations, *Am J Med Genet* 50:247, 1994.
12. Finlay AY, Marks R: An hereditary syndrome of lumpy scalp, odd ears, and rudimentary nipples, *Br J Dermatol* 99:423, 1978.
13. Wilson MG: Absent nipples, *Humangenetik* 15:268, 1972.
14. Hindano A, Kobayishi T: Adnexal polyp of neonatal skin, *Br J Dermatol* 92:659, 1975.
15. Millns JL, Dickin CH: Hereditary acrolabial telangiectasia, *Arch Dermatol* 115:474, 1979.
16. Bergbrant IM: Seborrhoeic dermatitis and *Pityrosporum* yeasts, *Curr Top Med Mycol* 6:95, 1995.
17. Tschen JA, Ramsdell WM: Disciform erythrasma, *Cutis* 31:541, 1983.
18. Cianchini G et al: Acral Darier's disease successfully treated with adapalene, *Acta Derm Venereol* 81:57, 2001.
19. Knulst AC, De La Faille HB, Van Vloten WA: Topical 5-fluorouracil in the treatment of Darier's disease, *Br J Dermatol* 133:463, 1995.
20. Levit F: Jogger's nipples, *N Engl J Med* 297:1127, 1977.
21. Perez EA, Campbell DL, Ryu JK: Radiation recall dermatitis induced by edatrexate in a patient with breast carcinoma, *Cancer Invest* 13:604, 1995.
22. Phillips KA, Urch M, Bishop JF: Radiation recall dermatitis in a patient treated with paclitaxel, *J Clin Oncol* 13:305, 1995 (letter).
23. Polgar C, Orosz Z, Fodor J: Is postirradiation angiosarcoma of the breast so rare and does breast lymphedema contribute to its development? *J Surg Oncol* 76:239, 2001.
24. Raghavan VT, Bloomer WD, Merkel DE: Taxol and radiation recall dermatitis, *Lancet* 341:1354, 1993 (letter).
25. Burstein HJ: Side effects of chemotherapy: radiation recall dermatitis from Gemcitabine, *J Clin Oncol* 18:693, 2000.
26. Levine EL, Ribeiro GG: Vitiligo and radiotherapy: the Koebner phenomenon demonstrated in patients with vitiligo undergoing radiotherapy for carcinoma of the breast, *Clin Oncol R Coll Radiol* 6:133, 1994.

27. Dekio S, Kawasaki Y, Jidoi J: Herpes simplex on nipples inoculated from herpetic gingivostomatitis of a baby, *Clin Exp Dermatol* 11:664, 1986.

28. Colome MI, Sanchez RL: Dermatomyofibroma: report of two cases, *J Cutan Pathol* 21:371, 1994.

29. Mentzel T, Calonje E, Fletcher CD: Dermatomyofibroma: additional observations on a distinctive cutaneous myofi-broblastic tumour with emphasis on differential diagnosis, *Br J Dermatol* 129:69, 1993.

30. DeFranzo AJ, Marasco P, Argenta LC: Warfarin-induced necrosis of the skin, *Ann Plast Surg* 34:203, 1995.

31. Selva A et al: Pyoderma gangrenosum-like ulcers associated with lupus anticoagulant, *Dermatology* 189:182, 1994.

32. Green RA, Dowden RV: Mondor's disease in plastic surgery patients, *Ann Plast Surg* 20:231, 1988.

33. Finkel LJ, Griffiths CE: Inflammatory breast carcinoma (carcinoma erysipeloides): an easily overlooked diagnosis, *Br J Dermatol* 129:324, 1993.

34. Cho S et al: Clinical and histologic features of 64 cases of steatocystoma multiplex, *J Dermatol* 29:152, 2002.

35. Kageyama N, Tope WD: Treatment of multiple eruptive hair cysts with erbium:YAG laser, *Dermatol Surg* 25:819, 1999.

36. Lever WF, Schaumburg-Lever G: Tumors and cysts of the epidermis. In Lever WF, Schaumberg-Lever G (eds): *Histopathology of the skin,* ed 7, Philadelphia, 1990, JB Lippincott.

37. Lundquist K, Kohler S, Rouse RV: Intraepidermal cytokeratin 7 expression is not restricted to Paget cells but is also seen in Toker cells and Merkel cells, *Am J Surg Pathol* 23:212, 1999.

38. Tsuji T: Mammary and extramammary Paget's disease: expression of Ca 15-3, Ka-93, Ca 19-9, and CD44 in Paget cells and adjacent normal skin, *Br J Dermatol* 132:7, 1995.

39. Jahn H et al: An electron microscopic study of clinical Paget's disease of the nipple, *APMIS* 103:628, 1995.

40. Sakorafas GH et al: Paget's disease of the breast, *Cancer Treat Rev* 27:9, 2001.

41. Dunn JM et al: Exfoliative cytology in the diagnosis of breast disease, *Br J Surg* 82:789, 1995.

42. Lucarotti ME, Dunn JM, Webb AJ: Scrape cytology in the diagnosis of Paget's disease of the breast, *Cytopathology* 5:301, 1994.

43. Thomas JM: Premalignant and malignant epithelial tumors. In Sams WM, Lynch J (eds): *Principles and practice of dermatology,* New York, 1990, Churchill Livingstone.

44. Lee YN, Sparks FC, Morton DL: Primary melanoma of the skin of the breast region, *Ann Surg* 185:17, 1977.

45. Roses DF et al: Cutaneous melanoma of the breast, *Ann Surg* 189:112, 1979.

46. National Institutes of Health Consensus Development Conference: *Diagnosis and treatment of early melanoma,* Bethesda, MD, 1992, National Institutes of Health.

47. Garbe C et al: Primary cutaneous melanoma: prognostic classification of anatomic location, *Cancer* 75:2492, 1995.

48. Papachristou DN et al: Melanoma of the nipple and areola, *Br J Surg* 66:287, 1979.

48a. Balch CM et al: Melanoma of the skin. In Greene FL et al (eds): *AJCC staging manual,* ed 6, New York, 2002, Springer-Verlag.

49. Carey WP Jr et al: Dysplastic nevi as a melanoma risk factor in patients with familial melanoma, *Cancer* 74:3118, 1994.

50. Goldstein AM, Tucker MA: Genetic epidemiology of familial melanoma, *Dermatol Clin* 13:605, 1995.

51. Lucchina LC et al: Familial cutaneous melanoma, *Melanoma Res* 5:413, 1995.

52. Newton JA: Genetics of melanoma, *Br Med Bull* 50:677, 1994.

53. Newton JA: Familial melanoma, *Clin Exp Dermatol* 18:5, 1993.

54. Shelley ED, Shelley WB, Kurczynski TW: Painful fingers, heat intolerance, and telangiectases of the ear: easily ignored childhood signs of Fabry disease, *Pediatr Dermatol* 12:215, 1995.

55. Calonje E, Fletcher CD: Sinusoidal hemangioma: a distinctive benign vascular neoplasm within the group of cavernous hemangiomas, *Am J Surg Pathol* 15:1130, 1991.

56. Meunier L, Barneon G, Meynadier J: Acquired progressive lymphangioma, *Br J Dermatol* 131:706, 1994.

57. Rosso R, Gianelli U, Carnevali L: Acquired progressive lymphangioma of the skin following radiotherapy for breast carcinoma, *J Cutan Pathol* 22:164, 1995.

58. Bonett A, Pagliari C, Morrica B: Postradiation angiosarcoma of the breast: a clinical case, *Tumori* 81:219, 1995.

59. Fineberg S, Rosen PP: Cutaneous angiosarcoma and atypical vascular lesions of the skin and breast after radiation therapy for breast carcinoma, *Am J Clin Pathol* 102:757, 1994.

60. Moskaluk CA et al: Low-grade angiosarcoma of the skin of the breast: a complication of lumpectomy and radiation therapy for breast carcinoma, *Hum Pathol* 23:710, 1992.

61. Chahin F et al: Angiosarcoma of the breast following breast preservation therapy and local radiation therapy for breast cancer, *Breast J* 7:120, 2001.

62. Dawn G et al: Bilateral symmetrical pilar leiomyomas on the breasts, *Br J Dermatol* 133:331, 1995.

63. Carney JA: Carney complex: the complex of myxomas, spotty pigmentation, endocrine overactivity and schwannomas, *Semin Dermatol* 14:90, 1995.

64. Mac Moune Lai F et al: Cutaneous Rosai-Dorfman disease presenting as a suspicious breast mass, *J Cutan Pathol* 21:377, 1994.

65. Gautier C, Vignolly B, Taieb A: Benign cutaneous lymphocy-toma of the breast areola and erythema chronicum migrans, *Arch Pediatr* 2:343, 1995.

VII

NATURAL HISTORY, EPIDEMIOLOGY, GENETICS, AND SYNDROMES OF BREAST CANCER

16

Epidemiology
of Breast Cancer

VICTOR G. VOGEL

Chapter Outline

Risk Factors for Breast Cancer

Few breast cancer risk factors are prevalent in more than 10% to 15% of the population, although some are associated with very large relative risks (e.g., mutated genes, cellular atypia). Common risk factors for breast cancer are shown in Table 16-1, along with the magnitude of their associated risks and the strength of the evidence that establishes them as risk factors for breast cancer. Traits associated with large relative risks are rare; common risk factors are associated with relative risks less than 2.0, so the attributable risk for any particular risk factor is small.[1] Estimates of the summary

population attributable risk for breast cancer range from only 21% to 55%, leaving most of the population attributable risk for the disease unexplained. It is instructive, nevertheless, to examine what is known regarding risk factors for breast cancer. This chapter concentrates on new and recently identified traits, factors, and exposures.

Age is one of the most important risk factors for breast cancer. The relationship of age to breast cancer incidence and death in U.S. women is shown in Table 16-2 and in Figure 16-1. Although age-adjusted incidence rates continue to rise, breast cancer mortality has fallen in the past decade in the United States (Figure 16-2).

TABLE 16-1   Epidemiologic Risk Factors for Breast Cancer

FACTORS OF PROVEN SIGNIFICANCE	STRENGTH OF THE ASSOCIATION	SIZE OF THE EFFECT	EVIDENCE FROM PROSPECTIVE, RANDOMIZED STUDIES	EVIDENCE FROM CASE-CONTROL OR OBSERVATIONAL STUDIES
FACTORS THAT INCREASE RISK				
Age	+++	++	X	X
Early age at menarche (<12 yr)	++	+	X	X
Late age at first live birth (>30 yr)	++	+	X	X
Genetic mutations	+++	+++	X	X
Benign breast disease (proliferation ± atypia)	+++	++	X	X
Elevated levels of endogenous sex hormones	+++	+	X	X
Estrogen metabolism	+	+		X
Hormone replacement therapy	+++	++	X	X
Environmental factors				
Alcohol	++			X
Smoking	+?			X
Ionizing radiation	+++			X
Large body size (height and weight)	+	+		X
FACTORS THAT DECREASE RISK OR CAUSE NO CHANGE				
Lactation	++	—		X
Oral contraceptives	No effect	0		X
Induced abortion	No effect	0		X
Weight loss	+?	—		X
Exercise	+?	—		X
Dietary factors				
Fat	No effect	0	X	X
Red meat	No effect	0		X
Dietary fiber	No effect	0		X
Caffeine	No effect	0		X
Micronutrients				
Vitamin A	No effect	0		X
Vitamin C	No effect	0		X
Vitamin E	No effect	0		X
Selenium	No effect	0		X
Organochlorines	No effect	0		X
Phytoestrogens	+?	—		X

| TABLE 16-2 | Estimated Incidence of In Situ and Invasive Breast Cancer and Breast Cancer Deaths in U.S. Women, 2001 |

AGE	IN SITU CASES	%	INVASIVE CASES	%	DEATHS	%
<30	100	0.2	900	0.5	100	0.2
30-39	1,600	3.4	8,000	4.2	1,200	3.0
40-49	10,800	22.9	35,400	18.4	5,000	12.5
50-59	12,500	26.5	46,800	24.3	7,300	18.3
60-69	9,400	19.9	33,100	17.2	5,900	14.6
70-79	9,400	19.9	43,000	22.4	9,800	24.3
80+	3,300	7.0	25,000	13.0	10,900	27.2
Total	47,100	100.0	192,200	100.0	40,200	100.0

Data from the American Cancer Society, 2002.

BENIGN BREAST DISEASE

A history of benign breast disease is associated with a 57% increase (95% confidence interval [CI], 43% to 73%) in cumulative risk of breast cancer by age 70.[2] The presence of proliferative changes further increases risk, especially if the changes are associated with cellular atypia.

INDUCED ABORTION

In a cohort of 1.5 million women (28.5 million person-years) and after adjustment for known risk factors, induced abortion was not associated with an increased risk of breast cancer. No increases in risk were found in subgroups defined according to age at abortion, parity,

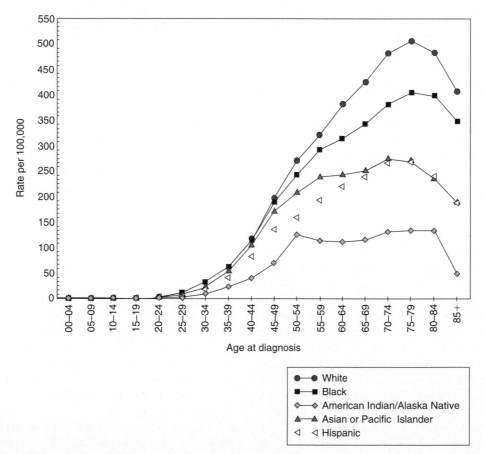

FIG. 16-1 Age-specific incidence of breast cancer by race for U.S. women. *(From the Surveillance, Epidemiology, and End Results [SEER] Program Public-Use Data [1973-1999], National Cancer Institute, DCCPS, Surveillance Research Program, Cancer Statistics Branch, released April 2002, based on November 2001 submission.)*

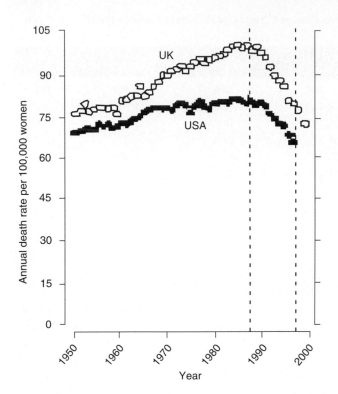

FIG. **16-2** Breast cancer mortality among women between the ages of 50 and 69 in the United States and United Kingdom through 1999. *(From Peto R et al: Lancet 355:1822, 2000.)*

time since abortion, or age at diagnosis of breast cancer.[3] The relative risk of breast cancer increased with increasing gestational age of the fetus at the time of the most recent induced abortion: at less than 7 weeks, 0.81 (95% CI, 0.58 to 1.13); at greater than 12 weeks, 1.38 (1.00 to 1.90) (reference category, 9 to 10 weeks). Induced abortions appear to have no overall effect on the risk of breast cancer.

GENETIC PREDISPOSITION

Many genes are known to affect the risk of developing breast cancer; among them are *BRCA1*[4,5] and *BRCA2*.[6] Women who inherit a deleterious mutation in *BRCA1* or *BRCA2* have an increased lifetime risk of breast and ovarian cancer and possibly colon cancer. Men are at increased risk of breast cancer (primarily *BRCA2*) and prostate cancer. The prevalence of deleterious *BRCA1* mutations is estimated to be 1 per 800 in the general population. Several mutations in *BRCA1* and *BRCA2* have been observed to occur with a higher frequency among individuals of Ashkenazi Jewish descent. These mutations include 185delAG and 5382insC for *BRCA1* and 6174delT for *BRCA2*. A study of more than 5000 individuals of Ashkenazi Jewish descent observed a prevalence of 2.3% for these three mutations,

which were associated with lifetime risks of 56% for breast cancer and 16% for ovarian cancer and prostate cancer.[7]

Estimates of the lifetime risk of breast cancer among women with *BRCA1* or *BRCA2* mutations vary from 56% to as high as 80% to 85%.[7-9] The variations in estimates of risk are related to differences in study populations and mutations evaluated. Other genes and nongenetic factors may affect a deleterious mutation carrier's cancer risk.

The percentage of inherited forms of breast cancer susceptibility in very-high-risk families that may be attributed to deleterious mutations in *BRCA1* was initially estimated to be 45%, with a smaller proportion attributable to the less common *BRCA2* mutations. Breast cancers among women who carry an altered *BRCA1* or *BRCA2* gene tend to occur at younger ages than in other women. The probability of detecting a deleterious mutation is higher when there is a family history of both breast and ovarian cancer, compared with women with a family history of breast cancer without ovarian cancer[10]; in addition, the ages of onset of breast cancers are important, with younger ages of onset being more likely associated with a deleterious mutation, especially a mutation in *BRCA1*.[11] Women who carry an abnormal ataxia telangiectasia (AT) gene may be at increased risk of breast cancer, but it is unclear whether these women are at increased risk of early-onset breast cancer (diagnosed at age 40 or younger).[12,13]

Mutations in either the *BRCA1* or *BRCA2* gene are found in 15% to 20% of individuals referred for testing, including 20% of women with breast cancer and 34% of women with ovarian cancer. The prevalence of mutations is correlated with specific features of the personal and family histories of the individuals tested. Mutations are as prevalent in high-risk women of African (19%) and other non-Ashkenazi ancestries as those of European ancestry (16%) and are significantly less prevalent in women diagnosed before age 50 with ductal carcinoma in situ than with invasive breast cancer (13% versus 24%). Among mutations identified in individuals of Ashkenazi ancestry through full sequence analysis of both *BRCA1* and *BRCA2*, about 20% are nonfounder mutations.[14] Among men with breast cancer, about 25% carry mutations, of which more than one third occur in *BRCA1*. Specific features of personal and family history can be used to assess the likelihood of identifying a mutation in *BRCA1* or *BRCA2* in individuals tested in a clinical setting.

The average age of breast cancer diagnosis is earlier in *BRCA2* mutation carriers (32.1 years) than in women with *BRCA1* mutations.[15] *BRCA1* mutations are detected in 45.5% of families with ovarian cancer and

75% of families with both breast and ovarian cancer in a single individual. Significantly fewer *BRCA2* mutations are detected in families with ovarian cancer. *BRCA1* mutations appear to be three times more prevalent than *BRCA2* mutations in families with male breast cancer. Breast cancer diagnosis before age 50, ovarian cancer, breast and ovarian cancer in a single individual, and male breast cancer are all significantly more common in families with *BRCA1* and *BRCA2* mutations, but none of these factors distinguishes between *BRCA1* and *BRCA2* mutations. Some evidence suggests that reduced breast cancer penetrance is associated with the *BRCA2* mutation 6174delT.

ORAL CONTRACEPTIVES

Oral contraceptive use is weakly associated with breast cancer risk in the general population, but the association among women with a familial predisposition to breast cancer is less clear. In one study that evaluated the effect of oral contraceptives on women with a family history of the disease, a total of 394 sisters and daughters of the probands, 3002 granddaughters and nieces, and 2754 women who married into the families were studied.[16] After accounting for age and birth cohort, ever having used oral contraceptives was associated with significantly increased risk of breast cancer among sisters and daughters of the probands (relative risk 3.3; 95% CI 1.6 to 6.7), but not among granddaughters and nieces of the probands or among those who married into the family. The results were essentially unchanged after adjustment for parity, age at first birth, age at menarche, age at menopause, oophorectomy, smoking, and education. The elevated risk among women with a first-degree family history of breast cancer was most evident for oral contraceptive use during or before 1975, when formulations were likely to contain higher dosages of estrogen and progestins.

These results suggest that women who have ever used earlier formulations of oral contraceptives and who also have a first-degree relative with breast cancer may be at increased risk for breast cancer. Population-based studies of the risk of breast cancer among former and current users of oral contraceptives do not suggest, however, that these drugs increase risk.[17] The relative risk is not increased for women who are currently using oral contraceptives or for those who have previously used them. The relative risk does not increase consistently with longer periods of use or with higher dosages of estrogen, and the results are similar among white and black women. Use of oral contraceptives by women with a family history of breast cancer is not associated with an increased risk of breast cancer, nor is the initiation of oral contraceptive use at a young age.

Some single cohort studies do not show any association between oral contraceptive use and breast cancer (relative risk 1.0; 95% CI 0.9 to 1.1). However, a 1996 meta-analysis of data from 54 epidemiologic studies of oral contraceptive use and the risk of breast cancer showed that women had a slightly increased risk of breast cancer while taking oral contraceptives, as compared with the risk among nonusers. The Collaborative Group on Hormonal Factors in Breast Cancer analyzed the worldwide epidemiologic evidence on the relation between breast cancer risk and use of hormonal contraceptives.[18] Individual data on 53,297 women with breast cancer from 54 studies conducted in 25 countries were collected, checked, and analyzed.

While women are taking combined oral contraceptives and in the 10 years after stopping, there is a 24% increase in the relative risk of having breast cancer diagnosed in current users (relative risk 1.24; 95% CI 1.15 to 1.33). The risk declines with increasing years since stopping use. Reassuringly, there is no significant excess risk of having breast cancer diagnosed 10 years or more after stopping use of oral contraceptives.

Features of hormonal contraceptive use, such as duration of use, age at first use, and the dose and type of hormone within the contraceptives, have little effect on breast cancer risk, once recency of use is taken into account. Women who begin use before age 20 have higher relative risks of having breast cancer diagnosed while they are using combined oral contraceptives and in the 5 years after stopping than do women who begin use at older ages; however, the higher relative risks apply at ages when breast cancer is rare, and for a given duration of use, earlier use does not result in more cancers being diagnosed than use beginning at older ages.

Because breast cancer incidence rises steeply with age, the estimated excess number of cancers diagnosed in the period between starting use and 10 years after stopping increases with age at last use is only 0.5 to 5.0 cases among 10,000 women who use oral contraceptives, depending on age of use. The risk of breast cancer increases with the use of oral contraceptives at older ages. Up to 20 years after cessation of use, the difference between ever-users and never-users appears in their clinical presentation, with the breast cancers diagnosed in ever-users being less advanced clinically than those diagnosed in never-users. There is no evidence of an increase in the risk of having breast cancer diagnosed 10 years or more after cessation of use of oral contraceptives, and the cancers diagnosed then are less advanced clinically than the cancers diagnosed in never-users.

HORMONE REPLACEMENT THERAPY

More extensive data link the use of hormone replacement therapy (HRT) after menopause to the risk of developing breast cancer, as shown in Table 16-3. The Collaborative Group on Hormonal Factors in Breast Cancer[21] brought together and reanalyzed about 90% of the worldwide epidemiologic evidence on the relation between risk of breast cancer and use of HRT. The main analyses were based on nearly 54,000 postmenopausal women with a known age at menopause, of whom 17,830 (33%) had used HRT at some time. The median age at first use was 48 years, and 34% of ever-users had used HRT for 5 years or longer. Estimates of the relative risk of breast cancer associated with the use of HRT were obtained after stratification of all analyses by study, age at diagnosis, time since menopause, body mass index (BMI),

parity, and the age a woman was when her first child was born. Among current users of HRT or those who ceased use 1 to 4 years previously, the risk of having breast cancer diagnosed increased by 2.3% for each year of use; the relative risk was 1.35 for women who had used HRT for 5 years or longer. This increase is comparable with the effect on breast cancer of delaying menopause, as evidenced by the fact that among never-users of HRT, the relative risk of breast cancer increases by a factor of 2.8% for each year older they are at menopause. Five or more years after cessation of HRT use, there was no significant excess of breast cancer overall or in relation to duration of use.

TABLE 16-3 | Studies Evaluating the Risk of Breast Cancer in Relation to Hormone Replacement Therapy

YEAR	REFERENCES	STUDY TYPE	PARTICIPANTS	HORMONES	RESULTS	OTHER NOTES
1989	Adami et al[19]	Cohort	23,244	E	Increases risk 10%	Average follow-up 6.7 yr
1995	Colditz et al[20] (Nurses' Health Study)	Cohort	69,586	E, E + P	E alone increases risk 32%; E + P increases risk 41%	Average follow-up 10.4 yr
1997	Collaborative Group[21]	Meta-analysis	52,705 cases 108,411 controls	E, E + P	Incidence of breast cancer increases with increasing duration of use	Effect nearly disappears 5 yr after stopping
1999	Greendale et al[22] (Postmenopausal Estrogen/Progestin Interventions [PEPI])	Randomized	307	E, E + P	Increased breast density during first year of use for both E alone and E + P	High breast density increases breast cancer risk; increases in breast density among more women in E + P group than E alone
1999	Schairer et al[23]	Cohort	2,614	E	Reduces mortality when continued after cancer diagnosis	Mortality results determined 14-22 yr after diagnosis
2000	Ross et al[24]	Case-control	3,534	E, E + P	Increases risk approximately 10% for each 5 yr of use	Greater increase in risk among E + P users than E alone
2000	Schairer et al[25]	Cohort	46,355	E, E + P	Increases risk 1% to 8% for each year of use	Greater increase in risk among E + P users than E alone
2000	Colditz and Rosner[26] (Nurses' Health Study)	Cohort	58,520	E, E + P	Five or more years of use increases risk 40%	Greater increase in risk among E + P users than E alone; increased risk disappears 2-5 yr after discontinuation of use
2001	O'Meara et al[27]	Cohort	2,755	E, E + P	Reduces recurrence and mortality when continued after cancer diagnosis	79% of hormone users used E alone; results determined 2-19 yr after diagnosis
2002	Women's Health Initiative[28]	Randomized	16,608	E + P	Increases risk 26%	5.2 yr of follow-up

Courtesy Ms. Nancy Nelson, National Cancer Institute Office of Cancer Communication.
E, Estrogen; E + P, estrogen plus progestin.

Of the many factors examined that might affect the relation between breast cancer risk and use of HRT, only weight and BMI had a material effect: The increase in the risk of breast cancer associated with long durations of use in current and recent users was greater for women of lower than of higher weight or BMI. There were no marked variations in the results according to hormonal type or dose, but little information was available about long durations of use of any specific preparations. Cancers diagnosed in women who ever use HRT tend to be less advanced clinically than those diagnosed in never-users. In North America and Europe, the cumulative incidence of breast cancer between the ages of 50 and 70 in never-users of HRT is about 45 per 1000 women. The cumulative excess numbers of breast cancers diagnosed between these ages per 1000 women who began use of HRT at age 50 and used it for 5, 10, and 15 years, respectively, are estimated to be 2, 6, and 12. Whether HRT affects mortality from breast cancer is unknown, although some data suggest a more favorable outcome among users of HRT following a diagnosis of breast cancer.[27]

To assess the major health benefits and risks of the most commonly used combined hormone preparation in the United States, the National Heart, Lung and Blood Institute conducted the Women's Health Initiative, a randomized controlled primary prevention trial in which 16,608 postmenopausal women aged 50 to 79 with an intact uterus at baseline were recruited.[28] Participants received conjugated equine estrogens, 0.625 mg daily, plus medroxyprogesterone acetate, 2.5 mg daily, in 1 tablet ($n = 8506$) or placebo ($n = 8102$).

The primary outcome was coronary heart disease (CHD) (nonfatal myocardial infarction and CHD death), with invasive breast cancer as the primary adverse outcome. After slightly more than 5 years of follow-up, the risk of CHD increased by 29%, breast cancer by 26%, stroke by 41%, and pulmonary embolism by 213%. The risks of both colorectal cancer and hip fracture were both reduced by more than 30%. Absolute excess risks per 10,000 person-years attributable to estrogen plus progestin were seven more CHD events, eight more strokes, eight more pulmonary embolisms, and eight more invasive breast cancers, whereas absolute risk reductions per 10,000 person-years were six fewer colorectal cancers and five fewer hip fractures. Overall health risks exceeded benefits from use of combined estrogen plus progestin for an average 5-year follow-up among healthy, postmenopausal U.S. women.

ENDOGENOUS ESTROGEN LEVELS

Based on the association of hormonally related risk factors such as age at menarche and age at first live birth with the risk of developing breast cancer, differences in endogenous estrogen metabolism may also affect the risk of breast cancer. The relationship is uncertain, however. To test the hypothesis that serum concentrations of estradiol and testosterone predict risk for breast cancer, a prospective case-cohort study was conducted.[29] Participants were 97 white women with confirmed incident breast cancer and 244 randomly selected controls; all women were 65 years or older and were not receiving estrogen. Sex-steroid hormone concentrations were assayed by using serum that was collected at baseline. Risk factors for breast cancer were ascertained by questionnaire. The relative risk for breast cancer in women with the highest concentration of estradiol (≥6.83 pmol/L or 1.9 pg/mL) was 3.6, compared with women with the lowest concentration. The risk for breast cancer in women with the highest concentration of free testosterone compared with those with the lowest concentration was 3.3. The estimated incidence of breast cancer per 1000 person-years was 0.4 in women with the lowest levels of bioavailable estradiol and free testosterone, compared with 6.5 in women with the highest concentrations of these hormones. Traditional risk factors for breast cancer were similar in case-patients and controls, and adjustments for these risk factors had little effect on the results. Estradiol and testosterone levels may therefore play important roles in the development of breast cancer in older women. Some investigators have proposed that a single measurement of bioavailable estradiol and free testosterone may be used to estimate a woman's risk for breast cancer, but this concept has not been validated prospectively.

Both experimental and clinical evidence suggest that 16α-hydroxylated estrogen metabolites, biologically strong estrogens, are associated with increased breast cancer risk, whereas 2-hydroxylated metabolites, with lower estrogenic activity, are weakly related to the disease. Among premenopausal women, a higher ratio of 2-hydroxyestrone to 16α-hydroxyestrone at baseline has been associated with a reduced risk of breast cancer: In one study, women in the highest quintile of the ratio had an adjusted odds ratio for breast cancer of 0.58. The corresponding adjusted odds ratio in postmenopausal women was 1.29. These observations support the hypothesis that the estrogen metabolism pathway favoring 2-hydroxylation over 16α-hydroxylation is associated with a reduced risk of invasive breast cancer risk in premenopausal women.[30]

Similar results were obtained in another study of postmenopausal women. Those with the highest estradiol levels (≥12 pmol/L) had a twofold increased invasive breast cancer risk, compared with women with lower levels.[31] The selective estrogen receptor modulator raloxifene significantly reduced breast cancer risk in both the low- and high-estrogen subgroups for all risk factors examined. The women with the highest bone mineral density and those with a family history of breast cancer experienced a significantly greater therapeutic benefit with raloxifene, compared with the two thirds of patients with lower bone mineral density or those without a family history, respectively.

Taken together, these studies all suggest that increased lifetime endogenous estrogen exposure appears to increase breast cancer risk.

BODY SIZE AND ANTHROPOMETRY

The identification of potentially modifiable risk factors for breast cancer, such as dietary folate intake, alcohol consumption, physical activity, and certain anthropometric factors, provides opportunities for risk-reducing interventions both among women at average and high risk for breast cancer.[32]

Epidemiologic evidence implicating anthropometric risk factors in breast cancer etiology is accumulating.[33] For premenopausal women, breast cancer risk increases with increasing height but paradoxically decreases with higher weight or BMI, and no association with increased central adiposity exists. For postmenopausal women, however, an increased risk of breast cancer is found with increasing levels of all the anthropometric variables, including height, weight, BMI, waist/hip ratio, waist circumference, and weight gain. Weight loss appears to decrease risk, particularly if it occurs later in life.

Several hypothetical biologic mechanisms exist to explain how anthropometric factors influence breast cancer risk. Obesity may increase levels of circulating endogenous sex hormones, insulin and insulin-like growth factors that all, in turn, increase breast cancer risk. Genetic predisposition to obesity and to specific body fat distributions are also implicated. In one large epidemiologic, population-based study, however, there was no association with height, waist circumference, or waist/hip ratio or an increased risk of developing breast cancer.[34] Curiously, a linear trend of increasing risk with increasing waist/hip ratio has been reported among women with a family history of breast cancer but not among women with no family history.

As previously mentioned, BMI shows significant inverse and positive associations with breast cancer among premenopausal and postmenopausal women, respectively, and these associations are nonlinear.[35] Compared with premenopausal women with a BMI of less than 21 kg/m², women with a BMI exceeding 31 kg/m² have a relative risk of breast cancer of 0.54. In postmenopausal women, the relative risks do not increase further when BMI exceeds 28 kg/m². There is little evidence for interaction with other breast cancer risk factors. These data indicate that height is an independent risk factor for postmenopausal breast cancer, but in premenopausal women, this relation is less clear.

The association between BMI and breast cancer varies by menopausal status. Weight control may reduce the risk of breast cancer among postmenopausal women, but this hypothesis requires confirmation in prospective clinical trials.

EXERCISE AND PHYSICAL ACTIVITY

Whether physical activity reduces the risk of postmenopausal breast cancer is uncertain, and few studies have addressed this issue. Women reporting the highest level of physical activity at baseline compared with women with the lowest level of activity appear to have an age-adjusted relative risk of breast cancer less than 1.0.[36] Women reporting any regular leisure-time physical activity also have a relative risk of nearly 1.0, compared with those reporting no such regular physical activity. Adjustment for potential confounders does not appreciably alter the findings. There is little evidence, therefore, that physical activity later in life is associated to any appreciable extent with breast cancer incidence.

A population-based case-control study of incident breast cancer cases and controls was conducted in Alberta, Canada, to examine the effect of physical activity performed at different ages and life periods on breast cancer risk.[37,38] The frequency, duration, and intensity of occupational, household, and recreational activities were measured throughout lifetime with the Lifetime Total Physical Activity Questionnaire and cognitive interviewing methods. Breast cancer risk reductions were comparable when self-reported and assigned intensity values were used, although the results and trends were more evident with the assigned intensity data. Moderate-intensity occupational and household activities decreased breast cancer risk, whereas recreational activity, at any intensity level, did not contribute to a breast cancer risk reduction. Of the types of activity considered, the greatest risk reductions observed were for occupational and household activities. Breast cancer risk was most associated with a risk reduction for activity done later in life, particularly after menopause, for which the odds ratio was 0.70. For women who sustained physical activity throughout life, compared with those who were never active, the breast cancer risk reduction was 42%, suggesting that sustained activity throughout life, and particularly activity done later in life, may have the most benefit in reducing breast cancer risk.

Another population-based case-control study of New Mexican women used incident breast cancer cases aged 35 to 74 and matched controls.[39] Activity type and weekly duration of usual nonoccupational physical activity were used to calculate weekly metabolic equivalent (MET) hours of total and vigorous physical activity (≥5 METs). Vigorous physical activity was associated with reduced breast cancer risk in both

Hispanic and non-Hispanic white women. Women in the highest category of vigorous activity had lower risk of breast cancer (66% reduction for Hispanic women; 40% reduction for non-Hispanic white women), compared with women reporting no vigorous physical activity. Both premenopausal and postmenopausal Hispanic women showed decreasing risk with increasing level of activity. Physical activity was protective, however, only among postmenopausal non-Hispanic white women. The effects of physical activity were independent from reproductive factors, usual BMI, BMI at age 18, adult weight gain, and total energy intake.

DIET

In industrial countries, women often have excess metabolic energy due to high food consumption and low physical activity.[40] High lifetime energy availability results in high lifetime levels of ovarian steroid hormones. Estrogens and progesterone are hypothesized to play a crucial role in the development and prognosis of breast cancer. The risk of breast cancer is higher in industrial countries than in developing countries, where women are characterized with lower energy intake and higher energy expenditure. It is possible that the beneficial effects of physical activity and of negative energy balance are mediated by reduced levels of ovarian steroids. Although both weight loss and physical activity may have similar efficacy in suppressing ovarian function, and therefore in reducing the risk of breast cancer, it may be more advantageous for premenstrual women to achieve lifetime reduction in steroid levels by increasing their physical activity rather than by losing weight through caloric restriction alone.

No study of the relationship between diet and breast cancer shows a significant association with total fat intake observed when comparing the highest with the lowest category of total fat intake.[41] A collaborative pooled analysis of large prospective studies published through 1995 included a total of 4980 cases of breast cancer among 337,819 women[42] (Table 16-4). In addition to providing great statistical precision, the pooled analysis allowed standard analytic approaches to be applied to all studies, an examination of a wider range of fat intake, and a detailed evaluation of interactions with other breast cancer risk factors. Overall, no association was observed between intake of total, saturated, monounsaturated, or polyunsaturated fat and risk of breast cancer. No reduction in risk was seen even for fat intakes as low as 20% of energy. When the relatively few women with fat intake lower than 15% of energy were examined, their risk of breast cancer actually increased twofold; this could not be accounted for by other dietary or nondietary factors. A recent update of the pooled data has continued to support an overall lack of association. Prospective, randomized data from the National Institutes of Health's Women's Health Initiative should provide a definitive answer to this question in the next few years.

DIETARY MICRONUTRIENTS

The consumption of vegetables and fruit may protect against some types of cancer, but research evidence is not compelling for breast cancer. Carotenoids are pigments that are present in most plants and have known antioxidant properties. Blood concentrations of carotenoids have been proposed as integrated biochemical markers of consumed vegetable, fruit, and synthetic

TABLE 16-4 Results from Large Prospective Studies of Total and Saturated Fat Intake and Risk of Breast Cancer

STUDY	TOTAL NO. IN COHORT	YEARS OF FOLLOW-UP	NO. OF CASES	RELATIVE RISK (95% CONFIDENCE INTERVAL) (HIGH VERSUS LOW CATEGORY) TOTAL FAT	SATURATED FAT
Nurse's Health Study	89,494	8	1439	0.86 (0.67-1.08)	0.86 (0.73-1.02)
Canadian Study	56,837	5	519	1.30 (0.90-1.88)	1.08 (0.73-1.59)
New York State cohort	17,401	7	344	1.00 (0.59-1.70)	1.12 (0.78-1.61)
Iowa Women's Study	32,080	4	408	1.13 (0.84-1.51)	1.10 (0.83-1.46)
Dutch Health Study	62,573	3	471	1.08 (0.73-1.59)	1.39 (0.94-2.06)
Adventists Health Study	20,341	6	193		1.21 (0.81-0.81)
Swedish mammography screening cohort	61,471	6	674	1.00 (0.76-1.32)	1.09 (0.83-1.42)
Breast Cancer Detection Demonstration Project	40,022	5	996	1.07 (0.86-1.32)	1.12 (0.87-1.45)

From Willett WC et al: Epidemiology and nongenetic causes of breast cancer. In Harris JR et al (eds): *Diseases of the breast,* ed 2, Philadelphia, 2000, Lippincott Williams & Wilkins.

supplements. In one case-control study, the carotenoids lutein, zeaxanthin, beta-cryptoxanthin, lycopene, alpha-carotene, and beta-carotene were measured in archived serum samples using liquid chromatography.[43] There was an evident increase in the risk of breast cancer for decreasing beta-carotene, lutein, alpha-carotene, and beta-cryptoxanthin. The risk of breast cancer approximately doubled among subjects with blood levels of beta-carotene at the lowest quartile, as compared with those at the highest quartile. The risk associated with the other carotenoids was similar, varying between 2.1 for lutein and 1.7 for beta-cryptoxanthin. The odds ratio for the lower quartile of total carotenoids was 2.3. These observations offer evidence that a low intake of carotenoids, through poor diet and/or lack of vitamin supplementation, may be associated with increased risk of breast cancer and may have public health relevance for people with markedly low intakes.

Women in the lowest 10th percentile of folate intake from diet alone are at modestly increased risk of breast cancer relative to those above the 50th percentile.[44] The relative risk of breast cancer associated with low dietary folate intake is not increased among nondrinkers but is increased about 30% among moderate drinkers and 60% among heavy drinkers. These results suggest that the risks of postmenopausal breast cancer may be increased among women with low intakes of folate if they consume beverages that contain alcohol.

ALCOHOL CONSUMPTION

There are lingering questions regarding the relation between alcohol consumption and breast cancer risk in women.[45] A meta-analysis of epidemiologic studies carried out through 1999 examined the dose-response relation and assessed whether effect estimates differed according to various study characteristics. Overall, there was a monotonic increase in the relative risk of breast cancer with alcohol consumption, but the magnitude of the effect was small; in comparison with nondrinkers, women averaging 12 g of alcohol per day (approximately one typical drink) had a relative risk of 1.10. Estimates of relative risk were 7% greater in hospital-based case-control studies than in cohort studies or community-based case-control studies, 3% greater in studies published before 1990 than in studies published later, and 5% greater in studies conducted outside of the United States than in U.S. studies. The findings of five U.S. cohort studies published since 1990 yielded a relative risk of 1.06 for consumers of 12 g per day, as compared with nondrinkers. Cohort studies with less than 10 years of follow-up gave estimates 11% higher than cohort studies with longer follow-up periods. No meaningful difference was seen by menopausal status or type of beverage consumed.

PHYTOESTROGENS

Phytoestrogens are substances derived from plants that have estrogenic properties, but research on the relation between phytoestrogens and breast cancer risk has been limited in scope. Most epidemiologic studies have involved Asian women and have examined the effects of traditional soy foods (e.g., tofu), soy protein, or urinary excretion of phytoestrogens. In one study, African-American, Latino, and white women aged 35 to 79 who were diagnosed with breast cancer between 1995 and 1998 were compared with women selected from the general population.[46] Usual intake of specific phytoestrogenic compounds was assessed via a food frequency questionnaire and a nutrient database. Phytoestrogen intake was not associated with breast cancer risk. Results were similar for premenopausal and postmenopausal women, for women in each ethnic group, and for all seven phytoestrogenic compounds studied. Based on these data, phytoestrogens appear to have little effect on breast cancer risk at the levels commonly consumed by non-Asian U.S. women, an average intake equivalent to less than one serving of tofu per week. Whether greater consumption of phytoestrogens will reduce the incidence of breast cancer remains unknown.

BIOLOGIC GROWTH FACTORS

Transgenic animal experiments suggest that increased expression of transforming growth factor-β1 (TGF-β1) is protective against early breast cancer development. A thymine-to-cytosine transition in the twenty-ninth nucleotide in the coding sequence results in a leucine-to-proline substitution at the tenth amino acid and is associated with increased serum levels of TGF-β1. To determine whether an association exists between this TGF-β1 polymorphism and breast cancer risk, the relationship between the TGF-β1 genotype and the risk of breast cancer was evaluated in the Study of Osteoporotic Fractures, a prospective cohort study of white, community-dwelling women aged 65 or older.[47] Risk of breast cancer was similar in women with the T/T genotype and women with the T/C genotype but was significantly lower in women with the C/C genotype. In analyses that adjusted for age, age at menarche, age at menopause, estrogen use, parity, BMI, and bone mineral density, women with the C/C genotype had a significantly lower risk of developing breast cancer compared with women with the T/T or T/C genotype (hazard ratio = 0.36). There was no significant difference between the risk for women with the T/C genotype compared with women with the T/T genotype. The findings suggest that the TGF-β1 genotype is associated with risk of breast cancer in white women aged 65 or older. Because the T allele is the common variant and confers an increased risk, it may be associated with a large proportion of breast cancer cases.

Insulin resistance may also be a risk factor for breast cancer, possibly through increased levels of estrogens or insulin-like growth factor-I (IGF-I). Insulin resistance has been associated with obesity, hypertension, dyslipidemia, and impaired glucose tolerance. The insulin-like growth factor binding-protein family comprises six proteins with high affinity for insulin-like growth factors and several lower affinity proteins. Their production in the breast is controlled by hormones and other local regulators. In tumors, their production relates to the estrogen receptor status. Their functional activity can also be affected by various posttranslational modifications. Lower serum concentrations of IGF-I binding proteins are found in patients with breast cancer, thus increasing the bioavailability of IGF-I.[48]

In a prospective study of women without breast cancer, there was no association between IGF-I concentrations and breast cancer risk among the whole study group.[49] In postmenopausal women, there was no association between IGF-I concentrations and breast cancer risk. The relative risk of breast cancer among premenopausal women by tertiles of IGF-I concentration was 2.33. Among premenopausal women younger than 50 at the time of blood collection, the relative risk was 4.6. After further adjustment for plasma IGFBP-3 concentrations, these relative risks were 2.9 and 7.3, respectively. A positive relation between circulating IGF-I concentration and risk of breast cancer was found among premenopausal but not postmenopausal women, suggesting that plasma IGF-I concentrations may be useful in the identification of women at high risk of breast cancer and in the development of risk-reduction strategies.

SMOKING

The role of active and passive smoking in breast cancer remains controversial.[50] In the Nurses' Health Study, a total of 78,206 women were followed prospectively. For active smoking, a modest 20% increase in risk was confined to women who began smoking before age 17. These results suggest that passive smoking is unrelated to breast cancer. However, results for active smoking are compatible with a small increase in risk when smoking is initiated at young ages.

Some of the inconsistencies in the relationship between breast cancer and cigarette smoking may be due in part to heterogeneity in carcinogen metabolism. *N*-acetyltransferase-2 (NAT2) enzyme activity is believed to play a role in the activation of tobacco smoke carcinogens. One study examined the effect of NAT2 genetic polymorphisms on breast cancer risk from active and passive smoking.[51] There was no association between breast cancer risk and NAT2, smoking status (never, former, current), smoking duration, or cigarettes per day. There were also no effects of passive exposure among never-smokers. There were no statistical interactions between tobacco smoke exposure and NAT2. The results were similar when restricting the analysis to invasive cancers. These findings do not support the hypothesis that NAT2 is a risk factor for breast cancer or that it alters susceptibility to tobacco smoke.

Catechol-*O*-methyltransferase (COMT) catalyzes the *O*-methylation of catechol estrogens, using *S*-adenosylmethionine (SAM) as a methyl donor. Several studies have indicated that the val108met COMT polymorphism, which results in a threefold to fourfold decrease in activity, is associated with increased breast cancer risk. Folate, whose intake levels have also been associated with breast cancer risk, and other micronutrients in the folate metabolic pathway influence levels of SAM and *S*-adenosylhomocysteine (SAH), a COMT inhibitor generated by the demethylation of SAM. Because these micronutrients have been shown to alter SAM and SAH levels, they could also affect COMT-catalyzed methylation of catechol estrogens.[52] Although measurements of SAM and SAH were not initially collected, a secondary analysis of data from two nested case-control studies was performed to examine whether serum levels of folate, vitamin B_{12} (B_{12}), pyridoxal 5'-phosphate (PLP), cysteine and homocysteine, in conjunction with the COMT genotype, were associated with breast cancer risk. COMT (HH) (high-activity COMT homozygote) breast cancer cases had statistically significantly lower levels of homocysteine and cysteine and higher levels of PLP than COMT (HH) controls. In contrast, COMT (LL) (low-activity COMT homozygote) cases had higher levels of homocysteine than COMT (LL) controls. No associations were seen between B_{12}, COMT genotype, and breast cancer risk. An increasing number of COMT (LL) alleles was significantly associated with increased breast cancer risk in women with below-median levels of folate or above-median levels of homocysteine. These findings are consistent with a role for certain folate pathway micronutrients in mediating the association between COMT genotype and breast cancer risk.

Both COMT and glutathione-*S*-transferase (GST) genotypes modify individual breast cancer risk.[53] No significant increase in overall breast cancer risk was seen for any combinations of the studied genotypes in one large study. However, a substantially increased risk of breast cancer is seen for women who had used HRT and simultaneously carried the COMT-L allele containing genotypes and either the GSTP1 Ile/Ile or null genotypes. In those cases, the risk increases fourfold. These associations appear to be attributable to long-term users (>30 months) of HRT, in whom the risk of breast cancer rises sevenfold to eightfold. In addition, the combination of COMT-L allele containing genotypes with the

GSTM1 null genotype poses a nearly tenfold increased risk of breast cancer. These results suggest that the use of HRT could substantially increase the risk of breast cancer among women with specific combinations of the at-risk genotypes of COMT and GST genes.

ENVIRONMENTAL TOXINS

Whether environmental contaminants increase breast cancer risk is unknown. Experimental studies show that hormonal and nonhormonal activities of polychlorinated biphenyls (PCBs) are structurally dependent, suggesting that the breast cancer risk associated with PCBs may vary according to specific PCB congeners.[54] A case-control study investigated whether breast cancer risk was associated with body burden of PCBs or varied by PCB congeners. No individual congeners or groups of congeners were associated with a significantly increased risk of breast cancer. Further stratification by type of breast disease; menopausal, parity, and lactation status; and body size also showed no significant association with body levels of PCBs. These results suggest that environmental exposure to PCBs do not substantially affect breast cancer risk.

Several additional studies have sought to determine whether breast cancer risk is increased in relation to exposure to organochlorines, compounds with known estrogenic characteristics that were extensively used in some areas of the United States. Some reports do not support a strong association, although there have been concerns with high risks observed in some subgroups of women. In one study,[55] no substantial elevation in breast cancer risk was observed in relation to the highest quintile of lipid-adjusted serum levels of p,p'-bis(4-chlorophenyl)-1,1-dichloroethene (DDE), chlordane, dieldrin, the sum of the four most frequently occurring PCB congeners, and other PCB congener groupings. No dose-response relations were apparent, nor was risk increased in relation to organochlorines among women who had not breastfed or were overweight, postmenopausal, or long-term residents of the geographic area studied; or with whether the case was diagnosed with invasive rather than in situ disease, or with a hormone receptor-positive tumor. These findings do not support the hypothesis that organochlorines increase breast cancer risk.

To examine whether currently measurable aromatic hydrocarbon-induced damage to DNA increases breast cancer risk, a population-based case-control study was conducted as a component of the study just described.[56] Cases were women newly diagnosed with in situ and invasive breast cancer; controls were randomly selected women frequency matched to the age distribution of the cases. Blood samples were assayed for aromatic hydrocarbon-DNA adducts. The mean levels of DNA adducts was slightly, but not significantly, higher among cases than among controls. The age-adjusted odds ratio for breast cancer in relation to the highest quintile of adduct levels compared with the lowest was 1.51. There was no consistent elevation in risk with increasing adduct levels, nor was there a consistent association between adduct levels and two of the main sources of polycyclic aromatic hydrocarbons, active or passive cigarette smoking, or consumption of grilled and smoked foods. These data indicate that polycyclic aromatic hydrocarbon-DNA adduct formation may influence breast cancer development, although the association does not appear to be dose dependent and may have a threshold effect.

IONIZING RADIATION EXPOSURE

There is a well-established relationship between exposure to ionizing radiation and the risk of developing breast cancer.[57,58] Excess breast cancer risk is consistently observed in association with a variety of exposures, such as fluoroscopy for tuberculosis and radiation treatments for medical conditions. Although risk is inversely associated with age at radiation exposure, the manifestation of breast cancer risk occurs according to the usual age-related pattern. An estimate of breast cancer risk associated with medical radiology puts the figure at less than 1% of the total. It has been theorized that certain populations, however, such as AT heterozygotes, are at increased risk from the usual sources of radiation exposure.[59]

Women treated for Hodgkin's disease by age 16 may have a subsequent risk of developing breast cancer as high as 35% by age 40.[60,61] One study suggests that higher dosages of radiation (median dose, 40 Gy in breast cancer cases) and treatment between ages 10 and 16 correspond with higher risk. An earlier study suggests a high level of breast cancer risk in women treated for Hodgkin's disease, especially those treated before age 15 with radiation to the thorax and/or neck.[61] When radiation therapy was administered after age 14 but before age 30, the risk of developing breast cancer was also elevated, but to a lesser degree. Unlike the risk for secondary leukemia, the risk of treatment-related breast cancer did not abate with duration of follow-up.[60,62] In these studies, the great majority (85% to 100%) of patients who developed breast cancer did so either within the field of radiation or at the margin.[62] Whereas intensive mammographic screening has been advocated for this high-risk population, it is unknown whether the additional radiation exposure could produce additional risk.

In theory, breast cancer patients treated with lumpectomy and radiation therapy may be at increased risk for second breast or other malignancies, compared with those treated by mastectomy. Outcome studies after a median follow-up of 15 years show no difference, however, in the risk of second malignancies.[63]

REFERENCES

1. Vogel VG: Breast cancer risk factors and preventive approaches to breast cancer. In Kavanagh J et al (eds): *Cancer in women*, Cambridge, MA, 1998, Blackwell Scientific.

2. Colditz GA, Rosner B: Cumulative risk of breast cancer to age 70 years according to risk factor status: data from the Nurses' Health Study, *Am J Epidemiol* 152:950, 2000.

3. Melbye, M et al: Induced abortion and the risk of breast cancer, *N Engl J Med* 336:81, 1997.

4. Miki Y et al: A strong candidate for the breast and ovarian cancer susceptibility gene *BRCA1, Science* 266:66, 1994.

5. Futreal PA et al: BRCA1 mutations in primary breast and ovarian carcinomas, *Science* 266:120, 1994.

6. Wooster R et al: Localization of a breast cancer susceptibility gene, *BRCA2*, to chromosome 13q12-13, *Science* 265:2088, 1994.

7. Struewing JP et al: The risk of cancer associated with specific mutations of *BRCA1* and *BRCA2* among Ashkenazi Jews, *N Engl J of M* 336:1401, 1997.

8. Easton DF et al: Genetic linkage analysis in familial breast and ovarian cancer: results from 214 families, *Am J Hum Genet* 52:678, 1993.

9. Easton DF, Ford D, Bishop DT: Breast and ovarian cancer incidence in *BRCA1*-mutation carriers, Breast Cancer Linkage Consortium, *Am J Hum Genet* 56:265, 1995.

10. Couch FJ et al: *BRCA1* mutations in women attending clinics that evaluate the risk of breast cancer, *N Engl J of Med* 336:1409, 1997.

11. Berry DA et al: Probability of carrying a mutation of breast-ovarian cancer gene BRCA1 based on family history, *J Natl Cancer Inst* 89:227, 1997.

12. Athma P, Rappaport R, Swift M: Molecular genotyping shows that ataxia-telangiectasia heterozygotes are predisposed to breast cancer, *Cancer Genet Cytogenet* 92:130, 1996.

13. Fitzgerald MG et al: Heterozygous ATM mutations do not contribute to early onset of breast cancer, *Nat Genet* 15:307, 1997.

14. Frank TS et al: Clinical characteristics of individuals with germline mutations in *BRCA1* and *BRCA2*: analysis of 10,000 individuals, *J Clin Oncol* 20:1480, 2002.

15. Shih HA et al: *BRCA1* and *BRCA2* mutation frequency in women evaluated in a breast cancer risk evaluation clinic, *J Clin Oncol* 20:994, 2002.

16. Grabrick DM et al: Risk of breast cancer with oral contraceptive use in women with a family history of breast cancer, *JAMA* 284:1791, 2000.

17. Marchbanks PA et al: Oral contraceptives and the risk of breast cancer, *N Engl J Med* 346:2025, 2002.

18. Collaborative Group on Hormonal Factors in Breast Cancer: Breast cancer and hormonal contraceptives: collaborative reanalysis of individual data on 53,297 women with breast cancer and 100,239 women without breast cancer from 54 epidemiological studies, *Lancet* 347:1713, 1996.

19. Adami HO et al: Risk of cancer in women receiving hormone replacement therapy, *Int J Cancer* 44:833, 1989.

20. Colditz GA et al: The use of estrogens and progestins and the risk of breast cancer in postmenopausal women, *N Engl J Med* 332:1589, 1995.

21. Collaborative Group on Hormonal Factors in Breast Cancer: Breast cancer and hormone replacement therapy: collaborative reanalysis of data from 51 epidemiological studies of 52,705 women with breast cancer and 108,411 women without breast cancer, *Lancet* 350:1047, 1997.

22. Greendale GA et al: Effects of estrogen and estrogen-progestin on mammographic parenchymal density, *Ann Intern Med* 130:262, 1999.

23. Schairer C et al: Estrogen replacement therapy and breast cancer survival in a large screening study, *J Natl Cancer Inst* 91:264, 1999.

24. Ross RK et al: Effective hormone replacement therapy on breast cancer risk: estrogen versus estrogen plus progestin *J Natl Cancer Inst* 92:328, 2000.

25. Schairer C et al: Menopausal estrogen and estrogen-progestin replacement therapy and breast cancer risk, *JAMA* 283:485, 2000.

26. Colditz G, Rosner B: Cumulative risk of breast cancer to age 70 years according to risk factor status: data from the Nurses' Health Study, *Am J Epidemiol* 152:950, 2000.

27. O'Meara ES et al: Hormone replacement therapy after a diagnosis of breast cancer in relation to recurrence and mortality, *J Natl Cancer Inst* 93:754, 2001.

28. Writing Group for the Women's Health Initiative: Risks and benefits of combined estrogen and progestin in healthy postmenopausal women: principal results from the Women's Health Initiative randomized controlled trial, *JAMA* 288:321, 2002.

29. Cauley JA et al: Elevated serum estradiol and testosterone concentrations are associated with a high risk for breast cancer, Study of Osteoporotic Fractures Research Group, *Ann Intern Med* 130:270, 1999.

30. Muti P et al: Estrogen metabolism and risk of breast cancer: a prospective study of the 2:16 alpha-hydroxyestrone ratio in premenopausal and postmenopausal women, *Epidemiology* 11:635, 2000.

31. Lippman ME et al: Indicators of lifetime estrogen exposure: effect on breast cancer incidence and interaction with raloxifene therapy in the multiple outcomes of raloxifene evaluation study participants, *J Clin Oncol* 19:3111, 2001.

32. Brewster A, Helzlsouer K: Breast cancer epidemiology, prevention, and early detection, *Curr Opin Oncol* 13:420, 2001.

33. Friedenreich CM: Review of anthropometric factors and breast cancer risk, *Eur J Cancer Prev* 10:15, 2001.

34. Sellers TA et al: Interaction of waist-hip ratio and family history on the risk of hormone receptor-defined breast cancer in a prospective study of postmenopausal women, *Am J Epidemiol* 155:225, February 1, 2002.

35. Van den Brandt PA et al: Pooled analysis of prospective cohort studies on height, weight, and breast cancer risk, *Am J Epidemiol*, 152:514, 2000.

36. Moore DB et al: Physical activity and incidence of postmenopausal breast cancer, *Epidemiology* 11:292, 2000.

37. Friedenreich CM, Courneya KS, Bryant HE: Influence of physical activity in different age and life periods on the risk of breast cancer, *Epidemiology* 12:604, 2001.

38. Friedenreich CM, Courneya KS, Bryant HE: Relation between intensity of physical activity and breast cancer risk reduction, *Med Sci Sports Exer* 33:1538, 2001.

39. Gilliland FD et al: Physical activity and breast cancer risk in Hispanic and non-Hispanic white women, *Am J Epidemiol* 154:442, 2001.

40. Jasienska G, Thune I, Ellison PT. Energetic factors, ovarian steroids and the risk of breast cancer, *Eur J Cancer Prevent* 9:231, 2000.

41. Willett WC: Diet and breast cancer, *J Intern Med* 249:395, 2001.

42. Hunter DJ et al: Cohort studies of fat intake and the risk of breast cancer: a pooled analysis *N Engl J Med* 334:356, 1996.

43. Toniolo P et al: Serum carotenoids and breast cancer, *Am J Epidemiol* 153:1142, 2001.

44. Sellers TA et al: Dietary folate intake, alcohol, and risk of breast cancer in a prospective study of postmenopausal women, *Epidemiology* 12:420, 2001.

45. Ellison RC et al: Exploring the relation of alcohol consumption to risk of breast cancer, *Am J Epidemiol* 154:740, 2001.

46. Horn-Ross PL et al: Phytoestrogen consumption and breast cancer risk in a multiethnic population: the Bay Area Breast Cancer Study, *Am J Epidemiol* 154:434, 2001.

47. Ziv E et al: Association between the T29 C polymorphism in the transforming growth factor beta1 gene and breast cancer among elderly white women: the Study of Osteoporotic Fractures, *JAMA* 285:2859, 2001.

48. Zumkeller W: IGFs and IGFBPs: surrogate markers for diagnosis and surveillance of tumor growth? *Mol Pathol* 54:285, 2001

49. Hankinson SE et al: Circulating concentrations of insulin-like growth factor-I and risk of breast cancer, *Lancet* 351:1393, 1998.

50. Egan KM et al: Active and passive smoking in breast cancer: prospective results from the Nurses' Health Study, *Epidemiology* 13:138, 2002.

51. Delfino RJ et al: Breast cancer, passive and active cigarette smoking and N-acetyltransferase 2 genotype, *Pharmacogenetics* 10:461, 2000.

52. Goodman JE et al: COMT genotype, micronutrients in the folate metabolic pathway and breast cancer risk, *Carcinogenesis* 22:1661, 2001.

53. Mitrunen K et al: Combined COMT and GST genotypes and hormone replacement therapy associated breast cancer risk, *Pharmacogenetics* 12:67, 2002.

54. Zheng T et al: Breast cancer risk associated with congeners of polychlorinated biphenyls, *Am J Epidemiol* 152:50, 2000.

55. Gammon MD et al: Environmental toxins and breast cancer on Long Island. II. Organochlorine compound levels in blood, *Cancer Epid Biomarkers Prev* 11:686, 2002.

56. Gammon MD et al: Environmental toxins and breast cancer on Long Island. I. Polycyclic aromatic hydrocarbon DNA adducts, *Cancer Epid Biomarkers Prev* 11:677, 2002.

57. John EM, Kelsey JL: Radiation and other environmental exposures and breast cancer, *Epidemiol Rev* 15:157, 1993.

58. Evans JS, Wennberg JE, McNeil BJ: The influence of diagnostic radiography on the incidence of breast cancer and leukemia, *N Engl J Med* 315:810, 1986.

59. Swift M et al: Incidence of cancer in 161 families affected by ataxia-telangiectasia, *N Engl J Med* 325:1831, 1991.

60. Bhatia S et al: Breast cancer and other second neoplasms after childhood Hodgkin's disease, *N Engl J Med* 334:745, 1996.

61. Hancock SL, Tucker MA, Hoppe RT: Breast cancer after treatment of Hodgkin's disease, *J Natl Cancer Inst* 85:25, 1993.

62. Sankila R et al: Risk of subsequent malignant neoplasms among 1,641 Hodgkin's disease patients diagnosed in childhood and adolescence: a population-based cohort study in the five Nordic countries, *J Clin Oncol* 14:1442, 1996.

63. Obedian E, Fischer DB, Haffty BG: Second malignancies after treatment of early-stage breast cancer: lumpectomy and radiation therapy versus mastectomy, *J Clin Oncol* 18:2406, 2000.

17

Primary Prevention of Breast Cancer

ANDREW LAMAN

VICTOR G. VOGEL

Chapter Outline

Chemoprevention can be defined as the use of specific natural or synthetic chemical agents to reverse, suppress, or prevent carcinogenic progression to invasive cancer.[1-12] This definition excludes food compounds ingested as part of the normal diet. Epidemiologic data suggesting that breast cancer is preventable through drug intervention include time trends in cancer incidence and mortality, geographic variations and the effects of migration, identification of specific causative factors, and the observation that most human cancers do not show simple patterns of genetic inheritance. In this chapter we review the basic science and clinical data that direct us to potentially active agents for the reduction of breast cancer risk.

Hormonal Carcinogenesis in the Breast

The mammary gland is the only organ that is not fully developed at birth,[13,14] and it undergoes dramatic changes in size, shape, and function during growth, puberty, pregnancy, and lactation.[15] Russo and Russo have carefully described the developmental progression of the human breast and describe four distinct types of breast lobules. Type 1 lobules are the least differentiated ones; they are also called *virginal lobules* because they are present in the immature female breast before menarche. Type 2 lobules evolve from type I lobules and have a more complex morphology characterized by a higher number of ductal structures per lobule. Type 3 lobules are characterized by having an average of 80 ductules or alveoli per lobule; they are often seen in the breasts of women under hormonal stimulation or during pregnancy. The type 4 lobule has been described as being present during the lactational period.

Study of the pathogenesis of human breast cancer indicates that the type 1 lobules are the site of origin of preneoplastic lesions such as atypical ductal hyperplasia, which evolves to ductal carcinoma in situ (DCIS) and progresses to invasive carcinoma. Although ductal breast cancer originates in type 1 lobules, or terminal ductal lobular units,[16] the epidemiologic observation that nulliparous women exhibit a higher incidence of breast cancer than do parous women indicates that type 1 lobules in these two groups of women may be biologically different or exhibit different susceptibility to carcinogenesis.[17,18] Parous women undergo lobular differentiation, whereas nulliparous women seldom reach the type 3 lobular stage.

Type 1, 2, and 3 lobules also exhibit different cell kinetic characteristics: Type 1 and 2 lobules grow faster in vitro, possess higher DNA labeling indices, and demonstrate a shorter doubling time than type 3 lobules.[19,20] Correspondingly, the breasts of nulliparous women with and without cancer reveal a similar architecture. The breasts of parous women without cancer have the lowest percentage of type 1 lobules and a slightly higher percentage of type 2 lobules, whereas parous women in whom breast cancer develops have breasts that contain higher numbers of type 1 lobules.

The degree of breast development is important in the susceptibility to carcinogenesis. It has been suggested that parous women in whom breast cancer develops may exhibit a defective response to the differentiating effect of the hormones of pregnancy.[21] Breast tissue comprised almost exclusively of type 3 lobules exhibits a significantly lower number of mitotic doublings.[17] It is also recognized that the proliferative activity of the breast varies depending on the phase of the menstrual cycle: Cell proliferative activity has been shown to be consistently lower in the follicular than in the secretory phase.[22-24] This finding suggests a possible use of cell proliferation as an intermediate end point for assessing the effect of chemopreventive agents; however, this requires determining the exact location of the cells in which proliferative activity is measured.[25]

The repair of DNA damage is also important in the prevention of malignancy, and agents that increase mitotic activity increase the likelihood of converting DNA damage into mutations.[26,27] The breasts of nonpregnant, premenopausal women are not quiescent. The breast epithelium undergoes repetitive cycles of cell proliferation and apoptosis, and the key stimuli for these events are estrogen and progesterone.[28,29] In the terminal duct lobular unit of the premenopausal breast, cell proliferation is low during the follicular phase of the menstrual cycle. After ovulation, progesterone stimulates breast epithelial cell proliferation twofold to threefold, and if pregnancy ensues, proliferation increases even further. During the second half of pregnancy, cell proliferation decreases and differentiation occurs. These effects appear to be mediated through estrogen regulation of progesterone receptor, epidermal growth factor receptor, and transforming growth factor (TGF)-β_1.[30] In addition to these known effects, use of the 19-nortestosterone derivatives of progesterone in oral contraceptives (OCs) is associated with breast cancer incidence rates only half as great as those observed in women not using OCs.[31] A linear trend is observed for decreased RR of breast cancer with increasing duration of use of OCs.

An observation that may relate diet to circulating levels of steroid hormones is the presence of the isoflavone genistein in soy products. Genistein may lead to increased levels of dehydroepiandrosterone (DHEA), which is associated with a lower risk of breast cancer.[32] DHEA is produced by the adrenal glands and is a precursor of estrone and testosterone. In both retrospective and prospective epidemiologic studies, decreased circulating levels of DHEA and its metabolites have been associated with increased mammary cancer incidence.[33,34] This steroid is a potent noncompetitive inhibitor of mammalian glucose-6-phosphate dehydrogenase (G6PD). This inhibition has been proposed as the basis for DHEA's cancer chemopreventive activity; hereditary G6PD deficiency correlates with decreased cancer incidence. The enzyme pathway including G6PD is the source of the cofactor nicotinamide adenine dinucleotide phosphate (NADPH), which is necessary for many processes, including DNA precursor biosynthesis, cytochrome P-450 metabolism, and production of oxygen radicals by neutrophils and macrophages. Putative effects of DHEA include decreased activation of some carcinogens, reduced DNA synthesis (proliferation), inhibition of oxygen radical damage, and decreased prostaglandin production. The 16α-fluoro derivative fluasterone has been shown to be a more effective chemopreventive agent than DHEA, and it lacks the androgenic and liver toxicity of the parent compound. Fluasterone also inhibits carcinogenesis in the N-methyl-N-nitrosourea (MNU)–induced rat mammary cancer model, but clinical experience with the compound is limited.[34]

Hormonal Modulation of Experimental Carcinogenesis

Mammary carcinogenesis induced by 7,12-dimethylbenz[a] anthracene (DMBA) is significantly inhibited in rats that have undergone full-term pregnancy or pregnancy and lactation before exposure to the carcinogen.[35-38] The protective effect observed after pregnancy depends on permanent structural changes induced in the mammary parenchyma by these processes.

On the basis of studies evaluating the effect of pregnancy as a physiologic mechanism of breast cancer prevention, it is possible experimentally to reproduce the protective effect exerted by pregnancy by treating young virgin rats with human chorionic gonadotropin (hCG).[39-43] It is likely that lobular differentiation is the underlying mechanism responsible for this protection.[21,37,38,42] Analogous to pregnancy, hCG induces full differentiation of the mammary gland, which is manifested morphologically as a reduction in the number of terminal end buds as a result of profuse lobular development, depression in DNA synthesis, inhibition of the binding of the carcinogen to the cellular DNA, and increased ability of the cells to repair DNA damage.[44] Pregnancy and hCG treatment followed by a 21-day rest period before DMBA administration significantly depress both mammary tumorigenesis and carcinogenesis. Pregnant and hCG-treated animals develop significantly fewer tumors than their age-matched controls, indicating that the length of time after delivery or

termination of hormonal treatment does not ameliorate the protective effect of these two events.[44,45] The number of alveolar buds in control animals progressively decreases with aging, whereas treatment with hCG maintains their number between the first and tenth day of injection, decreasing sharply between the tenth and twenty-first days of injection when the number of lobules begins to rise. The morphologic pattern observed during hCG treatment is nearly identical to that seen during pregnancy.[44]

Treatment with hCG diminishes the proliferative activity in rat mammary terminal end buds as measured by DNA labeling indices. Carcinogen treatment induces 100% tumor incidence in the animals that receive DMBA alone, whereas tumor incidence and number are significantly attenuated in animals treated with hCG after DMBA administration. Published results indicate that hCG inhibits tumor progression because treatment with this hormone after carcinogen administration produces a significant reduction in the number of tumors and adenocarcinomas per animal. Therefore, because the latency period is not modified, hCG appears to act on the initiated foci, inhibiting their progression, not merely delaying the time of tumor appearance.[40] It is unknown whether the endocrine milieu induced by hCG results in inhibition of tumor progression or exerts this effect through inhibition of cell proliferation, induction of cell differentiation, or activation of programmed cell death.

The fact that hCG induces the mammary epithelium to synthesize inhibin,[46] a secreted protein with tumor suppressor activity,[47] may represent the local regulatory mechanism through which hCG mediates its effect on the mammary gland. The finding of inhibin subunit mRNA in nonreproductive tissues suggests a role for inhibin protein beyond the reproductive axis as an important regulator of cellular differentiation.[48-50] In addition, α-inhibin is an important negative regulator of cell proliferation.[51] Synthesis of inhibin by the ovary is stimulated by gonadotropic hormones, pregnant mare serum gonadotropin, and hCG,[48,52,53] hormones known to have a powerful differentiating effect on the mammary gland.[39-41,43] The mammary glands of virgin control rats do not show any immunoreactivity to inhibin,[46] but immunocytochemical reactivity to inhibin is observed in the mammary gland of pregnant and hCG-treated animals.

There are two mutually exclusive pathways of estrogen metabolism; one involves C-2 hydroxylation and the other involves C-16α hydroxylation.[54] Epidemiologic studies indicate that 16α-hydroxylation activity is a risk factor for breast cancer (16α-hydroxyestrone is genotoxic in mammary cells), whereas 2-hydroxylation activity is not (2-hydroxyestrone is not genotoxic and does not promote proliferation).[55] Markedly increasing 2-hydroxylation activity decreases the formation of 16α-hydroxylated metabolites. Indole-3-carbinol, a constituent of cruciferous vegetables, induces enzyme P-450 1A1, which is responsible for 2-hydroxylation. In clinical trials, indole-3-carbinol increased 2-hydroxyestrone levels in healthy women during 3 months of administration.[55] In addition, indole-3-carbinol inhibits both DMBA- and MNU-induced rat mammary tumors.[54] These preliminary studies indicate that additional investigation of estrogen metabolism pathways as targets for reducing the risk of breast cancer is warranted.

Chemoprevention in Humans

The need for effective breast cancer preventive strategies is apparent based solely on the number of women who are at increased risk for the disease.[56,57] More than 30 million women in the United States are older than 50 years, and at least 2 million of these women have first-degree relatives with breast cancer. At least 6 million postmenopausal women have undergone biopsy for benign breast disease, and one fourth of these women have proliferative changes. As many as 10 million older women are obese, and 1 in 6 women age 40 years or older is nulliparous. A substantial proportion of breast cancer will occur in women with these characteristics, and strategies to reduce their risk may have a significant effect on the burden of breast cancer in the United States.

There are three areas unique to the field of chemoprevention that must be considered in all stages of the clinical evaluation of a new chemopreventive agent.[58] First, the characteristics of the target population must be clearly defined. For breast cancer chemoprevention, the target is a group of healthy women who may have had a previous diagnosis of breast cancer or who may be known to have a condition that predisposes them to the development of breast cancer. Second, the frequency and severity of side effects of the chemopreventive agent should be acceptable to the individual and ethically justifiable in the target population. Third, the duration of use of the chemopreventive agent must be defined. For most preventable malignancies, this requires a sustained period of drug administration that may be lifelong.

Identifying suitable populations for breast cancer chemoprevention trials is difficult and costly.[57] The target population includes both individuals who perceive their risk to be high and those who are unaware that their risk is increased. Because the goal of chemoprevention, as in any prevention strategy, is to prevent disease, an individual who remains well may not recognize the benefit of the intervention, as opposed to a sick person who is treated and returns to health. Therefore recruiting patients to use chemopreventive drugs involves extensive education and targeting of individuals with identified risk factors. Because chemoprevention is applied to healthy individuals who will take the agent for prolonged periods, the drug that is to be used must have an excellent safety and toxicity profile or at least a favorable benefit/risk ratio. In addition, the agent must be relatively inexpensive because of the cumulative cost of prolonged administration to many individuals. Tamoxifen fulfills these criteria and serves as the prototypical agent for clinical breast cancer risk reduction.

TAMOXIFEN

Hormones, especially estrogens, have been linked to breast cancer,[59,60] with their role being attributed to their ability to stimulate cell proliferation. This cellular proliferation leads to the accumulation of random genetic errors that result in neoplastic transformation.[61] According to this concept, chemoprevention of breast cancer has been targeted to reducing the rate of cell proliferation through administration of hormonal modulators.[62] Tamoxifen activity has been shown to be species, tissue, and cell-type specific.[63] In the pubertal rat, tamoxifen is capable of promoting full ductal development in the mammary gland.[64] In the mature reproductive-age animal, tamoxifen acts as an estrogen antagonist, inducing atrophy of lobular structures.[65] In postmenopausal women, tamoxifen treatment results in upregulation of the proportion of ductal cells expressing estrogen receptor (ER).[66]

Epidemiologic studies indicate that estrogen-mediated events are integral in the development of breast cancer[67-69] and support the hypothesis that intact ovarian function is required to develop breast cancer. Prior investigations also indicate that oophorectomy or radiation-induced ovarian ablation can reduce the incidence of breast cancer by up to 75%.[70,71] These observations suggest that estrogen antagonists may be instrumental in the primary prevention of breast cancer.

Tamoxifen, a triphenylethylene compound, was synthesized in 1966 as a potential fertility agent. Demethylation to the active metabolite, N-desmethyl tamoxifen, is the principal metabolic pathway in humans. Maximum serum concentration of N-desmethyl tamoxifen is observed within 12 to 24 hours after dosing; its serum half-life is approximately 12 days.[72] The parent compound and conjugates (at least six metabolites) are excreted in the bile and undergo enterohepatic circulation. This enterohepatic circulation and large volume of distribution result in a terminal elimination half-life of 4 to 7 days.[73-76]

Tamoxifen suppresses the appearance of chemically induced breast tumors in laboratory animals.[77] Both DMBA and MNU induce hormone-responsive mammary tumors in rats, but DMBA-induced mammary carcinomas rarely develop in spayed animals or animals treated with androgens.[78,79] Experimentally, chemical initiation by DMBA is followed by a period of promotion with estrogen, prolactin, and progesterone, with the appearance of tumors 3 to 4 months later. The simultaneous administration of a large dose of tamoxifen and DMBA to 50-day-old female Sprague-Dawley rats results in a dramatic reduction (<10% of control rate) in the number and type of palpable mammary tumors.[80,81] Another dose of tamoxifen administered 30 days after DMBA administration inhibits tumorigenesis for up to 120 days. In rats, ovariectomy or the injection of antiestrogens after carcinogen administration results in the appearance of very few mammary tumors.[82,83]

Several mechanisms have been proposed regarding tamoxifen's ability to prevent or suppress breast carcinogenesis. These are listed in Table 17-1.

The effect of tamoxifen on growth factors may occur independently of an effect on growth factor receptors.[95,96] Tamoxifen interacts with cell membranes and affects the physical properties of the lipid bilayer.[97] These lipid-mediated physical effects may contribute to the inhibition of breast cancer cell proliferation. Not all effects of tamoxifen are beneficial, however. Prolonged administration of tamoxifen suppresses natural killer (NK) cell activity; this suppression may contribute to tamoxifen's inability to prevent breast tumors with complete efficiency. Resistance to the inhibitory effects of tamoxifen is also possible through several alternative mechanisms[98]: (1) through the production and local accumulation of an estrogenic metabolite(s) of tamoxifen, (2) through the loss of ER on precancerous or cancerous breast tissue, (3) through the production of mutated ER that produces an estrogenic stimulus to cells when bound with tamoxifen, or (4) through altered subcellular factors and altered signal transduction. Any of these or other mechanisms could explain tamoxifen's inability to prevent all newly emerging malignant breast clones.

A comprehensive assessment of tamoxifen's ability to prevent second primary breast cancers is found in the overview of the world's literature on tamoxifen as adjuvant therapy for breast cancer.[99] The meta-analysis includes data from 55 randomized comparisons of tamoxifen and placebo on more than 37,000 women. Information regarding contralateral second primary breast cancers is shown in Table 17-2. Among the 18,534 women who received placebo in these trials, 485 (2.6%) developed contralateral second primary breast cancers, whereas among 18,565 women who received tamoxifen adjuvant therapy, 369 (2.0%) developed second breast cancers. The 23% RR reduction (2.6 to 2.0/2.6) of a second primary breast cancer varied with the duration of tamoxifen adjuvant therapy. Among women who received less than 2 years of adjuvant therapy, the reduction in the odds was only 13%, compared with 26% among women who received exactly 2 years of therapy and 47% among women who received more than 2 years of adjuvant tamoxifen therapy. These data suggest a dose-response effect for tamoxifen's ability to prevent second primary breast cancers.

In the overview data, information was available from two thirds of the trials about deaths that occurred before a relapse from breast cancer. Among 900 non–breast cancer deaths, tamoxifen use was associated with a 12% ($p < .05$) reduction in all non–breast cancer deaths, a 25% ($p < .06$) reduction in deaths from vascular causes, and a significant 9% reduction in other causes of death, suggesting that the benefits from tamoxifen extend beyond its ability to prevent breast cancer.

Not all published studies demonstrate a reduction in the occurrence of second primary breast tumors among women receiving tamoxifen. In one trial, postmenopausal women with positive axillary lymph nodes, large primary tumors, or tumor invasion into the skin or fascia were randomized to receive postoperative radiation with or without tamoxifen 30 mg/day for 48 weeks.[100] After a median follow-up of 7.9 years, no protective effect of tamoxifen on the development of contralateral breast cancers was observed. It is possible that the biologic characteristics of the primary breast cancers in these patients diminished the ability of tamoxifen to prevent second breast cancers. More important, because tamoxifen was given for only 48 weeks, suppression of second tumors may have been compromised.

TABLE 17-1 Possible Mechanisms of Inhibition of Cell Proliferation by Tamoxifen

1. Modulating the production of transforming growth factors (TGF-α and TGF-β) that regulate breast cancer cell proliferation, including proliferation of estrogen receptor–negative cell lines[84-87]
2. Binding to cytoplasmic antiestrogenic binding sites, increasing intracellular drug levels[88]
3. Increasing sex-hormone–binding globulin (SHBG) levels, which may decrease the availability of free estrogen for diffusion into tumor cells[89]
4. Increasing levels of natural killer (NK) cells[90]
5. Decreasing circulating insulin-like growth factor-I (IGF-I) levels, which may modify the hormonal regulation of breast cancer cell kinetics[91-94]

95% CIs for these observations excluded 1.0 and were statistically significant. A benefit was also seen for women with a history of LCIS (risk ratio, 0.44; 95% CI 0.16 to 1.06). For women with a history of atypical lobular or ductal hyperplasia, the risk ratio was markedly diminished at 0.14 (95% CI 0.03 to 0.47). Reduced risk ratios were seen at all projected levels of risk and among women with one or more first-degree relatives with a history of invasive breast cancer.

EFFECT OF TAMOXIFEN IN CARRIERS OF PREDISPOSING GENETIC MUTATIONS

BRCA1 acts, in part, as a tumor-suppressor gene. Reduction in *BRCA1* expression in vitro results in the accelerated growth of breast and ovarian cell lines, although overexpression of *BRCA1* results in inhibited growth.[111,112] *BRCA1* serves as a substrate for certain cyclin-dependent kinases, and estradiol induces *BRCA1* through an increase in DNA synthesis, which suggests that *BRCA1* may serve as a negative modulator of estradiol-induced growth.[113,114]

Like *BRCA1*, *BRCA2* expression in the breast is induced during puberty and pregnancy and after treatment with estradiol and progesterone. In multiple fetal and adult tissues, the temporal expression of *BRCA2* mRNA is indistinguishable from *BRCA1*,[112,115] and it seems that both *BRCA1* and *BRCA2* expression may be regulated through similar pathways. Expression of both genes is differentially regulated by hormones during the development of specific target tissues, but the upregulation of mRNA expression in the breast by ovarian steroid hormones is greater for *BRCA1* than for *BRCA2*.

Although *BRCA1* mutation carriers are more likely to develop ER-negative tumors,[116,117] prophylactic oophorectomy reduces the risk of breast cancer by approximately 30% in women who carry mutations in either the *BRCA1* or *BRCA2* gene.[118] More important, Narod and colleagues[119] compared 209 women with bilateral breast cancer and *BRCA1* or *BRCA2* mutation (bilateral disease cases) with 384 women with unilateral disease and *BRCA1* or *BRCA2* mutation (controls) in a matched case-control study. The multivariate odds ratio for contralateral breast cancer associated with tamoxifen use was 0.50 (95% CI 0.28 to 0.89). Tamoxifen protected against contralateral breast cancer for carriers of *BRCA1* mutations (odds ratio, 0.38; 95% CI 0.19 to 0.74) and for those with *BRCA2* mutations (odds ratio, 0.63; 95% CI 0.20 to 1.50). The greater apparent benefit of tamoxifen in carriers of *BRCA1* mutations as compared with carriers of *BRCA2* mutations is paradoxical given the greater prevalence of ER-positive breast cancer reported among carriers of *BRCA2* mutations.[120] This observation needs to be validated in additional studies.

To evaluate the effect of tamoxifen on the incidence of breast cancer among women with inherited *BRCA1* or *BRCA2* mutations, genomic analysis of *BRCA1* and *BRCA2* was performed for 288 women who developed breast cancer after entry into the trial.[121] Of the 288 breast cancer cases, 19 (6.6%) inherited disease-predisposing *BRCA1* or *BRCA2* mutations. Of 8 patients with *BRCA1* mutations, 5 received tamoxifen and 3 received placebo (risk ratio, 1.67; 95% CI 0.32 to 10.70). Of 11 patients with *BRCA2* mutations, 3 received tamoxifen and 8 received placebo (risk ratio, 0.38; 95% CI 0.06 to 1.56).

Therefore tamoxifen reduced breast cancer incidence among healthy *BRCA2* carriers by 62%, similar to the reduction in incidence of ER-positive breast cancer among all women in the trial. In contrast, tamoxifen use did not reduce breast cancer incidence among healthy women with inherited *BRCA1* mutations. These results must be interpreted with caution, however, given the small number of women with mutations or either *BRCA1* or *BRCA2* who were identified in the trial. Larger prospective studies of women with predisposing mutations will be required to provide conclusive evidence of either protection or lack of effect by tamoxifen in women with these mutations.

OTHER OUTCOMES IN BCPT

Coronary Artery Disease and Fracture Outcomes in BCPT. Tamoxifen is known to have estrogen agonist-like effects on both bone mineral density and serum cholesterol levels in postmenopausal women.[122,123] Few ischemic heart disease events occurred (133 total events) during the BCPT, perhaps because only 30% of the participants were age 60 or older or perhaps because the median duration of follow-up at the time of the report of the trial was only approximately 4 years. The event rate was similar between the tamoxifen and placebo groups. More consistent with expected outcomes were a total of 955 women who experienced skeletal fractures. The incidence of osteoporotic fractures involving the hip, spine, or distal radius was reduced by 19% in the tamoxifen group (111 versus 137 events in the tamoxifen and placebo groups, respectively). There was a 45% reduction in fractures of the hip that failed to reach statistical significance because of the small number of events reported ($n = 34$) in a population whose median age at enrollment was 52 years. It is likely that tamoxifen has a significant effect on fractures in postmenopausal women, but additional data are required to confirm this observation. Preliminary data in premenopausal women suggest a potentially negative effect of tamoxifen on bone mineral density,[124,125] but additional observation is required before a definitive statement can be made about fracture outcomes in younger women taking tamoxifen for risk reduction.

OTHER UNFAVORABLE OUTCOMES IN BCPT

Tamoxifen is a drug with both estrogen agonist and estrogen antagonist properties. Women who received tamoxifen in the BCPT had a 2.5 times greater risk of developing invasive endometrial cancer than did women who received placebo; the average annual rate was 2.3 per 1000 women and 0.9 per 1000 women in the tamoxifen and placebo groups, respectively. This incidence rate is similar to that of women receiving tamoxifen as adjuvant therapy for breast cancer in the NSABP B-14 trial.[126] All 36 invasive endometrial cancers that occurred among women receiving tamoxifen in the BCPT were FIGO stages 0 or I and had excellent clinical prognoses, although it is premature to make definitive statements about the long-term outcome of these tumors.

In the BCPT an increased number of thromboembolic vascular events occurred among women receiving tamoxifen. Although only the event rate for pulmonary embolism achieved statistical significance, there is cause for concern with increased event rates for strokes, transient ischemic attacks, and deep venous thromboses, particularly among women age 50 and older.

In addition to these side effects, there was a statistically marginal increase of approximately 14% in the rate of cataract development among women who were free of cataracts at the time of entry into the BCPT. Event rates for cataract surgery were also increased for women taking tamoxifen when compared with those of women taking the placebo.

Bothersome hot flashes were reported by 46% of women in the tamoxifen group, compared with only 29% in the placebo group. Similarly, vaginal discharge reported as moderately bothersome or worse was observed in 29% of the tamoxifen group, compared with 13% of the placebo group.

Royal Marsden Hospital Tamoxifen Chemoprevention Trial

The Royal Marsden Hospital Tamoxifen Chemoprevention Trial was designed and initiated as a feasibility trial.[106] Between October 1986 and April 1996, 2494 women were randomized in a placebo-controlled, double-blind clinical trial to evaluate the effectiveness of tamoxifen 20 mg/day for 8 years for the prevention of breast cancer in women at increased risk of developing breast cancer. Women were eligible for participation in this trial if they were between the ages of 30 and 70 years with an increased risk of breast cancer based on family history (at least one first-degree relative with breast cancer diagnosed before age 50, one first-degree relative with bilateral breast cancer, or one first-degree relative of any age plus another

affected first- or second-degree relative). The median age of participants was 47 years (range, 30 to 70 years), and 66% of these women were premenopausal or perimenopausal. Hormone replacement therapy (HRT) was being taken by 16% of the women at the time of randomization, and an additional 26% of participants required HRT at some time after randomization. Throughout the trial, concomitant use of HRT and tamoxifen occurred during 13% of the tamoxifen medication period.

At the time of an interim analysis with a median follow-up of 70 months, 63% of women were taking tamoxifen after 5 years, compared with 73% of women taking placebo. Noncompliance because of toxicity occurred in 320 women taking tamoxifen, compared with 176 women taking placebo ($p < .0005$). At the time of the interim analysis, there was no difference in the incidence of breast cancer for women randomized to receive tamoxifen (34) or placebo (36) ($p = .8$). Eight patients, four from each group, had DCIS, and no interaction was identified between the use of HRT and the effect of tamoxifen on breast cancer incidence.

These results have been controversial, however, for several reasons: (1) Only 156 patients completed 8 years of treatment; 877 patients prematurely discontinued therapy, and 280 patients were lost to follow-up, raising uncertainties about the findings. (2) The trial permitted women to use HRT concomitantly with the study medication (336 women taking tamoxifen and 305 women taking placebo received estrogen), perhaps inhibiting the protective effect of tamoxifen on development of breast malignancy. (3) The statistical power of the trial to detect a difference was not large and was probably less than 50% to detect a reduction in ER-positive breast cancer.[127]

ITALIAN TAMOXIFEN PREVENTION TRIAL

A third trial examining the ability of tamoxifen to prevent breast cancer has been conducted at the European Institute of Oncology, the F. Addarii Cancer Institute at Bologna, and the Cancer Institute of Naples, Italy.[107] Between October 1992 and July 1997, 5408 women were randomized in a placebo-controlled, double-blind clinical trial to evaluate the effectiveness of tamoxifen 20 mg/day for 5 years for the prevention of breast cancer. Women were eligible for participation in this trial if they were between the ages of 35 and 70 and had undergone hysterectomy for benign disease. This group of women was at less-than-normal risk of breast cancer because some of them had undergone bilateral oophorectomy before menopause. Participants were not permitted to use HRT. The primary end points of the study were the reduction in the incidence of and mortality from breast cancer. Accrual to the trial was halted prematurely by the data-monitoring committee because of patient dropout (26.3% of women randomized) and the tamoxifen side effect profile (increased incidence of superficial phlebitis and hyper-triglyceridemia). No statistically significant difference in the incidence of breast cancer between the two arms of the trial was noted.

In the extended follow-up (median, 81.2 months; range, 66.0 to 87.2 months) of the Italian trial, tamoxifen did not significantly protect against breast cancer in women at usual or slightly reduced risk of the disease, according to the Italian investigators. Use of HRT increased the risk of breast cancer, and users of such treatment who were randomly allocated to tamoxifen had a rate of breast cancer that was close to that of never-users. The investigators concluded that "tamoxifen was not significantly protective against breast cancer in women at normal or slightly reduced risk of the disease," but the interpretation of the results of this trial has been controversial as well. The study population was young and at low risk for breast cancer, there was poor compliance with assigned treatment, and this trial (like the Royal Marsden trial) was also underpowered to detect a difference between the placebo and tamoxifen groups.

INTERNATIONAL BREAST CANCER INTERVENTION STUDY I

A larger trial with an appropriate design, the IBIS I, more closely replicated the findings in BCPT.[108] In the IBIS I, more than 7000 women aged 35 to 70 years (median, 50.7 years) at high risk for breast cancer were randomly assigned to receive tamoxifen or placebo. The primary end point was the incidence of breast cancer, including DCIS.

Among the patients randomized, 3574 received placebo and 3578 received tamoxifen. The median follow-up was 50 months, and the estimated compliance at 5 years was 77% in the placebo group and 67% among women taking tamoxifen. The women in the study had a fourfold increased risk of developing breast cancer compared with the usual population, in most cases because of family history. About 60% of participants had two or more first-degree relatives with breast cancer. One third of the women had had hysterectomies, and about 50% of women used HRT at some point during the trial. It is important to note that among women who took HRT during the trial, the reduction in the incidence of breast cancer was 27%, compared with 26% among women who had never taken HRT. The reduction in breast cancer incidence associated with tamoxifen was independent of age, and there was no difference between tamoxifen and placebo cases in nodal status, size, or grade of breast cancers diagnosed.

The summary odds ratio for breast cancer incidence in the BCPT, the Royal Marsden trial, and the Italian trial, when taken together, is 0.62, as it is for the reduction of second, contralateral breast malignancies in the Early Breast Cancer Trialists' overview of the world's literature on the use of tamoxifen for the adjuvant therapy of breast cancer.[99] The trials, when considered together and recognizing the limitations of the smaller studies, confirm an odds ratio of 0.62 (a risk reduction of 38%) for ER-positive tumors and no effect on ER-negative breast cancer when using tamoxifen for risk reduction.

Appropriate Candidates for Reduction of Breast Cancer Risk Using Tamoxifen

In response to findings from the Breast Cancer Prevention Trial, the U.S. Food and Drug Administration approved the use of tamoxifen to reduce the incidence of breast cancer in women at increased risk. The risks and benefits of using tamoxifen depend on age and race, as well as on a woman's specific risk factors for breast cancer. In particular, the absolute risks of endometrial cancer, stroke, pulmonary embolism, and deep venous thrombosis associated with tamoxifen use increase with age, as does the protective effect of tamoxifen on fractures. A strategy to weigh these risks and benefits in the setting of breast cancer risk reduction in a semiquantitative manner was developed at a national conference of breast cancer experts, and the methods and their recommendations have been published.[128] The conferees reviewed information on the incidence of invasive breast cancer and of in situ lesions, as well as on several other health outcomes, in the absence of tamoxifen treatment. Data on the effects of tamoxifen on these outcomes were also reviewed, and methods were developed to compare the risks and benefits of tamoxifen. Tables and aids were developed to describe the risks and benefits of tamoxifen and to identify classes of women for whom the benefits outweigh the risks. An increase in the rates of either thrombosis or endometrial cancer was not seen among premenopausal women in the BCPT. Consequently, tamoxifen is most beneficial for women age 50 or younger who have an elevated risk of breast cancer. The published quantitative analyses can assist both health care providers and women in weighing the risks and benefits of tamoxifen for reducing breast cancer risk.

Tamoxifen is approved for the reduction of breast cancer risk in women whose risk of developing breast cancer is equal to the minimum eligibility for the trial, that is, a probability of developing breast cancer of 1.66% or greater in 5 years as determined by the Gail model. The use of tamoxifen for the reduction of breast cancer risk requires consideration of a woman's absolute risk of breast cancer as determined by quantitative modeling or the presence of risk factors themselves known to increase the risk of breast cancer substantially (e.g., LCIS). It is also necessary to evaluate risk/benefit considerations that include the absolute reduction in the risk of breast cancer that is expected to accrue with the use of tamoxifen. The risk of developing breast cancer is the primary determinant of net benefit, with greater net benefits accruing to women with the highest risk of breast cancer. Weighting the relative risks and benefits associated with tamoxifen has a modest effect on calculated net benefits. Both age and the presence of factors that increase the risk of toxicity have the greatest effect on the net benefit associated with tamoxifen.

The model developed by Gail and colleagues[110] is an accurate method of quantifying a woman's risk of developing breast cancer. The model allows estimation of the likelihood that a woman of a given age with certain risk factors will develop breast cancer over a specified interval. It was derived using 4496 matched pairs of subjects from the Breast Cancer Detection and Demonstration Project, a mammography screening project carried out between 1973 and 1980 that involved more than 280,000 women. The risk factors were adjusted simultaneously for the presence of the other risk factors, and only six factors were shown to be significant predictors of the lifetime risk of breast cancer:

1. Current age
2. Age at menarche
3. Number of breast biopsies
4. Age at first live birth (or nulliparity)
5. Family history of breast cancer in first-degree relatives
6. Race

A previous diagnosis of atypical lobular or ductal hyperplasia nearly doubles the estimated risk. Costantino and co-workers[129] used data from 5969 white women in the placebo arm of the BCPT who were screened annually to explore the accuracy of the Gail model. With an average follow-up period of 48.4 months, they compared the observed number of breast cancers with the predicted numbers from the model. The ratio of total expected to observed numbers of cancers was 1.03 (range, 0.88 to 1.21). The model tends to overestimate the risk for women classified at higher levels of predicted 5-year risk and to underestimate risk for those women with lower risk.

The validity of the Gail model was also evaluated in a cohort of 82,109 white women aged 45 to 71 years in the Nurses' Health Study. The model was applied to these women over a 5-year follow-up period to estimate a 5-year risk of invasive breast cancer. The model fit well

in the total sample (ratio of expected to observed numbers of cases, 0.94; 95% CI 0.89 to 0.99). Underprediction was slightly greater for younger women (<60 years), but in most age and risk factor strata, expected-to-observed ratios were close to 1.0.[130]

The Gail model can be accessed via the Internet.[131] A computer program disk that performs the calculations and prints an explanation for patients in lay language is also available from the National Cancer Institute. The patient's perception of her own risk should be elicited so that it can be compared with an objective risk estimate. This discussion might include her personal experience of breast cancer in family members and her beliefs and fears concerning cancer etiology and treatment. Clinicians should strive to ensure that the patient understands her objective risk and its implications for making a decision about the use of tamoxifen.

Women younger than 50 who are at increased risk for breast cancer tend to overestimate their risk, even as much as twentyfold.[132] Risk calculations should be used to estimate only the probability of developing the disease, not the risk of dying from breast cancer. Previous research suggests that discussion of risk of breast cancer may have unwanted psychologic effects,[133] so counseling should include an assessment of a woman's risk perception.[134]

Management of women at increased risk for breast cancer should include comprehensive quantitative risk assessment, counseling appropriate to the individual's risk, the opportunity for genetic testing when appropriate, and a specific management prescription.[101] The latter should include discussion of the risks and benefits of screening, prophylactic surgery when indicated, and risk reduction using approved chemopreventive agents.

Indications and contraindications for the use of tamoxifen for reduction of breast cancer risk are listed in Table 17-4. Absolute contraindications to the use of tamoxifen for risk reduction include a history of deep venous thrombosis or pulmonary embolism, a history of stroke or transient ischemic attack, a history of uncontrolled diabetes or hypertension, and/or a history of uncontrolled atrial fibrillation. Women currently taking estrogen, progesterone, androgens, or birth control pills should discontinue these medications before initiating tamoxifen therapy. Women who may be pregnant or may become pregnant should not take tamoxifen.

The optimal duration of risk-reducing therapy is unknown, but adjuvant therapy studies with tamoxifen indicate that therapy of less than 5 years' duration is not as effective as at least 5 years of therapy in reducing the incidence of second contralateral invasive breast cancer. Whether using tamoxifen for longer than 5 years is more effective in preventing the recurrence of breast cancer than using it for only 5 years is the subject of ongoing clinical trials; however, no trials are currently being conducted or planned to examine the ideal duration of

TABLE 17-4	Women in Whom Tamoxifen Should Be Considered for Reducing the Incidence of Invasive Breast Cancer

Women with a history of one of the following:
Lobular carcinoma in situ (LCIS)
Ductal carcinoma in situ (DCIS)
Atypical ductal or lobular hyperplasia
Premenopausal women with mutations in either the *BRCA1* or *BRCA2* genes
Premenopausal women ≥35 years with 5-year probability of breast cancer ≥1.66%
Women aged ≥60 years with Gail model 5-year probability of breast cancer ≥5%

therapy in the risk-reduction setting. The optimal age at which to start therapy is unknown, and tamoxifen cannot be used by women who are pregnant or attempting to become pregnant. Acceptance of tamoxifen may be poor among eligible subjects who will elect prophylactic surgery instead of a chemopreventive risk-reduction strategy, and toxicity is a concern among postmenopausal women. Additional data are needed from both ongoing adjuvant therapy trials and risk reduction trials, as well as from future trials that will examine the use of selective estrogen response modulators in the management of women who are at increased risk of developing breast cancer.

Lobular Carcinoma In Situ and Atypical Hyperplasia. Women with a history of LCIS experienced an annual risk for invasive breast cancer of 1.3% per year in the BCPT, and tamoxifen reduced this risk by approximately 55%. Women with atypical ductal or lobular hyperplasia experience an increased risk of subsequent invasive breast cancer, and tamoxifen reduced that risk by 86% in BCPT. Therefore women with either LCIS or atypical hyperplasia should be considered candidates for primary reduction of breast cancer risk with tamoxifen if there are no absolute contraindications to its use.

Recent Small Invasive Breast Cancers. Women with a history of invasive breast cancer have a risk of developing a second, contralateral, primary breast tumor of about 0.6% per year.[135] This figure corresponds to a 5-year risk of about 3%, which is greater than the risk of invasive breast cancer of 2.2% over 5 years that occurs among high-risk women experiencing incidence rates equal to those in the BCPT placebo arm. Consensus opinion suggests that adjuvant therapy with tamoxifen is not indicated for women with invasive breast tumors less than 1 cm in size with negative axillary lymph nodes.[136] However, these opinions were based on studies of tamoxifen as treatment for primary cancer rather than as a preventive agent against a second primary breast cancer. Because the risk of a second primary breast cancer approaches 20% over the life of a woman diagnosed with a first breast cancer at the age of 40 (which is similar to the risk for women in the BCPT), the use of tamoxifen for primary prevention may be a reasonable option, particularly for younger women. No data are available from studies designed to examine this question, but a review of data from NSABP trials and others showed that tamoxifen reduces the incidence of contralateral second primary breast cancers by roughly the same proportion as observed for primary breast malignancies in the BCPT.[137] Therefore preventive use of tamoxifen for women with small, node-negative invasive breast cancers may be justified in some cases in which there is doubt about its use as adjuvant therapy.

Another group of women for whom there is no definitive answer about the use of tamoxifen for prevention are women with no evidence of disease who were diagnosed with breast cancer 5 years or more previously and who were not treated with adjuvant tamoxifen. In several NSABP protocols, as noted previously, the subsequent risk of invasive breast cancer in women who had survived disease free for 5 years after an initial breast cancer diagnosis and who had not received adjuvant tamoxifen was 3.4%, which is close to the risk of 3.3% for invasive breast cancer in the placebo arm of the BCPT; the cumulative risk of all invasive breast cancer in such women was 14.4%. The decision to use tamoxifen for risk reduction in these patients must be informed by an assessment of the duration and quality of life remaining, the risks as well as potential benefits of tamoxifen, and the presence of competing morbidities that may weigh against the use of tamoxifen. For example, tamoxifen might be appropriate in a 50-year-old woman who is otherwise healthy, but it might be less suitable in a 68-year-old woman with a history of cataracts and deep venous thrombosis.

CONCERNS ABOUT ESTROGEN RECEPTOR–NEGATIVE BREAST CANCER

The reduction in the risk of invasive breast cancer was seen within the first year of the BCPT. Moreover, with up to 6 years of follow-up, lower incidence rates for women taking tamoxifen compared with those taking placebo were seen for each subsequent year of the trial. The distribution of primary tumor size and pathologic involvement of the axillary lymph nodes was not markedly different between women taking tamoxifen and those taking placebo. There was a substantial difference, however, when comparing the proportion of ER-positive tumors that occurred among women taking tamoxifen. The incidence rate of ER-positive breast cancers was 5 per 1000 women in the placebo group, compared with only 1.6 per 1000 women in the tamoxifen group, a 69% reduction. Concordant with this observation, rates of ER-negative tumors were not significantly different in the two treatment groups (1.46 per 1000 women in the tamoxifen group compared with 1.20 per 1000 women in the placebo group).

It is unclear from these data whether using tamoxifen promotes the development of ER-negative breast tumors, and no data to address this question are available in the setting of primary risk reduction. Limited information is available from women with a first breast cancer who are taking tamoxifen as adjuvant therapy. Using data from a population-based tumor registry that collects information on the ER status of breast tumors, Li and colleagues followed 8981 women residing in western Washington State who were diagnosed as having a primary unilateral invasive breast cancer from 1990 through 1998 to identify cases of contralateral breast cancer.[138] Their analyses were restricted to women who were at least 50 years old and whose first breast cancer had a localized or regional stage; women who received adjuvant hormonal therapy but not chemotherapy ($n = 4654$) were classified as tamoxifen users, and those who received neither adjuvant hormonal therapy nor chemotherapy ($n = 4327$) were classified as nonusers of tamoxifen. The risk of developing an ER-positive contralateral breast cancer as compared with an ER-negative contralateral breast cancer among tamoxifen users was 0.8 (95% CI 0.5 to 1.1) and 4.9 (95% CI 1.4 to 17.4), respectively, times that of nonusers of tamoxifen ($p < .0001$).

These data suggest that tamoxifen use may decrease the risk of ER-positive contralateral breast tumors while increasing the risk of ER-negative contralateral tumors, but the findings have been questioned. The findings are inconsistent with other data in the literature obtained by an overview analysis, by randomized comparisons, or by a population-based case-control study.[139] Because information about duration of tamoxifen use was not captured in the report,[138] it is possible that many of the patients included in that analysis took tamoxifen for less than 1 year, a treatment interval not known to be associated with a statistically significant decrease in contralateral breast cancer. No biologic data support the hypothesis that tamoxifen promotes ER-negative breast

cancer. A comprehensive review of ER expression in breast cancer[140] concludes that ER expression is a stable phenotype and that there is no phenotypic drift after treatment with tamoxifen. However, there may be a decreased expression of the ER. Breast cancer is heterogeneous and contains both ER-negative and ER-positive cells, which likely have different origins. It is more likely that when breast cancer is treated with tamoxifen, the ER-positive cells respond by decreasing proliferation and the ER-negative cells may continue to grow by selective pressure.

In the BCPT, tamoxifen affected only the incidence of ER-positive breast cancer; there was no suggestion of the induction or promotion of ER-negative breast cancers among the women exposed to the drug. Concerns about inducing invasive breast cancer with a poor prognosis as a result of exposure to tamoxifen at the time of diagnosis do not seem to be supported by the available data at this time.

CARRIERS OF *BRCA1* OR *BRCA2* MUTATIONS

Using a simulated cohort of 30-year-old women who tested positive for either *BRCA1* or *BRCA2* mutations, Grann and co-workers[141] estimated that a 30-year-old woman with a mutation of either gene could prolong survival by undergoing a bilateral oophorectomy and/or bilateral mastectomy, as compared with surveillance alone. In their simulation model, chemoprevention with tamoxifen increased survival time by 1.6 years (95% CI 1.0 to 2.1) and yielded more quality-adjusted life-years than did prophylactic surgery, even when treatment was delayed until age 40 or 50 years. All of these procedures were cost-effective or cost-saving procedures when compared with surveillance alone.

Others have calculated that, compared with surveillance alone, 30-year-old patients with early-stage breast cancer with *BRCA1* or *BRCA2* mutations gain 0.4 to 1.3 years of life expectancy from tamoxifen therapy, 0.2 to 1.8 years from prophylactic oophorectomy, and 0.6 to 2.1 years from prophylactic mastectomy. The magnitude of these gains is least for women with low-penetrance mutations and greatest for those with high-penetrance mutations.[142]

Clinical Monitoring of Women Taking Tamoxifen. Experience with appropriate clinical management and follow-up of women taking tamoxifen for primary prevention is limited to only a few studies, principally the BCPT. Surprisingly little published information is available from clinical trials that used tamoxifen to treat breast cancer. Endometrial hyperplasia and cancer were more frequent among women taking tamoxifen than among women taking placebo in the BCPT, but there was no statistically significant evidence of elevated risk from tamoxifen use in women younger than 50 (RR, 1.21

with a 95% CI 0.41 to 3.60). There is accumulating evidence to support a noninvasive surveillance strategy for the detection of endometrial cancer. The utility of endometrial cancer screening with either endometrial biopsy or transvaginal ultrasound in asymptomatic tamoxifen-treated women is limited and is not to be recommended outside of a clinical trial setting. Rather, women receiving tamoxifen should have annual gynecologic examinations with Pap tests and pelvic examinations. Any abnormal bleeding should be evaluated with appropriate diagnostic testing. Women should be counseled about the risk of benign and malignant conditions associated with tamoxifen.

Routine screening with hematologic or chemical blood tests is not indicated because no hematologic or hepatic toxicities attributable to tamoxifen were demonstrated in the BCPT or in clinical trials using tamoxifen as adjuvant therapy. Because of the modest increase in risk of cataracts (RR, 1.14) and cataract surgery among women using tamoxifen compared with women taking placebo,[109] women taking tamoxifen should be questioned about symptoms of cataracts during follow-up and should discuss with their health care provider the value of periodic eye examinations.

Ethical Considerations in the Use of Tamoxifen for Reduction of Breast Cancer Risk. Individuals with a family history of breast cancer, with or without an identified predisposing genetic mutation, constitute a unique target population for primary preventive interventions. It is difficult to determine whether these individuals should be considered "patients," "subjects," or "participants." Labeling healthy individuals as patients carries the potentially negative connotations of illness in all of the behavioral metaphors associated with illness.[143] Although cancer patients and their physicians may tolerate significant toxicity, or even death, as a consequence of therapy, it is unlikely that patients who do not yet have malignancy, even if they are at substantially increased risk of developing cancer, will find serious toxicity acceptable. The challenge in chemopreventive applications is to find agents that are both effective and safe.

Finally, the duration of treatment must be considered. Our current understanding of carcinogenesis is that it is a chronic process that must be suppressed with long-term drug administration. It is impossible at present to administer a single dose of a preventive agent and permanently reverse the tendency for the development of a malignancy. Each chronic suppressive approach requires daily administration of an active agent and creates the need for the healthy individual to remain in contact with the health care system throughout prolonged periods of drug administration. The effectiveness of tamoxifen in preventing primary breast cancer beyond 5 years of treatment is also uncertain.

CLINICAL DATA WITH RALOXIFENE

The Multiple Outcomes of Raloxifene Evaluation (MORE) trial was designed to test whether 3 years of raloxifene therapy reduces the risk of fracture in postmenopausal women with osteoporosis.[144] The study was a multicenter, randomized, double-blind trial in which women taking raloxifene or placebo were followed from 1994 through 1998 at 180 clinical centers composed of community settings and medical practices in 25 countries, including the United States and Europe. A total of 7705 postmenopausal women with osteoporosis, younger than 81 (mean age, 66 years), were enrolled. No prospective studies have been performed to examine the effect of raloxifene on the incidence of breast cancer. However, data regarding the effect of raloxifene on the subsequent development of breast cancer are available from the MORE trial.[145]

Following the publication of the results of the BCPT, the MORE investigators sought to determine whether women taking raloxifene have a lower risk of invasive breast cancer. After a median follow-up of 40 months, 13 cases of breast cancer were confirmed among the 5129 women assigned to raloxifene, versus 27 among the 2576 women assigned to placebo. The RR of breast cancer was 0.24 (95% CI 0.13 to 0.44; $p < .001$). Raloxifene decreased the risk of ER-positive breast cancer by 90%, but not ER-negative breast cancer.

Like tamoxifen, raloxifene increased the risk of venous thromboembolic disease threefold (RR, 3.1; 95% CI 1.5 to 6.2), but unlike tamoxifen, it did not increase the risk of endometrial cancer (RR, 0.8; 95% CI 0.2 to 2.7). However, this finding was based on only 10 total cases of invasive endometrial cancer (6 among those taking either 60 or 120 mg of raloxifene and 4 among those taking placebo) and requires additional years of observation. Endometrial cancer was a rare event, occurring at a rate of only 2 to 3 cases per 1000 person-years, and these results are based on only 25,000 total person-years of observation. It is possible that additional cases will occur in the future and alter the estimates of the risk of endometrial cancer associated with raloxifene. Raloxifene at either 60 or 120 mg/day was also associated with statistically significant increases in the incidence of influenza-like symptoms, hot flashes, leg cramps, and endometrial cavity fluid.

As endogenous estradiol increases, the risk of breast cancer increases. To test the hypothesis that raloxifene reduces breast cancer risk more in women with relatively high estradiol levels than in women with very low estradiol levels, the MORE investigators evaluated the effect of serum estradiol levels at entry into the trial on the subsequent risk of developing invasive breast cancer.[146] A total of 7290 postmenopausal women aged 80 years or younger with osteoporosis had baseline serum estradiol concentrations measured by a central laboratory using a sensitive assay. In the placebo group, women with estradiol levels greater than 10 pmol/L (2.7 pg/ml) had a 6.8-fold higher rate of breast cancer (3.0% per 4 years; 95% CI 1.8% to 4.1%) than that of women with undetectable estradiol levels (0.6% per 4 years; 95% CI, 0% to 1.1%; $p = .005$ for trend). Women with estradiol levels greater than 10 pmol/L in the raloxifene group had a rate of breast cancer that was 76% (95% CI 53% to 88%) lower than that of women with estradiol levels greater than 10 pmol/L in the placebo group (absolute rate reduction, 2.2%; 95% CI 1.0% to 3.5%). In contrast, women with undetectable estradiol levels had similar breast cancer risk, regardless of whether they were treated with raloxifene (risk difference, –0.1%; 95% CI, –0.8% to 0.6%; $p = .02$ for the interaction). These data suggest that measurement of estradiol level with a sensitive assay in postmenopausal women may identify those at high risk for breast cancer who may benefit most from risk-reduction interventions, but the results must be confirmed in additional prospective trials. If confirmed, measuring estradiol and treating women with high estradiol levels could substantially reduce the rate of breast cancer among postmenopausal women.

Other Effects of Raloxifene. In postmenopausal women taking raloxifene, the risk of venous thromboembolism is increased approximately threefold. This finding is virtually identical to the risk of thromboembolism seen with tamoxifen or HRT in postmenopausal women. Most of the thrombotic events reported with raloxifene occurred in the MORE study, in which the mean age of participants was 66 years. When patients with risk factors for thrombosis (e.g., immobilization, history of thrombotic event) are removed from this analysis, the risk drops to 1.7-fold.

Study of Tamoxifen and Raloxifene. The findings of the BCPT and IBIS I, coupled with the observations from the MORE trial, led the NSABP to design and launch the Study of Tamoxifen and Raloxifene (STAR) trial. Eligible women are at least 35 years old and postmenopausal, and they must have either LCIS or a 5-year risk of invasive breast cancer of at least 1.67% as determined by the Gail model. Subjects are randomly assigned to receive either tamoxifen 20 mg/day or raloxifene 60 mg/day in a double-blind, double-dummy design. No group of women in the trial receives placebo alone. The trial opened for subject accrual on July 1, 1999. It is designed to recruit a total of 22,000 postmenopausal women and is powered to demonstrate superior efficacy of either agent or their equivalence in reducing the incidence of primary breast cancer. Additional end points include the incidence of cardiovascular events and bone fractures. Thromboembolic

events and endometrial cancer are the predicted toxicities. Serum and lymphocytes are being collected for future studies after appropriate informed consent. Ancillary studies of cognitive function will also be performed.

After nearly 3 years of enrollment of eligible subjects at 193 clinical centers in North America, risk assessments have been performed in 116,669 women and 64,955 (56.7%) were eligible for the trial.[147] Of the eligible subjects, 13,416 have been randomized (21.8% of those eligible). The median age of randomized women is 58 years, and their median 5-year risk of developing invasive breast cancer is 3.3%. Recruitment will continue through 2005, and preliminary results are anticipated 1 or 2 years later. Until those results are available, the routine clinical use of raloxifene to reduce the incidence of invasive breast cancer is inappropriate. The drug is not approved for this indication in the United States, nor are there any safety or efficacy data related to the use of raloxifene in premenopausal women.

Future Developments

Tamoxifen is not the ideal drug to reduce the incidence of primary invasive breast cancer for a number of reasons, and it has neither the safety nor the efficacy desired to be the optimal agent. Because of this, several agents or classes of agents are being evaluated to identify a more suitable alternative to tamoxifen for reducing the risk of breast cancer in high-risk women.

ATAC TRIAL RESULTS

Aromatase inhibitors are a class of drugs shown to reduce circulating estrogen levels by approximately 90% in postmenopausal women.[148] Drugs of this class are approved for first-line treatment of advanced breast cancer that expresses ER protein in postmenopausal women. Many adjuvant therapy trials designed to evaluate the efficacy of the aromatase inhibitors in early breast cancer are currently being conducted. The ATAC (anastrazole, tamoxifen, alone and in combination) trial was the first such international, multicenter, randomized, double-blind trial to report preliminary results.[149] In the ATAC trial, 9366 postmenopausal patients with early-stage breast cancer were randomly assigned to one of three treatment arms: tamoxifen 20 mg/day, anastrazole 1 mg/day, or the combination for 5 years. Primary study end points include disease-free survival and safety/tolerability, and the development of new (contralateral) breast cancer primaries is a secondary end point.

In the ATAC trial, anastrazole, but not the anastrazole plus tamoxifen combination, was superior to tamoxifen in prolonging disease-free survival after 33 months of median follow-up. Importantly, anastrazole was associated with a statistically significant 58% reduction in new contralateral primary invasive breast cancers (RR, 0.42; 95% CI 0.22 to 0.79; for anastrazole compared with tamoxifen groups, $p < .0068$) based on 62 new invasive contralateral breast cancers that occurred in the ATAC trial through October 2001. Anastrazole was also associated with a significant excess of bone fractures related to osteoporosis when compared with tamoxifen. Substantial additional data will be required from future clinical trials before anastrazole (or any aromatase inhibitor) can be used safely to reduce the risk of breast cancer.

Hormone Replacement Therapy in Women at Increased Risk for Breast Cancer

HRT is typically avoided in women with a history of breast cancer because of concerns that estrogen will stimulate recurrence. In one study that sought to examine this question,[150] data were assembled from 2755 women aged 35 to 74 years who were diagnosed with incident invasive breast cancer while they were enrolled in a large health maintenance organization from 1977 through 1994. Pharmacy data identified 174 users of HRT after diagnosis. Each HRT user was matched to four randomly selected non-HRT users. The rate of breast cancer recurrence was 17 per 1000 person-years in women who used HRT after diagnosis and 30 per 1000 person-years in nonusers (adjusted RR for users compared with nonusers, 0.50; 95% CI 0.30 to 0.85). Breast cancer mortality rates were 5 per 1000 person-years in HRT users and 15 per 1000 person-years in nonusers (adjusted RR, 0.34; 95% CI 0.13 to 0.91). Total mortality rates were 16 per 1000 person-years in HRT users and 30 per 1000 person-years in nonusers (adjusted RR, 0.48; 95% CI 0.29 to 0.78). The relatively low rates of recurrence and death were observed in women who used any type of HRT (oral only, 41% of HRT users; vaginal only, 43%; both oral and vaginal, 16%). No trend toward lower relative risks was observed with increased dosage. The results suggest that HRT after breast cancer has no adverse effect on recurrence and mortality, but these results must be interpreted cautiously because of the small number of patients, the mix of hormone replacement regimens used, and the possible variable effects on ER-positive as compared with ER-negative breast cancer. It is also not yet known whether a similar result would be found among women who are at increased risk for breast cancer.

REFERENCES

1. Atiba JO, Meyskens FL: Chemoprevention of breast cancer, *Semin Oncol* 19:220, 1992.
2. Bertram JS, Kolonel LN, Meyskens FL: Rationale and strategies for chemoprevention of cancer in humans, *Cancer Res* 47:3012, 1987.
3. Boone CW, Kelloff GJ, Steele VE: Natural history of intraepithelial neoplasia in humans with implications for cancer chemoprevention strategy, *Cancer Res* 52:1651, 1991.
4. Costa A: Breast cancer chemoprevention, *Eur J Cancer* 29A:589, 1993.
5. Lippman SM et al: Biomarkers as intermediate end points in chemoprevention trials, *J Natl Cancer Inst* 82:555, 1990.
6. Lippman SM, Benner SE, Hong WK: Cancer chemoprevention, *J Clin Oncol* 12:851, 1994.
7. Lippman SM, Hong WK, Benner SE: The chemoprevention of cancer. In Greenwald P, Kramer BS, Weed DL (eds): *Cancer prevention and control,* New York, 1995, Marcel Dekker.
8. Moon RC, Mehta RG: Chemoprevention of experimental carcinogenesis in animals, *Prev Med* 18:576, 1989.
9. O'Shaughnessy JA: Chemoprevention of breast cancer, *JAMA* 275:1349, 1996.
10. Sporn MB: Carcinogenesis and cancer: different perspectives on the same disease, *Cancer Res* 51:6215, 1991.
11. Sporn MB et al: Prevention of chemical carcinogenesis by vitamin A and its synthetic analogs (retinoids), *Fed Proc* 35:1332, 1976.
12. Wattenberg LW: Chemoprevention of cancer, *Cancer Res* 45:1, 1985.
13. Russo J, Russo IH: Development of the human mammary gland. In Neville MD, Daniel C (eds): *The mammary gland,* New York, 1987, Plenum.
14. Vorher H: *The breast,* New York, 1974, Academic.
15. Russo J, Russo IH: Toward a physiological approach to breast cancer prevention, *Cancer Epidemiol Biomarkers Prev* 3:353, 1994.
16. Russo J, Lynch H, Russo IH: Mammary gland architecture as a determining factor in the susceptibility of the human breast to cancer, *Breast J* 7:278, 2001.
17. Russo J et al: Influence of human breast development of the growth properties of primary cultures, *In Vitro Cell Dev Biol* 25:643, 1989.
18. Russo J et al: Expression of phenotypical changes by human breast epithelial cells treated with carcinogens in vitro, *Cancer Res* 48:2837, 1988.
19. Russo IH, Calaf G, Russo J: Hormones and proliferative activity in breast tissue. In Stoll BA (ed): *Approaches to breast cancer prevention,* Dordrecht, 1990, Kluwer Academic.
20. Russo J et al: Developmental, cellular, and molecular basis of human breast cancer, *J Natl Cancer Inst Monogr* 27:17, 2000.
21. Russo IH, Russo J: Chorionic gonadotropin: a tumoristatic and preventive agent in breast cancer. In Teicher BA (ed): *Drug resistance in oncology,* New York, 1992, Marcel Dekker.
22. Anderson TJ et al: Oral contraceptive use influences breast proliferation, *Hum Pathol* 20:1139, 1989.
23. Longacre TA, Bartow SA: A correlative morphologic study of human breast and endometrium in the menstrual cycle, *Am J Surg Pathol* 10:382, 1986.
24. Potten CS et al: The effect of age and menstrual cycle upon proliferative activity of the normal human breast, *Br J Cancer* 58:163, 1988.
25. Russo IH, Russo J: Hormone prevention of mammary carcinogenesis: a new approach in anticancer research, *Anticancer Res* 8:1247, 1988.
26. Ames B: Mutagenesis and carcinogenesis: endogenous and exogenous factors, *Environ Mol Mutagen* 14:66, 1989.

27. Ames BN, Gold LS: Too many rodent carcinogens: mitogenesis increases mutagenesis, *Science* 249:970, 1990.

28. Bernstein L, Ross RK, Henderson BE: Prospects for the primary prevention of breast cancer, *Am J Epidemiol* 135:142, 1992.

29. Henderson BE et al: Endogenous hormones as a major factor in human cancer, *Cancer Res* 42:3232, 1982.

30. Spicer DV, Krecher EA, Pike MC: The endocrine prevention of breast cancer, *Cancer Invest* 13:495, 1995.

31. Plu-Bureau G et al: Progestogen use and decreased risk of breast cancer in a cohort study of premenopausal women with benign breast disease, *Br J Cancer* 70:270, 1994.

32. Persky V, Van Horn L: Epidemiology of soy and cancer: perspectives and directions, *J Nutr* 125:709S, 1995.

33. Kelloff GJ et al: Development of breast cancer chemopreventive drugs, *J Cell Biochem* 17G:2, 1993.

34. Schwarz AG, Lewbart ML, Pashko LL: Inhibition of tumorigenesis by dehydroepiandrosterone and structural analogs. In Wattenberg L et al (eds): *Cancer chemoprevention*, Boca Raton, 1992, CRC Press.

35. Dao TL, Bock FG, Greiner MJ: Mammary carcinogenesis by dimethylcholanthrene. II. Inhibitory effect of pregnancy and lactation on tumor induction, *J Natl Cancer Inst* 25:991, 1960.

36. Dao TL: The role of ovarian hormones in initiating the induction of mammary cancer in rats by polynuclear hydrocarbons, *Cancer Res* 22:973, 1962.

37. Russo IH, Russo J: Developmental stage of the rat mammary and as determinant of its susceptibility to 7,12-dimethylbenz (a) anthracene, *J Natl Cancer Inst* 61:1439, 1978.

38. Russo J, Russo IH: Biological and molecular bases of mammary carcinogenesis, *Lab Invest* 57:112, 1987.

39. Russo IH, Koszalka M, Russo J: Human chorionic gonadotropin and rat mammary cancer prevention, *J Natl Cancer Inst* 82:1286, 1990.

40. Russo IH, Koszalka M, Russo J: Effect of human chorionic gonadotropin on mammary gland differentiation and carcinogenesis, *Carcinogenesis* 11:1849, 1990.

41. Russo IH, Koszalka MS, Russo J: Protective effect of chorionic gonadotropin on DMBA-induced mammary carcinogenesis, *Br J Cancer* 62:243, 1990.

42. Russo IH, Russo J: Hormone prevention of mammary carcinogenesis: a new approach in anticancer research, *Anticancer Res* 8:1247, 1988.

43. Russo J: Basis of cellular autonomy in the susceptibility to carcinogenesis, *Toxicol Pathol* 11:149, 1983.

44. Russo IH, Koszalka M, Russo J: Comparative study of the influence of pregnancy and hormonal treatment on mammary carcinogenesis, *Br J Cancer* 64:481, 1991.

45. Chakravarty PK, Sinha DK: Pregnancy induced cytotoxicity of B-cell rich fraction against mammary adenocarcinoma cells in rats, *Carcinogenesis* 12:2499, 1992.

46. Alvarado MV, Russo J, Russo IH: Immunolocalization of inhibin in the mammary gland of rats treated with hCG, *J Histochem Cytochem* 41:29, 1993.

47. Matzuk MM et al: α-Inhibin is a tumour-suppressor gene with gonadal specificity in mice, *Nature* 360:313, 1992.

48. Davis SR et al: Inhibin A-subunit gene expression in the ovaries of immature female rats is stimulated by pregnant mare serum gonadotrophin, *Biochem Biophys Res Commun* 138:1191, 1986.

49. Erickson GF, Hsueh AJW: Secretion of inhibin by rat granulosa cells in vitro, *Endocrinology* 103:1960, 1978.

50. Steinberger A, Steinberger E: Secretion of an FSH-inhibiting factor by cultured Sertoli cells, *Endocrinology* 103:1960, 1978.

51. Mehta RG, Cerny WL, Moon RC: Distribution of retinoic acid binding protein in normal and neoplastic mammary tissues, *Cancer Res* 40:47, 1980.

52. Rivier C, Rivier J, Vale W: Inhibin-mediated feedback control of follicle-stimulating hormone secretion in the female rat, *Science* 234:205, 1986.

53. Robertson DM et al: Radioimmunoassay of rat serum inhibin: changes after PMSG stimulation and gonadectomy, *Mol Cell Endocrinol* 58:1, 1988.

54. Bradlow HL et al: Indole-3-carbinol: a novel approach to breast cancer prevention, *Ann NY Acad Sci* 768:180, 1995.

55. Bradlow HL et al: Long-term responses of women to indole-3-carbinol or a high fiber diet, *Cancer Epidemiol Biomarkers Prev* 3:591, 1994.

56. Harris JR et al: Breast cancer, *N Engl J Med* 327:319, 1992.

57. Vogel VG, Lippman SM, Boyd N: Is breast cancer preventable? *Can J Oncol* 1:28, 1991.

58. Goodman GE: The clinical evaluation of cancer chemoprevention agents: defining and contrasting phase I, II, and III objectives, *Cancer Res* 52:2752, 1992.

59. Henderson BE et al: Endogenous hormones as a major factor in human cancer, *Cancer Res* 42:3232, 1982.

60. Russo J, Russo IH: Toward a physiological approach to breast cancer prevention, *Cancer Epidemiol Biomarkers Prev* 3:353, 1994.

61. Henderson BE, Ross RK, Pike MC: Hormonal chemoprevention of cancer in women, *Science* 259:633, 1993.

62. Petrakis NL, Ernster VL, King MC: Breast. In Schottenfeld D, Fraumeni JF Jr (eds): *Cancer epidemiology and prevention*, Philadelphia, 1982, WB Saunders.

63. Furr BJ, Jordan VC: The pharmacology and clinical uses of tamoxifen, *Pharmacol Ther* 25:127, 1984.

64. Nicholson RI et al: Actions of oestrogens and anti-oestrogens on rat mammary gland development: relevance to breast cancer prevention, *J Steroid Biochem* 30:95, 1988.

65. Gotze S, Nishino Y, Neumann F: Anti-oestrogenic effects of tamoxifen on mammary gland and hypophysis in female rats, *Acta Endocrinol Copenh* 105:360, 1984.

66. Walker KJ et al: Influence of the antiestrogen on normal breast tissue, *Br J Cancer* 64:764, 1991.

67. Kelsey JL, Berkowitz GS: Breast cancer epidemiology, *Cancer Res* 48:5615, 1988.

68. Kelsey JL: A review of the epidemiology of human breast cancer, *Epidemiol Rev* 1:74, 1979.

69. Petrakis NL, Ernster VL, King MC: Breast. In Schottenfeld D, Fraumeni JF Jr (eds): *Cancer epidemiology and prevention*, Philadelphia, 1982, WB Saunders.

70. Hirayama T, Wynder E: Study of epidemiology of cancer of the breast: influence of hysterectomy, *Cancer* 15:28, 1962.

71. MacMahon B, Feinlieb M: Breast cancer in relation to nursing and menopausal history, *J Natl Cancer Inst* 24:733, 1960.

72. Adam HK, Petterson JS, Kemp JV: Studies on the metabolism and pharmacokinetics of tamoxifen in normal volunteers, *Cancer Treat Rep* 64:761, 1980.

73. Buckley MM, Goa KL: Tamoxifen: a reappraisal of its pharmacodynamic and pharmacokinetic properties and therapeutic use, *Drugs* 37:451, 1989.

74. Robinson SP et al: Metabolites, pharmacodynamics, and pharmacokinetics of tamoxifen in rats and mice compared to the breast cancer patient, *Drug Metab Dispos* 19:36, 1991.

75. Herrlinger C et al: Pharmacokinetics and bioavailability of tamoxifen in healthy volunteers, *Int J Pharmacol Ther Toxicol* 30:487, 1992.

76. Jordan VC, Murphy CS: Endocrine pharmacology of antiestrogens as antitumor agents, *Endocr Rev* 11:578, 1990.
77. Jordan VC: Chemosuppression of breast cancer with long-term tamoxifen therapy, *Prev Med* 20:3, 1991.
78. Briziarelli G: Effects of dosage and time of administration of testosterone propionate on 7,12-dimethylbenzanthracene mammary carcinogenisis in the rat, *Z Krebsforsch Klin Onkol* 66:517, 1965.
79. Terenius L: Effect of anti-estrogens on initiation of mammary cancer in the female rat, *Eur J Cancer* 7:65, 1971.
80. Jordan VC: Effect of tamoxifen (ICI 46,474) on initiation and growth of DMBA-induced rat mammary carcinomata, *Eur J Cancer* 12:419, 1976.
81. Jordan VC: Antitumor activity of the antiestrogen ICI 46,474 (tamoxifen) in the dimethylbenzanthracene (DMBA)-induced rat mammary carcinoma model, *J Steroid Biochem* 5:354, 1974.
82. Dao TL: The role of ovarian hormones in initiating the induction of mammary cancer in rats by polynuclear hydrocarbons, *Cancer Res* 22:973, 1962.
83. Tsai TLS, Katzenellenbogen BS: Antagonism of development and growth of 7,12-dimethylbenz(a) anthracene-induced rat mammary tumors by the antiestrogen U23,469 and effects on estrogen and progesterone receptors, *Cancer Res* 37:1537, 1977.
84. Noguchi S et al: Down regulation of transforming growth factor-α by tamoxifen in human breast cancer, *Cancer* 72:131, 1993.
85. Butta A et al: Induction of transforming growth factor β in human breast cancer in vivo following tamoxifen treatment, *Cancer Res* 52:4261, 1992.
86. Grainger DJ, Metcaffe JC: Tamoxifen: teaching an old drug new tricks? *Nat Med* 2:381, 1996.
87. Dickens T-A, Colletta AA: The pharmacological manipulation of members of the transforming growth factor beta family in the chemoprevention of breast cancer, *Bioessays* 15:71, 1993.
88. Murphy LC, Sutherland RL: Antitumor activity of clomiphene analogs in vitro: relationship to affinity for the estrogen receptor and another high affinity antiestrogen-binding site, *J Clin Endocrinol Metab* 57:373, 1983.
89. Jordan VC, Fritz NF, Tormey DC: Long term adjuvant therapy with tamoxifen: effects on sex hormone binding globulin and antithrombin III, *Cancer Res* 47:4517, 1987.
90. Berry J, Green BJ, Matheson DS: Modulation of natural killer cell activity by tamoxifen in stage I postmenopausal breast cancer, *Eur J Cancer Clin Oncol* 23:517, 1987.
91. Pollak MN, Huymh HT, Lefebre SP: Tamoxifen reduces serum insulin-like growth factor I (IGF-I), *Breast Cancer Res Treat* 22:91, 1992.
92. Friedl A, Jordan VC, Pollack M: Suppression of serum insulin-like growth factor-1 levels in breast cancer patients during adjuvant tamoxifen therapy, *Eur J Cancer* 29A:1368, 1993.
93. Lien EA et al: Influence of tamoxifen, aminoglutethimide and goserelin on human plasma IGF-I levels in breast cancer patients, *J Steroid Biochem Molec Biol* 41:541, 1992.
94. Lonning PE et al: Influence of tamoxifen on plasma levels of insulin-like growth factor β and insulin-like growth factor binding protein I in breast cancer patients, *Cancer Res* 52:4719, 1992.
95. Croxtall JD et al: Tamoxifen inhibits growth of oestrogen receptor-negative A549 cells, *Biochem Pharmacol* 47:197, 1994.
96. Vignon F, Bouton MM, Rochefort H: Antiestrogens inhibit the mitogenic effect of growth factors on breast cancer cells in the total absence of estrogens, *Biochem Biophys Res Comm* 146:1502, 1987.
97. Custodio JBA, Almeida LM, Madeira VMC: The anticancer drug tamoxifen induces changes in the physical properties of model and native membranes, *Biochim Biophys Acta* 1150:123, 1993.
98. Morrow M, Jordan VC: Molecular mechanisms of resistance to tamoxifen therapy in breast cancer, *Arch Surg* 128:1187, 1993.
99. Tamoxifen for early breast cancer: an overview of the randomised trials. Early Breast Cancer Trialists' Collaborative Group, *Lancet* 351:1451, 1998.
100. Andersson M, Storm HH, Morrisden HT: Incidence of new primary cancers after adjuvant tamoxifen therapy and radiotherapy for early breast cancer, *J Natl Cancer Inst* 83:1013, 1991.
101. Vogel VG: Chemoprevention: reducing breast cancer risk. In Vogel VG (ed): *Management of patients at high risk for breast cancer,* Malden, MA, 2001, Blackwell Science.
102. Vogel VG: High risk populations as targets for breast cancer prevention trials, *Prev Med* 20:86, 1991.
103. Vogel VG: Breast cancer risk factors and preventive approaches to breast cancer. In Kavanagh J et al (eds): *Cancer in women,* Cambridge, MA, 1998, Blackwell Scientific.
104. Greenwald P et al: Concepts in cancer chemoprevention research, *Cancer* 65:1483, 1990.
105. Malone WF et al: Chemoprevention and modern cancer prevention, *Prev Med* 18:553, 1989.
106. Powles TJ: The Royal Marsden Hospital (RMH) trial: key points and remaining questions, *Ann NY Acad Sci* 949:109, 2001.
107. Veronesi U et al, and Italian Tamoxifen Study Group: Tamoxifen for breast cancer among hysterectomised women, *Lancet* 359:1122, 2002.
108. Cuzick J: The prevention of breast cancer. Program and abstracts of the 3rd European Breast Cancer Conference, March 19-23, 2002, Barcelona, Spain.
109. Fisher B et al: Tamoxifen for prevention of breast cancer: report of the National Surgical Adjuvant Breast and Bowel Project P-1 Study, *J Natl Cancer Inst* 90:1371, 1998.
110. Gail MH et al: Projecting individualized probabilities of developing breast cancer for white females who are being examined annually, *J Natl Cancer Inst* 81:1879, 1989.
111. Lane TF et al: Expression of *BRCA1* is associated with terminal differentiation of ectodermally and mesodermally derived tissues in mice, *Dev Biol* 9:2712, 1995.
112. Rajan JV et al: Developmental expression of *BRCA2* co-localizes with *BRCA1* and is associated with proliferation and differentiation in multiple tissues, *Dev Biol* 184:385, 1997.
113. Marks JR et al: *BRCA1* expression is not directly responsive to estrogen, *Oncogene* 14:115, 1997.
114. Fan S et al: *BRCA1* inhibition of estrogen receptor signaling in transfected cells, *Science* 284:1354, 1999.
115. Marquis ST et al: The developmental pattern of *BRCA1* expression implies a role in differentiation of the breast and other tissues, *Nat Genet* 11:17, 1995.
116. Karp SE et al: Influence of *BRCA1* mutations on nuclear grade and estrogen receptor status of breast carcinoma in Ashkenazi Jewish women, *Cancer* 80:435, 1997.

117. Loman N et al: Steroid receptors in hereditary breast carcinomas associated with *BRCA1* or *BRCA2* mutations or unknown susceptibility genes, *Cancer* 83:310, 1998.
118. Rebbeck TR et al: Reduction in breast cancer risk after bilateral prophylactic oophorectomy in *BRCA1* mutation carriers, *J Natl Cancer Inst* 91:1475, 1999.
119. Narod SA et al: Tamoxifen and risk of contralateral breast cancer in *BRCA1* and *BRCA2* mutation carriers: a case-control study—Hereditary Breast Cancer Clinical Study Group, *Lancet* 356:1876, 2000.
120. Verhoog LC et al: Survival and tumour characteristics of breast-cancer patients with germline mutations of *BRCA1*, *Lancet* 251:316, 1998.
121. King M-C et al: Tamoxifen and breast cancer incidence among women with inherited mutations in *BRCA1* and *BRCA2*. National Surgical Adjuvant Breast and Bowel Project (NSABP-P1) Breast Cancer Prevention Trial, *JAMA* 286:2251, 2001.
122. Love RR et al: Effects of tamoxifen on bone mineral density in postmenopausal women with breast cancer, *N Engl J Med* 326:852, 1992.
123. Love RR et al: Effects of tamoxifen on cardiovascular risk factors in postmenopausal women, *Ann Intern Med* 115:860, 1991.
124. Jordan VC, Gapstur S, Morrow M: Selective estrogen receptor modulation and reduction in risk of breast cancer, osteoporosis, and coronary heart disease, *J Natl Cancer Inst* 93:1449, 2001.
125. Powles TJ et al: Tamoxifen preserves bone mineral density in post-menopausal women but causes loss of bone density in premenopausal women, *Proc Am Soc Clin Oncol* 14:165, 1995.
126. Fisher B et al: Endometrial cancer in tamoxifen-treated breast cancer patients: findings from the National Surgical Adjuvant Breast and Bowel Project (NSABP) B-14, *J Natl Cancer Inst* 86:527, 1994.
127. Costantino JP, Vogel VG: Results and implications of the Royal Marsden and other tamoxifen chemoprevention trials: an alternative view, *Clin Breast Cancer* 2:41, 2001.
128. Gail MH et al: Weighing the risks and benefits of tamoxifen treatment for preventing breast cancer, *J Natl Cancer Inst* 91:29, 1999.
129. Costantino JP et al: Validation studies for models projecting the risk of invasive and total breast cancer incidence, *J Natl Cancer Inst* 91:1541, 1999.
130. Rockhill B et al: Validation of the Gail et al model of breast cancer risk prediction and implications for chemoprevention, *J Natl Cancer Inst* 93:358, 2001.
131. National Cancer Institute: Breast Cancer Risk Assessment Tool. Available at: http://bcra.nci.nih.gov/brc. Accessed August 2001.
132. Black WC, Nease RF Jr, Tosteson A: Perceptions of breast cancer risk and screening effectiveness in women younger than 50 years of age, *J Natl Cancer Inst* 87:720, 1995.
133. Lerman C, Rimer BK, Engstrom PF: Cancer risk notification: psychological and ethical implications, *J Clin Oncol* 9:1275, 1991.
134. Lerman C, Schwartz M: Adherence and psychological adjustment among women at high risk for breast cancer, *Breast Cancer Res Treat* 28:145, 1993.
135. Vogel VG: Reducing the risk of breast cancer with tamoxifen in women at increased risk, *J Clin Oncol* 19:87s, 2001.
136. Adjuvant therapy for breast cancer, *NIH Consens Statement* 17:1, 2000.
137. Fisher B, Redmond C: New perspective on cancer of the contralateral breast: a marker for assessing tamoxifen as a preventive agent, *J Natl Cancer Inst* 83:1278, 1991.
138. Li CI et al: Tamoxifen therapy for primary breast cancer and risk of contralateral breast cancer, *J Natl Cancer Inst* 93:1008, 2001.
139. Swain SM: Tamoxifen and contralateral breast cancer: the other side, *J Natl Cancer Inst* 93:963, 2001.
140. Robertson JF: Oestrogen receptor: a stable phenotype in breast cancer, *Br J Cancer* 73:5, 1996.
141. Grann VR et al: Prevention with tamoxifen or other hormones versus prophylactic surgery in *BRCA1/2*-positive women: a decision analysis, *Cancer J Sci Am* 6:13, 2000.
142. Schrag D et al: Life expectancy gains from cancer prevention strategies for women with breast cancer and *BRCA1* or *BRCA2* mutations, *JAMA* 283:617, 2000.
143. Vogel VG, Parker LP: Ethical issues of chemoprevention-clinical trials, *Cancer Control* 4:142, 1997.
144. Ettinger B et al: Reduction of vertebral fracture risk in postmenopausal women with osteoporosis treated with raloxifene: results from a 3-year randomized clinical trial. Multiple Outcomes of Raloxifene Evaluation (MORE) Investigators, *JAMA* 282:637, 1999.
145. Cummings SR et al: The effect of raloxifene on risk of breast cancer in postmenopausal women: results from the MORE randomized trial. Multiple Outcomes of Raloxifene Evaluation, *JAMA* 281:2189, 1999.
146. Cummings SR et al: The Multiple Outcomes of Raloxifene Evaluation (MORE) Trial. Serum estradiol level and risk of breast cancer during treatment with raloxifene, *JAMA* 287:216, 2002.
147. Vogel VG et al: The study of tamoxifen and raloxifene: preliminary enrollment data from a randomized breast cancer risk reduction trial, *Clin Breast Cancer* 3:153, 2002.
148. Clemons M, Goss P: Estrogen and the risk of breast cancer, *N Engl J Med* 344:276, 2001.
149. The ATAC (Arimidex, Tamoxifen Alone or in Combination) Trialists' Group: Anastrazole alone or in combination with tamoxifen versus tamoxifen alone for adjuvant treatment of postmenopausal women with early breast cancer: first results of the ATAC randomized trial, *Lancet* 359:2131, 2002.
150. O'Meara ES et al: Hormone replacement therapy after a diagnosis of breast cancer in relation to recurrence and mortality, *J Natl Cancer Inst* 93:754, 2001.

18

Breast Cancer Genetics: Heterogeneity, Molecular Genetics, Syndrome Diagnosis, and Genetics Counseling

HENRY T. LYNCH

JOSEPH N. MARCUS

JANE F. LYNCH

CARRIE L. SNYDER

WENDY S. RUBINSTEIN

Approximately 1,334,100 new cases of cancer will occur in the United States in 2003 (675,300 males, 658,800 females), 212,600 of which involve the breast.[1] Using a conservative estimate that 5% of the total breast cancer burden is hereditary, in 2003, 10,630 new cases of breast cancer will fit a hereditary etiology. Most published estimates of the prevalence of BRCA1 mutations have used techniques with less than ideal sensitivities,[2] and up to 15% of BRCA1 and BRCA2 mutations may be undetectable by DNA sequencing[3]; thus the contribution of these genes to hereditary cancer is known somewhat imprecisely. As well, additional "breast cancer genes" continue to be reported.[4,5] As the knowledge gap narrows for genetic and environmental etiologies and these interactions are clarified, cancer control can be better targeted to a smaller fraction of the population at the highest risk.[6]

The etiology of breast cancer remains enigmatic. Madigan and colleagues[7] calculated incidence rates, relative risks (RRs), and population attributable risks (PARs) for breast cancer risk factors. They have extended these results to the U.S. population using data from the National Health and Nutrition Examination Survey (NHANES-I) and Epidemiologic Follow-up Study (NHEFS). Their findings disclosed that PAR estimates suggest that later age at first birth and nulliparity accounted for a large fraction, 29.5%, of U.S. breast cancer cases (95% confidence interval [CI] = 5.6% to 53.3%); higher income contributed 18.9% (95% CI = 4.3% to 42.1%); and family history of breast cancer accounted for 9.1% (95% CI = 3.0% to 15.2%). Taken together, these well-established risk factors accounted for approximately 47% (95% CI = 17% to 77%) of breast cancer cases in the NHEFS cohort and about 41% (95% CI = 2% to 80%) in the U.S. population. The authors concluded that the RRs in the majority of these risk factors were modest. However, their prevalence as a group was high, thereby suggesting that a large proportion of breast cancer cases in the United States can be explained by well-established risk factors.

Few systematic studies have defined these breast cancer risk factors in concert with primary genetic susceptibility to this disease. Narod and colleagues[8] studied the reproductive histories of 333 North American women who were found by haplotype analysis to carry BRCA1 mutations. An increased risk for breast cancer was associated with menarche below the age of 12 (RR 1.57), parity of less than three (RR 2.04), and year of birth after 1930 (RR 2.72). The risk of ovarian cancer (OC), however, increased with increasing parity and earlier age at last childbirth. Will BRCA1 germline mutation carriers who have had a late menarche, early age of onset of a full-term pregnancy, and a late menopause likely be protected from developing breast cancer or OC? Would such a patient experience a later age of cancer onset? Is tamoxifen an effective chemoprevention agent for women with germline mutations? In some instances, the effect of hormonal[9] and other[10] risk factors may actually be opposite of those seen for sporadic breast cancer. For example, BRCA1 and BRCA2 carriers who have children have an increased risk of breast cancer compared with nulliparous carriers.[9] These are the types of research questions genetic epidemiologists should pursue, and they may be answerable given the current ability to identify carriers of the BRCA1 mutation.

Our purpose in this chapter is to provide a comprehensive study of hereditary breast cancer (HBC), with particular attention given to its molecular genetic basis (when known), natural history, pathology, phenotypic and genotypic heterogeneity, as well as implications for its control through risk assessment, genetic counseling, and genetic testing.

History of Hereditary Breast Cancer

Research during the past several decades has taught us more about the genetic etiology of breast cancer than perhaps all of the knowledge that had accrued on the subject since Paul Broca, the famed French surgeon, first described his wife's pedigree in 1865 (Figure 18-1).[11] Her family showed four generations of breast cancer and occurrences of cancer of the gastrointestinal tract, making this the first report of the tumor heterogeneity of HBC.

The importance of genetic and clinical heterogeneity in HBC received very little attention until a century later, when Lynch and co-workers[12] described 34 families with two or more first-degree relatives affected with breast cancer in association with a variety of other cancer sites, including the first description of the now well-known hereditary breast/ovarian cancer (HBOC) syndrome. Thus, up to that time, breast cancer risk was computed primarily on the patient's position within the pedigree, often when there were multiple first- and second-degree relatives affected with breast cancer and/or OC. Therefore these publications, more than three decades ago, constituted the first reports of what is now known as the HBOC syndrome.[12,13] These studies also contributed to the identification of the profound heterogeneity in HBC (Figure 18-2).

Understanding of the genetic etiology of breast cancer advanced dramatically in 1990, when Hall and associates[14] identified linkage for early site-specific breast cancer on chromosome 17q. Shortly thereafter, Narod and co-workers[15] showed linkage to this same locus in

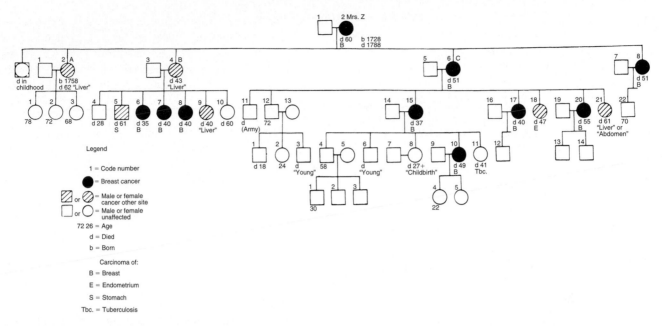

FIG. **18-1** Pedigree chart of Broca's family constructed from a review of his original paper published in 1866. *(From Lynch et al: JAMA 222:1631, 1972. Copyright 1972, American Medical Association.)*

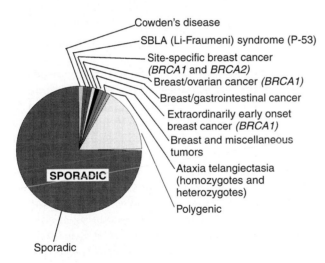

FIG. **18-2** Schematic depicting heterogeneity in breast cancer. *(From Lynch HT et al: Surg Clin North Am 70:753, 1990.)*

concert with OC in the HBOC syndrome. The gene, now known as *BRCA1*, has been cloned.[16] Subsequently, a second breast cancer gene, *BRCA2*, was shown to be linked to chromosome 13q[17] and has been identified.[18] These important events are discussed in greater detail throughout this chapter.

Family History of Cancer

The study of genealogy has become fashionable. However, gathering the family history and investigating causes of death or serious illnesses such as cancer may raise concerns about how one's heritage could affect cancer risk. The scientific advances in the clinical and molecular genetics of hereditary cancer that have been reported recently in the scientific and lay literature have piqued the interest of physicians as well as the general public.

Identification of familial susceptibility to cancer requires compiling a family history of cancer of *all* anatomic sites. A family history of congenital anomalies and benign growths can provide important clues. The patient should be queried about cancer information on both first-degree relatives (parents, siblings, and children) and second-degree relatives (grandparents, aunts, and uncles) from both maternal and *paternal* lineages (Figure 18-3). Information on older relatives is more genetically significant because most cancers are of adult onset, making the phenotypic expression more likely than in younger relatives (children, cousins, nephews, and nieces of probands). The compilation should include the age of cancer onset, the primary source, and the occurrence of multiple primary cancers (including bilaterality of paired organs). This detailed cancer family history, particularly when it is supported by medical and pathology records, is an integral component of the patient's medical workup. The identification of a hereditary cancer syndrome with its cancer control potential should be made available to all extended family members, although it must be kept in mind that patient confidentiality is a concern that needs to be addressed when cancer family history is shared.

Patient's Modified Nuclear Pedigree

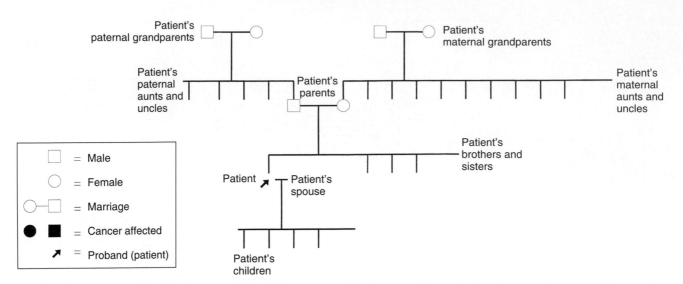

FIG. **18-3** Diagram representing a simple, modified nuclear pedigree for clinical use. *(From Lynch HT et al:* Surv Dig Dis *2:244, 1984. Copyright S. Karger AG, Basel.)*

However, our experience indicates that clinicians generally do not compile a family history of cancer in sufficient detail to diagnose a hereditary cancer syndrome, and if they do, primary and secondary at-risk relatives rarely benefit from this knowledge.

Lynch and colleagues[19] interviewed 200 consecutive cancer patients who were undergoing treatment in an oncology clinic. They noted numerous examples of familial cancer clusters, as well as several hereditary cancer syndromes. However, in the overwhelming majority of cases, the family history of cancer, as reported in patients' initial medical records, had either been entirely omitted or reported as negative, despite substantial evidence to the contrary. Furthermore, even when the family history was strongly positive, the information was not used to benefit either the patient or his or her close relatives. Subsequently, David and Steiner-Grossman[20] conducted a survey of 76 acute care, nonpsychiatric hospitals in New York City to determine the notation of family history of cancer in the medical charts. Only 4 of the 64 reporting hospitals reported any notation of cancer family history. Surprisingly, the American College of Surgeons and accrediting agencies of hospitals did not require this information.

SPORADIC, FAMILIAL, AND HEREDITARY BREAST CANCER

Definitions

Sporadic Breast Cancer. A breast cancer case with no other family history of breast carcinoma through two generations, including siblings, offspring, parents, and both maternal and paternal aunts, uncles, and grandparents, is considered sporadic.

Familial Breast Cancer. Familial breast cancer occurs when the patient has a positive family history, including one or more first- or second-degree relatives with breast cancer, that does not fit the HBC definition given later.

It is important to note that a patient with one or more first-degree relatives with breast cancer in this familial breast cancer category has a substantial excess lifetime breast cancer risk when compared with patients in the general population who do not have affected first-degree relatives. A collaborative reanalysis of data from 52 epidemiologic studies provides the largest data source for risk estimation in familial breast cancer.[21] This study found that risk ratios for breast cancer increase with increasing numbers of affected first-degree relatives (risk ratios 1.80, 2.93, and 3.90, respectively, for one, two, and three first-degree relatives) compared with women who had no affected relative. In countries where breast cancer is common, the lifetime excess incidence of breast cancer was found to be 5.5% for women with one first-degree relative with breast cancer and 13.3% for women with two affected first-degree relatives.

As yet, genetic and environmental causes of familial (as opposed to hereditary) cancer are incompletely described. Therefore genetic testing is not feasible in the setting of familial breast cancer. However, quantitative breast cancer risk assessment is extremely useful for this category of at-risk women[22] and guides medical

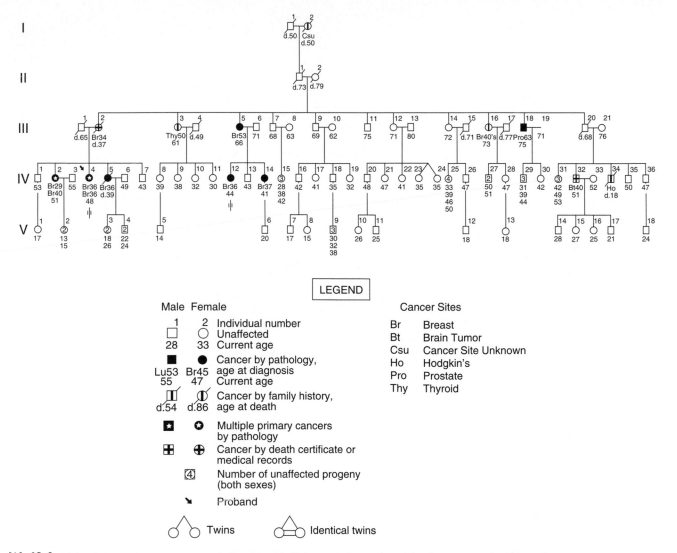

FIG. **18-4** A classic hereditary breast cancer family with eight cases (III-2, III-5, III-16, IV-2, IV-4, IV-5, IV-12, and IV-14) of breast cancer over two generations. Note the classic sign of bilateral breast cancer primaries in two cases (IV-2 and IV-4). (*Courtesy Tami Richardson-Nelson, BGS.*)

decision making about chemoprevention and prophylactic mastectomy (PM).

Hereditary Breast Cancer. HBC is characterized by a significantly earlier age of breast cancer onset (average age of onset, 45 years), an excess of bilateral breast cancer, a greater frequency of multiple primary cancer such as cancer of the breast and ovary in the HBOC syndrome, and an autosomal dominant inheritance pattern for cancer susceptibility.[23,24] Surveillance and management strategies for HBC must be in accord with these clinical features and address the risk to relatives, and therefore clearly differ from that required for sporadic cases.[23,24] Figure 18-4 shows the pedigree of a site-specific HBC family. Figures 18-5 and 18-6 are pedigrees for two classic HBOC syndrome families.[24]

Screening and Management Melded to Genetic and Natural History. The natural history of HBC mandates that high-risk patients (i.e., germline mutation carriers and first-degree relatives of women affected with breast cancer and/or OC) receive special attention when compared with the screening and management practices of patients who are at general population risk. Physicians must keep in mind that these high-risk women often have a heightened sense of fear of developing breast cancer and/or OC, which is likely amplified because the patient has lived with this fear for years and has seen loved ones become affected by, and sometimes succumb to, these cancers.

Genetic counseling is mandatory, particularly when germline mutation testing is considered. Such

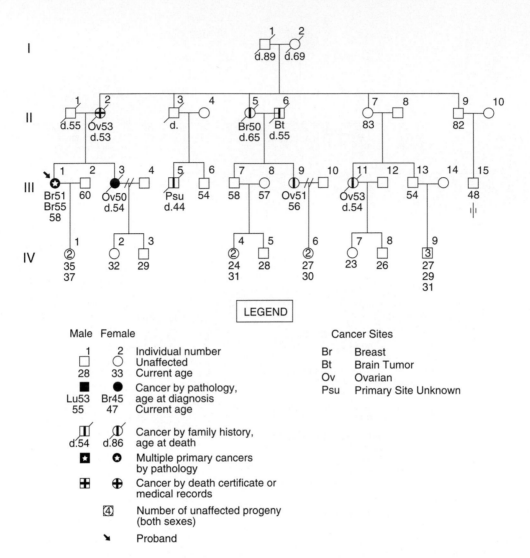

FIG. **18-5** A classic HBOC pedigree showing two breast cancer cases (II-5 and III-1) and four ovarian cancer cases (II-2, III-3, III-9, and III-11). Note the decreased penetrance in II-7 who remains unaffected with breast or ovarian cancer even though she is an obligate gene carrier with a daughter who developed ovarian cancer at 53. *(Courtesy Tami Richardson-Nelson, BGS.)*

counseling should be initiated before DNA collection and provided again, in person, when results are disclosed. All matters concerning psychologic issues, costs, potential insurance and/or employment discrimination, and confidentiality must be discussed with the patient.[25-29] Available options, such as prophylactic bilateral mastectomy[30] and prophylactic bilateral oophorectomy,[31] chemoprevention such as tamoxifen,[32] as well as the limitations of these preventive strategies, also need to be discussed in detail (Table 18-1).[33-35] PM may be discussed as an option for women with excessive fear of breast cancer, as well as those who may be noncompliant with screening because they fear finding a tumor or because fibrocystic disease has increased the difficulty of examination.[30,34] We also discuss ovarian screening procedures and their limitations, with the

option for prophylactic oophorectomy once procreation is completed.[36] The severe limitations of current OC screening merit priority attention to new technologies for early diagnosis of OC.[37-39]

Hereditary Breast Cancer

HEREDITARY BREAST/OVARIAN CANCER SYNDROME

HBC, inclusive of HBOC, is genotypically and phenotypically heterogeneous. It is estimated that approximately 45% of hereditary early-onset site-specific breast cancer and about 80% of HBOC kindreds show linkage to *BRCA1*. The majority of the remaining families are attributable to *BRCA2*. The predominant cancer types in

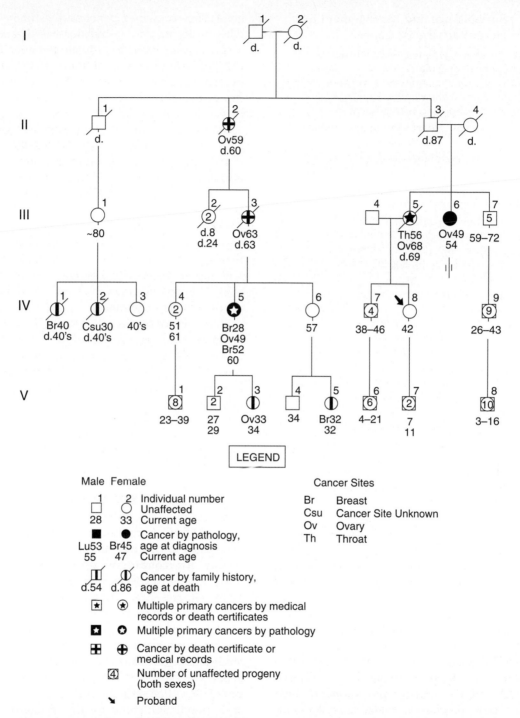

FIG. **18-6** A classic HBOC pedigree demonstrating four generations of ovarian cancer cases (II-2, III-3, IV-5, and V-3). Also note the very early onset of breast cancer in IV-5 and V-5. Individual II-3 is shown as an obligate gene carrier with two daughters (III-5 and III-6) being affected with ovarian cancer. *(Courtesy Tami Richardson-Nelson, BGS.)*

the HBOC syndrome are breast and ovary. The lifetime breast cancer risk in *BRCA1* and *BRCA2* carriers is estimated to be 85%.[40] The lifetime OC risk is estimated to be 40% to 60% for *BRCA1* carriers[41] and 15% for *BRCA2* carriers.[40,42] *BRCA2* is more highly associated

with male breast cancer than *BRCA1*; about one third of *BRCA* positive cases involve *BRCA1* and two thirds involve *BRCA2*.[43] The risk of a second female breast cancer in a putative gene carrier already affected with breast cancer was estimated to be 65% by age 70

TABLE 18-1	Surveillance and Management for Hereditary Breast Cancer

I.	Education about genetics, natural history, surveillance, and management—initiate midteens; genetic counseling can take place at age 18 and, when indicated, *BRCA1/2* mutation testing can take place at that age
II.	Instruction in self-breast examination–initiate age 18
III.	Clinical breast examination—begin at age 20 and repeat semiannually
IV.	Mammography—begin at age 25 and every 6-12 months after that[33,35]
V.	Ovarian cancer screening (transvaginal ovarian ultrasound, Doppler color blood flow imagery, CA 125, annual pelvic examinations)—begin age 30 and annually thereafter
VI.	Option for contralateral prophylactic mastectomy in patient with ipsilateral breast cancer, and bilateral prophylactic mastectomy and prophylactic oophorectomy—when family completed
VII.	Emphasis on clinical and self-breast examination in male carriers
VIII.	Consideration of tamoxifen or selective estrogen receptor modulator
IX.	Consideration of annual bilateral breast magnetic resonance imaging under research protocol
X.	Surveillance and chemoprevention for at-risk relatives; surgical prevention guided by results of gene testing

(95%; confidence limits 47% to 77%).[40] When allowing for the fact that such women have only one breast at risk, the corresponding penetrance estimate was 87% by age 70, with a CI of 72% to 95%. The corresponding estimate for OC was 44% by age 70, with a CI of 28% to 56%.

CANCER SYNDROMES

BRCA1. Easton and colleagues computed RRs for breast cancer and OC in *BRCA1* carriers and compared them with general population risks for England and Wales for 1978 to 1982. The RR for breast cancer based on the contralateral breast cancer data declined significantly with age, from more than 200-fold below age 40 to 15-fold in the 60- to 69-year-old age group (*p* trend <.0001). The RR for OC, based on the second cancer data, also declined significantly (*p* trend <.001), but it was not as dramatic as that for breast cancer.[40]

Ford and Easton[41] suggest that the majority of multiple-case families that segregate both breast cancer and OC in a dominant manner, consistent with the HBOC syndrome, manifest mutations in the *BRCA1*

gene. They combined penetrance estimates for *BRCA1* with results from two population-based genetic epidemiologic investigations to estimate the gene frequency of *BRCA1*. Using the assumption that the excess risk of ovarian carcinoma in first-degree relatives of breast cancer patients, and conversely that the breast cancer excess in relatives of OC patients are both entirely accounted for by *BRCA1*, they estimate that the *BRCA1* gene frequency is 0.0006 (95% CI 0.0002 to 0.001) and that the proportion of breast cancer cases in the general population caused by *BRCA1* is 5.3% for women younger than age 40, 2.2% for women between the ages 40 and 49, and 1.1% for women between the ages 50 and 70. The corresponding estimates for OC are 5.7%, 4.6%, and 2.1%, respectively. These investigators concluded that the occurrence of cancer in the majority of families with breast cancer with less than four cases and no OC is likely to be due either to chance or to more common genes of lower penetrance.

Ford and co-workers[44] examined cancers of other anatomic sites among individuals affected with breast cancer or OC and their first-degree relatives in *BRCA1*-linked families. They observed 87 cancers (other than breast or ovary) in individuals with breast cancer or OC and their first-degree relatives, compared with 69.3 cancers expected based on national incidence rates. Significant excesses were observed for colon cancer (estimated relative risk to gene carriers, 4.11 [95% CI 2.36 to 7.15]) and prostate cancer (3.33 [1.78 to 6.20]).

***BRCA1* and *BRCA2* and Ashkenazi Jews.** Struewing and co-workers[45] studied the frequency of the 185delAG frameshift mutation in *BRCA1* in 858 Ashkenazi Jewish individuals who had sought genetic testing for conditions unrelated to cancer. They observed the 185delAG mutation in 0.9% of Ashkenazi DNA samples (95% confidence limit 0.4% to 1.8%). They concluded that approximately 1 in 100 women of Ashkenazi descent may be at increased risk of developing breast or ovarian carcinoma, or both.[45] Subsequent studies have confirmed the increased prevalence of the 185delAG *BRCA1* mutation in the Ashkenazi Jewish population. Roa and co-workers[46] performed a large-scale population study for the 185delAG mutation in 3000 Ashkenazi Jewish blood samples collected for relatively common diseases among this population and found a carrier frequency of 1.09%.[46] Offit and colleagues evaluated the frequency of the 185delAG mutation in Ashkenazi Jewish women with early-onset breast cancer seen at medical oncology and genetic counseling clinics in New York. They found 20% of 80 women with breast cancer diagnosed before the age of 42 carry this mutation and concluded that screening for the 185delAG mutation in the Ashkenazi Jewish population may serve as a useful tool in the genetic counseling of these families.[47] In addition, Modan and co-workers identified an increased prevalence of the 185delAG mutation in OC cases in Israel compared with healthy controls.[48]

The specificity of 185delAG appears to be the result of a founder effect in the Ashkenazi Jewish population. Therefore Struewing and co-workers[45] reasoned that inherited breast cancer possibly represents a higher proportion of breast cancer in this population than in others.

Helmrich and colleagues[49] evaluated risk factors for breast cancer in a hospital-based case-control study of 1185 women with breast cancer (90% in the United States, 4% in Canada, 6% in Israel). Jewish ethnicity was associated with a relative risk of 2.8 compared with Catholics (95% CI 2.3 to 3.4) and was "not confounded materially" by parity, age at first birth, or years of education. The increased prevalence of 185delAG and more recently discovered founder mutations might partially explain the possibly increased risk of breast cancer among Jewish women.[45]

The BRCA2 mutation 6174delT has been identified as characteristic in Ashkenazi Jewish women and appears to have an approximately 1.5% prevalence rate in this population.[46,50] Therefore the 185delAG BRCA1 and 6174delT BRCA2 mutations appear to constitute the two most frequent mutation alleles predisposing to HBC among Ashkenazi Jewish women. The BRCA2 6174delT mutation is less penetrant than the BRCA1 185delAG mutation. It has been found less frequently in breast cancer–affected Ashkenazi Jewish women than the 185delAG mutation.[50] Phenotypic variation in BRCA2 has also been identified. Gayther and colleagues studied the distribution of BRCA2 mutations in 25 families with multiple cases of breast cancer, OC, or both and found mutations in families with a high proportion of OC to cluster in exon 11.[51] Mutations in the ovarian cancer cluster region (OCCR) appear to convey as high a risk of OC as do mutations in BRCA1. Furthermore, colorectal, stomach, pancreatic, and prostate cancer occurred in excess in first-degree relatives of carriers of OCCR mutations compared with mutations in other regions of BRCA2.[52]

Although these studies focused on Ashkenazi Jewish women, it is vital to keep in mind that Ashkenazi Jewish males can also carry these mutations.

MOLECULAR BIOLOGY AND MUTATIONS IN BRCA1

BRCA1 is a large gene that contains 22 coding exons that are distributed over approximately 100 kb of genomic DNA. It produces a protein of 1863 amino acids.

Most mutations that have been identified in BRCA1 are frameshifts, nonsense mutations, or splice mutations.[43,53,54] These mutations presumably lead to premature truncation of the BRCA1 protein. More than 800 distinct mutations, polymorphisms, and variants have been reported in BRCA1, of which 500 have been reported only once. For BRCA2, about 900 distinct mutations, polymorphisms, and variants have been reported, and about 600 are unique to one family (Breast Cancer Information Core [BIC] website: http://research.nhgri.nih.gov). Methods used to scan for mutations, including DNA sequencing, fail to identify large duplications, deletions, and rearrangements, which may account for approximately 10% of mutations,[55] but enhancement of testing to ascertain these types of mutations is in process.

Phenotypic Variation in BRCA1. Based on linkage analysis, Easton and co-workers[40] predicted the existence of two variants of families with BRCA1: (1) those showing a high penetrance of OC (84% by age 70); and (2) those showing a low penetrance of OC (32% by age 70).

Gayther and associates[56] studied 60 families with a history of breast or ovarian carcinoma, or both, for BRCA1 germline mutations. They found 22 different mutations detected in 32 families (53%). A significant correlation was observed between the location of the mutation in the gene and the ratio of breast cancer to OC incidence within each family. They suggested that mutations in the 3' third of the gene are associated with a lower proportion of OC.

BRCA2. A second susceptibility gene, BRCA2, was mapped to chromosome 13 in 1994[17] and was subsequently identified.[18] The majority of BRCA-associated cases of male breast cancer appear to be associated with BRCA2.[43] BRCA2 confers a high risk of breast cancer and a lower risk of OC (approximately 15%).

Figure 18-7 shows a BRCA2 family with three males affected with breast cancer; two of these males also developed prostate cancer. Note that in this family the proband's father (see Figure 18-7, III-1), paternal grandfather (see Figure 18-7, II-2), and paternal great-uncle (see Figure 18-7, II-3) each developed breast cancer, at ages 53, 57, and 60, respectively. Furthermore, the father and grandfather also developed prostate cancer at ages 64 and 79, respectively. A BRCA2 mutation has been identified in this family.

Wooster and colleagues[18] report on the identification of BRCA2 mutation in five different families with breast cancer. Each of these mutations was found to disrupt the open reading frame of the transcriptional unit.

In the course of the mutational screen of candidate coding sequences from the BRCA2 region, the first detected sequence variant that was predicted to this rough translation of an encoded protein was observed in a Creighton University breast cancer-prone family.

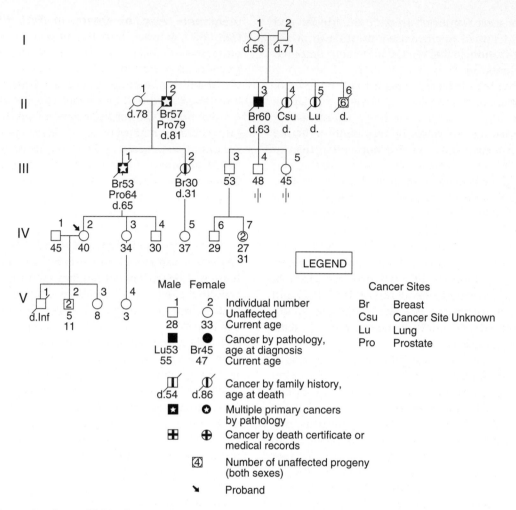

FIG. **18-7** Pedigree showing a *BRCA2* family with three males affected with breast cancer; two of these males also developed prostate cancer. *(Courtesy Tami Richardson-Nelson, BGS.)*

This family is strongly linked to *BRCA2* with a multipoint log of the odds (LOD) score of 3.01 using D13S260 and D13S267. Wooster and co-workers[18] reported a six-base pair deletion in this family resulting in a premature termination codon. This mutation has been detected in two other early-onset breast cancer cases in this family.

Estimated *BRCA1/2* Mutation Probabilities: Clinical Implications. Berry and colleagues[3] compared results for mutations involving *BRCA1* and *BRCA2* with estimated probabilities of harboring these mutations to assess sensitivity of genetic testing as well as the relevance of other susceptibility genes in familial breast cancer and OC. They employed BRCAPRO,[57,58] which is a computer program that implements a statistical model enabling the calculation of an individual's probability of harboring a *BRCA1* or *BRCA2* mutation. Neither of these, or even both, were based on the individual's cancer status in concert with the history of breast cancer and OC among that individual's first- and second-degree relatives. Data were collected and analyzed from

six high-risk genetic counseling clinics and focused on individuals from families containing at least one member who was tested for *BRCA1* and *BRCA2* mutations. Findings disclosed BRCAPRO "is an accurate counseling tool for determining the probability of carrying mutations of *BRCA1* and *BRCA2*. Genetic testing for *BRCA1* and *BRCA2* is highly sensitive, missing an estimated 15% of mutations. In the population studied, breast cancer susceptibility genes other than *BRCA1* and *BRCA2* either do not exist, are rare, or are associated with low disease penetrance."[3]

From a practical standpoint, BRCAPRO could be used in the clinical setting to assist in advising individuals whether they are sufficient candidates to undergo genetic testing. BRCAPRO also has important research potential, particularly as a guide to determine who to test and to judge the utility of such testing, as well as a substitute for testing. Thus a researcher "who contemplates genetic testing for subjects involved in a clinical trial or subjects in a research database can use BRCAPRO to determine the expected number of mutations in each subset of study participants. This allows for judging whether the scientific question can be addressed with sufficient statistical power."[3]

It also allows for selecting the most informative subset of individuals for testing in a setting where funds for genetic testing are limited.

Low-Penetrance Breast Cancer Susceptibility Mutations.

Meijers-Heijboer and associates[4] described a new low-penetrant breast cancer susceptibility locus, namely CHEK, which encodes a cell cycle checkpoint kinase that is implicated in the DNA repair process involving BRCA1 and p53. CHEK2*1100delC is a truncating variant that abrogates the kinase activity. It occurs in 1.1% of healthy individuals and in 5.1% of individuals with breast cancer. This finding is based on the study of 718 families that do not carry mutations in BRCA1 or BRCA2 (p = .00000003). Interestingly, 15.5% of individuals with breast cancer from families with male breast cancer and no mutations in BRCA1 or BRCA2 harbor CHEK2 (p = .00015).

It is estimated that CHEK2*1100delC variant results in an approximate twofold increase of breast cancer risk in females and an approximate tenfold increase of risk in males. The variant confers no increased cancer risk in carriers of BRCA1 or BRCA2 mutations. de Jong and colleagues[59] studied a large number of genes other than BRCA1 and BRCA2 that are involved in breast cancer susceptibility. An association with breast cancer at a 5% significance level was found for 13 polymorphisms in 10 genes described in more than one breast cancer study. These authors stressed the need to focus on further analysis of genetic polymorphisms and combinations of such polymorphisms, which may then facilitate the combination of population-attributable risks, understanding of gene-to-gene interactions, and improving estimates of genetic cancer risk.

Probabilistic Implications of Hereditary Cancer.

When evaluating families with hereditary cancer, it is important to realize that genetic information is probabilistic. Not all carriers of BRCA1 and BRCA2 germline mutations develop cancer (penetrance of the genes is about 85% to 90%), and conversely, some noncarriers do not remain cancer free because these cancers are relatively common in the general population. In addition, there is always uncertainty in a mutation carrier about whether and when cancer will occur. Given the fact that these cancers are common, affected individuals within a pedigree cannot invariably be assumed to be gene carriers because they may, in fact, represent a sporadic case. This consideration has importance for genetic counseling, selection of individuals for genetic testing, and ultimate medical management of the offspring of such sporadic cases.

Variable Age of Onset in Hereditary Breast Cancer.

Extremely early age of onset of breast cancer appears to be another example of heterogeneity in HBC (Figure 18-8). In this category, we see breast cancer clustering in the twenties and early thirties in certain families. In contrast, we see clustering of late age of onset in selected families (discussed subsequently).

We studied the relationship between age of onset of breast cancer in 328 breast cancer probands (consecutively ascertained patients from our oncology clinic) and breast cancer incidence and age of onset in their female relatives.[60] A family history of early-onset breast cancer was associated with a higher risk of early-onset breast cancer. A family history of early-onset breast cancer occurred more frequently among young (younger than 40 years) breast cancer probands than among older ones (older than 40 years) (odds ratio [OR] = 23; $p < .001$). This relationship was particularly evident when the analysis was restricted to HBC (OR = 3.3; $p < .001$). We also observed a positive family history of breast cancer (at any age) more frequently in young breast cancer probands than in older breast cancer probands (OR = 2.9; $p < .001$). These observations have important pragmatic implications for surveillance. Specifically, we recommend that intense surveillance for breast cancer be initiated *earlier* for women who have close relatives with early-onset breast cancer.[60] Such women are important candidates for intensive pedigree studies.

From a genetic and epidemiologic standpoint, there are two questions to address. Is earlier age at breast cancer onset more likely to predict genetic susceptibility than later age at onset? Are some families characterized by early-onset breast cancer, whereas others show familial aggregation of later age at onset? The case-control study by Claus and co-workers[61] (4730 histologically confirmed breast cancer cases aged 20 to 54 and 4688 controls) showed that a major factor influencing breast cancer risk in first-degree relatives of cases was the age at which the case was affected with breast cancer.

Mettlin and colleagues[62] suggest that some families are characterized by early-onset breast cancer, whereas others show familial aggregations of later age at onset of breast cancer. They hypothesized that breast cancers in younger and older women were distinct epidemiologic entities. Of interest is the finding that the occurrence of breast cancer in an immediate family member at an older age may increase the risk specifically for the disease to occur in a subject at older ages; conversely, it may be that it poses a risk in younger women only when the diagnosis of breast cancer occurs in a close relative at a young age.

The bulk of the literature on HBC has shown early age at onset to be an important predictor of breast cancer risk in the patient's primary relatives. Systematic

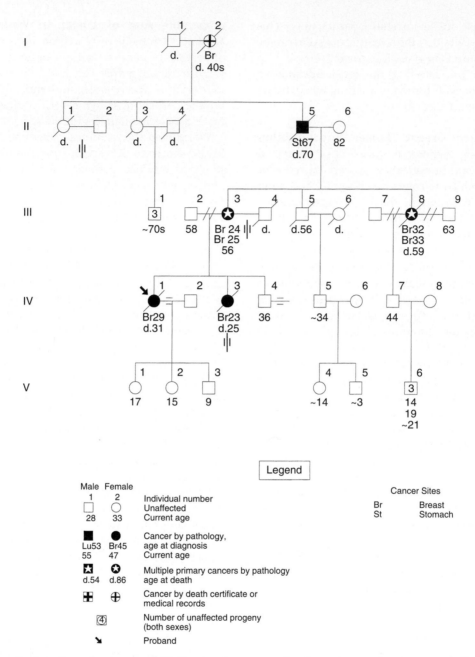

FIG. 18-8 Pedigree of a hereditary breast cancer family showing extraordinarily early age of cancer onset. (From Lynch HT et al: Neb Med J 73:97, 1988.)

investigation of familial clustering of late age at onset of breast cancer has been virtually ignored. However, we have identified a number of putative HBC kindreds characterized by late-onset breast cancer (Lynch HT, unpublished data). Perhaps the lack of attention to late age at onset is because it is more difficult to determine the genetic significance of a familial aggregation of patients with onset of breast cancer in the seventh, eighth, or ninth decade of life. For example, many high-risk relatives may have died from competing causes.

It is also much more difficult to secure documentation of cancer in the parents, aunts, uncles, and grandparents of these older-onset patients, many of whom may be deceased.

Survival in *BRCA1/BRCA2* Mutation Carriers.
Jóhannsson and colleagues[63] conducted a well-designed population-based study of survival of 71 *BRCA1*-associated cancer patients in southern Sweden using a population-based comparison group, as well as an age- and

stage-matched control group. Survival of *BRCA1* carriers was equal to or worse than the comparison group after adjustment for age and calendar year of diagnosis, as well as in comparison with an age- and stage-matched control group.

In a Finnish study of 359 familial breast cancer patients (32 patients from *BRCA1*-positive families, 43 patients from *BRCA2*-positive families, and 284 patients from *BRCA1/2*-negative breast cancer families), there was no difference in cumulative survival rates when compared with sporadic breast cancer (adjusted for age, stage, and year of diagnosis).[64] However, a study of 118 breast tumor blocks from Ashkenazi Jewish breast cancer patients with negative axillary lymph nodes found that *BRCA1* mutation carrier status was a significant prognostic factor of death (risk ratio 5.8, 95% CI 1.5 to 22, $p = .009$).[65] Furthermore, a French study of 183 women with breast cancer and a family history of breast cancer and/or OC found a worse prognosis for *BRCA1* carriers in terms of overall survival and metastasis-free interval.[66]

The current evidence, described subsequently, presents a paradox. *BRCA1* HBC has poor prognostic markers (aneuploidy, high grade, high cell proliferation rates) but better disease-free survival rates in some studies, whereas *BRCA2* HBC has neutral markers but poorer behavior. This paradox is as yet unexplained.

Glutathione-S Polymorphisms and Survival. Ambrosone and colleagues[67] discuss the role of polymorphisms in glutathione S-transferases (*GSTM1* and *GSTT1*) and survival following therapy for breast cancer. These are conjugating enzymes and *GSTM1* and *GSTT1* have deletion polymorphisms that result in an absence of enzyme activity. These authors studied the role of *GSTM1*- and *GSTT1*-null genotypes on disease-free and overall survival among 251 women after their therapy for incident, primary breast cancer. When age, race, and stage at diagnosis were adjusted for, those women with null genotypes for *GSTM1* and *GSTT1* "had reduced hazard of death (adjusted hazard ratio [HR], 0.59; 95% CI, 0.36-0.97; and HR, 0.51; CI, 0.29-0.90, respectively) in relation to those with alleles present. Furthermore, women who were null for both *GSTM1* and *GSTT1* had one-third the hazard of death of those with alleles for both genes present (adjusted HR, 0.28; 95% CI, 0.11-0.70). Similar relationships were noted for risk of recurrence." The authors concluded that interindividual differences in the activity of those enzymes that play a role in preventing therapy-generated reactive oxidant damage "may have an important impact on disease recurrence and overall survival."[67]

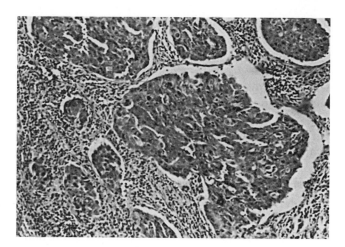

FIG. **18-9** Medullary breast carcinoma in a 24-year-old woman who, 1 year later, developed a "no special type" (NST) carcinoma in the contralateral breast. Note the expansive islands of large tumor cells with intervening stroma filled with lymphocytes. Medullary and atypical medullary carcinoma are common in *BRCA1* HBC. (×125.)

PATHOBIOLOGY OF *BRCA1* AND *BRCA2* HEREDITARY BREAST CANCER

Even before the discovery and isolation of the major breast cancer genes *BRCA1* and *BRCA2*, there were clues that the pathology of HBC differed from that of its sporadic counterpart.[68] Earlier work showed (1) more medullary carcinoma (Figure 18-9)—a proliferative, high-grade special type with good prognosis—in familial and HBC settings[69-72]; (2) a higher mitotic grade (Figure 18-10) in the no special type (NST, or ductal) invasive carcinoma in HBC[68,70]; (3) a statistically insignificant association of invasive lobular[73-75] or tubular[76,77] carcinomas in familial settings; and (4) conflicting positive[78,79] and negative[73] associations of lobular carcinoma in situ (LCIS) with family history. Only

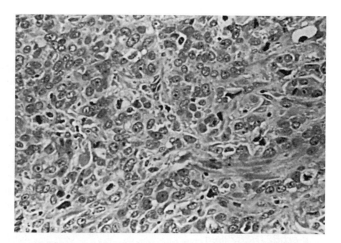

FIG. **18-10** NST (ductal) carcinoma with a high mitotic grade. Increased tumor cell proliferative rates are characteristic of *BRCA1* HBC. (×375.)

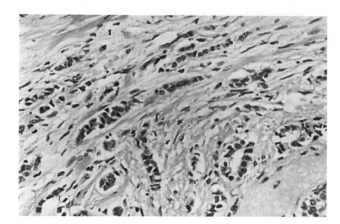

FIG. **18-11** Invasive tubular-lobular breast carcinoma. Note that the cancer cells form single "Indian files" like lobular carcinoma and tubules like tubular carcinoma. This histologic type is a member of the so-called tubular-lobular group (TLG) that includes lobular, tubular, and cribriform carcinoma. TLG carcinomas are decreased in *BRCA1* HBCs and possibly increased in *BRCA2* HBCs. (×400.)

As further evidence for a proliferative phenotype, we found that a high DNA S-phase fraction originally observed in the whole HBC cohort[93] was confined to the *BRCA1* subset.[68,80,82] Jóhannsson and colleagues[89] have confirmed this observation (see Table 18-2). The Creighton data also showed that *BRCA1* HBC is more prevalently aneuploid than non-HBC and that the average aneuploid DNA index is less compared with non-HBC (see Table 18-2).[80,82,83] *p53* tumor-suppressor protein is more frequently increased in *BRCA1* breast cancers compared with sporadic breast cancers.[87,94-96] This had been observed earlier in the Creighton breast-ovary HBC family cases,[97] most of which were later identified as *BRCA1* HBC. Overexpression of *p53*, almost always the result of a mutation in the *TP53* gene, has been observed in general in highly proliferating breast carcinomas.[98] The *TP53* mutations in *BRCA1* and *BRCA2* breast cancers are unusual in that most of them are not in usual "hotspots" and are distributed in a region of the protein on the opposite side of its DNA-binding surface.[99]

Jóhannsson and colleagues[89] showed that *BRCA1* HBCs have decreased expression of estrogen receptor, progesterone receptor, and *c-erb-B2* (Her2/neu) oncoprotein (see Table 18-2). These results have been confirmed by the Breast Cancer Linkage Consortium[95] and by us (Lehman N, unpublished data).

All of the evidence indicates a remarkable proliferative phenotype in *BRCA1* breast cancers. High proliferation rates are characteristic of the ovarian carcinomas in the Creighton families with breast-ovary (and mostly *BRCA1*) HBC as well.[100] The distinctive pathobiology of *BRCA1* HBC can be understood in context with a model of tumor genetic evolution. In the model,[101,102] intermediate and transformed cells suffer small losses or gains of chromosomal material while remaining near diploid in DNA content (DNA index = DI − 1). At some point, the chromosome complement duplicates to near-tetraploidy (DI − 2), continuing with a more severe segmental or complete chromosomal loss, which progressively lessens the DI. In this scenario, hyperdiploid breast cancers with $1.3 \leq DI \leq 1.7$, higher S-phase fractions, and *p53* mutations are among the most "evolved."[103-105] The *BRCA1* phenotype—aneuploidy, lower aneuploid DI (see Table 18-3), high proliferation, and *p53* overexpression—fits the profile of a genetically evolved tumor. To evolve genetically, the target cell must proliferate. In the model the *BRCA1* mutation would put the intermediate target cell[106,107] on a fast track of increased or unregulated proliferation, beginning near the time of menarche. At transformation, the intrinsic high proliferation rate is locked in to the tumor as a fossil phenotype of the intermediate cell.[108] The *BRCA1* protein fulfills the role required in this model. When mutated, its well-established antiproliferative function[109-111] is lost, which may send the target cells into unregulated proliferation.

The *BRCA2* HBC Phenotype. The *BRCA2* HBC phenotype is less well determined than that of *BRCA1* HBC because there are fewer cases and probably greater intrinsic heterogeneity, leading to less concordance in the literature. Most studies agree that the age of onset is significantly greater than in *BRCA1* HBC (see Table 18-3) but still considerably less than in non-HBC. All studies agree that there is a lesser propensity for the NST (ductal) carcinomas to form tubules (see Table 18-3), as in *BRCA1* HBC. The pathologists in the blinded Creighton studies[80,82,83] (Marcus JN, Page DL, unpublished data) have made special efforts to not under diagnose the TLG carcinomas. They find that TLG group carcinoma is a powerful discriminator between *BRCA1* and *BRCA2* HBC, scarce in the former but prevalent in the latter (see Table 18-3). Consistent with this result, Armes and colleagues[91] also find increased lobular carcinoma in *BRCA2* HBC, but other groups do not,[84,112] for reasons that may relate to differing diagnostic thresholds or to intrinsic differences in the data sets.

The Breast Cancer Linkage Consortium[84] claims a higher grade for *BRCA2* HBC than for the age-matched non-HBC controls, but this result is questionable. Higher nuclear, mitotic, and total grades are not seen in the large Creighton data set displayed in Table 18-3. The problem is that the Consortium *BRCA2* pathology data set is dominated by the Icelandic founder 999del5 mutation, which comprises nearly half (49%) of its cases. The pathology associated with this mutation, reported in a separate publication by non-Consortium pathologists,[112] is remarkable for very high grades that do not appear typical of the non-999del5 *BRCA2* cases in other data sets. Because the Consortium cases are so

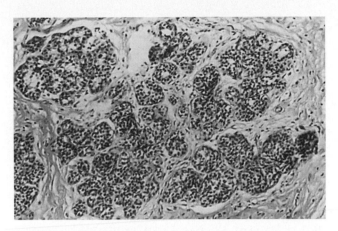

FIG. **18-12** Lobular carcinoma in situ (LCIS). Lobular neoplasia (LCIS and atypical lobular hyperplasia) is prevalent in affected members of this *BRCA2* family. (×200.)

heavily weighted with this specific mutation, its overall results may be skewed toward higher grade. Thus, despite its large size, the Consortium database may not be representative of *BRCA2* HBC at large. On the other hand, the fact that this argument can be made is itself evidence that *BRCA2* HBC phenotype, at least insofar as the 999del5 mutation is concerned, is heterogeneous.

In the Creighton *BRCA2* HBC data set, there is prevalent lobular neoplasia, defined as lobular carcinoma in situ or atypical lobular hyperplasia (Figure 18-12). In one *BRCA2* HBC family, 10 of 13 invasive breast carcinomas were associated with lobular neoplasia. Of interest, TLG carcinomas have a high prevalence of lobular neoplasia (see Marcus and colleagues[83] and references therein). The DNA cytometric characteristics of *BRCA2* HBC differ from those of *BRCA1* HBC (see Table 18-3): there is lesser aneuploidy and a lower mean aneuploid S-phase fraction, which is more in line with the characteristics of non-HBC (see Table 18-3). Estrogen receptor, progesterone receptor, p53, and HER2/neu proteins also appear to be expressed at levels comparable to those in non-HBC (see Table 18-2).[87,89,94-97,113-115]

CLINICAL IMPLICATIONS OF *BRCA1* AND *BRCA2* HBC PATHOPHENOTYPES

The decreased estrogen and progesterone receptor expression suggests that *BRCA1* breast cancer generally will not respond well to therapy with hormone receptor modulators such as tamoxifen. However, we have cautioned[116] that this supposition should not preclude consideration of such therapy in chemoprevention trials, for there is no evidence that the pretransformed target intermediate cell lacks receptors. Early data in the National Surgical Adjuvant Breast and Bowel Project prevention trial (NSABP-P1) indicate that tamoxifen may not reduce breast cancer incidence among *BRCA1* mutation carriers but may reduce the incidence among *BRCA2* mutation carriers, whose tumors are usually

estrogen receptor-positive when they develop (see Table 18-2).[117] However, the number of positive events in the trial currently is quite small and the results do not reach statistical significance for either *BRCA1* or *BRCA2* carriers. Clearly this and other trials with larger numbers of *BRCA1* and *BRCA2* mutation carriers and more extended follow-up times are needed before this issue can be properly addressed.

The prognosis of *BRCA1* HBC has been a matter of ongoing debate. The issue is important because it weighs in the decisions on prophylactic therapies. Most studies find no significant differences in survival in comparison with non-HBC,* but better[120] and worse[66,121] outcomes have also been reported. Methodologic differences may account in part for the variability in results.[122] Why the prognosis of *BRCA1*-related HBC, with its adverse pathology markers, would be no worse than non-HBC is a conundrum that is deepened by the observation that in the Creighton families, *BRCA1*-related HBC cases fare better than non–*BRCA1*-related HBC cases, which have neutral pathology indicators.[82,116] But there are clues that *BRCA1* HBC is not an ordinary high-grade breast cancer. As we have seen, it does not highly express *c-erbB2*, a marker of poor prognosis,[89,95] and a high proportion are medullary carcinomas,[80,82-84,91,92] which in pure forms are prognostically favorable, despite their high mitotic and nuclear grades.[123] Might genetic instability in *BRCA1* HBC—manifested by the prevalent aneuploidy, low aneuploid DNA index, and increased p53 expression previously described—indicate fragility and increased susceptibility to chemotherapy and radiation therapy? These observations and questions point to directions for future investigation.

Less is known about the prognosis of *BRCA2* HBC. The best available evidence from several studies is that survivals probably do not differ from non-HBC when adjusted for other variables such as stage.[124]

The pathobiologic features of *BRCA1* and *BRCA2* HBC summarized in Tables 18-2 and 18-3 offer some clues as to whether a patient in a family untested for the genes may be more susceptible to one or the other syndrome. However, these should not be regarded as sufficiently sensitive and specific to serve as a substitute for syndrome identification by direct genetic testing for germline mutations.

Recently, a small number of *BRCA1* HBC, *BRCA2* HBC, and non-HBC tumors were looked at for expression of 5361 genes by microarray technology.[125] The analysis disclosed 176 genes that were differentially expressed in tumors with *BRCA1* versus *BRCA2* mutations. The results also showed that the expression profiles could accurately classify the tumor as having arisen from a germline mutation in *BRCA1* or *BRCA2*.

---

*References 63, 82, 115, 116, 118, 119.

If these results can be confirmed with larger numbers of cases, this technology could become a powerful tool in diagnosing *BRCA1* or *BRCA2* mutation carrier status from the breast tumors directly.

RADIATION SENSITIVITY IN *BRCA1/2* MUTATION CARRIERS[126-138]

The *BRCA1* and *BRCA2* genes function in several important cellular pathways, including (1) mediating the cellular response to DNA damage, (2) serving as a cell cycle checkpoint protein, and (3) regulating transcription.[34,132,138] Of clinical concern is the substantial evidence that *BRCA1* and *BRCA2* are key components of the repair pathway for double-stranded DNA breaks, a form of damage induced by ionizing radiation. The main scenarios in which to consider the potential clinical impact of impaired DNA repair function are (1) low-dose exposure to ionizing radiation from screening mammography, particularly in young, high-risk women, and (2) the effect of radiotherapy in *BRCA* carriers with breast cancer who opt for breast-conserving therapy (BCT) (lumpectomy plus radiation) instead of mastectomy.

There is considerable biologic plausibility to support the concern that radiation from screening and diagnostic procedures may pose additional risks to *BRCA1* and *BRCA2* mutation carriers. *BRCA1* associates in nuclear dots with *Rad51*, which mediates the repair of double-stranded DNA breaks.[134] The *RAD51* gene has a single nucleotide polymorphism that increases the risk of breast cancer but not OC in *BRCA2* mutation carriers.[139] *BRCA1* is phosphorylated by the ataxia telangiectasia-mutated (ATM) protein kinase in response to DNA damage induced by gamma radiation. Epidemiologic evidence has suggested that ATM heterozygotes, who comprise about 1% of the population, may be at increased risk of breast cancer,[136] a theory confirmed by some but not all molecular studies.[128] Furthermore, *BRCA2*-deficient mouse embryos are acutely sensitive to ionizing radiation.[135] In surviving *BRCA2*-deficient mice with partial gene function, repair of double-stranded DNA is impaired.[130] The extreme sensitivity of human *BRCA2*-deficient cancer cells to agents that cause double-stranded DNA breaks[126] may ultimately serve as a specific molecular target for genotype-based therapy in mutation carriers.[127] Radiation sensitization may also be a viable strategy.[129]

It is difficult to predict the clinical impact of basic research findings. On one hand, radiation exposure could induce mutations that accumulate as a result of limited repair function, inducing a higher rate of cancer. On the other hand, radiation-induced damage could induce programmed cell death (apoptosis), limiting the potential for invasive cancer to develop. Although basic research helps frame the relevant clinical questions, medical decision making must be based on clinical studies on *BRCA* carriers. There are no controlled trials assessing the possible adverse effects of radiation from mammography screening in *BRCA* carriers. The hypothetical sequelae[131] must be balanced against the need for surveillance in high-risk individuals and the emerging evidence that mammographic screening is valuable.[35]

BCT and the potential consequences of radiation have been explored by Pierce and colleagues[133] and Turner and associates.[137] Pierce and colleagues[133] compared rates of radiation-associated complications, in-breast tumor recurrence, and distant relapse in 71 women with *BRCA1/2* mutations treated with BCT using radiotherapy with rates observed in 213 matched controls with sporadic breast cancer. Comparable rates of tumor control and 5-year survival rates were observed among the sporadic and germline cases, providing reassurance regarding the safety of administering radiotherapy to germline *BRCA1/2* mutation carriers.

Turner and associates[137] examined the rate of ipsilateral breast tumor recurrence (IBTR) in *BRCA* mutation carriers by estimating the frequency of *BRCA1/2* mutations in breast cancer patients with IBTR treated with BCT. Among 52 patients with IBTR, 8 (15%) had deleterious *BRCA1/2* mutations, compared with 6.6% of matched control patients without IBTR ($p = .03$). The median time to IBTR for mutation carriers was prolonged (7.8 years), compared with noncarriers (4.7 years) ($p = .03$). Considering the long time to recurrence, as well as histologic and clinical criteria, IBTRs in mutation carriers were interpreted as representing new primary breast cancers. These data suggest that radiation therapy is effective in treating primary breast cancers and highlight the risk of second primaries in *BRCA* mutation carriers, which may be best addressed at the time of initial diagnosis, if not before. However, the possible role of radiation in inducing second primary breast cancers is raised by the high rate of late IBTRs observed in the study. If so, the radiation therapist and medical oncologist must then become concerned about recommendations for lumpectomy followed by radiation therapy. It is clear that molecular genetic discoveries in HBC and their clinical implications have barely begun to be translated to patient care.

Heterogeneity: Multiple Breast Cancer Syndromes

SBLA (LI-FRAUMENI) SYNDROME

Lynch and colleagues[140] described an extended kindred that showed a broad spectrum of cancer: namely, sarcoma, breast cancer and brain tumors, lung and laryngeal cancer, leukemia, lymphoma, and adrenal cortical carcinoma (SBLA) syndrome. A limited description of the elements of this syndrome had been recognized previously in four nuclear kindreds by Li and Fraumeni,[141] who subsequently published a prospective observation of these families that covered a 12-year time frame (1969 through 1981).[142,143] Of interest was the fact that in 31 surviving family members, 16 additional cancers developed (the expected number was 0.5). Five of these were carcinomas of the breast, four were soft tissue sarcomas, and seven were cancers of other anatomic sites. Eight of the patients had multiple primary cancers. Four cancers occurred at sites of prior radiotherapy (three soft tissue sarcomas and one mesothelioma).

The SBLA syndrome has also been appropriately referred to as the *Li-Fraumeni syndrome*. This syndrome is pertinent to this chapter because of the occurrence of breast cancer (particularly with remarkably early age at onset), as well as recent reports of germ cell tumors of the ovary. The SBLA syndrome is caused by the *p53* germline mutation, which, like many cancer-prone genes, gives rise to a spectrum of cancers owing to its carcinogenic pleiotropic effects.[144,145]

The authors have continued to follow the SBLA syndrome kindred that they first described in 1978 (Figure 18-13).[140] They republished the pedigree in 1985, when children in the fifth generation began to develop cancer. The father (see Figure 18-13, IV-16) of these affected children did not have cancer when that study was first published. He was considered to be an obligate gene carrier. Since then, however, he developed colorectal cancer and died from this disease. A further update of this family has been noteworthy for a marked excess of brain tumors.[145]

SBLA is obviously an exceedingly complex syndrome and requires investigation of cancer of all anatomic sites with a vigorous effort to histopathologically verify cancer. Problems in pedigree analysis in the SBLA syndrome are compounded by the fact that in addition to reduced penetrance of the deleterious gene, two age-specific modes of cancer expression are encountered, one in childhood and the second in adult life.

COWDEN DISEASE

Brownstein and associates[146] described in detail a cancer-associated genodermatosis known as *Cowden disease*. This hereditary disorder, also known as *multiple hamartoma syndrome*, is inherited as an autosomal dominant trait and is characterized by distinctive mucocutaneous lesions and cancer of the breast, thyroid, and female genitourinary tract.

Germline mutations in the *PTEN* gene[147,148] are associated with Cowden disease, as well as Bannayan-Riley-Ruvalcaba syndrome. Because the major malignancies in Cowden disease, breast cancer and thyroid cancer, can be detected in early stages by surveillance, recognition of the syndrome is critical. The International Cowden Syndrome Consortium operational criteria for diagnosis are useful for weighting the pleiotropic manifestations according to major and minor criteria to make a formal diagnosis.[149,150]

The cutaneous manifestations of Cowden disease involve multiple trichilemmomas, the presence of which appears to be pathognomonic. These multiple cutaneous lesions are often located on the face (Figure 18-14) and on the dorsal and ventral aspects of the hands, feet, and forearms. These are hyperkeratotic, slightly brownish lesions, but they show the histologic pattern of benign keratoses. The stratum corneum is thick, compact, and largely orthokeratotic. The granular layer is prominent; the malpighian layer is papillomatous, acanthotic, and well differentiated but shows no distinguishing features. Additional skin features include multiple facial papules, acral and palmoplantar keratoses, multiple skin tags and subcutaneous lipomas. Cobblestone-like gingival and buccal mucosa papules, and papillomatous tongue, are hallmarks. Merkel cell carcinoma (primary neuroendocrine carcinoma of the skin) is a distinguishing feature.

In their review of the literature, Williard and coworkers[151] noted that 30% of women with Cowden disease manifested infiltrating ductal carcinoma of the breast, and a third of these individuals had bilateral primary breast carcinomas. The median age at breast cancer onset was 41 years, with a range of 20 to 62 years, leading some authors to recommend PM.[152] Williard and colleagues[151] suggest that those patients showing clinical manifestations of this disorder should be considered candidates for prophylactic bilateral total mastectomy. They suggest that this procedure be considered by the third decade of life. Should the patient decline surgical prophylaxis, then alternatively she should consider monthly breast self-examination (BSE), physician examination every 3 months (we recommend physician examination every 6 months), and bilateral mammograms every 6 to 12 months, with appropriate biopsy of suspicious lesions.

In addition to the susceptibility to breast cancer, women may show virginal hypertrophy of the breasts. Breast hamartomas, as well as an array of benign breast findings, may occur, including ductal hyperplasia, intraductal papillomatosis, adenosis, lobular atrophy, fibroadenomas, fibrocystic change, densely fibrotic hyalinized breast nodules, and nipple and areolar malformations.[153] The risk of fibrocystic breast disease may be as high as 67%. Males and females who have the cutaneous lesions may also manifest thyroid goiter,

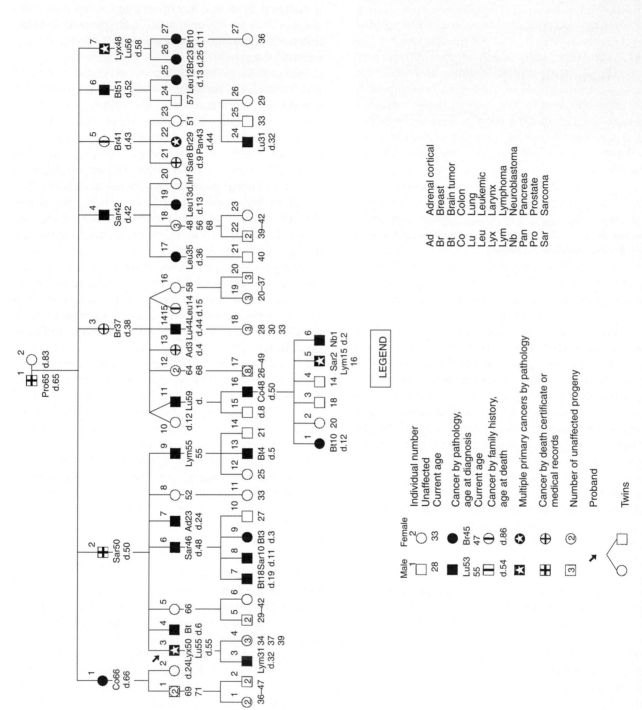

FIG. **18-13** An updated pedigree of an SBLA kindred showing cancer occurrences through five generations. *(From Lynch HT et al: Cancer 41:2055, 1978. Copyright 1978 American Cancer Society. Reprinted by permission of Wiley-Liss Inc., a subsidiary of John Wiley & Sons, Inc.)*

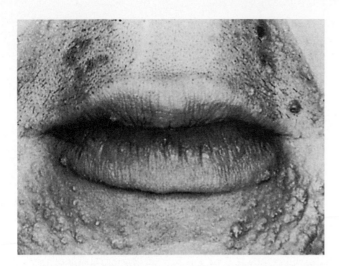

FIG. **18-14** Multiple trichilemmomas in a patient with Cowden's disease, which is often associated with breast cancer. *(From Brownstein MH: Breast cancer in Cowden's syndrome. In Lynch HT [ed]: Genetics and breast cancer, New York, 1981, Van Nostrand Reinhold.)*

thyroid adenoma, and hyperthyroidism or hypothyroidism, as well as carcinoma of the thyroid mainly of the follicular type. Thyroid disease is seen in 50% to 75% of individuals, and there is a 3% to 10% chance of epithelial thyroid carcinoma. Multiple, early-onset uterine leiomyomas are characteristic, and brain tumors (meningiomas, glioblastoma multiforme) also occur. Hamartomatous polyps are relatively common and have been observed throughout the gastrointestinal tract, including the esophagus. Adenocarcinoma of the colon has been reported in patients with Cowden disease but the risk is yet to be clearly defined.

Dysmorphic features are part of the Cowden phenotype and are especially useful for diagnosis.[149] The pleiotropic effects of the *PTEN* gene in development are highlighted by the numerous affected organ systems: neurologic (Lhermitte-Duclos disease, mild to moderate mental retardation in 12%, cerebellar gangliocytoma manifesting as seizure and tremor), head and neck (progressive macrocephaly, "birdlike" facies, high-arched palate, scrotal tongue), skeletal (pectus excavatum, scoliosis, kyphosis), and genitourinary (hydrocele, varicocele, vaginal and vulvar cysts, ovarian cysts, and leiomyomas). These are in addition to the endocrine, gastrointestinal, oncologic, and dermatologic features previously noted.

Although Cowden Syndrome is said to be rare, underdiagnosis is likely because of a lack of awareness of the syndrome, as well as its variable expressivity and sometimes subtle manifestations.[154] In addition, there may be a lack of family history as a result of de novo mutations. Yet, regardless of whether there is a family history, the risk of transmission by affected individuals is 50%; therefore institution of cancer surveillance is crucial in at-risk relatives.

ATAXIA TELANGIECTASIA

A mutated gene that is responsible for the rare childhood neurologic disorder ataxia telangiectasia (AT) has been identified on chromosome 11q.[155,156] AT is characterized by progressive cerebellar and neuromotor deterioration, telangiectasia of the conjunctivae and facial skin, cellular and humoral immune deficiencies, growth retardation, clinical and cellular hypersensitivity to ionizing radiation, and cancer.[157] The disease follows an autosomal recessive pattern of inheritance, with homozygous-affected individuals bearing a cancer risk 61 to 184 times greater than the general population.[158] Obligate heterozygous carriers of the gene have been found to be at threefold to fourfold the population risk for cancer.[159,160] Female carriers of the mutated AT gene (*ATM*) are at five times the population risk for developing breast cancers.[160]

In younger patients with AT, there is an increased frequency of lymphoreticular neoplasms or leukemia. However, an association with epithelial cancers is rare in young AT patients. In contrast, older patients with AT show an excess of epithelial neoplasms, but interestingly, lymphoreticular cancer and leukemia rarely occur in the older patients. At least two young patients with AT who developed dysgerminomas have been reported.[161,162]

It is estimated that as many as 1% of the general population carries the *ATM* gene,[163] which may predispose to as many as 9% to 18% of all breast cancers.[160] It is of interest that the *ATM* gene also seems to convey susceptibility to cancers of the lung, pancreas, gallbladder, and stomach, but in obligate heterozygous carriers of the gene, colorectal cancers are observed less frequently than expected.[159] This autosomal recessive disease and the somatic effects of the heterozygous carrier state of *ATM* are exceedingly important models for future study, and they present a dilemma to the physician for clinical management. Homozygotic individuals are excessively sensitive to the necrotizing effects of radiation therapy, and in vitro their cells show several repair and growth defects following radiation exposure. Heterozygotic carriers of *ATM*, however, are susceptible to early-onset breast cancers and therefore might benefit from screening mammography, yet it is speculated that they may be particularly susceptible to malignant transformation induced by this radiation exposure.[164] DNA screening for mutations is clinically feasible, although test sensitivity is imperfect. It is possible to identify those individuals who are at increased genetic risk for neoplasms associated with this specific genetic defect; however, clear screening guidelines have not been developed.

Psychologic Aspects of Familial Breast Cancer

QUALITY OF LIFE AND HEALTH BEHAVIOR

As our knowledge of breast cancer risk factors has increased, so has attention to the impact of risk assessment on women's quality of life. In one of the first empirical studies to examine this systematically, Kash and colleagues[165] showed that more than one fourth of women with a family history of breast cancer exhibited psychologic distress that warranted counseling. Significant distress was also reported in a subsequent population-based study of first-degree relatives of breast cancer patients.[166] In this study, 53% of women reported intrusive thoughts about breast cancer, 33% reported impairments in daily functioning related to breast cancer worries, and 20% reported sleep disturbance. Psychologic distress in high-risk women parallels that of women diagnosed with invasive breast cancer,[167] and it is increased significantly compared with women who do not have a family history of this disease.[168] Younger high-risk women, those aged 35 and younger, appear to be at greatest risk for cancer-related distress.[169,170]

In addition to its effects on quality of life, breast cancer–related distress can also influence health behavior in high-risk women. One adaptive aspect of distress is that it may motivate women to seek counseling about their breast cancer risk and options for prevention and surveillance. In a study of predictors of participation in a breast cancer health promotion trial, high-risk women who were more distressed about their risk were significantly more likely to participate than those with low levels of distress.[171] However, although distress may increase motivation for counseling, it may interfere with comprehension of the information provided during the counseling session. In the same study, Lerman and colleagues[172] found that women who had high levels of breast cancer–related distress before the risk counseling session were significantly less likely to improve in terms of their comprehension of personal risk. Moreover, anxieties and fears about breast cancer can lead some high-risk women to avoid breast cancer detection practices. Psychologic distress has been associated with decreased adherence to guidelines for clinical breast examination, BSE, and mammography.[165,166]

INTEREST IN GENETIC TESTING FOR BREAST CANCER SUSCEPTIBILITY

In anticipation of the widespread availability of genetic testing for breast cancer susceptibility, several studies have examined interest in testing and anticipated reactions to positive and negative test results. Overall, interest in genetic testing for inherited breast cancer risk has been reported to be very high. In a sample of women with a family history of OC, 75% said they would definitely want to be tested for mutations in the *BRCA1* gene and 20% said they probably would want to be tested.[171] Interest in testing was significantly greater among women who perceived themselves to be at higher risk for cancer and those who were more worried about their risk. Similar levels of interest have been observed among women in the general population,[173] women with a family history of breast cancer,[172] and female members of families with HBOC.[45,60] However, with the possible exception of the study by Lynch and colleagues,[60] these studies used hypothetical scenarios to assess interest in testing and actual test results were not available.

It is therefore possible that the actual demand for genetic testing for breast cancer susceptibility is not as great as that suggested by these preliminary studies. For example, before the initiation of predictive testing for Huntington's disease (HD), more than two thirds of persons at risk expressed interest in testing.[103] Since HD predictive testing has become available, less than 15% of those who initially expressed interest have come forward.[174,175] However, one critical difference between HD and breast cancer is that breast cancer can be treated and has the potential to be cured if it is found early. This potential for early detection and treatment of breast cancer and the high levels of anxiety about this disease has generated great demand for genetic testing now that it is commercially available.

For those persons who ultimately do decide to receive genetic testing for breast cancer susceptibility, there may be a significant burden associated with the knowledge that one is a carrier of a cancer-predisposing mutation. In the hypothetical studies described earlier, a substantial proportion of women indicated that they would become very depressed and anxious if they received positive results.[172,173] Interestingly, many women also anticipated adverse effects of negative results, including "survivor guilt" (i.e., that other family members had inherited the mutation but they had not) and continued worry.

An earlier descriptive report by Lynch and colleagues did not contain evidence for serious adverse emotional effects of disclosure of *BRCA1* mutation status in families with HBOC; however, the need for controlled trials of the impact of testing was acknowledged.[60]

Factors Associated with Use of *BRCA* Testing. In our study (Lynch HT, unpublished data), the reasons most often cited by family members for wanting *BRCA* testing were to learn about one's children's risks and to increase the use of cancer-screening tests. Of interest, almost half of individuals surveyed reported childbearing decisions as a very important reason for wanting *BRCA* testing. This is surprising because reproductive decision making generally is not a focus in genetic counseling for cancer susceptibility. Overall, fewer individuals reported strong reasons for not having testing. This is consistent with the high level of acceptance of testing in this population. However, concerns about the effect of testing on one's family and worries about insurance discrimination were cited most frequently as barriers to receiving *BRCA* test results.

We also examined whether persons who came forward for *BRCA* testing had different sociodemographic backgrounds than those who declined. Individuals who decided to be tested were predominantly female, younger than age 50, had at least a high school education, and had health insurance. *BRCA1* test decliners were mostly males older than age 50 who had not completed high school and had no health insurance. In a logistic regression model, the following factors were significant independent predictors of acceptance of testing: gender (OR = 3.8, CI = 1.8 to 8.1), age (OR = 2.9, CI = 1.3 to 6.2), education (OR = 3.4, CI = 1.1 to 11.2), and health insurance status (OR = 5.1, CI = 1.5 to 17.0). Females were almost four times more likely than males to request testing, individuals younger than age 50 were three times more likely than those who were older than age 50, and individuals with health insurance were about five times more likely to request testing than those who did not have insurance.

Prophylactic Bilateral Mastectomy and Oophorectomy in HBOC

PM and prophylactic oophorectomy on patients at inordinately high risk for HBOC were initially discussed by Lynch and colleagues in the early 1970s.[12,13,176-180] Prophylactic contralateral mastectomy in high-risk women with ipsilateral breast cancer was considered a logical option, given the enormous risk of bilaterality in hereditary cases.[181] This was predicated by the concern that women at inordinately high familial breast cancer and OC risk required special cancer-control measures. PM, for example, was suggested as an option for members of breast cancer–prone families wherein the risk to first-degree relatives of the proband "approach 50%, consistent with an autosomal dominant factor."[179] For example, a relative who developed a crippling cancer phobia resulting from her awareness of this disease in her family may express a strong desire to have what she correctly considers her extremely highly cancer-prone breast tissue excised.

Patients who were candidates for the option of PM included those who failed to comply with screening recommendations, often because of their fear of "finding" breast cancer.[177] Also included were women at high HBC risk who manifested severe fibrocystic breast disease that made it difficult for them and their physicians

to determine which palpable masses were significant.[179] Even in those "early days," counseling and consultation with a medical geneticist was recommended when weighing genetic risk factors relevant to considerations of prophylactic surgery.[177,180]

PM has long been a controversial issue, raising such questions as, "Will it work? Will patients accept it? Will physicians recommend it? Will insurance companies cover the cost? Will it effectively reduce breast cancer's and OC's morbidity and mortality? Is this considered a particularly radical medical and surgical concern, meaning that patients who harbor *BRCA1/2* germline mutations and who therefore may have an enormous lifetime risk for breast cancer (in the range of 70% to 85%) or some of their physicians may remain reluctant to advocate PM?"

RECENT SURGICAL PROPHYLAXIS STUDIES

Hartmann and colleagues[182] initially used "high-risk" criteria, such as the number of breast cancer-affected first- and second-degree relatives, for consideration of PM. They found that PM was effective in these high-risk women in that there was a 90% reduction in the risk of breast cancer, with a significant reduction in mortality.

Seven breast cancers occurred in their study after subcutaneous bilateral mastectomy; there were none after total mastectomy.[182] Subsequently,[30] they used genetic testing to distinguish the *BRCA1/2* mutation carriers in this cohort and proved that PM works in these *BRCA1/2* mutation carriers.[30] For example, breast cancer did not develop in any of the women with a confirmed *BRCA1* or *BRCA2* mutation after a median follow-up of 16 years.[30] Therefore PM appears to reduce the long-term risk of breast cancer in those women with a *BRCA1* or *BRCA2* mutation.

A prospective study by Meijers-Heijboer and colleagues[183] also showed significant benefit of PM among *BRCA1/2* mutation carriers. These investigators studied 139 women with a *BRCA1* or *BRCA2* mutation who were part of a prospective study of the effectiveness of PM in a breast cancer surveillance program at the Rotterdam Family Cancer Clinic in the Netherlands. Of these women, 76 eventually underwent PM, whereas 63 declined PM in preference to regular surveillance. Cox proportional-hazards method evaluated the incidence of breast cancer as a time-dependent covariate for the effect of mastectomy on the incidence of breast cancer. Findings disclosed an absence of breast cancer among those undergoing PM during a follow-up of 2.9 (±1.4) years, whereas, in comparison, eight breast cancers developed in those women who elected regular surveillance after a mean follow-up of 3.0 (±1.5) years ($p = .003$; HR, 0; 95% CI 0 to 0.36). The authors concluded that, "in women with a *BRCA1* or *BRCA2* mutation, prophylactic bilateral total mastectomy reduces the incidence of breast cancer at three years of follow-up." It was of particular interest that of the eight cancers identified in the screening group, four were identified between screening sessions, consonant with so-called interval cancers, and herein "the interval from screening to diagnosis was two to five months." Cancers in the remaining four patients were detected during a screening session. Thus it is possible that some were "missed lesions" versus accelerated breast carcinogenesis.

A significantly greater number of women in the PM group, as opposed to those in the surveillance group, had undergone a premenopausal oophorectomy (44 versus 24 [58% versus 38%], $p = .03$). Thus there was likely protective effect from prophylactic oophorecomy, consistent with the findings of Rebbeck and colleagues,[31] discussed subsequently.

Given the assumption that within 10 years breast cancer will develop in approximately 25% of the women undergoing regular surveillance, these authors[183] estimated that 10% to 20% of high-risk women who choose surveillance instead of PM will die of breast cancer within 20 years, and 35% to 50% of women under surveillance who develop primary breast cancer will die of distant metastases within 10 to 15 years.[115,184]

Meijers-Heijboer and colleagues[183] suggest that the use of high-resolution imaging, as well as more frequent screening, might be effective in early breast cancer detection among women with a BRCA1 or BRCA2 mutation. Specifically, in their study, magnetic resonance imaging (MRI) was performed in six women at the time of breast cancer diagnosis and it detected all six cancers. In contrast, mammography was diagnostic in only two of the eight women with breast cancer.

BILATERAL PROPHYLACTIC OOPHORECTOMY IN BRCA1 MUTATION CARRIERS

Recent studies[36,185] have provided prospective findings about the risk-reducing effects on both breast cancer and OC in patients who were harbingers of BRCA1 and BRCA2 and who underwent prophylactic salpingo-oophorectomy.

Rebbeck and colleagues[31] studied a cohort of women with BRCA1 mutations who underwent bilateral prophylactic oophorectomy (BPO) in order to test the hypothesis that decreases in ovarian hormone exposure following BPO may alter breast cancer risk in BRCA1 mutation carriers. This study showed a statistically significant reduction in breast cancer risk following BPO that was greater in women who were followed 5 to 10 years, or for at least 10 years, after surgery. BPO also provided a potential for reduction of risk for OC. Hormone replacement therapy did not negate this reduction in breast cancer risk following BPO. The study concluded that BPO "is associated with a reduced breast cancer risk in women who carry a BRCA1 mutation. The likely mechanism is reduction of ovarian hormone exposure."

Rebbeck and colleagues,[36] in a prospective study, evaluated 551 women with BRCA1 or BRCA2 germline mutations identified from registries, 259 of whom had undergone BPO and 292 who were matched controls who had not undergone the procedure. They then investigated these women for the occurrence of carcinoma of the breast and ovary. Among a subgroup of 241 women who lacked a history of carcinoma of the breast and of PM, the incidence of breast cancer was determined in 99 women who had undergone BPO and in 142 matched controls. Postoperative follow-up with both groups was at least eight years. Findings disclosed that, "Six women who underwent prophylactic oophorectomy (2.3%) received a diagnosis of stage I ovarian cancer at the time of the procedure; two women (0.8%) received a diagnosis of papillary serous peritoneal carcinoma, 3.8 and 8.6 years after bilateral prophylactic oophorectomy. Among the controls, 58 women (19.9 percent) received a diagnosis of ovarian cancer after a mean follow-up of 8.8 years. With the exclusion of the six women whose cancer was diagnosed at surgery, prophylactic oophorectomy significantly reduced the risk of coelomic epithelial cancer (hazard ratio, 0.04; 95 percent confidence interval, 0.01 to 0.16). Of 99 women who underwent bilateral prophylactic oophorectomy and who were studied to determine the risk of breast cancer, breast cancer developed in 21 (21.2 percent), as compared with 60 (42.3 percent) in the control group (hazard ratio, 0.47; 95 percent confidence interval, 0.29 to 0.77)." In conclusion, BPO reduced the risk of OC and breast cancer in those women who were harbingers of BRCA1 or BRCA2 germline mutations.

Kauff and colleagues[185] compared the effect of risk-reducing salpingo-oophorectomy to that of surveillance for OC on the incidence of carcinoma of the breast and OC in harbingers of BRCA mutations. They studied 170 women 35 years or older who had declined bilateral oophorectomy in preference to other surveillance for OC. Kaplan-Meier analysis and a Cox proportional-hazards model were used to compare the time to cancer in both groups. Herein, it was found that, "The time to breast cancer or BRCA-related gynecologic cancer was longer in the salpingo-oophorectomy group, with a hazard ratio for subsequent breast cancer or BRCA-related gynecologic cancer of 0.25 (95 percent confidence interval, 0.08 to 0.72)."

Grann and associates[186] found that women who were positive for BRCA1 or BRCA2 mutations "may derive greater survival and quality adjusted survival benefits than previously reported from chemoprevention, prophylactic surgery, or a combination. Observational studies and clinical trials are needed to verify the results of this analysis of the long-term benefits of preventive strategies among *BRCA1/2*-positive women."

We believe that third-party carriers should defray the expenses of not only surveillance but, moreover, PM and prophylactic salpingo-oophorectomy among women at inordinately high risk for carcinoma of the breast, inclusive of those who are harbingers of *BRCA1/BRCA2* germline mutations.

BRCA1/2 CONCERNS ABOUT PROPHYLACTIC SURGERY

We have identified the *BRCA1/BRCA2* germline mutation status of 1252 individuals from 95 families with HBOC (Lynch HT, unpublished data). To date, we have counseled 687 women from 83 of these families. Pertinent insights about their interest in surgical prophylaxis have emerged. For example, before receiving their DNA results, 362 women were asked if they would consider the option of PM. Of those 362 women, 138 (38%) said they would consider PM if they were positive for the mutation. Conversely, 5 of 307 (2%) said they would still consider PM even if they tested negative for the mutation, reflecting, in part, their concern about the 1:8 to 1:9 lifetime general-population breast cancer risk and personal experiences with breast cancer suggesting it cannot be survived. It may also reflect a lack of belief that a negative mutation finding would remove them from the greater HBOC lifetime breast cancer risk, given that they may have been labeled high-risk for years and/or that so many of their relatives may have been affected with breast cancer. If positive for the mutation, 172 (51%) of the 336 who answered the question said they would consider BPO and, if negative, 14 (5%) of 289 would still consider BPO. Following disclosure, our follow-up survey found that 27 of 142 (19%) mutation-positive women had undergone PM, whereas 46 of 131 (35%) had had a BPO.

Genetic counseling is mandatory when working with patients from high-risk families.[177] But will it make a difference? With the discovery of mutations in the *BRCA1* and *BRCA2* genes that predispose to breast cancer, we have been able to counsel these women with greater precision not only about their risk but also about screening and management options, including chemoprevention and prophylactic surgery.

ATTITUDES ABOUT PROPHYLACTIC SURGERY

Meiser and colleagues[187] showed that cancer worry as opposed to objective risk estimates strongly influences consideration of prophylactic oophorectomy. Lerman and associates[188] suggested that many women will likely postpone prophylactic surgery until they obtain results of their mutation status testing. Decisions about surgical prophylaxis are conditioned strongly by assessing the positive and negative issues surrounding the outcome of surgery.

Hallowell and colleagues[189] studied a cohort of women who had at least two first- or second-degree relatives with carcinoma of the ovary or breast and assessed the attitudes that influence decisions about prophylactic oophorectomy. Knowledge about *BRCA1* or *BRCA2* mutation status, before prophylactic surgery, was an important consideration. These findings were in accord with studies showing that many women undergo *BRCA1/BRCA2* testing to facilitate their decisions relevant to prophylactic surgery.[190,191] Hallowell and colleagues[189] also noted less anxiety among women who did not have close relatives with cancer, and none of the women in the screening group would, at the time of the study, absolutely exclude the possibility of prophylactic surgery at some future date.

Eisen and Weber[192] conclude that in considering the imperfect surveillance tools for early detection of OC, coupled with the difficult surgical choices for women with *BRCA1* and *BRCA2* mutations, it appears that PM is clearly "the right choice for some women. For the remainder, oophorectomy and tamoxifen in conjunction with intensive screening that includes MRI is a viable alternative. More important, ongoing and novel prospective studies to define the role of prophylactic surgery, new chemopreventive agents, and optimal screening strategies must be supported, and women at very high risk should be encouraged to participate."

PUBLIC HEALTH IMPACT OF SURGICAL PROPHYLAXIS

What will be the public health impact of the findings by Hartmann and colleagues,[30,182] Meijers-Heijboer and associates,[183] and Rebbeck and colleagues,[31,36] given the enormous magnitude of breast cancer in the general population, particularly in women in Western highly-industrialized nations? How will women determine if they are at high risk?[34] Will physicians take family histories that are sufficiently detailed to enable them to make hereditary cancer-risk determinations? Are there enough genetic counselors who are sufficiently knowledgeable about cancer genetics and the pros and cons of PM and BPO, particularly the potential physical and psychologic sequelae, to adequately and responsibly advise their consultants? Indeed, should offering such options be the responsibility of the nonmedically trained genetic counselor? Are the skills of these counselors being sufficiently used? Will insurers defray the cost of genetic counseling, genetic testing, and prophylactic surgery? Will there be insurance discrimination? Will women accept the loss of sexual stimulation following PM, particularly with sacrifice of the nipple/areola complex, and/or the change in their body image related to disfigurement? Will women accept the cardiovascular, osteoporotic, and physiologic/sexual risks of BPO? What will be the spouse response? Only time will tell!

TUBAL LIGATION AND OC RISK IN *BRCA1* OR *BRCA2* MUTATION CARRIERS

Narod and colleagues,[193] in a matched case-control study, assessed women with a pathogenic mutation in *BRCA1* or *BRCA2* to determine the potential reduction in the risk of OC through tubal ligation. Cases were 232 women with a history of invasive OC and controls were 232 women without OC who had both ovaries intact. Cases and controls were matched for year of birth and mutation (*BRCA1* or *BRCA2*) status. The OR for OC occurrence was estimated for tubal ligation with adjustment for parity, breast cancer history, oral contraceptive use, and ethnic background.

Findings disclosed that in an unadjusted analysis among *BRCA1* carriers "significantly fewer cases than controls had ever had tubal ligation (30 of 173 [18%] vs 60 of 173 [35%], odds ratio 0.37 [95% CI 0.21-0.63]; $p = 0.0003$). After adjustment for oral contraceptive use, parity, history of breast cancer, and ethnic group, the odds ratio was 0.39 ($p = 0.002$). Combination of tubal ligation and past use of an oral contraceptive was associated with an odds ratio of 0.28 (0.15-0.52). No protective effect of tubal ligation was seen among carriers of the *BRCA2* mutation."

It was therefore concluded that tubal ligation may be a feasible option for the reduction of OC in women with *BRCA1* mutations who have completed their childbearing. However, we consider it mandatory that genetic counselors emphasize the fact that these are statistical findings that need to be confirmed in additional studies, that the magnitude of protection is much less for tubal ligation than prophylactic oophorectomy, and that due caution must be exercised when considering tubal ligation as a preventive measure for reduction of OC risk in *BRCA1* carriers.

TAMOXIFEN AND RISK OF CONTRALATERAL BREAST CANCER IN *BRCA1* AND *BRCA2* MUTATION CARRIERS

Tamoxifen has been shown to protect against contralateral breast cancer in women with a prior history of estrogen receptor–positive breast cancer and to be protective for women without a prior history of breast cancer who are at increased risk. To evaluate the effect of tamoxifen on contralateral breast cancer in *BRCA1/2* mutation carriers, Narod and colleagues[32] compared 209 women with bilateral breast cancer and a *BRCA1* or *BRCA2* mutation with 384 women with unilateral breast cancer and *BRCA1* or *BRCA2* mutation (controls), in a matched case-control study. Findings disclosed that "the multivariate odds ratio for contralateral breast cancer associated with tamoxifen use was 0.50 (95% CI,

0.28-0.89). Tamoxifen protected against contralateral breast cancer for carriers of *BRCA1* mutations (odds ratio 0.38, 95% CI 0.19-0.74) and those with *BRCA2* mutations (0.63, 0.20-1.50). In women who used tamoxifen for 2-4 years, the risk of contralateral breast cancer was reduced by 75%. A reduction in risk of contralateral breast cancer was also seen with oophorectomy (0.42, 0.22-0.83) and with chemotherapy (0.40, 0.26-0.60)." It was therefore concluded that there was a reduction of contralateral breast cancer in women harboring *BRCA1* or *BRCA2* mutations, and herein the protective effect of tamoxifen appeared to be independent of that of oophorectomy.

ORAL CONTRACEPTIVES AND RISK OF HEREDITARY OC

Oral contraceptives have been shown to protect against OC in the general population. Narod and colleagues[194] showed that oral contraceptive use may provide a reduction in the risk of OC in women harboring *BRCA1* or *BRCA2* germline mutations.

Marchbanks and colleagues[195] studied oral contraceptive use in 4575 women affected with breast cancer and 4683 controls who were 35 to 64 years old. Conditional logistical regression for calculating ORs revealed the relative risk of 1.0 (95% CI 0.8 to 1.3) for women currently using oral contraceptives and 0.9 (95% CI 0.8 to 1.0) for those who had previously used oral contraceptives. Interestingly, there was no increase among women who had longer periods of use or who had higher doses of estrogen. There were no differences between white and black women.

In support of the results obtained by Narod and associates,[194] those obtained by Marchbanks and colleagues[195] showed that neither use of oral contraceptives nor the initiation of oral contraceptive use at a young age was associated with an increased risk of breast cancer in women with a family history of breast cancer.

Endocrine Signaling

The substantial interindividual variability in the occurrence of breast cancer among *BRCA1/2* mutation carriers has been partially attributed to endocrine signaling, which may modify the *BRCA1/2*-associated age-specific breast cancer penetrance.[196] This hypothesis was supported by the finding that women showed a significantly higher breast cancer risk "if they carried alleles with at least 28 or 29 polyglutamine repeats at *AIB1*, compared with women who carried alleles with fewer polyglutamine repeats [odds ratio (OR), 1.59; 95% confidence interval (CI), 1.03-2.47 and OR, 2.85; 95% CI, 1.64-4.96, respectively].....Women were at significantly increased risk if they were nulliparous or had a late age at first live birth and had *AIB1* alleles no shorter than 28 or 29 or more *AIB1* polyglutamine repeats (OR, 4.62; 95% CI, 2.02-10.56 and OR, 6.97; 95% CI, 1.71-28.43, respectively) than women with none of these risk factors." Clearly, endocrine signaling, as evidenced through *AIB1* genotype and reproductive history, may show a powerful effect on *BRCA1/2*-associated breast cancer risk.[196]

POLYMORPHIC ANDROGEN-RECEPTOR CAG REPEAT

As in the case of breast cancer risk modification in *BRCA1* and *BRCA2* mutation carriers by *AIB1* genotype and reproductive history, endocrine signaling in concert with the CAG repeat-length polymorphism found in exon 1 of the androgen-receptor *(AR)* gene *(AR-CAG)* may also modify the *BRCA1*-associated age-specific breast cancer risk. For example, Rebbeck and associates[197] found that all of the women who harbored at least one *AR-CAG* allele with 29 or more repeats had breast cancer. Results from this study supported the hypothesis that age at breast cancer diagnosis "is earlier among *BRCA1* mutation carriers who carry very long *AR-CAG* repeats....[indicating that] pathways involving androgen signaling may affect the risk of *BRCA1*-associated breast cancer."

Ductal Lavage: Implications for Early Breast Cancer Diagnosis in High-Risk Patients

The landmark paper by Dupont and Page[198] set the stage for understanding the significance of proliferative breast disease with and without atypical hyperplasia in concert with family history status. For example, women with proliferative breast disease without atypical hyperplasia harbored a breast cancer risk that was 1.9 times that for women with nonproliferative lesions. Those with atypical hyperplasia were at 5.3 times increased breast cancer risk than for women with nonproliferative lesions. In women with nonproliferative lesions, a family history of breast cancer had little effect. In contrast, the breast cancer risk in women with atypia and a family history of breast cancer showed a risk that was about nine times that in women who had nonproliferative lesions in the absence of a positive family history. Decision logic from these pioneering observations have contributed heavily to the recent interest in ductal lavage (DL) with cytologic studies of breast fluids.

O'Shaughnessy and colleagues,[199] in discussing the role of DL in the clinical management of women at inordinately high risk for carcinoma of the breast, show that collecting breast ductal epithelial cells for cytologic analysis is a minimally invasive office procedure. The efficacy of DL rests on the fact that breast carcinoma cells arise in the epithelial cells lining the milk ducts and lobules that comprise the ductal system. A microcatheter can be inserted into the nipple orifice with lavaging of the cannulated ductal system with normal saline. The collected lavage effluent can then be analyzed for normal, atypical, or malignant breast ductal cells.

The efficacy of DL is based on computer-reviewed data that demonstrated an elevated risk of developing breast carcinoma in concert with long-term follow-up of women with atypical ductal epithelial cells. O'Shaughnessy and colleagues[199] cite the work of Wrensch and associates,[200] which was based on the collection of ductal epithelial cells from 2701 women volunteers using nipple aspiration and analysis of these cells cytologically in concert with a prospective longitudinal follow-up on 2343 women over a period of 12.7 years. Findings showed that "women with cellular atypia in nipple aspirate fluid (NAF) had a relative risk of developing breast carcinoma that was 4.9 times greater than women whose breast did not yield NAF. Women with a family history of breast carcinoma and cellular atypia on NAF had an increase in their relative risk that was 18 times greater than that for women without cellular atypia on NAF"[200] (cited by O'Shaughnessy and colleagues[199]).

Fabian and associates[201] studied ductal epithelial cells from 480 high-risk women wherein they employed random, four-quadrant periareolar fine-needle aspiration (FNA) for cytologic analysis. The women were then prospectively followed for a median of 45 months. Importantly, 15% of those showing both atypical cytology and an elevated 10-year Gail risk, manifested carcinoma of the breast within the first 3 years of follow-up. In comparison to these findings, only 4% of women who were at an elevated 10-year Gail risk but who lacked atypical cytology manifested breast cancer within that same time period.

Given the safety of DL and its ability to provide additional information regarding breast cancer risk in women who are already at an elevated risk for this disease and who do not have a history of biopsy-proven atypical hyperplasia, the finding of cytologic atypia in DL "provides risk assessment information that is independent of her Gail risk. This information can assist the woman and her physician in weighing the risks and benefits of hormone replacement therapy, antiestrogen therapy, and, in very high-risk women, prophylactic mastectomies."[199] Thus DL provides additional information regarding breast cancer risk to these women, as well as their physicians, so that women can become more informed about physicians' advice, given the DL findings and, therein, can participate in a more informed manner with decision logic relevant to hormone replacement therapy and antiestrogen risk-reduction therapy.[199]

Dooley and colleagues[202] described a new procedure for collecting ductal cells with a microcatheter and compared this with nipple aspiration with respect to safety, tolerability, and the ability to detect abnormal breast epithelial cells. They found that DL detected abnormal intraductal breast cells 3.2 times more often than nipple aspiration (79 versus 25 breasts; McNemar's tests, p <.001). There was no report of any serious procedure-related adverse events. They concluded that large numbers of ductal cells can be collected by DL identifying atypical cellular changes in this safe and well-tolerated procedure, which they conclude is a more sensitive method for detecting cellular atypia when compared with nipple aspiration.

These methods of DL will merit meticulous examinations in a clinical trial setting, preferably involving women who are harbingers of *BRCA1* and *BRCA2* germline mutations, in order to test its efficacy. However, at this time, DL should not be considered a substitute for mammography, BSE, or clinical breast examination.

Racial and Sociocultural Variation in Breast Cancer Rates: A Genetic-Environmental Dilemma

The international variation in breast cancer incidence, particularly with respect to ethnic, racial, and socio-ethnic populations such as Ashkenazi Jews, must be considered when interpreting the etiologic role of hereditary factors in these disorders. For example, Deapen and colleagues[203] have shown marked fluctuation in breast cancer incidence rates over relatively short time spans among differing racial groups, particularly Asian-American women. These authors note that, overall, breast cancer incidence rates remained stable in the Los Angeles area during the late 1980s and early 1990s. However, data from the most recent 5-year period suggest that the breast cancer incidence may be increasing for Asian-American and non-Hispanic white women older than age 50.

These changes occurred in the face of little change in breast cancer incidence occurring among black and Hispanic women. Attention was given to sorting breast cancer rate differences among specific subsets of the Asian population. For example, Filipinas, who historically had higher rates of breast cancer than other Asian-American counterparts, were shown to not have as rapid a rate of increase as Japanese women; nevertheless,

they remain relatively high. Women of Japanese and Filipino ancestry had breast cancer rates that were twice that of Chinese and Korean women. Asian women, who commonly have low breast cancer rates in their native countries, typically experience increasing breast cancer incidence after immigrating to the United States. How much of this variation in breast cancer rates is attributable to host factors, environmental-culture exposures, and/or their interaction? Do *BRCA1* or *BRCA2* mutations behave differently with respect to such parameters as age of onset, bilaterality, virulence, or association with carcinomas of the ovary and other anatomic sites in these racial and ethnic population subtypes?

Expression Profiling of Breast Cancer

Novel scientific terms have been adopted into popular parlance, such as *DNA fingerprinting* and *genetic profiling*. This new technospeak attempts to explain the mystery of our biologic selves as being attributable to the result of our unique, individual genetic programs. When interaction with the outside world is added to the equation, we have the classic nature versus nurture theory (or more accurately, nature "plus" nurture). Our genetic blueprint, or DNA code, is essentially the same in each of our cells, yet our cells are visibly and functionally different. Lung, nerve, heart, and breast cells all have different functions and different morphologies reflecting that functionality. A particular set of genes from the master blueprint is activated and deactivated in specialized cells, which defines those cells. Although we can distinguish colonic epithelium from cerebral cortex with hematoxylin and eosin staining and a microscope, another approach would be to isolate the messenger RNA from each specimen, create a DNA copy (cDNA) of the RNA to work with (because RNA is highly degradable), and review the pattern of each sample. The set of genes turned on and off in each specimen would provide a colon or brain fingerprint, and we could tell the specimens apart.

Although pathologic specimens from different tissues are readily distinguished with the use of a microscope, histopathologic techniques have approached a limit in terms of discerning the finer steps of malignant progression from benign tissue to atypia to preinvasive lesions to invasive malignancies and metastases. A finer "microscope" is needed and comes in the form of discerning molecular techniques. The fingerprinting process previously described is termed *genetic expression profiling* and is technically feasible using "microarrays," which can analyze the expression of hundreds to thousands of genes on a small slide, or chip. Among the many applications of this technology is the potential to assess individual cancers for their genetic fingerprint. Genes of interest in oncogenic pathways are selected for analysis, printed onto slides, and then hybridized with the test sample (e.g., RNAs from different breast cancer specimens). Gene expression levels for each tumor are compared with a control or median level of expression among samples and color-coded (red = high, green = low). Samples are then compared using clustering algorithms, which assign a hierarchy of similarity (i.e., identify the closest neighbors).

The traditional approach in biology has been to evaluate one or two genes at a time and elucidate relevant pathways; microarray technology supplements this approach by discovering "molecular portraits" of tumors. This new approach has begun to lead toward a subclassification of tumors that cannot otherwise be distinguished using histopathologic techniques. First effectively applied to the subclassification of lymphomas, tumor profiling has defined breast cancer portraits as well.[204] Correlations between clinical outcomes and tumor profiles are beginning to emerge.[205,206] The divergence of breast cancer evolutionary pathways according to estrogen receptor status is confirmed by tumor profiling and does not strictly correlate with estrogen responsiveness.[207] The clinical need to distinguish between primary and secondary breast tumors is also amenable to molecular profiling analysis: distantly located metachronous ipsilateral breast tumors may be shown to be genetically related[208] and lymph node metastases can be confirmed to have arisen from the primary tumor.[204]

The delineation of molecular targets has led to a few success stories in targeted therapeutics, namely Herceptin for HER2/neu-positive breast cancers and STK571 for gastric intestinal stromal tumors. Initial work in breast tumor profiling demonstrates significant potential to identify new diagnostic and prognostic markers and therapeutic targets. For example, doxorubicin resistance correlates with a particular gene expression profile, which could theoretically be used for chemotherapy selection and to develop strategies to undermine resistance.[209] Expression profiling of disseminated breast tumor cells in peripheral blood may be a viable approach to early cancer detection.[208]

Prostate Cancer and *BRCA1/2* Mutations

Rosen and colleagues[210] described the possible etiologic relationship between *BRCA1* and prostate cancer. In their review, they found that a positive family history of prostate cancer confers an approximate twofold or threefold greater risk for prostate cancer to first-degree relatives of affected persons as opposed to men without a family history.[211-213] Rosen and colleagues[210] suggested that only a minority (<10%) of patients with prostate cancer are clearly familial in origin.[214] Their review[210] disclosed that certain epidemiologic studies documented a statistically significant linkage between prostate cancers and other tumor types such as carcinoma of the breast, ovary, and uterus.[212,215-218] In one such study involving 143 families with three or more cases of OC, males showed a 4.5-fold increase in the RR for prostate cancer, whereas females had a 2.5-fold increased risk for breast cancer and a 5-fold higher risk for uterine cancer.[216]

In the case of *BRCA1* and *BRCA2* mutations, investigators have shown an association between these mutations and prostate cancer in male probands and in these settings, the prostate cancers occurred at a younger age than in their sporadic counterparts. In the case of Ashkenazi Jews, a population-based study involving two *BRCA1* founder mutations (185delAG and 5382insC) showed an increased lifetime risk for prostate cancer.[219] Carriers of these mutations harbored risk estimates of 20% occurrence of prostate cancer by 70 years and 35% by 80 years, compared with 5% and 10%, respectively, for noncarriers. An increased proportion of *BRCA1* and *BRCA2* mutation carriers had a family history involving prostate cancer in first-degree relatives (14%) compared with noncarriers (8%) (*p* <.01).

Rosen and colleagues[210] suggest that genetic linkage studies support "the existence of a prostate tumor suppressor gene located on chromosome 17q at or near the BRCA1 locus (D17S855-D17S856).[220-222] Allelic loss at this location was observed in about 25-50% of localized prostate cancer cases in these studies. Furthermore, fragments of normal chromosomal region 17q that include the BRCA1 gene inhibited tumorigenicity of a human prostate cancer cell line.[223] A further analysis of sporadic localized prostate cancers suggests the existence of a second prostate tumor suppressor gene on chromosome 17q distal to BRCA1"[224] (quote is from Rosen and colleagues[210]).

Prostate cancer was the most common cancer type following carcinoma of the breast in seven Icelandic families who were characterized by HBOC.[225] Two of the families showed linkage to *BRCA1*, wherein 44% of the males harboring the putative breast cancer gene alleles had a history of prostate cancer.

Insurance Issues

The possibility of insurance discrimination against persons tested for cancer-predisposing genes is a concern raised in the genetics community[226,227] and also among persons considering testing.[228] In a sample of 88 individuals tested for *BRCA* mutations, 4 indicated problems in obtaining or maintaining insurance; however, in each of these cases, the difficulties predated receipt of test results. Of 38 individuals who tested positive, 4 indicated changes in their insurance since testing; however, these changes were unrelated to genetic testing. Although it may be too early to determine the actual rates of insurance discrimination among participants in genetic testing programs, our data indicate that the perception of insurance discrimination may have an effect on decisions to receive *BRCA* testing and on medical decision making. For example, 18% of mutation carriers indicated that insurance concerns affected their decisions about receiving prophylactic surgery. Thus it is critical that the potential for insurance discrimination be addressed during the pretest education session. In addition, as genetic testing programs become more widespread, it will be crucial to evaluate the extent to which participants are discriminated against in their employment or insurance and also to urge policy makers to pass legislation that would preclude these detrimental practices.

INSURANCE ADJUDICATION FAVORING PROPHYLACTIC OOPHORECTOMY IN HEREDITARY BREAST/OVARIAN CANCER

Many patients contemplating prophylactic surgery are concerned about whether their insurance will cover the costs for these procedures. We provide a case report that we hope will become a legal precedent in support of insurance coverage for indicated prophylactic surgery.[229]

The proband was from a classic HBOC family in which the *BRCA1* gene was subsequently identified. She met our criteria for prophylactic oophorectomy based on her estimated cancer risk status in an HBOC syndrome pedigree (Figure 18-15).[229] Payment for this procedure was initially denied by the insurer, and the decision was later upheld in a summary judgment issued by the District Court, which ruled in favor of the insurance company against the patient. On appeal, the Nebraska Supreme Court concluded that the patient did in fact suffer from a bodily disorder or disease.[230] The Nebraska Supreme Court's decision hinged on descriptions of the term *disease* that were used in several prior court decisions based, in part, on definitions of disease found in standard general and professional dictionaries. The Nebraska Supreme Court applied wording from court decisions concerning related cases, using these definitions to expand the criteria for identifying human conditions in which genetic aberrations result in the impairment of function or damage to tissue.[231-233]

Ethical, Legal, and Social Considerations and Genetic Testing

Burke and colleagues[234] discuss the ethical, legal, and social implications (ELSI) of genetic tests as part of the genetic counseling process, and the manner in which certain genetic testing decisions should be determined by personal values. These issues (genetic testing versus no testing) strike an important balance relevant to their potential benefits for ultimate treatment versus potential harms of "genetic labeling," which must be carefully weighed. Pertinent to HBC, there may exist uncertainty "concerning both clinical validity and effectiveness of treatment, as in the case of *BRCA1/2* mutation testing, the value of testing may vary according to different testing contexts. This approach to test categorization allows a rapid determination of the predominant ELSI concerns with different kinds of genetic tests and identifies the data most urgently needed for test evaluation." We must strive to include the patient as a responsible decision-making participant in this genetic testing decision process, which in fact is the art of medical judgment during the course of the genetic counseling process.

The Future of Research in Genetics in Hereditary Cancer

We have attempted to review what we consider the most salient clinical and research aspects of HBC. However, the reader will realize immediately that progress has been so rapid in this field that by the time this work is sent to the printer, new concepts and developments in all facets of HBC research will probably have taken place. Therefore the best use of material in this chapter is to provide background, much of which will become historical, thereby compelling the reader to search the current literature.

Society will have to find ways for DNA testing costs to be contained and, whenever possible, covered by third-party payers. Legislation may become necessary to prohibit employers or insurance companies from discrimination because an individual happens to have been found to harbor a deleterious cancer-prone gene. Clearly, the task will be an enormous one, but it must be initiated at this time because progress in the field of molecular genetics and cancer epidemiology is moving ahead at an almost logarithmic pace. The professional and lay literature is keeping abreast of these advances, and as a consequence, patient demand for genetic services, including DNA testing, has increased at almost exponential proportions.

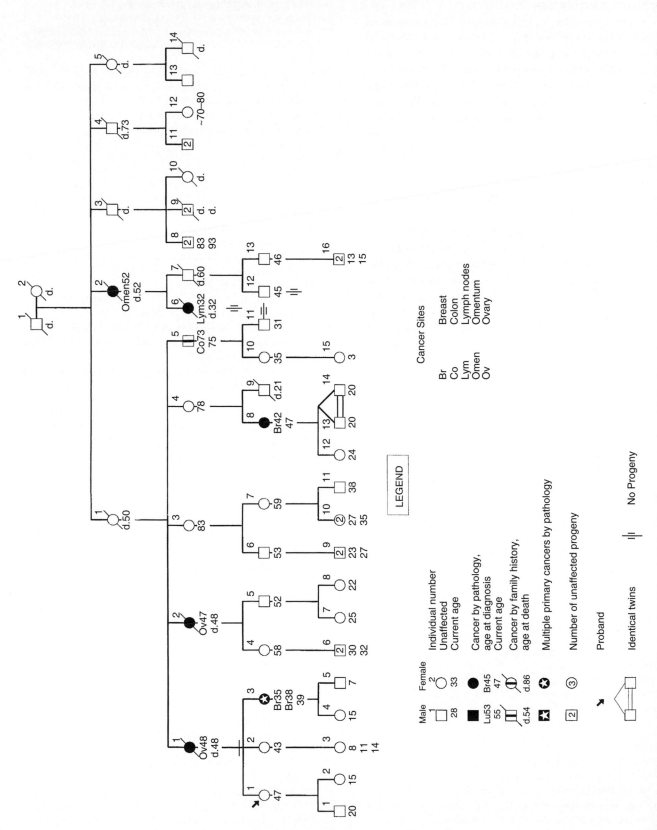

FIG. 18-15 Pedigree of a family showing linkage to *BRCA1* and clinical findings consistent with the hereditary breast and ovarian cancer syndrome. The proband initially was denied insurance coverage for prophylactic oophorectomy. *(From Lynch HT et al: Gynecol Oncol 57:23, 1995.)*

ACKNOWLEDGMENTS

We greatly appreciate funding support for the several research projects on hereditary breast cancer and OC that provided us material to include in this chapter. This includes revenue from Nebraska cigarette taxes awarded to Creighton University by the Nebraska Department of Health and Human Services. The chapter's contents are solely the responsibility of the authors and do not necessarily represent the official views of the State of Nebraska or the Nebraska Department of Health and Human Services.

Funding support was also provided through the following NIH/NCI Grants: 5 U01 CA86389; 1 U01 CZ 77165; and 1 RO1 CA 838555.

We gratefully acknowledge the painstaking effort provided by Trudy Shaw, M.A., throughout the updating of this chapter. We also extend our gratitude to the literally thousands of high-cancer-risk patients who have allowed us to study their families to learn about breast cancer genetics so that this knowledge could be used to write this chapter. These studies have allowed us to grasp some degree of understanding of this exceedingly complex subject.

REFERENCES

1. Jemal A et al: Cancer statistics, 2003, *CA Cancer J Clin* 53:5, 2003.
2. Eng C et al: Interpreting epidemiological research: blinded comparison of methods used to estimate the prevalence of inherited mutations in *BRCA1*, *J Med Genet* 38:824, 2001.
3. Berry DA et al: BRCAPRO validation, sensitivity of genetic testing of *BRCA1/BRCA2* and prevalence of other breast cancer susceptibility genes, *J Clin Oncol* 20:2701, 2002.
4. Meijers-Heijboer H et al: Low-penetrance susceptibility to breast cancer due to *CHEK2*1100delC in noncarriers of *BRCA1* and *BRCA2* mutations, *Nat Genet* 31:55, 2002.
5. Howlett NG et al: Biallelic inactivation of *BRCA2* in Fanconi anemia, *Science* 297:606, 2002.
6. Pharoah PD et al: Polygenic susceptibility to breast cancer and implications for prevention, *Nat Genet* 31:33, 2002.
7. Madigan MP et al: Proportion of breast cancer cases in the United States explained by well-established risk factors, *J Natl Cancer Inst* 87:1681, 1995.
8. Narod SA et al: Risk modifiers in carriers of BRCA1 mutations, *Int J Cancer (Pred Oncol)* 64:394, 1995.
9. Jernstrom H et al: Pregnancy and risk of early breast cancer in carriers of *BRCA1* and *BRCA2*, *Lancet* 354:1846, 1999.
10. Brunet J-S et al: Effect of smoking on breast cancer in carriers of mutant *BRCA1* or *BRCA2* genes, *J Natl Cancer Inst* 90:761, 1998.
11. Broca PP: *Traité des tumeurs*, vol 1, 2, Paris, 1866, Asselin.
12. Lynch HT et al: Tumor variation in families with breast cancer, *JAMA* 222:1631, 1972.
13. Lynch HT, Krush AJ: Carcinoma of the breast and ovary in three families, *Surg Gynecol Obstet* 133:644, 1971.
14. Hall JM et al: Linkage of early-onset breast cancer to chromosome 17q21, *Science* 250:1684, 1990.
15. Narod SA et al: Familial breast-ovarian cancer locus on chromosome 17q12-q23, *Lancet* 388:82, 1991.
16. Miki Y et al: A strong candidate for the breast and ovarian cancer susceptibility gene *BRCA1*, *Science* 266:66, 1994.
17. Wooster R et al: Localization of a breast cancer susceptibility gene, *BRCA2*, to chromosome 13q12-13, *Science* 265:2088, 1994.
18. Wooster R et al: Identification of the breast cancer susceptibility gene *BRCA2* [published erratum appears in *Nature* 379:749, 1996], *Nature* 378:789, 1995.
19. Lynch HT et al: Family history in an oncology clinic: implications for cancer genetics, *JAMA* 242:1268, 1979.
20. David KL, Steiner-Grossman P: The potential use of tumor registry data in the recognition and prevention of hereditary and familial cancer, *NY State J Med* 91:150, 1991.
21. Collaborative Group on Hormonal Factors in Breast Cancer: Familial breast cancer: collaborative reanalysis of individual data from 52 epidemiological studies including 58,209 women with breast cancer and 101,986 women without the disease, *Lancet* 358:1389, 2001.
22. O'Neill SM: Quantitative risk assessment. In Vogel VG (ed): *Management of women at high risk for breast cancer*, Malden, MA, 2000, Blackwell Science.
23. Lynch HT et al: Hereditary breast cancer and family cancer syndromes, *World J Surg* 18:21, 1994.
24. Lynch HT et al: DNA screening for breast/ovarian cancer susceptibility based on linked markers: a family study, *Arch Intern Med* 153:1979, 1993.
25. Kauff ND et al: Insurance reimbursement for risk-reducing mastectomy and oophorectomy in women with *BRCA1* or *BRCA2* mutations, *Genet Med* 3:422, 2001.
26. Lynch HT et al: A descriptive study of *BRCA1* testing and reactions to disclosure of test results, *Cancer* 79:2219, 1997.
27. Peters J: Familial cancer risk. Part I. Impact on today's oncology practice, *J Oncol Manage* 3:18, 1994.
28. Peters J: Familial cancer risk. Part II. Breast cancer risk counseling and genetic susceptibility testing, *J Oncol Manage* 3:14, 1994.
29. Peterson EA et al: Health insurance and discrimination concerns and *BRCA1/2* testing in a clinic population, *Cancer Epidemiol Biomarkers Prev* 11:79, 2002.
30. Hartmann LC et al: Efficacy of bilateral prophylactic mastectomy in *BRCA1* and *BRCA2* gene mutation carriers, *J Natl Cancer Inst* 93:1633, 2001.
31. Rebbeck TR et al: Breast cancer risk after bilateral prophylactic oophorectomy in *BRCA1* mutation carriers, *J Natl Cancer Inst* 91:1475, 1999.
32. Narod SA et al: Tamoxifen and risk of contralateral breast cancer in *BRCA1* and *BRCA2* mutation carriers: a case-control study, *Lancet* 356:1876, 2000.
33. Eisen A et al: Prophylactic surgery in women with a hereditary predisposition to breast and ovarian cancer, *J Clin Oncol* 18:1980, 2000.
34. Lynch HT, Lynch JF, Rubinstein WS: Prophylactic mastectomy: obstacles and benefits, *J Natl Cancer Inst* 93:1586, 2001.
35. Scheuer L et al: Outcome of preventive surgery and screening for breast and ovarian cancer in BRCA mutation carriers, *J Clin Oncol* 20:1260, 2002.
36. Rebbeck TR et al: Prophylactic oophorectomy in carriers of *BRCA1* or *BRCA2* mutations, *N Engl J Med* 346:1616, 2002.
37. Dyck HG et al: Autonomy of the epithelial phenotype in human ovarian surface epithelium: changes with neoplastic progression and with a family history of ovarian cancer, *Int J Cancer (Pred Oncol)* 69:429, 1996.

38. Hensley ML, Castiel M, Robson ME: Screening for ovarian cancer: what we know, what we need to know, *Oncology* 14:1601, 2001.

39. Petricoin EF et al: Use of proteomic patterns in serum to identify ovarian cancer, *Lancet* 359:572, 2002.

40. Easton DF et al: Breast and ovarian cancer incidence in *BRCA1* mutation carriers, *Am J Hum Genet* 56:265, 1995.

41. Ford D, Easton DF: The genetics of breast and ovarian cancer, *Br J Cancer* 72:805, 1995.

42. Easton DF et al: Genetic linkage analysis in familial breast and ovarian cancer: results from 214 families, *Am J Hum Genet* 52:678, 1993.

43. Frank TS et al: Clinical characteristics of individuals with germline mutations in *BRCA1* and *BRCA2*: analysis of 10,000 individuals, *J Clin Oncol* 20:1480, 2002.

44. Ford D et al: Risks of cancer in *BRCA1*-mutation carriers, *Lancet* 343:692, 1994.

45. Struewing JP et al: Detection of eight *BRCA1* mutations in 10 breast/ovarian cancer families, including one family with male breast cancer, *Am J Hum Genet* 57:1, 1995.

46. Roa BB et al: Ashkenazi Jewish population frequencies for common mutations in *BRCA1* and *BRCA2*, *Nat Genet* 14:185, 1996.

47. Offit K et al: Germline *BRCA1* 185delAG mutations in Jewish women with breast cancer, *Lancet* 347:1642, 1996.

48. Modan B et al: High frequency of *BRCA1* 185delAG mutation in ovarian cancer in Israel, *JAMA* 276:1823, 1996.

49. Helmrich SP et al: Risk factors for breast cancer, *Am J Epidemiol* 117:35, 1983.

50. Oddoux C et al: The carrier frequency of the *BRCA2* 6174delT mutation among Ashkenazi Jewish individuals is approximately 1%, *Nat Genet* 14:188, 1996.

51. Gayther SA et al: Variation of risks of breast and ovarian cancer associated with different germline mutations of the *BRCA2* gene, *Nat Genet* 15:103, 1997.

52. Risch HA et al: Prevalence and penetrance of germline *BRCA1* and *BRCA2* mutations in a population series of 649 women with ovarian cancer, *Am J Hum Genet* 68:700, 2001.

53. Serova O et al: A high incidence of *BRCA1* mutations in 20 breast/ovarian cancer families, *Am J Hum Genet* 58:42, 1996.

54. Shattuck-Eidens D et al: A collaborative survey of 80 mutations in the *BRCA1* breast and ovarian cancer susceptibility gene: implications for presymptomatic testing and screening, *JAMA* 273:535, 1995.

55. Bressac-de-Paillerets B et al: Comparative analysis of methods for detecting *BRCA1* rearrangements in breast/ovarian cancer families, *Am J Hum Genet* 69(suppl 4):248, 2001 (abstract #377).

56. Gayther SA et al: Germline mutations of the *BRCA1* gene in breast and ovarian cancer families provide evidence for a genotype-phenotype correlation, *Nat Genet* 11:428, 1995.

57. Parmigiani G, Berry DA, Aguilar O: Determining carrier probabilities for breast cancer-susceptibility genes *BRCA1* and *BRCA2*, *Am J Hum Genet* 62:145, 1998.

58. Parmigiani G et al: Modeling risk of breast cancer and decisions about genetic testing. In Gatsonis C et al (eds): *Case studies in Bayesian statistics IV*, New York, 1999, Springer.

59. de Jong MM et al: Genes other than *BRCA1* and *BRCA2* involved in breast cancer susceptibility, *J Med Genet* 39:225, 2002.

60. Lynch HT et al: Breast cancer family history as a risk factor for early-onset breast cancer, *Breast Cancer Res Treat* 11:263, 1988.

61. Claus EB, Risch N, Thompson WD: Age of onset as an indicator of familial risk of breast cancer, *Am J Epidemiol* 131:961, 1990.

62. Mettlin C et al: The association of age and familial risk in a case-control study of breast cancer, *Am J Epidemiol* 131:973, 1990.

63. Jóhannsson OT et al: Survival of *BRCA1* breast and ovarian cancer patients: a population-based study from southern Sweden, *J Clin Oncol* 16:397, 1998.

64. Eerola H et al: Survival of breast cancer patients in *BRCA1*, *BRCA2*, and non-*BRCA1/2* breast cancer families: a relative survival analysis from Finland, *Int J Cancer* 93:368, 2001.

65. Foulkes WD et al: Primary node negative breast cancer in *BRCA1* mutation carriers has a poor outcome, *Ann Oncol* 11:307, 2000.

66. Stoppa-Lyonnet D et al: Familial invasive breast cancers: worse outcome related to *BRCA1* mutations, *J Clin Oncol* 18:4053, 2000.

67. Ambrosone CB et al: Polymorphisms in glutathione S-transferases (*GSTM1* and *GSTT1*) and survival after treatment for breast cancer, *Cancer Res* 61:7130, 2001.

68. Marcus J et al: The pathobiology of *BRCA1*-linked and -unlinked hereditary breast cancer (HBC), *Modern Pathol* 7:18A, 1994 (abstract).

69. Claus EB et al: Relationship between breast histopathology and family history of breast cancer, *Am J Epidemiol* 131:961, 1990.

70. Marcus J et al: High mitotic grade in hereditary breast cancer, *Lab Invest* 56:61A, 1988 (abstract).

71. Mulcahy GM, Platt R: Pathologic aspects of familial carcinoma of the breast. In Lynch HT (ed): *Genetics and breast cancer*, New York, 1981, Van Nostrand Reinhold.

72. Rosen PP et al: Epidemiology of breast carcinoma III: relationship of family history to tumor type, *Cancer* 50:171, 1982.

73. Erdreich LS, Asal NR, Hoge AF: Morphologic types of breast cancer: age, bilaterality, and family history, *South Med J* 73:28, 1980.

74. LiVolsi VA et al: Effect of age at first childbirth on risk of developing specific histologic subtype of breast cancer, *Cancer* 49:1937, 1982.

75. Stalsberg H, Thomas DB, Noonan EA: The WHO collaborative study of neoplasia and steroid contraceptives. Histologic types of breast carcinoma in relation to international variation and breast cancer risk factors, *Cancer* 44:399, 1989.

76. Lagios MD, Rose MR, Margolin FR: Tubular carcinoma of the breast: association with multicentricity, bilaterality, and family history of mammary carcinoma, *Am J Clin Pathol* 73:25, 1980.

77. Mosimann S et al: Histopathological aspects of familial breast cancer. In Weber W, Laffer UT, Durig M (eds.): *Hereditary cancer and preventive surgery*, Basel, Switzerland, 1990, Karger.

78. Claus EB, et al: Relationship between breast histopathology and family history of breast cancer, *Cancer* 71:147, 1993.

79. Glebov OK et al: Frequent *p53* gene mutations and novel alleles in familial breast cancer, *Cancer Res* 54:3703, 1994.

80. Marcus JN et al: *BRCA1* and *BRCA2* hereditary breast carcinoma phenotypes, *Cancer* 80(suppl):543, 1997.

81. Marcus JN et al: The pathology and heredity of breast cancer in younger women, *J Natl Cancer Inst Monogr* 16:23, 1994.

82. Marcus JN, et al: Hereditary breast cancer: pathobiology, prognosis, and *BRCA1* and *BRCA2* gene linkage, *Cancer* 77:697, 1996.

83. Marcus JN et al: *BRCA2* hereditary breast cancer pathophenotype, *Breast Cancer Res Treat* 44:275, 1997.

84. Breast Cancer Linkage Consortium: Pathology of familial breast cancer: differences between breast cancers in carriers of *BRCA1* or *BRCA2* mutations and sporadic cases, *Lancet* 349:1505, 1997.

85. Eisinger F et al: Germ line mutation at *BRCA1* affects the histoprognostic grade in hereditary breast cancer, *Cancer Res* 56:471, 1996.

86. Lakhani SR et al: Multifactorial analysis of differences between sporadic breast cancers and cancers involving *BRCA1* and *BRCA2* mutations, *J Natl Cancer Inst* 90:1138, 1998.

87. Lynch BJ et al: Pathobiologic characteristics of hereditary breast cancer, *Hum Pathol* 29:1140, 1998.

88. Sobol H et al: Truncation at conserved terminal regions of *BRCA1* protein is associated with highly proliferating hereditary breast cancers, *Cancer Res* 56:3216, 1996.

89. Jóhannsson OT et al: Tumour biological features of *BRCA1*-induced breast and ovarian cancer, *Eur J Cancer* 33:362, 1997.

90. Rahman N, Stratton MR: The genetics of breast cancer susceptibility, *Annu Rev Genet* 32:95, 1998.

91. Armes JE et al: The histologic phenotypes of breast carcinoma occurring before age 40 years in women with and without *BRCA1* or *BRCA2* germline mutations: a population-based study, *Cancer* 83:2335, 1998.

92. Eisinger F et al: Mutations at *BRCA1*: the medullary breast carcinoma revisited, *Cancer Res* 58:1588, 1998.

93. Marcus J et al: High S phase fraction in hereditary breast carcinoma, *Cytometry* 14:34, 1993 (abstract).

94. Armes JE et al: Distinct molecular pathogeneses of early-onset breast cancers in *BRCA1* and *BRCA2* mutation carriers: a population-based study, *Cancer Res* 59:2011, 1999.

95. Lakhani SR et al: The pathology of familial breast cancer: predictive value of immunohistochemical markers estrogen receptor, progesterone receptor, HER-2, and p53 in patients with mutations in *BRCA1* and *BRCA2*, *J Clin Oncol* 20:2310, 2002.

96. Noguchi S et al: Clinicopathologic analysis of *BRCA1*- or *BRCA2*-associated hereditary breast carcinoma in Japanese women, *Cancer* 85:2200, 1999.

97. Thor AD et al: Accumulation of *p53* tumor suppressor gene protein: an independent marker of prognosis in breast cancers, *J Natl Cancer Inst* 84:845, 1992.

98. Meyer JS, He W: High proliferative rates demonstrated by bromodeoxyuridine labeling index in breast carcinomas with *p53* overexpression, *J Surg Oncol* 156:146, 1994.

99. Greenblatt M et al: *TP53* mutations in breast cancer associated with *BRCA1* and *BRCA2* germline mutations: distinctive spectrum and structural distribution, *Cancer Res* 61:4092, 2001.

100. Bewtra C et al: Hereditary ovarian cancer: a clinicopathological study, *Int J Gynecol Pathol* 11:180, 1992.

101. Hartwell LH, Kastan MB: Cell cycle control and cancer, *Science* 266:1821, 1994.

102. Shackney SE et al: Model for the genetic evolution of solid tumors, *Cancer Res* 49:3344, 1989.

103. Cornelisse CJ et al: Fractional allelic imbalance in human breast cancer increases with tetraploidization and chromosome loss, *Int J Cancer* 50:544, 1992.

104. Dutrillaux B et al: Breast cancer genetic evolution. I. Data from cytogenetics and DNA content, *Breast Cancer Res Treat* 19:245, 1991.

105. Remvikos Y et al: Proliferative activity of breast cancers increases in the course of genetic evolution as defined by cytogenetic analysis, *Breast Cancer Res Treat* 23:43, 1992.

106. Meyer JS: Cellular proliferation in normal human breast ducts, fibroadenomas, and other ductal hyperplasias measured by nuclear labeling with tritiated thymidine: effects of menstrual phase, age, and oral contraceptive hormones, *Hum Pathol* 8:67, 1977.

107. Russo J et al: Influence of age and gland topography on cell kinetics of normal human breast tissue, *J Natl Cancer Inst* 78:413, 1987.

108. Olsson H et al: Proliferation and DNA ploidy in malignant breast tumors in relation to early oral contraceptive use and early abortions, *Cancer* 67:1285, 1991.

109. Holt JT et al: Growth retardation and tumour inhibition by *BRCA1*, *Nat Genet* 12:298, 1996.

110. Jarvis EM, Kirk JA, Clarke CL: Loss of nuclear *BRCA1* expression in breast cancers is associated with a highly proliferative tumor phenotype, *Cancer Genet Cytogenet* 101:109, 1998.

111. Thompson ME et al: Decreased expression of *BRCA1* accelerates growth and is often present during sporadic breast cancer progression, *Nat Genet* 9:444, 1995.

112. Agnarsson BA et al: Inherited *BRCA2* mutation associated with high grade breast cancer, *Breast Cancer Res Treat* 47:121, 1998.

113. Karp SE et al: Influence of *BRCA1* mutations on nuclear grade and estrogen receptor status of breast carcinoma in Ashkenazi Jewish women, *Cancer* 80:435, 1997.

114. Loman N et al: Steroid receptors in hereditary breast carcinomas associated with *BRCA1* or *BRCA2* mutations or unknown susceptibility genes, *Cancer* 83:310, 1998.

115. Verhoog LC et al: Survival and tumour characteristics of breast-cancer patients with germline mutations of *BRCA1*, *Lancet* 351:316, 1998.

116. Watson P, Marcus JN, Lynch HT: Prognosis of *BRCA1* hereditary breast cancer, *Lancet* 351:304, 1998.

117. King M-C et al: Tamoxifen and breast cancer incidence among women with inherited mutations in *BRCA1* and *BRCA2*: National Surgical Adjuvant Breast and Bowel Project (NSABP-P1) breast cancer prevention trial, *JAMA* 286:2251, 2001.

118. Gaffney DK et al: Response to radiation therapy and prognosis in breast cancer patients with *BRCA1* and *BRCA2* mutations, *Radiotherapy Oncol* 47:129, 1998.

119. Hamann U, Sinn H-P: Survival and tumor characteristics of German hereditary breast cancer patients, *Breast Cancer Res Treat* 59:185, 2000.

120. Porter DE et al: Breast cancer incidence, penetrance and survival in probable carriers of *BRCA1* gene mutation in families linked to *BRCA1* on chromosome 17q12-21, *Br J Surg* 81:1512, 1994.

121. Foulkes WD et al: Germ-line *BRCA1* mutation is an adverse prognostic factor in Ashkenazi Jewish women with breast cancer, *Clin Cancer Res* 3:2465, 1997.

122. Phillips K-A, Andrulis IL, Goodwin PJ: Breast carcinomas arising in carriers of mutations in *BRCA1* or *BRCA2*: Are they prognostically different? *J Clin Oncol* 17:3653, 1999.

123. Ridolfi RL et al: Medullary carcinoma of the breast: a clinicopathologic study with 10-year follow-up, *Cancer* 40:1365, 1977.

124. Verhoog LC et al: Prognostic significance of germline *BRCA2* mutations in hereditary breast cancer patients, *J Clin Oncol* 18:119s, 2000.

125. Hedenfalk I et al: Gene expression profiles in hereditary breast cancer, *N Engl J Med* 344:539, 2001.

126. Abbott DW, Freeman ML, Holt JT: Double-strand break repair deficiency and radiation sensitivity in *BRCA2* mutant cancer cells, *J Natl Cancer Inst* 90:978, 1998.

127. Biggs PJ, Bradley A: A step toward genotype-based therapeutic regimens for breast cancer in patients with *BRCA2* mutations? *J Natl Cancer Inst* 90:951, 1998.

128. Broeks A et al: ATM-heterozygous germline mutations contribute to breast cancer susceptibility, *Hum Genet* 66:494, 2000.

129. Coleman CN: Molecular biology in radiation oncology. Radiation oncology perspective of *BRCA1* and *BRCA2*, *Acta Oncologica* 38(suppl):55, 1999.

130. Connor F et al: Tumorigenesis and a DNA repair defect in mice with a truncating *BRCA2* mutation, *Nat Genet* 17:423, 1997.

131. Friedenson B: Is mammography indicated for women with defective *BRCA* genes? Implications of recent scientific advances for the diagnosis, treatment, and prevention of hereditary breast cancer, Medscape Portals, Inc., Medscape General Medicine 2:2000, Available at: http://www.medscape.com/viewarticle/408048.

132. Harkin DP: Uncovering functionally relevant signaling pathways using microarray-based expression profiling, *Oncologist* 5:501, 2000.

133. Pierce LJ et al: Effect of radiotherapy after breast-conserving treatment in women with breast cancer and germline *BRCA1/2* mutations, *J Clin Oncol* 18:3360, 2000.

134. Scully R et al: Association of *BRCA1* with *Rad51* in mitotic and meiotic cells, *Cell* 88:265, 1997.

135. Sharan SK et al: Embryonic lethality and radiation hypersensitivity mediated by *Rad51* in mice lacking *BRCA2*, *Nature* 386:804, 1997.

136. Swift M et al: Incidence of cancer in 161 families affected by ataxia telangiectasia, *N Engl J Med* 325:1831, 1991.

137. Turner B et al: *BRCA1/BRCA2* germline mutations in locally recurrent breast cancer patients after lumpectomy and radiation therapy: implications for breast-conserving management in patients with *BRCA1/BRCA2* mutations, *J Clin Oncol* 17:3017, 1999.

138. Venkitaraman AR: Breast cancer genes and DNA repair, *Science* 286:1100, 1999.

139. Levy-Lahad E et al: A single nucleotide polymorphism in the *RAD51* gene modifies cancer risk in *BRCA2* but not *BRCA1* carriers, *Proc Natl Acad Sci USA* 98:3232, 2001.

140. Lynch HT et al: Genetic and pathologic findings in a kindred with hereditary sarcoma, breast cancer, brain tumors, leukemia, lung, laryngeal, and adrenal cortical carcinoma, *Cancer* 41:2055, 1978.

141. Li FP, Fraumeni JF: Soft-tissue sarcomas, breast cancer, and other neoplasms: a familial syndrome? *Ann Intern Med* 71:747, 1969.

142. Li FP, Fraumeni JF: Familial breast cancer, soft-tissue sarcomas, and other neoplasms, *Ann Intern Med* 83:833, 1975.

143. Li FP, Fraumeni JF: Prospective study of a family cancer syndrome, *JAMA* 247:2692, 1982.

144. Malkin D et al: Germ line *p53* mutations in a familial syndrome of breast cancer, sarcomas and other neoplasms, *Science* 250:1233, 1990.

145. Lynch HT et al: Predominance of brain tumors in an extended Li-Fraumeni (SBLA) kindred, including a case of Sturge-Weber syndrome, *Cancer* 88:433, 2000.

146. Brownstein MH, Wolf M, Bikowski JB: Cowden's disease: a cutaneous marker of breast cancer, *Cancer* 41:2393, 1978.

147. Liaw D et al: Germline mutations of the *PTEN* gene in Cowden disease, an inherited breast and thyroid cancer syndrome, *Nat Genet* 16:64, 1997.

148. Nelen MR et al: Germline mutations in the *PTEN/MMAC1* gene in patients with Cowden disease, *Hum Mol Genet* 6:1383, 1997.

149. Eng C: Cowden syndrome, *J Genet Counsel* 6:181, 1997.

150. Marsh DJ et al: Germline *PTEN* mutations in Cowden syndrome-like families, *J Med Genet* 35:881, 1998.

151. Williard W et al: Cowden's disease: a case report with analyses at the molecular level, *Cancer* 69:2969, 1992.

152. Walton BJ et al: A further indication for prophylactic mastectomy, *Surgery* 99:82, 1986.

153. Schrager CA et al: Clinical and pathological features of breast disease in Cowden's syndrome: an underrecognized syndrome with an increased risk of breast cancer, *Hum Pathol* 29:47, 1998.

154. Lynch ED et al: Inherited mutations in *PTEN* that are associated with breast cancer, Cowden disease, and juvenile polyposis, *Am J Hum Genet* 61:1254, 1997.

155. Gatti RA et al: Localization of an ataxia telangiectasia gene to chromosome 11q22-23, *Nature* 366:577, 1988.

156. Savitsky K et al: A single ataxia telangiectasia gene with a product similar to PI-3 kinase, *Science* 268:1749, 1995.

157. Swift M: Genetic aspects of ataxia telangiectasia, *Immunodefic Rev* 2:67, 1990.

158. Morrell D, Cromartic E, Swift M: Mortality and cancer incidence in 263 patients with ataxia telangiectasia, *J Natl Cancer Inst* 77:89, 1986.

159. Morrell D, Chase CL, Swift M: Cancers in 44 families with ataxia telangiectasia, *Cancer Genet Cytogenet* 50:119, 1990.

160. Swift M, Chase CL, Morrell D: Cancer predisposition of ataxia telangiectasia heterozygotes, *Cancer Genet Cytogenet* 46:21, 1990.

161. Buyse M, Hartman CT, Wilson MG: Gonadoblastoma and dysgerminoma with ataxia telangiectasia, *Birth Defects* 12:165, 1976.

162. Narita T, Takagi K: Ataxia telangiectasia with dysgerminomas of the right ovary, papillary carcinoma of the thyroid and adenocarcinoma of the pancreas, *Cancer* 54:1113, 1984.

163. Swift M et al: The incidence and gene frequency of ataxia telangiectasia in the United States, *Am J Hum Genet* 39:573, 1986.

164. Lavin MF et al: Defect in radiation signal transduction in ataxia telangiectasia, *Int J Radiat Biol* 66(suppl 6): S151, 1994.

165. Kash KM et al: Psychological distress and surveillance behaviors of women with a family history of breast cancer, *J Natl Cancer Inst* 84:24, 1992.

166. Lerman C et al: Mammography adherence and psychological distress among women at risk for breast cancer, *J Natl Cancer Inst* 85:1074, 1993.

167. Lerman C, Schwartz M: Adherence and psychological adjustment among women at high risk for breast cancer, *Breast Cancer Res Treat* 28:145, 1993.

168. Valdimarsdottir HB et al: Psychological distress in women with a familial risk of breast cancer, *Psycho-Oncology* 4:133, 1995.

169. Lerman C, Kash K, Stefanek M: Younger women at increased risk for breast cancer: perceived risk, psychological well-being, and surveillance behavior, *J Natl Cancer Inst Monogr* 16:171, 1994.

170. Schwartz M et al: Utilization of ovarian cancer screening by women at increased risk, *Cancer Epidemiol Biomarkers Prev* 4:269, 1995.

171. Lerman C et al: Recruiting high risk women into a breast cancer health promotion trial, *Cancer Epidemiol Biomarkers Prev* 3:271, 1994.

172. Lerman C et al: Effects of individualized breast cancer risk counseling: a randomized trial, *J Natl Cancer Inst* 87:286, 1995.

173. Chaliki H et al: Women's receptivity to testing for a genetic susceptibility to breast cancer, *Am J Public Health* 85:1133, 1995.

174. Bloch M et al: Predictive testing for Huntington disease II. Demographic characteristics, life-style patterns, attitudes, and psychosocial assessments of the first 51 test candidates, *Am J Med Genet* 32:217, 1989.

175. Craufurd D et al: Uptake of presymptomatic predictive testing for Huntington's disease, *Lancet* 2:603, 1989.

176. Lynch HT: Hereditary factors in carcinoma. In Lynch HT (ed): *Recent results in cancer research*, vol 12, New York, 1967, Springer-Verlag.

177. Lynch HT: *Dynamic genetics counseling for clinicians,* Springfield, IL, 1969, CC Thomas.

178. Lynch HT et al: Early age of onset in familial breast cancer: genetic and cancer control implications, *Arch Surg* 111:126, 1976.

179. Lynch HT, Krush AJ: Genetic predictability in breast cancer risk: surgical implications, *Arch Surg* 103:84, 1971.

180. Lynch HT et al: Hereditary cancer: ascertainment and management, *CA Cancer J Clin* 29:216, 1979.

181. Harris RE, Lynch HT, Guirgis HA: Familial breast cancer: risk to the contralateral breast, *J Natl Cancer Inst* 60:955, 1978.

182. Hartmann LC et al: Efficacy of bilateral prophylactic mastectomy in women with a family history of breast cancer, *N Engl J Med* 340:77, 1999.

183. Meijers-Heijboer H et al: Breast cancer after prophylactic bilateral mastectomy in women with a *BRCA1* or *BRCA2* mutation, *N Engl J Med* 345:159, 2001.

184. Verhoog LC et al: Survival in hereditary breast cancer associated with germline mutations of *BRCA2, J Clin Oncol* 17:3396, 1999.

185. Kauff ND et al: Risk-reducing salpingo-oophorectomy in women with a *BRCA1* or *BRCA2* mutation, *N Engl J Med* 346:1609, 2002.

186. Grann VR et al: Effect of prevention strategies on survival and quality-adjusted survival of women with *BRCA1/2* mutations: an updated decision analysis, *J Clin Oncol* 20:2520, 2002.

187. Meiser B et al: Attitudes toward prophylactic oophorectomy and screening utilization in women at increased risk of developing hereditary breast/ovarian cancer, *Gynecol Oncol* 75:122, 1999.

188. Lerman C et al: Prophylactic surgery decisions and surveillance practices one year following *BRCA1/2* testing, *Prev Med* 31:75, 2000.

189. Hallowell N et al: Surveillance or surgery? A description of the factors that influence high-risk premenopausal women's decisions about prophylactic oophorectomy, *J Med Genet* 38:683, 2001.

190. Droegemueller W: Screening for ovarian cancer: hopeful and wishful thinking, *Am J Obstet Gynecol* 170:1095, 1994.

191. National Institutes of Health Consensus Development Conference Statement: Ovarian cancer: screening, treatment, and follow-up, *Gynecol Oncol* 55:S4, 1994.

192. Eisen A, Weber BL: Prophylactic mastectomy for women with *BRCA1* and *BRCA2* mutations–facts and controversy, *N Engl J Med* 345:207, 2001.

193. Narod SA et al: Tubal ligation and risk of ovarian cancer in carriers of *BRCA1* or *BRCA2* mutations: a case-control study, *Lancet* 357:1467, 2001.

194. Narod SA et al: Oral contraceptives and the risk of hereditary ovarian cancer, *N Engl J Med* 339:424, 1998.

195. Marchbanks PA et al: Oral contraceptives and the risk of breast cancer, *N Engl J Med* 346:2025, 2002.

196. Rebbeck TR et al: Modification of *BRCA1*- and *BRCA2*-associated breast cancer risk by *AIB1* genotype and reproductive history, *Cancer Res* 61:5420, 2001.

197. Rebbeck TR et al: Modification of *BRCA1*-associated breast cancer penetrance by androgen receptor CAG repeat length variants, *Am J Hum Genet* 64:1371, 1999.

198. Dupont WD, Page DL: Risk factors for breast cancer in women with proliferative breast disease, *N Engl J Med* 312:146, 1985.

199. O'Shaughnessy JA et al: Ductal lavage and the clinical management of women at high risk for breast carcinoma: a commentary, *Cancer* 94:292, 2002.

200. Wrensch MR et al: Breast cancer incidence in women with abnormal cytology in nipple aspirates of breast fluid, *Am J Epidemiol* 135:130, 1992.

201. Fabian CJ et al: Short-term breast cancer prediction by random periareolar fine-needle aspiration cytology and the Gail risk model, *J Natl Cancer Inst* 92:1217, 2000.

202. Dooley WC et al: Ductal lavage for detection of cellular atypia in women at high risk for breast cancer, *J Natl Cancer Inst* 93:1624, 2001.

203. Deapen D et al: Rapidly rising breast cancer incidence rates among Asian-American women, *Int J Cancer* 99:747, 2002.

204. Perou CM et al: Molecular portraits of human breast tumours, *Nature* 406:747, 2000.

205. Sorlie T et al: Gene expression patterns of breast carcinomas distinguish tumor subclasses with clinical implications, *Proc Natl Acad Sci USA* 98:10869, 2001.

206. van't Veer LJ et al: Gene expression profiling predicts clinical outcome of breast cancer, *Nature* 415:530, 2002.

207. Gruvberger S et al: Estrogen receptor status in breast cancer is associated with remarkably distinct gene expression patterns, *Cancer Res* 61:5979, 2001.

208. Martin KJ et al: High sensitivity array analysis of gene expression for the early detection of disseminated breast tumor cells in peripheral blood, *Proc Natl Acad Sci USA* 98:2646, 2001.

209. Kudoh K et al: Monitoring the expression profiles of doxorubicin-induced and doxorubicin-resistant cancer cells by cDNA microarray, *Cancer Res* 60:4161, 2000.

210. Rosen EM, Fan S, Goldberg ID: *BRCA1* and prostate cancer, *Cancer Invest* 19:396, 2001.

211. Carter BS et al: Mendelian inheritance of familial prostate cancer, *Proc Natl Acad Sci USA* 89:3367, 1992.

212. Thiessen EU: Concerning a familial association between breast cancer and both prostatic and uterine malignancies, *Cancer* 34:1102, 1974.

213. Whittemore AS et al: Family history and prostate cancer risk in black, white, and Asian men in the United States and Canada, *Am J Epidemiol* 141:732, 1995.

214. Bishop DT, Kiemeney LA: Family studies and the evidence for genetic susceptibility to prostate cancer, *Semin Cancer Biol* 8:45, 1997.

215. Anderson DE, Badzioch MD: Familial breast cancer risks: effects of prostate and other cancers, *Cancer* 72:114, 2001.

216. Jishi MF et al: Risks of cancer among members of families in the Gilda Radner Familial Ovarian Cancer Registry, *Cancer* 76:1416, 1995.

217. Sellers TA et al: Familial clustering of breast and prostate cancers and risk of postmenopausal breast cancer, *J Natl Cancer Inst* 86:1860, 1994.

218. Tulinius H et al: Risk of prostate, ovarian, and endometrial cancer among relatives of women with breast cancer, *Br Med J* 305:855, 1992.

219. Struewing JP et al: The risk of cancer associated with specific mutations of BRCA1 and BRCA2 among Ashkenazi Jews [see comments], *N Engl J Med* 336:1401, 1997.

220. Brothman AR et al: Loss of chromosome 17 loci in prostate cancer detected by polymerase chain reaction quantitation of allelic markers, *Genes Chromosomes Cancer* 13:278, 1995.

221. Gao X et al: Localization of potential tumor suppressor loci to a <2 Mb region on chromosome 17q in human prostate cancer, *Oncogene* 11:1241, 1995.

222. Gao X et al: Loss of heterozygosity of the BRCA1 and other loci on chromosome 17q in human prostate cancer, *Cancer Res* 55:1002, 1995.

223. Murakami YS et al: Suppression of malignant phenotype in a human prostate cancer cell line by fragments of normal chromosome region 17q, *Cancer Res* 55:3389, 1995.

224. Williams BJ et al: Evidence for a tumor suppressor gene distal to BRCA1 in prostate cancer, *J Urol* 155:720, 1996.

225. Arason A, Barkardóttir RB, Egilsson V: Linkage analysis of chromosome 17q markers and breast/ovarian cancer in Icelandic families, and possible relationship to prostatic cancer. *Am J Hum Genet* 52:711, 1993.

226. Nuffield Council on Bioethics: *Genetic screening: ethical issues*, London, 1993, Nuffield Foundation.

227. Ostrer H et al: Insurance and genetic testing? Where are we now? *Am J Hum Genet* 52:565, 1993.

228. Lerman C et al: A randomized trial of breast cancer risk counseling: interacting effects of counseling, educational level, and coping style, *Health Psychol* 15:75, 1996.

229. Lynch HT et al: Insurance adjudication favoring prophylactic surgery in hereditary breast/ovarian cancer syndrome, *Gynecol Oncol* 57:23, 1995.

230. *Katskee v. Blue Cross/Blue Shield of Nebraska*, k. 1994; Nebraska Supreme Court No. S-92–1002.

231. *Beggs v. Pacific Mutual Life Insurance Company*, 171 Ga. App. 204, 218 S.E.2d 836, b. 1984.

232. *Cheney v. Bell National Life*, 315 Md. 761, 556 A.2d 1135 (1989), c. 1989.

233. *Silverstein v. Metropolitan Life Insurance Company*, 171 N.E. 914, s. 1930.

234. Burke W, Pinsky LE, Press NA: Categorizing genetic tests to identify their ethical, legal, and social implications, *Am J Med Genet (Semin Med Genet)* 106:233, 2001.

19

Patterns of Recurrence in Breast Cancer

MAHMOUD EL-TAMER

Chapter Outline

- Predictors of Recurrence
- Patterns of Local and Regional
  Recurrences

Regional Recurrences
Systemic Recurrences
Time of Recurrence

Breast cancer recurrence is the reappearance or return of the disease and is related to multiple factors. First and foremost, recurrences are intimately related to the type or characteristics of the tumor. These factors include the size of the tumor, the number of the axillary nodes involved, the stage of the tumor at presentation, and certain histologic and biologic parameters. The second predictor of recurrence is the type of treatment rendered to the patient: surgery, radiation, chemotherapy, or a combination thereof. The type and extent of surgical treatment has an impact on locoregional recurrence (positive margins, the omission of axillary node dissection, and the number of nodes dissected). The addition of radiation therapy has clearly shown better local control of the disease, and currently there is some debate about improvement in survival with radiation after mastectomy.[1,2] Adjuvant chemotherapy has proved its efficacy in improving survival by decreasing systemic and local recurrences, perhaps without affecting the pattern of recurrences. The previously reported trends of recurrences may not reflect the current or future patterns. This potential difference is related to variation in tumor presentation: type (in situ versus invasive), size, and stage, as well as the change in surgical treatment (breast preservation) and the widespread use of hormonal and adjuvant chemotherapy.

Recurrences can be local, regional, or systemic. Local recurrence (LR) depends on the type of surgical procedure performed. After a mastectomy, local recurrence is the return of the disease in the soft tissue of the chest wall at the site of the resected breast. After a breast-preserving procedure, a *recurrence* is defined as the reappearance of the disease in the same breast where the original cancer was located. A *regional recurrence* is defined as the recurrence of the disease in the ipsilateral axillary nodal basin. In the past a supraclavicular nodal recurrence was considered a regional recurrence. A change in the American Joint Commission on Cancer (AJCC) Staging System[3] upstaged supraclavicular nodal recurrence to systemic disease. Regional recurrence depends on the number of axillary lymph nodes dissected. With the new modality of sentinel lymph node biopsy, the incidence of regional recurrence may change. *Systemic recurrence* refers to evidence of metastatic breast cancer cells at any site other than local or regional but usually involves the bone, the liver, and the lungs.

Predictors of Recurrence

The stage at diagnosis, size of the primary tumor, and lymph node status are the most influential predictors of breast cancer recurrence.[4] As tumor size increases, the number of involved axillary lymph nodes increases accordingly. However, each factor is found independently to be a considerable predictor of locoregional recurrence (LRR) after correcting for the other. Patients with a tumor 5 cm or larger who have 20% or more involved lymph nodes face a greater risk of LRR. In addition, the percentage of involved axillary lymph nodes seems to be a more accurate predictor of the risk of LRR than the absolute number of involved nodes. This observation is a reflection of the direct relationship of the prognostic accuracy and the total number of nodes dissected.[4]

When the tumor is small and the axillary lymph nodes are negative, various other histologic and biologic factors have been shown to predict the risk of breast cancer recurrence. Among others, tumor grade, the presence of lymphovascular invasion, the absence of estrogen and progesterone receptors, and the overexpression of c-$erbB_2$/HER2/neu oncogene and mutant $p53$[5-7] have been shown to be indicators of poor clinical outcome. The detection of disseminated epithelial cells in the bone marrow at the time of primary diagnosis has been associated with poor clinical outcome in patients with breast cancer, but the literature is divided regarding whether the presence of these cells in the bone marrow can be a useful predictive marker for early distant recurrence of breast cancer.[8-10]

Patterns of Local and Regional Recurrences

Surgeons and radiotherapists have been particularly concerned with LRR following the primary treatment of breast cancer. Over the past 20 years, breast conservation therapy (BCT) has emerged as an established alternative to mastectomy as a surgical treatment for breast cancer. Several prospective, randomized controlled trials have reported similar rates of distant disease-free and overall survival, as well as local control following both treatments (Table 19-1). Although the incidence of LRR has not changed with the shift in primary surgical therapy, the pattern of local recurrence did.

After mastectomy the most common local recurrences present as a cutaneous or subcutaneous mass palpated on physical examination. If left undiagnosed, the mass tends to grow and involve the overlying skin and/or the underlying pectoralis muscle and chest wall. The recurrence may become symptomatic as it ulcerates, bleeds, and produces foul-smelling odors as a result of superimposed infection and tissue necrosis. Occasionally, recurrences may present as a widespread skin and dermal infiltration with or without inflammation. Such extensive skin recurrences are known as *carcinoma en cuirasse.*

Most series in the literature report local and regional recurrences together; hence it is sometimes difficult to

| TABLE 19-1 | Incidence of Locoregional Recurrence after Mastectomy and Breast Conservation Therapy in Prospective Randomized Trials |

TRIAL	STAGE	n	FOLLOW-UP (YR)	LRR (%) BCT	LRR (%) MASTECTOMY
Milan[11]	I	701	20	8.8	2.3
IGR[12]	I	179	10	7	10
NSABP-B-06[13]	I-II	1219	20	12.8	14.7
NCI[14]	I-II	237	10	18	10
EORTC 10801[15]	I-II	874	8	13	9
DBCG[16]	I-III	904	6	3	4

BCT, Breast conservation therapy; *DBCG*, Danish Breast Cancer Group; *EORTC*, European Organization for Research and Treatment of Cancer; *IGR*, Institut Gustave Roussy; *LRR*, locoregional recurrence; *NCI*, National Cancer Institute; *NSABP*, National Surgical Adjuvant Breast and Bowel Project.

separate these two sites. Furthermore, some studies do not distinguish between isolated local and regional failure and LRR presenting with metastasis. The reported incidence of LRR after radical or modified radical mastectomy ranges from 3% to 48%.[17,18] The incidence of LRR without distant metastasis is clearly lower.

In an extensive review of the literature, Clemons and colleagues[19] approximated the incidence of LRR 10 years after mastectomy to 13% (interquartile range [IQR], 9% to 26%). Approximately 35% (IQR, 21% to 52%) of women who have an LRR after mastectomy present with prior or synchronous systemic disease. After mastectomy, more than 70% of LRRs involve the mastectomy scar or the skin flaps. From 80% to 90% of isolated LRRs occur in the first 5 years after surgery, with almost all of the remaining LRRs occurring 5 to 10 years after mastectomy.[20-22] Local recurrences 10 years after mastectomy have been infrequently reported.[23]

The predictors of LRR after mastectomy are directly related to the T stage of the primary tumor. They include size larger than 4 to 5 cm, skin or chest wall involvement, and the presence of inflammatory changes. Other established predictors of LRR include the number of lymph nodes involved and evidence and extent of extranodal involvement. Histologic type, tumor features (grade, estrogen receptor, HER2/*neu* oncogene, and *p53* status), and certain patient characteristics have been associated with an increased risk of LRR.

Radiation therapy is a well-established measure to decrease the incidence of LRR after mastectomy in patients with T_3 and T_4 tumors, as well as in patients with a large number of positive nodes. It is also thought to act synergistically with chemotherapy and perhaps improve survival.[1,2]

A recent review from MD Anderson[24] included 1031 patients who were part of five prospective studies. The primary treatment of these patients included mastectomy and postoperative doxorubicin-based chemotherapy without radiation. This review included only patients with stage II and IIIA breast cancer and had a median follow-up of 116 months. Over 10 years, 124 patients developed LRRs without distant metastasis (isolated LRRs) and 55 patients presented with LRRs with metastasis (total LRRs) for a total of 179 patients. The actuarial incidence of isolated and total LRRs was 14% and 19%, respectively. Of the patients with isolated LRRs, 98% had chest wall involvement. The regional involvement was divided into supraclavicular, infraclavicular, axillary, and internal mammary; these sites were part of the isolated LRR in 33%, 17%, 8%, and 0% of patients, respectively. Among all patients with LRRs who presented with or without distant metastasis, the chest wall was part of the failure in 68% of the patients, followed by the supraclavicular area (40%), axillary (14%), infraclavicular (7%), and internal mammary nodal failure (8%). The median interval to chest wall recurrence was 27 months, whereas for supraclavicular, axillary, and infraclavicular nodes the median interval was 35, 40, and 63 months, respectively. The predictors of LRR in a Cox multivariate analysis were T stage, number of involved nodes, and extranodal extension 2 mm or larger.

After BCT, local recurrence most commonly presents as a lesion in the breast that is detected with routine mammography or as a palpable clinical finding. True recurrences are located in the same quadrant of the breast as the original primary tumor. However, any ipsilateral breast recurrence arising in a different quadrant from the original primary tumor is usually considered a new breast cancer. In reviewing the experience of the Joint Center for Radiation Therapy, Recht and co-workers[25] classified recurrences following BCT as true recurrences (TRs), marginal miss (MM), or new primaries. TRs occur in the original tumor bed, whereas MM is a recurrence in the same quadrant of the original primary tumor. New primaries are recurrences that occur several centimeters from the boosted volume. Occasionally, recurrences after BCT may present as a widespread skin involvement or carcinoma en cuirasse. TRs, MM, new primaries, and skin recurrences occurred in 50%, 22.4%, 18%, and 10% of patients, respectively. Gage and associates[26] updated the same series 10 years later. They found the annual incidence rate of LRs following BCT to be relatively constant during the first 10 years. TR/MM was the most common type of ipsilateral breast cancer recurrence and was highest during years 2 through 7. The risk of a recurrence elsewhere in the breast increased with longer follow-up and was highest during years 8 through 10. The study notes that any decrease in ipsilateral breast tumor recurrence (IBTR) is not due to patterns of LR but rather to improvements in mammographic and pathologic evaluation, patient selection, and increased use of the reexcision technique.

The incidence of IBTR in the literature has been variable and clearly depends on many factors, including the size of the primary tumor, adequacy of resection, status of margins, addition of radiation therapy, boost dose, and tumor, as well as patient characteristics. In the 15-year update of the findings of the National Surgical Adjuvant Breast and Bowel Project (NSABP) Protocol B-06,[6] Fisher and colleagues assessed 31 pathologic and 6 clinical features that were observed in 1039 patients with breast cancer to determine their value in predicting IBTR and survival rates. In addition to nodal status and nuclear grade, factors that were correlated with a greater risk of breast cancer recurrence that have not yet been mentioned were race (African American descent), histologic tumor type, and detection of tumoral blood vessel extension.

In an extensive review of the literature, Clemons and associates[19] approximated the incidence of LRR 10 years after BCT and radiation therapy as being 12% (IQR, 7% to 15%). The incidence of IBTR is approximately 1.5% to 2% per year for the first 7 to 8 years. At 10 to 15 years of follow-up, IBTR stabilizes at an incidence of 10% to 20%.[27,28] Approximately 10% (IQR, 6.5% to 22%) of patients with IBTR after BCT and radiation therapy present with prior or synchronous systemic disease.[19]

The impact of radiation therapy on local recurrence patterns after BCT was studied carefully in the NSABP-B-06 trial. At 12 years of follow-up, the incidence of IBTR was 10% with radiation, compared with 35% without radiation. Other studies reported a similar reduction in IBTR with radiotherapy.[29-33]

Many studies have reported worse survival rates in patients with LR after a mastectomy than after BCT; however, some raised the possibility of bias because women who are generally treated with mastectomies tend to have larger and more aggressive tumors. To avoid the bias of differences in prognostic profiles, Janni and colleagues[34] completed a matched-pair analysis of 134 patients and reported a worse prognosis for LR after mastectomy compared with LR after BCT. They also

concluded that early-onset recurrence in the chest wall was the highest independent risk for cancer-associated death.[34]

REGIONAL RECURRENCES

Regional recurrences are considered recurrences in the regional nodal basins and are divided into axillary, supraclavicular, infraclavicular, and internal mammary nodal basins. The delineation between level III axillary nodes, Rotter's nodes, and infraclavicular nodes is not clear, and perhaps all are lumped together under the broad subheading of infraclavicular nodes. Most studies continue to include supraclavicular node metastasis as regional recurrence. In the absence of other systemic disease, many clinicians treat patients with supraclavicular node metastases as if they have stage IIIB disease.[35] Although this treatment decision does not conform to AJCC staging, patients with supraclavicular node metastasis seem to have an outcome similar to that of patients with stage IIIB disease.[36]

Regional recurrences most commonly arise from tumor tissue left behind in the axilla. Occasionally, regional recurrences may be related to metastasis from a local recurrence. Axillary lymph node dissection (ALND) has traditionally been performed as part of the treatment of invasive breast cancer. Large patient series are required to compile data about the risk factors of axillary recurrence because it is an uncommon event following ALND, with an incidence of 0.25% to 3%.[37-39] The incidence of axillary recurrence is directly related to the extent of initial axillary dissection or the number of lymph nodes removed. With complete node dissection, Haagensen[39] noticed two axillary recurrences in 794 patients. The Danish Breast Cancer Group reviewed 3128 patients and found a direct relationship between the number of negative lymph nodes sampled and the incidence of axillary recurrence. Over 5 years the risk of axillary recurrence varied from 19% when no node dissection was performed, 10% when fewer than three nodes were removed, 5% following removal of fewer than five nodes, to 3% when more than five negative axillary nodes were dissected.[40] Later, the same group recommended the removal of a minimum of 10 axillary nodes to achieve optimal regional control of the disease.[41]

Similar findings were noticed in the NSABP-B-04 trial, where patients had been randomized into three arms: radical mastectomy, total mastectomy (TM) with axillary radiation, and TM alone. Axillary recurrence in the TM arm was directly related to the number of axillary nodes removed. The incidence of axillary recurrence was 21% when no axillary nodes were dissected, 12% when 6 or fewer nodes were dissected, and 0.3% when more than 10 nodes were excised.[42] In this prospective randomized study, 40% of patients in the radical mastectomy arm had histologically positive axillary nodes. It is assumed that a similar number in the TM arm would have histologically positive nodes left behind. Only 17.8% of the 365 patients in the TM arm who had no axillary treatment underwent a delayed axillary node dissection for isolated axillary recurrences. The median time for axillary recurrence from mastectomy was 14.7 months (range, 3 to 112.6). Most recurrences (78.5%) occurred within 24 months of mastectomy.[43]

The supraclavicular fossa is clearly not addressed surgically during mastectomy or BCT. In the NSABP-B-04 trial, the 10-year incidence of supraclavicular recurrence following radical mastectomy with clinically negative axilla was 1.1% and 5.8% for patients with clinically positive axilla. In the TM and radiation arms, the supraclavicular recurrence incidence was 0.3% in patients with clinically negative axilla and 0% for patients with clinically positive axilla. This drop in recurrence rate is attributed to the addition of a supraclavicular field in the radiation group. In the literature review done by Clemons and co-workers,[19] the authors estimate the incidence of supraclavicular nodal recurrence after 5 years to be 14% (IQR, 9% to 28%) following mastectomy and 7% (3% to 10%) following BCT. The incidence of infraclavicular and isolated internal mammary node recurrence is reported to be extremely low.

With the shift in axillary management and the widespread application of sentinel node biopsy, the number of axillary recurrences may increase over the next 10 years. Sentinel node biopsy has a false-negative rate of about 5% in the best of hands. In the NSABP-B-04 trial, only 50% of patients with untreated axilla and presumed residual axillary disease had presented with isolated axillary recurrences over 10 years. If we extrapolate from this finding, an axillary recurrence of about 2.5% after sentinel node biopsy can be anticipated. However, irradiation to the breast is an integral part of BCT, and the field of radiation may include part of the axilla, hence further reducing the incidence of axillary recurrences to perhaps less than 1%. In a recent review, Guiliano and colleagues[44] reported a 0% recurrence after 4 years of follow-up.

SYSTEMIC RECURRENCES

Systemic recurrences in patients with breast cancer can occur in any organ of the body but primarily present in the bone, the liver, and the lungs. *Metastasis* is the invasion of cancer into healthy tissue. Scientists have known for more than 100 years that metastasis is not a random phenomenon. Cancer cells preferentially grow in organs that promote and provide an adequate environment: the "soil and seed theory." More recently, the "homing theory" postulates that different organs have the ability to attract or arrest cancer cells through specific chemotactic factors.[45] Currently, studies have focused on the role of chemokines in cancer metastasis. Chemokines are a large family of proteins crucial to the function and circulation of leukocytes. Muller and associates[46] found increased levels of two chemokine receptor genes in human breast cancer cells. In addition, extracts of organs consistently targeted by breast cancer metastasis (lungs, liver, bone marrow, and lymph nodes) were found to have chemotactic ability for breast cancer cells that could be neutralized by antibodies against one of the chemokines. Mundy and Gallwitz[47] related the proliferation of breast cancer cells in bone to the production of transforming growth factor (TGF)-β and insulin-like growth factor-I (IGF-I) by the osteoclastic bone resorption process, as well as parathyroid hormone-related peptide (PTHrP) by the cancer cells.

Patterns of systemic recurrence are derived from different types of studies. Historically, studies have relied on data collected from autopsy series performed on patients who have been diagnosed as having breast cancer (Table 19-2). The most common cause of death in these series is assumed to be breast cancer. Such data do not reflect the site of first recurrence or the time or interval to such events. However, autopsy data are an accurate assessment of the final pattern of metastasis at death. Lee[51] reviewed the American experience between 1943 and 1977 and concluded that the pattern of metastasis did not change over the 35-year span. The reported median incidence in the six most common sites were as follows: lung, 71% (57% to 77%); bone, 71% (49% to 74%); lymph nodes, 67% (50% to 67%); liver, 62% (50% to 71%);

| TABLE **19-2** | Site of Metastasis of Breast Cancer: Autopsy Series |

AUTHOR	YEAR	n	LUNG (%)	PLEURA (%)	LIVER (%)	BONE (%)	SKIN/SOFT TISSUE (%)	CNS (%)	GI (%)
Walther[48]	1948	186	62	—	35	73	19	—	—
Trauth[49]	1978	116	71	46	59	59	21	—	—
Cifuentes and Pickren[50]	1979	676	67	50	62	71	—	44	16
Lee[51]*	1983	2147	71	50	62	71	—	—	—
Hagemeister[52]	1980	166	75		71	67	30	38	—
Haagensen[53]	1986	100	69	51	65	71	30	22	18

CNS, Central nervous system; *GI*, gastrointestinal.
*Lee summarized the data from American series from 1943 to 1977.

pleura, 50% (36% to 65%); and adrenal glands, 41% (30% to 54%). Similar observations were documented in Europe.[48,49]

The pattern of recurrence in breast cancer is perhaps better derived from longitudinal observational studies documenting the first site of recurrence (Table 19-3). In many of these studies, multiple sites of first recurrences were included as separate first sites; hence the total percentage may have exceeded 100%. The most common site of recurrences was systemic, with bone being the most common organ, followed by LRR, the lung, and the liver. Such data are limited by many factors, including their retrospective nature. Furthermore, the first site of recurrence is dependent on the type and intensity of screening during follow-up. Extensive screening may entail a frequent detailed history and physical examination only or may include blood testing (alkaline phosphatase, liver function tests, and tumor markers), bone scans, liver scan or ultrasound, chest films or computed tomography (CT) scan, CT scans of the abdomen and pelvis, as well as CT scans or magnetic resonance imaging (MRI) of the brain. It has been documented that such extensive screening may detect metastasis before the development of any symptoms.

The incidence of recurrences and perhaps the pattern may vary with the stage of disease and administration of adjuvant chemotherapy. Breast cancer is increasingly being diagnosed at an earlier stage, and the indication for adjuvant chemotherapy has changed. Furthermore, histologic tumor type has been shown to affect the pattern of recurrence. In a study comparing the metastatic patterns of invasive lobular carcinoma to invasive ductal carcinoma of the breast, Borst and Ingold[62] retrospectively examined 2605 cases of invasive lobular and ductal carcinoma. Their findings, as well as those of others, have demonstrated that invasive lobular carcinoma has a higher incidence of metastasis to the gastrointestinal system, gynecologic organs, peritoneum and retroperitoneum, adrenal glands, and bone marrow, whereas invasive ductal carcinoma has been found to have a higher incidence of metastasis to the lungs and pleura. In both histologic types the incidence of metastasis to the axillary lymph nodes, liver, central nervous system, and soft tissue have been shown to be similar.[63-65]

A more reliable representation of the first site of metastasis can be seen in the prospective clinical trials shown in Table 19-4. Similarly, these studies have shown the bone to be the most common first site of recurrence in up to 35% of the patients with metastasis, followed by LRR, the lungs, and the liver. Two recent studies investigating the value of intensive follow-up are valuable in describing the pattern of recurrences. In a study by the Interdisciplinary Group for Cancer Care Evaluation (GIVIO) investigators, a total of 1320 women diagnosed as having stage I to III breast cancer, with the exclusion of T_4N_2, were followed up either intensively or regularly and the difference in outcome was examined based on the type of survival. The intensive follow-up group had a chest film every 6 months and a bone scan and liver sonogram yearly. LRRs and distant metastases were reviewed, whereas new primaries, contralateral disease, and deaths from other causes were ignored. A total of 322 such events occurred in both groups, with a distribution detailed in Table 19-4. At a median follow-up of 71 months, no difference was apparent in overall survival between the two groups. Bone was the most common site of first recurrence, consisting of 32.6% of the total events, followed by LRR, the lungs, and the pleura, as well as the liver.[62]

In a study by Roselli Del Turco[68] and colleagues, 1243 women with stage I to III (no exclusion) breast cancer who had undergone BCT were studied to assess whether the early detection of intrathoracic and bone metastases was effective in reducing mortality in patients with breast cancer. All patients were given a physical examination and underwent mammography, but patients in the intensive follow-up group received a chest x-ray study and a bone scan every 6 months. After 5 years, 393 patients had developed a similar pattern of metastasis as those in the GIVIO study

| TABLE **19-3** | The Site of First Recurrence in Retrospective Studies Presented as Percentages |

AUTHOR	YEAR	n	LOCOREGIONAL (%)	BONE (%)	LUNG AND PLEURA (%)	LIVER (%)	SOFT TISSUE (%)	BRAIN (%)
Hatschek et al.[54]	1989	81	36	30	22	11	—	—
Tomin and Donegan[55]	1987	248	32	28	16	5	—	—
Kamby et al.[56]	1988	401	65	31	29	15	—	2
Rutgers, van Slooten, and Kluck[57]	1989	194	23	62	26	22	—	—
Stierer and Rosen[58]	1989	133	30	29.3	21	5.25	5.5	2.25
Zwaveling et al.[59]	1987	128	11	43	18	15	—	—
Hannisdal et al.[60]	1993	126	29	43.7	24	10	—	5.5
Mirza et al.[61]*	2001	261	47.9	26.4	20.3	13.4	—	3.0

*Locoregional recurrences without systemic disease were excluded.

| TABLE **19-4** | Pattern of Recurrences in Prospective Series |

AUTHOR	YEAR	FOLLOW-UP (YR)	STAGE	LOCOREGIONAL (%)	BONE (%)	LUNG/PLEURA (%)	LIVER (%)	MULTIPLE (%)	OTHER (%)
Veronesi et al.[66]	1981	5	I-II	27	50	38	15	Listed separately	8
NSABP-B-04[43]	1985	10	I-III	23.9	22.3	16.9	—	22.9	14
GIVIO[67]	1994	5	I-III	21.1	32.6	7.8	13.9	9.6	14.3
Roselli Del Turco, Palli, and Cariddi[68]	1994	5	I-III	26.5	34.8	11.7	—	16	10.9

(see Table 19-4). Relapse-free survival was significantly better for the clinical follow-up group ($p = .01$), probably attributable to lead-time bias because the overall survival over 5 years was the same for both groups (18.6% versus 19.5%).[63]

TIME OF RECURRENCE

Although there is no cutoff period beyond which patients are assumed cured from breast cancer, most systemic recurrences occur within the first 10 years. Most studies have noted a peak in LRRs and distant recurrences during the first to fifth years after diagnosis and initiation of treatment. There has been a uniform observation that most recurrences plateau after the first decade, although they continue to occur at a much smaller rate. Demicheli and colleagues[69] from the Milan Cancer Institute reviewed the incidence of recurrence at a given time in 1173 patients with breast cancer who had undergone mastectomy by using the cause-specific hazard function. The results produced a graph with two peaks, demonstrating a hazard function for first failure at approximately 18 months after surgery, followed by another peak at approximately 60 months, and tapering off with a plateaulike tail extending up to 15 years. A similar pattern for LR and distant metastases was observed in all tumors, but the size of the tumor was shown to be a determinant in the time frame of LR or distant recurrence. The risk of early LR and distant recurrences was lower for T_1 tumors than for larger tumors, whereas the risk of late recurrence was similar for all tumors regardless of size. Demonstrating an increased risk of LR and distant recurrence, node-positive patients showed peaks four to five times higher than node-negative patients. The division of node-positive patients into those with one to three positive nodes and those with more than three positive nodes did not substantially affect the general time frame of tumor recurrence, although the height of the peaks was double for those with more than three positive nodes. Data regarding recurrences in premenopausal and postmenopausal patients resulted in hazard functions that were virtually superimposable, showing no difference in the rates of local or distant recurrence on the basis of menopausal status. The time frame for distant metastasis was reported to be similar for 2233 patients with breast cancer who underwent BCT.[69]

In a follow-up article, Demicheli and co-workers[70] compared the risk of recurrence over time for the 877 patients who were given 6 or 12 cycles of adjuvant cyclophosphamide/methotrexate/fluorouracil (CMF) therapy against 575 who received no adjuvant treatment. The recurrence risk for this group of patients was estimated based on the event-specific hazard rate to ascertain the time of first failure and distant metastases, and following Efron, hazard rates were fitted with logistic regression models. Again a double-peaked pattern was observed for both treated patients and controls, with the first hazard peak occurring at approximately 18 to 24 months after surgery (defined as early metastases), a second minor peak occurring at the fifth to sixth year, and a tapered, plateaulike tail extending over 10 years after surgery (late metastases). Compared with the previous trial, the recurrence risk of CMF-treated patients was lower than the corresponding risk of patients who had undergone only surgery—an expected result. However, the difference between recurrence risks was highly evident only for early recurrences and disappeared after approximately 2 years.[70]

Models of tumor growth play a key role in understanding breast cancer as a systemic disease. Demicheli[71] disagrees with the exponential Gompertzian model—(i.e., the explanation of uncontrolled tumor growth as a result of tumor seeding). He rejects this theory because of the inadequacy of the model in explaining clinical findings concerning the long-lasting recurrence risk, as well as the time distribution of the first treatment failure and mortality for patients undergoing mastectomy. According to Demicheli, the theory of tumor dormancy provides a more reasonable description of the natural history of breast cancer, assuming that for some patients during the preclinical phase, micrometastases present in the breast do not grow for a given time interval that is dependent on tumor and/or host characteristics. Using the tumor dormancy model facilitates the treatment of patients with recurrent disease. If the recurrence is related to the growth of micrometastases that were latent during adjuvant chemotherapy, the patient can be considered previously untreated and full-treatment options are available. This model explains the response of patients who had a recurrence more than 1 year after the end of adjuvant CMF to the same chemotherapy, an observation consistent with the hypothesis that the metastases were dormant and had not yet been treated.[71]

The pattern of recurrence of breast cancer provides a valuable insight into the behavior of the disease and may direct future research in the prevention of such occurrences. Based on the concept previously described, the "soil and seed theory" as it relates to breast cancer metastasis to the bone, Mundy and Gallwitz[47] decreased tumor burden in bone of metastatic breast cancer model using bisphosphonates. The role of bisphosphonates in breast cancer bone metastasis was explored in a recent prospective randomized study in humans.[72] This study had shown that bisphosphonates significantly decreased the incidence of bony metastasis compared with placebo, although only during the 2-year medication period. This significant advantage was lost after the medication was stopped (patients were followed up for the total 5-year study period). A better understanding of the tumor dormancy concept and tumor-host interaction may change the therapeutic strategies and result in different treatment modalities than cytotoxic chemotherapeutic agents.

REFERENCES

1. Overgaard M et al: Postoperative radiotherapy in high-risk premenopausal women with breast cancer who receive adjuvant chemotherapy. Danish Breast Cancer Cooperative Group 82b Trial, *N Engl J Med* 337:949, 1997.
2. Ragaz J et al: Adjuvant radiotherapy and chemotherapy in node-positive premenopausal women with breast cancer, *N Engl J Med* 337:956, 1997.
3. Beahrs OH, Myers MH (eds): *Manual for the staging of cancer*, ed 2, Philadelphia, 1983, JB Lippincott.
4. Katz A et al: Recursive partitioning analysis of locoregional recurrence patterns following mastectomy: implications for adjuvant irradiation, *Int J Radiat Oncol Biol Phys* 50:397, 2001.
5. Bundred NJ: Prognostic and predictive factors in breast cancer, *Cancer Treat Rev* 27:137, 2001.
6. Fisher ER et al: Fifteen-year prognostic discriminants for invasive breast carcinoma: National Surgical Adjuvant Breast and Bowel Project Protocol-06, *Cancer* 91:1679, 2001.
7. Turner BC et al: Mutant P53 protein over-expression in women with ipsilateral breast tumor recurrence following lumpectomy and radiation therapy, *Cancer* 88:1091, 2000.
8. Janni W et al: The fate and prognostic value of occult metastatic cells in the bone marrow of patients with breast carcinoma between primary treatment and recurrence, *Cancer* 92:46, 2001.
9. Ooka, M et al: Bone marrow micrometastases detected by RT-PCR for mammaglobin can be an alternative prognostic factor of breast cancer, *Br Cancer Res Treat* 67:169, 2001.
10. Gebauer G et al: Epithelial cells in bone marrow of breast cancer patients at time of primary surgery: clinical outcome during long-term follow-up, *J Clin Oncol* 19:3669, 2001.
11. Veronesi U et al: Twenty-year follow-up of a randomized study comparing breast conserving surgery with radical mastectomy for early breast cancer, *N Engl J Med* 347:1227, 2002.
12. Sarrazin D et al: Ten-year results of a randomized trial comparing a conservative treatment to mastectomy in early breast cancer, *Radiother Oncol* 14:177, 1989.
13. Fisher B et al: Twenty-year follow-up of a randomized trial comparing total mastectomy, lumpectomy, and lumpectomy plus irradiation for the treatment of invasive breast cancer, *N Engl J Med* 347:1233, 2002.
14. Jacobson JA et al: Ten-year results of a comparison of conservation with mastectomy in the treatment of stage I and II breast cancer, *N Engl J Med* 332:907, 1995.
15. vanDongen JA et al: Randomized clinical trial to assess the value of breast-conserving therapy in stage I and II breast cancer. EORTC 10801 trial, *Monogr Natl Cancer Inst* 11:15, 1992.
16. Blichert-Toft M et al: Danish randomized trial comparing breast conservation therapy with mastectomy: six years of life table analysis, *Monogr Natl Cancer Inst* 11:19, 1992.
17. Maddox WA et al: A randomized prospective trial of radical (Halsted) mastectomy versus modified radical mastectomy in 311 breast cancer patients, *Ann Surg* 198:207, 1983.
18. Patterson R, Russell MH: Clinical trials in malignant diseases. Part III–Breast Cancer; evaluation of postoperative radiotherapy, *J Faculty Radiologists* 10:174, 1959.
19. Clemons M et al: Locoregionally recurrent breast cancer: incidence, risk factors and survival, *Cancer Treat Rev* 27:67, 2001.
20. Donegan WL, Perez-Meza CM, Watson FR: A biostatistical study of locally recurrent breast carcinoma, *Surg Gynecol Obstet* 122:529, 1966.
21. Karaball-Damamaga S et al: Natural history and prognosis of recurrent breast cancer, *BMJ* 2:730, 1978.
22. Zimmerman KW, Montague ED, Fletcher GH: Frequency, anatomical distribution and management of local recurrences after definitive therapy for breast cancer, *Cancer* 19:67, 1966.
23. Danckers U, Hamann A, Savage J: Postoperative recurrence of breast cancer after thirty-two years: a case report and review of the literature, *Surgery* 47:656, 1960.
24. Katz A et al: Locoregional recurrence patterns after mastectomy and doxorubicin-based chemotherapy: Implication for postoperative radiation, *J Clin Oncol* 18:2817, 2000.
25. Recht A et al: Time-course of local recurrence following conservative surgery and radiotherapy for early stage breast cancer, *Int J Radiat Oncol Biol Phys* 15:255, 1988.
26. Gage I et al: Long-term outcome following breast-conserving surgery and radiation therapy, *Int J Radiat Oncol Biol Phys* 33:245, 1995.
27. Hafty BG et al: Ipsilateral breast tumor recurrence as a predictor of distant disease: implication for systemic therapy at the time of local relapse, *J Clin Oncol* 14:52, 1996.
28. Fourquet A et al: Prognostic factors of breast recurrences in the conservative management of early breast cancer: a 25-year follow-up, *Int J Radiat Oncol Biol Phys* 17:719, 1989.
29. Lijegren G et al: Sector resection with or without postoperative radiation therapy for stage I breast cancer: five year results of a randomized trial. Uppsala-Orebro breast cancer study group, *J Natl Cancer Inst* 86:717, 1994.
30. Veronesi U et al: Radiotherapy after breast preserving surgery in women with localized cancer of the breast, *N Engl J Med* 328:1587, 1993.
31. Clark RM et al: Randomized clinical trial of irradiation following lumpectomy and axillary dissection of node-negative

breast cancer: an update. Ontario Clinical Oncology Group, *J Natl Cancer Inst* 88:1659, 1996.

32. Forest AP et al: Randomized controlled trial of conservative therapy for breast cancer: 6-year analysis of the Scottish trial. Scottish Cancer Trial Breast Group, *Lancet* 348:708, 1996.

33. Renton SC et al: The importance of resection margin in conservative surgery for breast cancer, *Eur J Surg Oncol* 22:17, 1996.

34. Janni W et al: Matched pair analysis of survival after chestwall recurrence compared to mammary recurrence: a longterm follow up, *J Cancer Res Clin Oncol* 127:455, 2001.

35. Update: NCCN practice guidelines for the treatment of breast cancer. National Comprehensive Cancer Network, *Oncology* 13:41, 1999.

36. Brito RA et al: Long term results of combined modality therapy for locally advanced breast cancer with ipsilateral supraclavicular metastases: the University of Texas M.D. Anderson Cancer Center experience, *J Clin Oncol* 19:628, 2001.

37. Newman LA et al: Presentation, management and outcome of axillary recurrence from breast cancer, *Am J Surg* 180:252, 2000.

38. de Boer R et al: Detection, treatment and outcome of axillary recurrence after axillary clearance for invasive breast cancer, *Br J Surg* 88:118, 2001.

39. Haagensen CD: The surgical treatment of mammary carcinoma. In *Diseases of the breast,* ed 2, Philadelphia, 1971, WB Saunders.

40. Graversen H et al: Breast cancer: Risk of axillary recurrence in node negative patients following partial dissection of the axilla, *Eur J Surg Oncol* 14:407, 1988.

41. Axelsson CK et al: Axillary dissection of level I and II lymph nodes is important in breast cancer classification. The Danish Breast Cancer Cooperative Group (DBCG), *Eur J Cancer* 28A:1415, 1992.

42. Fisher B et al: The accuracy of clinical nodal staging and of limited axillary dissection as a determinant of histologic nodal status in carcinoma of the breast, *Surg Gynecol Obstet* 152:765, 1981.

43. Fisher B et al: Ten-year results of a randomized clinical trial comparing radical mastectomy and total mastectomy with or without radiation, *N Engl J Med* 312:674, 1985.

44. Giuliano AE et al: Prospective observational study of sentinel lymphadenectomy without further axillary dissection in patients with sentinel node-negative breast cancer, *J Clin Oncol* 18:2553, 2000.

45. Murphy PM: Chemokines and the molecular basis of cancer metastasis, *N Engl J Med* 345:833, 2001.

46. Muller A et al: Involvement of chemokine receptors in breast cancer metastasis, *Nature* 410:50, 2001.

47. Mundy G, Gallwitz W: Breast cancer metastasis to bone: pathophysiology and new therapeutic approaches, *Bone* 29:296, 2001.

48. Walther H, Kerbsmetastasen. In Walther H (ed): *Kerbsmetastasen,* Basel, 1948, Schwabe.

49. Trauth H: Zur pathologie der hamatogenen metastasierung des mammakarzinoms. In *Pathologieder Brustedruse,* Berlin, 1978, Springer.

50. Cifuentes N, Pickren JW: Metastases from carcinoma of the mammary gland: an autopsy study, *J Surg Oncol* 11:193, 1979.

51. Lee Y-T: Breast carcinoma: pattern of metastases at autopsy, *J Surg Oncol* 23:175, 1983.

52. Hagemeister FB et al: Causes of death in breast cancer, *Cancer* 46:162, 1980.

53. Haagensen C: *Diseases of the breast,* Philadelphia, 1986, WB Saunders.

54. Hatschek T et al: Influence of S-phase fraction on metastatic pattern and post-recurrence survival in a randomized mammography screening trial, *Breast Cancer Res Treat* 14:321, 1989.

55. Tomin R, Donegan WL: Screening for recurrent breast cancer—its effectiveness and prognostic value, *J Clin Oncol* 5:62, 1987.

56. Kamby C et al: Metastatic pattern in recurrent breast cancer, *Cancer* 62:2226, 1988.

57. Rutgers E, van Slooten EA, Kluck H: Follow-up after treatment of primary breast cancer, *Br J Surg* 76:187, 1989.

58. Steirer M, Rosen HR: Influence of early diagnosis on prognosis of recurrent breast cancer, *Cancer* 64:1128, 1989.

59. Zwaveling A et al: An evaluation of routine follow up for detection of breast cancer recurrences, *J Surg Oncol* 34:194, 1987.

60. Hannisdal E et al: Follow-up of breast cancer patients stage I-II: a baseline strategy, *Eur J Cancer* 29:992, 1993.

61. Mirza N et al: Predictors of systemic recurrence and impact of local failure among early stage breast cancer patients treated with breast conserving therapy, Abstracts of 24th Annual San Antonio Breast Cancer Symposium, San Antonio, December 2001.

62. Borst MJ, Ingold JA: Metastatic patterns of invasive lobular versus invasive ductal carcinoma of the breast, *Surgery* 114:637, 1993.

63. Lamovec J, Bracko M: Metastatic pattern of infiltrating lobular carcinoma of the breast: an autopsy study, *J Surg Oncol* 48:28, 1991.

64. Harris M et al: A comparison of the metastatic pattern of infiltrating lobular carcinoma and infiltrating duct carcinoma of the breast, *Br J Cancer* 50:23, 1984.

65. Weiss MC et al: Outcome of conservative therapy for invasive breast cancer by histologic subtype, *Int J Radiat Oncol Biol Phys* 23:941, 1992.

66. Veronesi U et al: Comparing radical mastectomy with quadrantectomy, axillary dissection, and radiotherapy in patients with small cancer of the breast, *N Engl J Med* 305:6, 1981.

67. The GIVIO Investigators: Impact of follow-up and testing on survival and health related quality of life in breast cancer patients: a multicenter randomized controlled trial, *JAMA* 271:1587, 1994.

68. Roselli Del Turco M, Palli D, Cariddi A: Intensive diagnostic follow-up after treatment of primary breast cancer: a randomized trial, *JAMA* 271:1593, 1994.

69. Demicheli R et al: Time distribution of the recurrence risk for breast cancer patients undergoing mastectomy: further support about the concept of tumor dormancy, *Breast Cancer Res Treat* 41:177, 1996.

70. Demicheli R et al: Comparative analysis of breast cancer recurrence risk for patients receiving or not receiving adjuvant cyclophosphamide, methotrexate, fluorouracil (CMF). Data supporting the occurrence of 'cures', *Breast Cancer Res Treat* 53:209, 1999.

71. Demicheli R: Tumour dormancy: findings and hypotheses from clinical research on breast cancer, *Semin Cancer Biol* 11:297, 2001.

72. Powles TJ et al: A randomized placebo controlled trial to evaluate the effect of the bisphosphonate, clodronate, on the incidence of metastases and mortality in patients with primary operable breast cancer, *Breast Cancer Res Treat* 69:209, 2001.

VIII

STAGING OF BREAST CANCER

20

Assessment and Designation of Breast Cancer Stage

CHRISTINA J. KIM

KIRBY I. BLAND

TIMOTHY J. YEATMAN

Chapter Outline

Staging Past, Present, and Future

Classification schemas and staging of cancers are useful for determining the extent of disease, predicting overall survival, and providing guidance for therapy. This process requires objective analysis of pertinent, well-organized clinical and pathologic data.

In the past, the cancer staging system was quite simplistic. Neoplasms were staged on the basis of clinical evaluation alone as operable or inoperable and classified as local, regional, or metastatic. However, there were limitations of clinical staging in accurately predicting the outcome in patients, and therefore the importance of deriving a more sophisticated staging system has been realized. Its predictive power is largely based on simple physical measurements such as size or extent of anatomic spread of the disease to regional lymph nodes and distant organ sites at the time of diagnosis. These measurements are static and permit only limited evaluation of an ever-changing, heterogeneous neoplasm that often has been in existence for years before the initiation of the staging process.

Furthermore, advancements in breast cancer research and the development of new therapies have led to more treatment options (e.g., systemic chemotherapy, hormonal and other novel biologic therapies). In addition, the impact of treatment on long-term prognosis is not incorporated. Even today, the classification schemas for staging patients are limited by the inability to accurately assess the biologic behavior of tumors and only minimal levels of molecular data are available.

Breast cancers, in general, are considered relatively indolent tumors with a long natural history. However, breast cancer in different patients progresses at different rates, despite similarities in the clinical parameters at the time of diagnosis. The growth rate may range from a few to as many as 25 years, making it difficult to predict the biologic behavior of each tumor. The rate of tumor progression depends on a number of factors, such as size and lymph node status, histologic type, DNA ploidy, and others that we have not yet identified.

Future staging systems will likely include new technologies and in-depth molecular and pathologic analysis of the tissue specimen. The introduction of the sentinel lymph node technique has the potential of allowing more accurate staging with much less morbidity to the patient compared with a complete axillary node dissection. With improvements in the sensitivity of detection methods, including histopathologic assays and molecular techniques, microscopic and submicroscopic tumor metastases can be detected. The recent rapid expansion of genetic knowledge associated with the Human Genome Project has provided a large number of molecular tools that may prove valuable in the evaluation of tumor progression. Molecular staging using reverse transcriptase polymerize chain reaction (RT-PCR), microarray analysis, and proteomics to identify unique gene and protein expression profiles may allow the detection of occult cancer before it becomes clinically evident and may provide more accurate information to help determine prognosis and survival with minimal morbidity to the patient.

Clinical, Pathologic, and Molecular Makers/Factors in Determining Prognosis

Central to any staging system are identifiable objective tumor and host characteristics that are prognostic of tumor progression. A number of clinical and pathologic factors have been identified that may predict the long-term outcome in patients with breast cancer. Generally accepted prognostic factors include age, tumor size, lymph node status, histologic tumor type and grade, mitotic rate, and hormone receptor. A number of other biologic factors have also been studied and provide information regarding the potential for aggressive behavior of tumors (Table 20-1).

TABLE 20-1   Prognostic Factors in Breast Cancer

CLINICAL HISTOPATHOLOGIC FACTORS	BIOLOGIC FACTORS
Age	Angiogenesis (VEGF)
Tumor size	Proliferation (MIBI/Ki67/TLI)
Lymph node status	Growth factor receptor (EGFR/*cerbB2/neu*)
Tumor histology	Cell cycle regulators (*p53/c-myc/*cyclins)
Tumor grade	Proteases (urokinase/plasminogen activator/cathepsin D)
Hormone receptor status	Metastasis proteins (Laminin 67-kDa receptor/nm23)
Vascular invasion	Heat shock proteins (pS2)
	Others

From Bundred NJ: *Cancer Treat Rev* 27:137, 2001.

Clinical and pathologic staging systems are both useful in providing prognostic information. Clinical parameters historically have been used to predict survival because of the simplicity in obtaining the data. The clinical system may serve to guide initial therapy based on all available preoperative data that include history, physical and laboratory examinations, and biopsy material. However, we are now detecting tumors at very early stages before they become clinically evident; as a result, histopathologic staging based on the primary tumor and local/regional lymph nodes status has proved to be more accurate in predicting survival. The pathologic system, because of its ability to precisely define the histology and the extent of disease, is more accurate for grouping of patients with similar prognoses and for planning subsequent therapies.

CLINICAL FACTORS

Clinical staging is based on a thorough physical examination of the breast tissue, skin overlying the breasts, and the regional lymph nodes (axillary, infraclavicular, supraclavicular, cervical) and various imaging modalities. On physical examination, important characteristics to note are the tumor size, whether there is extension into the chest wall, involvement of the overlying skin (e.g., erythema, induration, edema) and the regional lymph nodes. Mobility of the involved regional lymph nodes is important to note as a prognosticating indicator, with fixed nodes having a worse prognosis.

Imaging modalities such as mammograms, ultrasound, and computed tomography (CT) scans are available and useful as an adjunct to the physical examination. Newer imaging modalities that are currently under clinical investigation as a diagnostic screening tool include digital mammography, magnetic resonance imaging (MRI) scans, and positron emission tomography (PET).

PRIMARY TUMOR CHARACTERISTICS

Tumor Size. Tumor size is defined as the maximal size of the invasive component of the primary tumor

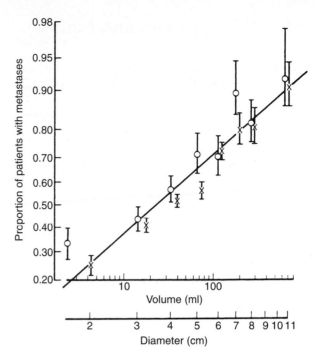

FIG. **20-1** A linear relationship exists between tumor size (volume or diameter) and potential for metastasis. *(From Koscielny S et al: Br J Cancer 49:709, 1984.)*

on pathologic specimen. Clinical evaluation of tumor size has been included in many staging systems as an independent predictor of survival.[1-4] The potential for metastasis increases in a linear relationship with the size of the primary tumor[2] (Figure 20-1). Metastasis does not occur in 50% of the cases until the primary tumor reaches a size of 3.6 cm in diameter. Furthermore, there is a distinct relationship between increasing tumor size and the probability of axillary nodal metastasis.[5] These investigators demonstrated that tumor size must reach 3.1 to 4.0 cm in diameter to generate axillary metastasis in 50% of patients (Table 20-2). Fisher[6] has likewise shown that tumor size correlates with disease-free survival at 10 years, even when controlled for nodal metastases

TABLE **20-2**   Relationship between Tumor Size and Axillary Metastases

TUMOR DIAMETER (cm)	NO. OF PATIENTS	AXILLARY NODE-NEGATIVE (%)	AXILLARY NODE-POSITIVE (%)
0.1-0.5	147	71.4	28.6
0.6-1.0	960	75.3	24.7
1.1-2.0	4044	65.9	34.1
2.1-3.0	3546	57.3	42.1
3.1-4.0	1917	49.9	50.1
4.1-5.0	1135	43.5	56.5
>5.0	1232	35.5	64.5

Modified from Nemoto T et al: *Cancer* 45:2917, 1980.

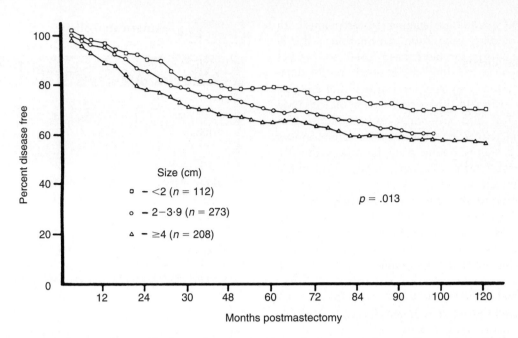

FIG. **20-2** Primary tumor size correlates with disease-free survival in patients undergoing curative surgery. *(From Fisher ER: NCI Monogr 1:29, 1986.)*

(Figure 20-2). Tumor size is particularly useful as a prognostic tool in patients with no involvement of regional lymph nodes. Tumor size alone may alter adjuvant treatment options. Patients with small tumors (<1 cm) who have node-negative disease have an excellent overall prognosis.[7,8] It is also true, however, that patients with small tumors can have metastasis to the axillary lymph nodes, and conversely, more than one third of patients with tumors greater than 6 cm in palpable diameter have negative lymph nodes, thus demonstrating the limited predictiveness of tumor size alone.[3]

Tumor Location. The location of the tumor within the breast may have some prognostic importance for patients with negative nodes. Although the risk of axillary lymph node metastasis is greater for lateral versus medial breast cancers, one study by Fisher and colleagues[9] showed that patients with medial tumors fare more poorly than those with lateral tumors because of a greater risk of local recurrence. Another study[10] demonstrated that the prognosis is quite similar between groups of patients with tumors in the medial or lateral half of the breast. More recently, other investigators[11,12] have found that medial and central locations of tumors are associated with up to a twofold increase in the risk of developing systemic relapse and breast cancer–related death compared with the lateral location. They postulated that this may be attributed to the risk of occult spread to the internal mammary nodes (IMNs).

Tumor Histology. The most commonly used classification of tumor types is shown in Table 20-3.[13] The World Health Organization has classified tumors into six major groups, with epithelial tumors being the most common. Of the malignant epithelial tumors, there are three subtypes: noninvasive, invasive, and Paget's disease of the nipple. Next to inflammatory carcinoma, which has a 5-year survival rate of 11%, the invasive ductal carcinoma (the most common subtype) carries the worst prognosis, with 5-year survival rates of approximately 59%.[14] Medullary, papillary, and colloid subtypes have a better prognosis than do ductal invasive cancers (Table 20-4).[15]

Attempts have been made to stage tumors based on histologic characteristics alone. Hoge and colleagues[16] described four classes of tumors after analyzing tumor specimens from 3902 patients. Class A tumors (5% of the total) included all in situ lesions and carried a 5-year survival rate of 91%. Class B tumors (41% of the total) consisted of medullary, mucinous, tubular, and adenoid cystic carcinomas and were associated with a 75% survival rate. Class C tumors (85% of the total) included the most common tumor types, infiltrating ductal and infiltrating lobular carcinomas, and had a reduced 5-year survival rate of 66%. Class D tumors (4.3% of the total) consisted of high-risk lesions such as inflammatory and undifferentiated carcinomas and had the worst survival rate of 33%.

Tumor Grade. Histologic grading based on criteria established by Bloom and Richardson[17] incorporates

TABLE 20-3	Histologic Classification of Breast Tumors

I. Epithelial tumors
  A. Benign
    1. Intraductal papilloma
    2. Adenoma of the nipple
    3. Adenoma
      a. Tubular
      b. Lactating
  B. Malignant
    1. Noninvasive
      a. Intraductal carcinoma
      b. Lobular carcinoma in situ
    2. Invasive
      a. Invasive ductal carcinoma
      b. Invasive ductal carcinoma with a predominant intraductal component
      c. Invasive lobular carcinoma
      d. Mucinous carcinoma
      e. Medullary carcinoma
      f. Papillary carcinoma
      g. Tubular carcinoma
      h. Adenoid cystic carcinoma
      i. Secretory (juvenile) carcinoma
      j. Apocrine
      k. Carcinoma with metaplasia
        i. Squamous type
        II. Spindle-cell type
        iii. Cartilaginous and osseous type
        iv. Mixed type
      l. Others
    3. Paget's disease of the nipple
II. Mixed connective tissue and epithelial tumors
  A. Fibroadenoma
  B. Phyllodes tumor (cystosarcoma phyllodes)
  C. Carcinosarcoma
III. Miscellaneous tumors
  A. Soft tissue tumors
  B. Skin tumors
  C. Tumors of hematopoietic and lymphoid tissues
IV. Unclassified tumors
V. Mammary dysplasia/fibrocystic disease
VI. Tumor like lesions
  A. Duct ectasia
  B. Inflammatory pseudotumors
  C. Hamartoma
  D. Gynecomastia
  E. Others

From *WHO International Histological Classification of Tumors, No. 2. Histological Typing of Breast Tumors,* ed 2, Geneva, 1981, World Health Organization.

TABLE 20-4	American College of Surgeons 1979 Survey of Infiltrating Breast Cancer

	NO. OF CASES	PERCENT OF TOTAL	PERCENT 5-YR SURVIVAL
Histologic type			
Lobular	700	3	70
Ductal	2,845	56	59
Paget's	122	0.5	61
Scirrhous	2,438	11	60
Medullary	735	3	66
Colloid	442	2	69
Comedo	236	1	65
Inflammatory	117	0.5	11
All cases	22,989	100	58

Modified from Hutter RVP: *Cancer* 46:961, 1980.

cytoplasmic and nuclear characteristics such as size, shape, and hyperchromatism along with the percentage and number of mitotic figures and tubules. Other systems of grading based on nuclear characteristics alone have also been developed.[18] Hutter[15] has reviewed this topic and reports that overall survivorship is related to differentiation of tumor cells. Survival at 20 years was estimated to be 41% for grade I (well differentiated), 29% for grade II (moderately differentiated), and 21% for grade III (poorly differentiated). Fisher and colleagues[19] examined histologic grade in relationship to 5-year treatment failures and found that there is a significant correlation between these two factors in patients with absent nodal metastases or with four or more positive lymph nodes.

Histopathologic Features of Tumor. Fisher and colleagues[20] examined the relationship of 32 pathologic seven clinical characteristics to 5-year survival in 1000 patients treated with radical mastectomy. Although they found that pathologic nodal status was the most dominant influence on treatment failure rates and corresponding survival, they also identified a number of other important predictors of short-term (<24 months) treatment failure (Table 20-5). Characteristics such as noncircumscription, perineural invasion, tumor necrosis, absence of sinus histiocytosis, and other parameters correlated with poor long-term survival.

Other histologic characteristics have also been found to bear prognostic information. These include blood vessel invasion, lymphatic extension, elastosis, glycogen staining, and the presence or absence of numerous host inflammatory responses. These and other histologic characteristics often can be identified in many patients. Unfortunately, histologic criteria can rarely be used to modify the management of a patient by stratification

TABLE 20-5	Factors Associated with Short-Term Treatment Failure

FEATURE	TIME TO FAILURE (mo)
Clinically positive axillas	6, 12, 18, 24
>4 pathologically positive nodes	6, 12, 18, 24
Size >4.1 cm	6, 12, 18, 24
Noncircumscribed (gross and micro)	12, 18, 24
Lymphatic extension in quadrants	12, 18
Proliferative fibrocystic disease in quadrants	12, 18
Age 20-54 years	18, 24
Nipple involvement	6
Absent or slight/moderate cell reaction to tumor	6
Absent sinus histiocytosis	12
Skin involvement	12
Perineural extension	18
Black race	18
Nuclear grade 1	24
Marked tumor necrosis	24
Glycogen present	24

Modified from Fisher ER, Redmond C, Fisher B: *Cancer* 46:908, 1980.

into different substages; when these characteristics are present, the prognosis is usually guarded.

Estrogen and Progesterone Receptors. Both estrogen receptors (ERs) and progesterone receptors (PRs) are important prognostic indicators in patients with breast cancer, and they also predict which patients might benefit from antihormonal therapies. ER and PR positivity generally correlates with a better prognosis and a better response to chemotherapy, with or without the concomitant use of tamoxifen. Knight and colleagues,[21] Stewart and Rubens,[22] and Osborne and McGuire[23] have shown that ER status affects survival independent of axillary nodal status.

Similarly, another study[24] has demonstrated longer survivorship for PR-positive patients than for PR-negative patients. Reports of the beneficial use of chemotherapy and/or tamoxifen have suggested that receptor status may be important in patients with known systemic disease, as well as in patients without axillary metastases

Tumor Growth Rate and Kinetics. Anatomic methods for staging breast cancer have withstood the test of time and remain the gold standard; however, these methods often provide only a static or instantaneous view of what is actually occurring at the molecular and cellular level. Attempts at measuring dynamic

characteristics (clinical and pathologic) have also been predictive of tumor progression. Clinical measurements of flux of tumor volume over time and pathologic determinations of cell kinetics have both been useful.

Charlson and Feinstein[25] developed a clinical index of growth rate based on the first clinical manifestation of disease and then on subsequent unfavorable transition events. Their methods were used in conjunction with the anatomic tumor, node, metastasis (TNM) system to better predict which subgroups of patients would have predictably good 10-year survival rates despite poor anatomic status. Conversely, patients with rapidly progressing lesions could be identified despite favorable anatomic staging.

Measurement of tumor doubling time, although not clinically practical, has been shown to correlate with prognosis (see Chapter 32). Multiple studies have demonstrated a wide range of doubling times, not only between patients but also within the same patient over time.[26-28] This heterogeneity is typical of breast cancer. Serial mammography has also been used for this purpose and has shown that shorter doubling times correlate with diminished survival.[29]

Studies of tumor cell kinetics through the use of tritium-labeled thymidine (^{3}H-TdR) incorporation into DNA have demonstrated some promise in their ability to identify aggressive, rapidly growing tumors. This method is more sensitive than standard histologic tests that enumerate the relative number of mitoses. Tumor cells are sampled from the specimen and then incubated with ^{3}H-TdR, which is taken up by cells in the DNA synthetic or S phase. Measuring ^{3}H-TdR uptake then permits the estimation of the percentage of cells in the S phase (labeling index). Tubiana and associates[30] demonstrated a correlation between the thymidine labeling index and the long-term prognosis in 128 patients. Labeling indices signifying a low level of cell replication (<0.25) were predictive of low rates of relapse (25%) and death (30%) at 10 years, whereas high indices ($\geq$3.84) correlated with high rates of relapse (62%) and death (37%). With multivariate analysis, the labeling index has been found to be independent of clinical and pathologic staging factors such as the presence of axillary node involvement and primary tumor size. This index does, however, correlate with histologic characteristics such as tumor grade and may be important in the staging of node-negative patients.[31]

Because ^{3}H-TdR uptake assays can be tedious and time consuming, flow cytometry has recently been used to estimate cellular kinetics and to detect the presence of aneuploidy. Flow cytometry permits rapid, single-cell analysis of DNA content per cell, enabling the determination of the fraction of cells within the S phase and the ploidy levels within a tumor cell population. This type

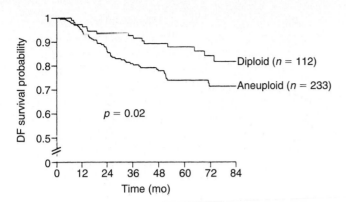

FIG. **20-3** Aneuploid tumors have poorer disease-free *(DF)* survival probabilities than diploid tumors. *(From Clark GM et al: N Engl J Med 320:627, 1989.)*

of analysis has been used in multiple studies to predict future survival.[32-34]

Knowing that 50% to 60% of patients with breast cancer have disease confined to the breast at the time of diagnosis, Clark, Dressler, and Owens[35] studied 395 specimens of node-negative breast cancer using aliquots of frozen breast tissue. Of these tumors, 68% were aneuploid, with an associated 5-year survival of 74%, and 32% were diploid, with an 88% survival rate (Figure 20-3). The S-phase fraction of cells was also an important predictor of disease-free survival in patients with diploid tumors. Five-year survival rates of 90% and 70% were measured for tumors with low and high S-phase fractions, respectively.

BIOLOGIC MARKERS

With the development of monoclonal antibody technology, antibodies specific for breast cancer have been developed.[36] These antibodies can be used to detect microscopic disease not easily seen on routine histopathology by using immunoperoxidase technology and radioimmunoassay. They may be useful in accurately staging the anatomic extent of axillary disease and distant disease such as tumor infiltration of bone marrow.[37] Newer technology may also permit preoperative staging of the axilla and the internal mammary chain through the use of handheld probes that detect radiolabeled tumor cells. Tumor markers, such as carcinoembryonic antigen (CEA), pregnancy-associated glycoprotein, human tissue polypeptide antigen, and C-reactive protein, are not very specific for breast cancer and are unpredictably secreted by heterogeneous breast carcinomas.[38]

Oncogenes may be related to the complex phenomenon of human breast cancer initiation and progression through the processes of gene amplification, mutation, chromosomal breakage, or insertion of retroviral promoters near oncogenes.[39] With current technology, both their number and their expressed gene products

may be measured. Amplification of the *HER2/neu* oncogene has recently been found to portend a poor prognosis, correlating with axillary lymph node and steroid receptor status along with the nuclear grade.[40,41] This oncogene, however, has prognostic significance only in patients with node-positive breast cancer.[41] Other oncogenes, such as *myc*, are also under current study and have been associated with poor prognosis.[42]

Although studies of individual oncogenes and tumor-suppressor genes may prove fruitful in identifying poor patient prognosis, recent studies evaluating panels of oncogenes have shown promise in providing greater accuracy in predicting outcomes. Bland and colleagues[43] examined 85 breast cancer cases of various stages (I through IIB) using a panel of monoclonal antibodies directed at oncogene products such as FOS, MYC, and HRAS and the mutated tumor-suppressor gene *P53*. Interestingly, they found that although expression of one to two oncogenes was not useful in predicting recurrence, coexpression of three or more oncogenes identified poor survival. Further multiparameter studies of oncogene expression may be warranted based on these preliminary findings. (See Chapter 25 for a more comprehensive discussion of oncogenes and growth regulation of normal breast and breast cancer.)

LYMPH NODE STATUS

In the late nineteenth century, Halsted[44] described how breast cancer spreads systematically from the primary breast tissue to the ipsilateral axilla and is finally disseminated into the systemic circulation. The presence of axillary nodal metastasis was considered a poorer prognostic factor compared with improvement in survival with a more radical operation. However, this theory has been challenged over the years when it became evident that more extensive mastectomies proved to have survival benefit equal to that of less extensive, breast-conserving operations.[45,46] Furthermore, up to 30% of patients with node-negative disease will eventually develop recurrent metastatic disease.[47] However, once the diagnosis of breast cancer has been established, the lymph nodes status remains the most powerful predictor for long-term survival.[48] Not only does the lymph node status give prognostic information, it is important in making therapeutic decisions.

Physical examination, however, is notoriously inaccurate in preoperative assessment of the presence of lymph node metastasis. In fact, microscopic evidence of tumor can be demonstrated in one third of patients in the absence of palpable axillary lymph nodes. Clinical examination has a false-positive rate for detection of axillary metastases ranging from 25% to 31%. False-negative rates range from 27% to 33%.[49,50]

| TABLE 20-6 | Survival of Patients with Breast Cancer Relative to Histologic Stage |

HISTOLOGIC STAGING	CRUDE SURVIVAL (%)		5-YR DISEASE-FREE SURVIVAL (%)
	5 yr	10 yr	
All patients	64	46	60
Negative	78	65	82
Positive axillary lymph nodes	46	25	35
1-3 positive axillary lymph nodes	62	38	50
>4 positive axillary lymph nodes	32	13	21

Modified from Henderson IC, Canellos GP: *N Engl J Med* 302:17, 1980. Copyright 1980. Massachusetts Medical Society.

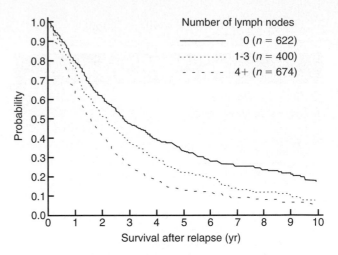

FIG. 20-4 Survival after first relapse by the number of positive axillary lymph nodes.[53]

Axillary Nodal Disease. In a 10-year clinical trial, Fisher, Fisher, and Redmond,[51] reporting for the National Surgical Adjuvant Breast and Bowel Project (NSABP), found that crude and disease-free survival correlated directly with the number of positive lymph nodes. Patients with negative axillary lymph nodes had 5- and 10-year survival rates of 78% and 65%, respectively (Table 20-6). Similarly, the number of positive nodes correlated with the 5- and 10-year treatment failures. Zero positive nodes were associated with a 20% treatment failure rate at 10 years, whereas more than four positive nodes were associated with a 71% treatment failure rate. More than 13 positive nodes increased the failure rate even further to 87% (Table 20-7). Diab and associates[52] have shown that the presence of more than 10 positive lymph nodes is associated with an increased risk in locoregional and distant failure rates. Not only is axillary lymph node metastasis a time-dependent variable, but it also seems to be a marker for a more aggressive tumor phenotype. Jatoi and associates[53] have shown that patients with four or more involved lymph nodes at the time of initial diagnosis have a significantly worse outcome after their first recurrence (Figure 20-4).

The location of the positive axillary lymph nodes is important. Involvement of apical axillary (level 3) or infraclavicular lymph nodes carries a grim prognosis.[54] Another issue is the level of axillary lymph nodes that must be removed to obtain accurate prognostic information. Certainly, complete dissection of all three levels of lymph nodes (Patey dissection) not only provides the maximum amount of prognostic information but also clears the axilla of gross disease and obviates the need for axillary irradiation. In fact, total axillary clearance has been supported by some authors as the only acceptable method of assessing axillary nodal status.[55] Several studies, however, have addressed this topic and have concluded that, in certain cases, a level 1 dissection can be predictive of the actual involvement of the remaining nodal basin. Boova, Bonanni, and Rosato[56] examined the contents of 200 consecutive mastectomy and total axillary dissection specimens. The average number of lymph nodes recovered from each level was 14 at level 1, 11 at level 2, and 8 at level 3. Of the patients, 40% had axillary metastases, with half of these involving only level 1 (Table 20-8). Interestingly, 7 patients (3.5% of all patients and 8.7% of those with lymph node metastases) had positive nodes at level 2 and/or 3 without positive nodes at level 1 (skip metastasis). These authors concluded that level 1 dissections can be accurate predictors of the status of the entire axillary lymph node basin, assuming that an adequate number of lymph nodes has been sampled. Fisher and colleagues have also suggested that dissection of levels 1 and 2 is more

| TABLE 20-7 | Nodal Status and 5- and 10-Year Treatment Failure |

NO. OF POSITIVE NODES	NO. OF PATIENTS (n = 614)	TREATMENT FAILURE (%)	
		5 yr	10 yr
0	279	13	20
1-3	160	39	47
4+	175	69	71
4-6	65		59
7-12	55		69
13+	55		87

Modified from Fisher ER: *NCI Monogr* 1:29, 1986.

TABLE 20-8	Patterns of Axillary Nodal Involvement: Levels 1, 2, and 3

NODE STATUS	NO. OF PATIENTS (%)
All levels negative	120 (60.0)
Level 1 positive	39 (19.5)
Levels 1 and 2 positive	19 (9.5)
Levels 1, 2, and 3 positive	11 (5.5)
Levels 1 and 3 positive	4 (2.0)
Level 2 positive*	5 (2.5)
Level 3 positive*	1 (0.5)
Levels 2 and 3 positive*	1 (0.5)

From Boova RS, Roseann B, Rosato F: *Ann Surg* 196:642, 1982.
*Skip metastasis group.

than adequate in most cases to accurately predict prognosis. Their report found that qualitative disease (positive versus negative) in the axilla could be determined equally well by studying 3 to 5 or 27 or more lymph nodes; however, to quantitatively determine the true axillary involvement, sampling of more than 10 lymph nodes is required.[50] The current standard of care for a complete axillary lymph node dissection includes both level 1 and level 2 lymph nodes with procurement of at least 10 lymph nodes. Sentinel lymph node technique is also changing our current standard of nodal staging in breast cancer patients.

Sentinel Lymph Node Mapping. The recent introduction of sentinel lymph node mapping technology has challenged the classic approach to breast cancer staging that involves routine axillary lymph node dissection. This methodology, first tested and proved effective for nodal staging in patients with melanoma,[57-60] has been shown to be an accurate means of nodal staging in patients with breast cancer.[61] Sentinel lymph nodes mapping is emerging as an alternative method to complete axillary lymph node dissection, thereby offering patients accurate staging information with minimal or no morbidity.[62]

The sentinel lymph node concept supports the notion that breast cancer cells spread in an orderly fashion via a direct lymphatic communication from the primary tumor to the sentinel lymph node. Therefore the sentinel lymph node is the most likely to be the first site metastasis within the lymph node basin and should accurately predict the tumor status of the remaining lymph node basin. On average, one to three sentinel lymph nodes may be found within an axillary basin. A number of large, single and multiinstitutional trials have now demonstrated the accurate predictability of the sentinel lymph node technique in staging the

axilla in breast cancer patients by using various injection techniques with technetium sulfur colloid, isosulfan blue, or a combination of both agents.[61,63-69] These studies have shown a success rate in identification of 65% to 92%, with an accuracy rate of 96% to 100% and a false-negative rate of approximately 2%. Long-term follow-up is needed to define the true false-negative rate, that is, to identify axillary recurrences in breast cancer patients with negative sentinel lymph node and no complete axillary node dissections.

In addition, the accuracy of sentinel lymph node mapping technique is enhanced by the ability to improve upon the histologic examination of the lymph node when 1 to 3 lymph nodes, as opposed to 15 to 20 lymph nodes in a complete node dissection, are submitted for a more detailed examination. Routine histologic examination with serial step sectioning and hematoxylin and eosin (H&E) staining is performed to identified tumor deposits within the lymph node. Furthermore, immunohistochemistry (IHC; cytokeratin assays) shows an increased rate of detection of occult micrometastatic disease, further improving the accuracy of the technique.[70] Cote and colleagues[71] have shown the importance of IHC and serial sectioning for accurate evaluation of sentinel lymph nodes. Occult nodal metastases were detected in 7% of patients with H&E sections and in 20% with IHC. Others investigators have also shown the increase in detection of rate of occult micrometastatic disease in patients who were determined to be node negative based on routine histologic methods.[72-75] In a study by Schreiber and colleagues,[76] up to 9.4% of the patients were upstaged with the addition of IHC and serial sectioning. However, to date, the clinical significance of identifying micrometastatic and submicrometastatic disease as a prognostic variable is unknown.

Molecular staging using techniques such as RT-PCR is allowing the detection of one tumor cell in the background of a million. These studies have been performed for the detection of melanoma cells in sentinel lymph nodes,[77,78] and the techniques are currently under investigation for breast cancer.

Internal Mammary Nodal Disease. The status of the IMNs has been a point of controversy since the time of Halsted in the 1890s. Prospective randomized trials have failed to demonstrate a benefit in survival for women who had complete IMN dissections (extended radical mastectomy) while incurring significant operative morbidity. However, other studies have shown a prognostic significance of metastasis to the IMNs.[79-81] Veronesi and associates[82] reported a decrease in 5-year overall survival rate in patients with positive IMN disease (44%) compared with 78% in IMN negative disease. When considering IMN disease, one must also consider whether there is synchronous involvement of the axillary lymph nodes. There is some evidence to suggest that patients who have positive axillary and IMNs have a worse prognosis.[79,81] Positive IMNs can be found in up to 8.9% of cases when axillary nodes are negative and in as many as 26% of cases when the primary tumor location is medial.[83] The emergence of the lymphatic mapping technique may lead to the ability to sample IMNs with minimal morbidity to provide additional staging information.

Supraclavicular Nodal Disease. Historically, supraclavicular lymph nodes involved with tumor indicated advanced disease and were associated with a poor prognosis. Positive supraclavicular lymph nodes were considered to have survival rates similar to those with distant spread rather than of regional nodal disease.[84,85] More recent studies suggest that the outcomes of these patients are comparable to the outcomes of those with locally advanced disease rather than those with distant metastatic disease.[86]

Currently, routine scalene lymph node biopsies are not indicated. In the prechemotherapy era, scalene lymph nodes biopsy was done to determine operability of breast cancer patients with advanced local disease but without evidence of distant metastases. It was noted by Papaioannou and Urban,[87] however, that when scalene lymph nodes were pathologically positive, despite the use of radical mastectomy with adjuvant radiotherapy, no patients were disease free after 1 year and more than 50% were dead with disease in 3 years. These data once again suggest that metastases to lymph node beds other than regional (axillary, clavicular, and internal mammary) suggest the presence of distant systemic disease.[87]

Pathologic Assessment of Lymph Nodes. Although routine pathologic examination of lymph nodes is more accurate than physical examination, exhaustive studies of lymph nodes with thin section techniques have demonstrated occult micrometastases in patients with lymph nodes initially reported as histologically negative.[19] Similarly, it has been estimated by Wilkinson and Lawrence[88] that commonly used methods of sectioning lymph nodes can result in greater than 30% false-negative rate. The prognostic implication of micrometastases, however, is not yet clear because the survival of patients is not different from that of patients with negative nodes when the same pathologic technique is used. Recent studies concerning the treatment of node-negative patients with adjuvant therapies have further complicated this issue.

Other indices that portend an unfavorable prognosis for breast cancer relate to the presence of gross rather than microscopic disease in the lymph nodes[35] and/or the presence of extranodal disease.[89,90]

Evolution of Staging Systems

Early staging systems for breast cancer were based on the feasibility of operative intervention. Most tumors were classified as either operable or inoperable; however, this grouping did not offer any significant prognostic information. In 1905 Steinthal[91] recommended three different classifications for patients with breast cancer: (1) tumors not larger than "a plum" and clinically not associated with skin or axillary lymph node involvement; (2) large tumors adherent to the skin with palpably enlarged axillary lymph nodes; and (3) large tumors diffusely involving the breast with skin, deep muscle, and supraclavicular lymph node involvement. This classification was based on clinical factors that were perceived as important in predicting prognosis. Early on, it was clear that surgeons had identified some of the most ominous prognostic indicators for breast cancer. It is also interesting to note the inclusion of primary tumor size in this primitive staging scheme. An unpopular but insightful system was proposed by Lee and Stubenbord[92] in 1928. Their system included an index of the rate of tumor growth. This method was the first to attempt assessment of the biology of individual tumors and their potential for progression.

In 1940 the four-stage Manchester classification was introduced (Table 20-9).[93] It permitted staging based solely on clinical criteria, including the extent of local

TABLE 20-9	The Manchester System
Stage I	The tumor is confined to the breast. Involvement of the skin may be present, provided the area is small in relation to the size of the breast.
Stage II	The tumor is confined to the breast and associated lymph nodes are present in the axilla.
Stage III	The tumor extends beyond the breast as demonstrated by the following: a. Skin invasion or fixation of a large area in relation to the size of the breast or skin ulceration. b. Tumor fixation to the underlying muscle or fascia; mobile axillary nodes
Stage IV	The tumor extends beyond the breast as shown by the following: a. Fixation or matting of the axillary nodes b. Fixation of tumor to chest wall c. Deposits in supraclavicular nodes or in the opposite breast d. Satellite nodules or distant metastases

From Patterson R: *The treatment of malignant disease by radium and x-rays*, London, 1948, Edward Arnold.

TABLE 20-10 Portmann Classification

Stage I		
−	Skin—not involved	
+	Tumor—localized to breast, mobile	
−	Metastases—none	
Stage II		
−	Skin—not involved	
+	Tumor—localized to breast, mobile	
+	Metastases—few axillary lymph nodes involved in microscopic evaluation; no other metastases	
Stage III		
−	Skin—edematous; brawny red induration and inflammation not obviously caused by infection; extensive ulceration; multiple secondary nodules	
++	Tumor—diffusely infiltrating breast; fixation of tumor or breast to chest wall; edema of breast; secondary tumors	
++	Metastases—many axillary lymph nodes involved or fixed; no clinical or roentgenologic evidence of distant metastases	
Stage IV		
+/−	Skin—involved or not involved	
+/++	Tumor—localized or diffuse	
+++	Metastases—axillary and supraclavicular lymph nodes extensively involved, and clinical or roentgenological evidence of more distant metastases	

Modified from Portmann UV: *Cleve Clin Q* 10:41, 1943.

involvement by the primary tumor, the presence and mobility of palpably enlarged axillary lymph nodes, and the presence of distant metastases. Neither pathologic information nor tumor size were included in this system.

In 1943 Portmann[94] described a staging system that incorporated clinical, pathologic, and roentgenographic characteristics of breast cancers and evaluated each lesion based on three categories: skin involvement, the location and mobility of the primary tumor, and the extent of local and distant metastases (Table 20-10). Haagensen and Stout[95] evaluated 568 patients with breast cancer who were treated with radical mastectomy. In 1943 they published the following criteria of inoperability, which were based on the clinical characteristics of patients who were clearly incurable by aggressive surgery alone:

1. Extensive edema of the skin overlying the breast or edema of the arm
2. Satellite nodules of the breast or parasternal tumor nodules
3. Inflammatory carcinoma
4. Supraclavicular or distant metastases

5. Two or more of the "grave signs" of locally advanced cancer:
   a. Breast skin edema
   b. Breast skin ulceration
   c. Tumor fixation to chest wall
   d. Axillary lymph node fixation to skin or deep tissues
   e. Enlarged axillary lymph nodes larger than 2.5 cm in diameter

Haagensen and Stout also advocated the use of biopsy material in the determination of inoperability. Their proposed "triple biopsy" included sampling the primary tumor, apical axillary nodes, and IMNs as part of the pretreatment evaluation. This represented the first attempt at including pathologic data in the staging process.

Although largely derived from Haagensen and Stout's criteria of inoperability, the Columbia Clinical Classification (CCC) ignored the use of tumor size and any biopsy material or other pathologic data. It has, however, been successfully used to separate different groups of patients with distinctly different survival rates.[96] Staging was determined on the basis of physical examination and other roentgenographic information in an attempt to simplify and streamline the staging process. Four stages were defined (Table 20-11). Stages A and B were both used to describe operable cancers, but stage B patients had palpably enlarged, unfixed axillary lymph nodes (presumed to represent regional metastases). Based on the five "grave signs" listed previously, stage C defined a group of patients with cancers that were locally advanced. In stage D patients, the tumors were considered inoperable as defined by the "criteria of inoperability." Stage A and B patients were treated with radical mastectomy, whereas stage C and D patients underwent radiation therapy.

Despite initial acceptance, the CCC has since been replaced by the current TNM system, which incorporates both clinical and pathologic features. This system was adopted for many reasons, including its initial simplicity, clinical applicability, and universal utility. Moreover, it is clear that in the last decade, because of the widespread use of screening mammography and public education, breast cancers are being detected earlier, with smaller delays in diagnosis. This has necessarily shifted the contemporary population of patients being studied to earlier stages at diagnosis. In turn, the need for elaborate classification schemes based on generally advanced clinical criteria has become obsolete. At present, patients need to be stratified into groups based on more subtle, less advanced characteristics of disease progression. This is necessary not only because many women now have small or nonpalpable tumors but also because not all small tumors have the same biologic behavior (e.g., growth, metastases).

TABLE 20-11	Columbia Clinical Classification

Stage A	No skin involvement or fixation of the tumor to the chest wall. Axillary nodes are not palpable.
Stage B	No skin involvement or fixation of the tumor to the chest wall. Clinically palpable nodes, but <2.5 cm in transverse diameter and not fixed to overlying skin or deeper structures of the axilla.
Stage C	Any one of the five grave signs of advanced breast carcinoma: 1. Limited edema of the skin involving less than one third of the skin over the breast 2. Skin ulceration 3. Fixation of the tumor to the chest wall 4. Massive involvement of axillary lymph nodes measuring >2.5 cm in transverse diameter 5. Fixation of the axillary nodes to overlying skin or deeper structures of the axilla
Stage D	Any patients with signs of advanced breast carcinoma: 1. A combination of any two or more of the five grave signs listed under stage C 2. Extensive edema of the skin (involving more than one third of the skin over the breast) 3. Satellite skin nodules 4. The inflammatory type of carcinoma 5. Clinically involved supraclavicular lymph nodes 6. Internal mammary metastases as evidenced by a parasternal tumor 7. Edema of the arm 8. Distant metastases

From Haagensen CD: Clinical classification of the stage of advancement of breast carcinoma. In *Diseases of the breast,* Philadelphia, 1986, WB Saunders.

The TNM system for classification of malignant tumors was first conceived by Denoix in 1943.[97] In 1958 the International Union Against Cancer (UICC) described the first recommendations for the staging of breast cancer and for the presentation of results. Since then, four separate editions of the TNM manual for classification of malignant tumors have been published. Simultaneously, the American Joint Committee on Cancer (AJCC) has produced four editions of their *Manual for Staging of Cancer.* The proposals of the AJCC have undergone somewhat parallel and confluent evolutionary changes to those of the UICC, meaning that in 1987, for the first time, a truly universal staging system was developed. The current UICC[98] and AJCC[99] staging systems for breast cancer are now identical. This alliance will now permit collaboration in multiinstitutional trials on an international level.

Rationale Behind the TNM System

The TNM system was originally conceived to be a simple system that would classify patients into various groups, each with a different survival rate and prognosis. There were binary choices for each evaluable patient/tumor characteristic: T_0 represented the absence of tumor; T_1 represented the presence of tumor. Similarly, N_0/M_0 and N_1/M_1 represented the absence or presence of regional or distant metastatic disease. Thus using three different determinants (T, N, and M) with two possible choices (0 or 1), $2^3 (= 8)$ permutations were possible. Any patient could be rapidly classified into one of eight possible groups that could then be stratified into any number of stages based on observed survival frequencies. Such a classification system would have been simple, logical, and easy to commit to memory for future use.

Although the TNM system was originally simple in design, modifications were necessary to improve prognostic power and stage definition. A large number of clinical and pathologic prognostic indicators have been identified since the inception of the TNM system (see section on clinical and pathologic correlates with prognosis). The TNM staging system, to date, is the only system that has successfully incorporated many of these factors. For this reason, despite the observation that this method of staging for breast cancer is the most complicated, it is also highly practical and adaptable. It provides more prognostic information and better stratifies patients for the purpose of guiding therapy than do other systems that are based largely on clinical criteria alone.

The more precisely the clinician is able to define specific groups of patients who should undergo equivalent therapeutic regimens, the greater is the probability that medical scientists should be able to reduce the number of patients with aggressive disease who are undertreated and those with limited disease who are overtreated. As more and more prognostic indices are identified and successful therapeutic modalities discovered, more subcategories will be required; for this reason, binary choices have become quaternary (N_0, N_1, N_2, N_3) or greater (T_0, Tis, T_1, T_2, T_3, T_4). Further delineation within each subcategory has also been added.

CURRENT STAGING SYSTEM

Currently, the most popular staging system is the TNM system, based on the AJCC, sponsored by the American Cancer Society and the American College of Surgeons (ACS). Although the TNM system lacks simplicity, its gains in prognostic power and accuracy have never been surpassed. The updated version represents the culmination of many years of evolution of the AJCC and ACS. Despite these unified efforts, however, the current system will certainly undergo future changes. The best staging system will be flexible and continue to evolve with new prognostic data.

The current staging system requires microscopic confirmation and histologic typing of the tumor before attempting any stage classification. Any patient with documented breast cancer may then be staged by clinical (preoperative) or pathologic criteria (postoperative, designated by a "p" prefix).

The clinical-diagnostic staging process requires a complete physical examination, with determination of the extent of ipsilateral and contralateral neoplastic involvement of skin, breast tissue, regional and distant lymph nodes, and underlying muscles. The microscopic diagnosis of breast cancer must be confirmed by examination of breast tissue. Routine laboratory examinations, chest x-ray films, and bilateral mammograms are also recommended.

The pathologic classification uses all the data used in clinical staging; however, this more definitive staging system can be implemented only after the resection of the primary tumor and regional lymph nodes. It requires that no gross tumor be present at the margins of resection and that at least the level 1 axillary lymph nodes (usually six or more in number) be resected and histologically examined. Should tumor be present at the margins on gross examination of the resected specimen, the code T_X is applied, indicating that the pathologic stage cannot yet be determined. The current TNM staging system based on the sixth edition of the AJCC staging manual[99] is summarized in the following sections

T Stage (Tumor Size). Clinical tumor stage is the size of the tumor (reported in centimeters) based on the physical examination and various imaging modalities (e.g., mammogram, ultrasound, CT scans, MRI scans). The pathologic T stage is based on the tumor size on the final pathologic specimen measuring only the invasive component. For multiple synchronous ipsilateral primary carcinomas, the largest tumor is used for the T classification and the physician should document that there are multiple primaries with their corresponding sizes and characteristics. Bilateral synchronous breast cancers are staged separately as separate primaries (Table 20-12).

Tis includes ductal carcinoma in situ (DCIS), lobular carcinoma in situ (LCIS), or Paget's disease of the nipple with no invasive tumor. Paget's disease of the nipple with an associated invasive tumor is classified based on the invasive component. Although there is controversy regarding LCIS—whether this is a merely a marker for increased risk of developing breast cancer or a precursor of invasive lobular carcinoma—LCIS is reported as a malignancy. T_1 is designated for tumors that are 2 cm or smaller and subclassified as T_{1mic}, T_{1a}, T_{1b}, and T_{1c}. Microinvasive breast cancer is defined as a focus of tumor less than or equal to 0.1 cm in greatest dimension. When there are multiple foci of microinvasion, the T designation is based on the largest of the foci and not the additive sum of these. T_2 tumors are between 2 and 5 cm, and T_3 tumors larger than 5 cm. Tumors with direct invasion into the chest wall or skin are designated as T_4 tumors, with subclassification based on edema, skin ulceration, peau d'orange, or inflammation.

N Stage. Clinical nodal staging is based on physical examination or imaging studies, including CT scans and ultrasound but excluding lymphoscintigraphy. If the regional lymph nodes cannot be assessed clinically (previously removed or not removed for pathologic examination), they are designated N_X. If no regional lymph nodes are involved with tumor, it is designated as N_0. Categorization of clinical regional lymph node involvement is based on whether the lymph nodes are mobile (N_1) or fixed (N_{2a}) and evidence of involvement of the ipsilateral IMNs (N_{2b}) and ipsilateral infraclavicular lymph nodes (N_{3a}). Metastasis to ipsilateral IMNs in the presence of axillary nodal disease is classified as N_{3b}. Ipsilateral supraclavicular lymph node disease was considered to have a prognosis similar to that for patients with distant disease; however, the overall survival is better and was changed to stage N_{3c} in the revised 2002 AJCC staging system.

Sentinel lymph node biopsy techniques have dramatically changed the pathologic staging of patients with breast cancer. Patients are now being diagnosed at earlier tumor stages with the detection of microscopic and submicroscopic metastatic tumor deposits. This is reflected and incorporated into the revised 2002 AJCC pathologic staging system for the first time. This revised system also incorporates the assessment of microscopic disease based on IHC and molecular techniques (RT-PCR).

Pathologic staging of lymph nodes is based on biopsies taken from sentinel lymph node or complete axillary lymph node dissections. If the regional lymph nodes cannot be assessed pathologically (previously removed or not removed for pathologic examination),

TABLE **20-12**	AJCC TNM Clinical Staging System
T_X	Primary tumor cannot be assessed
T_0	No evidence of primary tumor
Tis	Carcinoma in situ
Tis (DCIS)	Ductal carcinoma in situ
Tis (LCIS)	Lobular carcinoma in situ
Tis Paget's disease	Paget's disease of the nipple with no tumor
T_1	Tumors ≤2 cm in greatest dimension
T_{1mic}	Microinvasion ≤0.1 cm in greatest dimension
T_{1a}	Tumor >0.5 cm but not more than 1 cm in greatest dimension
T_{1c}	Tumor >1 cm and not more than 2 cm in greatest dimension
T_2	Tumor >2 cm and not more than 5 cm in greatest dimension
T_3	Tumor >5 cm in greatest dimension
T_4	Tumor of any size with direct extension to (a) chest wall or (b) only as described below
T_{4a}	Extension to chest wall, not including pectoralis muscle
T_{4b}	Edema (including peau d'orange) or ulceration of the skin of the breast or satellite skin nodules confined to the same breast
T_{4c}	Both T_{4a} and T_{4ba}
T_{4d}	Inflammatory carcinoma

REGIONAL LYMPH NODES (N)

N_X	Regional lymph nodes cannot be assessed (e.g., previously removed)
N_0	No regional lymph node metastasis
N_1	Metastasis to movable axillary lymph node(s)
N_2	Metastasis in ipsilateral axillary lymph nodes fixed or matted, or clinically apparent ipsilateral internal mammary nodes in the absence of clinically evident axillary lymph node metastasis
N_{2a}	Metastasis to ipsilateral axillary lymph nodes fixed to one another (matted) or to other structures
N_{2b}	Metastasis only in clinically apparent ipsilateral internal mammary nodes and in the absence of clinically evident axillary lymph node metastasis
N_3	Metastasis in ipsilateral infraclavicular lymph node(s) or clinically apparent ipsilateral internal mammary node(s) and in the presence of clinically evident axillary lymph node metastasis; or metastasis in ipsilateral supraclavicular lymph node(s) with or without axillary or internal mammary lymph node involvement
N_{3a}	Metastasis in ipsilateral infraclavicular lymph node(s) and axillary lymph node(s)
N_{3b}	Metastasis in ipsilateral internal mammary node(s) and axillary lymph node(s)
N_{3c}	Metastasis in ipsilateral supraclavicular lymph node(s)

PATHOLOGIC CLASSIFICATION (PN)

pN_X	Regional lymph nodes cannot be assessed (e.g., previously removed or not removed for pathologic studies)
pN_0	No regional lymph node metastasis histologically, no additional examination for isolated tumor cells (ITC)

Note: ITC are defined as single tumor cells or small cell clusters not greater than 0.2 mm, usually detected with immunohistochemistry (IHC) or molecular methods but that may be verified with H&E stains. ITCs do not usually show evidence of metastatic activity (e.g., proliferation or stromal reaction).

$pN_0(i-)$	No regional lymph node metastasis histologically, negative IHC
$pN_0(i+)$	No regional lymph node metastasis histologically, positive IHC, no IHC cluster >0.2 mm
$pN_0(mol-)$	No regional lymph node metastasis histologically, negative molecular findings (RT-PCR)
$pN_0(mol+)$	No regional lymph node metastasis histologically, positive molecular findings (RT-PCR)
pN_{1mi}	Micrometastasis (>0.2 mm, none >2 mm)
pN_1	Metastasis in 1-3 axillary lymph nodes and/or in internal mammary nodes with microscopic disease detected by sentinel lymph node dissection but not clinically apparent
pN_{1a}	Metastasis in 1-3 axillary lymph nodes

| TABLE 20-12 | AJCC TNM Clinical Staging System—cont'd |

PATHOLOGIC CLASSIFICATION (PN)—cont'd

pN_{1b}	Metastasis in internal mammary lymph nodes with microscopic disease detected with sentinel lymph node dissection but not clinically apparent
pN_{1c}	Metastasis in 1-3 axillary lymph nodes and in internal mammary lymph nodes with microscopic disease detected with sentinel lymph node dissection but not clinically apparent (if associated with >3 positive axillary lymph nodes, the internal mammary nodes are classified as pN_{3b} to reflect increased tumor burden)
pN_2	Metastasis in 4-9 axillary lymph nodes or in clinically apparent internal mammary lymph nodes in the absence of axillary lymph node metastasis
pN_{2a}	Metastasis in 4-9 lymph nodes (at least 1 tumor deposit >2.0 mm)
pN_{2b}	Metastasis in clinically apparent internal mammary lymph nodes in the absence of axillary lymph node metastasis
pN_3	Metastasis to ≥10 axillary lymph nodes, in infraclavicular lymph nodes, or in clinically apparent ipsilateral internal mammary lymph nodes in the presence of ≥1 positive axillary lymph nodes; or in ≥3 axillary lymph nodes with clinically negative microscopic metastasis in internal mammary lymph nodes; or in ipsilateral supraclavicular lymph nodes
pN_{3a}	Metastasis in ≥10 axillary lymph nodes (at least 1 tumor deposit >2.0 mm) or metastasis to the infraclavicular lymph nodes
pN_{3b}	Metastasis in clinically apparent ipsilateral internal mammary lymph nodes in the presence of ≥1 positive axillary lymph nodes; or in >3 axillary lymph nodes and in internal mammary lymph nodes with microscopic disease detected with sentinel lymph node dissection but not clinically apparent
pN_{3c}	Metastasis in ipsilateral supraclavicular lymph nodes

DISTANT METASTASIS (M)

M_X	Distant metastasis cannot be assessed
M_0	No distant metastasis
M_1	Distant metastasis

H&E, Hematoxylin and eosin; *RT-PCR,* reverse transcriptase polymerize chain reaction.

they are designated pN_X. If no regional lymph nodes are involved with tumor, it is designated as pN_0. Further subclassification of pN_0 allows the distinction between the identification of microscopic cells based on IHC or molecular techniques (RT-PCR). Isolated tumor cells (ITCs) are defined as single tumor cells or small clusters not greater than 0.2 mm, usually detected with IHC or molecular methods but that may be verified on H&E stains. ITCs usually show no evidence of metastatic activity. Pathologic node positivity is based on the number of lymph nodes involved (pN). pN_1 is divided into four categories, including pN_{1mic} (>0.2 mm, <2.0 mm), pN_1 (1 to 3 positive nodes, microscopic IMNs positive as determined with sentinel lymph node dissection), pN_2 (4 to 9 positive nodes, positive IMNs with at least one tumor deposit greater than 2.0 mm), and pN_3 (more than 10 nodes, or positive infraclavicular lymph nodes or both internal mammary and axillary nodes positive). In the previous AJCC 1997 staging system, the designation of fixed, matted nodes were separate categories. In the revised AJCC 2002 staging system, there is not a distinction for fixed or matted lymph nodes.

One of the major changes in the revised staging system was to subclassify internal mammary nodal metastasis. This is, for the most part, dependent on sentinel lymph node biopsies, because small metastatic tumor burden within the IMNs is difficult to detect clinically and routine IMN dissection is not performed. IMN disease without evidence of axillary disease is designated as pN_{1b} and pN_{1c} with the presence of synchronous axillary disease.

M Stage. Distant metastatic disease is designated as M_1 disease. Ipsilateral supraclavicular lymph node disease is no longer considered distant metastatic disease but rather locally advanced disease (N_3). Evidence of metastatic disease may be based on clinical history and physical examination, with or without the assistance of various imaging modalities and biochemical markers.

Stage Grouping. There are five stage groupings (O, I, II, III, and IV) in the new TNM staging system, with stage II being subdivided into A and B and stage III into A, B, and C (Table 20-13). Stage O (Tis N_0 M_0) refers

TABLE 20-13 Stage Grouping

Stage 0	$T_{is} N_0 M_0$
Stage I	$T_1^* N_0 M_0$
Stage IIA	$T_0 N_1 M_0$
	$T_1^* N_1 M_0$
	$T_2 N_0 M_0$
Stage IIB	$T_2 N_1 M_0$
	$T_3 N_0 M_0$
Stage IIIA	$T_0 N_2 M_0$
	$T_1^* N_2 M_0$
	$T_2 N_2 M_0$
	$T_3 N_1 M_0$
	$T_3 N_2 M_0$
Stage IIIB	$T_4 N_0 M_0$
	$T_4 N_1 M_0$
	$T_4 N_2 M_0$
Stage IIIC	Any T $N_3 M_0$
Stage IV	Any T Any N M_1

*T_1 includes T_{1mic}.

to preinvasive cancers (carcinoma in situ) that have not penetrated the basement membrane or the ductule or lobule. There are no regional or distant metastasis, and the prognosis is excellent, nearly 100% curable. Stage I ($T_{1mic} N_0 M_0$) refers to tumors that are micrometastatic; these patients also have an excellent prognosis. Stage I cancers are localized to the breast and are small. Stage IIA ($T_0 N_1, M_0, T_{1mic} N_1 M_0, T_2 N_0 M_0$) and stage IIB ($T_2 N_1 M_0, T_3 N_0 M_0$) are reserved for cases with regional lymph node metastases and carry a worse prognosis. Stage IIIA ($T_0 N_2 M_0, T_1 N_2 M_0, T_2 N_2 M_0, T_3 N_1 M_0, T_3 N_2 M_0$), stage IIIB ($T_4 N_0 M_0, T_4 N_1 M_0, T_4 N_2 M_0$), and stage IIIC (any T $N_3 M_0$) refer to larger tumors that are locally advanced and a worse prognosis. Stage IV (any T any N M_1) refers to distant systemic spread of disease with a significantly poor survival (Figure 20-5).

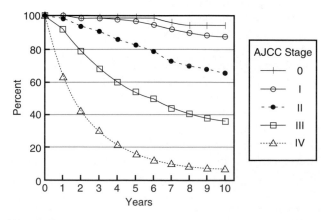

FIG. 20-5 The relative survival for breast cancer patients according to the American Joint Committee on Cancer (AJCC) stage group. (From Bland KI et al: Cancer 86:1262, 1998.)

TABLE 20-14 Histopathologic Grading System

G_X	Grade cannot be assessed
G_1	Low combined histologic grade (favorable)
G_2	Intermediate combined histologic grade (moderately favorable)
G_3	High combined histologic grade (unfavorable)

Histopathologic Grade. The AJCC recommended histologic grading system is based on the Nottingham combined histologic grade[100,101] (Table 20-14). The grade "G" of the tumor is designated based on the morphologic features of the primary tumor (tubule formation, nuclear pleomorphism, and mitotic count) by assigning a value of 1 to 3 (1, favorable; 3, unfavorable). The scores are added together for each feature. Grade 1 tumors have a combined score of 3 to 5 points; grade 2, 6 to 7 points; and grade 3, 8 to 9 points. Primary tumors may also be assigned to one of the three basic histopathologic types (ductal, lobular, or nipple) (Table 20-15).

Future Trends

Detection of circulating tumor cells in the bone marrow[102-104] and the peripheral blood using IHC

TABLE 20-15 Histopathologic Types

IN SITU CARCINOMAS
NOS (not otherwise specified)
Intraductal
Papillary intraductal, noninfiltrating
Paget's disease and intraductal

INVASIVE CARCINOMAS
NOS (not otherwise specified)
Ductal
Inflammatory
Medullary, NOS
Medullary with lymphoid stroma
Mucinous
Papillary (dominantly micropapillary pattern)
Tubular
Lobular
Paget's disease and infiltrating
Undifferentiated
Squamous
Adenoid cystic
Secretory
Cribriform

methods or RT-PCR and real-time RT-PCR techniques may be useful as a prognostic indicator in breast cancer. New technology using microarray analysis for gene expression allows screening of large numbers of expressed genes, more than 30,000 in one experiment. This powerful tool not only is useful in identifying the important genes that are responsible for the malignant potential of a cell, but has a variety of applications. Gene expression profiles can be used to predict prognosis and to classify tumors in a manner that is distinct from the standard method of histopathology.[105] In breast cancer, it has been shown that gene expression profiles are valuable tools for accurately predicting the clinical status, such as ER status and lymph node status.[106] Furthermore, the ability to assess and predict the axillary nodal status of a patient with breast cancer based on the gene expression of the primary tumor could potentially obviate the need to perform lymph node dissections. Proteomics is a novel, powerful approach in identifying differential protein expression in tumor cells. Used together with gene expression analysis, this new technology may allow the molecular classification of tumors and may dramatically improve our current methodology of predicting prognosis in patients with breast cancer.[107,108]

REFERENCES

1. McGuire WL, Clark GM: Prognostic factors and treatment decisions in axillary-node-negative breast cancer, *N Engl J Med* 326:1756, 1992.
2. Koscielny S et al: Breast cancer: relationship between the size of the primary tumour and the probability of metastatic dissemination, *Br J Cancer* 49:709, 1984.
3. Fisher B, Slack NH, Bross ID: Cancer of the breast: size of neoplasm and prognosis, *Cancer* 24:1071, 1969.
4. Carter CL, Allen C, Henson DE: Relation of tumor size, lymph node status, and survival in 24,740 breast cancer cases, *Cancer* 63:181, 1989.
5. Nemoto T et al: Management and survival of female breast cancer: results of a national survey by the American College of Surgeons, *Cancer* 45:2917, 1980.
6. Fisher ER: Prognostic and therapeutic significance of pathological features of breast cancer, *NCI Monogr* 29, 1986.
7. Rosen PP, Groshen S, Kinne DW: Survival and prognostic factors in node-negative breast cancer: results of long-term follow-up studies, *J Natl Cancer Inst Monogr* 11:159, 1992.
8. Mirza AN et al: Prognostic factors in node-negative breast cancer: a review of studies with sample size more than 200 and follow-up more than 5 years, *Ann Surg* 235:10, 2002.
9. Fisher B et al: Location of breast carcinoma and prognosis, *Surg Gynecol Obstet* 129:705, 1969.
10. Nemoto T et al: Breast cancer in the medial half: results of 1978 National Survey of the American College of Surgeons, *Cancer* 51:1333, 1983.
11. Lohrisch C et al: Relationship between tumor location and relapse in 6,781 women with early invasive breast cancer, *J Clin Oncol* 18:2828, 2000.
12. Zucali R et al: Early breast cancer: evaluation of the prognostic role of the site of the primary tumor, *J Clin Oncol* 16:1363, 1998.
13. *WHO International Histological Classification of Tumors N: histologic typing of breast tumors,* Geneva, 1981, World Health Organization.
14. Vana J et al: American College of Surgeons Commission on Cancer: final report on long-term patient care evaluation study for carcinoma of the female breast, *Am Coll Surg* 1979.
15. Hutter RV: The influence of pathologic factors on breast cancer management, *Cancer* 46(suppl 4):961, 1980.
16. Hoge AF et al: Histologic and staging classification of breast cancer: implications for therapy, *South Med J* 75:1329, 1982.
17. Bloom H, Richardson W: Histologic grading and prognosis in breast cancer: a study of 1409 cases of which 359 have been followed 15 years, *Br J Cancer* 11:359, 1957.
18. Black M, Speer F: Nuclear structure in cancer tissues, *Surg Gynecol Obstet* 105:97, 1957.
19. Fisher ER et al: Detection and significance of occult axillary node metastases in patients with invasive breast cancer, *Cancer* 42:2025, 1978.
20. Fisher ER et al: The pathology of invasive breast cancer: a syllabus derived from findings of the National Surgical Adjuvant Breast Project (Protocol No. 4), *Cancer* 36:1, 1975.
21. Knight WA et al: Estrogen receptor as an independent prognostic factor for early recurrence in breast cancer, *Cancer Res* 37:4669, 1977.
22. Stewart J, Rubens R: General prognostic factors. In Bonadonna G (ed): *Breast cancer: diagnosis and management,* Chichester, 1984, John Wiley.
23. Osborne CK, McGuire WL: Current use of steroid hormone receptor assays in the treatment of breast cancer, *Surg Clin North Am* 58:777, 1978.
24. Pichon MF et al: Relationship of presence of progesterone receptors to prognosis in early breast cancer, *Cancer Res* 40:3357, 1980.
25. Charlson ME, Feinstein AR: A new clinical index of growth rate in the staging of breast cancer, *Am J Med* 69:527, 1980.
26. Gershon-Cohen J, Berger S, Klickstein H: Roentgenography of breast cancer moderating the concept of biologic predeterminism, *Cancer* 16:961, 1963.
27. Lee Y: The lognormal distribution of growth rates of soft tissue metastases of breast cancer, *J Surg Oncol* 4:81, 1972.
28. Phillippe E, Gal YL: Growth of 78 recurrent mammary carcinomas, *Cancer* 21:461, 1968.
29. Heuser LS et al: The association of pathologic and mammographic characteristics of primary human breast cancers with "slow" and "fast" growth rates and with axillary lymph node metastases, *Cancer* 53:96, 1984.
30. Tubiana M et al: The long-term prognostic significance of the thymidine labelling index in breast cancer, *Int J Cancer* 33:441, 1984.
31. Schwartz GF, Feig SA, Patchefsky AS: Significance and staging of nonpalpable carcinomas of the breast, *Surg Gynecol Obstet* 166:6, 1988.
32. Ewers SB et al: Flow-cytometric DNA analysis in primary breast carcinomas and clinicopathological correlations, *Cytometry* 5:408, 1984.
33. Hedley DW, Friedlander ML, Taylor IW: Application of DNA flow cytometry to paraffin-embedded archival material for the study of aneuploidy and its clinical significance, *Cytometry* 6:327, 1985.
34. Moran RE et al: Correlation of cell-cycle kinetics, hormone receptors, histopathology, and nodal status in human breast cancer, *Cancer* 54:1586, 1984.

35. Clark GM et al: Prediction of relapse or survival in patients with node negative breast cancer by DNA flow cytometry, *N Engl J Med* 320:627, 1989.

36. Buckman R et al: Some clinical uses of biologic markers. In Bonadonna G (ed): *Breast cancer: diagnosis and management,* Chichester, 1984, John Wiley.

37. Redding WH et al: Detection of micrometastasis in patients with primary breast cancer, *Lancet* 2:1271, 1983.

38. Hillyard JW et al: Biochemical aids to the staging of breast cancer, *Clin Biochem* 15:9, 1982.

39. Cline MJ, Battifora H, Yokota J: Proto-oncogene abnormalities in human breast cancer: correlations with anatomic features and clinical course of disease, *J Clin Oncol* 5:999, 1987.

40. Berger MS et al: Correlation of c-erbB-2 gene amplification and protein expression in human breast carcinoma with nodal status and nuclear grading, *Cancer Res* 48:1238, 1988.

41. Slamon DJ et al: Human breast cancer: correlation of relapse and survival with amplification of the *HER-2/neu* oncogene, *Science* 235:177, 1987.

42. Varley JM et al: Alterations to either c-erbB-2(neu) or c-myc proto-oncogenes in breast carcinomas correlate with poor short-term prognosis, *Oncogene* 1:423, 1987.

43. Bland KI et al: Oncogene protein co-expression: value of Ha-ras, c-myc, c-fos, and p53 as prognostic discriminants for breast carcinoma, *Ann Surg* 221:706, 1985.

44. Halstead WS: A clinical and histologic study of certain adenocarcinoma of the breast and a brief consideration of the supraclavicular operation and of the results of operation for cancer of the breast from 1889 to 1898 at the Johns Hopkins Hospital, *Ann Surg* 28:557, 1898.

45. Fisher B et al: Ten-year results of a randomized clinical trial comparing radical mastectomy and total mastectomy with or without radiation, *N Engl J Med* 312:674, 1985.

46. Cancer Research Campaign (King's/Cambridge) trial for early breast cancer: a detailed update at the tenth year. Cancer Research Campaign Working Party, *Lancet* 2:55, 1980.

47. Bonadonna G: Evolving concepts in the systemic adjuvant treatment of breast cancer, *Cancer Res* 52:2127, 1992.

48. Fisher B, Slack NH: Number of lymph nodes examined and the prognosis of breast carcinoma, *Surg Gynecol Obstet* 131:79, 1970.

49. Wallace IW, Champion HR: Axillary nodes in breast cancer, *Lancet* 1:692, 1972.

50. Fisher B et al: The accuracy of clinical nodal staging and of limited axillary dissection as a determinant of histologic nodal status in carcinoma of the breast, *Surg Gynecol Obstet* 152:765, 1981.

51. Fisher B, Fisher ER, Redmond C: Ten-year results from the National Surgical Adjuvant Breast and Bowel Project (NSABP) clinical trial evaluating the use of L-phenylalanine mustard (L-PAM) in the management of primary breast cancer, *J Clin Oncol* 4:929, 1986.

52. Diab SG et al: Radiation therapy and survival in breast cancer patients with 10 or more positive axillary lymph nodes treated with mastectomy, *J Clin Oncol* 16:1655, 1998.

53. Jatoi I et al: Significance of axillary lymph node metastasis in primary breast cancer, *J Clin Oncol* 17:2334, 1999.

54. Adair F et al: Long term follow-up of breast cancer patients: the 30 year report, *Cancer* 33:1145, 1974.

55. Davies GC, Millis RR, Hayward JL: Assessment of axillary lymph node status, *Ann Surg* 192:148, 1980.

56. Boova RS, Bonanni R, Rosato FE: Patterns of axillary nodal involvement in breast cancer: predictability of level one dissection, *Ann Surg* 196:642, 1982.

57. Albertini JJ et al: Intraoperative radio-lympho-scintigraphy improves sentinel lymph node identification for patients with melanoma, *Ann Surg* 223:217, 1996.

58. Morton DL et al: Technical details of intraoperative lymphatic mapping for early stage melanoma, *Arch Surg* 127:392, 1992.

59. Ross MI, Reintgen D, Balch CM: Selective lymphadenectomy: emerging role for lymphatic mapping and sentinel node biopsy in the management of early stage melanoma, *Semin Surg Oncol* 9:219, 1993.

60. Reintgen DS: Emerging evidence for a survival benefit associated with regional lymph node dissection for melanoma, *Ann Surg Oncol* 7:75, 2000.

61. Albertini JJ et al: Lymphatic mapping and sentinel node biopsy in the patient with breast cancer, *JAMA* 276:1818, 1996.

62. Ivens D et al: Assessment of morbidity from complete axillary dissection, *Br J Cancer* 66:136, 1992.

63. Krag DN et al: Surgical resection and radiolocalization of the sentinel lymph node in breast cancer using a gamma probe, *Surg Oncol* 2:335, 1993.

64. Giuliano AE et al: Lymphatic mapping and sentinel lymphadenectomy for breast cancer, *Ann Surg* 220:391, 1994.

65. Borgstein PJ et al: Sentinel lymph node biopsy in breast cancer: guidelines and pitfalls of lymphoscintigraphy and gamma probe detection, *J Am Coll Surg* 186:275, 1998.

66. Veronesi U et al: Sentinel-node biopsy to avoid axillary dissection in breast cancer with clinically negative lymph-nodes, *Lancet* 349:1864, 1997.

67. Kern KA: Sentinel lymph node mapping in breast cancer using subareolar injection of blue dye, *J Am Coll Surg* 189:539, 1999.

68. Giuliano AE et al: Sentinel lymphadenectomy in breast cancer, *J Clin Oncol* 15:2345, 1997.

69. Cox CE et al: Lymphatic mapping in the treatment of breast cancer, *Oncology (Huntingt)* 12:1283, 1998.

70. Giuliano AE et al: Prospective observational study of sentinel lymphadenectomy without further axillary dissection in patients with sentinel node-negative breast cancer, *J Clin Oncol* 18:2553, 2000.

71. Cote RJ et al: Role of immunohistochemical detection of lymph-node metastases in management of breast cancer: International Breast Cancer Study Group, *Lancet* 354:896, 1999.

72. Hainsworth PJ et al: Detection and significance of occult metastases in node-negative breast cancer, *Br J Surg* 80:459, 1993.

73. Hsueh EC, Giuliano AE: Sentinel lymph node technique for staging of breast cancer, *Oncologist* 3:165, 1998.

74. Turner RR et al: Histopathologic validation of the sentinel lymph node hypothesis for breast carcinoma, *Ann Surg* 226:271, 1997.

75. van Diest PJ et al: Pathological investigation of sentinel lymph nodes, *Eur J Nucl Med* 26(suppl 4):S43, 1999.

76. Schreiber RH et al: Microstaging of breast cancer patients using cytokeratin staining of the sentinel lymph node, *Ann Surg Oncol* 6:95, 1999.

77. Shivers SC et al: Molecular staging of malignant melanoma: correlation with clinical outcome, *JAMA* 280:1410, 1998.

78. Li W et al: Clinical relevance of molecular staging for melanoma: comparison of RT-PCR and immunohistochemistry staining in sentinel lymph nodes of patients with melanoma, *Ann Surg* 231:795, 2000.

79. Veronesi U et al: Risk of internal mammary lymph node metastases and its relevance on prognosis of breast cancer patients, *Ann Surg* 198:681, 1983.

80. Cody HS III, Urban JA: Internal mammary node status: a major prognosticator in axillary node-negative breast cancer, *Ann Surg Oncol* 2:32, 1995.

81. Sugg SL et al: Should internal mammary nodes be sampled in the sentinel lymph node era? *Ann Surg Oncol* 7:188, 2000.

82. Veronesi U et al: The dissection of internal mammary nodes does not improve the survival of breast cancer patients: 30-year results of a randomised trial, *Eur J Cancer* 35:1320, 1999.

83. Morrow M, Foster RS Jr: Staging of breast cancer: a new rationale for internal mammary node biopsy, *Arch Surg* 116:748, 1981.

84. Kiricuta IC et al: The prognostic significance of the supraclavicular lymph node metastases in breast cancer patients, *Int J Radiat Oncol Biol Phys* 28:387, 1994.

85. Debois JM: The significance of a supraclavicular node metastasis in patients with breast cancer: a literature review, *Strahlenther Onkol* 173:1, 1997.

86. Brito RA et al: Long-term results of combined-modality therapy for locally advanced breast cancer with ipsilateral supraclavicular metastases: The University of Texas M.D. Anderson Cancer Center experience, *J Clin Oncol* 19:628, 2001.

87. Papaioannou A, Urban J: Scalene node biopsy in locally advanced primary breast cancer of questionable operability, *Cancer* 17:1006, 1964.

88. Wilkinson E, Lawrence H: Probability of lymph node sectioning, *Cancer* 33:1269, 1974.

89. Mambo N, Gallagher H: Carcinoma of the breast: the prognostic significance of extranodal extension of axillary disease, *Cancer* 320:485, 1977.

90. Pierce LJ et al: Microscopic extracapsular extension in the axilla: is this an indication for axillary radiotherapy? *Int J Radiat Oncol Biol Phys* 33:253, 1995.

91. Steinthal C: Dauerheilung des brustkrebses, *Beitr Z Klin Chir* 47:226, 1905.

92. Lee B, Stubenbord J: Clinical index of malignancy for carcinoma of the breast, *Surg Gynecol Obstet* 47:812, 1928.

93. Patterson R: *Treatment of malignant diseases by radium and x-rays*, London, 1948, Edward Arnold.

94. Portman U: Clinical and pathological criteria as a basis for classifying cases of primary cancer of the breast, *Cleve Clin Q* 10:41, 1943.

95. Haagensen C, Stout A: Carcinoma of the breast: criteria for operability, *Ann Surg* 118:859, 1943.

96. Haagensen C et al: Treatment of early mammary carcinoma: a cooperative international study, *Ann Surg* 170:875, 1969.

97. Denoix P: *Bull Inst Nat Hyg (Paris)* 1:1, 1944.

98. Hermanek P, Sobin L (eds): *UICC TNM classification of malignant tumors*, ed 4, Berlin, 1987, Springer-Verlag.

99. Beahrs O, Hensen D, Hutter R (eds): *American Joint Committee on Cancer: manual for staging breast cancer*, Philadelphia, 1992, JB Lippincott.

100. Elston CW, Ellis IO: Pathological prognostic factors in breast cancer. I. The value of histological grade in breast cancer: experience from a large study with long-term follow-up, *Histopathology* 19:403, 1991.

101. Fitzgibbons PL et al: Prognostic factors in breast cancer: College of American Pathologists Consensus Statement 1999, *Arch Pathol Lab Med* 124:966, 2000.

102. Funke I, Schraut W: Meta-analyses of studies on bone marrow micrometastases: an independent prognostic impact remains to be substantiated, *J Clin Oncol* 16:557, 1998.

103. Relihan N et al: Combined sentinel lymph-node mapping and bone-marrow micrometastatic analysis for improved staging in breast cancer, *Lancet* 354:129, 1999.

104. Schlimok G et al: Micrometastatic cancer cells in bone marrow: in vitro detection with anti-cytokeratin and in vivo labeling with anti-17-1A monoclonal antibodies, *Proc Natl Acad Sci USA* 84:8672, 1987.

105. Sorlie T et al: Gene expression patterns of breast carcinomas distinguish tumor subclasses with clinical implications, *Proc Natl Acad Sci USA* 98:10869, 2001.

106. West M et al: Predicting the clinical status of human breast cancer by using gene expression profiles, *Proc Natl Acad Sci USA* 98:11462, 2001.

107. Hondermarck H et al: Proteomics of breast cancer for marker discovery and signal pathway profiling, *Proteomics* 1:1216, 2001.

108. Wulfkuhle JD et al: New approaches to proteomic analysis of breast cancer, *Proteomics* 1:1205, 2001.

IX

PROGNOSTIC FACTORS FOR BREAST CANCER

CHAPTER

21

Clinically Established Prognostic Factors in Breast Cancer

WILLIAM C. WOOD

TONCRED M. STYBLO

Chapter Outline

Prognostic factors have grown in importance as the options for the treatment of breast cancer have increased. By definition, *prognostic factors* (Table 21-1) are quantifiable data about the tumor or host that provide information about the expected outcome of a population of patients with similar defining characteristics in the absence of systemic therapy. Several facts that follow from this definition are often overlooked in clinical medicine. The first is that the prognostic value, which may be clearly defined for a population, bears only limited application to any individual within that population. Patients should not be terrorized by membership in a high-risk population, nor should they be made to feel invincible by membership in a favorable risk group. The second fact is that with the broad application of systemic therapy, less and less information will become available about prognostic factors in the absence of such therapy. The best example of a prognostic factor is lymph node status, the degree to which the axillary lymph nodes have been colonized by metastatic breast cancer.[1-5]

Some parameters of a tumor that were measured and originally described as prognostic factors are now considered primarily *predictive factors* (see Table 21-1). The best example of a predictive factor is estrogen receptor (ER) status. It is of great clinical importance as a predictor of response to hormonal therapy. Certain tumor parameters, such as hormone receptor status, are both prognostic factors and predictive factors and may be considered separately for their contributions to each of these areas.

In the past, prognostic indicators were valued both for their ability to offer a glimpse of risk—desired by both the patient and the physician—and in a related way, the importance of systemic adjuvant therapy. Prognostic factors can be used to define a population of patients at so little risk of progression or recurrence of breast cancer that systemic therapy may be avoided.[6,7] This is recognized as increasingly important now that the series of overviews from the Early Breast Cancer Trialists' Collaborative Group have demonstrated that

the *relative* value of adjuvant therapy applies to all women with breast cancer.[8-11] Only those with truly minimal risk can be dismissed from consideration because the *absolute* benefit is so small. On the other hand, studies of the adverse effects of adjuvant therapy that were initially focused on dose-limiting toxicities are beginning to quantify other toxicities, such as neurocognitive dysfunction associated with cytotoxic chemotherapy.[12-14] With the recognition that an improvement in survival accruing to 2% to 3% of certain subgroups may be achieved at a cost of toxicity accruing to 20% or more of the patients, the need for more precise prognostic factors has grown. Can we divide the most favorable groups of women into those at greater and lesser risk in the future? And of at least as great importance, can we identify predictive factors that will allow us to determine—independent of risk—whether the contemplated therapy will be effective against her tumor?

Clinically established prognostic factors are those that meet the following criteria:

- Are reproducibly associated with a better or worse prognosis at a level of clinical utility
- Provide independent information not available by more easily measured parameters (this requires multivariate analysis with other established factors)
- Are reproducible in multiple clinics or laboratories
- Have demonstrated prognostic value in prospective trials

The literature of prognostic and predictive factors is replete with retrospective analysis of data sets. Although these are useful in generating hypotheses, any of multiple parameters may relate to outcome by play of chance in a given data set. If the data set is large, the statistical significance value of such chance associations may appear great. It is only when evaluated prospectively, at best, or in multiple other data sets retrospectively, that prognostic value may be validated. Of such prognostic values, some may be associated with other values, such as nodal status or tumor size. Unless significant additional prognostic information is added, as evaluated with multivariate statistical methods, they lack clinical utility.

The two best-established prognostic factors form the basis of clinical and pathologic staging as discussed in Chapter 20. Both nodal status and tumor size represent a summation of biologic effects in both the host and tumor that relate to the rate of tumor progression and the time from the initiation of the tumor or the development of its blood supply. Thus a very indolent cancer biologically, long undetected, may present at an identical stage to an extremely biologically aggressive tumor present for a lesser time. Other prognostic factors, such

TABLE 21-1	Prognostic and Predictive Factors for Breast Cancer

STANDARD PROGNOSTIC FACTORS
Lymph node status
Tumor size
Histologic grade
Age
PREDICTIVE FACTORS
Estrogen and/or progesterone receptor status
HER2 overexpression

as markers of proliferation, may distinguish between these two scenarios in a specific individual.

The most powerful adjuvant therapy demonstrated to date—tamoxifen in a receptor-positive individual—achieved only a 50% reduction in annual risk of recurrence.[10] Although the ability to identify individuals who lack ERs or progesterone receptors (PRs) and who will consequently not benefit at all from tamoxifen therapy is a great triumph, greater still will be the ability to define predictive factors that will identify the responders from the nonresponders in the receptor-positive population. This is even more true in the case of cytotoxic chemotherapy.[6,15] Dose-dense therapy is associated with greater population benefit than less intensive chemotherapy in clinical adjuvant trials. Certain data suggest that this benefit accrues from a subpopulation of individuals who require this greater dose density and that many other individuals would do as well with less aggressive chemotherapy.[6,15] Predictive factors that will reproducibly define these subpopulations are the subject of active investigation.

Prognostic Factors

AXILLARY LYMPH NODES

The degree of involvement of axillary lymph nodes by metastatic tumor cells is the dominant prognostic factor for later systemic disease.[2] Oncologists believe that virtually all women with axillary lymph node involvement should receive adjuvant systemic therapy.[16-18] Other prognostic factors and combinations of such factors have repeatedly been shown to be of equal or greater value in a given retrospective database, but when such factors or combination of factors have been tested prospectively, axillary lymph node status has been shown to be more predictive. This is understandable because any parameters of the primary tumor are surrogates for the likelihood of metastatic involvement. The potential for metastatic spread also depends on interaction with host resistance. Axillary lymph node status reflects actual end-results data on the interaction between tumor aggressiveness and host defense mechanisms. Therefore it is not surprising that it provides the most important prognostic measure available in clinical decision making.

Clinical staging of axillary lymph nodes is notoriously inaccurate: The difference is 33% in clinical evaluation of axillary nodes, even by experienced clinicians. Cutler and Connelly[19] found that among patients who have clinically negative nodes, 38% had evidence of nodal metastases on pathologic examination and in those who had clinically suspicious nodes, the nodes were pathologically negative 38% of the time. Fisher and colleagues reported that the false-positive and

false-negative clinical evaluation rates for axillary nodes were 24% and 39%, respectively, and the overall error in clinical staging was 32%.[20,21] Smart, Myers, and Gloeckler[22] reported that 35% of clinically negative lymph nodes had metastases detected on pathologic examination, and 87% of those considered clinically positive contained metastases. Because the clinical staging of axillary nodes is so inaccurate and accurate staging is so important, histopathologic axillary lymph node staging is necessary to stage patients accurately and assign population risks for considering adjuvant therapy. To avoid the consequences of axillary dissection for those with negative axillae, a variety of radiologic and nuclear medicine techniques for diagnosis have been attempted. They have all proved less than accurate in predicting the presence or absence of small axillary nodal metastases, even though some of the techniques (e.g., positron emission tomography) may surpass clinical examination in accuracy. The use of sentinel lymph node biopsy to limit axillary dissection in those with nodal metastases has revolutionized axillary lymph node staging.

The adoption of sentinel lymph node biopsy has, however, introduced other areas of controversy in prognostic factor research. The first issue concerns the additional value of the number of involved lymph nodes in planning adjuvant systemic therapy. If a patient has a clinically node positive, the risk of systemic failure is roughly 70% at 10 years.[23] Independent of the question of control of axillary disease is the question of additional prognostic information related to the number of involved lymph nodes. Clinical trials are under way to better define this question.

The identification of a limited number of sentinel lymph nodes invited a focused pathologic examination of these nodes. This has included multiple histologic sections (versus one or two),[24] the use of immunohistochemistry (IHC) with cytokeratin stains to identify tiny foci of breast cancer cells that escape notice on hematoxylin and eosin (H&E) staining,[25,26] and the use of polymerase chain reaction (PCR) to search for "breast cancer RNA" in these lymph nodes. Complicating this question is the pervasive use of core needle biopsy for diagnosis with the introduction of tumor cell clumps into local lymphatics. This has been demonstrated to lead to *in transit* cell clumps in the subcapsular spaces of axillary lymph nodes. Although this is clearly different than an established metastasis in an axillary lymph node, it may also reflect tumor volume, lack of tumor cellular adhesion, or other factors that may be of prognostic influence.

Micrometastases to axillary lymph nodes, defined as metastases less than 2 mm in diameter, have been found in some studies to have the same prognostic significance as negative nodes.[3,27,28] Other authors have suggested a worse prognosis.[29-31] However, any difference in outcome between the populations is not dramatic and calls into question whether this is additional prognostic information that should influence individual therapeutic decision making. Cells seen in lymph nodes with IHC but not with H&E are similarly of uncertain significance. The present consensus is that axillary micrometastases identified only with IHC should be noted but that the patient be staged as "node negative." Any such clinical consensus is fragile.

Because virtually all women with axillary lymph nodes involved by breast cancer metastases will be offered adjuvant systemic therapy, it is in advising node-negative patients concerning adjuvant therapy decisions that all the other prognostic and predictive factors are considered.

TUMOR SIZE

Tumor size is probably the most important single, secondary prognostic factor for risk of recurrence and consequent benefit from systemic therapy in axillary node–negative breast cancer. Tumor size also affects axillary node involvement: Axillary nodes were involved in 15% of patients with tumors smaller than 1.1 cm in diameter and in 60% of those with tumors 5.5 cm in diameter or larger. Small tumors associated with positive nodes had a better prognosis than large tumors with positive nodes. Survival decreased with increasing tumor size in all node categories (Figure 21-1).[32] There is a clear relationship between the size of the primary tumor and recurrence and survival rates. Tumor size 1 cm or smaller was associated with a very favorable prognosis in studies by Rosen and colleagues[28] and Carter, Allen, and Henson.[33] Subsequent

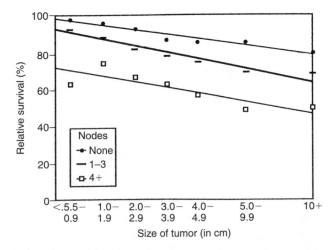

FIG. 21-1 Invasive female breast cancer. Five-year relative survival rates by tumor size and number of positive regional lymph nodes, excluding cases with further extension or distant metastasis. SEER 1977 to 1982.

studies have reinforced the importance of a prognostic break at 1 cm for node-negative tumors with 98% to 99% distant disease-free outcomes.[7,34] Node-negative patients with tumors 1 cm or smaller should receive adjuvant systemic therapy only on investigative protocols. Patients with tumors larger than 2 cm benefit significantly from adjuvant therapy, and those with tumors measuring 1 to 2 cm should be evaluated for risks and benefits based on careful examination of other prognostic factors.

HISTOLOGIC GRADING SYSTEM

Histolopathologic analysis is based on individual characteristics such as nuclear grade, gland formation (e.g., tumor grading), or the clustering of various cytologic and histologic features into special types of breast carcinoma. Several histologic grading systems have been described and have prognostic value in the evaluation of breast carcinoma. Two commonly used grading systems were those of Scarff, Blume, Richardson, and Fisher and co-workers.[35] Both evaluated architectural arrangement of cells or tubule formation, degree of nuclear differentiation, and mitotic rate, although each system used distinct and differently weighted histologic criteria. These grading systems have been shown to be poorly reproducible and to have marked interobserver variation. Today the Nottingham combined histologic grade is recommended.[36] Nuclear grading is also subjective, but there is more concordance on grade I of III and grade III of III.

Regardless of the grading system used, grade I or its equivalent identifies a small subset of axillary node–negative patients at very low risk of recurrence and death from breast cancer. Grade I cancers up to 2 cm in diameter have a systemic failure rate of only 2% at 5 years.[37]

In addition to nuclear grade, another important indicator of favorable prognosis is histologic tumor type. A number of classifications are aimed at grouping breast cancer according to the histologic growth pattern and structural characteristics.[38-40] Breast cancers generally arise from the two major functional units of the breast: lobules and ducts. Invasive ductal and invasive lobular histologies behave similarly, and the differentiation has no particular prognostic significance. They are further classified as *noninvasive* or *cancers in situ* if the malignant cells fail to traverse the basement membrane and as *infiltrating* or *invasive* if the malignant cells do invade the basement membrane.

Certain histologic types of breast cancer, even though they are invasive, have a more favorable prognosis. About 20% to 30% of all breast cancers are classified as *special*, and their frequency has increased as a result of mammographic detection of smaller carcinomas.[41] The histologic features that define special types of carcinomas are present homogeneously throughout more than 90% of the lesion; however, when these features are present throughout only 75% to 90% of the carcinoma, the prognosis may be only slightly better. The three special types of invasive breast cancer are tubular, mucinous (or colloid), and medullary.

Tubular carcinoma has an excellent prognosis.[42,43] It accounts for some 3% to 5% of all breast cancers but may be the most prevalent of the special breast cancers. It is associated with a favorable prognosis when it occurs in its pure form and meets the histologic criteria. Invasive cribriform carcinoma is very similar, both histologically and biologically, to tubular carcinoma.

Colloid carcinoma is a glandular papillary or glandular cystic tumor that demonstrates a high degree of maturity and prominent mucin surrounding the cellular aggregates. It has also been called *mucinous* or *gelatinous carcinoma*. A favorable prognosis is associated with colloid carcinoma only when it occurs in the pure form. It accounts for 2% to 4% of all invasive breast cancers and usually affects older women. Women who have pure mucinous carcinomas have a 10-year survival rate of about 90%. It is more often seen in the mixed form and, in that context, does not have the favorable prognosis.[21,44-48] Generally, special-type carcinomas are low grade. An exception is medullary carcinoma.

Medullary carcinoma is a parenchyma-rich tumor with little stroma that shows a marked lymphoid infiltrate. These tumors have a favorable prognosis despite a high degree of cellular pleomorphism and a high mitotic rate. Generally, the tumors are well circumscribed and may be large, but size does not seem to affect prognosis adversely.[49-51] Medullary carcinomas account for 5% to 7% of all breast cancers. Bloom, Richardson, and Field,[52] in a 20-year follow-up, reported a 74% survival rate for patients with medullary carcinoma, as compared with 14% for those who had other types. Typical medullary breast carcinoma is a favorable histologic type of breast carcinoma with very good prognosis for pathologically node-negative patients.[53]

Pure infiltrating *papillary carcinoma* is rare: It accounts for only 0.3% to 1.5% of all breast cancers. Intraductal papillary growth is a common component of breast cancer of many other histologic types, and like colloid carcinoma, unless the papillary carcinoma is present in the pure form, it is not associated with a more favorable prognosis.[54]

Adverse histologic features such as lymphatic vessel or blood vessel invasion may be noted at the time of diagnosis. These findings are strongly related to the presence of lymph node metastases and are consequently of moderate prognostic significance. Despite their association with increased risk, they are not of independent significance sufficient for them to influence clinical decision making regarding such things as systemic therapy.

AGE

Age at diagnosis has proved to be an important prognostic factor. Younger age is a major risk factor for bad outcome in breast cancer. A multivariate analysis of more than 4000 women younger than 50 demonstrated that the hazard ratio set at 1.0 for women 40 to 44 and 45 to 49, was 1.8 for those younger than 30 years, 1.7 for women 30 to 34, and 1.5 for those 35 to 39. These differences were highly statistically significant.[55]

Predictive Factors

STEROID RECEPTORS

The measurement of ERs and PRs has become standard practice in the evaluation of patients with primary breast cancer. The measurement can be performed accurately on paraffin-embedded sections of formaldehyde-fixed breast tissue by using immunohistochemical assay, and results correlate well with those of the biochemical (Dextran-coated charcoal) assay. Results from paraffin-embedded sections agree very closely with those from frozen sections, so frozen tissue is not needed for optimal results.[56]

Although there is a modest prognostic effect of receptor status, it disappears by 5 years. Much data on the prognostic significance of hormone receptor assays is confounded by the predictive value of receptor positivity. Data from both the National Surgical Adjuvant Breast Project (NSABP) and the National Cancer Institute (NCI) Breast Intergroup have been confirmed by the Early Breast Cancer Trialists' Collaborative Overview of all randomized trials.[10] These all show that the benefits of tamoxifen, the most potent therapy in preventing systemic failure of breast cancer, is confined to patients with receptor-positive tumors. Thus the treatment benefit prediction confounds the prognostic value except when it is measured in patients who have not received systemic therapy.

DNA AND S PHASE

Proliferative rate can be determined by studying the percentage of cells in the DNA synthetic phase of the cell cycle (S phase). It does not require fresh tissue but can be performed on frozen or formalin-fixed paraffin-embedded material. Cell proliferation can also be assessed with an immunohistochemical assay that detects and quantifies cellular proteins unique to proliferating cells in either single cells or tissue sections. Proliferation-dependent antigens have been identified, including Ki-67 and proliferating cell nuclear antigen (PCNA).[57] Recent reports demonstrate that an increased percentage of S phase predicts early recurrence or poor survival for breast cancer patients who are either axillary node negative or axillary node positive. This is the

48. Nemoto T et al: Management of survival of female breast cancer: results of a national survey by the American College of Surgeons, *Cancer* 45:2917, 1980.

49. Moore OS, Foote FW Jr: The relatively favorable prognosis of medullary carcinoma of the breast, *Cancer* 2:635, 1949.

50. Richardson WW: Medullary carcinoma of the breast: a distinctive tumor type with a relatively good prognosis following radical mastectomy, *Br J Cancer* 10:415, 1956.

51. Ridolfi RL et al: Medullary carcinoma of the breast: a clinico-pathologic study with a ten-year follow-up, *Cancer* 40:1365, 1977.

52. Bloom HJG, Richardson WW, Field JR: Host resistance and survival in carcinoma of the breast: study of 104 cases of medullary carcinoma in a series of 1411 cases of breast cancer followed for twenty years, *BMJ* 3:181, 1970.

53. Reinfuss M et al: Typical medullary carcinoma of the breast: a clinical and pathological analysis of 52 cases, *J Surg Oncol* 60:89, 1995.

54. McDivitt RW, Stewart FW, Berg JW: Tumors of the breast. In Firminger HI (ed): *Atlas of tumor pathology*, Washington, DC, 1968, Armed Forces Institute of Pathology.

55. Bernstein V et al: How young is too young? The impact of age on premenopausal breast cancer prognosis, *Breast Cancer Res Treat* 76:A137, 2002.

56. Miller RT, Hapke MR, Greene GL: Immunocytochemical assay for estrogen receptor with monoclonal antibody in routinely processed formaldehyde-fixed breast tissue: Comparison with frozen section assay with monoclonal antibody, *Cancer* 71:3541, 1993.

57. Oza AM, Tannock IF: Clinical relevance of breast cancer biology, *Hematol Oncol Clin North Am* 8:1, 1994.

58. Lupu R et al: Growth control of normal and malignant breast epithelium. In Lippman M, Mihich E (eds): *The therapeutic implications of the molecular biology of breast cancer,* Rome, 1991, John Libbey.

59. Plowman GD et al: Ligand-specific activation of HER4, *Proc Natl Acad Sci USA* 90:1746, 1993.

60. Harris AL et al: Epidermal growth factor receptor and other oncogenes as prognostic markers, *J Natl Cancer Inst Monogr* 11:181, 1992.

61. Anderson BO et al: Improved survival in young women with breast cancer, *Ann Surg Oncol* 2:5, 407, 1995.

62. Nicholson S et al: Expression of epidermal growth factor receptors associated with lack of response to endocrine therapy in recurrent breast cancer, *Lancet* i:182, 1989.

63. Wright C et al: Expression of c-*erbB-2* oncoprotein: a prognostic indicator in breast cancer, *Cancer Res* 49:2087, 1989.

64. Petrek JA: Breast cancer during pregnancy, *Cancer* 74(suppl):518, 1994.

CHAPTER

22

Investigational Molecular Prognostic Factors for Breast Carcinoma

S. EVA SINGLETARY

Chapter Outline

TABLE **22-2** | Genetic Events Related to Breast Tumorigenesis

PATHWAY	GENETIC EVENTS ASSOCIATED WITH PATHWAY
DH → ADH*	HER2/*neu* amplification ↑ (5%-10%)
	p53 mutation ↑ (8%)
	Retinoblastoma gene product ↓
ADH → ncDCIS	*p53* mutation ↑ (10%-20%)
	Cyclin D1 ↑ (ER+)
	Cyclin E ↑ (ER−)
	Cyclin D2 ↓
	HER2/*neu* expression ↑
	Vascular endothelial growth factor ↑
	Thrombospondin ↓
	Telomerase ↑
ncDCIS → cDCIS	HER2/*neu* expression ↑ (60%-80%)
	p53 mutation ↑ (40%)
	Insulin-like growth factor-II receptor ↑ (22%)
	bcl-2 ↓ (ER−)
cDCIS → IDC	*c-myc* amplification ↑
	h-ras mutation ↑
	HER2/*neu* ↓ (23%-40%)
	p53 mutation ↓ (30%)
IDC → mIDC	Vimentin ↑
	nm23 ↓
	Reticulocalbin ↑
	Lysyl oxidase (extracellular matrix crosslinks) ↑
	Zinc finger proteins ↑
	Heterochromatin-binding protein-1 ↓
	S100A4 ↑
	Progression elevated gene-3 ↑ (?)

Adapted from Figure 1 in Singletary SE: *J Am Coll Surg* 194:202, 2002.
ADH, Atypical ductal hyperplasia; *cDCIS,* comedo ductal carcinoma in situ; *DH,* ductal hyperplasia; *ER,* estrogen receptor; *IDC,* invasive ductal carcinoma; *mIDC,* metastatic invasive ductal carcinoma; *ncDCIS,* noncomedo ductal carcinoma in situ.
*X → Y: The genetic change(s) indicated is (are) found in stage Y but not in stage X.

following indirect evidence. First, hyperplastic and neoplastic noninvasive lesions are statistically associated with an increased risk for the later development of breast cancer.[12] Patients with ductal hyperplasia (DH), atypical ductal hyperplasia (ADH), or DCIS have been shown to have 2 times, 5 times, or 10 times the RR of developing invasive ductal carcinoma than patients without these lesions. Second, cancerous breasts are more likely to contain ADH than are noncancerous breasts.[13-15] Invasive carcinoma is commonly found side-by-side with hyperplastic lesions or DCIS, and they occasionally are continuous with the noninvasive lesion.[16] Third, autopsy studies have shown that DH, ADH, and DCIS are more often present in the breasts of women who died of the breast cancer than in women who died of other causes.[17] Fourth, loss of heterozygosity (LOH) (i.e., deletion of one of the two alleles that make up a gene) at specific genetic loci has been found in 50% of hyperplastic lesions and 80% of DCIS that were found to coexist in the breasts with invasive cancer.[18] Finally, a retrospective pathologic study of benign breast biopsy samples showed that patients whose specimens were found on reexamination to have DCIS had a 25% chance of developing invasive cancer in the same breast.[19,20]

Although this evidence is indirect, it makes a strong case for using the model shown in Table 22-2 for the evolution of invasive breast cancer. As is true for the mouse model, however, each lesion in the model might best be considered as a nonobligatory precursor of the next. Some lesions may arise independently with respect to the preceding stage, whereas others may not progress to the next stage.

Genetic Changes in Neoplastic versus Normal Breast Tissue

A common approach to studying the genetic basis of tumorigenesis involves comparing genetic changes in neoplastic breast lesions with the genetic characteristics of normal tissue. The development of immunohistochemical and molecular techniques for the identification of specific genes and gene products in archived tissue samples has made a broad patient base available to study the genetic basis of breast cancer. With the understanding that some genes may have multiple roles in tumorigenesis, such studies have looked at specific genes implicated in the early stages of tumor development, including oncogenes, tumor-suppressor genes, growth factor receptor genes, genes associated with regulation of the cell cycle, and genes involved in apoptosis. In addition, researchers are attempting to identify specific genes that mark a cell's progression from early, nonaggressive cancer to aggressive metastatic disease. This process includes an increase in invasiveness, the ability to migrate and evade the immune system, and the development of angiogenesis. Finally, LOH studies have implicated specific genetic loci with currently unknown function as being associated with breast tumorigenesis.

Oncogenes

Oncogenes can be broadly defined as genes that can act to increase cell replication and decrease differentiation. Oncogene activation, which occurs through mutation, amplification, or rearrangement, has been widely associated with the process of tumorigenesis, but the exact role for these genes has been difficult to define. In the colon, mutation of the *ras* oncogene seems to be associated with progression from early- to intermediate-grade adenoma, a precursor of carcinoma.[7] In the breast, early studies reported that *ras* gene expression was widespread in both normal and neoplastic breast tissue, indicating that it might be a marker for certain cell types rather than for malignancy.[21,22] On the other hand, a study by Mizukami and colleagues[23] found that *ras* gene expression in normal tissue, benign lesions, and DCIS was either absent or present at very low levels, but expression levels were high in more than half (62%) of patients with invasive disease. Liu and colleagues[24] hypothesized that *ras* gene mutations were associated with a more aggressive tumor phenotype occurring late in the course of a disease, and Czerniak and colleagues reported that *ras* expression was associated with axillary lymph node metastases.[25] More recently, Von Lintig and co-workers[26] reported that *ras* is abnormally activated in breast cancers that overexpress receptors for epidermal growth factor or HER2 and that *ras* is highly activated in 55% of cancers relative to its levels in benign tissue. From these studies, it seems likely that *ras* activation would not be an initiating event in breast tumorigenesis, but rather it would be involved in the later progression of the disease.

Amplification of the *c-myc* gene can be detected in only 4% to 6% of patients with DCIS, mostly in high-grade DCIS.[27,28] Deming and colleagues,[29] in a meta-analysis of 29 studies of invasive breast tumors, reported *c-myc* amplification in an average of 16% of patients. They found weak but statistically significant associations between *c-myc* amplification and the presence of lymph node metastases, as well as risk of relapse and death from disease. This picture is similar to that seen for *ras* activation, indicating a role for *c-myc* in tumor progression rather than initiation.

Tumor-Suppressor Genes

Tumor-suppressor genes were first identified in studies of hereditary cancers. In such cases (e.g., retinoblastoma), cancers cluster in specific pedigrees and are characterized clinically by early onset, bilateral occurrence, and multiple foci. The genetic mechanism, as originally formulated in the "two-hit" hypothesis of Knudsen,[30] involves a germline mutation of one copy of the gene (the first hit) followed by somatic mutation or deletion of the second copy (the second hit). Although, first identified in association with hereditary cancers, the same genes are now thought to be involved in many sporadic cancers as well.

One of the best-studied tumor-suppressor genes associated with breast cancer is *p53*. Located at 17p13, this gene is mutated in individuals with Li-Fraumeni syndrome, which is characterized by a high incidence of breast cancers and other tumors. The wild-type p53 protein in normal cells is an important "gatekeeper," preventing the propagation of cells containing damaged DNA through its effects on cell cycle arrest and apoptosis.[31-33] Arresting the progress of a damaged cell through the cell cycle before mitosis sometimes makes it possible for the DNA to be repaired before the cell can replicate. If the damage to the cell is too severe, a separate program is triggered, sending the cell into apoptosis and death. If *p53* function is disrupted through mutation or degradation of the protein product, the DNA damage can be passed on to daughter cells, leading to an accumulation of mutations that may contribute to tumorigenesis.

The wild-type p53 protein is involved in the transcriptional activation of *gadd45*, a DNA repair gene,[34] and *p21INK*, a cyclin-dependent kinase inhibitor,[35] among others. As described later in this chapter, the induction of apoptosis in severely damaged cells may be accomplished through the downregulation of *bcl-2* by *p53*.[36]

Mutation of *p53* causes downregulation of thrombospondin, a naturally occurring inhibitor of angiogenesis[37]; *p53* mutations may also be involved in the increased expression of *MDR-1*, a multiple-drug resistance gene.[38] Because mutated p53 protein tends to accumulate in cells, it can be quantified with immunohistochemical staining.

Millikan and colleagues[39] studied *p53* mutations in biopsy samples of benign breast lesions exhibiting atypical epithelial proliferation or fibroadenoma. In 60 such samples examined, 5 samples showed mutations in *p53* and 14 samples exhibited immunoreactivity to the p53 protein. These findings indicate that although *p53* mutation can occur as an early event in breast tumorigenesis, it is clearly not universal. In DCIS, which has been proposed as being a later stage in tumorigenesis, there is a marked difference in *p53* immunoreactivity between high-grade (comedo) DCIS and low-grade (noncomedo) DCIS. Using 5% of nuclei staining for *p53* as a negative/positive cutoff point, Querzoli and colleagues[40] found that 42.1% cases of comedo DCIS were *p53* positive, as compared with 23.5% of cases of noncomedo DCIS. This finding is consistent with an earlier report from Allred, O'Connell, and Fuqua,[41] who reported *p53* positivity in only 10% of noncomedo DCIS lesions, compared with 40% of comedo DCIS lesions.

Other tumor-suppressor genes have been implicated in the development of breast carcinoma. Loss of the retinoblastoma gene, *Rb,* may be relatively common in primary breast tumors (approximately 36%),[42,43] but this loss is believed to be a progression event rather than an initiating event in breast cancer.[44] The gene for the insulin-like growth factor-II receptor, located on chromosome arm 6q, activates transforming growth factor (TGF)-β1, a potent growth inhibitor. Abnormal expression of this gene has not been reported in low-grade DCIS, but it occurs in approximately 22% of high-grade DCIS.[45] Additional genes of interest include *NF1, APC, VHL, NSH2,* the familial breast cancer genes *BRCA1* and *BRCA2,* and *nm23.* The *nm23* gene is thought to be associated with the development of the metastatic phenotype; an association has been found between reduced *nm23* expression and aggressive tumor behavior.[46,47]

Epidermal Growth Factor Receptor Genes

The epidermal growth factor receptor (EGFR) family consists of four closely related tyrosine kinases: EGFR, HER2 (ERB-2), HER3 (ERB-3), and HER4 (ERB-4).[48] Of these proteins, HER2 has received the most attention,

showing amplification or overexpression in up to 40% of primary breast tumors.[49] In a study by Stark and colleagues,[50] HER2 amplification was seen in 4.5% to 9.5% of benign breast lesions (typical or atypical hyperplasia) and was associated with an increased risk of future breast cancer development. HER2 overexpression has not been reported to occur in benign breast disease, and it seems not to occur until the transition from hyperplasia to DCIS.[41,50] HER2 overexpression is more often seen in comedo DCIS than in noncomedo DCIS. Querzoli and colleagues[40] reported HER2 positivity (defined as >10% of cells stained) in 73% of comedo DCIS versus 13% of noncomedo DCIS; these finding are consistent with those of Allred and co-workers,[41] who found HER2 positivity in 80% and 10% of cases, respectively. Interestingly, both researchers observed greater amounts of HER2 protein in comedo DCIS than in invasive carcinomas. This may indicate that not all HER2-positive DCIS lesions develop into invasive cancers or that some invasive cancers do not arise from a DCIS precursor. Alternatively, Kim and Muller[51] suggest that efficient transformation of cells may require the coexpression of HER2 and another member of the EGFR family. In studies of normal fibroblasts, expression of individual EFGR family members was not sufficient for transformation in cells that lacked other EGFR family members.[52]

Ligands that bind to various members of the EGFR family may also play roles in the development of breast cancer. TGF-α, EGF, *neu* differentiation factor, and Heregulin are EGF family ligands that have been implicated in human breast tumorigenesis.[53-56]

Genes Associated with Regulation of the Cell Cycle

CYCLINS AND CDK INHIBITORS

Replication of mammalian cells proceeds in phases, from G_1 through S to mitosis, and that progression is regulated by changes in cyclins, cyclin-dependent kinases (CDKs), and CDK inhibitors. CDKs are expressed uniformly throughout the cell cycle, whereas cyclin levels are mediated by growth signals and vary from phase to phase. Cyclins D and E are expressed early in the cell cycle and are likely to be involved with the G_1-S phase checkpoint.[57] Normally, these cyclins merge with and activate specific CDKs, leading to a cascade of protein phosphorylation that ultimately triggers the onset of S phase.[58]

When a cell is damaged, CDK inhibitors are involved in arresting the cell cycle, thereby preventing the replication of a damaged template. The best-studied CDK inhibitor is p21, which is a primary mediator of the *p53*-dependent G_1 arrest that is triggered by cell damage.[59] Other CDK inhibitors (e.g., p27, p16) may also be associated with response to *p53*-mediated response to G_1 cell damage.

In tumor cells the balance between cyclins, CDKs, and CDK inhibitors is disrupted. Cyclin D1 normally activates CDK4 and CDK6,[60] leading to the phosphorylation of the retinoblastoma gene products (pRb).[61,62] These complexes can be inactivated by the CDK inhibitor p16.[63] Loss of normal controls on cell growth can occur through overexpression of cyclin D1 or inactivation of pRb or p16. Cyclin E activates CDK2, and formation of this complex, possibly mediated by the formation of a cyclin D1/cdk4/6 complex, may be the rate-limiting step in the G_1 to S transition.[64] Cyclin E normally accumulates at the G_1 to S boundary and is promptly degraded as the cells progress through S phase.[65]

Cyclin D1 and cyclin E can both be overexpressed in breast cancer, but the exact type of overexpression may be a function of ER status. In ER-positive cells, estrogen-induced mitogenic activity is associated with overexpression of cyclin D1.[66-68] In ER-negative cells, on the other hand, cyclin D1, CDK4, and CDK6 are not overexpressed and transformation is more commonly associated with overexpression of cyclin E.[66,69,70] Keyomarsi and colleagues demonstrated in a series of studies that overexpression of cyclin E can lead to pRb phosphorylation and cell cycle progression even when cyclin D1 complexes are inactivated by p16.[64,70] Overexpression of cyclin E is associated with aggressive disease and a significantly increased risk of recurrence or death.[69] It has also been seen in combination with poor differentiation, high proliferative index, presence of mutant *p53*, and increased chromosomal instability (presumably as a result of impairment of S-phase progression).[66]

Umekita and Yoshida[68] examined cyclin D1 levels in a range of breast epithelial cell types thought to represent progression ranging from normal breast cells to invasive ductal carcinoma. They found no evidence of increased cyclin D1 expression in normal cells, DH, or ADH; however, 72% of cases of DCIS (57 of 79) were positive for increased cyclin D1, compared with 50% of cases of predominantly intraductal carcinoma (44 of 88) and 44% of cases of invasive ductal carcinoma (92 of 201). In all cell types, increased cyclin D1 expression was strongly correlated with ER status. Zhou and colleagues[71] also reported cyclin D1 overexpression in 80% of DCIS cases and little or no overexpression in ADH or benign proliferative lesions. Although some investigators have reported increased cyclin D1 expression in ADH,[72,73] this finding may reflect differences in procedure; for example, Gillett and colleagues[74] reported only 1 of 9 cases of ADH as being positive when they used the same antibody as did Umekita and Yoshida.[68] Cyclin E expression seems to vary in the same way as does cyclin D1.[75]

Another cyclin, D2, has been implicated as a negative regulator of cell division.[58] In phenotypically normal human cells, D2 is upregulated under conditions of growth arrest. In contrast, cyclin D2 mRNA and protein are absent in almost all breast cancer cell lines that have been examined to date.[76,77] Loss of cyclin D2 expression has also been reported in 44% of DCIS cases, indicating that this may be an early event in tumor progression.[58]

TELOMERASE

Telomeres are short tandem-repeat DNA sequences found at the ends of eukaryotic chromosomes. Telomeres are believed to stabilize the otherwise "sticky" ends of the chromosomes during DNA replication and cell division. Because chromosomes lose some telomeric subunits from their ends during each cell division, theoretically there exists a maximum number of cell division cycles possible for normal cells unless the subunits can be replaced.

Telomerase is a ribonucleoprotein complex that adds telomeric repeats to the ends of chromosomes. Telomerase is activated in dividing embryonic cells but is repressed in most differentiated somatic cells. Reactivation or increased expression of telomerase prevents the progressive telomeric shortening that normally occurs during cell division and is thought to be a key component of cell immortalization.

Sugino and colleagues[78] used a polymerase chain reaction–based assay to analyze telomerase activity in fine-needle aspirates from human breast tissue. Samples were obtained from 17 fibrocystic lesions, 15 fibroadenomas, 71 primary breast carcinomas, and 6 normal breast tissue samples. These investigators found no detectable telomerase in normal or fibrocystic tissue and found telomerase activity in only 1 of 15 fibroadenoma samples. In comparison, telomerase activity was found in 52 of 71 (73%) invasive breast carcinomas. These findings were replicated in a 1997 study by Bednarek and colleagues,[79] who found telomerase activity in 99 of 104 (95%) breast cancer samples and in 1 of 5 (20%) fibroadenomas but found no activity in any of 10 nonmalignant breast tissue samples. Of special interest, they also detected telomerase activity in all 6 DCIS samples tested, and the level of telomerase activity in those samples was positively correlated with nuclear grade.

More recently, Kolquist and colleagues[80] examined telomerase expression at the single-cell level by using in situ hybridization to detect expression of the telomerase catalytic subunit gene *TERT*. Using this technology, 17 of 18 cases of carcinoma in situ (both ductal and lobular) were found to have moderate to high levels of *TERT* expression. *TERT* expression was also seen in some cells lining the terminal ducts (low levels) and in cells located more distally in the terminal duct-lobular units (high levels). Both of these normal cell types typically undergo repeated cycles of proliferation in response to physiologic stimuli. This finding suggests that in some cases, tumorigenesis may occur in cells that normally express telomerase rather than the abnormal induction of telomerase expression being a precipitating event.

GENES ASSOCIATED WITH APOPTOSIS: THE *bcl* GENE FAMILY

Tumors can increase in size through increasing cell division, decreasing cell death, or both. Apoptosis is the programmed cell death that occurs as part of the normal processes of embryogenesis or cell turnover in normal tissues. It is regulated by members of the *bcl* gene family, which include cell-death suppressors (*bcl-2, Bcl-XbMCLI*) and cell-death promoters (*Bax, Bcl-Xs, Bak*).

The cell-death suppressor *bcl-2*, the best-studied gene in the *bcl* gene family, is located at 18q21. In the adult female breast, the expression of *bcl-2* is most apparent in the lobular cells, peaking at the midpoint of the menstrual cycle and decreasing sharply at the end of the cycle.[81] This rise and fall in *bcl-2* expression reflects the alternating rounds of proliferation and apoptosis that occur in end-bud epithelial tissue in response to cyclic hormonal stimuli.

Expression of *bcl-2* has been reported in 96% of normal ductal epithelial cells, in 69% of DCIS, and in 45% of invasive carcinomas.[82] In DCIS, *bcl-2* expression is correlated with histologic grade. Several researchers have reported detectable *bcl-2* in 100% of well-differentiated DCIS lesions, compared with only 33% of poorly differentiated DCIS.[83,84] Expression of *bcl-2* in DCIS is also positively correlated with ER status. Quinn and colleagues[85] reported that 47 of 57 patients with DCIS who were positive for *bcl-2* were also ER positive and that 49 of 51 patients who were negative for *bcl-2* were ER negative. Similar results have been found in invasive ductal carcinoma.[86,87] Leek and colleagues[86] reported that 70 of 88 *bcl-2*–positive tumors were also ER positive, compared with only 7 of 23 *bcl-2*–negative tumors; that group also found that *bc1-2* expression was negatively correlated with expression of *p53* and *c-erbB-2*. Bhargava, Kell, and van de Rijn[87] also reported that 23 of 24 carcinomas that were *bcl-2* positive were also ER positive and that 14 of 15 *bcl-2*–negative tumors were also ER negative. Thus *bcl-2* expression seems to be related to hormonal regulation, and loss of *bcl-2* expression is associated with a range of molecular markers of poor prognosis in breast carcinoma.

It seems paradoxical that decreased *bcl-2* expression, which would normally be associated with increased cell death through apoptosis, is associated with increased oncogenic potential (presumably associated with increased cell growth) in breast epithelial cells. This paradox may be clarified by considering the relationship between *bcl-2* and *p53* in breast tumorigenesis in ER-negative cells. The expression of *bcl-2* tends to be inversely correlated with mutated *p53* expression.[86,88] Normal levels of immunohistochemically detectable *bcl-2* are found in noncomedo DCIS, and those levels decrease in comedo DCIS and invasive carcinoma in conjunction with increasing values of mutant *p53*.[82,83,88] Siziopiku and Schnitt[89] examined the cellular proliferation index in DCIS in relation to the expression of *bcl-2* and *p53*. They found that low-grade DCIS tended to have a low proliferation index and tended to be associated with a *bcl-2*–positive/*p53*-negative phenotype. In contrast, high-grade DCIS tended to have abnormal combinations of *bcl-2* and *p53*, with the highest proliferation index seen in patients who were *bcl-2* negative and *p53* positive.

Liu and colleagues[36] hypothesized that abnormal *bcl-2/p53* phenotypes result in dysregulation of the normal apoptosis pathways. In wild-type cells, *p53* responds to DNA damage either by causing G_1 arrest, thus enabling DNA repair, or by shunting the cell to apoptosis by downregulating *bcl-2*. They speculate that mutant *p53* may not be able to function in G_1 arrest but may still be able to downregulate *bcl-2*. Thus as reported by Megha and colleagues,[90] *p53*-positive/*bcl-2*–negative DCIS lesions are characterized by high values of both mitotic index and apoptotic index, whereas the reverse is true of *p53*-negative/*bcl-2*–positive lesions.

The occurrence of necrotic areas in high-grade comedo DCIS may serve to illustrate the relationship between dysregulation of normal apoptosis and increasing tumorigenicity. Such lesions are characterized by increased risk of recurrence and poor outcome. Gandhi and colleagues[91] found that increased apoptotic index, increased proliferation index, and decreased *bcl-2* were all significantly associated with high-grade comedo necrosis in DCIS lesions.

Genetic Changes Related to the Development of the Metastatic Phenotype

Although some transformed cells result in small, nonaggressive tumors, others develop into aggressive lesions characterized by the development of the ability to invade and metastasize. Are specific genetic mutations associated with these advanced tumorigenic characteristics? Do these mutations occur late in tumor development, or are cells programmed to become aggressive and metastatic when they are first transformed? Various studies involving both tissue culture models and examination of breast tissue have examined these questions.

Liu, Brattain, and Appert[92] used the technique of differential display analysis to identify genes involved in invasion and metastasis in well-characterized breast epithelial cell lines of different metastatic capability. Comparison of *MDA-MB-435* cells (invasive, metastatic) with *MCF-7* cells (poorly invasive, nonmetastatic) revealed the upregulation of five genes. Four of these genes had unknown functions, but one coded for reticulocalbin, a protein with six calcium domains. These investigators also detected that the transition from an epithelial to a mesenchymal type of cellular matrix was marked by the expression of vimentin intermediate filaments in addition to cytokeratin. In vitro tests have shown that breast carcinoma cells that express both vimentin and cytokeratin have a high invasive potential.[93]

In a subsequent study with the highly invasive and metastatic *MDA-MB-231* cell line, Kirschmann and colleagues[94] identified abnormal expression of two possible transcription regulators: upregulation of zinc finger protein (which presumably binds DNA) and downregulation of HP1, a heterochromatin-binding protein that is known to silence gene expression in the fruit fly *Drosophila melanogaster*. They also found increased expression of lysyl oxidase, an extracellular copper enzyme important in maintaining the stability of the extracellular matrix. Interestingly, lysyl oxidase expression has been shown to be decreased in cell lines derived from other types of human cancer (e.g., fibrosarcoma, melanoma). The increased expression shown by breast cancer cells in this study may mean that lysyl oxidase has additional functions (not related to the extracellular matrix) that contribute to the metastatic phenotype.

Tumor growth and metastasis both depend on angiogenesis. This process is normally regulated by wild-type p53 through the induction of thrombospondin, a naturally occurring inhibitor of angiogenesis. The presence of non–wild-type p53, especially those molecules characterized by insertions, deletions, and stop-codon mutations, is associated with decreased levels of thrombospondin and increased levels of vascular endothelial growth factor (VEGF).[95] In addition to increasing angiogenesis, VEGF increases vessel permeability and activates proteolytic enzymes involved in cellular invasion.

However, a VEGF-associated increase in angiogenesis is not restricted to invasive carcinoma cells undergoing metastatic conversion; it is also commonly found in DCIS. Guidi and co-workers[96] found that VEGF expression in DCIS was greater than that in adjacent benign epithelial cells in 96% of cases; they also found that increased VEGF levels were associated with increased angiogenesis. Brown and colleagues[97] also studied the expression of VEGF in DCIS, invasive ductal carcinoma, and metastatic carcinoma. In all cases they found strong tumor cell expression of VEGF and strong endothelial cell expression of VEGF receptors. This raises the possibility that rather than invading into normal stroma, tumor cells invade into vascular stroma, stroma that they themselves have induced in their immediate environment. Thus a DCIS cell could initially become invasive, or an already-invasive cell could metastasize to a new site through the preinduction of a suitable vascular environment.

The S100A4 protein has been shown in many cancer types to be specifically associated with high invasive and metastatic potential. In rodent breast cancer models, S100A4 can induce metastasis in transformed cells. Grigorian and colleagues[98] reported that S100A4 binds to the end of the c-terminal regulatory domain of *p53*, resulting in differential expression of genes influenced by *p53* (p21, *Bax*, *bcl-2*, thrombospondin, *MDR-2*). They hypothesize that the ability of S100A4 to enhance *p53*-dependent apoptosis through its effect on the *bcl-2* gene family may result in the preferential loss of those cells that still carry wild-type p53, thereby contributing to a more aggressive phenotype. The S100A4 protein and the gene product from the putative metastasis-suppressor gene *nm23* have also been shown to alter cytoskeletal dynamic.[99]

In humans, nearly half of stage I and II primary breast cancers are positive for S1004A, as detected with immunohistochemical staining.[100] High levels of S100A4 are associated with metastatic spread to regional lymph nodes.

The multiple downstream effects of S100A4 on the cytoskeleton and on *p53*-related genetic elements support the idea that a very limited number of genetic mutations may trigger a cascade of events leading to metastasis. This idea has been explored by Fisher and others at Columbia University, who have isolated a gene (progression elevated gene-3, or *PEG-3*) that seems to be strongly correlated with tumor progression in a variety of rodent and human cell types.[101] Although *PEG-3* lacks classic oncogenic potential and does not transform normal cells, its overexpression results in aggressive tumorigenic properties. Fisher and colleagues hypothesize that *PEG-3* mutation may involve constitutive induction of DNA damage response pathways, leading to genomic instability and a more aggressive phenotype.

Summary

Evidence about the time course of genetic events in breast tumorigenesis is summarized in Table 22-2. Data from two types of human breast cancer studies (those using normal and neoplastic breast tissue samples and those using human mammary epithelial cell lines) have been combined under the assumption that the transition from immortalized cells to transformed cells occurs after the development of atypical hyperplasia and low-grade DCIS. This assumption is based on several observations, namely that genetic changes associated with cell immortalization (e.g., telomerase activation) have been reported in low-grade DCIS, whereas changes associated with cell transformation (e.g., increased expression of *h-ras*) are associated with high-grade DCIS or invasive cancer but not usually with earlier stages of tumorigenesis.* Most patients with hyperplasia and low-grade DCIS, although they are at increased risk, do not develop invasive carcinoma.[12]

The early stages of tumorigenesis in breast cancer (DH, ADH, and low-grade DCIS correlated here with the immortalization process) are marked by activation of telomerase[79,80,102,103]; increased frequency of *p53* mutations[39-41,104]; and dysregulation of HER2,[40,41,50] Rb,[105,106] and cyclins D1, D2, and E.[58,66,68-70] It should be noted that the increased mutation of *p53* and amplification/expression of HER2 are seen in only a few cases of ADH (<10%). There is a slight increase in the proportion of lesions that are positive for these markers in low-grade DCIS, followed by a large increase (to a proportion of 40% for *p53*, 60% to 80% for HER2) seen in high-grade DCIS. Interestingly, the frequency with which lesions are positive for *p53* and HER2 is much lower in invasive ductal carcinoma (30% *p53* positive and 40% HER2 positive) and remains at similar levels in metastatic invasive ductal carcinoma.[40,41,49,107] This finding may be interpreted to mean that not all high-grade DCIS ultimately develop into invasive carcinoma or, more likely, as suggested previously by Allred and colleagues,[41] that some invasive carcinomas may arise de novo without the intervening developmental steps described in this model.

The expression pattern of genetic markers is very different in low-grade versus high-grade DCIS. Aside from increases in the frequency of *p53* mutation and HER2 expression, a comparison of low-grade to high-grade DCIS also shows a significant increase in the receptor for insulin-like growth factor-II and a decrease (in ER-negative lesions) in *bcl-2* expression.[83,84] Does this mean that the transition from low-grade to high-grade DCIS is a particularly significant gateway in breast tumorigenesis? Perhaps. It certainly seems likely that many cases of high-grade DCIS represent a further developmental stage of low-grade DCIS, a stage marked by additional genetic mutations. However, Leong and colleagues[108] have suggested that some cases of low-grade DCIS may develop directly into low-grade invasive ductal carcinoma, whereas high-grade DCIS represents the precursor of high-grade invasive ductal carcinoma. They based this hypothesis on two observations: first, that the pattern of biologic markers differs between the different grades of DCIS, and second, that there is a positive correlation between the markers expressed in DCIS and those expressed in concurrent invasive ductal carcinoma, suggesting a clonal relationship between the two lesions.

Mutation of the *h-ras* oncogene and accumulation of the *c-myc* oncogene are seen in the transition to invasive carcinoma, along with decreases in the frequency of *p53* mutation and HER2 expression as described earlier.[109]

The development of aggressive, metastatic properties in an invasive lesion is associated with a number of markers, but the exact mechanisms involved have yet to be defined.* Of special interest is the observation that several factors that might be assumed to be closely associated with the metastatic process (e.g., VEGF, thrombospondin, vimentin) have been observed at abnormal levels in certain cases of DCIS.[95-97,108] On the one hand, this observation may provide support for a previously described hypothesis from Vogelstein's work that although a certain number of genetic changes must be accumulated for the development of metastatic breast cancer, there is no fixed order in which they must occur.[7] Alternatively, this observation may provide additional support for Leong's theory that different genetic variants of DCIS are destined to evolve into different types of invasive ductal carcinoma.

Although the picture that has emerged is complex, several tentative conclusions can be made relative to breast tumorigenesis. First, very early stages of breast carcinogenesis (up to and including low-grade DCIS) are probably best characterized by activation of telomerase and dysregulation of the cyclins. Although *p53* and HER2 levels may be affected in these early lesions, changes in the expression of these markers are seen in, at best, 20% of cases and thus these would not make useful biomarkers in early-stage lesions. High-grade DCIS, on the other hand, shows mutation of *p53* in up to 40% of cases and increased expression of HER2 in 60% to 80% of cases, thus making these markers more appropriate for this type of lesion. Second, the apoptosis-related marker *bcl-2* shows a significant decrease in high-grade DCIS, but only in ER-negative lesions.[83,84] Although relevant data are not available for all of the markers discussed here, several important ones are significantly different in ER-positive versus ER-negative lesions. In addition to *bcl-2*, cyclin D1 increases associated with DCIS are seen only in ER-positive lesions,[68] whereas cyclin E increases are seen in patients with ER-negative lesions.[65,69,70] It is not surprising that important markers for breast tumorigenesis should be strongly affected by ER status, given the estrogen-dependent nature of many breast cancers and the numerous observations of biologic differences between ER-positive and ER-negative breast tumors. Third, the transition from DCIS to invasive ductal carcinoma is poorly understood, and markers that may be associated with this change (e.g., *myc, ras*) should be interpreted with caution. Finally, although various markers are associated with development of the metastatic phenotype, some of these markers, including several associated with increased angiogenesis, may be present in earlier lesions such as DCIS.

---

*References 23, 24, 79, 80, 102, 103.

*References 46, 47, 92, 100, 101, 103.

Well-designed trials will need to consider the biologic importance of biomarkers in terms of the time course of genetic changes in breast tumorigenesis, viewed against the background of the hormonal and biochemical status of the patient.

ACKNOWLEDGMENT

I thank Laura Gardner for her contribution in preparing this chapter.

REFERENCES

1. Fitzgibbons PL et al: Prognostic factors in breast cancer. College of American Pathologists consensus statement, *Arch Pathol Lab Med* 124:966, 2000.
2. Henderson IC, Patek AJ: The relationship between prognostic and predictive factors in the management of breast cancer, *Breast Cancer Res Treat* 52:261, 1998.
3. American Society of Clinical Oncology: Clinical practice guidelines for the use of tumor markers in breast and colorectal cancer, *J Clin Oncol* 14:2843, 1996.
4. American Society of Clinical Oncology: 1997 update of recommendations for the use of tumor markers in breast and colorectal cancer, *J Clin Oncol* 16:793, 1998.
5. Singletary SE, AJCC Task Force: Breast. In Greene FL et al (eds): *AJCC cancer staging manual*, ed 6, New York, 2002, Springer-Verlag.
6. Mirza AN et al: Prognostic factors in node-negative breast cancer: a review of studies with sample size >200 and follow-up >5 years, *Ann Surg* 235:10, 2002.
7. Fearon EF, Vogelstein B: A genetic model for colorectal tumorigenesis, *Cell* 61:759, 1990.
8. Polyak K: Early alteration of cell-cycle-regulated gene expression in colorectal neoplasia, *Am J Pathol* 149:381, 1996.
9. Vogelstein B et al: Genetic alterations during colorectal tumor development, *N Engl J Med* 319:525, 1988.
10. Peto R et al: Cancer and aging in mice and man, *Br J Cancer* 21:411, 1975.
11. DeOme KB et al: Development of mammary tumors from hyperplastic alveolar nodules transplanted into gland free mammary fat pads of female C3H mice, *Cancer Res* 19:515, 1959.
12. Dupont WD, Page DL: Risk factors for breast cancer in women with proliferative breast disease, *N Engl J Med* 312:146, 1985.
13. Ryan JA, Coady CJ: Intraductal epithelial proliferation in the human breast: a comparitive study, *Can J Surg* 5:12, 1962.
14. Karpas CM et al: Relationship of fibrocystic disease to carcinoma of the breast, *Ann Surg* 162:1, 1995.
15. Kern WH, Brooks RN: Atypical epithelial hyperplasia associated with breast cancer and fibrocystic disease, *Cancer* 24:668, 1969.
16. Lakhani SR: The transition from hyperplasia to invasive carcinoma of the breast, *J Pathol* 187:272, 1999.
17. Bartow SA et al: Prevalence of benign, atypical, and malignant breast lesions in populations at different risk for breast cancer: a forensic autopsy study, *Cancer* 60:2751, 1987.
18. O'Connell P et al: Molecular genetic studies of early breast cancer evolution, *Breast Cancer Res Treat* 32:5, 1994.
19. Betsil WLJ et al: Intraductal carcinoma: long term follow-up after treatment by biopsy alone, *JAMA* 239:1863, 1987.
20. Page DL et al: Intraductal carcinoma of the breast: follow-up after biopsy only, *Cancer* 49:751, 1982.
21. Candlish W, Kerr IB, Simpson HW: Immunocytochemical demonstration and significance of p21 *ras* family oncogene product in benign and malignant breast disease, *J Pathol* 150:163, 1986.
22. Ghosh AK, Moore M, Harris M: Immunohistochemical detection of *ras* oncogene p21 product in benign and malignant mammary tissue in man, *J Clin Pathol* 39:428, 1986.
23. Mizukami Y et al: Immunohistochemical study of oncogene product *ras* p21, *c-myc*, and growth factor EGF in breast carcinomas, *Anticancer Res* 11:1485, 1991.
24. Liu E et al: Molecular lesions involved in the progression of a human breast cancer, *Oncogene* 3:323, 1988.
25. Czerniak B et al: Expression of *ras* oncogene p21 protein in relation to regional spread of human breast carcinomas, *Cancer* 63:2008, 1989.
26. Von Lintig FC et al: *Ras* activation in human breast cancer, *Breast Cancer Res Treat* 62:51, 2000.
27. Glockner S et al: Amplification of growth regulatory genes in intraductal breast cancer is associated with higher nuclear grade but not with the progression to invasiveness, *Lab Invest* 81:565, 2001.
28. Vos CB et al: Genetic alterations on chromosome 16 and 17 are important features of ductal carcinoma in situ of the breast and are associated with histologic type, *Br J Cancer* 81:1410, 1999.
29. Deming SL et al: *C-myc* amplification in breast cancer: a meta-analysis of its occurrence and prognostic relevance, *Br J Cancer* 83:1688, 2000.
30. Knudsen AG: Mutation and cancer: statistical study of retinoblastomas, *Proc Natl Acad Sci USA* 68:820, 1971.
31. Kern SE: *p53*: tumor suppression through control of the cell cycle, *Gastroenterology* 106:1708, 1994.
32. Kastan MB et al: Participation of *p53* protein in the cellular response to DNA damage, *Cancer Res* 51:6304, 1991.
33. Kuerbitz SJ: Wild-type *p53* is a cell cycle checkpoint determinant following irradiation, *Proc Natl Acad Sci USA* 89:7491, 1992.
34. Smith ML et al: Interaction of the *p53*-regulated protein gadd45 with proliferating cell nuclear antigen, *Science* 266:1376, 1994.
35. Peter M, Herskowitz E: Joining the complex: cyclin-dependent kinase inhibitory proteins and the cell cycle, *Cell* 79:181, 1994.
36. Liu Q-L: *bcl-2*: role in epithelial differentiation and oncogenesis, *Hum Pathol* 27:102, 1996.
37. Linderholm BK et al: *P53* and vascular-endothelial-growth factor expression predicts outcome in 833 patients with primary breast carcinoma, *Int J Cancer* 89:51, 2000.
38. Lee E: Tumor suppressor genes and their alterations in breast cancer, *Semin Cancer Biol* 6:119, 1995.
39. Millikan R et al: *P53* mutations in benign breast tissue, *J Clin Oncol* 13:2293, 1995.
40. Querzoli P et al: Modulation of biomarkers in minimal breast carcinoma, *Cancer* 83:89, 1998.
41. Allred DC, O'Connell P, Fuqua S: Biomarkers in early breast neoplasia, *J Cell Biochem* 17G:125, 1993.
42. Borg A et al: The retinoblastoma gene in breast cancer: allele loss is not correlated with loss of gene protein expression, *Cancer Res* 52:2991, 1992.
43. Trudel M et al: Retinoblastoma and *p53* gene product expression in breast carcinoma: immunohistochemical analysis and clinicopathologic correlation, *Hum Pathol* 23:1388, 1992.

44. Cox LA, Chen G, Lee Y-HP: Tumor suppressor genes and their roles in breast cancer, *Breast Cancer Res Treat* 32:19, 1994.

45. Chappell SA et al: Loss of heterozygosity at the mannose-6-phosphate insulin-like growth factor 2 receptor gene correlates with poor differentiation in early breast carcinomas, *Br J Cancer* 76:1558, 1997.

46. Bevilacqua G et al: Association of low nm23 RNA levels in human primary infiltrating ductal breast carcinomas with lymph node involvement and other histopathological indicators of high metastatic potential, *Cancer Res* 49:5185, 1989.

47. Hennessy C et al: Expression of the antimetastatic gene nm23 in human breast cancer: an association with good prognosis, *J Natl Cancer Inst* 83:281, 1991.

48. Hynes NE, Stern DF: The biology of erb-2/*neu*-HER-2 and its role in cancer, *Biochem Biophys Acta* 1198:165, 1994.

49. Dhingra K, Hittelman WN, Hortobagyi GN: Genetic changes in breast cancer—consequences for therapy? *Gene* 159:59, 1995.

50. Stark A et al: HER2/*neu* amplification in benign breast disease and the risk of subsequent breast cancer, *J Clin Oncol* 18:267, 2000.

51. Kim H, Muller WJ: The role of the epidermal growth factor receptor family in mammary tumorigenesis and metastasis, *Exp Cell Res* 253:78, 1999.

52. Cohen BD, Kiener PA, Green JM: The relationship between human epidermal growth-like factor expression and cellular transformation in NIH3T3 cells, *J Biol Chem* 271:30897, 1996.

53. Normanno N et al: Epidermal growth factor-related peptides in the pathogenesis of human breast cancer, *Breast Cancer Res Treat* 29:11, 1994.

54. Salomon DS, Bianco C, De Santis M: Cripto: a novel epidermal growth factor-related peptide in mammary gland development and neoplasia, *Bioessays* 21:61, 1999.

55. Kenney NJ et al: Detection of amphiregulin and cripto-1 in mammary tumors from transgenic mice, *Mol Carcinog* 15:44, 1996.

56. Peles E, Yarden Y: *Neu* and its ligands: from an oncogene to neural factors, *Bioessays* 15a:815, 1993.

57. Hartwell LH, Kastan MB: Cell cycle control and cancer, *Science* 266:1821, 1994.

58. Evron E et al: Loss of cyclin D2 expression in the majority of breast cancers is associated with promoter hypermethylation, *Cancer Res* 61:2782, 2001.

59. Elledge SJ, Harper JW: Cdk inhibitors: on the threshold of checkpoints and development, *Curr Opin Cell Biol* 6:847, 1994.

60. Hunter T, Pines J: Cyclins and cancer II: cyclin D and Cdk inhibitors come of age, *Cell* 779:573, 1994.

61. Hinds PW et al: Regulation of retinoblastoma protein functions by ectopic expression of human cyclins, *Cell* 70:993, 1992.

62. Kato JY et al: Direct binding of cyclin D to the retinoblastoma gene product and pRb phosphorylation by the cyclin D-dependent kinase, Cdk4, *Genes Dev* 7:331, 1993.

63. Medema RH et al: Growth suppression by p16inkH requires functional retinoblastoma protein, *Proc Natl Acad Sci USA* 92:6289, 1995.

64. Harwell RM et al: Processing of cyclin E differs between normal and tumor breast cells, *Cancer Res* 60:481, 2001.

65. Spruck CH, Won KA, Reed SI: Deregulated cyclin E induces chromosome instability, *Nature* 401:297, 1999.

66. Scott KA, Walker RA: Lack of cyclin E immunoreactivity in non-malignant breast and association with proliferation in breast cancer, *Br J Cancer* 76:1288, 1997.

67. Foster JS et al: Multifaceted regulation of cell cycle progression by estrogen: regulation of Cdk inhibitors and Cdc25A independent of cyclin D1-Cdk4 function, *Mol Cell Biol* 21:794, 2001.

68. Umekita Y, Yoshida H: Cyclin D1 expression in ductal carcinoma in situ, atypical ductal hyperplasia and usual ductal hyperplasia: an immunohistochemical study, *Pathol Int* 50:527, 2000.

69. Nielsen NH et al: Cyclin E overexpression, a negative prognostic factor in breast cancer with strong correlation to oestrogen receptor status, *Br J Cancer* 74:874, 1996.

70. Gray-Bablin J et al: Cyclin E, a redundant cyclin in breast cancer, *Proc Natl Acad Sci USA* 93:15215, 1996.

71. Zhou Q et al: Cyclin D1 overexpression in a model of human breast premalignancy: preferential stimulation of anchorage-independent but not anchorage dependent growth is associated with increased cdk2 activity, *Breast Cancer Res Treat* 59:27, 2000.

72. Alle KK: Cyclin D1 protein is overexpressed in hyperplasia and intraductal carcinoma of the breast, *Clin Cancer Res* 4:847, 1998.

73. Mommers ECM et al: Expression of proliferation and apoptosis-related proteins in usual ductal hyperplasia of the breast, *Hum Pathol* 29:1539, 1998.

74. Gillett CE et al: Cyclin D1 and associated proteins in mammary ductal carcinoma in situ and atypical ductal hyperplasia, *J Pathol* 184:396, 1998.

75. Steeg PS, Zhou Q: Cyclins and breast cancer, *Breast Cancer Res Treat* 52:17, 1998.

76. Buckley MF et al: Expression and amplification of cyclin genes in human breast cancer, *Oncogene* 8:2127, 1993.

77. Lukus J et al: Cyclin D2 is a moderately oscillating nucleoprotein required for G_1 phase progression in specific cell types, *Oncogene* 10:2125, 1995.

78. Sugino T et al: Telomerase activity in human breast cancer and benign breast lesions: diagnostic applications in clinical specimens, including fine needle aspirates, *Int J Cancer* 69:301, 1996.

79. Bednarek AK et al: Analysis of telomerase activity levels in breast cancer: positive detection at the in situ breast carcinoma stage, *Clin Cancer Res* 3:11, 1997.

80. Kolquist KA et al: Expression of TERT in early premalignant lesions and a subset of cells in normal tissues, *Nature* 19:182, 1998.

81. Sabourin JC et al: *bcl-2* expression in normal breast tissue during the menstrual cycle, *Int J Cancer* 59:1, 1994.

82. Zhang GJ et al: Correlation between the expression of apoptosis-related *bcl-2* and *p53* oncoproteins and the carcinogenesis and progression of breast carcinomas, *Clin Cancer Res* 3:2329, 1997.

83. Siziopikou KP et al: *bcl-2* expression in the spectrum of preinvasive breast lesions, *Cancer* 77:499, 1996.

84. Zaugg K, Bodis S: Is there a role for molecular prognostic factors in the clinical management of ductal carcinoma in situ of the breast? *Radiother Oncol* 55:95, 2000.

85. Quinn CM et al: Loss of *bcl-2* expression in ductal carcinoma in situ of the breast relates to poor histological differentiation and to expression of *p53* and c-erbB-2 proteins, *Histopathology* 33:531, 1998.

86. Leek RD et al: *bcl-2* in normal human breast and carcinoma, association with oestrogen receptor-positive, epidermal growth factor receptor-negative tumors and in situ cancer, *Br J Cancer* 69:135, 1994.

87. Bhargava V, Kell DL, van de Rijn M: *bcl-2* immunoreactivity in breast carcinoma correlated with hormone receptor positivity, *Am J Pathol* 145:535, 1994.

88. Shen KL et al: The extent of proliferative and apoptotic activity in intraductal and invasive ductal breast carcinomas detected by Ki67 labeling and terminal deoxynucleotidyl transferase-mediated digoxigenin-11dUTP nick end labeling, *Cancer* 82:2373, 1998.

89. Siziopikou KP, Schnitt SJ: MIB-1 proliferation index in ductal carcinoma in situ of the breast: relationship to the expression of the apoptosis-regulating proteins *bcl-2* and *p53*, *Breast J* 6:400, 2000.

90. Megha T et al: Cellular kinetics and expression of *bcl-2* and *p53* in ductal carcinoma of the breast, *Oncol Rep* 7:473, 2000.

91. Gandhi A et al: Evidence of significant apoptosis in poorly differentiated ductal carcinoma in situ of the breast, *Br J Cancer* 78:788, 1998.

92. Liu X-L, Brattain MH, Appert H: Differential display of reticulocalbin in the highly invasive cell line, MDA-MB-435, versus the poorly invasive cell line, MCF-7, *Biochem Biophys Res Comm* 231:283, 1997.

93. Sommers CL et al: Differentiation state and invasiveness of human breast cancer cell lines, *Breast Cancer Res Treat* 31:325, 1994.

94. Kirschmann DA et al: Differentially expressed genes associated with the metastatic phenotype in breast cancer, *Breast Cancer Res Treat* 55:127, 1999.

95. Linderholm BK et al: The expression of vascular endothelial growth factor correlates with mutant *p53* and poor prognosis in human breast cancer, *Cancer Res* 61:2256, 2001.

96. Guidi AJ et al: Vascular permeability factor (vascular endothelial growth factor) expression and angiogenesis in patients with ductal carcinoma in situ of the breast, *Cancer* 80:1945, 1997.

97. Brown LF et al: Vascular stroma formation in carcinoma in situ, invasive carcinoma, and metastatic carcinoma of the breast, *Clin Cancer Res* 5:1041, 1999.

98. Grigorian M et al: Tumor suppressor p53 protein is a new target for the metastasis-associated Mts1/S100A4 protein: functional consequences of their interaction, *J Biol Chem* 276:22699, 2001.

99. Albertazzi E et al: Expression of metastasis-associated genes h-mts1 and nm23 in carcinoma of breast is related to disease progression, *DNA Cell Biol* 17:335, 1998.

100. Rudland PS et al: Prognostic significance of the metastasis-inducing protein S100A4 in human breast cancer, *Cancer Res* 60:1595, 2000.

101. Su Z-Z et al: PEG-3, a nontransforming cancer progression gene, is a positive regulator of cancer aggressiveness and angiogenesis, *Proc Natl Acad Sci USA* 96:15115, 1999.

102. Russo J, Russo IH: The pathway of neoplastic transformation of human breast epithelial cells, *Radiat Res* 155:151, 2001.

103. Ratsch SB et al: Multiple genetic changes are required for efficient immortalization of different subtypes of normal human mammary epithelial cells, *Rad Res* 155:143, 2001.

104. Scheffner M et al: The E6 oncoprotein encoded by human papilloma-virus types 16 and 18 promotes the degradation of *p53*, *Cell* 63:1129, 1990.

105. Dyson N et al: The human papilloma virus-16 E7 oncoprotein is able to bind to the retinoblastoma gene product, *Science* 2443:934, 1989.

106. Banks L, Edmonds, Vousden KH: Ability of the HPV 16 E7 protein to bind RB and induce DNA synthesis is not sufficient for efficient transforming activity, *Oncogene* 5:1283, 1990.

107. Nieto Y et al: Evaluation of the predictive value of Her2/*neu* overexpression and *p53* mutations in high-risk primary breast cancer patients treated with high-dose chemotherapy and autologous stem cell transplantation, *J Clin Oncol* 18:2070, 2000.

108. Leong A S-Y et al: Biologic markers in ductal carcinoma in situ and concurrent infiltrating carcinoma, *Am J Clin Pathol* 115:709, 2001.

109. Russo J et al: Critical steps in breast carcinogenesis, *Ann NY Acad Sci USA* 698:1, 1993.

23

Risk Factors for Breast Carcinoma in Women with Proliferative Breast Disease

WILLIAM D. DUPONT

DAVID L. PAGE

Chapter Outline

The histology of benign breast biopsies is highly variable, and biopsied tissue may vary from the physiologically normal at one extreme to in situ carcinoma at the other. It thus made sense to subdivide these lesions into biologically meaningful categories and to attempt to determine the cancer risk associated with these different categories. This task has proved to be difficult because the studies must be large and there have been numerous classification schemes by authors of studies addressing this question. Many of these authors[1-6] have performed concurrent studies in which the malignant potential of benign lesions was judged by the frequency of their association with breast carcinoma in the same biopsy. The problem with such studies is that it is impossible to infer whether the implicated benign lesions are true precursor lesions for cancer, markers of risk elevation, or themselves a consequence of the malignancy. Thus, to prove that a benign lesion increases a woman's breast cancer risk, it is necessary to establish a temporal relationship between the occurrence of the benign lesion and the later development of breast cancer. Several investigators have performed such studies, most notably Kodlin and colleagues,[7] Black and associates,[8] Hutchinson and colleagues,[9] and our own group studying the Nashville cohort.[10-19] In addition, other studies have assessed Page's histologic classification scheme in other cohorts of women using other pathologists.[20-23] These studies are discussed later.

The other major challenge with studies of premalignant breast disease is that of establishing reproducible and biologically meaningful diagnoses. Our approach to this problem has been, first, through extensive pretesting to devise a preliminary classification scheme that can distinguish between fine differences in breast morphology and cytology and yet be reproducible. This classification scheme was first evaluated in 1978.[15] After revision, it was then applied to more than 10,000 benign breast biopsies, and follow-up from a suitable sample of the women who had undergone biopsies was obtained. Relative risk estimates associated with the different benign lesions were derived and compared. Our published benign disease categories represent groupings of preliminary classifications that are associated with consistent and clinically meaningful levels of cancer risk. These categories and the cancer risks associated with them have been endorsed by the College of American Pathologists (CAP).[24] The results of our studies are discussed in the next section. The relationship between our results and those of other investigators is described subsequently.

The Nashville Studies

We reevaluated 10,366 consecutive benign breast biopsies that were performed between 1950 and 1968 at three hospitals in Nashville, Tennessee[11] (Table 23-1).

These analyses indicated that 70% of women who undergo biopsy revealing benign breast tissue are not at increased risk of breast cancer. The remaining 30% of the 10,000 evaluated biopsies contained proliferative lesions. These lesions are characterized by at least moderate hyperplasia[26] and are associated with an approximate twofold increase in breast cancer risk. The lesions within this disease category include, most prominently, hyperplasia of usual type (ductal) of moderate and florid degree and sclerosing adenosis and papillomas. Also constituting a minor component of this category are mild or poorly developed examples of atypical hyperplasia (AH). This latter category was created primarily to provide a clear lower boundary for the criteria needed to diagnose AH. Mild hyperplasia of usual type is excluded from the proliferative disease category because it is not associated with increased cancer risk and thus is not considered a disease. Clinical correlates of proliferative disease are unproved, except for dense mammographic patterns that are positively correlated with the presence of proliferative disease.[27]

The proliferative lesions can be further dichotomized into those with and without atypia. The former (AH) are characterized by meeting some, but not all, of the criteria needed for a diagnosis of carcinoma in situ. These lesions are rare, having a prevalence of 4% in our consecutive series of benign biopsies, and are associated with a fourfold to fivefold increase in breast cancer risk. There are two morphologically distinct subtypes of AH: lobular (ALH) and ductal (ADH) (see Chapter 7). However, women with these lesions have roughly comparable breast cancer risks.[16] Minor differences include a shorter average period between biopsy and invasive carcinoma diagnosis for ADH (8 years) than for ALH (12 years). There are also differences in the age distribution,[16,22] with both types predominating in the perimenopausal period but with ALH even less common in younger and older women. Proliferative disease without atypia (PDWA) was associated with a 60% increase in breast cancer risk (1.6 times) when compared with women from the Third National Cancer Survey and was associated with a 90% increase (1.9 times) when compared with women without such changes from our study. The CAP Consensus Conference[24] stated that this slight elevation in risk ranged from 1.5 to 2 times that of the general population.

Tables 23-1 and 23-2 are adapted from Dupont and Page.[11] In reading these tables it is important to bear in mind that the estimated relative risks may differ from their true values owing to chance by the amount indicated in the 95% confidence intervals. The p values given in these tables are with respect to the null hypothesis that the true relative risk equals 1. Table 23-1 shows the effect of family history, calcification, and age on

| TABLE 23-1 | Relative Risk of Breast Cancer in Women Who Have Undergone Benign Breast Biopsy | | | | |

	NO. OF WOMEN	NO. OF CANCERS	RELATIVE RISK*	95% CONFIDENCE INTERVAL	p VALUE
All women	3303	134	1.5	1.3-1.8	<.0001
Proliferative disease	1925	103	1.9	1.6-2.3	<.0001
No proliferative disease	1378	31	0.89	0.62-1.3	.51
Family history†	369	26	2.5	1.7-3.7	<.0001
No family history	2934	108	1.4	1.2-1.7	.0007
Proliferative disease and					
Family history	234	22	3.2	2.1-4.9	<.0001
No family history	1691	81	1.7	1.4-2.2	<.0001
Calcification	359	23	2.4	1.6-3.6	<.0001
No calcification	1566	80	1.8	1.5-2.3	<.0001
Age‡ 20-45	1205	57	1.9	1.5-2.5	<.0001
Age 46-55	563	35	1.9	1.3-2.6	.0002
Age >55	157	11	2.2	1.2-4.0	.007
No proliferative disease and					
Family history	135	4	1.2	0.43-3.1	.78
No family history	1243	27	0.86	0.59-1.3	.43
Calcification	174	4	0.80	0.30-2.1	.66
No calcification	1204	27	0.90	0.62-1.3	.59
Age 20-45	1025	23	0.99	0.66-1.5	.96
Age 46-55	247	7	0.83	0.40-1.8	.63
Age >55	106	1	0.30	0.04-2.2	.21
Family history and					
Cysts	246	21	3.0	1.9-4.5	<.0001
No cysts	123	5	1.6	0.65-3.7	.32
No family history and					
Cysts	1808	73	1.5	1.2-1.9	.0008
No cysts	1126	35	1.2	0.88-1.7	.23

Modified from Dupont WD, Page DL: *N Engl J Med* 312:146, 1985. Follow-up was obtained on 3303 of these women, representing 84% of eligible subjects. This sample was weighted in favor of patients with proliferative disease. The median length of follow-up was 17 years.
*Risk relative to women from Atlanta survey[25] adjusted for age at biopsy and length of follow-up.
†Mother, sister, or daughter with breast cancer.
‡Age at benign breast biopsy.

breast cancer risk in women with and without proliferative disease. Study subjects with a mother, sister, or daughter who developed breast cancer were at 2.5 times the risk of women in the general population, whereas study subjects without such a history had only a 40% increase in cancer risk. This 40% increase reflects the average of our entire study group. A family history of breast cancer had little effect on breast cancer risk in women without proliferative disease. However, among women with proliferative disease, a family history almost doubled breast cancer risk. This interaction is much stronger for AH (see Table 23-2). Similarly, the presence of calcification was of some importance in women with proliferative disease, but it had no effect on cancer risk among women lacking proliferative lesions.

The interaction between proliferative disease and age at biopsy is particularly interesting. Women with proliferative disease are at approximately twice the breast cancer risk of women of similar age from the general population, regardless of whether they are in the premenopausal, perimenopausal, or postmenopausal age group. In contrast, the relative breast cancer risk falls with increasing age among patients without proliferative disease, with postmenopausal patients having about one third the risk of postmenopausal women in general. This result suggests that women undergoing senile involution whose breasts lack any hyperplastic activity may be at reduced risk of breast cancer.

Table 23-2 shows how breast cancer risk varies among women with proliferative breast disease. Note the marked interaction between family history and AH.

Figure 23-1 shows the absolute risk of breast cancer associated with the disease categories discussed previously as a function of time since benign biopsy. These

TABLE 23-2 Relative Risk of Breast Cancer in Women With Proliferative Breast Disease

	NO. OF WOMEN	NO. OF CANCERS	RELATIVE RISK*	95% CONFIDENCE INTERVAL	p VALUE
Proliferative disease without atypia	1693	73	1.6	1.3-2.0	.0001
Atypical hyperplasia	232	30	4.4	3.1-6.3	<.0001
Calcification	533	27	1.8	1.3-2.7	.001
Proliferative disease without atypia and					
Family history†	195	12	2.1	1.2-3.7	.009
No family history	1498	61	1.5	1.2-1.9	.002
Calcification	321	16	1.9	1.2-3.1	.012
No calcification	1372	57	1.5	1.2-1.9	.002
Atypical hyperplasia and					
Family history	39	10	8.9	4.8-17	<.0001
No family history	193	20	3.5	2.3-5.5	<.0001
Calcification	38	7	6.5	3.1-14	<.0001
No calcification	194	23	4.0	2.7-6.1	<.0001

Modified from Dupont WD, Page DL: *N Engl J Med* 312:146, 1985.
*Risk relative to women from Atlanta survey,[25] adjusted for age at biopsy and length of follow-up.
†Mother, sister, or daughter with breast cancer.

curves emphasize the considerable variation in cancer risk associated with these lesions. Patients with both AH and a first-degree family history have a breast cancer incidence of about 20% in the first 15 years after their biopsy. This level of risk is comparable to that of women with in situ carcinoma (see Chapter 79). Traditionally, all patients in our study cohort would have been diagnosed as having fibrocystic disease. It is clear from Figure 23-1 that this term has little prognostic value and should be replaced by more precise terminology. When an imprecise indication is useful, the term *fibrocystic change* may be preferred.

Evaluation of Page's Histologic Classification Scheme by Other Authors

Page's histologic classification scheme has been evaluated in four other studies.[20-23] Dupont and colleagues[20] studied women who underwent benign biopsy as part of the Breast Cancer Detection Demonstration Project (BCDDP). London and associates[21] studied women from Harvard's Nurses Health Study, and Palli and co-workers[23] conducted a nested case-control study of a cohort of Italian women. In the studies by Dupont and colleagues and London and associates, the study pathologists reviewed a training set of biopsies with Page in person before conducting their study reviews. Page was not consulted during the pathology review of either of these studies. In Palli and co-workers' study, the study pathologist used

Page's published criteria without any direct interaction with Page himself. The results of these studies are summarized in Figure 23-2. These studies have overlapping confidence intervals within each diagnostic category and are consistent with AH being associated with a fourfold to fivefold elevation in breast cancer risk, whereas PDWA approximately doubles breast cancer risk. The fact that other pathologists have found similar levels of breast cancer risk associated with these lesions supports the reproducibility and credibility of our findings.

Marshall and colleagues[22] have studied the difference in breast cancer risk between women with ALH and

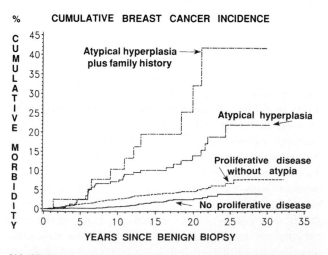

FIG. 23-1 Proportion of patients who have developed invasive breast cancer as a function of time since their benign breast biopsy. (*Modified from Dupont WD, Page DL: Hum Pathol 20:723, 1989.*)

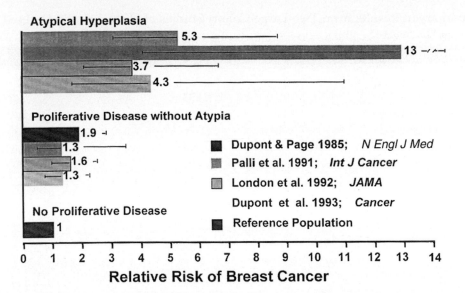

Atypical Hyperplasia

5.3

13

3.7

4.3

Proliferative Disease without Atypia

1.9

1.3

1.6

1.3

■ Dupont & Page 1985; *N Engl J Med*
■ Palli et al. 1991; *Int J Cancer*
□ London et al. 1992; *JAMA*
   Dupont et al. 1993; *Cancer*
■ Reference Population

No Proliferative Disease

1

0 1 2 3 4 5 6 7 8 9 10 11 12 13 14

Relative Risk of Breast Cancer

FIG. **23-2** Estimated relative risks of breast cancer associated with atypical hyperplasia and proliferative disease without atypia that have been reported in the literature. The studies shown are those that have used Page's histologic criteria. These studies suggest that different pathologists can identify subgroups of patients with benign breast disease who have similar levels of breast cancer risk.

ADH. The estimate of the relative risk of breast cancer in women with ALH was 5.3 (95% confidence interval 2.7 to 10.4), whereas for women with ADH this risk was 2.4 (95% confidence interval 1.3 to 4.5). Although the estimated risk was higher for women with ALH than for those with ADH, the confidence intervals are wide and these estimates are not significantly different from each other. The researchers also observed a higher estimated relative risk for premenopausal women with ALH than for postmenopausal women with this lesion.

Relationship between the Histologic Classification Schemes of Different Authors

The results of our studies should be compared with those of Kodlin and colleagues[7] and Hutchinson and associates.[9] Kodlin and colleagues used a scheme devised by Black and Chabon[28] that classifies lesions by their location in the breast and by their degree of proliferation. Black and Chabon's method of grouping lesions by location has not proved to be useful in distinguishing between different levels of breast cancer risk, and authors who have used their system have emphasized the component of this system that quantifies the degree of proliferation. This system consists of an atypia score in which *1* denotes normal epithelium, *2* denotes hyperplasia, *3* and *4* denote different degrees of atypia, and *5* denotes in situ carcinoma. The major results of the study by Kodlin and colleagues[7] are summarized in Table 23-3. This was a retrospective cohort study of

women in a health maintenance organization. It is important to note that 11% of their patients had atypia scores of 3 or 4, as compared with 4% of our patients with AH. Thus it is clear that the criteria for atypia in the Black-Chabon system are broader than those in our own. It would appear, however, that their grade 4 atypia is roughly comparable to our AH. As a group, the patients in Kodlin's cohort were at considerably higher breast cancer risk than the women in our study. This discrepancy may be the result of several factors, including different selection biases between the studies.

Table 23-3 also shows the results of the retrospective cohort study by Hutchinson and co-workers.[9] In this study, as in Kodlin's and our own, the benign breast biopsies of the study patients were reanalyzed using a predefined classification scheme. The discussion of the classification scheme is brief, making it difficult to compare their results with those of other investigators. They found a threefold elevation in cancer risk associated with epithelial hyperplasia or papillomatosis. This risk was not appreciably affected by the presence or absence of atypia. They did find that calcification substantially increased the risk of breast cancer associated with epithelial hyperplasia or papillomatosis. This result is consistent with our finding of increased risk associated with calcification and proliferative disease.

Haagensen and associates[29] have reported an increased risk of breast cancer associated with cysts. This result is in partial agreement with our finding that the presence of cysts increased cancer risk among women with a first-degree family history of breast cancer. This association was not present among women without such a history (see Table 23-1). Dixon and colleagues[30] observed a

| TABLE 23-3 | Summary of Results from Two Large Cohort Studies of Histologically Defined Benign Breast Disease | | |

HISTOLOGIC DIAGNOSES	NO. OF PATIENTS	RELATIVE RISK*
Kodlin et al.[7]		
Entire group	2931	2.7
Black-Chabon atypia score 4	49	6.0
Black-Chabon atypia score 3	262	2.4
Black-Chabon atypia score 1-2	2092	2.3
Fibroadenoma	849	7.0
Adenosis or fibrosing adenosis	177	5.0
Intraductal papilloma	80	5.0
Hutchinson et al.[9]		
Entire group	1356	2.2
Epithelial hyperplasia or papillomatosis	466	2.8
With atypia	33	2.9
Without atypia	433	2.8
With calcification†	102	5.3
Without calcification†	190	2.8
Fibroadenoma with fibrocystic disease	122	3.8

*Calculated with respect to the general population. Different external reference populations were used in each study.
†Women with main lesion type other than epithelial hyperplasia or papillomatosis were excluded.

modest elevation in breast cancer risk for women with palpable cysts. The relative risk of breast cancer associated with cysts in this study was higher in premenopausal women than in postmenopausal women.

Complex Fibroadenoma and Proliferative Breast Disease

Fibroadenomas exhibit a wide range of cytologic and histologic patterns, with the histologic component of these lesions varying from nonexistent to carcinoma in situ. Also, although fibroadenomas have traditionally been thought to be unrelated to breast cancer risk, several authors have reported that women with these lesions have a mildly elevated risk of breast cancer.[9,31-35] This led us to investigate whether different histologic types of fibroadenomas were associated with different levels of breast cancer risk.[12] We obtained follow-up on 1835 patients from our Nashville study hospitals who were diagnosed as having fibroadenoma between 1950 and 1968. These women represented 90% of eligible subjects. The histologic slides of study subjects were reclassified without knowledge of subsequent cancer outcome. The risk of breast cancer in fibroadenoma patients was 2.17 times that of women from a sister-in-law control group. This risk increased to 3.1 in patients with complex fibroadenomas that contained either cysts, sclerosing adenosis, epithelial calcifications, or papillary apocrine changes. Breast cancer risk was also elevated in patients whose adjacent parenchyma

contained proliferative disease (Table 23-4). Breast cancer risk was further enhanced in patients with a first-degree family history of breast cancer and either complex fibroadenoma or adjacent proliferative disease. These women had a cumulative 25-year incidence of breast cancer of about 20% (Figure 23-3). Two thirds of study subjects had simple fibroadenomas and no family history of breast cancer. These patients did not have a significant elevation in breast cancer risk compared with women from the general population. We have also studied the importance of ALH or ADH within fibroadenomas.[10] These findings are rare, being found in 0.8% of fibroadenomas. Atypia within fibroadenomas cannot be used to predict the presence of atypia in the adjacent parenchyma and does not impart a clinically meaningful elevation in breast cancer risk over that associated with fibroadenoma alone.

The clinical implications of these results are most important in women with a first-degree family history of breast cancer. For these women the presence of either adjacent proliferative disease or complex fibroadenomas adds to the magnitude of their breast cancer risk. Although it is inappropriate to unduly concern young women with a family history, a complex fibroadenoma diagnosis should be a further encouragement for regular mammographic surveillance by age 35 or 40 years. Although it may occasionally be technically difficult, the inclusion of some adjacent parenchyma when fibroadenomas are surgically removed seems appropriate and will more often reduce anxiety than increase it. Women with noncomplex fibroadenomas who have neither adjacent

| TABLE 23-4 | Relative Risks of Invasive Breast Cancer in Fibroadenoma Patients |

RISK FACTOR	NO. OF WOMEN	NO. OF CANCERS	CONNECTICUT CONTROLS RELATIVE RISK*	CONNECTICUT CONTROLS 95% CONFIDENCE INTERVAL	SISTER-IN-LAW CONTROLS RELATIVE RISK*	SISTER-IN-LAW CONTROLS 95% CONFIDENCE INTERVAL
All patients	1835	87	1.61	1.3-2.0	2.17	1.5-3.2
Internal diagnosis†						
Not complex	1413	58	1.42	1.1-1.8	1.89	1.3-2.9
Complex	422	29	2.24	1.6-3.2	3.10	1.9-5.1
External diagnosis‡						
No parenchyma	477	21	1.59	1.0-2.5	1.89	1.1-3.2
No proliferative disease (no PD)	1177	51	1.48	1.1-1.9	2.07	1.4-3.2
PD without atypia	162	12	2.16	1.2-3.8	3.47	1.8-6.8
Atypical hyperplasia	19	3	4.77	1.5-15	7.29	2.2-24
Total PD	181	15	2.43	1.5-4.0	3.88	2.1-7.2

*Risks are relative to women from Connecticut and to sister-in-law controls. The Connecticut risks are adjusted for age at diagnosis, year of diagnosis, and length of follow-up. The sister-in-law risks are adjusted for age at diagnosis, length of follow-up, parity, age of first birth, and age of menarche. (The age of diagnosis for each sister-in-law was the age at which her matched in-law's fibroadenoma was diagnosed.)
†Complex fibroadenomas contain either cysts, sclerosing adenosis, epithelial calcifications, or papillary apocrine change.
‡Diagnosis of parenchyma adjacent to the fibroadenoma.

proliferative disease nor a family history of breast cancer are not at elevated breast cancer risk. It should be emphasized that two thirds of patients with fibroadenoma have neither a complex lesion nor a family history, and they may be reassured with the knowledge that their breast cancer risk is not appreciably affected by their tumor.

We believe that there is clinical value in defining *proliferative breast disease* to mean lesions that have been shown to be markers approaching a twofold to threefold elevation in breast cancer risk. When this definition is used, complex fibroadenomas should be included among the proliferative breast lesions.

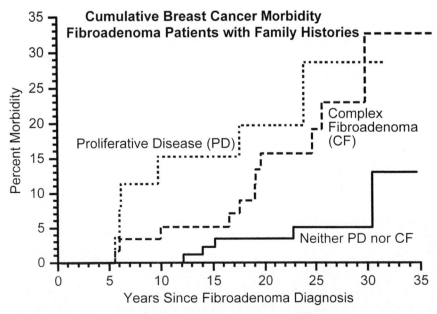

FIG. 23-3 Cumulative incidence of invasive breast cancer among patients with fibroadenoma who have a first-degree family history of breast cancer (FH). Among fibroadenoma patients with FH, women with complex fibroadenomas (CF) or adjacent proliferative disease (PD) had significantly greater cancer incidence than women without CF (*p* = 0.004) or PD (*p* = 0.001), respectively. The cumulative incidence after 25 years for women with FH and either CF or PD was about 20%. (*Modified from Dupont WD et al: N Engl J Med 331:10, 1994. Copyright 1994 Massachusetts Medical Society. All rights reserved.*)

Effect of Time Since Biopsy on Breast Cancer Risk

Most relative risk estimates from longitudinal studies are derived under the assumption that each patient's relative risk remains constant over time. It is possible, however, for the relative risk of an individual patient to vary as a function of either age or time since initial diagnosis. An example of such a change can be found in our studies of benign breast disease. We have previously reported that women who have undergone breast biopsy that reveals AH have 5.3 times the breast cancer risk of women who underwent biopsy but lacked proliferative disease and that the corresponding relative risk for women with PDWA is 1.9.[11] These results were obtained using a proportional hazards regression model that assumes that relative risk remains constant over time. Figure 23-4, however, shows an alternative analysis of these same data. The risk estimates were derived from a hazard regression model that uses time-dependent covariates.[36,37] Figure 23-4 shows that the breast cancer risk for women with both AH and PDWA is greatest in the first 10 years after benign breast biopsy. Women with PDWA who remain free of breast cancer for 10 years are at no greater risk than are women of similar age who do not have such a history. The relative risk of breast cancer in women with AH is halved if they remain free of breast cancer for 10 years after their initial biopsy. This supports the hypothesis that the AHs are not obligate precursor lesions for breast cancer and that these lesions may

progress to cancer, remain unchanged, or possibly regress over a substantial period. Their presence at time of biopsy may be best regarded as a marker of increased risk.

Krieger and Hiatt[32] have reported similar findings of the effect of time since biopsy on breast cancer risk. Women whose benign breast lesions had a Black-Chabon[28] score of 1 or 2 had a twofold elevation in breast cancer risk that varied little with time since biopsy. For women with a Black-Chabon score of 4, however, breast cancer relative risks of 3.5, 2.4, and 1.7 were reported for follow-up intervals of 0 to 17, 10 to 17, and 15 to 17 years, respectively.

The absolute risk for all the women in our study group[11] seems to be approximately evenly distributed over the 17-year period of follow-up (see Figure 23-1). The knowledge that invasive carcinomas were fairly evenly distributed over this time, combined with the fact that approximately half the invasive carcinomas had occurred by year 10, would have led us to predict the finding just described. Thus an approximately constant cancer incidence over a 17-year age span, together with a rising age-specific incidence in women without proliferative disease (the denominator of the relative risk statistic), implies that a woman's relative risk of breast cancer must fall with increasing time since biopsy. Whether relative risk will continue to drop with further follow-up is, of course, yet to be determined. This time-dependent analysis does suggest that one should not presume the constancy of relative risk figures through an entire lifetime when making clinical decisions.

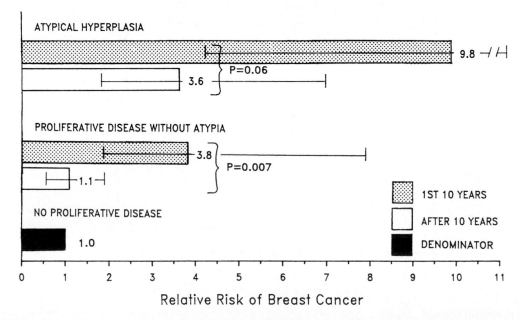

FIG. 23-4 Relative risk of breast cancer in women with proliferative disease. Risks of patients with and without atypia are contrasted with risks of women who underwent biopsy and who did not have proliferative disease. Breast cancer relative risks drop substantially in women who remain free of breast cancer for 10 years following their proliferative disease biopsy. (*From Dupont WD, Page DL: Hum Pathol 20:723, 1989.*)

RADIAL SCAR

Jacobs and colleagues[38] studied the association between radial scars in benign breast biopsies and breast cancer risk. They found that women with radial scars had 1.8 (95% confidence interval 1.1 to 2.9) times that of women without radial scars. This risk was increased to 3.0 (95% confidence interval 1.7 to 5.5) in women with both radial scars and PDWA compared with women with neither lesion. In our cohort, radial scar is highly correlated with PDWA but does not appear to be an independent risk factor for breast cancer.[39]

HORMONAL REPLACEMENT THERAPY IN WOMEN WITH PROLIFERATIVE DISEASE

A question of great importance to women and their physicians is whether hormonal replacement therapy (HRT) can be safely given to women with a history of proliferative breast disease. This question has been studied by us[40] and by Byrne and colleagues.[41] Both of these studies found no evidence that breast cancer risk in women with either PDWA or AH was further increased by taking HRT. While these findings are reassuring it must be noted that the power of both studies to detect a moderate elevation in risk related to this therapy was fairly low. Hence, these studies cannot rule out such an increase. Also, the majority of women in both studies took HRT for less than 5 years. Hence, the question of risk in these women associated with long-term HRT use cannot be adequately addressed.

It should also be noted that a clinical trial conducted by the Women's Health Initiative[42] found HRT to be associated with a relative risk of breast cancer of 1.26 (95% confidence interval 1.00 to 1.59). In this trial, women were enrolled after menopause. Therapy consisted of conjugated equine estrogens plus a progestin, which study subjects took for an average duration of 5.2 years. Breast cancer risk was entirely restricted to women who had taken HRT before enrolling in this study. The relative risk of breast cancer among women with no prior HRT exposure was 1.06 (95% confidence interval 0.81 to 1.38). Hence, the Women's Health Initiative provides no evidence that taking HRT for a few years to wean women from their endogenous estrogen increases breast cancer risk. This study also did not address breast cancer risk in women with a history of benign breast disease. However, in light of these results, it would be prudent for women with a history of AH to avoid taking HRT for more than 5 years.

REDUCED EXPRESSION OF TRANSFORMING GROWTH FACTOR-β TYPE II RECEPTORS IN WOMEN WITH PROLIFERATIVE DISEASE

We have studied the effect on breast cancer risk of reduced expression of the transforming growth factor (TGF)-β type II receptors (TβRII) in women with epithelial hyperplasia lacking atypia (EHLA).[13] We found that among women with these lesions, breast cancer risk increased with decreasing expression of this receptor. Women with EHLA and 25% to 75% TβRII positive cells had 1.98 times the breast cancer risk of women with EHLA and normal TβRII expression (>75% TβRII-positive cells). Women with EHLA and less than 25% TβRII-positive cells had 3.41 times the breast cancer risk of women with EHLA and normal TβRII expression (test for trend = 0.008). This finding is biologically plausible because the normal role of TGF-β is to downregulate cellular proliferation. A reasonable hypothesis that is consistent with these results is that proliferative lesions that cannot "hear" this downregulating TGF-β signal are more likely to progress to cancer than are lesions with normal TβRII expression that are at least aware of this signal.

REFERENCES

1. Foote FW, Stewart FW: Comparative studies of cancerous versus noncancerous breasts, *Ann Surg* 121:197, 1945.
2. Frantz VK et al: Incidence of chronic cystic disease in so-called "normal breasts," *Cancer* 4:762, 1951.
3. Jensen HM, Rice JR, Wellings SR: Preneoplastic lesions in the human breast, *Science* 191:295, 1976.
4. Kramer WM, Rush BF Jr: Mammary duct proliferation in the elderly: a histopathologic study, *Cancer* 31:130, 1973.
5. Sandison AT: *An autopsy study of the adult human breast.* National Cancer Institute Monograph No. 8, DHEW PHS, Washington, DC, 1962, US Government Printing Office.
6. Sasano N, Tateno H, Stemmermann GN: Volume and hyperplastic lesions of breasts of Japanese women in Hawaii and Japan, *Prev Med* 7:196, 1978.
7. Kodlin D et al: Chronic mastopathy and breast cancer: a follow-up study, *Cancer* 39:2603, 1977.
8. Black MM et al: Association of atypical characteristics of benign breast lesions with subsequent risk of breast cancer, *Cancer* 29:338, 1972.
9. Hutchinson WB et al: Risk of breast cancer in women with benign breast disease, *J Nat Cancer Inst* 65:13, 1980.
10. Carter BA et al: No elevation in long-term breast carcinoma risk for women with fibroadenomas that contain atypical hyperplasia, *Cancer* 92:30, 2001.
11. Dupont WD, Page DL: Risk factors for breast cancer in women with proliferative breast disease, *N Engl J Med* 312:146, 1985.
12. Dupont WD et al: Long-term risk of breast cancer in women with fibroadenoma, *N Engl J Med* 331:10, 1994.
13. Gobbi H et al: Transforming growth factor-beta and breast cancer risk in women with mammary epithelial hyperplasia, *J Natl Cancer Inst* 91:2096, 1999.
14. Jensen RA et al: Invasive breast cancer risk in women with sclerosing adenosis, *Cancer* 64:1977, 1989.
15. Page DL et al: Relation between component parts of fibrocystic disease complex and breast cancer, *J Nat Cancer Inst* 61:1055, 1978.
16. Page DL et al: Atypical hyperplastic lesions of the female breast: a long-term follow-up study, *Cancer* 55:2698, 1985.

17. Page DL et al: Lobular neoplasia of the breast: higher risk for subsequent invasive cancer predicted by more extensive disease, *Hum Pathol* 22:1232, 1991.

18. Page DL, Dupont WD, Jensen RA: Papillary apocrine change of the breast: associations with atypical hyperplasia and risk of breast cancer, *Cancer Epidemiol Biomarkers Prev* 5:29, 1996.

19. Page DL et al: Subsequent breast carcinoma risk after biopsy with atypia in a breast papilloma, *Cancer* 78:258, 1996.

20. Dupont WD et al: Breast cancer risk associated with proliferative breast disease and atypical hyperplasia, *Cancer* 71:1258, 1993.

21. London SJ et al: A prospective study of benign breast disease and the risk of breast cancer, *JAMA* 267:941, 1992.

22. Marshall LM et al: Risk of breast cancer associated with atypical hyperplasia of lobular and ductal types, *Cancer Epidemiol Biomarkers Prev* 6:297, 1997.

23. Palli D et al: Benign breast disease and breast cancer: a case-control study in a cohort in Italy, *Int J Cancer* 47:703, 1991.

24. Fitzgibbons PL, Henson DE, Hutter RV: Benign breast changes and the risk for subsequent breast cancer: an update of the 1985 consensus statement. Cancer Committee of the College of American Pathologists, *Arch Pathol Lab Med* 122:1053, 1998.

25. Cutler SJ, Young JL (eds): *Third national cancer survey: incidence data.* Publication No. (NIH) 75-787. Bethesda, MD, 1975, National Cancer Institute.

26. Page DL, Anderson TJ, Rogers LW: Epithelial hyperplasia. In Page DL, Anderson TJ (eds): *Diagnostic histopathology of the breast,* Edinburgh, 1987, Churchill Livingstone.

27. Friedenreich C et al: Risk factors for benign proliferative breast disease, *Int J Epidemiol* 29:637, 2000.

28. Black MM, Chabon AB: In situ carcinoma of the breast. In Sommers SC (ed): *Pathology annual,* New York, 1969, Appleton-Century-Crofts.

29. Haagensen CD, Bodian C, Haagensen DEJ: *Breast cancer risk and detection,* Philadelphia, 1981, WB Saunders.

30. Dixon JM et al: Risk of breast cancer in women with palpable breast cysts: a prospective study. Edinburgh Breast Group, *Lancet* 353:1742, 1999.

31. Carter CL et al: A prospective study of the development of breast cancer in 16,692 women with benign breast disease, *Am J Epidemiol* 128:467, 1988.

32. Krieger N, Hiatt RA: Risk of breast cancer after benign breast diseases: variation by histologic type, degree of atypia, age at biopsy, and length of follow-up, *Am J Epidemiol* 135:619, 1992.

33. Levi F et al: Incidence of breast cancer in women with fibroadenoma, *Int J Cancer* 57:681, 1994.

34. McDivitt RW et al: Histologic types of benign breast disease and the risk for breast cancer. The Cancer and Steroid Hormone Study Group, *Cancer* 69:1408, 1992.

35. Moskowitz M et al: Proliferative disorders of the breast as risk factors for breast cancer in a self-selected screened population: pathologic markers, *Radiology* 134:289, 1980.

36. Dupont WD, Page DL: Relative risk of breast cancer varies with time since diagnosis of atypical hyperplasia, *Hum Pathol* 20:723, 1989.

37. Kalbfleisch JD, Prentice RL: *The statistical analysis of failure time data,* New York, 1980, Wiley.

38. Jacobs TW et al: Radial scars in benign breast-biopsy specimens and the risk of breast cancer, *N Engl J Med* 340:430, 1999.

39. Sanders ME et al: Interdependence of radial scar and proliferative disease with respect to invasive breast cancer risk in benign breast biopsies, *Mod Pathol* 15:50A, 2002.

40. Dupont WD et al: Estrogen replacement therapy in women with a history of proliferative breast disease, *Cancer* 85:1277, 1999.

41. Byrne C et al: Mammographic features and breast cancer risk: effects with time, age, and menopause status, *J Nat Cancer Inst* 87:1622, 1995.

42. Rossouw JE et al: Risks and benefits of estrogen plus progestin in healthy postmenopausal women: principal results from the Women's Health Initiative randomized controlled trial, *JAMA* 288:321, 2002.

CHAPTER

24

Steroid Hormone Receptors

RUTH M. O'REGAN

SUNIL BADVE

WILLIAM J. GRADISHAR

Chapter Outline

More than 100 years ago the association between breast cancer and ovarian function was first recognized. Based on the observation that removal of the ovaries in animals could affect lactation, Beatson decided to treat a premenopausal woman with advanced breast cancer by removing her ovaries, which had a dramatic response.[1] Based on this report, Boyd[2] published data on 46 premenopausal women with advanced breast cancer who were treated with oophorectomy. He observed that approximately one third of these women had responses to oophorectomy. At that time, it was unclear why the remaining two thirds of women did not respond to removal of their ovaries.

Following the chemical characterization of estrogen,[3] Jensen and Jacobson synthesized radioactive estradiol.[4] By injecting radioactive estradiol into immature female rats, they noted that estradiol was retained only in the estrogen target tissues, uterus and vagina, suggesting that a receptor for estrogen must be present in these tissues. In 1966, the estrogen receptor (ER) protein was identified and the concept of estrogen target tissues containing ER was developed. Jensen then discovered in the laboratory that some breast cancers contain ER. Based on this finding, the initial clinical trials using endocrine maneuvers in breast cancer established that only breast cancers containing ER would regress.[5] Subsequently, ER determination was widely used to predict the likelihood that patients with breast cancer would respond to endocrine therapies. In addition, the presence of progesterone receptors (PRs) on breast tumors has proven to be important in determining the likelihood of response to endocrine therapies. PR synthesis is increased in estrogen-responsive tissues, including breast cancer, and it is believed that PR expression may be a better indicator of tumor endocrine responsiveness than ER alone because its presence may indicate a functioning ER.[6] Approximately 25% to 30% of breast cancers are negative for both ER and PR, whereas about 40% are positive for both. About 30% of breast cancers express ER alone, but less than 5%

express PR alone.[7] In advanced breast cancer, patients with tumors expressing both receptors respond to hormonal therapy in more than 60% of cases, whereas those with tumors expressing neither receptor respond in less than 10% of patients. Patients with ER-/PR- breast cancers are generally not offered hormonal therapy.[8] Patients with advanced breast cancer whose breast tumors express either ER or PR respond in about 30% of cases.

Estrogen Receptor Structure and Function

ESTROGEN RECEPTOR-α

The human ER is a member of the family of nuclear hormone receptors that can initiate or enhance the transcription of genes containing specific hormone response elements (Figure 24-1). The ER protein consists of 595 amino acids with a molecular weight of 66 kDa[9] and is separated into 6 different functional domains.[10,11] The human ER is located on chromosome 6q.[12]

The six functional domains of the ER are regions that have been defined based on the putative functions that are contained in each area. There are two activating function domains, AF-1 and AF-2, which activate transcription.[13] The AF-1 region is located in the A/B region, acts in a cell type-specific fashion, and its activation appears independent of the presence of ligand.[14,15] The AF-2 region is located in the E region, which contains the hormone-binding domain (HBD) and is thought to be involved in ligand-specific activation.[14,15] The C region contains the DNA binding domain (DBD) and a dimerization domain. The DBD is the most highly conserved region within the superfamily of nuclear hormone receptors. The DBD consists of 2 zinc fingers,[16] which are essential components of the ER, because it has been demonstrated that when the ER lacks the DBD, it can not bind DNA in vitro or in vivo.[11,17] The E region, or HBD, contains the AF-2 region, heat shock protein 90 binding function, and a dimerization domain. The HBD is responsible for specific ligand recognition.

Estrogen diffuses through the plasma membrane and binds to the ER within the cell nucleus.[18] On binding estrogen, heat shock proteins dissociate from the ER and homodimerization occurs.[19] Following dimerization, the ER binds to estrogen response elements (ERE) present in the promoter regions of genes, which results in gene transcription.

ESTROGEN RECEPTOR-β

In 1996, a second ER, ERβ, was discovered[20] (see Figure 24-1). ERα and ERβ have homology in the DNA binding domain, but only 55% homology in the ligand binding domain. It is possible that different levels

Estrogen Receptor (α and β)

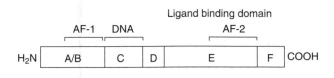

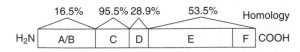

FIG. 24-1 Homology between α and β estrogen receptors.

of ERα and ERβ in target tissues may explain the target site-specific actions of tamoxifen. In addition it has been demonstrated that estradiol may act through an ERE signal transduction pathway via ERβ,[21] whereas tamoxifen may act through a different activating protein-1 (AP-1) pathway.[22] It is likely that coactivator/corepressor expression in target tissues may be also important in the target site-specific actions of tamoxifen and other selective estrogen receptor modulators. Despite the preclinical interest in ERβ, it is not a currently standard practice to measure tumor levels in patients with breast cancer.

Receptor Analysis

TISSUE PROCUREMENT FOR RECEPTOR ANALYSIS

Procedures for tissue handling and procurement of tumor samples were an important issue when ligand binding assays were used to assess steroid hormone receptors. With this type of assay, it was necessary to identify and isolate relatively "pure" samples of tumor. Presence of nontumoral breast tissue or necrotic tissue would significantly alter the results of the assay. In addition, it was critical that this tumor sample (at least 200 mg and usually 400 to 500 mg of tumor) be frozen and transported to the pathology laboratory. Degradation of tumor cells could occur because of delays in transportation or poor quality of storage before conducting the assay (Figure 24-2).

With the current widespread use of immunohistochemistry to detect steroid hormone receptors, tissue procurement has become a less critical issue. However, it remains important to ensure rapid transportation of tissue specimens to the pathology laboratory from the surgery suites (or mammography center). False-negative results due to improper fixation are still a significant problem.

Currently, a significant fraction of new cases of breast cancer are detected as a result of mammographic abnormalities. The excision of these lesions takes place after mammographic localization. It is often necessary to send the excised specimen to mammography to confirm that the mammographic abnormality has been excised. On occasion, this can lead to inordinate delay in fixing the specimen in formalin. One of the ways of circumventing some of the problems associated with fixation is to perform estimations of steroid hormone receptors on needle core biopsies done for diagnostic purposes. Better preservation stemming from a greater tissue/fixative ratio leads to superior results.[23]

ASSAYS FOR HORMONE RECEPTOR

The original methods of identification of steroid hormone receptors involved examination of cell fractions. Using this method, the ER was detected in the cytosol fraction. This led to the belief that these receptors were

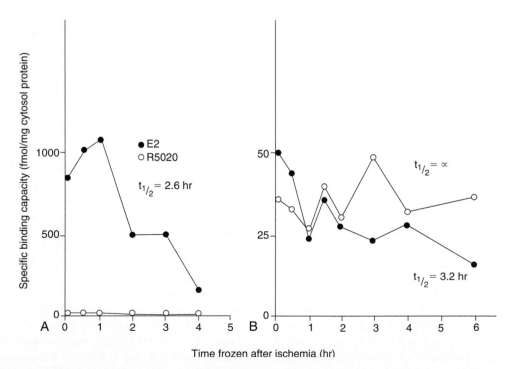

FIG. 24-2 Time course of steroid receptor decay in surgical biopsies of breast cancer. The half-life of each receptor (● for estrogen and ○ for progestin) is highly tissue dependent. *(From an unpublished study by Wittliff JL and Olson J.)*

located in the cell cytoplasm. After binding to their respective ligand, the ER was thought to relocate to the nucleus to bind to a specific segment of the DNA. This belief was first questioned because of the identification of the receptor protein predominantly within the nucleus of enucleated rat pituitary cells and little if any receptor protein within the cytosol. The development of immunohistochemical (IHC) methods confirmed the nuclear localization of the receptor protein.[24-26] The biochemical processing for steroid hormone receptors apparently results in diffusion of the receptor protein from the nucleus to the cytosol and it is the latter that is measured by these methods.

Early on, three types of estrogen binding sites were thought to exist.[27-30] Type I binding sites, also known as estrophilin, were present in low concentrations in the breast epithelial cell nuclei and have the highest affinity for estrogen, achieving saturation at 10^{-9} M estradiol. Type II binding sites, with intermediate affinity, were thought to be a group of different proteins located in the nucleus and cytoplasm that become fully bound to estrogen when its concentration reached 10^{-7} M.[27] Type III binding sites, the most abundant but with low affinity for estrogens, included membrane as well as cytoplasmic proteins. These sites were occupied at estrogen levels well above 10^{-7} M.[27] The working framework of more than one binding site was also used as an argument against the use of monoclonal antibodies to detect ER.[31]

The principal methods currently used to determine the expression of ER are biochemical methods and IHC methods. The standard biochemical methods for the detection and measurement of ER and PR in breast cancers are dextran-coated charcoal (DCC)[32] and sucrose gradient assay. Both of these methods require collection and freezing of a portion of fresh tumor tissue. This piece is homogenized, a buffer is added, and the mixture is ultracentrifuged. The sediment is discarded, and the supernatant cytosol is used for estimation of receptor levels. Radiolabeled steroid is added to the cytosol and the amount of specifically bound protein is measured.

ADVANTAGES OF THE BIOCHEMICAL METHODS OF ASSAY

Ligand binding assays had been the gold standard for ER determination for a long time. The levels of ER as determined by these methods have been shown to have good correlation with survival and response rates to hormonal therapy. Tumors with low levels (<3 fmol/mg), in general, are unlikely to respond to endocrine therapy. The major advantage of these methods is that they provide a quantitative assessment of the receptor as a function of its capacity to bind with estrogenic molecules. Conversely, IHC methods provide immunologic recognition of the receptor molecule rather than assessing their functional binding capacity.

DISADVANTAGES OF THE BIOCHEMICAL METHODS OF ASSAY

The biochemical assays measure the amount of steroid hormone receptor protein in the cytosol. The nuclear fraction usually forms part of the sediment, which is not examined. The measurement is dependent on the amount of receptor protein that translocates to the cytosol, an artifact of processing.

Another important determinant is the nature of the tissue examined. The tumor sample is a mixture of several different cell types and includes benign and malignant elements. These include nontumoral breast tissue as well as supporting stroma that contains fibroblasts, endothelial cells, nerves, and variety of inflammatory cells. Thus the ratios of tumor tissue to benign tissue and tumor tissue to stromal tissue could contribute significantly to the final estimation of ER and PR. These ratios were difficult to determine because few laboratories examined the frozen tissues under a microscope to determine the amount of tumor tissue in a given sample. The presence of stromal fibrosis or prior surgery on occasion could lead to complete absence of tumor in the submitted sample. Necrotic tissue could also interfere with the assay. Davidson's marking inks, which are used to aid assessment of margins, also have been shown to interfere with the assays.

The inconsistent reproducibility of biochemical assays was also an issue. King and colleagues divided each of 9 solid tumors and each of 10 common tumor cytosols among five laboratories for ER assay.[33] Except for one tumor, a fibrosarcoma, and a sample of plasma purposefully labeled as cytosol on which all five laboratories reported no measurable receptor, the results on all breast cancers were highly variable ranging from "not measurable" to several hundred fentomoles per milligram protein on the same tumor. However, the overall coefficient of variance is thought to be in the range of 5%,[34] whereas that for different laboratories is 7% to 19% for ER and 19% to 28% for PR.[35]

The advent of screening methods such as mammography has lead to a significant decrease in the average size of tumors. It has become increasingly difficult to provide a sizable piece of tumor tissue required for the biochemical assays. Most biochemical assays ideally require between 250 mg and 1.0 g of tumor tissue. As the receptor proteins are labile, it is critical that the tumor tissue is isolated immediately after surgery and is snap frozen to ensure proper preservation. This is not always possible for a variety of reasons. A pathologist may not be immediately available to examine the specimen and isolate the tumor tissue. Smaller hospitals and clinics may lack the facility to freeze tissues. A more common problem is the size of needle localization specimens. Currently, a significant number of cases of breast cancer are detected as mammographic abnormalities and excision of these lesions takes place after mammographic localization. It is often necessary to send the excised specimen to mammography to confirm that the mammographic abnormality has been excised. This can occasionally lead to inordinate delay for the specimen to reach the pathology laboratory, which is not conducive to proper tissue procurement for biochemical assays.

The interpretation of the assay requires Scatchard plot analysis to distinguish between specific and non-specific binding and can be difficult. As these assays are based on radioactivity, disposal of waste requires special attention. Biochemical assays also require specially trained personnel and expensive, highly specialized equipment; thus the performance is limited to large medical centers and reference laboratories. Only a limited number of assays can be performed at a given time and the turn around time may be long. Lastly, as the binding capacity of the tissue sample is measured, interference caused by other hormones or oral/menstrual cycle–related estrogens can occur.[36]

IMMUNOHISTOCHEMICAL ASSAYS

History. To circumvent the problems associated with ligand binding assays, attempts were made to use IHC methods for demonstrating ER in situ. Nenci and colleagues[37] report that 17B-estradiol, a natural estrogen, taken up by free viable breast cancer cells could be demonstrated by using indirect immunofluorescence technique. The antiestradiol rabbit serum used detected a nuclear fluorescence, which could be blocked by prior incubation with antiestrogenic drugs, such as nafoxidine and tamoxifen.[38] The major disadvantages of this technique were the time required for preparation and washing of cell suspensions and the difficulty in recognizing cancer cells in suspensions. Pertschuk[39] used polyestradiol phosphate to trace cancer cells in frozen sections. The sections were incubated in 1% polyestradiol phosphate for 1 hour before exposure to antiestradiol antibodies, the latter being tagged with fluorescent markers. The reaction could be blocked by preincubation with high quantities of antiestrogen, CI-628 (Parke-Davis). Although this technique permitted identification of ER expression within tumor cells, the relatively poor binding of polyestradiol to the cells resulted in weak staining.

Kurzon and Sternberger were the first to use the immunoperoxidase technique, instead of a fluorescent dye, as a tag to identify ER in the rat uterine cervix.[40] Lee[41-44] developed a more direct method that linked estrogen with a fluorescent protein carrier that could be directly applied to frozen sections. This was the first commercially available histochemical assay for detecting ER in situ. Because fluorescence fades with time, peroxidase was later substituted as the tag. The

generation of specific anti-ER antibodies made the use of these estrogen-labeled tags redundant.

Greene and associates[45,46] produced a monoclonal antibody by immunizing Lewis rats with estrophilin isolated from MCF-7 cells and by hybridizing the rat spleen cells with mouse myeloma cells. The generation of anti-ER in the Greene's laboratory was soon followed by several similar attempts elsewhere.[47,48] Miller and colleagues[49] and Garancis and associates[50] using a similar method to the Greene's laboratory generated the H222 monoclonal antibody, which was commercially available from Abbott Laboratories as the ER by immunocytochemistry assay (ER-ICA) kit. This antibody bonds to the steroid binding domain of the receptor.[51] However, H222 antibody worked reliably only on frozen tissues and did poorly on paraffin-embedded tissues. Shimada and associates[52] applied this antibody at high concentration (10 μg/ml) for 30 minutes at 37°C to material fixed for 24 hours at 4°C and then rinsed overnight in sodium phosphate buffer. A concordance of 82% was obtained with DCC assays and 86% with frozen section IHC. However, the requirement of cold formalin for 24 hours differs markedly from the conventional fixation. Using Bouin's fixed tissue, Poulsen and co-workers[53] detected ER positivity in approximately half of the biochemically positive tumors tested and suggested that the fixation process may reduce the immunoreactivity of ER proteins. To improve staining, Andersen and colleagues[54] applied full-strength H222 antibody for 16 hours at 4°C following trypsinization to routinely fixed breast sections. Agreement between DCC and IHC was obtained in 30 of 35 cases. Shintaku and Said[55] described a method of enzymatic digestion of paraffin sections with deoxynuclease (DNase) to obtain 94% concordance, whereas Hiort and associates[56] used both trypsin and DNase for antigen retrieval to obtain similar results. They also used cobalt chloride to enhance the color obtained with the reaction product. Cheng and co-workers[57] compared all the aforementioned techniques and reported the best result with digestion by pronase enzyme (Calbiochem, San Diego, CA). De Rosa and colleagues[58] used another monoclonal antibody D75 (from Greene's labortory[45,46]) on Bouin's solution fixed tissue and in tissues fixed in cold (4°C) formalin to obtain greater than 90% concordance. The generation of a second generation of monoclonal antibodies (Mabs) was a significant improvement. al Saati and associates[59] generated a monoclonal IgG1 antibody, 1D5, which produced against human ER using splenocytes of BALB/c mice immunized with recombinant ER. It recognized the A/B region of the N-terminal domain of ER and performed well on paraffin, which improved following heat-induced antigen retrieval. Several Mabs are now commercially available that have been shown to provide good concordance with ligand binding assays. However, different Mabs recognize different epitopes on the ER protein and do not give identical results.

Immunohistochemical Assay Technique. IHC assays can be performed on fresh frozen tissues or paraffin-embedded material. The basic process of paraffin processing includes fixation of tissues in formalin or alcoholic-based fixatives. This process causes precipitation of proteins and prevents tissue degeneration. The fixed tissue is then dehydrated and permeabilized with paraffin using graded levels of alcohol and xylene. The hardened tissue is then covered with excess paraffin to generate the paraffin block. Sections 4 microns thick are cut from the paraffin block and transferred to glass slides. The glass slides are often coated with egg albumin or silane ("plus" slides) to make the glass more "sticky" and to ensure adhesion of the tissues to the glass.

Fixation is an important issue and faulty preparation is the cause for most false-negative receptor analyses.[60] Some amount of degeneration of the tissue antigens is expected with fixation (therefore the need for antigen retrieval). In general, alcohol-based fixatives are better at preservation of the ER epitope. It is important to use buffered formalin (pH 7.0) as lowering of the pH results in loss of immunoreactivity and in the appearance of background and cytoplasmic staining. Several parameters, including temperature, pH, and duration in fixative, affect fixation.[58]

The IHC assay consists of several steps, which are important to understand to prevent erroneous results.[61] These steps include the following:

1. Blocking to prevent nonspecific binding
2. Antigen retrieval to unmask the epitopes that may have been altered during fixation
3. Incubation with primary antibody directed against the target antigen
4. Amplification of the reaction product and detection of the amplified product using tagged reagents to visualize the presence and localization of the product
5. The last step before microscopic examination is to coverslip the slide to prevent damage to section during examination or storage
6. Microscopic examination

Blocking. IHC reactions are usually detected by tagging the amplified product using enzymes. Biotin is the most commonly used agent for amplification, whereas horseradish peroxidase and alkaline phosphatase are commonly used tags. Although enzymes not present in human tissues, such as glucose oxidase, can be used as tags, these are rarely used in clinical practice. In general,

interference is a greater problem on frozen sections than on paraffin sections because routine fixation and processing significantly destroy enzyme activity.

Biotin is widely distributed in nature and more importantly in the human body. Its levels in the breast are low; therefore interference is not usually an issue. However, in certain tissues, such as the liver, it can cause major problems. Nonspecific binding because of the presence of biotin can give rise to high background and at times false-positive staining.[62-64] It can be detected by the presence of staining in the negative control slides. Preincubation with commercially available blocking agents is one way of ameliorating the problem. Alternatively, one can make use of non–biotin-based amplification systems such as the Envision kit (DAKO, Carpinteria, CA).

Peroxidase and peroxidase-like activity (catalase and cytochrome oxidase) is present in a number of normal cells, including red and white blood cells and hepatocytes.[61] These cells will routinely be stained if some form of blocking procedure is not performed. Incubation for 5 to 30 minutes in hydrogen peroxide (H_2O_2), in aqueous or alcoholic form, is usually used to block this endogenous activity.[61,65,66] Use of other agents, such as cyclopropanone hydrate, also has been described.

Isoenzymes of alkaline phosphatase are widely distributed throughout human tissues, with high concentrations detected in intestinal mucosa, proximal tubules of the kidney, and osteoblasts. Although concentrations of the enzyme in the breast are low, interference in the form staining of the endothelial cells may be seen. Levamisole added to the enzyme substrate solution in the concentration of 0.1 M blocks endogenous phosphatase activity. The rationale for this approach is that levamisole easily suppresses human phosphatases but has no effect on the calf intestinal phosphatases[67] used in the preparation of antibody conjugates. In some protocols, the tissue is heated to 65°C for up to 15 minutes to destroy the endogenous enzyme activity.

Antigen Retrieval. Antigen retrieval is a process by which antigenic sites, which may have been altered during fixation, are unmasked and made available for IHC reactions.[68] This process tends to compensate for a variety of the insults the protein epitopes receive during fixation and processing. Although a variety of antigen retrieval protocols exist, the most commonly used protocols for ER consist of heating the slides in buffer (either pH 6 or 8) using a microwave, pressure cooker, or steamer.[68,69] Protease digestion was required before incubation for some of the older ER antibodies; this occasionally was a source of erroneous results.

Antigen-Antibody Interaction. For an immune reaction to occur, the target antigen and the antitarget specific antibody must be exposed to each other.

The incubation time can vary from a few hours (either at room temperature or 35°C) to overnight incubation (usually at 4°C) with the primary antibody directed against the antigen. The concentration of the antibody needs to be titrated to achieve optimal results and to avoid a prozone phenomenon. It is necessary to use control slides (positive and negative) to ascertain the veracity of the reaction. Although it is common to use normal breast tissues for positive controls, other tissues such as breast tumors, cervix, and leiomyomas have also been used with equal or better results. Cell line controls are extremely useful in the assessment of HER2/neu expression. Substitution of primary antibody with serum, which has similar immunoglobulin isotype as the primary antibody, serves as a better control than buffer solutions (usually phosphate-buffered saline). Interference due to heterophilic antibodies can be detected using isotypic antibodies.

Amplification. The interaction between two molecules, in this case antigen and antibody, is difficult to detect by light microscopy. Therefore it is necessary to amplify the reaction product and use tagged reagents to visualize the presence and localization of the product. Most commonly used systems employ the strong specific binding between avidin and biotin for these purposes (hence the necessity for biotin block), although non–biotin-based kits are also commercially available.

A variety of chromogens that enable visualization of the amplified product are available. The most commonly used chromogen is diaminobenzidine (DAB). It is preferred because the brown reaction product is alcohol-fast and thus is suitable for a wide range of counterstains and mountants.[61] Amino-ethyl carbazole (AEC) is another chromogen, which gives a red product. It is thought to be a lower risk carcinogen than DAB but has the disadvantage of being alcohol soluble; thus an aqueous mounting medium, such as glycerol, must be used.

Coverslipping and Storage. The last step before microscopic examination is to coverslip the slide to prevent damage to the section during examination or storage. The major advantage of the peroxide-based systems is that the reaction product is not water-soluble. Thus it is possible to dehydrate and coverslip the slides as would be done for hematoxylin and eosin sections. The crisper staining results obtained with the alkaline phosphatase method is associated with one major disadvantage: The reaction product is water soluble, hence the sections must be mounted in glycerine or equivalent mounting medium. Storage of these slides can be problematic and the intensity of staining also tends to fade with time.

Microscopic Examination. Microscopic examination of the test sample should always be done after examination of both positive and negative controls.

This permits recognition of the staining artifacts and misinterpretation of the results. A variety of methods[70-74] have been used to score the IHC-stained slides, including measurements of the intensity of staining or percentage of positive cells or a combination of the two. The College of American Pathologists (CAP) does not recommend the use of intensity alone as a scoring method.[75] The most commonly used methods are the Quick score,[76] H score,[77,78] total score,[79] and percentage positivity. Quick score assigns a value to both intensity (0 to 3) and percentage (0, 1% to 25%, 26% to 50%, 51% to 75%, and 76% to 100%) of positive cells. The final score is obtained by adding the two values to get a range of 0 to 7. The H score uses a formula based on percentage of nuclei that stain and the intensity of the staining reaction as follows:

$$H \text{ score} = 3(\% \text{ nuclei stained intensity})$$
$$+ 2(\% \text{ nuclei stained moderately})$$
$$+ 1(\% \text{ nuclei stained weakly})$$

The total score method also assigns values for intensity from 0 to 3 and takes into account the average intensity but evaluates proportion of positive cells in a different manner (0, 1 = <1%, 2 = 1% to 10%, 3 = 11% to 33%, 4 = 34% to 66%, 5 = >67%). The percentage methods tend to take into account only the medium and strong intensity-stained cells and use 1% or 10% or even 20% as cutoff values to denote positivity.

Image analysis methods have also been used to assess ER expression. Several image analysis systems are commercially available that can provide an accurate and precise quantitation of the level of expression of ER. Lehr and colleagues[80] have reported the use of the Photoshop program to perform quantification. Most[80-85] but not all[86,87] of these studies have found computerized quantitation to be better than semiquantitative visual analysis. The main reason for this is the difficulty in distinguishing IHC staining and nuclear staining using two different binary images. Kohlberger and colleagues[88] used modified true-color computer assistance to overcome the problem. In one of the early studies, Sklarew and associates[81] in 1990 measured median optical density (MOD) and integrated optical density (IOD) of the tumor cells. They were able to distinguish four MOD patterns (I-IV) and four different contour plots (A-D). They found that the patients responding to endocrine therapy tended to display a type I or type III MOD pattern with either a type A, B, or D contour plot.

Advantages of Immunohistochemistry. The main advantage of the IHC methods is that they permit correlation of ER expression with morphology. The sections from the tumor mass can thus be screened for the amount of invasive tumor cell population.

Expression of ER is analyzed within the nuclei of these cells. Any interference caused by in situ component or adjoining benign elements or necrotic tissue can be easily excluded. The adjoining benign elements additionally serve as good internal control to confirm that the assay has worked.

Another advantage of IHC is that it does not require any special preanalysis manipulation or special tissue procurement. Analysis of ER status can be performed on frozen and paraffin-embedded tissues. The latter enables assessment of receptor status in cases with small incidentally diagnosed carcinomas as well as analysis in a retrospective manner. The antigenicity of the ER is preserved in the paraffin block with deterioration of antigens being an issue only in cut slides. The IHC methodology is relatively inexpensive and does not require any special instrumentation. A large number of cases can be simultaneously analyzed. Very little specialized training is required, particularly with currently available semiautomated immunostainers.

Disadvantages of Immunohistochemistry. Although tissue procurement is not as important as in ligand binding assays, care must be taken to ensure proper and timely fixation of the breast tissues. Because most fixatives are aqueous solutions, they poorly penetrate the predominantly fatty breast tissues. This can result in loss or degradation of the receptor protein.

Alterations in antigenic sites during initial tissue preparation (i.e., fixation, processing, and preparation of the tissue sections) are the commonest causes of false-negative ER results.[89] Tissue fixation involves a number of variables including type, concentration, pH and osmolarity of the fixative,[90] and the duration and temperature of the fixation process. Other factors that have been reported to affect fixation and therefore possibly IHC results are volume of fixative, delayed fixation, or secondary fixation by alcohol either during fixation by methanol, which is added as a preservative, or in alcohol during processing if fixation is incomplete.[91,92] Alcohol-based fixatives or mixtures of formalin and alcohol give better preservation of ER than pure aqueous buffered formalin. However, one problem commonly encountered with alcohol fixatives is associated with the determination of *HER2/neu*. The superior quality of fixation permits visualization of *HER2/neu* even in normal tissues. One solution to this problem is to use higher dilution of *HER2/neu* antibody to achieve negative result with normal breast tissues. However, this procedure deviates from the approved protocol of the U.S. Food and Drug Administration (FDA).

With the use of enclosed tissue processor systems in most laboratories, problems for both tissue and antigen preservation have been reported. This could be caused by the carryover of reagents from one step to the other, particularly xylene used in the cleaning cycle to the first step of the cycle (fixation).[93] Recycling of xylene was also shown to affect antigenicity. The type of reagents used, the timing and temperature used for each step of the processing (dehydration, clearing, and wax infiltration with vacuum) have been reported to affect IHC results.[94-96]

Even after the paraffin blocks are made, variations in air-drying the slides (both duration and temperature) can affect antigenicity.[97] ERs are particularly sensitive to air exposure, and there is a rapid deterioration of antigenicity once the slides are cut from a paraffin block.[98-100] Complete loss of antigenicity has been shown to occur within 3 to 4 weeks of storage of the cut slides. This is an irreversible process and antigenicity cannot be recovered even after antigen retrieval.

The availability of large numbers of primary antibodies and reagent detection kits for ER estimation is associated with variability in techniques for determination of steroid hormone receptors. Very few studies exist that have performed a head-to-head comparison of these reagents. As a result of variations in techniques, the coefficient of variance among laboratories is greater (13.3% to 23.6% for ERs and 25.8% to 35.9% for PRs) than for ligand binding assays.[101]

The final analysis of the slides is an important issue. A number of different methods have been used to evaluate the IHC-stained slides. A variety of cutoff points ranging from any positive cell to more than 20% positive cells have been used to determine positivity. These variations could lead to false-negative reporting, depriving the patient of endocrine therapy.

QUALITY CONTROL ISSUES

Immunohistochemistry: External and Internal. Ligand binding assays were performed in clinical chemistry laboratories, which were used for both internal and external quality control. The European Organization for the Research and Treatment of Cancer played a prominent role in ensuring reproducibility of these assays.[102,103] The IHC studies are less amenable to vigorous quality control. It is therefore even more important to be aware of the issues. Internal quality control involves running of proper positive and negative controls with each test and examining the test clinical sample slide for internal controls. The positive control is composed of tissue(s) that are similarly fixed and processed and contain a population of cells reactive to the antibody in question. It is important for this tissue to be an admixture of positive and negative elements to detect false positivity. The commonly used controls of ER include normal and malignant breast tissues and uterine cervix. The use of leiomyomas as controls is not recommended. In some cases, particularly for *HER2*, the use of cell lines is recommended, in which the controls are grouped together on one slide.

The clinical sample should be examined for internal positive and negative controls. The block to use for ER determinations should ideally contain some normal breast tissue. Normal breast tissue shows variable ER positivity, which is greater in postmenopausal than in premenopausal patients. For negative controls, it is important to use an isotypic immunoglobulin from the same species as the primary antibody to identify interference caused by heterophilic antibodies. They are also useful in identifying false-positive reactions due to other proteins including biotin.

The CAP plays a critical role in ensuring external quality control in the United States, whereas the National External Quality Assessment Scheme for Immunocytochemistry (NEQAS-ICC) provides a similar function in the United Kingdom. The CAP survey[104] of 467 participants in 2001 found that there were at least 15 different antibodies being used for each ER and PR determinations, although 3 antibodies (each) were used in more than 90% of the laboratories. In this survey, 97% of the laboratories correctly identified the test tumor sample as ER positive. Under the NEQAS scheme, Rhodes and colleagues[105] examined interlaboratory variance in detection of ER by 200 laboratories participating in the scheme. They found that although more than 80% of the laboratories could demonstrate positivity in tumors expressing moderate or high levels of ER, only one third could do so in tumors with low expression.

Clinical Relevance of Steroid Receptors in Breast Cancer

ESTROGEN RECEPTOR

The steroid receptors, ER and PR, have both prognostic and predictive value in the management of breast cancer. In general, the absence of both ER and PR is associated with early recurrence and poor survival rates in patients with breast cancer. This is probably a reflection of the intrinsic biologic behavior of receptor-positive tumors, in that ER-positive and PR-positive tumors are more likely to be well differentiated, to be diploid, and to have lower proliferative rates than receptor-negative tumors.[106,107]

Of more importance, however, is the value of ER and PR in predicting benefit from endocrine therapies. In advanced breast cancer, patients with breast tumors expressing neither ER nor PR respond to endocrine therapies in less than 10% of cases (Figure 24-3).[108] In contrast, patients with metastatic breast cancer whose tumors express both receptors can respond to endocrine therapy in up to 70% of cases.[108] PR status seems to be of equal and perhaps greater importance compared with ER in predicting response rates to endocrine

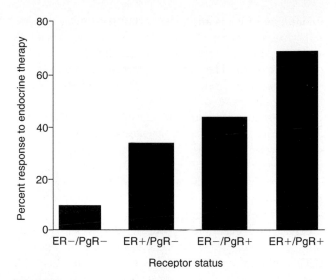

FIG. **24-3** Response to endocrine therapy in advanced breast cancer depends on hormone receptor status of the tumor.

therapy, and it has been hypothesized that the presence of PR indicates an intact endocrine response pathway and that PR is, in fact, a product of estrogen action.[6] In patients with tumors expressing discordant receptors, response rates in advanced breast cancer range from 35% to 45%, with patients whose tumors are PR positive and ER negative responding in a slightly higher percent of cases than those whose tumors are ER positive and PR negative.[108]

Similar to the findings for advanced breast cancer, ER status is predictive of outcome with adjuvant endocrine therapy, namely tamoxifen, in early-stage breast cancer. In general, regardless of the duration of tamoxifen treatment, recurrence rates in patients with ER-positive tumors with early-stage breast cancer receiving tamoxifen are significantly less compared with patients not receiving tamoxifen, although this finding is most definitive in patients receiving 5 years of tamoxifen therapy.[109] In patients with ER-positive tumors, 5 years of tamoxifen use reduces breast cancer recurrence by 50% and mortality by 28% (Figure 24-4).[109] For patients taking tamoxifen there appears to be a correlation between the degree of ER positivity and breast cancer outcome. In patients with tumors expressing high levels of ER (i.e., at least 100 fmol receptor per milligram cytosol protein), tamoxifen reduces recurrence and mortality rates by 60% and 36%, compared with 43% and 23%, respectively, for patients whose tumors express less ER.[109] In the Oxford Overview Analysis, PR was of little additional use in predicting outcome, in that recurrence rates with tamoxifen therapy were not significantly different in patients with ER-positive, PR-poor tumors, compared with patients whose tumors expressed both receptors.[109] However, the number of patients whose PR status was known was small and

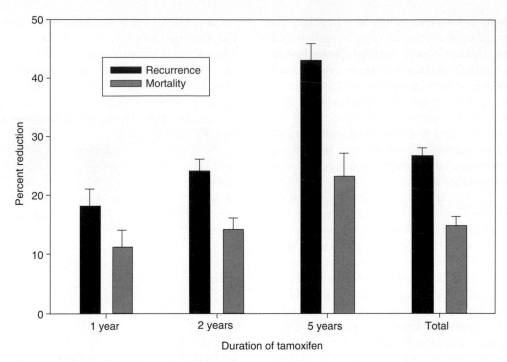

FIG. **24-4** Five years of tamoxifen significantly reduces mortality and recurrence from early-stage breast cancer. *(From Early Breast Cancer Trialists' Collaborative Group:* Lancet *351:1451, 1998.)*

patients whose tumors were ER positive and PR negative clearly benefited from 5 years of tamoxifen therapy.[109] Regardless of treatment duration, tamoxifen reduced breast cancer recurrence by only 10% and mortality by only 6% in patients with ER-poor breast tumors, with no evidence of improved outcome with longer treatment durations (see Figure 24-4). Recently, the results of the first clinical trial in which an aromatase inhibitor was used in the treatment of early-stage breast cancer were presented. The Arimidex, Tamoxifen and Combination (ATAC) trial, with a short follow-up of 3 years, shows improved disease-free survival (DFS) and a reduced rate of contralateral breast cancers in postmenopausal patients with ER-positive early-stage breast cancer treated with anastrozole alone compared with tamoxifen alone (Figure 24-5).[110]

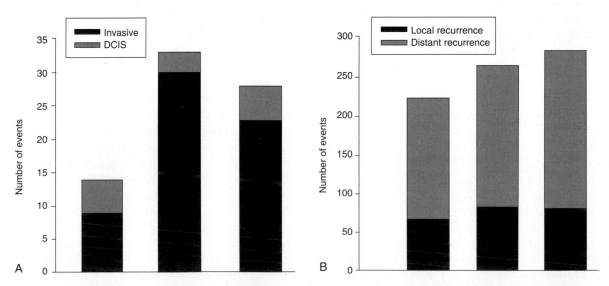

FIG. **24-5** Anastrozole is superior to tamoxifen and the combination of tamoxifen and anastrozole in postmenopausal women with early-stage breast cancer: disease-free survival **(A)** and contralateral breast cancer **(B)**. *(Modified from ATAC Trialists Group:* Lancet *359:2131, 2002.)*

Tamoxifen reduces breast cancer by 50% in women at high risk for the disease[111] and has been approved as a breast cancer preventive. Not surprisingly, according to the National Surgical Adjuvant Breast and Bowel Project P-1 (NSABP-P-1) prevention trial, tamoxifen appears to prevent only ER-positive breast cancers (69% reduction). Importantly, contrary to other reports,[112] tamoxifen did not appear to increase the incidence of ER-negative breast tumors. No statistically significant difference in the rate of ER-negative tumors was observed in the NSABP-P-1 trial.[111]

PROGESTERONE RECEPTOR

PR synthesis is increased in estrogen-responsive tissue, including breast tissue. PR positivity may be a better predictive factor for response to hormonal therapy, because its expression may reflect a functioning ER pathway.[6] Overall, about 30% of breast tumors overexpress ER but not PR, whereas less than 5% express PR but not ER. PR levels are higher in premenopausal women compared with postmenopausal women.[106] As seen with ER expression, PR expression is more commonly seen with well-differentiated breast tumors.

In general, very few ER-positive tumors become ER negative.[113] In contrast, it is not uncommon for tumors that are initially PR positive to become PR negative, and this loss of PR expression heralds a more aggressive phenotype, with poor survival rates.[114]

PR exists as two isoforms, PRA and PRB, each of which can bind hormone and DNA and can function as a transcription factor. There is evidence suggesting that PRA has repressor activity, whereas PRB has more activator functions.[13,115] Therefore it is possible that the relative expression of these two isoforms may be useful in predicting response to hormonal therapy.[7]

Progesterone Receptor as a Prognostic Factor. As with ER, the prognostic significance of PR is unclear, particularly because most patients with PR-positive tumors are treated with endocrine therapy. It seems likely that, like ER, PR holds more value as a predictive factor rather than a prognostic factor.

Progesterone Receptor as a Predictive Factor. A number of studies have demonstrated the importance of PR expression in predicting response to endocrine therapy in metastatic breast cancer.[7] A large, prospective trial demonstrated that elevated PR levels were associated with increased likelihood of responding to tamoxifen, as well as conferring a longer DFS and overall survival, by multivariate analysis.[116] Overall, patients with advanced breast cancer whose tumors express only PR respond in slightly more cases that those whose tumors express ER alone, but less than patients whose tumors express both receptors.[8]

The value of PR is less clear in the adjuvant setting. The Oxford Overview analysis failed to demonstrate that PR expression is an independent predictive factor for response to tamoxifen in patients with ER-positive tumors.[109] However, based on the data in patients with advanced breast cancer, most oncologists use tamoxifen in patients with early-stage breast cancer whose tumors express PR, but not ER.

The NSABP-P-1 prevention trial clearly demonstrates that tamoxifen reduced only the incidence of ER-positive tumors.[111] There is no data from this trial evaluating the effect of tamoxifen in preventing PR-positive breast tumors. In summary, PR expression appears to be as important as ER expression in predicting response to endocrine therapy, particularly tamoxifen, in advanced breast cancer. The importance of PR is less clear in early-stage breast cancer and the prevention setting, likely because of a paucity of data from adjuvant and prevention trials.

What Is Estrogen Receptor Positivity?: Interpretation of Results

The presence of ER in breast tissue is primarily determined with IHC or with LBA. When LBA was used, ER was said to be negative if the binding capacity was 3 fmol/mg or less.[117] Although in Europe it is more common to use 10 fmol/mg as a cutoff, other workers have used a cutoff of 20 fmol/mg.[118] When the LBA method was used, most of the ER-positive tumors were likely to respond to endocrine therapy. However, a percentage of ER-negative tumors (approximately 10%) also responded to these agents. The explanation for this phenomenon was that the ER in these cases had been falsely read as negative because of methodologic issues.

The definition of ER positivity based on IHC methods is less well defined. Several different methods of assessing ER have been reported, with the proponents of each regarding that method as the best. Most methods in common usage employ some combination of staining intensity and percentage positivity. By nearly all definitions, a tumor exhibiting high-intensity expression in 10% or more of tumor cell nuclei will be considered ER positive. When any of the methods are used, greater than 90% of the tumors are either clearly ER positive or ER negative. The question is essentially about the small number of cases in which ER expression is seen in only some (<10%) of the nuclei. In these situations, analysis of PR expression is extremely useful.

In many cases the presence of ER is not detected by IHC despite indirect evidence that these tumors are ER positive. The reasons for this phenomenon are unknown but could include multiple factors, such as tissue preservation. In these cases the presence of PR can serve as a surrogate marker for the presence of ER. ER-negative tumors that express PR are likely to respond to endocrine therapy. The San Antonio Group analyzed more than 25,000 cases by LBA, revealing the incidence of ER-negative, PR-positive tumors to be 4%. In an analysis of IHC results of 7016 breast cancer cases from multiple institutions, Rhodes and colleagues[101,119] found the incidence of the phenotype (ER–/PR+) to be 3.2%. In a recent review of more than 550 cases of needle core biopsies of breast cancer fixed using alcoholic formalin, we found the incidence to be approximately 1%.[120]

In our experience, the percentage of tumors that express low levels of ER (>10 fmol/mg) and that are also PR negative is approximately 1%. Whether 1% error is allowable in ER determination is debatable. The argument in favor of an all-inclusive definition (any positive cell) points out that 1% false negative translates into 2000 women per year (assuming the annual incidence of breast cancer to be 200,000). Labeling these women as ER negative would deprive them the benefit of endocrine therapy, one of the most effective and least toxic treatments for breast cancer. A major hurdle to finding the correct answer to the question of low-level expression of receptors is that most studies to date have used ER as a categorical parameter (positive or negative) rather than a continuous variable. Until the time such analyses are performed in well-established databases that contain patients treated with similar protocols, this question is likely to remain unanswered and will continue to be a topic of debate.

FACTORS INFLUENCING RECEPTOR STATUS

Premenopausal-Postmenopausal Status. Age has a significant effect on tumor morphology and incidence of ER-positive tumors in the breast. Tumors in postmenopausal patients are more likely to be better differentiated and ER positive than tumors arising in premenopausal women. Bauer-Marsh and colleagues[121] found that ER expression strongly correlated with tumor size in postmenopausal women but not in premenopausal women. As ER expression is strongly related to tumor grade, it is unknown whether the higher incidence of ER positivity in the postmenopausal group is a reflection of the grade or if it is an independent parameter. In a recent study, Talley and co-workers[122] compared the effects of age on the association between grade and ER expression. They found that irrespective of grade, premenopausal women are more likely to have lower ER expression and higher proliferative index.

Endogenous Hormone Levels. The measured ER level of a tumor is unlikely to be influenced by endogenous estrogen levels in premenopausal women because physiologic circulating levels of estrogen are not high enough to saturate all of the ER sites resulting in a false-negative ER assay. On the other hand, the measured PR level may be falsely negative if the measurement is taken during the luteal phase of the menstrual cycle when the circulating levels of progesterone are particularly high.

Exogenous Hormones. Exogenous hormones can take the form of oral contraceptives, hormone replacement therapy (HRT), and breast cancer treatment such as antiestrogens or estrogens. The estrogen dose administered in HRT may mask the ER; similarly, antiestrogens, such as tamoxifen, may also occupy the ER resulting in false-negative assay.[117,123] The latter may be most relevant in the setting in which a patient develops disease recurrence while receiving treatment with tamoxifen. An immediate biopsy to reconfirm the receptor status of the tumor may be falsely negative, because it requires at least 2 months for all of the tamoxifen to vacate receptors in the tumor. A similar scenario can be envisioned for a patient receiving high doses of estrogen as treatment for advanced breast cancer. A report by Hull and colleagues[117] confirms that false-negative assessment of ER status can result in patients receiving tamoxifen.

Older biochemical assay methods could be influenced by exogenous hormones, because these methods measure only unbound receptors present in the cytosol compartment. More commonly used IHC methods are not influenced by endogenous or exogenous hormones.

Tumor Grade. There is a strong inverse relation between ER and overall tumor grade, with low-grade tumors showing high frequency of ER positivity. In a retrospective analysis of more than 550 consecutive cases of infiltrating duct carcinoma, we found ER positivity in more than 95% of grade 1 tumors, more than 90% of grade 2 tumors, and slightly less than 50% of grade 3 tumors.[120] In our experience, it is extremely unusual to find lack of ER expression in grade 1 (and grade 2) tumors[120] and in classical lobular carcinoma. It is reasonable to repeat the stains (perhaps on a different specimen) when this finding excludes technical problems.

Receptors in Male Breast Cancer

ESTROGEN AND PROGESTERONE RECEPTORS

In women with breast cancer, 60% to 70% of tumors are ER positive or PR positive. In contrast, up to 91% of male breast cancers (MBCs) express ER and 96% express PR.[124,125] The expression of ER and PR may provide a growth advantage; at least one study suggests that ER+/PR+ tumors have higher proliferative activity than ER–/PR– tumors.[126]

ANDROGEN RECEPTOR

Androgen receptor (AR) expression is detected in 34% to 95% of breast cancers in men.[125-128] However, no association between AR expression and other clinicopathologic features or measures of outcome has been reported.[127]

Mutations in the AR gene have been implicated in the development of MBC.[129,130] These mutations have been identified in the DNA-binding domain, in an area responsible for transcriptional control. However, the contribution of AR mutations to tumorigenesis is not completely clear. In one series, AR mutations were not detected in tumor material from 11 men with MBC.[131]

Receptors in Other Breast Diseases

The expression of ER is low in normal breast tissues. In premenopausal breast tissues, ER-expressing cells are scattered within the lobule. This pattern changes with age with postmenopausal tissues exhibiting clusters of ER-positive cells within the lobules.[132] Sloane's group[133] analyzed the expression of ER in a variety of benign breast lesions. They found that the expression was increased in sclerosing adenosis, radial scars, papillomas, fibroadenomas and phyllodes tumors, but not in apocrine metaplasia (no ER-positive cells) or duct ectasia. As in the normal breast, the number of ER-positive cells increased with age in all the lesions with the exception of fibroadenomas. ER-positive cells in the normal breast do not constitute the proliferative compartment; however, the proportion of ER+/Ki67+ proliferating cells is increased in all "risk-associated lesions" of the breast. The percentage of ER+/Ki67+ proliferating cells is increased in all "risk-associated lesions" of the breast. The percentage of ER+/Ki67+ proliferating cells increases from normal breast lobules through hyperplasia to in situ carcinoma and invasive carcinoma.[132-135] In a more recent publication, Shaaban and colleagues[136,137] were able to show that patients who subsequently developed carcinoma had a greater population of cells that showed ER and Ki67 expression in the hyperplastic lesions than patients without carcinoma after a follow-up of 20 years.

Epidermal Growth Factor Receptor Family

Another receptor family, the epidermal growth factor receptor (EGFR) family, is becoming increasingly important in breast cancer. The EGFR family is made up of four receptors—ErbB-1 (also referred to as *HER1* or *EGFR*), ErbB-2 (or *HER2/neu*), ErbB-3 (or *HER3*), and ErbB-4 (or *HER4*)—each of which has an extracellular domain and an intracellular tyrosine kinase domain.[138] Natural ligands, predominantly heregulins,[139] have been identified for all of the receptors except ErbB-2.[140] However, when activated by ligands, it is clear that both homodimerization[141] and heterodimerization[142] between receptors of the family occurs. The member of this receptor family that has been most important in breast cancer research to date is ErbB-2, although the possible role of EGFR is becoming increasingly recognized.

OVEREXPRESSION OF ErbB-2 IN BREAST CANCER

Overexpression of ErbB-2 is seen in approximately 20% to 30% of breast cancer cases.[143] For a breast cancer to be deemed ErbB-2 positive, it must exhibit gene amplification and membrane protein overexpression. Protein overexpression is generally assessed by measuring IHC antibodies. Based on IHC alone, approximately one third of breast cancers are deemed ErbB-2 positive.[143] Gene amplification is generally measured by means of a fluorescence in situ hybridization (FISH) test and is believed to correlate with true ErbB-2 positivity.[144] Approximately 20% of breast cancers are positive for c-ErbB-2 on FISH testing.[145] ErbB-2 positivity appears to correlate with more aggressive phenotype and to portend a worse prognosis.[143,146,147]

ErbB-2 as a Predictive Factor. Expression of ErbB-2 has clear value as a predictive factor. Trastuzumab is a monoclonal antibody, which was developed against the extracellular domain of ErbB-2. Trastuzumab, used as monotherapy, results in response rates of approximately 40% in previously untreated patients,[144] and 20% in patients previously treated with chemotherapy,[148] with advanced ErbB-2–positive breast cancer. The highest response rates have been observed in patients whose tumors were ErbB-2 positive by FISH testing. Preclinical data suggested that although trastuzumab clearly had activity when used alone in ErbB-2–positive breast tumors, it was synergistic with a number of chemotherapy agents in vitro and in vivo.[149,150] This observation led to a large clinical trial that randomized patients with advanced ErbB-2–positive breast cancer to chemotherapy alone or chemotherapy plus trastuzumab.[151] Patients in this trial who received trastuzumab in combination with chemotherapy had a significantly better outcome than those treated with chemotherapy alone, which led to the FDA approval of this agent. Unexpectedly, there was an increase in cardiac failure in patients treated with trastuzumab in this trial, particularly in patients treated with concomitant anthracyclines.[151] Trastuzumab is currently being evaluated as an adjuvant therapy in patients with early-stage breast cancer.

ErbB-2 as a Predictor of Tamoxifen Resistance.
There is evidence suggesting that breast tumors that overexpress hormone receptors and ErbB-2 are more resistant to endocrine therapy, or at least tamoxifen, than hormone receptor–positive tumors that are ErbB-2 negative. The first suggestion of this was noted when MCF-7, ER-positive breast cancer cells were transfected with ErbB-2 and injected into athymic mice.[152] The ErbB-2–transfected MCF-7 breast tumors grew more quickly with estrogen compared with the wild type tumors, and more important, tamoxifen had no inhibitory effects on the growth of the ErbB-2–transfected tumors, but inhibited growth of the wild type MCF-7 tumors.[152] A meta-analysis of retrospective trials examining the outcome of patients with metastatic breast cancer treated with endocrine therapy based on ErbB-2 status of the tumors revealed that patients whose breast tumors were *HER-2/neu* negative were 2.6 times less likely to have progressed at 6 months, compared with ErbB-2–positive tumors.[153] In 6 of 7 of these trials, the endocrine therapy administered was tamoxifen. A clinical trial that compared the aromatase inhibitor, letrozole, with tamoxifen as preoperative therapy in postmenopausal women with locally advanced breast cancer demonstrated reduced response rates for the tamoxifen-treated patients, but not for the letrozole-treated patients, whose tumors overexpressed ErbB-2.[154] However, another clinical trial randomized patients with advanced breast cancer to letrozole or tamoxifen.[155] A retrospective analysis of this trial correlated elevated levels of serum ErbB-2 as a surrogate marker of ErbB-2 positivity.[156] Despite finding higher response rates and a longer time to disease progression in the overall population of patients treated with letrozole compared with those treated with tamoxifen, in the subgroup of patients with elevated serum ErbB-2 levels, there was no significant difference in response rate or time to progression between the two agents.[156]

Based on these data it is unclear what the optimum endocrine therapy should be for patients whose tumors overexpress hormone receptors and ErbB-2 or whether such tumors are resistant to endocrine therapy. There is evidence suggesting that targeting the estrogen receptor pathway and the ErbB-2 pathway decrease the proliferation of breast cancer cells overexpressing ER and ErbB-2 in vitro.[157]

EPIDERMAL GROWTH FACTOR RECEPTOR IN BREAST CANCER

In contrast to ErbB-2, there is less information about the importance of ErbB-1 (EGFR) in breast cancer. Several small molecules that target the intracellular tyrosine kinase domain of ErbB-1 are in clinical development.[158] Like trastuzumab, however, these agents may have greater antitumor activity if combined with chemotherapy or other active antitumor agents.

There are preclinical data suggesting that Iressa may prevent the development of tamoxifen resistance in ER-positive, MCF-7 breast cancer cells in vitro.[159] Wild type MCF-7 breast cancer cells express low levels of ErbB-1. However, after prolonged tamoxifen exposure in vitro, tamoxifen resistance develops and this has been shown to be associated with an upregulation of ErbB-1 at both protein and mRNA levels.[159] In addition, concomitant administration of tamoxifen and Iressa appears to prevent tamoxifen resistance in vitro[159] and in vivo.[160]

REFERENCES

1. Beatson GT: On the treatment of inoperable cases of carcinoma of the mamma: suggestions for a new method of treatment with illustrative cases, *Lancet* 2:104, 1896.
2. Boyd S: On oophorectomy in cancer of the breast, *BMJ* 2:1161, 1900.
3. Allen E, Doisy EA: An ovarian hormone: preliminary report of its localization, extraction, and partial purification and action in test animals, *JAMA* 81:819, 1923.
4. Jensen EV, Jacobson HI: Basic guides to the mechanism of estrogen action, *Recent Prog Horm Res* 18:387, 1962.
5. Jensen EV et al: Estrogen receptors and breast cancer response to adrenalectomy, *Natl Cancer Inst Monogr* 34:55, 1971.
6. Horwitz KB et al: Predicting response to endocrine therapy in human breast cancer: a hypothesis, *Science* 189:726, 1975.
7. Osborne CK: Steroid hormone receptors in breast cancer management, *Breast Cancer Res Treat* 51:227, 1998.
8. Horwitz KB: The structure and function of progesterone receptors in breast cancer, *J Steroid Biochem* 27:447, 1987.
9. Green S et al: Human oestrogen receptor cDNA: sequence, expression and homology with v-erb, *Nature (Lond)* 320:134, 1986.
10. Kumar V et al: Localization of the estradiol binding and putative DNA-binding domains of the estrogen receptor, *EMBO J* 5:9931, 1986.
11. Kumar V et al: Functional domains of the estrogen receptor, *Cell* 51:941, 1987.
12. Menasce LP et al: Localization of the estrogen receptor locus (ESR) to chromosome 6q25.1 by FISH and a simple post-FISH banding technique, *Genomics* 17:263, 1993.
13. Gronemeyer H: Transcription activation by estrogen and progesterone receptors, *Annu Rev Genet* 25:89, 1991.
14. Berry M, Metzger D, Chambon P: Role of the two activating domains of the estrogen receptor in the cell-type and promoter-context dependent agonist activity of the anti-oestrogen 4-hydroxytamoxifen, *EMBO J* 9:2811, 1990.
15. Webster NJG et al: The hormone-binding domains of the estrogen receptor and glucocorticoid receptors contain an inducible transcription activation function, *Cell* 54:199, 1988.
16. Schwabe JW et al: The crystal structure of the estrogen receptor DNA-binding domain bound to DNA: how receptors discriminate between their response elements, *Cell* 65:567, 1993.
17. Kumar V, Chambon P: The estrogen receptor binds tightly to its responsive element in a ligand-induced homodimer, *Cell* 55:145, 1988.

18. Rao GS: Mode of entry of steroid and thyroid hormones into cell, *Mol Cell Endocrinol* 21:97, 1981.

19. MacGregor JI, Jordan VC: Basic guide to the mechanisms of antiestrogen action, *Pharmacol Rev* 50:151, 1998.

20. Kuiper GG et al: Cloning of a novel estrogen receptor expressed in rat prostate and ovary, *Proc Natl Acad Sci USA* 93:5925, 1996.

21. Webb P et al: Tamoxifen activation of the estrogen receptor/AP-1 pathway: potential origin for the cell-specific estrogen-like effects of antiestrogens, *Mol Endocrinol* 9:443, 1995.

22. Paech K et al: Differential ligand activation of estrogen receptors ERα and ERβ at AP-1 sites, *Science* 277:1508, 1997.

23. Teicher I et al: Effect of operative devascularization on estrogen and progesterone receptor levels in breast cancer specimens, *Surgery* 98:784, 1985.

24. King WJ, Greene GL: Monoclonal antibodies localize oestrogen receptor in the nuclei of target cells, *Nature* 307:745, 1984.

25. Greene GL et al: Immunochemical studies of estrogen receptors, *J Steroid Biochem* 20:51, 1984.

26. Jensen EV: Intracellular localization of estrogen receptors: implications for interaction mechanism, *Lab Invest* 51:487, 1984.

27. Chamness GC, Mercer WD, McGuire WL: Are histochemical methods for estrogen receptor valid? *J Histochem Cytochem* 28:792, 1980.

28. Underwood JC et al: Biochemical assessment of histochemical methods for oestrogen receptor localization, *J Clin Pathol* 35:401, 1982.

29. Clark JH et al: Heterogeneity of estrogen binding sites in the cytosol of the rat uterus, *J Biol Chem* 253:7630, 1978.

30. Panko WB, Watson CS, Clark JH: The presence of a second, specific estrogen binding site in human breast cancer, *J Steroid Biochem* 14:1311, 1981.

31. Pascal RR et al: Immunohistologic detection of estrogen receptors in paraffin-embedded breast cancers: correlation with cytosol measurements, *Hum Pathol* 17:370, 1986.

32. Mauriac L et al: Inflammatory breast cancers: correlation between anatomopathology and steroid receptor assay, *Bull Cancer* 70:160, 1983.

33. King RJB et al: Measurement of oestrogen receptors by five institutions on common tissue samples. In King RJB (ed): *Steroid receptor assays in human breast tumors: methodological and clinical aspects*, Cardiff, 1979, Alpha Omega Publishing.

34. Goussard J et al: Comparison of monoclonal antibodies and tritiated ligands for estrogen receptor assays in 241 breast cancer cytosols, *Cancer Res* 46(suppl 8):4282s, 1986.

35. Romain S et al: Steroid receptor distribution in 47,892 breast cancers: a collaborative study of 7 European laboratories—the EORTC Receptor Study Group, *Eur J Cancer* 31A:411, 1995.

36. Parl FF, Posey YF: Discrepancies of the biochemical and immunohistochemical estrogen receptor assays in breast cancer, *Hum Pathol* 19:960, 1988.

37. Nenci I et al: Detection and dynamic localisation of estradiol-receptor complexes in intact target cells by immunofluorescence technique, *J Steroid Biochem* 7:505, 1976.

38. Nenci I: Receptor and centriole pathways of steroid action in normal and neoplastic cells, *Cancer Res* 38:4204, 1978.

39. Pertschuk LP: Detection of estrogen binding in human mammary carcinoma by immunofluorescence: a new technic utilizing the binding hormone in a polymerized state, *Res Commun Chem Pathol Pharmacol* 14:771, 1976.

40. Kurzon RM, Sternberger LA: Estrogen receptor immunocytochemistry, *J Histochem Cytochem* 26:803, 1978.

41. Lee SH: Cytochemical study of estrogen receptor in human mammary cancer, *Am J Clin Pathol* 70:197, 1978.

42. Lee SH: Cancer cell estrogen receptor of human mammary carcinoma, *Cancer* 44:1, 1979.

43. Lee SH: Cellular estrogen and progesterone receptors in mammary carcinoma, *Am J Clin Pathol* 73:323, 1980.

44. Lee SH: The histochemistry of estrogen receptors, *Histochemistry* 71:491, 1981.

45. Greene GL et al: Monoclonal antibodies to human estrogen receptor, *Proc Natl Acad Sci USA* 77:5115, 1980.

46. Greene GL, Fitch FW, Jensen EV: Monoclonal antibodies to estrophilin: probes for the study of estrogen receptors, *Proc Natl Acad Sci USA* 77:157, 1980.

47. Moncharmont B, Su JL, Parikh I: Monoclonal antibodies against estrogen receptor: interaction with different molecular forms and functions of the receptor, *Biochemistry* 21:6916, 1982.

48. Traish AM et al: Development and characterization of monoclonal antibodies to a specific domain of human estrogen receptor, *Steroids* 55:196, 1990.

49. Miller LS et al: Hybridomas producing monoclonal antibodies to human estrogen receptor, *Fed Proc* 41:520, 1982.

50. Garancis JC et al: Immunoperoxidase localization of estrogen receptors in human breast carcinoma, *Cancer Detect Prev* 6:235, 1983.

51. Kumar V et al: Functional domains of the human estrogen receptor, *Cell* 51:941, 1987.

52. Shimada A et al: Immunocytochemical staining of estrogen receptor in paraffin sections of human breast cancer by use of monoclonal antibody: comparison with that in frozen sections, *Proc Natl Acad Sci USA* 82:4803, 1985.

53. Poulsen HS et al: The use of monoclonal antibodies to estrogen receptors (ER) for immunoperoxidase detection of ER in paraffin sections of human breast cancer tissue, *J Histochem Cytochem* 33:87, 1985.

54. Andersen J, Orntoft T, Poulsen HS: Semiquantitative oestrogen receptor assay in formalin-fixed paraffin sections of human breast cancer tissue using monoclonal antibodies, *Br J Cancer* 53:691, 1986.

55. Shintaku IP, Said JW: Detection of estrogen receptors with monoclonal antibodies in routinely processed formalin-fixed paraffin sections of breast carcinoma: use of DNase pretreatment to enhance sensitivity of the reaction, *Am J Clin Pathol* 87:161, 1987.

56. Hiort O, Kwan PW, DeLellis RA: Immunohistochemistry of estrogen receptor protein in paraffin sections: effects of enzymatic pretreatment and cobalt chloride intensification. *Am J Clin Pathol* 90:559, 1988.

57. Cheng L et al: Demonstration of estrogen receptors by monoclonal antibody in formalin-fixed breast tumors, *Lab Invest* 58:346, 1988.

58. DeRosa et al: Immunohistochemical assessment of estrogen and progesterone receptors in stored imprints and cryostat sections of breast carcinomas, *Ann Surg* 210:224, 1989.

59. al Saati T et al: Production of monoclonal antibodies to human estrogen-receptor protein (ER) using recombinant ER (RER), *Int J Cancer* 55:651, 1993.

60. Williams JH, Mepham BL, Wright DH: Tissue preparation for immunocytochemistry, *J Clin Pathol* 50:422, 1997.

61. Taylor CR, Shi SR: Fixation, processing and special applications. In Taylor CR, Cote RJ (eds): *Immunomicroscopy: a*

diagnostic tool for the surgical pathologist: major problems in pathology, ed 2, Philadelphia, 1994, WB Saunders.

62. Dodson A, Campbell F: Biotin inclusions: a potential pitfall in immunohistochemistry avoided, *Histopathology* 34:178, 1999.

63. Nayler SJ, Goetsch S, Cooper K: Biotin inclusions: a potential pitfall in immunohistochemistry, *Histopathology* 33:87, 1998.

64. Bussolati G et al: Retrieved endogenous biotin: a novel marker and a potential pitfall in diagnostic immunohistochemistry, *Histopathology* 31:400, 1997.

65. Streefkerk JG: Inhibition of erythrocyte pseudoperoxidase activity by treatment with hydrogen peroxide following methanol, *J Histochem Cytochem* 20:829, 1972.

66. Heyderman E, Neville AM: A shorter immunoperoxidase technique for the demonstration of carcinoembryonic antigen and other cell products, *J Clin Pathol* 30:138, 1977.

67. Borges M: The cytochemical application of new potent inhibitors of alkaline phosphatases, *J Histochem Cytochem* 21:812, 1973.

68. Shi SR, Key ME, Kalra KL: Antigen retrieval in formalin-fixed, paraffin-embedded tissues: an enhancement method for immunohistochemical staining based on microwave oven heating of tissue sections, *J Histochem Cytochem* 39:741, 1991.

69. Gown AM, de Wever N, Battifora H: Microwave-based antigenic unmasking: a revolutionary technique for routine immunohistochemistry, *Appl Immunohistochem Molecul Morphol* 1:256, 1993.

70. Berger U et al: Correlation of immunocytochemically demonstrated estrogen receptor distribution and histopathologic features in primary breast cancer, *Hum Pathol* 18:1263, 1987.

71. Allred DC et al: Prognostic and predictive factors in breast cancer by immunohistochemical analysis, *Mod Pathol* 11:155, 1998.

72. Kinsel LB et al: Immunocytochemical analysis of estrogen receptors as a predictor of prognosis in breast cancer patients: comparison with quantitative biochemical methods, Cancer Res 49:1052, 1989.

73. Reiner A et al: Immunocytochemical localization of estrogen and progesterone receptor and prognosis in human primary breast cancer, *Cancer Res* 50:7057, 1990.

74. Remmele W, Schicketanz KH: Immunohistochemical determination of estrogen and progesterone receptor content in human breast cancer: computer-assisted image analysis (QIC score) vs. subjective grading (IRS), *Pathol Res Pract* 189:862, 1993.

75. Fitzgibbons PL et al: Prognostic factors in breast cancer: College of American Pathologists Consensus Statement 1999, *Arch Pathol Lab Med* 124:966, 2000.

76. Reiner A et al: Immunocytochemical localization of estrogen and progesterone receptor and prognosis in human primary breast cancer, *Cancer Res* 50:7057, 1990.

77. Berger U et al: Correlation of immunocytochemically demonstrated estrogen receptor distribution and histopathologic features in primary breast cancer, *Hum Pathol* 18:1263, 1987.

78. Kinsel LB et al: Immunocytochemical analysis of estrogen receptors as a predictor of prognosis in breast cancer patients: comparison with quantitative biochemical methods, *Cancer Res* 49:1052, 1989.

79. Allred DC et al: Prognostic and predictive factors in breast cancer by immunohistochemical analysis, *Mod Pathol* 11:155, 1998.

80. Lehr HA et al: Application of Photoshop-based image analysis to quantification of hormone receptor expression in breast cancer, *J Histochem Cytochem* 45:1559, 1997.

81. Sklarew RJ, Bodmer SC, Pertschuk LP: Quantitative imaging of immunocytochemical (PAP) estrogen receptor staining patterns in breast cancer sections, *Cytometry* 11:359, 1990.

82. Charpin C et al: Multiparametric evaluation (SAMBA) of growth fraction (monoclonal Ki67) in breast carcinoma tissue sections, *Cancer Res* 48:4368, 1988.

83. Charpin C: Multiparametric analysis (SAMBA 200) of the progesterone receptor immunocytochemical assay in nonmalignant and malignant breast disorders, *Am J Pathol* 132:199, 1988.

84. Franklin WA et al: Quantitation of estrogen receptor content and Ki-67 staining in breast carcinoma by the microTICAS image analysis system, *Anal Quant Cytol Histol* 9:279, 1987.

85. Bacus S et al: The evaluation of estrogen receptor in primary breast carcinoma by computer-assisted image analysis, *Am J Clin Pathol* 90:233, 1988.

86. Remmele W, Schicketanz KH: Immunohistochemical determination of estrogen and progesterone receptor content in human breast cancer: computer-assisted image analysis (QIC score) vs. subjective grading (IRS), *Pathol Res Pract* 189:862, 1993.

87. Schultz DS et al: Comparison of visual and CAS-200 quantitation of immunocytochemical staining in breast carcinoma samples, *Anal Quant Cytol Histol* 14:35, 1992.

88. Kohlberger PD et al: Modified true-color computer-assisted image analysis versus subjective scoring of estrogen receptor expression in breast cancer: a comparison, *Anticancer Res* 19:2189, 1999.

89. Battifora H: Assessment of antigen damage in immunohistochemistry: the vimentin internal control, *Am J Clin Pathol* 96:669, 1991.

90. Drury R, Wallington E: *Preparation and fixation of tissues, Carleton's histological technique,* ed 5, Oxford, 1980, Oxford University Press.

91. Elias JM et al: Quality control in immunohistochemistry: report of a workshop sponsored by the Biological Stain Commission, *Am J Clin Pathol* 92:836, 1989.

92. Larsson L-I: Tissue preparation methods for light microscopic immunohistochemistry, *Appl Immunohistochem* 1:2, 1993.

93. Slater D: Enclosed tissue system problem, *IMLS Gazette* 32:83, 1988.

94. Brain EB: Infiltration histological specimens with paraffin wax under vacuum: basic factors and a new approach, *Br Dent J* 128:71, 1970.

95. Horikawa M et al: Effect of stirring during fixation upon immunofluorescence: results with distribution of albumin-producing cells in liver, *J Histochem Cytochem* 24:926, 1976.

96. Matthews JB: Influence of clearing agent on immunohistochemical staining of paraffin-embedded tissue, *J Clin Pathol* 34:103, 1981.

97. Wakins J et al: Enhancement of immunostaining, *Histopathology* 17:185, 1990.

98. Bromley C, Palechek P, Benda J: Preservation of estrogen receptor in paraffin sections, *J Histotechnol* 17:115, 1994.

99. Prioleau J, Schnitt SJ: p53 antigen loss in stored paraffin slides, *N Engl J Med* 332:1521, 1995.

100. Jacobs TW et al: Loss of tumor marker-immunostaining intensity on stored paraffin slides of breast cancer, *J Natl Cancer Inst* 88:1054, 1996.

101. Rhodes A et al: Frequency of oestrogen and progesterone receptor positivity by immunohistochemical analysis in 7016 breast carcinomas: correlation with patient age, assay sensitivity, threshold value, and mammographic screening, *J Clin Pathol* 53:688, 2000.

102. Koenders A, Thorpe SM: Standardization of steroid receptor assays in human breast cancer—II: samples with low receptor content, *Eur J Cancer Clin Oncol* 19:1467, 1983.

103. Romain S et al: Steroid receptor distribution in 47,892 breast cancers: a collaborative study of 7 European laboratories. The EORTC Receptor Study Group, *Eur J Cancer* 31A:411, 1995.

104. College of American Pathologists, Immunohistochemistry Survey MK-2001 A. Used with permission.

105. Rhodes A et al: Reliability of immunohistochemical demonstration of oestrogen receptors in routine practice: interlaboratory variance in the sensitivity of detection and evaluation of scoring systems, *J Clin Pathol* 53:125, 2000.

106. Clark GM, Osborne CK, McGuire WL: Correlations between estrogen receptor, progesterone receptor and patient characteristics in breast cancer, *J Clin Oncol* 2:1102, 1984.

107. Clark GM, McGuire WL. Steroid receptors and other prognostic factors in primary breast cancer, *Semin Oncol* 15(suppl 1):20, 1988.

108. Steroid receptors in breast cancer: an NIH Consensus Development Conference, Bethesda, Maryland, June 27-29, 1979, *Cancer* 46(suppl 12):2759, 1980.

109. Early Breast Cancer Trialists' Collaborative Group: Tamoxifen for early breast cancer: an overview of the randomized trials, *Lancet* 351:1451, 1998.

110. ATAC Trialists Group: Anastrozole alone or in combination with tamoxifen versus tamoxifen alone for adjuvant treatment of postmenopausal women with early breast cancer: first results of the ATAC randomized trial, *Lancet* 359:2131, 2002.

111. Fisher B et al: Tamoxifen for prevention of breast cancer: report of the National Surgical Adjuvant Breast and Bowel Project P-1 Study, *J Natl Cancer Inst* 90:1371, 1998.

112. Li CI et al: Tamoxifen therapy for primary breast cancer and risk of contralateral breast cancer, *J Natl Cancer Inst* 93:1008, 2001.

113. Hull DF et al: Multiple estrogen receptor assays in human breast cancer, *Cancer Res* 43:413, 1983.

114. Gross GE et al: Multiple progesterone receptor assays in human breast cancer, *Cancer Res* 44:836, 1984.

115. Wen DX et al: The A and B forms of human progesterone receptor operate through distinct signaling pathways within target cells, *Mol Cell Biol* 14:8356, 1994.

116. Ravdin PM et al: Prognostic significance of progesterone receptor levels in estrogen receptor-positive patients with metastatic breast cancer treated with tamoxifen: results of a prospective Southwest Oncology Group study, *J Clin Oncol* 10:1284, 1992.

117. Hull DF III et al: Multiple estrogen receptor assays in human breast cancer, *Cancer Res* 43:413, 1983.

118. Barnes DM et al: Immunohistochemical determination of oestrogen receptor: comparison of different methods of assessment of staining and correlation with clinical outcome of breast cancer patients, *Br J Cancer* 74:1445, 1996.

119. Rhodes A et al: Reliability of immunohistochemical demonstration of oestrogen receptors in routine practice: interlaboratory variance in the sensitivity of detection and evaluation of scoring systems, *J Clin Pathol* 53:125, 2000.

120. Hill K, Wiley E, Badve S: Histologic grade and ER/PgR status in breast carcinoma, *Breast Cancer Treat Res* 64:18, 2000 (abstract).

121. Bauer-Marsh E et al: Is expression of *p*53 and *Her-2* related to estrogen receptor status in infiltrating ductal carcinoma of the breast, *Mod Pathol* 13:17A, 2000 (abstract).

122. Talley LI et al: Hormone receptors and proliferation in breast carcinomas of equivalent histologic grades in pre- and postmenopausal women, *Int J Cancer* 98:118, 2002.

123. Isaksson E et al: Expression of sex steroid receptors and IGF-1 mRNA in breast tissue—effects of hormonal treatment, *J Steroid Biochem Mol Biol* 70:257, 1999.

124. Donegan WL, Redlich PN: Breast cancer in men, *Surg Clin North Am* 76:343, 1996.

125. Rayson D et al: Molecular markers in male breast carcinoma, *Cancer* 83:1947, 1998.

126. Munoz de Toro MM et al: Proliferative activity and steroid hormone receptor status in male breast carcinoma, *J Steroid Biochem Mol Biol* 67:333, 1998.

127. Pich A et al: Androgen receptor expression in male breast carcinoma: lack of clinicopathological association, *Br J Cancer* 79:959, 1999.

128. Bezwoda WR et al: Breast cancer in men: clinical features, hormone receptor status, and response to therapy, *Cancer* 60:1337, 1987.

129. Wooster R et al: A germline mutation in the androgen receptor gene in two brothers with breast cancer and Reifenstein syndrome, *Nat Genet* 2:132, 1992.

130. Lobaccaro JM et al: Androgen receptor gene mutation in male breast cancer, *Hum Mol Genet* 2:1799, 1993.

131. Hiort O et al: The role of androgen receptor gene mutations in male breast carcinoma, *J Clin Endocrinol Metab* 81:3404, 1996.

132. Shoker BS et al: Estrogen receptor-positive proliferating cells in the normal and precancerous breast, *Am J Pathol* 155:1811, 1999.

133. Shoker BS et al: Abnormal regulation of the oestrogen receptor in benign breast lesions, *J Clin Pathol* 53:778, 2000.

134. Shoker BS et al: Oestrogen receptor expression in the normal and pre-cancerous breast, *J Pathol* 188:237, 1999.

135. Iqbal M et al: Subgroups of non-atypical hyperplasia of breast defined by proliferation of oestrogen receptor-positive cells, *J Pathol* 193:333, 2001.

136. Shaaban AM et al: Histopathologic types of benign breast lesions and the risk of breast cancer: case-control study, *Am J Surg Pathol* 26:421, 2002.

137. Shaaban AM et al: Breast cancer risk in usual ductal hyperplasia is defined by estrogen receptor-alpha and Ki-67 expression, *Am J Pathol* 160:597, 2002.

138. Salamon DS et al: Epidermal growth factor-related peptides and their receptors in human malignancies, *Crit Rev Oncol Hematol* 19:183, 1995.

139. Todaro GJ et al: Cellular and viral ligands that interact with the EGF receptor, *Semin Cancer Biol* 1:257, 1990.

140. Hung MC, Lau YK: Basic science of *HER-2/neu:* a review, *Semin Oncol* 26(4 suppl 12):51, 1999.

141. Carpenter G: Receptors for epidermal growth factor and other polypeptide antigens, *Annu Rev Biochem* 56:881, 1987.
142. Ullrich A, Schlessinger J: Signal transduction by receptors with tyrosine kinase activity, *Cell* 61:203, 1990.
143. Slamon DJ et al: Studies of the *HER-2/neu* proto-oncogene in human breast and ovarian cancer, *Science* 244:707, 1989.
144. Vogel CL et al: Efficacy and safety of trastuzumab as a single agent in first-line treatment of *HER2*-overexpressing metastatic breast cancer, *J Clin Oncol* 20:719, 2002.
145. Mass R et al: The concordance between clinical trials assay and fluorescence in situ hybridization in Herceptin pivotal trials, *Proc Am Soc Clin Oncol* 19:75a, 2000 (abstract).
146. Slamon DJ et al: Human breast cancer: correlation of relapse and survival with amplification of the *HER2/neu* oncogene, *Science* 235:177, 1987.
147. Press MF et al: *HER-2/neu* expression in node-negative breast cancer: direct tissue quantitation by computerized image analysis and association of overexpression with increased risk of recurrent disease, *Cancer Res* 53:4960, 1993.
148. Cobleigh MA et al: Multinational study of the efficacy and safety of humanized anti*HER2* monoclonal antibody in women who have *HER2*-overexpressing metastatic breast cancer that has progressed after chemotherapy for metastatic disease, *J Clin Oncol* 17:2639, 1999.
149. Pegram M et al: Inhibitory effects of combinations of *HER2/neu* antibody and chemotherapeutic agents used for treatment of human breast cancers, *Oncogene* 18:2241, 1999.
150. Konecny G et al: Therapeutic advantage of chemotherapy drugs in combination with Herceptin against human breast cancer cells with *HER2/neu* over-expression, *Breast Cancer Treat Res* 57:114, 1999 (abstract).
151. Slamon DJ et al: Use of chemotherapy plus a monoclonal antibody against *HER2* for metastatic breast cancer that overexpresses *HER2*, *N Engl J Med* 344:783, 2001.
152. Benz CC et al: Estrogen-dependent, tamoxifen-resistant tumorigenic growth of MCF7 cells transfected with her2/neu, *Breast Cancer Res Treat* 24:85, 1993.
153. De Laurentis M, Bianco A, Placido S: A meta-analysis of the interaction between her2 expression and response to endocrine treatment in advanced breast cancer, *Biol Treat Breast Cancer* 2:11, 2000.
154. Ellis MJ et al: Letrozole is more effective neoadjuvant endocrine therapy for ErbB-1 and/or ErbB-2-positive, estrogen receptor-positive primary breast cancer: evidence from a phase III randomized trial, *J Clin Oncol* 19:3808, 2001.
155. Mouridsen H et al: Superior efficacy of letrozole versus tamoxifen as first-line therapy for postmenopausal women with advanced breast cancer: results from a phase III study of the International Letrozole Breast Cancer Group, *J Clin Oncol* 15:2596, 2001.
156. Lipton A et al: Elevated serum *HER2/neu* level predicts decreased response to hormone therapy in metastatic breast cancer, *J Clin Oncol* 20:1467, 2002.
157. Witters LM et al: Enhanced anti-proliferative activity of the combination of tamoxifen plus her2/neu antibody, *Breast Cancer Res Treat* 42:1, 1997.
158. Woodburn JR et al: ZD 1839, an epidermal growth factor receptor tyrosine kinase inhibitor selected for clinical development, *Proc Am Assoc Cancer Res* 38:633, 1997 (abstract).
159. Nicholson RI et al: Oestrogen and growth factor cross-talk and endocrine insensitivity and acquire resistance in breast cancer, *Br J Cancer* 82:501, 2000.
160. Massarweh S et al: Inhibition of epidermal growth factor/*HER2* receptor signaling using ZD183 ("Iressa") restores tamoxifen sensitivity and delays resistance to estrogen deprivation in HER2-overexpressing breast tumors, *Proc Am Soc Clin Oncol* 21:33a, 2002 (abstract).

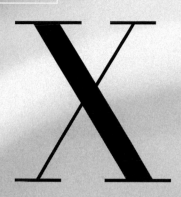

X

MOLECULAR BIOLOGY OF BREAST CARCINOGENESIS AND METASTASIS

CHAPTER

25

Molecular Oncology of Breast Cancer

MINETTA C. LIU
ROBERT B. DICKSON
MARC E. LIPPMAN
EDWARD P. GELMANN

Chapter Outline

Cancer is a genetic disease. The genes mutated during the process that changes a normal cell to a cancer cell are called *oncogenes*. The number of known oncogenes has dramatically increased over the past two decades, but the classification of these genes has essentially remained the same; the products of these genes may disrupt the regulation of cell growth, interrupt programmed cell death, or affect the susceptibility of the cell to DNA damage. The progression of breast cancer through its various stages of malignancy undoubtedly involves multiple genetic events. One class of breast cancers is initiated by an underlying genetic predisposition as a result of the inherited loss of a *BRCA1* or *BRCA2* allele. Other breast cancers begin by one or more sporadic gene mutations and then are promoted by estrogens and alterations of other molecules that activate growth and survival signals in the breast cancer cell.[1] As tumors grow from a few hundred or a few thousand cells, they undergo further genetic changes that cause them to diversify phenotypically. This process is called *malignant progression* and may include the development of mutations in response to such selective pressures as chemotherapy exposure. Studies of tumor cell populations also suggest that subpopulations of ever-changing, genetically distinct cancer cells can arise within an individual tumor,[2,3] preferentially survive, and overtake other, less progressed tumor and normal cells. These surviving subpopulations are mitigated by several selective pressures: host defenses, competition for nutrients, exposure to chemohormonal therapeutic agents, and alterations in the environment after metastatic spread.[4,5]

Early precancerous disturbances in the proliferation of mammary epithelial cells probably perturb only slightly the growth pathways that are normally controlled by specific steroid hormones and growth factors. These early disorders of proliferation induce benign breast disease or premalignant atypical ductal or lobular carcinoma, the molecular basis of which is now being elucidated with the use of cDNA microarray analysis.[6-8] Although the number of genetic lesions in early breast cancer foci may be minimal, the changes in gene expression patterns can differentiate early non-invasive cancer from the surrounding normal tissue.[9-12] The genetic events involved in the progression of cancer include the activation of dominant oncogenes and the inactivation of cancer-suppressive genes. Other genes may also play an important role via altered expression by protein-protein interactions, gene methylation, or loss of heterozygosity (LOH). Evidence from a number of tumor types suggests that tumorigenesis also requires multiple, sequential gene changes, leading to the concept of the gatekeeper oncogene. Because the first gene mutated in a cancer, the gatekeeper is required to initiate the oncogenic program.[13] For example, *APC* is disrupted in 85% of colon cancers that originate in

polyps, and mice deficient in *APC* develop widespread intestinal neoplasia reminiscent of the polyposis seen in human kindreds with *APC* mutations.

To date, a single gatekeeper for breast cancer has not been found. It is conceivable that breast cancer may result from several different oncogenic programs that each result in a similar disease with subtle differences in clinical behavior and prognosis. For example, the clinical characteristics of breast cancers that arise in women with inherited *BRCA1* hemizygosity are subtly different from those that arise sporadically in women without inherited gene mutations.[14-16] Further evidence of the identity of gatekeeper mutations may reside in common patterns of cytogenetic alterations in breast tumors.[11,17] However, the identity of these genes has not been established.

Mammary Gland Development and Mutagenesis

CONTROL OF MAMMARY GLAND DEVELOPMENT

Extensive insight into the biology of mammary epithelium and the mechanism of neoplastic growth has come from studies with animal models, particularly the mouse. Detailed studies of the earliest steps in breast organogenesis and the differentiation of mammary lobules and ducts have provided a platform on which to study effects in genetically altered mice. Development of the normal murine mammary gland results from the interaction between mammary epithelium and the surrounding stromal cells. Communication between the epithelium and stroma is facilitated by paracrine signaling and cell surface contact, both of which result in the activation of signaling pathways.[18,19] Breast development and carcinogenesis in female mice depend on two separate developmental programs that are under the control of steroid hormones and the subsequent activation of the corresponding steroid hormone receptors.

One breast development program occurs in the neonate and leads to the development of an immature breast with primitive ducts and end-buds. The embryonic mammary epithelium develops as a "bud" within the mammary fat pad. Fetal development is thought to proceed through epithelial-stromal (mesenchymal) interactions. The role of steroid hormones at this early stage is not well established,[20,21] however, because receptors for both androgen and estrogen are present in the murine mammary stroma but not in the primitive epithelial components.[22,23] A primitive gland duct is formed by day 19 of the female embryo but does not further develop until the postnatal period.[20] In the male, in contrast, the developing fetal testes secrete testosterone, which inhibits epithelial development, between days 13 and 15 through a stromal-epithelial interactive process.[22,24]

The second development program occurs during puberty and pregnancy as the mammary ducts undergo further lobuloalveolar development. After birth, the mouse mammary gland consists of the primary duct and a few branching ducts. Further development occurs later with the onset of puberty, and cyclical growth and regression occur during successive reproductive cycles. Glandular regression involves the active induction of cell death or apoptosis. Hormonal stimuli alter the tissue milieu by affecting both epithelial and stromal cells in the breast, leading to the expansion of mammary ducts as well as the formation and differentiation of lobules to produce milk proteins. Further studies with a number of animal models have shown that epithelial-stromal interactions are critical for the development and maintenance of the normal mammary ductal architecture. For example, work with monkeys, rabbits, and guinea pigs revealed that the local application of estrone to one nipple promotes lobuloalveolar growth at the site of application but not in untreated glands.[22-27] The local delivery of estradiol to the developing murine mammary gland has also shown that normal development is restricted to the glandular region adjacent to the area of hormone delivery or application.[28] Immunohistochemical analysis for estrogen receptor (ER) in breast specimens from nonlactating women demonstrated a lack of ER expression in stromal cells and only 7% positivity in epithelial cells scattered throughout the lobules.[29]

Estradiol is essential for the ductal phases of mammary gland development in both mice and humans.[30] The end-buds of the developing ducts appear to be the most rapidly proliferating regions. Quiescent ductal end-buds synthesize DNA and undergo ductal elongation in response to estradiol.[31] This process requires the presence of a functioning pituitary gland, a circumstance suggesting that it is not dependent solely on steroid hormones.[32-34] Estrogen and growth hormone partially reverse end-bud regression in animals whose ovaries, pituitaries, and adrenals have been removed, but they cannot fully prevent end-bud involution. This finding suggests that additional survival factors are essential for the maintenance of mammary gland integrity.[34] Data from in vitro studies with normal mammary epithelial cell cultures also suggest that the effects of estrogen are mediated by the local or paracrine effects of other cells,[35,36] because estrogen-induced epithelial cell proliferation has been observed only in cocultures with mammary stromal cells.[37,38] In addition, studies of both rat mammary glands and human reduction mammoplasty specimens have demonstrated that normal breast epithelial cells that express ER and progesterone receptor (PR) are separate from the population of proliferating cells, which were detected by assessment of Ki67 expression.[39] Taken together, these various findings further substantiate the hypothesis that estrogen and progesterone affect cell proliferation by an indirect mechanism.

Estradiol appears to induce glandular development and sustain glandular architecture through the induction of growth factor secretion by both stromal and epithelial cells. Hormonal priming of immature murine mammary gland cultures alters their sensitivity to other steroids such as aldosterone and hydrocortisone and to peptides such as insulin and prolactin.[40] The gland contains the epidermal growth factor (EGF) receptor that can be simulated by EGF or transforming growth factor-α (TGF-α), both of which are able to promote local lobuloalveolar development in vitro when implanted as slow-release pellets into the mammary gland.[18,41] Isolated murine ductal end-buds also require EGF for growth in culture.[42] The expression of EGF receptors is programmed at different times in stromal and epithelial cells,[41] and in vitro studies with cell lines derived from normal breast epithelium,[43] myoepithelial cells,[44] and immortalized epithelium[45-49] support the notion that the mitogenic effects of estradiol may be at least partially mediated by peptide growth factors. In fact, many of these cells do not express ER or do not respond to estrogens, but proliferating cultures of normal or immortalized mammary epithelial cells usually express high levels of the EGF receptor (EGFR) and TGF-α.[46,50] In low-density culture, the ER-negative mammary epithelial cells require multiple survival factors, including EGF (or TGF-α), insulin, transferrin, isoproterenol (or cholera toxin, PGE_1, or phosphodiesterase inhibitors, which stimulate cyclic adenosine monophosphate [cAMP] production or accumulation), hydrocortisone, and bovine pituitary extract (whose active ingredient is not yet known).[51] It should be noted, however, that none of these studies described isolation of the rare ER-positive mammary epithelial cells; thus there may have been selection bias in that the ER-negative cells were favored for in vitro growth.

EPITHELIAL MUTAGENESIS

Like the normal epithelial cells from which they are derived, many breast cancer cells are sensitive to estrogen-stimulated growth via either direct or indirect mechanisms. For example, studies in murine model systems have shown that estrogen can control breast tumor growth by inducing the synthesis and secretion of prolactin from the pituitary gland. Estrogen may also act by cooperating with other growth stimulators or by allowing breast cancers to overcome growth inhibitors.[52-54] Physiologic concentrations of estrogen can induce a large number of enzymes and other proteins involved in cell survival and nucleic acid synthesis, including DNA polymerase, MYC,[55] cyclin D1,[56] thymidine and uridine kinases, thymidylate synthetase, carbamyl phosphate synthetase, aspartate transcarbamylase, dihydroorotase, glucose-6-phosphate dehydrogenase, lactate dehydrogenase,[57] and dihydrofolate reductase.[58-61] For example, estrogen regulates thymidine kinase and dihydrofolate reductase at the mRNA level,[62,63] and it regulates thymidine kinase at the transcriptional level as well.[64] In addition, a screen of 41 protein kinases was recently created with a cloning technique based on reverse transcriptase–polymerase chain reaction (RT-PCR) technology.[65] The majority of the identified proteins do not have a currently recognized role in mammary development or carcinogenesis, but most were shown to have distinct patterns of expression, suggestive of a role in developmental regulation. In fact, this screen led to the identification of the hormonally upregulated NEU-associated kinase (HUNK), a serine/threonine kinase whose expression is associated with early pregnancy and treatment with estrogen and progesterone, as well as proper mammary epithelial proliferation and differentiation, in animal models.[66]

An elevated risk of human breast cancer has been associated with such reproductive factors as early menarche, late onset of menopause, nulliparity, and older age at first full-term pregnancy. Early pregnancy, however, is protective, which suggests that factors associated with pregnancy can induce changes in the tumorigenic response of breast cells. This theory has been substantiated by observations that mammary carcinogenesis in rats can be significantly reduced by both parity[67] and the exogenous administration of the placental hormone chorionic gonadotropin.[68]

Investigations into the hormonal control of breast cancer growth have been facilitated by the availability of cancer cell lines, which are typically derived from the pleural or ascitic fluid of patients with metastatic disease. Several estrogen-responsive cell lines exist, including MCF-7, T47D, MDA-MB-134, ZR-75-1, PMC42, and CAMA-1. MCF-7 is probably the most well characterized, and it has an absolute requirement for estrogenic stimulation in the in vivo model of tumor formation in athymic (nude) mice.[69] PMC42 has also been described as a well-differentiated, estrogen-responsive breast cancer cell line that has a relatively unique feature in that monoclonal antibodies prepared against its surface antigens can cross-react with specimens containing ductal carcinoma in situ.[70,71] At the other end of the spectrum, numerous estrogen-independent breast cancer lines exist as well, including the adenocarcinoma cell line MDA-MB-231 and the carcinosarcoma cell line Hs578T. Although existing cell lines can be ordered according to their ER state, nearly all were derived from metastatic sites in patients and are

fully malignant in that sense. Therefore controls, on metastatic behavior have been difficult to address.

Molecular Genetic Changes in Breast Carcinogenesis

DOMINANT AND RECESSIVE ONCOGENES

The activation of dominant oncogenes often involves specific mutations that change the functional control of growth-promoting proteins or gene amplification that increases protein expression. Dominant oncogenes influence the cancer process despite the presence of the normal contralateral allele. Genes that affect DNA repair tend to be included in this category because inactivation of a single allele of a DNA repair gene can reduce the level of repair in a dominant fashion and predispose to tumor formation. Recessive oncogenes, however, require the inactivation of both alleles to initiate or promote development of the cancer phenotype. The paradigm for suppressor oncogene inactivation is that one allele is lost by gross chromosomal rearrangement and the second is disrupted by a more subtle event such as a point mutation.[72] These so-called tumor-suppressor genes normally act to control cell growth or promote cell death.

CYTOGENETIC ABNORMALITIES IN BREAST CANCER

Analysis of chromosomes in cancer cells has provided important insights into the location and identification of oncogenes. Historically, the careful karyotypic analysis of cancer cells resulted in the implication of chromosomal regions in cancer pathogenesis. Karyotypic studies using chromosomal banding techniques initially implicated chromosomes 1, 3, 6, 7, 9, and 11 in breast tumors.[73-75] In particular, the loss of variable lengths of one arm of chromosome 1 has been significantly associated with grade III histology, distant metastasis, and the hormone receptor–negative phenotype. Cellular aneuploidy has also been related to increased rates of tumor proliferation and ER negativity.[76] Although several other specific genetic changes occur with high frequency and proven relevance in breast cancer, there are certainly many more important genetic changes to be fully elucidated.

Newer methodologies have enabled some of these advances. Studies of LOH, for example, have led to the identification of specific genetic regions that are commonly rearranged, amplified, or otherwise altered in breast cancer. These regions include chromosomes 1, 3, 6, 7, 8, 9, 11, 13, 15, 16, 17, 18, and 20.[77] Consistent loss of a single chromosomal locus in a given tumor type often indicates the presence of a suppressor gene at that locus. We know that the progression of breast cancer may involve LOH on 13q and 17p, corresponding to the *BRCA1* and *BRCA2* loci as well as the tumor-suppressor genes *RB1* and *P53,* respectively. In addition, the cell cycle inhibitor *P16 (MTS1, CDKN2)* was found to be disrupted in a subset of breast cancers by LOH on chromosome 9p.[78] Other suspected tumor-suppressor genes may reside on 7q, 9p, 11p, 11q, 17q, and 18q, and DNA losses are common on chromosomes 20 and 22 as well. However, more studies are needed before definitive conclusions can be made. Such data may in fact result from work with the evolving technique of comparative genomic hybridization (CGH), which provides even greater sensitivity in the search for chromosomal loci consistently altered in human cancers.[11,79-81] This technique allows rapid analysis of genomic imbalances within even very small regions, and it has enabled the additional implication of chromosomes 10, 12, and 22[11] in breast carcinogenesis as well as the observation that aneuploid breast tumors contain far more chromosomal aberrations than their diploid counterparts.[11]

Finally, gene amplifications have also been identified with cytogenetic analysis. An amplified genetic unit (amplicon) is thought to be initially much larger than the actual size of the principal gene of biologic importance to tumorigenesis. For this reason, genes may be coamplified with the target gene and still be silent because they are not expressed. Gene amplification activates the *HER2* and *MYC* oncogenes in breast cancer, as well as the gene encoding the cell cycle kinase regulatory protein cyclin D1. Other common DNA gains include those involving chromosomes 1q, 6p, 13q, and 16p, but in each of these cases the specific genes affected have not been identified.[11]

TRANSGENIC MODELS OF BREAST CARCINOGENESIS

Transgenic mice are created by introducing foreign DNA into murine blastocysts that are implanted into pseudopregnant females and allowed to complete gestation. Oncogenic transgenes are often placed under the control of gene promoters that control tissue-specific expression and may regulate the timing or level of gene expression. The evolution of cancer in this predictable model system provides information about the oncogenic potential of a particular transgene, whose influence on carcinogenesis and tumor progression can be directly measured. The combined effects of more than one transgene can then be observed by mating single transgenic mice to obtain offspring with two oncogenic transgenes, both of which are driven by tissue-specific promoters. In this way, a model system can be created to assess the transforming capacity of a series of oncogenes with targeted, tissue-specific expression.

To study the pathogenesis of breast cancer, transgenic mouse models have been created with two different tissue-specific promoters to target oncogene expression to the breast. One promoter is the murine mammary tumor virus long terminal repeat (MMTV-LTR), which contains a steroid-responsive promoter that can be activated by estrogen. Models including the MMTV promoter to drive oncogene expression typically yield breast cancers after one or more pregnancies, suggesting that the very high levels of estrogen associated with pregnancy are required to drive sufficient oncogene expression for neoplastic transformation. The MMTV promoter is not entirely mammary specific, however; it directs expression in a variety of secretory tissues, including the salivary gland and the harderian gland, a retrobulbar apocrine gland whose enlargement manifests clinically as exophthalmos.[82,83] This is in contrast to the promoter for the milk component whey acid protein (WAP), whose activity is essentially restricted to mammary epithelial cells during pregnancy and lactation.[84] The hormone-dependent MMTV and WAP promoters function in the setting of pregnancy and lactation, such that the resultant phenotype does not reflect the effects of gene expression changes in nonpregnant and nonlactating mammary tissue. In addition, and perhaps more important, the transgene is expressed in almost all mammary epithelial cells, contradicting the theory that sporadic human cancers originate from a single aberrant cell. Despite these possible shortcomings, however, transgenic animals continue to provide informative models for breast cancer pathogenesis. With the development of new therapies targeted at particular oncogenes and with the focus of prevention strategies on individual oncogenic pathways, these mice may be used more widely as preclinical models of breast cancer treatment or prevention.

The *MYC* and *RAS* models serve as classic examples of transgenic models for breast cancer. Mice transgenic for *MYC* under the control of the MMTV promoter or the WAP promoter develop mammary cancers after the second or third pregnancy or within 1 to 2 months after lactation, respectively.[85,86] Because these tumors appeared singly and were clonal, it was apparent that *MYC* contributed to, but was not sufficient for, the development of mammary cancer and that *MYC* expression driven by a heterologous promoter could be seen in histologically normal mammary glands. In contrast, the *HRAS* oncogene with its activating codon 12 mutation was introduced as a transgene under the control of the WAP promoter. These mice developed tumors of the breast and salivary glands after a latency period of nearly 200 days.[87] The combination of *MYC* and activated *HRAS* was therefore bred into mice by mating animals with the two individual transgenes, both under control of the MMTV promoter. The double-transgenic mice developed focal mammary tumors with a median latency of 46 days, compared with 168 days for the

MMTV-*HRAS* transgenic mice and 325 days for the MMTV-*MYC* transgenic mice.[82] The transgenic model results were therefore consistent with our understanding that breast carcinogenesis is a multistep process that can be accelerated by introducing oncogene expression in breast tissue.

The hormone-responsiveness of the MMTV-LTR was first demonstrated by the fact that the murine mammary tumor virus activated cellular oncogenes to promote breast cancer in mice.[88,89] The identification of the *int-1* and *int-2* genes shed light on the fact that both the *WNT* signaling and the fibroblast growth factor pathways could influence the development of mammary cancer. The ability of the *WNT-1* gene to mediate mammary carcinogenesis was underscored by reports of breast cancers in MMTV–*WNT-1* transgenic mice and enhanced breast carcinogenesis caused by the deletion of *P53* in the presence of *WNT-1* transgene expression.[90,91]

Important insight into the interaction of genes that can cause human breast cancer has also come from mouse models. The mouse homolog of the hereditary breast cancer gene *BRCA1* is essential for murine development. To establish a mouse breast cancer model that depended on inactivation of *BRCA1*, the gene was targeted by

mammary-specific expression of a prokaryotic recombinase that specifically inactivates *BRCA1* in mammary cells during pregnancy and lactation. Targeted disruption of *BRCA1* in the murine mammary gland predisposes to breast cancer development.[92-94] Moreover, loss of *P53* can cooperate with targeted disruption of *BRCA1* to enhance mammary tumor formation in mice.[95]

Cyclin D1 is essential for normal mammary gland development, and it is also overexpressed in about half of the cases of ductal carcinoma of the breast. Cyclin D1–deficient mice were immune to mammary carcinogenesis induced by *RAS* or *neu* transgenes but not by activated *MYC* or *WNT-1* transgenes.[96] Such data help elucidate oncogene pathways, identify which genes cooperate in the program that leads to breast cancer, and emphasize the importance of cyclin D1 overexpression in human breast cancer.

Cellular Growth Control Pathways in Breast Carcinogenesis

CELL CYCLE CONTROL AND APOPTOSIS

As illustrated in Figure 25-1, the cell cycle is under the direct regulation of an orderly series of cyclin-dependent

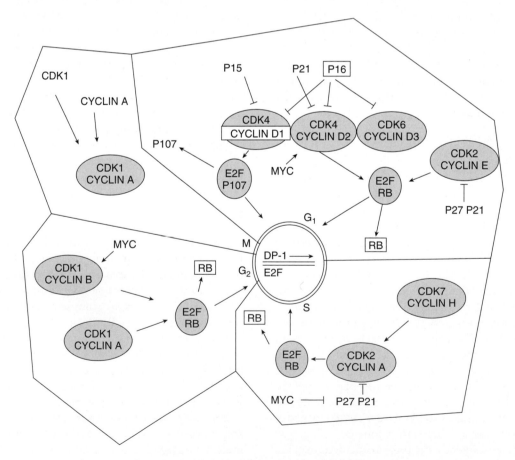

FIG. **25-1** Relationship of the factors participating in direct regulation of cell cycle progression.

kinases (CDKs), their positive regulatory subunits or cyclins, and their negative regulatory subunits or cyclin-dependent kinase inhibitors. There is growing evidence that cell cycle dysregulation plays a role in breast cancer pathogenesis. Of particular interest are alterations in those proteins that regulate the progression through the G_1 and S phases. The early G_1 phase of the cell cycle is driven by the relative expression of cyclins D1, D2, and D3, which preferentially bind to CDK4 and CDK6.[97,98] The cyclin E–CDK2 complex subsequently controls the transition between the G_1 and S phases,[99-101] cyclin A–CDK2 controls the passage through S phase,[102] and cyclin A–CDK2 and cyclin B–CDK2 control the transition between the G_2 and M phases.[103] These cyclins and their associated CDKs are tightly controlled through the coordinated activity of inducers and suppressors. The expression of cyclin D1, for example, is suppressed by MYC and induced by RAS,[104,105] the sex steroids, and various tyrosine kinase receptor–acting growth factors (e.g., EGF). CDK4, however, is inhibited by TGF-β, and cyclin D1–CDK4 is inhibited by P15[INK4], P16 (MTS1), and P21[WAF1/CIP1]. In the G_1 and S transition, the *MYC* gene product induces cyclin E, and P21[WAF1/CIP1] and P27[KIP1] both inhibit the cyclin E–CDK2 complex.[106]

Cyclin D1. Almost all human carcinomas are characterized by the disruption of one or more cell cycle control genes, including *P16[INK4]*, any of the cyclins, and *RB*. Cyclin D1 in particular has been implicated as an important oncogene in breast cancer. The cyclin D1 gene *CCND1* has been shown to function as a mammary cancer–inducing transgene when driven by the hormone-responsive MMTV-LTR promoter in a mouse model. Cyclin D1 overexpression is part of a carcinogenic program that includes *neu* and *RAS*.[107,108] Conversely, targeted disruption of murine *CCND1* in the mouse results in the dramatic suppression of lobuloalveolar development of the mammary gland.[109] *CCND1* amplification occurs in approximately 30% of breast cancer cases, and the incidence of cyclin D1 mRNA and/or protein overexpression is reported to be as high as 80%.[110-117] Cyclin D1 overexpression also correlates with the expression of ER in breast cancer,[114,118,119] consistent with the findings that cyclin D1 can bind to and activate the ER.[120,121] Whether cyclin D1 amplification or overexpression has independent prognostic significance, however, has not yet been shown.[122-125] Finally, there is also some evidence that the cyclin-dependent kinase inhibitors act as tumor suppressors. For example, the gene coding for *p16/MTS1* is not deleted or mutated in breast cancers.[126-129] However, *p16* expression may be affected by gene methylation[130-132] or dysregulation, resulting in cytoplasmic localization of the protein.[126,132,133]

Retinoblastoma *(RB)* **Gene.** CDK4 and CDK6 activation by the D cyclins results in the phosphorylation and inactivation of RB, a cell cycle regulatory molecule that interacts with members of the E2F family of transcription factors to regulate transition from the G_1 to S phase of the cell cycle.[134-136] Although RB appears to be present in most cell types, its inactivation directly and specifically results in tumors of the retina and an increased predisposition to osteosarcomas. Despite the selective association between RB inactivation and the predisposition for specific tumor types, most human cancers have been associated with some form of dysregulation of the RB signaling pathway.

The *RB* gene is located on chromosome 13q14.1, and it was the first cancer gene identified with positional cloning, facilitated by linkage analysis of families affected with retinoblastoma. Because chromosome 13 is a common site for LOH in breast cancer, the status of the *RB* gene was investigated.[137,138] Deletions and rearrangements of *RB* were seen in a number of breast cancer cell lines,[139,140] and *RB* gene structure was altered by deletion or rearrangement in about one fifth of primary tissue samples.[134,141-143] Paradoxically, the RB protein product was seen in almost all breast cancer samples,[144-146] and the presence of LOH at the region of the *RB* gene did not correlate with the low levels of RB protein expression detected with immunohistochemistry.[147] Therefore, although there is evidence of *RB* gene disruption in breast cancer tissues, it is unclear how this finding translates into loss of the RB protein product and its corresponding suppressor oncogene function. One possible explanation for this discrepancy is that the loss of tumor-suppressor function results from increased phosphorylation and inactivation of RB, as opposed to loss of the protein product itself. Estrogen-induced cell growth, for example, is associated with increased cyclin D1 activity and increased phosphorylation of RB. Antiestrogens induce the opposite effects.[148-150]

P53. P53 is an oligomeric phosphoprotein that binds to a specific recognition sequence on DNA and can activate transcription.[151] P53 protein responds to DNA damage and other cell injury as a cell cycle checkpoint, causing a pause in the cell cycle if DNA damage is present. P53 was first described as a 53-kDa coimmunoprecipitate with the T-antigen of the SV40-transforming DNA virus. It is a cellular protein encoded by a 20-kb gene that maps to chromosome 17p13.1.[152,153] The expression and function of P53 are controlled by a variety of posttranslational mechanisms that allow for rapid changes in protein levels and activity. This protein is involved in a broad range of cellular processes, including apoptosis, DNA damage repair, and cell cycle arrest (see reference 154 for review).

Regions of the *P53* gene are highly conserved throughout evolution.[155] These regions are the most common sites for mutations that inactivate *P53* in cancers. Point mutations in *P53* have been extensively characterized in a variety of human tumors and reflect the chemical nature of the carcinogenic insult.[156] Because roughly 60% of *P53* mutations in breast cancer are transitions (purine/purine—guanine/adenine and pyrimidine/pyrimidine—cytosine/thymine), it is likely that the carcinogenic mechanism in this malignancy differs from that of such malignancies as hepatocellular carcinoma and esophageal carcinoma, in which there is a direct link to chemical carcinogens that cause nucleotide transversions (purine/pyrimidine) in *P53*. Irrespective of their etiology, various mutations in *P53* can be used as molecular markers of clonality to study breast cancer progression from in situ to invasive carcinoma. A subset of cases of ductal carcinoma in situ do, in fact, contain *P53* mutations, suggesting that *P53* is mutated relatively early during breast carcinogenesis.[157-159] Mutations of *P53* were even found in histologically benign human breast tissue.[160] Moreover, in one case the same *P53* mutation was found in both ductal carcinoma in situ and the adjacent infiltrating ductal carcinoma, proving that the invasive cancer was derived from the in situ disease.[159]

P53 mutations initially were detected with nucleic acid analysis for single-strand conformational polymorphisms, followed by nucleotide sequencing of the polymorphic bands. It was then shown that *P53* mutations alter binding of the P53 protein to heat shock protein (HSP) 70, thus prolonging the half-life of P53.[161,162] Because of its short half-life, P53 protein is not normally detectable in tissue sections by immunohistochemical staining. Therefore positive staining for P53 has become a surrogate for the presence of a mutant protein. The assumption that detection of P53 in a tissue section represents a *P53* mutation is correct for about 80% to 90% of breast cancer specimens.[163-165]

The topic of P53 expression in breast cancer has been reviewed by Harris.[166] Approximately 30 reports have described P53 protein staining or *P53* mutational analysis in series of breast cancer specimens. The total number of tissues studied exceeds 4000. Some general conclusions can be drawn from these studies.[157,158,165,167-187] Overall, 20% to 30% of breast cancer specimens stain positively for P53 expression; a few studies have shown P53-positivity rates as high as 45%, but these may be due to differences in staining techniques and antibody reagents. The fraction of breast cancer specimens that stain positively for P53 correlates well with the fraction of breast cancer specimens that have identifiable *P53* mutations.

There is consensus that P53 expression in breast cancer correlates with high tumor grade, indices of proliferation such as S-phase fraction and proliferating cell nuclear antigen (PCNA) staining, aneuploidy, and absence of ER and PR. Because these parameters are associated with shortened disease-free and overall survival, it is not surprising that P53 staining would also be associated with poor prognosis. Fewer than half of the studies, however, demonstrated a correlation between P53 positivity and shortened disease-free or overall survival, but the results of many of these studies could have been confounded by small sample size. In terms of treatment response, there is no conclusive evidence of a relation between P53 status and response to anti-estrogen therapy, anthracycline-based chemotherapy regimens, or non–anthracycline-based chemotherapy regimens.[188,189] Although some studies suggest that P53 abnormalities are predictive of resistance,[164,190-195] others suggest that they are predictive of responsiveness[192] or not predictive at all.[193,194] For these reasons, the 1999 Consensus Statement of the College of American Pathologists ranked P53 as a category II prognostic factor in breast cancer, whose clinical utility must be validated more rigorously in statistically sound studies.[196]

The *P53* gene was the first gene to be identified as predisposing to hereditary breast cancer. This became apparent when mutations in *P53* were found in the germ lines of families with the Li-Fraumeni syndrome.[197] Li and Fraumeni described the syndrome after identifying four children with sarcomas who were first-degree relatives of other children with rhabdomyosarcoma.[198] They subsequently observed that the mothers of these children had a high incidence of early breast cancer. They also found that the kindreds had a high incidence of leukemias, lymphomas, osteosarcomas, and adrenocortical carcinomas. Germ line *P53* mutations in a substantial number of Li-Fraumeni kindreds cluster around codons 240 to 248, and other kindreds have mutations affecting other codons.[198,199] The data from the Li-Fraumeni syndrome, combined with findings of *P53* mutations in histologically normal breast tissue, strongly suggest that *P53* mutations can occur early in breast carcinogenesis.

The presence of *P53* mutations in breast cancer has also been correlated with LOH at chromosome 17p13.1. In contrast to findings with colon cancer, in which there is a high correlation between 17p13.1 LOH and *P53* mutations,[72] there is a consistently higher fraction of tumors with chromosome 17p13.1 LOH than with *P53* mutations in breast cancer. Although all cases with *P53* mutations can be expected to demonstrate LOH at 17p13.1, the reverse is not true. About 50% to 60% of breast cancers have LOH at 17p13, indicating that there is a second breast cancer oncogene located in that region of the chromosome.[165,200-203]

BCL-2 Family Proteins. Programmed cell death, or apoptosis, is a physiologic process that provides for the destruction and elimination of senescent cells. It is critical for the development and homeostasis of all organs, including the breast. The reduced levels of estrogen, progesterone, and prolactin after each reproductive cycle and after lactation lead to apoptosis of mammary epithelial cells and physiologic involution of the breast as a whole. In several experimental systems, estrogen acts to suppress apoptosis by inducing transcription of BCL-2, an antiapoptotic protein critical for blocking the activation of cell death pathways that originate in the mitochondria.[204] BCL-2 belongs to a family of proteins with structural similarities that have either proapoptotic or antiapoptotic functions. These proteins are involved in a complex relationship that involves dimerization of proapoptotic and antiapoptotic family members to regulate their function.[205-211]

The *BCL-2* gene was first identified in a reciprocal chromosomal translocation in human B-cell lymphoma.[212] BCL-2 localizes to the mitochondrial membrane and blocks the egress of cytochrome c, which is a major precipitant of programmed cell death or apoptosis.[213] It is one member of a family of regulatory proteins that includes BCL-X, BCL-X$_L$, BCL-X$_S$, BAX, BAK, and BAD.[214] The ratio of proapoptotic and antiapoptotic proteins determines a cell's fate, and it is this delicate balance that directs normal mammary gland development during puberty and pregnancy. Because of the central role of BCL-2 in maintaining tissue homeostasis, a number of investigators have studied BCL-2 expression in breast tumor tissues. In general, BCL-2 expression is associated with a prognostically favorable phenotype[215-223] and correlates with the presence of ER.[204,219,221,224-230] Estrogen regulates *BCL-2* gene expression,[56] possibly through estrogen-responsive elements within the *BCL-2* coding region.[231] Consistent with this theory is the clinical observation that ER-positive, BCL-2–positive tumors are more likely than ER-positive, BCL-2–negative tumors to be more responsive to tamoxifen. In addition, both chemotherapy and radiation exert their tumoricidal effects by the induction of apoptosis. Consequently, BCL-2 expression is an important determinant of chemotherapy and radiation resistance in many tumor types.[232-235] There has been particular interest about BCL-2 expression as a marker for response to the taxanes because both paclitaxel and docetaxel can effect the phosphorylation and inactivation of the BCL-2 protein, a biochemical action that is proapoptotic.[236]

BCL-X has significant structural homology with *BCL-2*.[237] Differential splicing yields two distinct species of mRNA that encode the antiapoptotic BCL-X$_L$ and proapoptotic BCL-X$_S$ proteins; the latter acts as a dominant negative inhibitor of both BCL-2 and BCL-X$_L$.

BCL-X$_L$ appears to be ubiquitously expressed,[238] although its exact role in many tissue types remains to be determined. With respect to breast cancer, its upregulation has been associated with the promotion of cell growth in selected breast cancer cell lines[239] and an increase in metastatic potential in xenograft models.[240] BCL-X$_L$ overexpression in primary breast cancers has been documented as well,[241,242] and some data support an association with axillary lymph node positivity and high tumor grade.[242]

GROWTH FACTORS AND THEIR RECEPTORS

Epidermal Growth Factor Receptor Family. Dominant oncogenes transduce proliferative and antiapoptotic signals that most commonly originate with cell-surface receptor molecules and are transmitted via activated kinases that sequentially phosphorylate downstream elements in the signaling pathway to shift the balance between cell death and cell growth. The signal transduction cascade often activated in human breast cancer is initiated by the EGFR family of receptor tyrosine kinases (RTKs). EGFR and its three homologous family members (HER2, HER3, and HER4) are transmembrane ligand–binding proteins with a cytoplasmic tyrosine kinase domain as well as SRC-homology domains (SH2 and SH3) that mediate interactions with other proteins. The interaction of EGFR and its family members with other cytoplasmic proteins is regulated by the phosphorylation of C-terminal tyrosine residues. These receptors share a similar structural organization and bind ligands in the EGF family, including EGF, heregulin, and cripto-1 or amphiregulin. On ligand binding, these proteins dimerize and activate their intracytoplasmic tyrosine kinases. The members of the family can also form heterodimers in a complex series of interactions that result in transphosphorylation and concerted regulation of the involved family members.

Epidermal Growth Factor Receptor (EGFR; HER1). EGF binding to EGFR triggers a series of molecular events that lead to activation of nuclear transcription factors and cell division. A schematic diagram of the EGFR is shown in Figure 25-2. Important intermediaries in this signal transduction cascade from cell membrane to nucleus are members of the *RAS* family of oncogenes that are not often mutated in human breast cancer and are discussed later. After two EGFR family molecules dimerize in response to ligand binding, C-terminal tyrosine residues become phosphorylated, either by autophosphorylation or by an *SRC*-related kinase. Next, the SH2 domain of the receptor is bound by GRB2, a RAS adaptor protein. The protein complex is then joined by SOS, a guanine nucleotide exchange factor that binds through its own proline-rich C-terminus to the SH3 domain of EGFR. The complex is now able to exchange a GTP for a GDP complexed to the RAS protein, and the signal transduction cascade proceeds downstream from RAS. RAS, which is activated by GTR binding, in turn, activates phosphatidylinositol-3-kinase to initiate signaling by the biochemical pathways that are triggered by diacylglycerol production and protein kinase C activation. RAS also activates a series of cytoplasmic serine and threonine kinases, beginning with RAF, that sequentially phosphorylate the protein immediately downstream in the cascade. RAF is a MAP kinase kinase kinase; therefore it phosphorylates MEK, a MAP kinase kinase. MEK then phosphorylates members of the MAP kinase family, for example, ERK 1 and 2. MAP kinases, in turn, phosphorylate nuclear proteins to trigger transcriptional activation. The signal transduction cascade that includes several protooncogenes is shown in Figure 25-2. EGFR signaling also activates other pathways in the cell including protein kinase C, the Janus kinase (JAK)/signal transduction activators of transcription (STAT) pathways, and phosphoinositol-3-kinase.[243,244]

Various mouse models suggest that EGFR is required for ductal morphogenesis in the development of the mammary gland.[245] Six EGF-like ligands are known to bind and activate EGFR: EGF itself, TGF-α, amphiregulin (cripto-1, or CR-1), heparin-binding EGF (HB-EGF), betacellulin (BTC), and epiregulin (EPR).[246,247] As in the case of other growth factors and growth factor receptors implicated in tumorigenesis, possible mechanisms of EGFR pathway activation include overexpression and/or decreased turnover of the receptor, the presence of excessive ligand, decreased phosphatase activity, and the development of receptors with aberrant ligand-binding or tyrosine kinase activity. The capacity of EGFR overexpression to contribute to cell transformation was underscored by in vitro transfection studies that resulted in overexpression of normal EGFR in cell lines and transformation of the recipient cells.[248-250] A number of mutant EGFRs have also been identified in human cancers, the most common of which is EGFRvIII.[251] This truncated form of EGFR is constitutively activated and thus able to stimulate cell proliferation in the absence

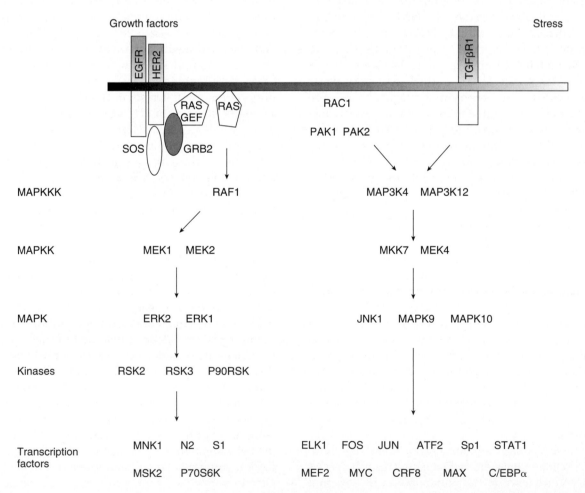

FIG. 25-2 Schematic diagram of the signal transduction cascades activated by the epidermal growth factor receptor and the transforming growth factor-α receptor.

of ligand.[252] It has been detected in malignant gliomas, non–small cell lung cancers, and ovarian cancers, and its transforming ability has been demonstrated in multiple cell lines.[253,254] There is also recent evidence of a high incidence of wild-type EGFR and mutant EGFRvIII coexpression in invasive breast cancer tissue.[255] The mutant form is not expressed in normal tissue, which suggests that it may be an ideal target for directed breast cancer therapies. A monoclonal antibody called *Y10* has specificity for murine and human EGFRvIII, and it has demonstrated antineoplastic activity in vitro and in animal models thus far.[256]

The germ line inactivation of various EGFR ligands impairs normal mammary gland development,[257] and transgenic mouse models have independently demonstrated that EGFR[258] and TGF-α[259,260] play roles in the development of mammary tumors. EGFR activation therefore appears to be critical for the development of normal mammary epithelium as well as mammary tumors. Several hundred thousand copies of EGFR may be present per cell in breast cancer cell lines,[261,262] and the *EGFR* gene is known to be amplified in at least one breast cancer cell line, MDA-MB-468. A substantial fraction of human breast cancers overexpress this receptor. However, *EGFR* does not fit the rigorous definition of an oncogene in any but a very few human breast cancers, because there is only rare evidence of *EGFR* amplification and no evidence of an activating gene mutation in breast cancer. The discussion of EGFR is included, however, because of substantial interest in the importance of EGFR in breast cancer, because of the structural similarities between EGFR and HER2, and because EGFR, like HER2, is a potential target of antibody-mediated therapy for breast cancer.

Because *EGFR* is rarely a breast cancer oncogene, there is no qualitative genetic criterion to identify tumors in which *EGFR* may play a causative role. *EGFR* amplification has been found to occur up to 14% of tumor specimens,[263-265] but EGFR is found to be overexpressed in approximately half of all breast cancers. EGFR levels can be determined by binding studies, immunohistochemical staining, and mRNA quantification. Despite a lack of consensus regarding the criteria for EGFR overexpression, a large number of studies on EGFR in breast cancer agree on the fraction of tumors that overexpress the receptor. One literature review tabulated 40 studies that had analyzed more than 5000 patient samples for EGFR expression.[266] Overall, 48% of all samples were identified as positive for EGFR expression,[266-308] and there was little difference between the fraction of EGFR-positive tumors detected with immunologic versus biochemical techniques. The majority of investigations have revealed a negative correlation between EGFR and ER expression, as well as a negative correlation between EGFR expression and relapse-free

survival. Because of limitations in the duration of follow-up, three reports demonstrated a relationship between EGFR expression and decreased overall survival,[275,289,307] but only one study determined this relationship to be significant on multivariate analysis.[275] A prospective study of 459 patients has also been done that reported highly significant correlations between EGFR expression and both disease-free and overall survival.[309] Notably, one other study suggests a particularly strong correlation between EGFR expression and invasive lobular carcinoma: all subjects with this histologic subtype died within 2 years of follow-up.[277] This time frame represents much shorter survival than for patients with other histologic subtypes and EGFR expression levels, suggesting that EGFR expression may be a particularly important prognostic marker in invasive lobular as opposed to invasive ductal carcinomas.

As stated earlier, there is an inverse correlation between EGFR expression and ER expression in breast cancer. This is reflected in the finding that EGFR expression predicts a poor response to tamoxifen therapy.[310] Because normal breast epithelial cells more frequently display simultaneous expression of EGFR and ER, the inverse correlation of the expression of these two receptors in cancer may reflect a biologic difference between malignant and nonmalignant breast epithelia.[295] Immunohistochemistry was retrospectively performed on 1029 frozen breast cancer specimens from patients followed for a mean of 46 months. EGFR overexpression was found in about 27% of samples in one cohort, and it was associated with decreased disease-free and overall survival in both node-negative and node-positive patients with an ER-negative phenotype.[311] In studies with cultured breast cancer cells, simultaneous expression of high levels of EGFR and ER was not seen.[262] Moreover, transfection of the *EGFR* gene into ER-positive cell lines results in transient expression of EGFR that is unstable in the presence of estradiol.[312] A similar phenomenon was observed after transfection of TGF-α into ER-positive cells.[313] Therefore the biologic data are consistent with the clinical observations that EGFR and ER expression are often mutually exclusive. One possible mechanism by which this inverse correlation is maintained in ER-positive breast cancer cells involves the direct suppression of EGFR transcription in the presence of an estrogen stimulus.[314] Such findings suggest that EGFR and ER represent the gateways to alternative pathways of growth regulation, such that therapy targeted against EGFR may prove particularly effective in conjunction with antiestrogen therapy for hormone receptor–positive invasive breast cancer. There is also evidence of cross-talk between EGFR and ER: EGF has been shown to effect the phosphorylation of specific residues on ERα in COS-7 and

MCF-7 breast cancer cell lines.[315] There is even evidence of an interaction between estrogen and the EGFR signaling pathway through activation of one of the G protein–coupled receptors in ER-negative cells.[316]

High expression of EGFR on the cell surface suggests that EGFR could be a target for antibody-mediated therapies in breast cancer and other malignancies. EGFR can be targeted therapeutically with a variety of approaches, including the use of monoclonal antibodies and small-molecule tyrosine kinase inhibitors.[317] Antibodies against EGFR may block growth signals to breast cancer cells, and this has been demonstrated with various breast cancer cell lines in culture.[318,319] These findings led to the development of the chimeric monoclonal antibody IMC-C225 (cetuximab; Erbitux), inhibits EGF-induced autophosphorylation,[320] promotes the dimerization and internalization of EGFR,[321] leads to the development of G_1 cell cycle arrest through increased expression of the P27^{KIP1} cyclin–dependent kinase inhibitor,[322] and inhibits tumor-induced angiogenesis.[323] Clinical trials with this agent are ongoing. Of the small-molecule tyrosine kinase inhibitors, the quinazoline derivatives ZD1839 (gefitinib; Iressa) and OSI-774 (erlotinib; Tarceva) appear to be the most promising. Both agents are oral, selective, reversible inhibitors of the EGFR tyrosine kinase that inhibit autophosphorylation of EGFR,[324,325] lead to G_1 cell cycle arrest through increased expression of the p27^{KIP1} cyclin–dependent kinase inhibitor,[324] and promote apoptosis.[317] IMC-C225, ZD1839, and OSI-774 are currently under investigation or have been approved for clinical use. They have been demonstrated to have clinical benefit with minimal toxicity in phase I and II trials involving a variety of solid tumors, including breast cancer; synergism with certain chemotherapeutic agents and with ionizing radiation has been demonstrated as well.

HER2 (ERBB2). By the mid-1990s, research on HER2 had had a greater impact on breast cancer research and treatment than any other molecule except ER. *HER2* was discovered independently by Weinberg and colleagues, who characterized the neu oncoprotein on the cell surface of carcinogen-induced neural tumors in weanling rats, and by Yamamoto and co-workers, who cloned *HER2* on the basis of sequence homology with the *ERBB* oncogene.[326-329] Both the neu oncogene and the *HER2* oncogene were ultimately found to be homologous to *EGFR*, and a carcinogen-induced mutation was identified at an amino acid in the transmembrane domain that caused dimerization and spontaneous activation of the erbB2 cytoplasmic tyrosine kinase.[330-332] It was soon discovered that some cancer cell lines, particularly several breast cancer cell lines, manifested overexpression and gene amplification of *HER2*.[333,334]

Tissue samples from human adenocarcinomas were shown to contain amplified copies of the *HER2* gene as well,[335] and later studies with a larger number of clinical specimens suggested a correlation between *HER2* amplification and poor prognosis for patients with early stage breast cancer.[334,336]

No naturally occurring, activating *HER2* mutation has been identified in the human gene. This is in contrast to mouse models, in which a point mutation erbB2 causes a valine–to–glutamic acid substitution ultimately results in selective overexpression of the activated *neu* locus.[337] However, an alternatively spliced variant of *HER2* mRNA was recently discovered in transgenic mice, and its presence in human cell lines and human breast tumors has been confirmed.[338,339] This variant lacks a portion of the juxtamembrane extracellular domain and is therefore able to constitutively form stable dimers. Although these findings suggest that this HER2 variant has a role in the pathogenesis of breast cancer, the exact nature of this role remains to be defined.

Unlike the other ERBB receptor tyrosine kinases, HER2 has no identifiable ligand. Rather, it forms heterodimers with the other EGFR family members, such that its activity is modulated by transphosphorylation by activated EGFR, ERBB3, or ERBB4.[340-344] Heterodimerization appears to be essential for effective receptor function, as evidenced by observations that fibroblast transformation occurs when ERBB2 and EGFR are coexpressed,[345,346] that mammary epithelial cell transformation occurs when ERBB2 and ERBB3 are coexpressed,[347] and that activation and expression of EGFR alone are inadequate for transformation.[348] The oncogenic effects of HER2 overexpression are likely related to the activation of other signaling pathways that are not yet fully defined. Preclinical data from the HER2-overexpressing BT474 breast cancer cell line reveal increased levels of the cyclin-dependent kinase inhibitor P27^{KIP1} as well as inactivation of the cyclin E–CDK2 complex in response to the specific inhibition of HER2 by monoclonal antibody (Mab) 4D5.[349] Other studies indicate that mammary tumorigenesis via HER2 activation may be linked to the SRC family of tyrosine kinases[350] and the mitogen-activated protein kinase ERK/MAPK pathway.[351]

Subsequent to the initial report that *HER2* was amplified in a fraction of breast cancer cases, more than 40 reports were published. Most of these reports confirmed that *HER2* amplification correlates with the presence of poor prognostic factors, with diminished response to therapy, and with shortened disease-free and overall survival for patients with node-positive breast cancer (see references 352 to 354 for reviews). Studies involving node-negative patients were also performed but required longer periods of follow-up because of the better prognosis associated with node-negative breast cancer; it is now clear, however, that the prognosis for node-negative patients with *HER2*-amplified breast cancer is poorer than that for patients without gene amplification.[355-360] The reports of *HER2* in breast cancer include more than 5000 cases that were characterized either for gene amplification or for overexpression, as detected by Southern blotting, immunohistochemical staining for HER2 protein, Western blotting for protein, and northern blotting for *HER2* mRNA. Overall, results with all the different detection techniques agreed within a few percent. Gene amplification, coupled with the resultant overexpression of EGFR-related HER2 protein, occurs in approximately 25% of cases of human breast cancer,[361] and either finding is associated with a somewhat shorter disease-free survival and poorer prognosis. In addition, the shed extracellular domain of HER2 protein may also represent a useful antigenic blood-borne marker of breast cancer burden.[362]

Among the subtypes of invasive breast cancer, only invasive ductal carcinoma has demonstrated *HER2* amplification. HER2 activation is generally not seen in invasive lobular carcinoma. Moreover, lobular carcinoma in situ (LCIS) has not been shown to involve HER2 overexpression.[363,364] In contrast, the comedo subtype of ductal carcinoma in situ is characterized by a greater than 90% prevalence of HER2 overexpression[363-368] as a result of gene amplification, suggesting that *HER2* gene amplification is an early genetic event in this type of breast cancer.[366] Moreover, because *HER2* amplification was detected in a substantially higher fraction of in situ as opposed to invasive ductal carcinoma, *HER2* amplification may be important for the induction of specific subtypes of in situ disease.

Not only has HER2 expression provided useful information about the natural history of a subset of breast cancer patients, but it also has provided information about the potential of patients to respond to therapy. In one study, the presence of elevated HER2 antigen in serum correlated with a diminished response to hormonal therapy among patients who were ER positive, ER unknown, or ER negative/PR positive.[25] There is also evidence correlating strong HER2 overexpression and/or *HER2* amplification with decreased responsiveness to endocrine therapy[369,370] and CMF chemotherapy[371] but increased responsiveness to anthracycline-based[372] and taxane-based[373] chemotherapy regimens. It is also possible that the interaction of HER2 with EGFR may affect signaling downstream from ER. Consistent with this notion was the finding that the aromatase inhibitor letrozole is superior to tamoxifen for the induction of clinical response in ER-positive women with EGFR or HER2 overexpression. Therefore estrogen depletion rather than receptor inhibition may be the preferable clinical strategy for ER-positive breast cancers that involve pathologic activation of the EGFR pathway.[370]

HER2 overexpression in tumor specimens may also identify a population of patients who will benefit from higher-dose anthracycline chemotherapy. Women with node-positive breast cancer randomized to receive one of three adjuvant chemotherapy regimens containing cyclophosphamide, doxorubicin, and fluorouracil in different doses and intensities had improved disease-free and overall survival with the highest-dose regimen if they were HER2 positive. Patients who were HER2 negative had the same disease-free and overall survival, regardless of the intensity of the doses they received.[372] Although this finding needs to be confirmed, it presents a compelling argument for oncogene analysis to help identify a population of patients with early-stage breast cancer who require more intensive adjuvant chemotherapy.

In addition to its importance as a prognostic marker, the *HER2* oncogene is becoming a therapeutic target in breast cancer. The rationale for anti-*HER2* therapy came from the observation that cultured breast cancer cells that had *HER2* amplification were growth inhibited by antibodies to HER2.[374-376] Moreover, it was shown that HER2 expression was critical for growth of those cell lines with an amplified *HER2* gene because antisense oligonucleotides inhibited growth of cell lines with HER2 amplification but had no effect on cell lines with diploid *HER2* copy number.[377] Therefore therapy directed at HER2 on the surface of breast cancer cells could employ agents that either downregulate the receptor or exploit it as a specific high-concentration target to deliver toxic compounds to the breast cancer cell.[378] Trastuzumab (Herceptin) is a humanized monoclonal antibody that binds tightly to the extracellular domain of the *HER2* receptor to block transmission of the growth signal and thus inhibit the growth of tumor cells overexpressing HER2. Phase I trials showed that the agent was well tolerated.[379] On the basis of preclinical data that trastuzumab could potentiate cytotoxicity induced by chemotherapeutic agents such as cisplatin, both single-agent and combination therapies were tested in subsequent phase II studies.[380-382]

Initial phase II trials revealed an overall response rate of 15% for trastuzumab monotherapy.[383] In a subsequent trial for patients with metastatic breast cancer, subjects were randomized to receive chemotherapy alone (doxorubicin/cyclophosphamide or paclitaxel) or in combination with trastuzumab; there was a statistically significant increase in overall response (50% versus 32%) and overall survival (25.1 versus 20.3 months) in the subgroups that received chemotherapy plus trastuzumab.[384] These results support synergism between the antiproliferative effects of the monoclonal antibody and the cytotoxic effects of the respective chemotherapeutic agents. As a result, trastuzumab monotherapy or combination therapy with paclitaxel is often used in the treatment of patients with HER2-positive metastatic breast cancer.[385] Conversely, the concurrent administration of doxorubicin and trastuzumab is not recommended because of the increased incidence of cardiotoxicity observed with this combination.

Currently, trastuzumab is indicated for use in metastatic breast cancer characterized by strong HER2 overexpression or *HER2* amplification. The most responsive tumors are those with *HER2* gene amplification, as seen by interphase-fluorescence in situ hybridization.[386,387] The administration of trastuzumab is often started upon the diagnosis of metastatic disease, but there are no set guidelines for the initiation or termination of treatment with this agent. In addition to the pivotal study in which paclitaxel or doxorubicin/cyclophosphamide was administered, studies of combination regimens with various cytotoxic agents (e.g., vinorelbine, docetaxel, carboplatin, liposomal doxorubicin), endocrine therapies (e.g., letrozole, anastrozole), and immunomodulators (e.g., interleukin-2, CpG7909) are ongoing. Preclinical data also suggest synergy with the EGFR tyrosine kinase inhibitor ZD1839 (Iressa)[388,389] and have led to a phase I clinical trial of trastuzumab plus ZD1839 in patients with metastatic breast cancer. In addition, the clinical benefits of trastuzumab in the management of metastatic disease are such that investigations into the role of this monoclonal antibody in the adjuvant or neoadjuvant therapy for high-risk or advanced breast cancer have been initiated as well.

Transforming Growth Factor-α. Breast cancer cells also produce ligands that activate the EGFR family of RTKs. Conditioned medium from MCF-7 cells, other breast cancer cell lines, and extracts of breast tumors have been studied to identify the growth-stimulatory activities present. Cell lines secrete stimulatory factors for MCF-7 and murine 3T3 fibroblast monolayer cultures, and these factors have "transforming growth activity," as determined by the stimulation of anchorage-independent colonies of rodent NRK and AKR/2B fibroblasts in soft agar culture.[390-394] Breast cancer cells produce factors with multiple levels of transforming activity in NRK fibroblasts.

Although initially described as a product of oncogene-transformed rodent fibroblasts,[395,396] TGF-α and several of its family members have now been identified in many proliferating normal and malignant human tissues. The prototypic family member EGF was first characterized as expressed from rodent salivary glands[397] and now appears to be more widely expressed

in well-differentiated normal tissues and a few malignant human tissues. Human EGF was originally known as urogastrone, a placental product. TGF-α is now known to exist in 25-, 21-, and 17- to 19-kDa precursor forms[398] that are usually pro-cessed to a 7-kDa form. EGF also appears to be pro-cessed from a very large precursor (130 kDa) formed with multiple polypeptide products.[399] EGF, TGF-α, and a related protein from vaccinia virus all appear to form a functional family of at least a dozen growth factors that use EGFR to carry out their many functions.[400] TGF-α mRNA species have been detected in MCF-7 and other human breast cancer cell lines and breast tumors,[390] ranging from low to high ER content. The ER-negative breast carcinosarcoma cell line Hs578T, in contrast, does not contain detectable levels of TGF-α protein or its mRNA.[390,394] No correlation of TGF-α mRNA expression was observed with ER status; at least 70% of the adenocarcinomas contained TGF-α mRNA.[390]

HER3 and HER4. Unlike EGFR and HER2, which are expressed during ductal morphogenesis, HER3 and HER4 appear to be preferentially expressed during alveolar morphogenesis and lactation.[245] These receptors directly interact with heregulins, resulting in the formation of HER2-HER3 and HER2-HER4 heterodimers and the subsequent tyrosine phosphorylation of HER2.[343] The heregulins, HER3, and HER4 have been implicated in breast cancer pathogenesis and treatment response by a number of investigators.[401-404] The heregulins are represented by several isoforms that are derived from the alternative splicing of four known genes.[405,406] Despite their structural similarity with the EGF-like family of ligands, the heregulins exclusively bind HER3 and HER4. This is in contrast to other EGF-like peptides such as heparin-binding HB-EGF,[407] betacellulin,[408] and EPR,[409] which are EGF-like proteins shown to interact with HER4 and EGFR. Last, the neural and thymus-derived activators for ERBB kinases (NTAK) are derived by alternative splicing and interact with HER3 and HER4 to transactivate EGFR and HER2 through heterodimer formation.[410] These peptides can stimulate the growth of cultured breast cancer cells.

Fibroblast Growth Factor Family. Members of the fibroblast growth factor (FGF) family were initially classified as "competency" factors, acting early in the G_1 phase of the cell cycle to stimulate the growth of mesenchymal cells. More recently, however, they have been appreciated as more widely functional in the normal and malignant growth control of the mammary epithelium. Twenty factors, designated FGF-1 through FGF-20, have been identified thus far, and the most well characterized are acidic FGF (aFGF, FGF-1), basic FGF (bFGF, FGF-2), Int-2 (FGF-3), and Kaposi FGF (kFGF,

FGF-4, HST-1 [human stomach tumor oncogene-1]) (see reference 411 for review). The FGFs function within the extracellular matrix through high-affinity extracellular receptors, and most of the FGFs are secreted via the classic polypeptide secretion pathway. Although FGF-1, FGF-2, and FGF-9 are also present in the extracellular space, they do not possess the classic signal sequence for extracellular transport and therefore must be secreted by alternative mechanisms that remain to be elucidated. FGF-1 and FGF-2 have also been found to have nuclear localization signals, the significance of which is unknown.[412,413]

Structure rather than function is the defining feature of this family, and it is this common primary structure that allows for the strong binding affinity for heparin and the heparan-like glucosaminoglycans, two major components of the extracellular matrix. The interaction between the FGFs and heparin is functionally relevant in two ways. First, it appears to protect the FGFs from degradation by circulating proteases.[414,415] Second, it creates a stable and localized reservoir of growth factors that can be readily mobilized for use in development and neovascularization and efficiently targeted to fibroblasts, epithelial cells, and endothelial cells. FGF activity is mediated by four receptor tyrosine kinases, designated FGFR-1, FGFR-2, FGFR-3, and FGFR-4.[416] Variants of these receptors are necessary to provide for the diversity of function associated with the FGFs, and such diversity is maintained through the alternative splicing of FGFR mRNA[416-418] and the coexpression of different FGFR genes to form transphosphorylating homodimers and heterodimers.[419] FGFR-mediated signal transduction has been shown to involve at least two independent pathways: the PLCγ pathway and the RAS-MEK-MAPK pathway (see reference 411 for review). Although various theories have been proposed, the exact role of heparin and the heparn-like glucosaminoglycans in facilitating the FGF receptor-ligand interaction is unknown. It appears that ligand binding is facilitated and/or stabilized in the presence of heparin cofactors, thus promoting the formation of a complex that contains two FGFs and two FGFRs.[420-423]

FGF has been shown to be a requirement for normal mouse mammary cells in culture. It is present in the pituitary extract used for culturing mouse and human mammary myoepithelial and epithelial cells.[424] FGF is a potent angiogenic substance,[425] and it is likely that FGF family members stimulate a variety of targets in the normal mammary gland, including myoepithelium and stroma.[426] Whereas FGF-1 and FGF-4 are expressed in luminal ductal epithelial cells during the ductal growth phase of the mouse mammary gland, expression of FGF-2 and FGF-7 are primarily stromal. Studies of the human mammary gland have localized FGF-1 and FGF-2 to myoepithelial and epithelial cells. Given

the diversity of FGF targets and the association between the FGFRs and major signal transduction pathways, dysregulation of FGF activity is likely to play an important role in tumorigenesis. In terms of breast cancer, unregulated cell proliferation appears to result from FGFR overexpression, FGF overexpression, or increased recruitment of FGF from the extracellular matrix; no activating mutations have been identified in any of the known ligands, and the activating point mutations that have been identified in the receptors are associated with developmental abnormalities as opposed to neoplasia (see reference 411 for review). FGF-1, FGF-2, and FGF-7 have been detected in preneoplastic mammary epithelium, mammary tumors, and breast cancer cell lines but not at significantly elevated levels. FGF-2 is capable of acting as an oncogene when expressed in fibroblasts.[427,428] In vitro studies have also implicated FGF-2 as an autocrine growth factor in immortalized human mammary epithelial cells.[429] FGF-3, the human homolog of murine Int-2, is a well-known oncogenic growth factor activated in the mouse mammary gland by insertional mutagenesis.[430,431] FGF-4 was initially identified because of its transforming ability,[432,433] and it is notable that this growth factor has been associated with metastasis of the mouse mammary tumors.[434] Finally, overexpression of FGF-1 and FGF-4 has been shown to induce an estrogen-independent phenotype in estrogen-dependent cell lines,[435,436] consistent with hypotheses that activation of cell signal pathways can free ER-positive tumors from estrogen control.

Clinical investigations of the role of FGF signaling in human breast cancer have primarily focused on FGF-1 and FGF-2 as the traditional FGFs and on FGF-8 as the steroid hormone–sensitive growth factor (androgen-induced growth factor [AIGF]). Comparisons of malignant versus benign breast epithelium have yielded conflicting reports: Some note that FGF-1 expression is detected only in malignant tissue,[437] and others note that FGF-1 expression is greatly reduced in malignant tissue.[438] The data on FGF-2 appear to be more consistent, suggesting that FGF-2 expression in breast cancer is associated with an earlier stage of disease, a more differentiated and less invasive phenotype, hormone receptor positivity, and a better prognosis.[439-443] FGF-8, on the other hand, is also expressed at higher levels in malignant versus normal and benign breast epithelium,[444,445] but it appears to be associated with increased tumor growth and invasiveness.[446] FGFR-1 through FGFR-4 have been localized to human breast cancer cells,[437,447,448] and there is evidence of protein overexpression and/or gene amplification. Amplification of the genes encoding FGF-3 and FGF-4 has been observed in human breast cancer, but protein expression has been difficult to detect in human breast cancer tissues and the two genes may be bystanders in coamplification with adjacent cyclin D1.[449,450]

Transforming Growth Factor-β. TGF-β is a 25-kDa polypeptide that was purified from platelets and various normal tissues and then found to be produced autonomously by oncogene-transformed fibroblasts.[451] It was originally described as required (along with other growth factors) for full induction of the transformed phenotype in fibroblasts. *TGF-β* is a member of a multigene family that includes müllerian-inhibiting substance, inhibins, activins,[451] a T-cell–suppressor factor,[452] and a *Drosophila* morphogenesis–controlling gene known as *decapentaplegic*.[453]). In contrast to TGF-α and many other growth factors, TGF-β is growth inhibitory, differentiation promoting, or apoptosis inducing for most epithelial cells.[454-456]

The family of at least three growth factors, termed TGF-β, is present in normal and malignant mammary epithelium and in human milk.[457-459] Receptors for the TGF-β family comprise a related series of heterodimeric serine/threonine kinases.[460] TGF-β family member expression is suppressed by estrogen and progesterone. The three TGF-β isoforms are detected at the mRNA level in the developing mouse mammary epithelium, and TGF-β expression targeted to the pregnant mammary epithelium with an MMTV promoter results in the inhibition of both alveolar development and lactation.[461] These three isoforms have been detected in the human mammary gland, and their distribution is similar to that observed in the mouse. TGF-β production increases with progression of malignancy in breast cancer; its accumulation therefore may have significance in the development of the characteristic fibrous desmoplastic stroma of the disease,[462] tumor angiogenesis, and immune suppression.[463] It therefore appears that while serving a growth inhibitory role in the normal gland, progression to cancer may be associated with desensitization of this pathway. TGF-β overexpression may thus contribute to aberrant tumor-host interactions in breast cancer.[458,462,464,465] At least in some cell lines in vitro, TGF-β may even stimulate tumor cell invasion.[466]

Another member of the TGF-β family, TGF-β$_2$, forms either a homodimeric complex or a heterodimeric complex with TGF-β. It appears to bind to the same 280-kDa TGF-β receptor, but it has a lower affinity for the 65- and 85-kDa receptor species.[467-469] The two are equipotent in inhibiting epithelial cell proliferation and adipogenic differentiation, but only TGF-β has been shown to inhibit hematopoietic progenitor cell proliferation.[470] The high-affinity 280-kDa TGF-β receptors are expressed at higher levels in ER-negative breast cancer cell lines. However, both ER-positive and ER-negative cells have been reported to contain receptors and undergo growth inhibition when exposed to TGF-β or TGF-β$_2$.[471,472] Despite the presence of TGF-β receptors, cell growth inhibition by TGF-β is abrogated by the expression of HRAS or SV40T in immortalized breast epithelial cells.[473]

RAS. There are at least four distinct *RAS* genes in the human genome. They code for proteins whose amino termini and specific internal regions are highly conserved among the group and whose carboxyterminal regions are more variable. The four well-characterized human genes are *HRAS* on chromosome 11,[474,475] *KRAS1* and *KRAS2* on chromosome 12,[474,475] *NRAS* on chromosome 1,[474-476] and *RRAS* on chromosome 19.[477] The *RAS* genes have similar exon structures, which suggests that they arose from a common ancestral precursor. *RAS* genes have been identified in yeast[478-480] and in higher organisms. The primary structure of the yeast *RAS* genes shows remarkable preservation of the aminoterminal protein sequence, compared with that of the *RAS* genes of higher organisms.[481] In mammalian cells, RAS proteins belong to the larger family of 21-kDa G proteins that bind guanine nucleosides. RAS is a critical component in the signal transduction pathway that transmits signals from growth factor receptors at the cell surface. Ligand-mediated signals from growth factor receptors influence the degree of RAS activity by regulating RAS protein association with GTP and RAS cleavage of GTP to GDP, which renders RAS inactive. Active RAS proteins interact with downstream targets such as protein kinase C and RAF, a serine-threonine kinase that initiates the MAP kinase cascade that activates mitosis.[482-484]

Activated *RAS* oncogenes have been detected in a number of human tumors, as determined by transformation of NIH/3T3 cells with human tumor DNA. The transformed cells lose contact inhibition and can form tumors in nude mice. The activation of *RAS* may be achieved by point mutation or by enhanced gene expression.[485] Point mutations in *RAS* genes occur predominantly at amino acids 12, 13, and 61. These mutations disrupt RAS protein interaction with GTPase-activating protein (GAP) and thus render the RAS protein constitutively "on" by virtue of GTP binding without hydrolysis to GDP.

The region downstream from the *HRAS* gene is a minisatellite locus because it contains repetitive DNA sequences of variable length. Four common forms of the *HRAS* minisatellite locus vary in size from 1000 to 2500 base pairs. Mutations of any one of these tandem repeats are associated with an increased risk of several cancers, including breast cancer.[486] Minisatellites are not found in animals below the level of primates. Therefore it is unlikely that they play a critical role in the transcription of the *HRAS* gene, although they could still be involved in DNA-protein interactions in that they do have some influence on the transcription of adjacent genes.[487]

RAS mutations have been detected in a variety of human cancers, but breast cancers have been under-represented on this list. No breast carcinoma has been found to have a point mutation in the *HRAS* protoonco-gene, but the breast carcinosarcoma cell line HS578T contains an Asp[12] mutation of the *HRAS* gene.[488] In terms of *KRAS*, a point mutation at codon 12 has been identified in one human breast carcinoma cell line as well as one case of human breast cancer.[489] A different mutation was identified at codon 13 in another breast cancer cell line.[490] At the genetic level, breast cancer is often characterized by the decreased frequency of normal *HRAS* alleles and increased frequency of rare alleles, suggesting rearrangements. No relationship has been detected between *HRAS* gene rearrangements and ER content.[491] Nevertheless, in vitro studies suggest that *RAS* expression may contribute to increased tumor invasion and metastasis,[492] polypeptide growth factor output,[493,494] and genetic mutability,[495] all potentially leading to increased malignant progression. When the *HRAS* gene was inserted and overexpressed in MCF-7 estrogen-dependent breast cancer cells, their capacity to form tumors in the nude mouse,[496] their capacity for invasion of an artificial basement membrane in vitro,[497] and their secretion of polypeptide growth factors[498,499] all increased. *RAS* expression may act at many stages of the tumorigenic process and cooperate with other oncogenes and hormones.

Although not commonly activated in human breast cancer, the *HRAS* protooncogene is commonly overexpressed in tumors compared with normal or benign lesion controls.[500] This factor may be important for breast cancer pathogenesis or progression, because elevated levels of *RAS* protooncogene expression at the mRNA[501-504] and protein[505-507] levels can transform NIH/3T3 cells in vitro.[485] Expression of RAS-p21 was found on immunohistochemistry to be higher in invasive mammary carcinoma than in hyperplastic lesions.[500] Expression of p21 in mammary cancers was heterogeneous among primary and metastatic lesions, with a trend toward higher expression in postmenopausal patients and no correlation with ER status. In 18 patients with hyperplastic lesions who had been followed for up to 15 years, p21 expression tended to decrease slightly over time. Of the 18 patients with mammary hyperplasia, the 5 who developed carcinoma had significantly higher levels of p21 expression at the time of first biopsy than did the 13 patients who did not develop carcinoma.

Genetic variation in a region of tandem 28-nucleotide repeats located 1000 base pairs downstream from the polyadenylation signal of the *HRAS* gene has been linked to an increased risk of breast cancer.[508] Structural heterogeneity and certain genetic polymorphisms in the 3′ flanking region of the human *HRAS* gene are disproportionately found in breast cancer patients.[491,504]

TRANSCRIPTION REGULATORS

MYC. The *MYC* oncogene was first identified in the avian MC-29 acutely transforming retrovirus.[509] In separate studies of the fowl disease called *avian leukosis*, it was shown that the avian *MYC* was the target of insertional activation by avian leukosis virus that integrated near the *MYC* protooncogene and induced transcriptional activation that contributed to clonal bursal lymphomas.[510] *MYC* mapped to human chromosome 8q22[511] and was found to be involved in translocations with chromosomes 2, 8, and 22 in Burkitt's lymphoma.[512-515] MYC is a nuclear protein that binds to DNA and is regulated during the cell cycle.[516] The MYC oncoprotein is a multipotent cellular regulator of gene expression; it promotes cell growth, facilitates apoptosis in the absence of survival-promoting factors, inhibits differentiation, and modulates cell adhesion and immune recognition.[517-519] Proliferation appears to be modulated at the molecular level by MYC induction of initiation of DNA replication. The MYC oncoprotein can also confer immortality to fibroblasts[520] and can alter responsiveness of fibroblasts to growth factors.[521,522] In addition, MYC deregulation in vitro induces DNA damage; abrogates the DNA damage–induced cell cycle checkpoints at G_1/S, G_2/M, and post M; and promotes chromosomal instability.[523-526]

An unusual aspect of *MYC* oncogene activation was that the protein-coding region of the gene was never altered; rather, the gene was disrupted in DNA sequences that controlled gene expression. Therefore the contribution of *MYC* to malignant transformation could occur just by the deregulated expression of the gene. *MYC* has two closely related homologs that are important in human cancer. *MYCN* was found to be amplified in neuroblastoma,[527] and *MYCL* is frequently amplified in lung cancers.[528] Of the three *MYC* protooncogenes, only *MYC* has been found to be altered in human breast cancer. The association of *MYC* with human breast cancer was first defined by *MYC* gene amplification in SKBr-3 and SW6B-5 breast cancer cell lines.[529,530]

The *MYC* gene product heterodimerizes with the MAX protein (sometimes termed Myn in the mouse) to modulate genes through a different consensus sequence in their promoters. MAX also binds a number of other regulatory proteins, itself, and MAD to block MYC–MAX dimer–induced transcription.[531] The MYC protein may also bind the retinoblastoma tumor-suppressor gene product RB complex and modulate its growth-inhibitory action.[532] With use of antisense oligonucleotides complementary to the *MYC* mRNA, the MYC protein was shown to be necessary for estrogen induction of proliferation of breast cancer.[532] The MYC protein is also of particular importance in human breast cancer because its gene is amplified in approximately 20% to 30% of cases.

The *MYC* gene has three initiation sites, resulting in three major transcripts, corresponding to the MYC1, MYC2, and MYCS proteins.[533-535] MYC1 and MYC2 are full-length proteins, and the latter represents the major protein product, referred to as a MYC in most studies. All three proteins can individually heterodimerize with the MAX transcription factor to form a complex that activates or represses the transcription of specific genes with the appropriate recognition sequence.[533,534] Target genes for the MYC/MAX heterodimers include *CDK4* (cyclin-dependent kinase 4),[536] *CYCLIN D1*,[537] *CYCLIN D2*,[538] *GADD45*,[539] *P21*[WAF1/CIP1],[540] and *hTERT* (human telomerase transcription gene),[541] accounting for the tissue-specific role of MYC in cell growth, proliferation, metabolism, and apoptosis.[542]

Expression of MYC appears to be necessary in the cell cycle; it is induced by growth factor treatment of quiescent fibroblasts just before S-phase entry, and it is reported to be a component of the DNA replication complex.[543] *MYC* is an avian retroviral oncogene and is commonly affected by characteristic chromosomal translocations, as in Burkitt's lymphoma.[544,545] For example, one study has shown that in human breast cancer, *MYC* is commonly rearranged and/or amplified and that its RNA may be overexpressed in primary tumors, compared with hyperplastic and normal breast controls.[546] MYC protein levels are difficult to measure, and no relationship has been observed between MYC changes and ER status. It is not yet known whether MYC expression bears a causal relationship to malignant progression of breast cancer, although as previously mentioned, animal models suggest this possibility.

The most common *MYC* gene abnormalities in human breast cancer are amplification, overexpression, or both. *MYC* gene amplification has been detected in 4% to 41% of samples tested.[1,547-555] Differences in degrees of amplification detected in different studies may reflect technical differences in protocols used by different laboratories. In addition, some investigators defined amplification as a greater-than-twofold increase in gene copy number; others had higher thresholds. Moreover, tissue heterogeneity may have played a role in the wide variation in findings of *MYC* gene amplification.[546] An enhanced *MYC* copy number or overexpression correlates with metastases and poor prognosis,

and as a prognostic marker for breast cancer, it is equivalent to or better than *HER2* amplification.[552,555-557] That MYC is overexpressed in both benign and malignant breast lesions suggests that its role is early in the development of breast cancer.[558,559] Nonetheless, there is great variability in reports of the incidence of *MYC* amplification[560] and overexpression in human breast cancer,[542] ranging from 1% to 94% and 22% to 100%, respectively. Such variability also extends to the clinical significance of gene amplification and protein overexpression; study findings have supported an association with poor outcomes,[552,557,560-565] an association with improved survival,[566,567] and no association with prognosis at all.[568,569]

BRCA1 is now known to repress MYC-mediated transcription by binding directly to the MYC protein.[570] There is also evidence that PTEN (phosphate and tensin homolog deleted on chromosome 10) directly suppresses *MYC* transcription itself.[571] These findings support the putative central role of MYC in tumorigenesis and indicate that tumor-suppressor genes may function by effecting decreased protein activity or downregulated gene transcription.

Despite evidence of a link between MYC and the steroid hormones, the exact nature and relevance of their interaction remains unclear. The three nuclear protooncogenes *FOS, JUN,* and *MYC* are responsive to transcriptional activation by both estrogen and progesterone in breast cancer,[572,573] but the promoter region of *MYC* that is associated with this activation does not contain the classic estrogen-responsive element.[574] Other confounding observations include data that *MYC* amplification and overexpression appear to correlate more with hormone receptor–negative breast cancer and data that they are inhibited with the administration of antiestrogen therapy in hormone receptor–positive disease.[575,576] At least three nuclear protooncogenes, *MYC, FOS,* and *JUN,* are induced by both estrogen and progesterone in breast cancer. In addition, progestins induce a *JUN*-related protooncogene known as *JUNB*.[577] The protein products of the *FOS* and *JUN* genes dimerize to form a complex that interacts with a gene promoter consensus sequence termed AP-1.[578]

Estrogen Receptors (ERα and ERβ). In the late 1950s, work by Jensen[579] focused attention on high-affinity, estrogen-binding components in estrogen target tissues. Initial cell localization studies using radiolabeled estrogen demonstrated long-term retention of estrogen by the rodent uterus. The principal binding component, ER, has now been fully characterized.

On the basis of subcellular fractionation results, investigators in early studies proposed that the unoccupied ER was located in the cellular cytoplasm.

Following ligand binding, the receptor affinity for chromatin increased (a process called *activation* or *transformation*), and a "translocation" to the nucleus was proposed to occur.[580] However, others observed "unoccupied" nuclear receptors in MCF-7 breast cancer cells, a finding inconsistent with the translocation hypothesis.[581] Although work by Edwards and colleagues[582] called into question the existence of unoccupied nuclear receptors in the intact cells, this receptor form is now generally accepted on the basis of two other lines of evidence. Following the characterization of monoclonal anti-ER antibodies, nuclear immunolocalization of the unoccupied ER was reported, further suggesting that the nuclear translocation model was incorrect.[583] Similar results were obtained with a cell enucleation procedure.[584] Both unoccupied and occupied ERs are now believed to reside largely in the nucleus, although probably in different biochemical complexes. Even if ER does not translocate to the nucleus in response to ligand occupancy, it must traverse the nuclear membrane at some point in its existence, because it is synthesized on cytoplasmic ribosomes. Indeed, its primary sequence, like that of the glucocorticoid receptor, for example, encodes two short series of amino acid residues that serve as nuclear transfer domains.

When not bound by ligand, ERα is sequestered in the cytoplasm bound to chaperones such as HSP90.[585,586] Upon binding to ligand, the receptor translocates to the nucleus, binds to DNA, and initiates transcription.[587] Recent data suggest that a cytoplasmic or perhaps cell surface–associated ER can play a physiologic role. It has been shown that cytoplasmic ERα can interact not only with estradiol but also with androgens to affect cellular events such as growth and apoptosis.[588] There is growing evidence of a membrane-bound ER that is capable of signal transduction, but there is debate about whether it originates from the same transcript as the intracellular nuclear forms[589] or is completely distinct from them.[590] Support for the latter, however, comes from the recent finding that estrogen can act through the G protein–coupled receptor GPR30 to trigger opposing G protein–dependent signaling cascades and thus regulate the activity of the extracellular signal-regulated kinases ERK-1 and ERK-2.[31]

ER is a member of the steroid hormone receptor family of proteins that have a common domain structure, including a regulatory N-terminal domain, a central DNA-binding region that determines the specificity of binding to DNA response elements,[591] and a C-terminal ligand-binding domain. Following expression in transfected cells or after in vitro translation, the protein product of the ER gene is able to bind estrogen with high affinity.[592,593] The activity of ER and other steroid hormone receptors can be regulated by phosphorylation, which is mediated by a number of growth-regulatory cellular kinases (see reference 493 for review).

A possible role of phosphorylation in the action of ER initially focused on phosphotyrosine and later on phosphoserine residues. Auricchio and colleagues initially purified tyrosine kinase and phosphatase activities from calf and rodent uteri and demonstrated that the purified ER is a substrate; the state of tyrosine phosphorylation was associated with the ability of the receptor to bind E_2 in in vitro assays.[594-596] These investigators initially proposed that a phosphorylation-dephosphorylation cycle might exist in intact cells to regulate receptor binding and nuclear localization. Another early study reported that cAMP decreased and cyclic guanine monophosphate (cGMP) increased estrogen binding in cytosol fractions of endometrial cancer cells.[597] However, this study did not directly evaluate receptor phosphorylation. Later work by other investigators, using intact MCF-7 cells and ER immunoprecipitation following metabolic labeling with radioactive phosphate, failed to show either high levels of phosphotyrosine or changes in receptor binding following treatment of cells with activators of adenylate cyclase. However, phorbol ester treatment of MCF-7 cells resulted in reduction of ER binding activity and cell proliferation and was associated with a loss of estrogen inducibility of proliferation and PR.[598,599] Phosphorylation of ER appeared to occur much more rapidly than did receptor loss.[587] Very recent studies have identified a kinase in growth factor pathways of signal transduction (the MAP kinase, described later) as the kinase responsible for this. Thus the current consensus appears to be that tyrosine and serine/threonine phosphorylation are important regulators of ER function and that ERα engages in substantial cross-talk with MAPK signaling pathways (see reference 493 for review).

Studies of ER expression in breast cancer specimens have been greatly facilitated by the availability of monoclonal antibodies to the receptor.[600] These antibodies, some available in commercial detection kits, allow radioimmunoassay in cytosolic or nuclear extracts of tissue and also allow detection of receptor-positive cells in tissue sections. One important caveat of these assay systems would appear to be their selectivity for estrogen-occupied receptor over ligand-unoccupied receptor.[601] Nevertheless, numerous studies have demonstrated the comparability of ligand binding assays and antibody-detection assays for ER.[602,603] Use of the immunohistochemical assay has supported the conclusion that normal breast epithelium is low (but with intermittent positive cells) in ER content. Another important advance in receptor analysis has been the development of two radioactive affinity labels for the ER: the antiestrogen tamoxifen aziridine and the estrogen ketononestrol aziridine.[604,605] Both of these compounds attach to and label the same 66-kDa ER in receptor-containing tissue extracts. Furthermore, tamoxifen aziridine and one monoclonal antibody (H222/Spγ) recognized the same 6-kDa tryptic fragment and 28-kDa V8 protease fragment of the receptor.[606]

ER binds to promoter regions in DNA by recognizing short, palindromic elements termed *estrogen-responsive elements* (EREs). Like other steroid hormone receptors, ER undergoes a conformational change when ligand is bound that allows the receptor to dimerize.[607-610] Ligand binding also affects conformation of the C-terminal helix 12 to open a groove for binding of proteins collectively called p160 coactivators that are critical for amplifying the transcriptional signals of steroid hormone receptors by recruiting CREB-binding protein/p300[611] and RNA polymerase II[612] to a transcriptional complex, as illustrated in Figure 25-3. Recent studies have identified alternatively spliced and mutated forms of ER in breast cancer and some normal tissues such as the brain and the uterus.[587,613]

ERβ was identified in 1996 as the second intracellular ER to mediate the biologic effects of estradiol.[614] It is encoded by a unique gene[615] and has a different spectrum of expression compared with ERα (i.e., the original ER). ERα predominates in the breast, uterus, cervix, and vagina, whereas ERβ predominates in the ovary, prostate, testis, hypothalamus, lung, and thymus; both receptors are expressed to varying degrees in different regions of the brain.[616] Both molecules are members of the steroid hormone superfamily of nuclear receptors, and they exhibit a high degree of homology in their DNA-binding and ligand-binding domains[617]; ERα and ERβ heterodimers therefore have been reported as well.[618]

The role of ERβ in the human breast remains unclear, and the discovery of splice variants that code for additional receptor proteins ERβcx and ERβ2 has only increased the complexity of ER signaling. These two isoforms form heterodimers, and both appear to modulate the activity of ERα.[619,620] ERβcx, for example, is a dominant negative repressor of ERα that itself has no apparent affinity for estradiol.[620] This finding supports the concept that ERβ modulates the activity of ERα and suggests that estrogen responsiveness may be determined by the ratio of isoforms present in a specific target tissue.[621] A determination of ERα and ERβ expression patterns will therefore prove important in increasing our understanding of ER signaling. Expression of ER isoforms in breast cancer is also complex. ERα was prominent in invasive ductal cancers but barely detected in normal tissue or benign breast disease. Conversely, ERβ was present in all three tissue types. Notably, grade 1 invasive ductal carcinomas were characterized by high levels of ERα but absent ERβ. Such variation in expression of ER isoforms may have clinical implications in the future treatment of breast cancer. The agonist versus antagonist activity of the various selective ER modulators, for example, could be determined by the ER isoforms to which they bind.[622]

ERα transcriptional activity is mediated by interactions with a number of molecules that amplify or repress the transcriptional signals initiated by ligand-binding and receptor dimerization. The receptor proteins interact with other proteins via two activation function (AF) domains: the constitutive AF-1 domain within the N terminus and the hormone-dependent AF-2 domain within the ligand-binding domain.[623] AF-2 is the site where members of the p160 coactivator family of molecules bind to ER via LXXLL peptide motifs in the coactivators. The gene on chromosome 20q for one of these coactivators, steroid receptor coactivator (SRC)–3, was found to be amplified in some breast cancer tissues. For this reason a second name for *SRC-3* is *AIB1*, for "amplified in breast cancer 1." *AIB1* gene amplification has been demonstrated in 5% to 10% of breast cancers,[624,625] increased *AIB1* mRNA in up to 60% of breast cancers,[624] and increased AIB1 intracellular protein in approximately 10% of tumors.[626] *AIB1* mRNA undergoes alternate splicing to generate an isoform that has greater transcription promoting activity than the wild-type protein.[627] In addition, AIB1 overexpression has been linked with the estrogen-dependent transcription of cyclin D1.[628]

Enhanced coactivation by an AIB1 isoform should sensitize ER to agonists and decrease the antagonist effects of ER modulators. In a retrospective analysis, the 5-year disease-free survival rates in a cohort of breast cancer patients who received no adjuvant therapy was highest for those patients whose tumors had elevated expression of AIB1.[629] In a group of women treated with tamoxifen, high AIB1 levels correlated with a worse 5-year disease survival, particularly in the

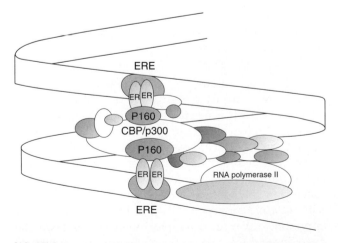

FIG. **25-3** Structural relationship of the transcriptional complex formed upon activation and dimerization of the estrogen receptor.

setting of concurrent HER2 overexpression.[629] Therefore AIB1 may be associated with a good prognosis in the absence of systemic therapy but predictive of a poorer prognosis for those receiving adjuvant tamoxifen.

Progesterone Receptor. The PR is induced by estrogen[630] and plays a major role in the breast and other tissues. Estrogen promotes cell proliferation, and progesterone influences cell differentiation in both normal and neoplastic breast epithelium. Progestins are partially growth-inhibitory for human breast cancer while inducing a specific protein of 48 kDa.[631] The presence of PR is generally coupled to functional growth regulation by estrogens in vivo and in vitro. Thus the PR content of breast tumors is used in addition to ER as a marker for estrogen and antiestrogen responsiveness in clinical therapy. Widespread exceptions to the coexpression of these two receptors do exist, however, both in vitro with T47D and MD-MB-134[630,632] and in vivo in some human tumors.[633] Estrogen appears to induce PR at the mRNA level.[634,635]

In contrast to ER, a single gene encodes three different isoforms of the PR subunit in mammary tissue, resulting in both homodimeric and heterodimeric forms of this receptor.[636-638] The multiple ER and PR isoforms in breast cancer may allow for significant variations in patterns of dimerization and in resultant variations in specificity of ligand recognition with respect to agonist versus antagonist and differential regulation of target genes.[639,640] Superimposed on this complexity, each receptor is able to adopt multiple conformations, depending on the characteristics of interaction of the steroid (or nonsteroid ligand) with the receptor-binding pocket. ER, for example, can adopt at least three distinct conformations, depending on the antiestrogen bound.[641]

Conclusions

Although it has been suggested that a very large number of genetic and phenotypic alterations occur in breast cancer, only a handful have been fully identified and brought to clinical study. It is encouraging that studies of each of these genes and phenotypic changes continue to provide their own unique perspectives on the biology of the disease. However, we must take advantage of this knowledge to improve the clinical outlook for patients with breast cancer. Improved methodologies for the determination of prognosis and response to therapy may be a realistic hope for the future.[642] Development of more accurate and rapid methods for the characterization of oncogenes, suppressor genes, and related proteins is under way. Determination of markers in serum or plasma is

also of interest. For example, current studies are examining HER2, in addition to the more classic tumor markers CA15.3, carcinoembryonic antigen (CEA), and erythrocyte sedimentation rate (ESR), for determining prognosis and response to therapy. Historically, detection of ER and PR in tumors has led the way for integration of molecular markers into clinical decisions regarding prognosis and response to therapy.[643] Detection of the HER2 oncoprotein has also proved its value for characterization of tumors associated with a poor prognosis, as well as those that are likely to respond poorly to adjuvant hormonal and chemotherapy. Although it is technically more difficult to measure, the EGF receptor is also of interest for future study of tumors likely to be associated with a poor prognosis and poor response to hormonal therapy. Because expression or overexpression of these two receptors commonly occurs in breast cancer, they are targets of new experimental therapies that include the use of antibodies to their extracellular domains, some of which are coupled or gene fused to toxic moieties.

REFERENCES

1. Cline MJ, Battifora H, Yokota J: Proto-oncogene abnormalities in human breast cancer: correlations with anatomic features and clinical course of disease, *J Clin Oncol* 5:999, 1987.
2. Teixeira C, Reed JC, Pratt MA: Estrogen promotes chemotherapeutic drug resistance by a mechanism involving *Bcl-2* proto-oncogene expression in human breast cancer cells, *Cancer Res* 55:3902, 1995.
3. Wang TT, Phang JM: Effects of estrogen on apoptotic pathways in human breast cancer cell line MCF-7, *Cancer Res* 55:2487, 1995.
4. Nicolson GL: Tumor cell instability, diversification, and progression to the metastatic phenotype: from oncogene to oncofetal expression, *Cancer Res* 47:1473, 1987.
5. Nunez AM et al: Characterization of the estrogen-induced pS2 protein secreted by the human breast cancer cell line MCF-7, *Endocrinology* 121:1759, 1987.
6. Desai KV et al: Initiating oncogenic event determines gene-expression patterns of human breast cancer models, *Proc Natl Acad Sci USA* 99:6967, 2002.
7. Jiang Y et al: Discovery of differentially expressed genes in human breast cancer using subtracted cDNA libraries and cDNA microarrays, *Oncogene* 21:2270, 2002.
8. Zajchowski DA et al: Identification of gene expression profiles that predict the aggressive behavior of breast cancer cells, *Cancer Res* 61:5168, 2001.
9. Lizard-Nacol S et al: Benign breast disease: absence of genetic alterations at several loci implicated in breast cancer malignancy, *Cancer Res* 55:4416, 1995.
10. Parham DM, Jankowski J: Transforming growth factor alpha in epithelial proliferative diseases of the breast, *J Clin Pathol* 45:513, 1992.
11. Ried T et al: Comparative genomic hybridization of formalin-fixed, paraffin-embedded breast tumors reveals different patterns of chromosomal gains and losses in fibroadenomas and diploid and aneuploid carcinomas, *Cancer Res* 55:5415, 1995.

12. Mellick AS et al: Differential gene expression in breast cancer cell lines and stroma-tumor differences in microdissected breast cancer biopsies revealed by display array analysis, *Int J Cancer* 100:172, 2002.

13. Kinzler KW, Vogelstein B: Lessons from hereditary colorectal cancer, *Cell* 87:159, 1996.

14. de Bock GH et al: Clinical and pathological features of *BRCA1* associated carcinomas in a hospital-based sample of Dutch breast cancer patients, *Br J Cancer* 85:1347, 2001.

15. Carter RF: *BRCA1, BRCA2* and breast cancer: a concise clinical review, *Clin Invest Med* 24:147, 2001.

16. Garcia-Patino E et al: Germ-line *BRCA1* mutations in women with sporadic breast cancer: clinical correlations, *J Clin Oncol* 16:115, 1998.

17. Callahan R et al: Genetic and molecular heterogeneity of breast cancer cells, *Clin Chim Acta* 217:63, 1993.

18. Vonderhaar BK: Local effects of EGF, alpha-TGF, and EGF-like growth factors on lobuloalveolar development of the mouse mammary gland in vivo, *J Cell Physiol* 132:581, 1987.

19. Vonderhaar BK: Regulation of development of the normal mammary gland by hormones and growth factors, *Cancer Treat Res* 40:251, 1988.

20. Balinsky BI: On the pre-natal growth of the mammary gland rudiment in the mouse, *J Anatomy* 84:227, 1950.

21. Raynaud A: Recherches experimentales sur le developpement de l'appareil genital et fonctionnement des glandes endocrines des foetus de souris et de mulot, *Arch Anat Microse Morphol Exp* 39:518, 1950.

22. Drews U, Drews U: Regression of mouse mammary gland anlagen in recombinants of Tfm and wild-type tissues: testosterone acts via the mesenchyme, *Cell* 10:401, 1997.

23. Narbaitz R, Stumpf WE, Sar M: Estrogen receptors in mammary gland primordia of fetal mouse, *Anat Embryol (Berl)* 158:161, 1980.

24. Raynaud A: Morphogenesis of the mammary gland. In Kon SA, Cowie AT (eds): *Milk, the mammary gland and its secretion,* New York: 1961, Academic Press.

25. Chamberlin TL, Gardener WU, Allen E: Local responses of the sexual skin and mammary glands of monkeys to cutaneous application of estrogen, *Endocrinology* 28:753, 1941.

26. Lyons WR, Suko Y: Direct action of estrone on the mammary gland, *Recent Progr Horm Res* 14:398, 1940.

27. Nelson W: Growth of the mammary gland following local application of estrogenic hormone, *Am J Physiol* 133:398, 1941.

28. Daniel CW, Silberstein GB, Strickland P: Direct action of 17 beta-estradiol on mouse mammary ducts analyzed by sustained release implants and steroid autoradiography, *Cancer Res* 47:6052, 1987.

29. Petersen OW, Hoyer PE, Van Deurs B: Frequency and distribution of estrogen receptor-positive cells in normal, nonlactating human breast tissue, *Cancer Res* 47:5748, 1987.

30. Kratochwil K: Epithelium-mesenchyme interactions in the fetal mammary gland. In Medina D et al (eds): *Cellular and molecular biology of mammary cancer,* New York, 1987, Plenum.

31. Bresciani F: Topography of DNA synthesis in mammary gland of the C3H mouse and its control by ovarian hormones: an autoradiographic study, *Cell Tissue Kinet* 1:51, 1968.

32. Lieberman ME, Maurer RA, Gorski J: Estrogen control of prolactin synthesis in vitro, *Proc Natl Acad Sci USA* 75:5946, 1978.

33. Sirbasku DA: New concepts in control of estrogen-responsive tumor cell growth, *Banbury Rep* 8:425, 1981.

34. Nandi S: Endocrine control of mammary gland development in the C3H/He Crg1 mouse, *J Natl Cancer Inst* 21:1039, 1958.

35. Stampfer MR, Bartley J: Growth and transformation of human mammary epithelial cells in culture. In Medina D et al (eds): *Cellular and molecular biology of mammary cancer,* New York, 1987, Plenum Press.

36. Yang J et al: Primary culture of mouse mammary tumor epithelial cells embedded in collagen gels, *In Vitro* 16:502, 1980.

37. Haslam SZ et al: Estrogen responsiveness of normal mouse mammary cells in primary cell culture: association of mammary fibroblasts with estrogenic regulation of progesterone receptors, *Endocrinology* 116:1835, 1985.

38. McGrath CM: Augmentation of the response of normal mammary epithelial cells to estradiol by mammary stroma, *Cancer Res* 43:1355, 1983.

39. Russo J et al: Pattern of distribution of cells positive for estrogen receptor alpha and progesterone receptor in relation to proliferating cells in the mammary gland, *Breast Cancer Res Treat* 53:217, 1999.

40. Topper YJ, Freeman CS: Multiple hormone interactions in the developmental biology of the mammary gland, *Physiol Rev* 60:1049, 1980.

41. Daniel CW, Silberstein GP: Postnatal development of the rodent mammary gland. In Daniel CW, Neville MC (eds): *The mammary gland: development, regulation, and function,* New York, 1987, Plenum Press.

42. Richards J et al: Growth of mouse mammary gland end buds cultured in a collagen gel matrix, *Exp Cell Res* 141:433, 1982.

43. Stampfer MR: Isolation and growth of human mammary epithelial cells, *J Tissue Cult Methods* 9:107, 1985.

44. Hackett AJ et al: Two syngeneic cell lines from human breast tissue: the aneuploid mammary epithelial (Hs578T) and the diploid myoepithelial (Hs578Bst, Cell lines), *J Natl Cancer Inst* 58:1795, 1977.

45. Briand P, Petersen OW, Van Deurs B: A new diploid nontumorigenic human breast epithelial cell line isolated and propagated in chemically defined medium, *In Vitro Cell Dev Biol* 23:181, 1987.

46. Caron DF et al: Epithelial HBL-100 cell line derived from milk of an apparently healthy woman harbours SV40 genetic information, *Exp Cell Res* 160:83, 1985.

47. Chang SE et al: Establishment and characterization of SV40-transformed human breast epithelial cell lines, *Cancer Res* 42:2040, 1982.

48. Chang SE: In vitro transformation of human epithelial cells, *Biochim Biophys Acta* 823:161, 1986.

49. Stampfer MR, Bartley JC: Induction of transformation and continuous cell lines from normal human mammary epithelial cells after exposure to benzo[a]pyrene, *Proc Natl Acad Sci USA* 82:2394, 1985.

50. Rudland PS: Stem cells in mammary development and cancer. In Medina D et al (eds): *Cellular and molecular biology of mammary cancer,* New York, 1987, Plenum Press.

51. Levay-Young BK et al: Primary culture systems for mammary biology studies. In Medina D et al (eds): *Cellular and molecular biology of mammary cancer,* New York, 1987, Plenum Press.

52. Devleeschouwer N et al: Estrogen conjugates and serum factors mediating the estrogenic trophic effect on MCF-7 cell growth, *Cancer Res* 47:5883, 1987.

53. Lykkesfeldt AE, Briand P: Indirect mechanism of oestradiol stimulation of cell proliferation of human breast cancer cell lines, *Br J Cancer* 53:29, 1986.

54. Soto AM, Sonnenschein C: Cell proliferation of estrogen-sensitive cells: the case for negative control, *Endocr Rev* 8:44, 1987.

55. Dubik D, Dembinski TC, Shiu RP: Stimulation of *c-myc* oncogene expression associated with estrogen-induced proliferation of human breast cancer cells, *Cancer Res* 47:6517, 1987.

56. Gompel A et al: Hormonal regulation of apoptosis in breast cells and tissues, *Steroids* 65:593, 2000.

57. Burke RE, Harris SC, McGuire WL: Lactate dehydrogenase in estrogen-responsive human breast cancer cells, *Cancer Res* 38:2773, 1987.

58. Aitken SC, Lippman ME: Hormonal regulation of de novo pyrimidine synthesis and utilization in human breast cancer cells in tissue culture, *Cancer Res* 43:4681, 1983.

59. Aitken SC, Lippman ME: Effect of estrogens and antiestrogens on growth-regulatory enzymes in human breast cancer cells in tissue culture, *Cancer Res* 45:1611, 1985.

60. Dickson RB, Aitken S, Lippman ME: Assay of mitogen-induced effects on cellular incorporation of precursors for scavenger, de novo, and net DNA synthesis, *Methods Enzymol* 146:329, 1987.

61. Edwards DP, Murthy SR, McGuire WL: Effects of estrogen and antiestrogen on DNA polymerase in human breast cancer, *Cancer Res* 40:1722, 1980.

62. Cowan KH et al: Dihydrofolate reductase gene amplification and possible rearrangement in estrogen-responsive methotrexate-resistant human breast cancer cells, *J Biol Chem* 257:15079, 1982.

63. Keating MT, Williams LT: Autocrine stimulation of intracellular PDGF receptors in v-sis-transformed cells, *Science* 239:914, 1988.

64. Kasid A et al: Transcriptional control of thymidine kinase gene expression by estrogen and antiestrogens in MCF-7 human breast cancer cells, *J Biol Chem* 261:5562, 1986.

65. Chodosh LA et al: Protein kinase expression during murine mammary development, *Dev Biol* 219:259, 2000.

66. Gardner HP et al: Developmental role of the SNF1-related kinase Hunk in pregnancy-induced changes in the mammary gland, *Development* 127:4493, 2000.

67. Russo J, Tay LK, Russo IH: Differentiation of the mammary gland and susceptibility to carcinogenesis, *Breast Cancer Res Treat* 2:5, 1982.

68. Russo IH, Koszalka M, Russo J: Comparative study of the influence of pregnancy and hormonal treatment on mammary carcinogenesis, *Br J Cancer* 64:481, 1991.

69. Soule HD, McGrath CM: Estrogen responsive proliferation of clonal human breast carcinoma cells in athymic mice, *Cancer Lett* 10:177, 1980.

70. Dempsey PJ et al: Development of monoclonal antibodies to the human breast carcinoma cell line PMC42, *J Natl Cancer Inst* 7:1, 1986.

71. Whitehead RH et al: A new human breast carcinoma cell line (PMC42) with stem cell characteristics. III. Hormone receptor status and responsiveness, *J Natl Cancer Inst* 73:643, 1984.

72. Baker SJ et al: Chromosome 17 deletions and *p53* gene mutations in colorectal carcinomas, *Science* 244:217, 1989.

73. Teixeira MR, Pandis N, Heim S: Cytogenetic clues to breast carcinogenesis, *Genes Chromosomes Cancer* 33:1, 2002.

74. Monni O et al: From chromosomal alterations to target genes for therapy: integrating cytogenetic and functional genomic views of the breast cancer genome, *Semin Cancer Biol* 11:395, 2001.

75. Trent JM: Cytogenetic and molecular biologic alterations in human breast cancer: a review, *Breast Cancer Res Treat* 5:221, 1985.

76. Fisher ER et al: The pathology of invasive breast cancer: a syllabus derived from findings of the National Surgical Adjuvant Breast Project (protocol no. 4), *Cancer* 36:1, 1975.

77. Cropp CS et al: Loss of heterozygosity on chromosomes 17 and 18 in breast carcinoma: two additional regions identified, *Proc Natl Acad Sci USA* 87:7737, 1990.

78. Brenner AJ, Aldaz CM: Chromosome 9p allelic loss and *p16/CDKN2* in breast cancer and evidence of *p16* inactivation in immortal breast epithelial cells, *Cancer Res* 55:2892, 1995.

79. Tachdjian G et al: Cytogenetic analysis from DNA by comparative genomic hybridization, *Ann Genet* 43:147, 2000.

80. Rooney PH et al: Comparative genomic hybridization and chromosomal instability in solid tumours, *Br J Cancer* 80:862, 1999.

81. Kallioniemi OP et al: Comparative genomic hybridization: a rapid new method for detecting and mapping DNA amplification in tumors, *Semin Cancer Biol* 4:41, 1993.

82. Sinn E et al: Coexpression of MMTV/v-Ha-ras and MMTV/c-myc genes in transgenic mice: synergistic action of oncogenes in vivo, *Cell* 49:465, 1987.

83. Bouchard L et al: Stochastic appearance of mammary tumors in transgenic mice carrying the *MMTV/c-neu* oncogene, *Cell* 57:931, 1989.

84. Pittius CW et al: A milk protein gene promoter directs the expression of human tissue plasminogen activator cDNA to the mammary gland in transgenic mice, *Proc Natl Acad Sci USA* 85:5874, 1998.

85. Schoenenberger CA et al: Targeted *c-myc* gene expression in mammary glands of transgenic mice induces mammary tumours with constitutive milk protein gene transcription, *EMBO J* 7:169, 1988.

86. Stewart TA, Pattengale PK, Leder P: Spontaneous mammary adenocarcinomas in transgenic mice that carry and express MTV/myc fusion genes, *Cell* 38:627, 1984.

87. Andres AC et al: *Ha-ras* oncogene expression directed by a milk protein gene promoter: tissue specificity, hormonal regulation, and tumor induction in transgenic mice, *Proc Natl Acad Sci USA* 84:1299, 1987.

88. Nusse R et al: Mode of proviral activation of a putative mammary oncogene *(int-1)* on mouse chromosome 15, *Nature* 307:131, 1984.

89. Dickson C et al: Tumorigenesis by mouse mammary tumor virus: proviral activation of a cellular gene in the common integration region int-2, *Cell* 37:529, 1984.

90. Donehower LA et al: Deficiency of p53 accelerates mammary tumorigenesis in Wnt-1 transgenic mice and promotes chromosomal instability, *Genes Dev* 9:882, 1995.

91. Tsukamoto AS et al: Expression of the *int-1* gene in transgenic mice is associated with mammary gland hyperplasia and adenocarcinomas in male and female mice, *Cell* 55:619, 1988.

92. Deng CX: Tumor formation in Brca1 conditional mutant mice, *Environ Mol Mutagen* 39:171, 2002.

93. Deng CX: Tumorigenesis as a consequence of genetic instability in Brca1 mutant mice, *Mutat Res* 477:183, 2001.

94. Ludwig T et al: Tumorigenesis in mice carrying a truncating Brca1 mutation, *Genes Dev* 15:1188, 2001.

95. Xu X et al: Genetic interactions between tumor suppressors *Brca1* and *p53* in apoptosis, cell cycle and tumorigenesis, *Nat Genet* 28:266, 2001.

96. Yu Q, Geng Y, Sicinski P: Specific protection against breast cancers by cyclin D1 ablation, *Nature* 411:1017, 2001.

97. Bates S et al: Cdk6 (Plstire) and Cdk4 (Psk-J3) are a distinct subset of the cyclin-dependent kinases that associate with cyclin D1, *Oncogene* 9:71, 1994.

98. Peters G: The D-type cyclins and their role in tumorigenesis, *J Cell Science* 18:89, 1994.

99. Dulic V, Lees E, Reed SI: Association of human cyclin-e with a periodic G(1)-S phase protein-kinase, *Science* 257:1958, 1992.

100. Koff A et al: Human cyclin-E, a new cyclin that interacts with 2 members of the *Cdc2* gene family, *Cell* 66:1217, 1991.

101. Koff A et al: Formation and activation of a cyclin E-Cdk2 complex during the G(1)-phase of the human cell-cycle, *Science* 257:1689, 1992.

102. Fotedar A et al: Role for cyclin A-dependent kinase in DNA replication in human S phase cell extracts, *J Biol Chem* 271:31627, 1996.

103. Pines J: The cell cycle kinases, *Semin Cancer Biol* 5:305, 1994.

104. Filmus J et al: Induction of cyclin D1 overexpression by activated Ras, *Oncogene* 9:3627, 1994.

105. Liu JJ et al: Ras transformation results in an elevated level of cyclin D1 and acceleration of G(1) progression in Nih 3T3 cells, *Mol Cell Biol* 15:3654, 1995.

106. Darbon JM, Fesquet D, Cavadore JC: New cell-cycle regulators: the Cdk-cyclins modulatory proteins, *Med Sci* 11:349, 1995.

107. Lee RJ et al: Cyclin D1 is required for transformation by activated Neu and is induced through an E2F-dependent signaling pathway, *Mol Cell Biol* 20:672, 2000.

108. Yu Q, Geng Y, Sicinski P: Specific protection against breast cancers by cyclin D1 ablation, *Nature* 411:1017, 2001.

109. Sicinski P et al: Cyclin D1 provides a link between development and oncogenesis in the retina and breast, *Cell* 82:621, 1995.

110. Bartkova J et al: Cyclin D1 protein expression and function in human breast-cancer, *Int J Cancer* 57:353-361, 1994.

111. Buckley MF et al: Expression and amplification of cyclin genes in human breast-cancer, *Oncogene* 8:2127, 1993.

112. Dickson C et al: Amplification of chromosome band 11Q13 and a role for cyclin D1 in human breast-cancer, *Cancer Lett* 90:43, 1995.

113. Gillett CE et al: Cyclin D1 and associated proteins in mammary ductal carcinoma in situ and atypical ductal hyperplasia, *J Pathol* 184:396, 1998.

114. Michalides R et al: A clinicopathological study on overexpression of cyclin D1 and of p53 in a series of 248 patients with operable breast cancer, *Br J Cancer* 73:728, 1996.

115. Oyama T et al: Frequent overexpression of the cyclin D1 oncogene in invasive lobular carcinoma of the breast, *Cancer Res* 58:2876, 1998.

116. Gillett C et al: Amplification and overexpression of cyclin D1 in breast cancer detected by immunohistochemical staining, *Cancer Res* 54:1812, 1994.

117. Zukerberg LR et al: Cyclin D1 (PRAD1) protein expression in breast cancer: approximately one-third of infiltrating mammary carcinomas show overexpression of the cyclin D1 oncogene, *Mod Pathol* 8:560, 1995.

118. Seshadri R et al: Cyclin DI amplification is not associated with reduced overall survival in primary breast cancer but may predict early relapse in patients with features of good prognosis, *Clin Cancer Res* 2:1177, 1996.

119. van Diest PJ et al: Cyclin D1 expression in invasive breast cancer: correlations and prognostic value, *Am J Pathol* 150:705, 1997.

120. Neuman E et al: Cyclin D1 stimulation of estrogen receptor transcriptional activity independent of cdk4, *Mol Cell Biol* 17:5338, 1997.

121. Zwijsen RM et al: CDK-independent activation of estrogen receptor by cyclin D1, *Cell* 88:405, 1997.

122. Jares P et al: Cyclin D1 and retinoblastoma gene expression in human breast carcinoma: correlation with tumour proliferation and oestrogen receptor status, *J Pathol* 182:160, 1997.

123. Gillett C et al: Cyclin D1 and prognosis in human breast cancer, *Int J Cancer* 69:92, 1996.

124. Nielsen NH et al: Deregulation of cyclin E and D1 in breast cancer is associated with inactivation of the retinoblastoma protein, *Oncogene* 4:295, 1997.

125. Kenny FS et al: Overexpression of cyclin D1 messenger RNA predicts for poor prognosis in estrogen receptor-positive breast cancer, *Clin Cancer Res* 5:2069, 1999.

126. Cairns P et al: Frequency of homozygous deletion at p16/CDKN2 in primary human tumours, *Nat Genet* 11:210, 1995.

127. Quesnel B et al: Analysis of p16 gene deletion and point mutation in breast carcinoma, *Br J Cancer* 72:351, 1995.

128. Berns EM et al: Infrequent *CDKN2 (MTS1/p16)* gene alterations in human primary breast cancer, *Br J Cancer* 72:964, 1997.

129. Xu L et al: Mutational analysis of *CDKN2 (MTS1/p16ink4)* in human breast carcinomas, *Cancer Res* 54:5262, 1994.

130. Nielsen NH et al: Methylation of the *p16(Ink4a)* tumor suppressor gene 5'-CpG island in breast cancer, *Cancer Lett* 163:59, 2001.

131. Woodcock DM et al: DNA methylation in the promoter region of the *p16 (CDKN2/MTS-1/INK4A)* gene in human breast tumours, *Br J Cancer* 79:251, 2001.

132. Brenner AJ et al: Preferential loss of expression of *p16(INK4a)* rather than *p19(ARF)* in breast cancer, *Clin Cancer Res* 2:1993, 1996.

133. Emig R et al: Aberrant cytoplasmic expression of the p16 protein in breast cancer is associated with accelerated tumour proliferation, *Br J Cancer* 78:1661, 1998.

134. Kaelin WG Jr: Functions of the retinoblastoma protein, *Bioessays* 21:950, 1998.

135. Morris EJ, Dyson NJ: Retinoblastoma protein partners, *Adv Cancer Res* 82:1, 2001.

136. Sellers WR, Kaelin WG Jr: Role of the retinoblastoma protein in the pathogenesis of human cancer, *J Clin Oncol* 15:3301, 1997.

137. Lundberg C et al: Loss of heterozygosity in human ductal breast tumors indicates a recessive mutation on chromosome 13, *Proc Natl Acad Sci USA* 84:2372, 1987.

138. Sato T et al: Allelotype of breast cancer: cumulative allele losses promote tumor progression in primary breast cancer, *Cancer Res* 50:7184, 1990.

139. Lee EY et al: Inactivation of the retinoblastoma susceptibility gene in human breast cancers, *Science* 241:218, 1988.

140. T'Ang A et al: Structural rearrangement of the retinoblastoma gene in human breast carcinoma, *Science* 242:263, 1988.

141. Berns EM et al: Association between *RB-1* gene alterations and factors of favourable prognosis in human breast cancer, without effect on survival, *Int J Cancer* 64:140, 1995.

142. Bieche I, Lidereau R: Loss of heterozygosity at 13q14 correlates with *RB1* gene underexpression in human breast cancer, *Mol Carcinog* 29:151, 2000.

143. Varley JM et al: The retinoblastoma gene is frequently altered leading to loss of expression in primary breast tumours, *Oncogene* 4:725, 1989.

144. Pietilainen T et al: Expression of retinoblastoma gene protein (Rb) in breast cancer as related to established prognostic factors and survival, *Eur J Cancer* 31A:329, 1995.

145. Sawan A et al: Retinoblastoma and *p53* gene expression related to relapse and survival in human breast cancer: an immunohistochemical study, *J Pathol* 168:23, 1992.

146. Spandidos DA et al: Expression of ras Rb1 and p53 proteins in human breast cancer, *Anticancer Res* 12:81, 1992.

147. Borg A et al: The retinoblastoma gene in breast cancer: allele loss is not correlated with loss of gene protein expression, *Cancer Res* 52:2991, 1992.

148. Hurd C et al: Regulation of tumor suppressor proteins, p53 and retinoblastoma, by estrogen and antiestrogens in breast cancer cells, *Oncogene* 15:991, 1997.

149. Watts CK et al: Antiestrogen inhibition of cell cycle progression in breast cancer cells in associated with inhibition of cyclin-dependent kinase activity and decreased retinoblastoma protein phosphorylation, *Mol Endocrinol* 9:1804, 1995.

150. Alban P et al: Differential regulation of retinoblastoma protein by hormonal and antihormonal agents in T47D breast cancer cells, *J Steroid Biochem Mol Biol* 77:135, 2001.

151. Donehower LA, Bradley A: The tumor suppressor *p53*, *Biochim Biophys Acta* 1155:181, 1993.

152. Lane DP, Crawford LV: T antigen is bound to a host protein in SV40-transformed cells, *Nature* 278:261, 1979.

153. vanTuinen P et al: Molecular detection of microscopic and submicroscopic deletions associated with Miller-Dieker syndrome, *Am J Hum Genet* 43:587, 1988.

154. Liu MC, Gelmann EP: *P53* gene mutations: case study of a clinical marker for solid tumors, *Semin Oncol* 29:246, 2002.

155. Soussi T, Caron DF, May P: Structural aspects of the p53 protein in relation to gene evolution, *Oncogene* 5:945, 1990.

156. Hollstein M et al: p53 mutations in human cancers, *Science* 253:49, 1991.

157. Poller DN et al: p53 protein expression in human breast carcinoma: relationship to expression of epidermal growth factor receptor, c-erbB-2 protein overexpression, and oestrogen receptor, *Br J Cancer* 66:583, 1992.

158. Walker RA et al: Expression of p53 protein in infiltrating and in-situ breast carcinomas, *J Pathol* 165:203, 1991.

159. Davidoff AM et al: Maintenance of p53 alterations throughout breast cancer progression, *Cancer Res* 51:2605, 1991.

160. Millikan R et al: p53 mutations in benign breast tissue, *J Clin Oncol* 13:2293, 1995.

161. Gannon JV et al: Activating mutations in p53 produce a common conformational effect: a monoclonal antibody specific for the mutant form, *EMBO J* 9:1595, 1990.

162. Finlay CA et al: Activating mutations for transformation by *p53* produce a gene product that forms an hsc70-p53 complex with an altered half-life, *Mol Cell Biol* 8:531, 1988.

163. Umekita Y et al: Nuclear accumulation of p53 protein correlates with mutations in the *p53* gene on archival paraffin-embedded tissues of human breast cancer, *Jpn J Cancer Res* 85:825, 1994.

164. Faille A et al: p53 mutations and overexpression in locally advanced breast cancers, *Br J Cancer* 69:1145, 1994.

165. Thompson AM et al: p53 allele losses, mutations and expression in breast cancer and their relationship to clinicopathological parameters, *Int J Cancer* 50:528, 1992.

166. Harris AL: p53 expression in human breast cancer, *Adv Cancer Res* 59:69, 1992.

167. Faille A et al: p53 mutations and overexpression in locally advanced breast cancers, *Br J Cancer* 69:1145, 1994.

168. Ciesielski D et al: p53 expression in breast cancer related to prognostic factors, *Neoplasma* 42:235, 1995.

169. Colecchia M et al: p53 protein expression in fine-needle aspirates of breast cancer: an immunocytochemical assay for identifying high-grade ductal carcinomas, *Diagn Cytopathol* 13:128, 1995.

170. Benini E et al: Detection of P53 expression and S-phase cell fraction in paraffin-embedded tissue by a double-labeling technique, *J Histochem Cytochem* 43:999, 1995.

171. Rosanelli GP et al: Mutant p53 expression and DNA analysis in human breast cancer comparison with conventional clinicopathological parameters, *Anticancer Res* 15:581, 1995.

172. Shiao YH et al: Racial disparity in the association of *p53* gene alterations with breast cancer survival, *Cancer Res* 55:1485, 1995.

173. Schimmelpenning H et al: Association of immunohistochemical *p53* tumor suppressor gene protein overexpression with prognosis in highly proliferative human mammary adenocarcinomas, *World J Surg* 18:827, 1994.

174. Wiltschke C et al: Coexpression of HER-2/neu and p53 is associated with a shorter disease-free survival in node-positive breast cancer patients, *J Cancer Res Clin Oncol* 120:737, 1994.

175. Marks JR et al: Overexpression of p53 and HER-2/neu proteins as prognostic markers in early stage breast cancer, *Ann Surg* 219:332, 1994.

176. Elledge RM et al: Tumor biologic factors and breast cancer prognosis among white, Hispanic, and black women in the United States, *J Natl Cancer Inst* 86:705, 1994.

177. Friedrichs K et al: Overexpression of p53 and prognosis in breast cancer, *Cancer* 72:3641, 1993.

178. Hassapoglidou S, Diamandis EP, Sutherland DJ: Quantification of p53 protein in tumor cell lines, breast tissue extracts and serum with time-resolved immunofluorometry, *Oncogene* 8:1501, 1993.

179. Silvestrini R et al: p53 as an independent prognostic marker in lymph node-negative breast cancer patients, *J Natl Cancer Inst* 85:965, 1993.

180. Barbareschi M et al: p53 and c-erbB-2 protein expression in breast carcinomas: an immunohistochemical study including correlations with receptor status, proliferation markers, and clinical stage in human breast cancer, *Am J Clin Pathol* 98:408, 1992.

181. Isola J et al: Association of overexpression of tumor suppressor protein p53 with rapid cell proliferation and poor prognosis in node-negative breast cancer patients, *J Natl Cancer Inst* 84:1109, 1992.

182. Mazars R et al: p53 mutations occur in aggressive breast cancer, *Cancer Res* 52:3918, 1992.
183. Sommer SS et al: Pattern of *p53* gene mutations in breast cancers of women of the midwestern United States, *J Natl Cancer Inst* 84:246, 1992.
184. Iwaya K et al: Nuclear p53 immunoreaction associated with poor prognosis of breast cancer, *Jpn J Cancer Res* 82:835, 1991.
185. Davidoff AM et al: Relation between p53 overexpression and established prognostic factors in breast cancer, *Surgery* 110:259, 1991.
186. Tarpley WG et al: Reduced hormone-stimulated adenylate cyclase activity in NIH-3T3 cells expressing the EJ human bladder *ras* oncogene, *Proc Natl Acad Sci USA* 83:3703, 1986.
187. Cattoretti G et al: *P53* expression in breast cancer, *Int J Cancer* 41:178, 1988.
188. Elledge RM, Allred DC: Prognostic and predictive value of *p53* and *p21* in breast cancer, *Breast Cancer Res Treat* 52:79, 1998.
189. Hamilton A, Piccart M: The contribution of molecular markers to the prediction of response in the treatment of breast cancer: a review of the literature on *HER-2*, *p53* and *BCL-2*, *Ann Oncol* 11:647, 2000.
190. Aas T et al: Specific *P53* mutations are associated with de novo resistance to doxorubicin in breast cancer patients, *Nat Med* 2:811, 1996.
191. Bergh J et al: Complete sequencing of the *p53* gene provides prognostic information in breast cancer patients, particularly in relation to adjuvant systemic therapy and radiotherapy, *Nat Med* 1:1029, 1995.
192. Stal O et al: *p53* expression and the result of adjuvant therapy of breast cancer, *Acta Oncol* 34:767, 1995.
193. Linn SC et al: Expression of drug resistance proteins in breast cancer, in relation to chemotherapy, *Int J Cancer* 71:787, 1997.
194. Rozan S et al: No significant predictive value of *c-erbB-2* or *p53* expression regarding sensitivity to primary chemotherapy or radiotherapy in breast cancer, *Int J Cancer* 79:27, 1998.
195. Elledge RM et al: Accumulation of p53 protein as a possible predictor of response to adjuvant combination chemotherapy with cyclophosphamide, methotrexate, fluorouracil, and prednisone for breast cancer, *J Natl Cancer Inst* 87:1254, 1995.
196. Fitzgibbons PL et al: Prognostic factors in breast cancer: College of American Pathologists Consensus Statement 1999, *Arch Pathol Lab Med* 124:966, 2000.
197. Malkin D et al: Germ line *p53* mutations in a familial syndrome of breast cancer, sarcomas, and other neoplasms, *Science* 250:1233, 1990.
198. Li FP, Fraumeni JF Jr: Soft-tissue sarcomas, breast cancer, and other neoplasms: a familial syndrome? *Ann Intern Med* 71:747, 1969.
199. Birch JM et al: Prevalence and diversity of constitutional mutations in the *p53* gene among 21 Li-Fraumeni families, *Cancer Res* 54:1298, 1994.
200. Chen YH et al: Detection of loss of heterozygosity of *p53* gene in paraffin-embedded breast cancers by non-isotopic PCR-SSCP, *J Pathol* 177:129, 1995.
201. Chen LC et al: Loss of heterozygosity on the short arm of chromosome 17 is associated with high proliferative capacity and DNA aneuploidy in primary human breast cancer, *Proc Natl Acad Sci USA* 88:3847, 1991.
202. Davidoff AM et al: Genetic basis for *p53* overexpression in human breast cancer, *Proc Natl Acad Sci USA* 88:5006, 1991.
203. Coles C et al: Evidence implicating at least two genes on chromosome 17p in breast carcinogenesis, *Lancet* 336:761, 1990.
204. Silvestrini R et al: The Bcl-2 protein: a prognostic indicator strongly related to p53 protein in lymph node-negative breast cancer patients, *J Natl Cancer Inst* 86:499, 1994.
205. Elledge RM, Lee WH: Life and death by *p53*, *Bioessays* 17:923, 1995.
206. Hanada M et al: Structure-function analysis of Bcl-2 protein: identification of conserved domains important for homodimerization with Bcl-2 and heterodimerization with Bax, *J Biol Chem* 270:11962, 1995.
207. Oltvai ZN, Milliman CL, Korsmeyer SJ: Bcl-2 heterodimerizes in vivo with a conserved homolog, Bax, that accelerates programmed cell death, *Cell* 74:609, 1993.
208. Otter I et al: The binding properties and biological activities of Bcl-2 and Bax in cells exposed to apoptotic stimuli, *J Biol Chem* 273:6110, 1998.
209. Ottilie S et al: Dimerization properties of human BAD: identification of a BH-3 domain and analysis of its binding to mutant BCL-2 and BCL-XL proteins, *J Biol Chem* 272:30866, 1997.
210. Sedlak TW et al: Multiple Bcl-2 family members demonstrate selective dimerizations with Bax, *Proc Natl Acad Sci USA* 92:7834, 1995.
211. Yang E et al: Bad, a heterodimeric partner for Bcl-XL and Bcl-2, displaces Bax and promotes cell death, *Cell* 80:285, 1995.
212. Tsujimoto Y et al: Cloning of the chromosome breakpoint of neoplastic B cells with the t(14;18) chromosome translocation, *Science* 226:1097, 1984.
213. Hockenbery D et al: Bcl-2 is an inner mitochondrial membrane protein that blocks programmed cell death, *Nature* 348:334, 1990.
214. Kumar R, Vadlamudi RK, Adam L: Apoptosis in mammary gland cancer, *Endocrine-Related Cancer* 7:257, 2000.
215. Alsabeh R et al: Expression of bcl-2 by breast cancer: a possible diagnostic application, *Mod Pathol* 9:439, 1996.
216. Daidone MG et al: Clinical studies of Bcl-2 and treatment benefit in breast cancer patients, *Endocrine-Related Cancer* 6:61, 1999.
217. Elledge RM et al: Bcl-2, p53, and response to tamoxifen in estrogen receptor-positive metastatic breast cancer: a Southwest Oncology Group study, *J Clin Oncol* 15:1916, 1997.
218. Kobayashi S et al: Clinical significance of *bcl-2* gene expression in human breast cancer tissues, *Breast Cancer Res Treat* 42:173, 1997.
219. Le MG et al: c-myc, p53 and bcl-2, apoptosis-related genes in infiltrating breast carcinomas: evidence of a link between bcl-2 protein over-expression and a lower risk of metastasis and death in operable patients, *Int J Cancer* 84:562, 1999.
220. Mauri FA et al: Prognostic value of estrogen receptor status can be improved by combined evaluation of p53, Bcl2 and PgR expression: an immunohistochemical study on breast carcinoma with long-term follow-up, *Int J Oncol* 15:1137, 1999.
221. Nakopoulou L et al: bcl-2 protein expression is associated with a prognostically favourable phenotype in breast cancer irrespective of p53 immunostaining, *Histopathology* 34:310, 1999.

222. Schorr K et al: *Bcl-2* gene family and related proteins in mammary gland involution and breast cancer, *J Mammary Gland Biol Neoplasia* 4:153, 1999.

223. Villar E et al: bcl-2 Expression and apoptosis in primary and metastatic breast carcinomas, *Tumour Biol* 22:137, 2001.

224. Doglioni C et al: The prevalence of BCL-2 immunoreactivity in breast carcinomas and its clinicopathological correlates, with particular reference to oestrogen receptor status, *Virchows Arch* 424:47, 1994.

225. Gee JM et al: Immunocytochemical localization of BCL-2 protein in human breast cancers and its relationship to a series of prognostic markers and response to endocrine therapy, *Int J Cancer* 59:619, 1994.

226. Hurlimann J, Larrinaga B, Vala DL: Bcl-2 protein in invasive ductal breast carcinomas, *Virchows Arch* 426:163, 1995.

227. Leek RD et al: Bcl-2 in normal human breast and carcinoma, association with oestrogen receptor-positive, epidermal growth factor receptor-negative tumours and in situ cancer, *Br J Cancer* 69:135, 1994.

228. Nathan B et al: Expression of BCL-2 in primary breast cancer and its correlation with tumour phenotype. For the International (Ludwig) Breast Cancer Study Group, *Ann Oncol* 5:409, 1994.

229. Sierra A et al: Bcl-2 expression is associated with lymph node metastasis in human ductal breast carcinoma, *Int J Cancer* 60:54, 1995.

230. Jalava PJ et al: Bcl-2 immunostaining: a way to finding unresponsive postmenopausal N+ breast cancer patients, *Anticancer Res* 20:1213, 2000.

231. Perillo B et al: 17Beta-estradiol inhibits apoptosis in MCF-7 cells, inducing bcl-2 expression via two estrogen-responsive elements present in the coding sequence, *Mol Cell Biol* 20:2890, 2000.

232. Dole M et al: Bcl-2 inhibits chemotherapy-induced apoptosis in neuroblastoma, *Cancer Res* 54:3253, 1994.

233. Hickman JA: Apoptosis induced by anticancer drugs, *Cancer Metastasis Rev* 11:121, 1992.

234. Teixeira C, Reed JC, Pratt MA: Estrogen promotes chemotherapeutic drug resistance by a mechanism involving *Bcl-2* proto-oncogene expression in human breast cancer cells, *Cancer Res* 55:3902, 1995.

235. Yang QF et al: Expression of Bcl-2 but not Bax or p53 correlates with in vitro resistance to a series of anticancer drugs in breast carcinoma, *Breast Cancer Res Treat* 61:211, 2000.

236. Haldar S, Basu A, Croce CM: Bcl2 is the guardian of microtubule integrity, *Cancer Res* 57:229, 1997.

237. Korsmeyer SJ: Bcl-2 initiates a new category of oncogenes: regulators of cell death, *Blood* 80:879, 1992.

238. Krajewski S et al: Immunohistochemical analysis of in vivo patterns of Bcl-X expression, *Cancer Res* 54:5501, 1994.

239. Simoes-Wust AP et al: Bcl-xl antisense treatment induces apoptosis in breast carcinoma cells, *Int J Cancer* 87:582, 2000.

240. Fernandez Y et al: Inhibition of apoptosis in human breast cancer cells: role in tumor progression to the metastatic state, *Int J Cancer* 101:317, 2002.

241. Krajewski S et al: Prognostic significance of apoptosis regulators in breast cancer, *Endocr Relat Cancer* 6:29, 1999.

242. Olopade OI et al: Overexpression of BCL-x protein in primary breast cancer is associated with high tumor grade and nodal metastases, *Cancer J Sci Am* 3:230, 1997.

243. Wallasch C et al: Heregulin-dependent regulation of HER2/neu oncogenic signaling by heterodimerization with HER3, *EMBO J* 14:4267, 1995.

244. Zhong Z, Wen Z, Darnell JE Jr: Stat3: a STAT family member activated by tyrosine phosphorylation in response to epidermal growth factor and interleukin-6, *Science* 264:95, 1994.

245. Troyer KL, Lee DC: Regulation of mouse mammary gland development and tumorigenesis by the ERBB signaling network, *J Mammary Gland Biol Neoplasia* 6:7, 2001.

246. Lee DC et al: Transforming growth factor alpha: expression, regulation, and biological activities, *Pharmacol Rev* 47:51, 1995.

247. Normanno N et al: Epidermal growth factor-related peptides in the pathogenesis of human breast cancer, *Breast Cancer Res Treat* 29:11, 1994.

248. Di Fiore PP et al: Overexpression of the human EGF receptor confers an EGF-dependent transformed phenotype to NIH 3T3 cells, *Cell* 51:1063, 1987.

249. Velu TJ et al: Epidermal-growth-factor-dependent transformation by a human EGF receptor proto-oncogene, *Science* 238:1408, 1987.

250. Kokai Y et al: Synergistic interaction of p185c-neu and the EGF receptor leads to transformation of rodent fibroblasts, *Cell* 58:287, 1989.

251. Pedersen MW et al: The type III epidermal growth factor receptor mutation: biological significance and potential target for anti-cancer therapy, *Ann Oncol* 12:745, 2001.

252. Moscatello DK et al: Transformational and altered signal transduction by a naturally occurring mutant EGF receptor, *Oncogene* 13:85, 1996.

253. Tang CK et al: Epidermal growth factor receptor vIII enhances tumorigenicity in human breast cancer, *Cancer Res* 60:3081, 2000.

254. Batra SK et al: Epidermal growth factor ligand-independent, unregulated, cell-transforming potential of a naturally occurring human mutant EGFRvIII gene, *Cell Growth Differ* 6:1251, 1995.

255. Ge H, Gong X, Tang CK: Evidence of high incidence of EGFRvIII expression and coexpression with EGFR in human invasive breast cancer by laser capture microdissection and immunohistochemical analysis, *Int J Cancer* 98:357, 2002.

256. Sampson JH et al: Unarmed, tumor-specific monoclonal antibody effectively treats brain tumors, *Proc Natl Acad Sci USA* 97:7503, 2000.

257. Luetteke NC et al: Targeted inactivation of the EGF and amphiregulin genes reveals distinct roles for EGF receptor ligands in mouse mammary gland development, *Development* 126:2739, 1999.

258. Brandt R et al: Mammary gland specific hEGF receptor transgene expression induces neoplasia and inhibits differentiation, *Oncogene* 19:2129, 2000.

259. Matsui Y et al: Development of mammary hyperplasia and neoplasia in MMTV-TGF alpha transgenic mice, *Cell* 61:1147, 1990.

260. Sandgren EP et al: Overexpression of TGF alpha in transgenic mice: induction of epithelial hyperplasia, pancreatic metaplasia, and carcinoma of the breast, *Cell* 61:1121, 1990.

261. Filmus J et al: MDA-468, a human breast cancer cell line with a high number of epidermal growth factor (EGF) receptors, has an amplified EGF receptor gene and is growth inhibited by EGF, *Biochem Biophys Res Commun* 128:898, 1985.

262. Davidson NE et al: Epidermal growth factor receptor gene expression in estrogen receptor-positive and negative human breast cancer cell lines, *Mol Endocrinol* 1:216, 1987.

263. Guerin M et al: Structure and expression of c-erbB-2 and EGF receptor genes in inflammatory and non-inflammatory breast cancer: prognostic significance, *Int J Cancer* 43:201, 1989.

264. Ro J et al: Amplified and overexpressed epidermal growth factor receptor gene in uncultured primary human breast carcinoma, *Cancer Res* 48:161, 1988.

265. Lacroix H et al: Overexpression of erbB-2 or EGF receptor proteins present in early stage mammary carcinoma is detected simultaneously in matched primary tumors and regional metastases, *Oncogene* 4:145, 1989.

266. Klijn JG et al: The clinical significance of epidermal growth factor receptor (EGF-R) in human breast cancer: a review of 5232 patients, *Endocr Rev* 13:3, 1992.

267. Fitzpatrick SL et al: Epidermal growth factor binding by breast tumor biopsies and relationship to estrogen receptor and progestin receptor levels, *Cancer Res* 44:3448, 1984.

268. Peyrat JP et al: EGF receptors in human breast cancer: relation to hormonal receptors [in French], *Ann Endocrinol (Paris)* 45:412, 1984.

269. Perez R et al: Epidermal growth factor receptors in human breast cancer, *Breast Cancer Res Treat* 4:189, 1984.

270. Skoog L et al: Receptors for EGF and oestradiol and thymidine kinase activity in different histological subgroups of human mammary carcinomas, *Br J Cancer* 54:271, 1986.

271. Macias A et al: Receptors for epidermal growth factor in human mammary carcinomas and their metastases, *Anticancer Res* 6:849, 1986.

272. Macias A et al: Prognostic significance of the receptor for epidermal growth factor in human mammary carcinomas, *Anticancer Res* 7:459, 1987.

273. Rios MA et al: Receptors for epidermal growth factor and estrogen as predictors of relapse in patients with mammary carcinoma, *Anticancer Res* 8:173, 1988.

274. Sainsbury JR et al: Presence of epidermal growth factor receptor as an indicator of poor prognosis in patients with breast cancer, *J Clin Pathol* 38:1225, 1985.

275. Sainsbury JR et al: Epidermal-growth-factor receptor status as predictor of early recurrence of and death from breast cancer, *Lancet* 1:1398, 1987.

276. Nicholson S et al: Quantitative assays of epidermal growth factor receptor in human breast cancer: cut-off points of clinical relevance, *Int J Cancer* 42:36, 1988.

277. Sainsbury JR et al: Epidermal growth factor receptor status of histological sub-types of breast cancer, *Br J Cancer* 58:458, 1988.

278. Nicholson S et al: Expression of epidermal growth factor receptors associated with lack of response to endocrine therapy in recurrent breast cancer, *Lancet* 1:182, 1989.

279. Nicholson S et al: Epidermal growth factor receptor (EGFr) as a marker for poor prognosis in node-negative breast cancer patients: neu and tamoxifen failure, *J Steroid Biochem Mol Biol* 37:811, 1990.

280. Wyss R et al: Phorbol ester and epidermal growth factor receptors in human breast cancer, *Anticancer Res* 7:721, 1987.

281. Costa S et al: Predictive value of EGF receptor in breast cancer, *Lancet* 2:1258, 1988.

282. Pekonen F et al: Receptors for epidermal growth factor and insulin-like growth factor I and their relation to steroid receptors in human breast cancer, *Cancer Res* 48:1343, 1988.

283. Delarue JC et al: Epidermal growth factor receptor in human breast cancers: correlation with estrogen and progesterone receptors, *Breast Cancer Res Treat* 11:173, 1988.

284. Spyratos F et al: Prognostic value of a solubilized fraction of EGF receptors in primary breast cancer using an immunoenzymatic assay: a retrospective study, *Breast Cancer Res Treat* 29:85, 1994.

285. Battaglia F et al: Receptors for epidermal growth factor and steroid hormones in human breast cancer, *Oncology* 45:424, 1988.

286. Battaglia F et al: Epidermal growth factor receptor in human breast cancer: correlation with steroid hormone receptors and axillary lymph node involvement, *Eur J Cancer Clin Oncol* 24:1685, 1988.

287. Cappelletti V et al: Simultaneous estimation of epidermal growth factor receptors and steroid receptors in a series of 136 resectable primary breast tumors, *Tumour Biol* 9:200, 1988.

288. Grimaux M et al: Prognostic value of epidermal growth factor receptor in node-positive breast cancer, *Breast Cancer Res Treat* 14:77, 1989.

289. Foekens JA et al: Prognostic value of receptors for insulin-like growth factor 1, somatostatin, and epidermal growth factor in human breast cancer, *Cancer Res* 49:7002, 1989.

290. Fekete M et al: Characteristics and distribution of receptors for [D-TRP6]-luteinizing hormone-releasing hormone, somatostatin, epidermal growth factor, and sex steroids in 500 biopsy samples of human breast cancer, *J Clin Lab Anal* 3:137, 1989.

291. Toi M et al: Immunocytochemical and biochemical analysis of epidermal growth factor receptor expression in human breast cancer tissues: relationship to estrogen receptor and lymphatic invasion, *Int J Cancer* 43:220, 1989.

292. Toi M et al: Role of epidermal growth factor receptor expression in primary breast cancer: results of a biochemical study and an immunocytochemical study, *Breast Cancer Res Treat* 29:51, 1994.

293. Bauknecht T et al: The occurrence of epidermal growth factor receptors and the characterization of EGF-like factors in human ovarian, endometrial, cervical and breast cancer: EGF receptors and factors in gynecological carcinomas, *J Cancer Res Clin Oncol* 115:193, 1989.

294. Zeillinger R et al: HER-2 amplification, steroid receptors and epidermal growth factor receptor in primary breast cancer, *Oncogene* 4:109, 1989.

295. Barker S et al: Epidermal growth factor receptor and oestrogen receptors in the non-malignant part of the cancerous breast, *Br J Cancer* 60:673, 1989.

296. Llorens MA et al: Epidermal growth factor receptors in human breast and endometrial carcinomas, *J Steroid Biochem* 34:505, 1989.

297. Bolla M et al: Estimation of epidermal growth factor receptor in 177 breast cancers: correlation with prognostic factors, *Breast Cancer Res Treat* 16:97, 1990.

298. Formento JL et al: Epidermal growth factor receptor assay: validation of a single point method and application to breast cancer, *Breast Cancer Res Treat* 17:211, 1991.

299. Koenders PG et al: Epidermal growth factor receptor-negative tumors are predominantly confined to the subgroup of estradiol receptor-positive human primary breast cancers, *Cancer Res* 51:4544, 1991.

300. Bolufer P et al: Epidermal growth factor receptor in human breast cancer: correlation with cytosolic and nuclear ER

receptors and with biological and histological tumor characteristics, *Eur J Cancer* 26:283, 1990.

301. Reubi JC, Torhorst J: The relationship between somatostatin, epidermal growth factor, and steroid hormone receptors in breast cancer, *Cancer* 64:1254, 1989.

302. Walker RA, Cowl J: The expression of c-fos protein in human breast, *J Pathol* 163:323, 1991.

303. Wrba F et al: Expression of epidermal growth factor receptors (EGFR) on breast carcinomas in relation to growth fractions, estrogen receptor status and morphological criteria: an immunohistochemical study, *Pathol Res Pract* 183:25, 1988.

304. Betta PG et al: Expression of epidermal growth factor receptor in human breast carcinoma and its correlation with morphological and biological features of tumour aggressiveness, *Pathologica* 81:425, 1989.

305. Moller P et al: Expression of epidermal growth factor receptor in benign and malignant primary tumours of the breast, *Virchows Arch A Pathol Anat Histopathol* 414:157, 1989.

306. Grimaux M et al: A simplified immuno-enzymetric assay of the epidermal growth factor receptor in breast tumors: evaluation in 282 cases, *Int J Cancer* 45:255, 1990.

307. Lewis S et al: Expression of epidermal growth factor receptor in breast carcinoma, *J Clin Pathol* 43:385, 1990.

308. Tsutsumi Y et al: Neu oncogene protein and epidermal growth factor receptor are independently expressed in benign and malignant breast tissues, *Hum Pathol* 21:750, 1990.

309. Koenders PG et al: Epidermal growth factor receptor and prognosis in human breast cancer: a prospective study, *Breast Cancer Res Treat* 25:21, 1993.

310. Nicholson RI et al: Epidermal growth factor receptor expression in breast cancer: association with response to endocrine therapy, *Breast Cancer Res Treat* 29:117, 1994.

311. Tsutsui S et al: Prognostic value of epidermal growth factor receptor (EGFR) and its relationship to the estrogen receptor status in 1029 patients with breast cancer, *Breast Cancer Res Treat* 71:67, 2002.

312. Miller DL et al: Emergence of MCF-7 cells overexpressing a transfected epidermal growth factor receptor (EGFR) under estrogen-depleted conditions: evidence for a role of EGFR in breast cancer growth and progression, *Cell Growth Differ* 5:1263, 1994.

313. Clarke R et al: The effects of a constitutive expression of transforming growth factor-alpha on the growth of MCF-7 human breast cancer cells in vitro and in vivo, *Mol Endocrinol* 3:372, 1989.

314. Yarden RI, Wilson MA, Chrysogelos SA: Estrogen suppression of EGFR expression in breast cancer cells: a possible mechanism to modulate growth, *J Cell Biochem* 81:232, 2001.

315. Marquez DC et al: Epidermal growth factor receptor and tyrosine phosphorylation of estrogen receptor, *Endocrine* 16:73, 2001.

316. Filardo EJ et al: Estrogen-induced activation of Erk-1 and Erk-2 requires the G protein-coupled receptor homolog, GPR30, and occurs via trans-activation of the epidermal growth factor receptor through release of HB-EGF, *Mol Endocrinol* 14:1649, 2000.

317. Ciardiello F, Tortora G: A novel approach in the treatment of cancer: targeting the epidermal growth factor receptor, *Clin Cancer Res* 7:2958, 2001.

318. Ennis BW et al: Anti-epidermal growth factor receptor antibodies inhibit the autocrine-stimulated growth of MDA-468 human breast cancer cells, *Mol Endocrinol* 3:1830, 1989.

319. Arteaga CL, Coronado E, Osborne CK: Blockade of the epidermal growth factor receptor inhibits transforming growth factor alpha-induced but not estrogen-induced growth of hormone-dependent human breast cancer, *Mol Endocrinol* 2:1064, 1988.

320. Goldstein NI et al: Biological efficacy of a chimeric antibody to the epidermal growth factor receptor in a human tumor xenograft model, *Clin Cancer Res* 1:1311, 1995.

321. Fan Z et al: Antibody-induced epidermal growth factor receptor dimerization mediates inhibition of autocrine proliferation of A431 squamous carcinoma cells, *J Biol Chem* 269:27595, 1994.

322. Peng D et al: Anti-epidermal growth factor receptor monoclonal antibody 225 up-regulates *p27KIP1* and induces G1 arrest in prostatic cancer cell line DU145, *Cancer Res* 56:3666, 1996.

323. Perrotte P et al: Anti-epidermal growth factor receptor antibody C225 inhibits angiogenesis in human transitional cell carcinoma growing orthotopically in nude mice, *Clin Cancer Res* 5:257, 1999.

324. Moyer JD et al: Induction of apoptosis and cell cycle arrest by CP-358,774, an inhibitor of epidermal growth factor receptor tyrosine kinase, *Cancer Res* 57:4838, 1997.

325. Wakeling AE et al: Specific inhibition of epidermal growth factor receptor tyrosine kinase by 4-anilinoquinazolines, *Breast Cancer Res Treat* 38:67, 1996.

326. Schechter AL et al: The *neu* oncogene: an *erb*-B-related gene encoding a 185,000-Mr tumour antigen, *Nature* 312:513, 1984.

327. Yamamoto T et al: Similarity of protein encoded by the human *c-erb-B-2* gene to epidermal growth factor receptor, *Nature* 319:230, 1986.

328. Akiyama T et al: The product of the human *c-erbB-2* gene: a 185-kilodalton glycoprotein with tyrosine kinase activity, *Science* 232:1644, 1986.

329. Schechter AL et al: The *neu* gene: an *erbB*-homologous gene distinct from and unlinked to the gene encoding the EGF receptor, *Science* 229:976, 1985.

330. Coussens L et al: Tyrosine kinase receptor with extensive homology to EGF receptor shares chromosomal location with *neu* oncogene, *Science* 230:1132, 1985.

331. Bargmann CI, Hung MC, Weinberg RA: The *neu* oncogene encodes an epidermal growth factor receptor-related protein, *Nature* 319:226, 1986.

332. Bargmann CI, Hung MC, Weinberg RA: Multiple independent activations of the *neu* oncogene by a point mutation altering the transmembrane domain of *p185*, *Cell* 45:649, 1986.

333. King CR, Kraus MH, Aaronson SA: Amplification of a novel *v-erbB*-related gene in a human mammary carcinoma, *Science* 229:974, 1985.

334. Zhou D et al: Association of multiple copies of the *c-erbB-2* oncogene with spread of breast cancer, *Cancer Res* 47:6123, 1987.

335. Yokota J et al: Amplification of *c-erbB-2* oncogene in human adenocarcinomas in vivo, *Lancet* 1:765, 1986.

336. Slamon DJ et al: Human breast cancer: correlation of relapse and survival with amplification of the *HER-2/neu* oncogene, *Science* 235:177, 1987.

337. Andrechek ER et al: Amplification of the *neu/erbB-2* oncogene in a mouse model of mammary tumorigenesis, *Proc Natl Acad Sci USA* 97:3444, 2000.

338. Siegel PM et al: Elevated expression of activated forms of *Neu/ErbB-2* and *ErbB-3* are involved in the induction of mammary tumors in transgenic mice: implications for human breast cancer, *EMBO J* 18:2149, 1999.

339. Kwong KY, Hung MC: A novel splice variant of *HER2* with increased transformation activity, *Mol Carcinog* 23:62, 1998.

340. Riese DJ, Stern DF: Specificity within the EGF family/ErbB receptor family signaling network, *Bioessays* 20:41, 1998.

341. Graus-Porta D et al: ErbB-2, the preferred heterodimerization partner of all ErbB receptors, is a mediator of lateral signaling, *EMBO J* 16:1647, 1997.

342. Karunagaran D et al: ErbB-2 is a common auxiliary subunit of NDF and EGF receptors: implications for breast cancer, *EMBO J* 15:254, 1996.

343. Pinkas-Kramarski R et al: Neu differentiation factor/neuregulin isoforms activate distinct receptor combinations, *J Biol Chem* 271:19029, 1996.

344. Tzahar E et al: A hierarchical network of interreceptor interactions determines signal transduction by Neu differentiation factor/neuregulin and epidermal growth factor, *Mol Cell Biol* 16:5276, 1996.

345. Brennan PJ et al: *HER2/neu:* mechanisms of dimerization/oligomerization, *Oncogene* 19:6093, 2000.

346. Kumagai T et al: The role of distinct *p185neu* extracellular subdomains for dimerization with the epidermal growth factor (EGF) receptor and EGF-mediated signaling, *Proc Natl Acad Sci USA* 98:5526, 2001.

347. Alimandi M et al: Cooperative signaling of ErbB3 and ErbB2 in neoplastic transformation and human mammary carcinomas, *Oncogene* 10:1813, 1995.

348. Cohen BD et al: The relationship between human epidermal growth-like factor receptor expression and cellular transformation in NIH3T3 cells, *J Biol Chem* 271:30897, 1996.

349. Lane HA et al: ErbB2 potentiates breast tumor proliferation through modulation of *p27(Kip1)*-Cdk2 complex formation: receptor overexpression does not determine growth dependency, *Mol Cell Biol* 20:3210, 2000.

350. Muthuswamy SK, Muller WJ: Activation of Src family kinases in Neu-induced mammary tumors correlates with their association with distinct sets of tyrosine phosphorylated proteins in vivo, *Oncogene* 11:1801, 1995.

351. Keshamouni VG, Mattingly RR, Reddy KB: Mechanism of 17-beta-estradiol-induced Erk1/2 activation in breast cancer cells: a role for HER2 AND PKC-delta, *J Biol Chem* 277:22558, 2002.

352. Yarden Y: Biology of HER2 and its importance in breast cancer, *Oncology* 61(suppl 2):1, 2001.

353. Pegram MD, Konecny G, Slamon DJ: The molecular and cellular biology of *HER2/neu* gene amplification/overexpression and the clinical development of Herceptin (trastuzumab) therapy for breast cancer, *Cancer Treat Res* 103:57, 2000.

354. Kurebayashi J: Biological and clinical significance of HER2 overexpression in breast cancer, *Breast Cancer* 8:45, 2001.

355. Allred DC et al: HER-2/neu in node-negative breast cancer: prognostic significance of overexpression influenced by the presence of in situ carcinoma, *J Clin Oncol* 10:599, 1992.

356. Gullick WJ et al: C-erbB-2 protein overexpression in breast cancer is a risk factor in patients with involved and uninvolved lymph nodes, *Br J Cancer* 63:434, 1991.

357. Ro JS et al: c-erbB-2 amplification in node-negative human breast cancer, *Cancer Res* 49:6941, 1989.

358. Richner J et al: c-erbB-2 protein expression in node negative breast cancer, *Ann Oncol* 1:263, 1990.

359. Paterson MC et al: Correlation between c-erbB-2 amplification and risk of recurrent disease in node-negative breast cancer, *Cancer Res* 51:556, 1991.

360. Press MF et al: Her-2/neu expression in node-negative breast cancer: direct tissue quantitation by computerized image analysis and association of overexpression with increased risk of recurrent disease, *Cancer Res* 53:4960, 1993.

361. Hynes NE, Stern DF: The biology of erbB-2/neu/HER-2 and its role in cancer, *Biochim Biophys Acta* 1198:165, 1994.

362. Langton BC et al: An antigen immunologically related to the external domain of gp185 is shed from nude mouse tumors overexpressing the *c-erbB-2 (HER-2/neu)* oncogene, *Cancer Res* 51:2593, 1991.

363. Ramachandra S et al: Immunohistochemical distribution of c-erbB-2 in in situ breast carcinoma: a detailed morphological analysis, *J Pathol* 161:7, 1990.

364. Gusterson BA et al: Immunohistochemical distribution of c-erbB-2 in infiltrating and in situ breast cancer, *Int J Cancer* 42:842, 1988.

365. Iglehart JD et al: Increased *erbB-2* gene copies and expression in multiple stages of breast cancer, *Cancer Res* 50:6701, 1990.

366. Liu E et al: The *HER2 (c-erbB-2)* oncogene is frequently amplified in in situ carcinomas of the breast, *Oncogene* 7:1027, 1992.

367. Maguire HC Jr et al: Expression of c-erbB-2 in in situ and in adjacent invasive ductal adenocarcinomas of the female breast, *Pathobiology* 60:117, 1992.

368. van de Vijver MJ et al: Neu-protein overexpression in breast cancer: association with comedo-type ductal carcinoma in situ and limited prognostic value in stage II breast cancer, *N Engl J Med* 319:1239, 1988.

369. Carlomagno C et al: C-erb B2 overexpression decreases the benefit of adjuvant tamoxifen in early-stage breast cancer without axillary lymph node metastases, *J Clin Oncol* 14:2702, 1996.

370. Ellis MJ et al: Letrozole is more effective neoadjuvant endocrine therapy than tamoxifen for ErbB-1- and/or ErbB-2-positive, estrogen receptor-positive primary breast cancer: evidence from a phase III randomized trial, *J Clin Oncol* 19:3808, 2001.

371. Gusterson BA et al: Prognostic importance of c-erbB-2 expression in breast cancer. International (Ludwig) Breast Cancer Study Group, *J Clin Oncol* 10:1049, 1992.

372. Muss HB et al: C-erbB-2 expression and response to adjuvant therapy in women with node-positive early breast cancer, *N Engl J Med* 330:1260, 1994.

373. Gianni L: Future directions of paclitaxel-based therapy of breast cancer, *Semin Oncol* 24(suppl 17):91, 1997.

374. Drebin JA et al: Down-modulation of an oncogene protein product and reversion of the transformed phenotype by monoclonal antibodies, *Cell* 41:697, 1985.

375. Hudziak RM et al: p185HER2 monoclonal antibody has antiproliferative effects in vitro and sensitizes human breast tumor cells to tumor necrosis factor, *Mol Cell Biol* 9:1165, 1989.

376. Shepard HM et al: Monoclonal antibody therapy of human cancer: taking the *HER2* protooncogene to the clinic, *J Clin Immunol* 11:117, 1991.

377. Colomer R et al: ErbB-2 antisense oligonucleotides inhibit the proliferation of breast carcinoma cells with *erbB-2* oncogene amplification, *Br J Cancer* 70:819, 1994.

378. Di Lazzaro C et al: Immunotoxins to the *HER-2* oncogene product: functional and ultrastructural analysis of their cytotoxic activity, *Cancer Immunol Immunother* 39:318, 1994.

379. Valone FH et al: Phase Ia/Ib trial of bispecific antibody MDX-210 in patients with advanced breast or ovarian cancer that overexpresses the proto-oncogene *HER-2/neu*, *J Clin Oncol* 13:2281, 1995.

380. Hancock MC et al: A monoclonal antibody against the c-erbB-2 protein enhances the cytotoxicity of cis-diamminedichloroplatinum against human breast and ovarian tumor cell lines, *Cancer Res* 51:4575, 1991.

381. Pegram M et al: Inhibitory effects of combinations of HER-2/neu antibody and chemotherapeutic agents used for treatment of human breast cancers, *Oncogene* 18:2241, 1999.

382. Pegram MD et al: Phase II study of receptor-enhanced chemosensitivity using recombinant humanized anti-p185HER2/neu monoclonal antibody plus cisplatin in patients with HER2/neu-overexpressing metastatic breast cancer refractory to chemotherapy treatment, *J Clin Oncol* 16:2659, 1998.

383. Cobleigh MA et al: Multinational study of the efficacy and safety of humanized anti-HER2 monoclonal antibody in women who have HER2-overexpressing metastatic breast cancer that has progressed after chemotherapy for metastatic disease, *J Clin Oncol* 17:2639, 1999.

384. Slamon DJ et al: Use of chemotherapy plus a monoclonal antibody against HER2 for metastatic breast cancer that overexpresses HER2, *N Engl J Med* 344:783, 2001.

385. Baselga J: Herceptin alone or in combination with chemotherapy in the treatment of HER2-positive metastatic breast cancer: pivotal trials, *Oncology* 61(suppl 2):14, 2001.

386. Press M et al: Improved clinical outcomes for Herceptin (R)-treated patients selected by fluorescence in situ hybridization (FISH), *Mod Pathol* 15:47A, 2002.

387. Vogel CL et al: First-line Herceptin monotherapy in metastatic breast cancer, *Oncology* 61:37, 2001.

388. Normanno N et al: Cooperative inhibitory effect of ZD1839 (Iressa) in combination with trastuzumab (Herceptin) on human breast cancer cell growth, *Ann Oncol* 13:65, 2002.

389. Moulder SL et al: Epidermal growth factor receptor (HER1) tyrosine kinase inhibitor ZD1839 (Iressa) inhibits HER2/neu (erbB2)-overexpressing breast cancer cells in vitro and in vivo, *Cancer Res* 61:8887, 2001.

390. Bates SE et al: Expression of transforming growth factor alpha and its messenger ribonucleic acid in human breast cancer: its regulation by estrogen and its possible functional significance, *Mol Endocrinol* 2:543, 1988.

391. Dickson RB et al: Induction of epidermal growth factor-related polypeptides by 17beta-estradiol in MCF-7 human breast cancer cells, *Endocrinology* 118:138, 1986.

392. Nickell KA, Halper J, Moses HL: Transforming factors in solid human malignant neoplasms, *Cancer Res* 43:1966, 1983.

393. Salomon DS et al: Presence of transforming growth factors in human breast cancer cells, *Cancer Res* 44:4069, 1984.

394. Dickson RB et al: Characterization of estrogen responsive transforming activity in human breast cancer cell lines, *Cancer Res* 46:1707, 1986.

395. De Larco JE, Todaro GJ: Growth factors from murine sarcoma virus-transformed cells, *Proc Natl Acad Sci USA* 75:4001, 1978.

396. Roberts AB, Sporn MB: Growth factors and transformation, *Cancer Surv* 5:405, 1986.

397. Cohen S: Isolation of a mouse submaxillary gland protein accelerating incisor eruption and eyelid opening in the newborn animal, *J Biol Chem* 237:1555, 1962.

398. Bringman TS, Lindquist PB, Derynck R: Different transforming growth factor-alpha species are derived from a glycosylated and palmitoylated transmembrane precursor, *Cell* 48:429, 1987.

399. Scott J et al: Structure of a mouse submaxillary messenger RNA encoding epidermal growth factor and seven related proteins, *Science* 221:236, 1983.

400. Carpenter G et al: Antibodies to the epidermal growth factor receptor block the biological activities of sarcoma growth factor, *Proc Natl Acad Sci USA* 80:5627, 1983.

401. Bodey B et al: Clinical and prognostic significance of the expression of the c-erbB-2 and c-erbB-3 oncoproteins in primary and metastatic malignant melanomas and breast carcinomas, *Anticancer Res* 17:1319, 1997.

402. Kew TY et al: C-erbB-4 protein expression in human breast cancer, *Br J Cancer* 82:1163, 2000.

403. Knowlden JM et al: C-erbB3 and c-erbB4 expression is a feature of the endocrine responsive phenotype in clinical breast cancer, *Oncogene* 17:1949, 1998.

404. Peles E, Yarden Y: *Neu* and its ligands: from an oncogene to neural factors, *Bioessays* 15:815, 1993.

405. Chang H et al: Ligands for ErbB-family receptors encoded by a neuregulin-like gene, *Nature* 387:509, 1997.

406. Harari D et al: Neuregulin-4: a novel growth factor that acts through the ErbB-4 receptor tyrosine kinase, *Oncogene* 18:2681, 1999.

407. Elenius K et al: Activation of HER4 by heparin-binding EGF-like growth factor stimulates chemotaxis but not proliferation, *EMBO J* 16:1268, 1997.

408. Riese DJ et al: Betacellulin activates the epidermal growth factor receptor and erbB-4, and induces cellular response patterns distinct from those stimulated by epidermal growth factor or neuregulin-beta, *Oncogene* 12:345, 1996.

409. Komurasaki T et al: Epiregulin binds to epidermal growth factor receptor and ErbB-4 and induces tyrosine phosphorylation of epidermal growth factor receptor, ErbB-2, ErbB-3 and ErbB-4, *Oncogene* 15:2841, 1997.

410. Higashiyama S et al: A novel brain-derived member of the epidermal growth factor family that interacts with ErbB3 and ErbB4, *J Biochem (Tokyo)* 122:675, 1997.

411. Powers CJ, McLeskey SW, Wellstein A: Fibroblast growth factors, their receptors and signaling, *Endocrine-Related Cancer* 7:165, 2000.

412. Bugler B, Amalric F, Prats H: Alternative initiation of translation determines cytoplasmic or nuclear localization of basic fibroblast growth factor, *Mol Cell Biol* 11:573, 1991.

413. Imamura T et al: Recovery of mitogenic activity of a growth factor mutant with a nuclear translocation sequence, *Science* 249:1567, 1990.

414. Lobb RR: Thrombin inactivates acidic fibroblast growth factor but not basic fibroblast growth factor, *Biochemistry* 27:2572, 1988.

415. Sommer A, Rifkin DB: Interaction of heparin with human basic fibroblast growth factor: protection of the angiogenic protein from proteolytic degradation by a glycosaminoglycan, *J Cell Physiol* 138:215, 1989.

416. Johnson DE, Williams LT: Structural and functional diversity in the FGF receptor multigene family, *Adv Cancer Res* 60:1, 1993.

417. Ezzat S et al: A soluble dominant negative fibroblast growth factor receptor 4 isoform in human MCF-7 breast cancer cells, *Biochem Biophys Res Commun* 287:60, 2001.

418. Johnson DE et al: The human fibroblast growth factor receptor genes: a common structural arrangement underlies the mechanisms for generating receptor forms that differ in their third immunoglobulin domain, *Mol Cell Biol* 11:4627, 1991.

419. Bellot F et al: Ligand-induced transphosphorylation between different FGF receptors, *EMBO J* 10:2849, 1991.

420. Ornitz DM et al: Heparin is required for cell-free binding of basic fibroblast growth factor to a soluble receptor and for mitogenesis in whole cells, *Mol Cell Biol* 12:240, 1992.

421. Plotnikov AN et al: Structural basis for FGF receptor dimerization and activation, *Cell* 98:641, 1999.

422. Stauber DJ, DiGabriele AD, Hendrickson WA: Structural interactions of fibroblast growth factor receptor with its ligands, *Proc Natl Acad Sci USA* 97:49, 2000.

423. Venkataraman G et al: Molecular characteristics of fibroblast growth factor-fibroblast growth factor receptor-heparin-like glycosaminoglycan complex, *Proc Natl Acad Sci USA* 96:3658, 1999.

424. Smith JA, Winslow DP, Rudland PS: Different growth factors stimulate cell division of rat mammary epithelial, myoepithelial, and stromal cell lines in culture, *J Cell Physiol* 119:320, 1984.

425. Thomas KA et al: Pure brain-derived acidic fibroblast growth factor is a potent angiogenic vascular endothelial cell mitogen with sequence homology to interleukin 1, *Proc Natl Acad Sci USA* 82:6409, 1985.

426. Rudland PS: Stem cells and the development of mammary cancers in experimental rats and in humans, *Cancer Metastasis Rev* 6:55, 1987.

427. Rogelj S et al: Basic fibroblast growth factor fused to a signal peptide transforms cells, *Nature* 331:173, 1988.

428. Sasada R et al: Transformation of mouse BALB/c 3T3 cells with human basic fibroblast growth factor cDNA, *Mol Cell Biol* 8:588, 1988.

429. Souttou B, Hamelin R, Crepin M: FGF2 as an autocrine growth factor for immortal human breast epithelial cells, *Cell Growth Differ* 5:615, 1994.

430. Dickson C et al: Tumorigenesis by mouse mammary tumor virus: proviral activation of a cellular gene in the common integration region *int-2*, *Cell* 37:529, 1984.

431. Hajitou A et al: Progression in MCF-7 breast cancer cell tumorigenicity: compared effect of FGF-3 and FGF-4, *Breast Cancer Res Treat* 60:15, 2000.

432. Delli BP et al: An oncogene isolated by transfection of Kaposi's sarcoma DNA encodes a growth factor that is a member of the FGF family, *Cell* 50:729, 1987.

433. Sakamoto H et al: Transforming gene from human stomach cancers and a noncancerous portion of stomach mucosa, *Proc Natl Acad Sci USA* 83:3997, 1986.

434. Coleman-Krnacik S, Rosen JM: Differential temporal and spatial gene expression of fibroblast growth factor family members during mouse mammary gland development, *Mol Endocrinol* 8:218, 1994.

435. Kern FG et al: Transfected MCF-7 cells as a model for breast-cancer progression, *Breast Cancer Res Treat* 31:153, 1994.

436. McLeskey SW et al: Fibroblast growth factor 4 transfection of MCF-7 cells produces cell lines that are tumorigenic and metastatic in ovariectomized or tamoxifen-treated athymic nude mice, *Cancer Res* 53:2168, 1993.

437. Yoshimura N et al: The expression and localization of fibroblast growth factor-1 (FGF-1) and FGF receptor-1 (FGFR-1) in human breast cancer, *Clin Immunol Immunopathol* 89:28, 1998.

438. Bansal GS et al: Expression of fibroblast growth factor 1 is lower in breast cancer than in the normal human breast, *Br J Cancer* 72:1420, 1995.

439. Blanckaert VD et al: Basic fibroblast growth factor receptors and their prognostic value in human breast cancer, *Clin Cancer Res* 4:2939, 1998.

440. Blanckaert VD et al: Distribution and prognostic value of the fibroblast growth factor-2 low-affinity binding sites in human breast cancer, *Anticancer Res* 20:3913, 2000.

441. Korah RM et al: Basic fibroblast growth factor confers a less malignant phenotype in MDA-MB-231 human breast cancer cells, *Cancer Res* 60:733, 2000.

442. Smith K et al: Upregulation of basic fibroblast growth factor in breast carcinoma and its relationship to vascular density, oestrogen receptor, epidermal growth factor receptor and survival, *Ann Oncol* 10:707, 1999.

443. Yiangou C et al: Fibroblast growth factor 2 in breast cancer: occurrence and prognostic significance, *Br J Cancer* 75:28, 1997.

444. Marsh SK et al: Increased expression of fibroblast growth factor 8 in human breast cancer, *Oncogene* 18:1053, 1999.

445. Tanaka A et al: High frequency of fibroblast growth factor (FGF) 8 expression in clinical prostate cancers and breast tissues, immunohistochemically demonstrated by a newly established neutralizing monoclonal antibody against FGF 8, *Cancer Res* 58:2053, 1998.

446. Ruohola JK et al: Enhanced invasion and tumor growth of fibroblast growth factor 8b-overexpressing MCF-7 human breast cancer cells, *Cancer Res* 61:4229, 2001.

447. Adnane J et al: BEK and FLG, two receptors to members of the FGF family, are amplified in subsets of human breast cancers, *Oncogene* 6:659, 1991.

448. McLeskey SW et al: MDA-MB-134 breast carcinoma cells overexpress fibroblast growth factor (FGF) receptors and are growth-inhibited by FGF ligands, *Cancer Res* 54:523, 1994.

449. Champeme MH et al: Int-2/FGF3 amplification is a better independent predictor of relapse than c-myc and c-erbB-2/neu amplifications in primary human breast cancer, *Mod Pathol* 7:900, 1994.

450. Katoh M: *WNT* and *FGF* gene clusters, *Int J Oncol* 21:1269, 2002 (review).

451. Sporn MB et al: Some recent advances in the chemistry and biology of transforming growth factor-beta, *J Cell Biol* 105:1039, 1987.

452. Wrann M et al: T cell suppressor factor from human glioblastoma cells is a 12.5-kd protein closely related to transforming growth factor-beta, *EMBO J* 6:1633, 1987.

453. Padgett RW et al: A transcript from a Drosophila pattern gene predicts a protein homologous to the transforming growth factor-beta family, *Nature* 325:81, 1987.

454. Chakrabarty S et al: Induction of carcinoembryonic antigen secretion and modulation of protein secretion/expression

and fibronectin/laminin expression in human colon carcinoma cells by transforming growth factor-beta, *Cancer Res* 48:4059, 1988.

455. Ignotz RA, Massague J: Cell adhesion protein receptors as targets for transforming growth factor-beta action, *Cell* 51:189, 1987.

456. Tucker RF et al: Growth inhibitor from BSC-1 cells closely related to platelet type beta transforming growth factor, *Science* 226:705, 1984.

457. McCune BK et al: Localization of transforming growth factor-beta isotypes in lesions of the human breast, *Hum Pathol* 23:13, 1992.

458. Sairenji M et al: Transforming growth factor activity in pleural and peritoneal effusions from cancer and noncancer patients, *Jpn J Cancer Res* 78:814, 1987.

459. Wakefield LM et al: Roles for transforming growth factors-beta in the genesis, prevention, and treatment of breast cancer, *Cancer Treat Res* 61:97, 1992.

460. Wrana JL et al: Mechanism of activation of the TGF-beta receptor, *Nature* 370:341, 1994.

461. Mieth M et al: Transforming growth factor-beta inhibits lactogenic hormone induction of beta-casein expression in HC11 mouse mammary epithelial cells, *Growth Factors* 4:9, 1990.

462. Stampfer MR et al: TGF beta induction of extracellular matrix associated proteins in normal and transformed human mammary epithelial cells in culture is independent of growth effects, *J Cell Physiol* 155:210, 1993.

463. Arteaga CL et al: Anti-transforming growth factor (TGF)-beta antibodies inhibit breast cancer cell tumorigenicity and increase mouse spleen natural killer cell activity: implications for a possible role of tumor cell/host TGF-beta interactions in human breast cancer progression, *J Clin Invest* 92:2569, 1993.

464. Travers MT et al: Growth factor expression in normal, benign, and malignant breast tissue, *BMJ (Clin Res Ed)* 296:1621, 1988.

465. Zugmaier G et al: Transforming growth factor beta 1 induces cachexia and systemic fibrosis without an antitumor effect in nude mice, *Cancer Res* 51:3590, 1991.

466. Welch DR, Fabra A, Nakajima M: Transforming growth factor beta stimulates mammary adenocarcinoma cell invasion and metastatic potential, *Proc Natl Acad Sci USA* 87:7678, 1990.

467. Cheifetz S et al: The transforming growth factor-beta system, a complex pattern of cross-reactive ligands and receptors, *Cell* 48:409, 1987.

468. Ikeda T, Lioubin MN, Marquardt H: Human transforming growth factor type beta 2: production by a prostatic adenocarcinoma cell line, purification, and initial characterization, *Biochemistry* 26:2406, 1987.

469. Segarini PR et al: Membrane binding characteristics of two forms of transforming growth factor-beta, *J Biol Chem* 262:14655, 1987.

470. Ohta M et al: Two forms of transforming growth factor-beta distinguished by multipotential haematopoietic progenitor cells, *Nature* 329:539, 1987.

471. Knabbe C et al: Evidence that transforming growth factor-beta is a hormonally regulated negative growth factor in human breast cancer cells, *Cell* 48:417, 1987.

472. Zugmaier G et al: Transforming growth factors type beta 1 and beta 2 are equipotent growth inhibitors of human breast cancer cell lines, *J Cell Physiol* 141:353, 1989.

473. Valverius EM et al: Production of and responsiveness to transforming growth factor-beta in normal and oncogene-transformed human mammary epithelial cells, *Cancer Res* 49:6269, 1989.

474. O'Brien SJ et al: Dispersion of the ras family of transforming genes to four different chromosomes in man, *Nature* 302:839, 1983.

475. Ryan J et al: Chromosomal assignment of a family of human oncogenes, *Proc Natl Acad Sci USA* 80:4460, 1983.

476. Hall A et al: Identification of transforming gene in two human sarcoma cell lines as a new member of the *ras* gene family located on chromosome 1, *Nature* 303:396, 1983.

477. Lowe DG et al: Structure of the human and murine R-ras genes, novel genes closely related to ras proto-oncogenes, *Cell* 48:137, 1987.

478. DeFeo-Jones D et al: *ras*-related gene sequences identified and isolated from Saccharomyces cerevisiae, *Nature* 306:707, 1983.

479. Kataoka T et al: Genetic analysis of yeast *RAS1* and *RAS2* genes, *Cell* 37:437, 1984.

480. Tatchell K et al: Requirement of either of a pair of ras-related genes of Saccharomyces cerevisiae for spore viability, *Nature* 309:523, 1984.

481. Powers S et al: Genes in *S. cerevisiae* encoding proteins with domains homologous to the mammalian ras proteins, *Cell* 36:607, 1984.

482. Marais R et al: Ras recruits Raf-1 to the plasma membrane for activation by tyrosine phosphorylation, *EMBO J* 14:3136, 1995.

483. Marshall MS: Ras target proteins in eukaryotic cells, *FASEB J* 9:1311, 1995.

484. Russell M, Lange-Carter CA, Johnson GL: Direct interaction between Ras and the kinase domain of mitogen-activated protein kinase kinase kinase (MEKK1), *J Biol Chem* 270:11757, 1995.

485. Chang EH et al: Tumorigenic transformation of mammalian cells induced by a normal human gene homologous to the oncogene of Harvey murine sarcoma virus, *Nature* 297:479, 1982.

486. Krontiris TG et al: An association between the risk of cancer and mutations in the *HRAS1* minisatellite locus, *N Engl J Med* 329:517, 1993.

487. Krontiris TG: Minisatellites and human disease, *Science* 269:1682, 1995.

488. Kraus MH, Yuasa Y, Aaronson SA: A position 12-activated *H-ras* oncogene in all HS578T mammary carcinosarcoma cells but not normal mammary cells of the same patient, *Proc Natl Acad Sci USA* 81:5384, 1984.

489. Prosperi MT et al: Point mutation at codon 12 of the *Ki-ras* gene in a primary breast carcinoma and the MDA-MB-134 human mammary carcinoma cell line, *Cancer Lett* 51:169, 1990.

490. Kozma SC et al: The human *c-Kirsten ras* gene is activated by a novel mutation in codon 13 in the breast carcinoma cell line MDA-MB231, *Nucleic Acids Res* 15:5963, 1987.

491. Lidereau R et al: High frequency of rare alleles of the human *c-Ha-ras-1* proto-oncogene in breast cancer patients, *J Natl Cancer Inst* 77:697, 1986.

492. Greig RG et al: Tumorigenic and metastatic properties of "normal" and ras-transfected NIH/3T3 cells, *Proc Natl Acad Sci USA* 82:3698, 1985.

493. Dickson RB, Lippman ME: Growth factors in breast cancer, *Endocr Rev* 16:559, 1995.

494. Salomon DS et al: Loss of growth responsiveness to epidermal growth factor and enhanced production of alpha-transforming growth factors in ras-transformed mouse mammary epithelial cells, *J Cell Physiol* 130:397, 1987.

495. Stenman G et al: Transfection with plasmid pSV2gptEJ induces chromosome rearrangements in CHEF cells, *Proc Natl Acad Sci USA* 84:184, 1987.

496. Kasid A et al: Transfection of v-rasH DNA into MCF-7 human breast cancer cells bypasses dependence on estrogen for tumorigenicity, *Science* 228:725, 1985.

497. Albini A et al: 17 beta-estradiol regulates and v-Ha-ras transfection constitutively enhances MCF7 breast cancer cell interactions with basement membrane, *Proc Natl Acad Sci USA* 83:8182, 1986.

498. Dickson RB et al: Activation of growth factor secretion in tumorigenic states of breast cancer induced by 17 beta-estradiol or *v-Ha-ras* oncogene, *Proc Natl Acad Sci USA* 84:837, 1987.

499. Kasid A, Knabbe C, Lippman ME: Effect of *v-rasH* oncogene transfection on estrogen-independent tumorigenicity of estrogen-dependent human breast cancer cells, *Cancer Res* 47:5733, 1987.

500. Ohuchi N et al: Expression of the 21,000 molecular weight ras protein in a spectrum of benign and malignant human mammary tissues, *Cancer Res* 46:2511, 1986.

501. Agnantis NJ et al: Comparative study of Harvey-*ras* oncogene expression with conventional clinicopathologic parameters of breast cancer, *Oncology* 43:36, 1986.

502. Clair T, Miller WR, Cho-Chung YS: Prognostic significance of the expression of a ras protein with a molecular weight of 21,000 by human breast cancer, *Cancer Res* 47:5290, 1987.

503. Spandidos DA, Agnantis NJ: Human malignant tumours of the breast, as compared to their respective normal tissue, have elevated expression of the Harvey *ras* oncogene, *Anticancer Res* 4:269, 1984.

504. Theillet C et al: Loss of a *c-H-ras-1* allele and aggressive human primary breast carcinomas, *Cancer Res* 46:4776, 1986.

505. DeBortoli ME et al: Amplified expression of p21 ras protein in hormone-dependent mammary carcinomas of humans and rodents, *Biochem Biophys Res Commun* 127:699, 1985.

506. Hand PH et al: Monoclonal antibodies of predefined specificity detect activated *ras* gene expression in human mammary and colon carcinomas, *Proc Natl Acad Sci USA* 81:5227, 1984.

507. Tanaka T et al: Expression of p21 ras oncoproteins in human cancers, *Cancer Res* 46:1465, 1986.

508. Kasperczyk A, DiMartino NA, Krontiris TG: Minisatellite allele diversification: the origin of rare alleles at the *HRAS1* locus, *Am J Hum Genet* 47:854, 1990.

509. Roussel M et al: Three new types of viral oncogene of cellular origin specific for haematopoietic cell transformation, *Nature* 281:452, 1979.

510. Hayward WS, Neel BG, Astrin SM: Activation of a cellular *onc* gene by promoter insertion in ALV-induced lymphoid leukosis, *Nature* 290:475, 1981.

511. Neel BG et al: Two human c-onc genes are located on the long arm of chromosome 8, *Proc Natl Acad Sci USA* 79:7842, 1982.

512. Adams JM et al: Cellular *myc* oncogene is altered by chromosome translocation to an immunoglobulin locus in murine plasmacytomas and is rearranged similarly in human Burkitt lymphomas, *Proc Natl Acad Sci USA* 80:1982, 1983.

513. Croce CM et al: Transcriptional activation of an unrearranged and untranslocated *c-myc* oncogene by translocation of a C lambda locus in Burkitt, *Proc Natl Acad Sci USA* 80:6922, 1983.

514. Dalla-Favera R et al: Human *c-myc onc* gene is located on the region of chromosome 8 that is translocated in Burkitt lymphoma cells, *Proc Natl Acad Sci USA* 79:7824, 1982.

515. Dalla-Favera R et al: Translocation and rearrangements of the *c-myc* oncogene locus in human undifferentiated B-cell lymphomas, *Science* 219:963, 1983.

516. Abrams HD, Rohrschneider LR, Eisenman RN: Nuclear location of the putative transforming protein of avian myelocytomatosis virus, *Cell* 29:427, 1982.

517. Jones N: Structure and function of transcription factors, *Semin Cancer Biol* 1:5, 1990.

518. Meichle A, Philipp A, Eilers M: The functions of Myc proteins, *Biochim Biophys Acta* 1114:129, 1992.

519. Prendergast GC, Lawe D, Ziff EB: Association of Myn, the murine homolog of max, with c-Myc stimulates methylation-sensitive DNA binding and ras cotransformation, *Cell* 65:395, 1991.

520. Kelekar A, Cole MD: Immortalization by c-myc, H-ras, and Ela oncogenes induces differential cellular gene expression and growth factor responses, *Mol Cell Biol* 7:3899, 1987.

521. Leof EB, Proper JA, Moses HL: Modulation of transforming growth factor type beta action by activated ras and c-myc, *Mol Cell Biol* 7:2649, 1987.

522. Stern DF et al: Differential responsiveness of myc- and ras-transfected cells to growth factors: selective stimulation of myc-transfected cells by epidermal growth factor, *Mol Cell Biol* 6:870, 1986.

523. Li Q, Dang CV: c-Myc overexpression uncouples DNA replication from mitosis, *Mol Cell Biol* 19:5339, 1999.

524. Sheen JH, Dickson RB: Overexpression of c-Myc alters G(1)/S arrest following ionizing radiation, *Mol Cell Biol* 22:1819, 2002.

525. Taylor C, Mai S: c-Myc-associated genomic instability of the dihydrofolate reductase locus in vivo, *Cancer Detect Prev* 22:350, 1998.

526. Vafa O et al: c-Myc can induce DNA damage, increase reactive oxygen species, and mitigate *p53* function: a mechanism for oncogene-induced genetic instability, *Mol Cell* 9:1031, 2002.

527. Schwab M et al: Amplified DNA with limited homology to *myc* cellular oncogene is shared by human neuroblastoma cell lines and a neuroblastoma tumour, *Nature* 305:245, 1983.

528. Nau MM et al: *L-myc*, a new *myc*-related gene amplified and expressed in human small cell lung cancer, *Nature* 318:69, 1985.

529. Kozbor D, Croce CM: Amplification of the *c-myc* oncogene in one of five human breast carcinoma cell lines, *Cancer Res* 44:438, 1984.

530. Modjtahedi N et al: Increased level of amplification of the *c-myc* oncogene in tumors induced in nude mice by a human breast carcinoma cell line, *Cancer Res* 45:4372, 1985.

531. Hurlin PJ et al: The Max transcription factor network: involvement of Mad in differentiation and an approach to identification of target genes, *Cold Spring Harb Symp Quant Biol* 59:109, 1994.

532. Rustgi AK, Dyson N, Bernards R: Amino-terminal domains of c-myc and N-myc proteins mediate binding to the retinoblastoma gene product, *Nature* 352:541, 1991.

533. Facchini LM, Penn LZ: The molecular role of Myc in growth and transformation: recent discoveries lead to new insights, *FASEB J* 12:633, 1998.

534. Henriksson M, Luscher B: Proteins of the Myc network: essential regulators of cell growth and differentiation, *Adv Cancer Res* 68:109, 1996.

535. Xiao Q et al: Transactivation-defective c-MycS retains the ability to regulate proliferation and apoptosis, *Genes Dev* 12:3803, 1998.

536. Hermeking H et al: Identification of CDK4 as a target of c-MYC, *Proc Natl Acad Sci USA* 97:2229, 2000.

537. Daksis JI et al: Myc induces cyclin D1 expression in the absence of de novo protein synthesis and links mitogen-stimulated signal transduction to the cell cycle, *Oncogene* 9:3635, 1994.

538. Perez-Roger I et al: Cyclins D1 and D2 mediate myc-induced proliferation via sequestration of *p27(Kip1)* and *p21(Cip1)*, *EMBO J* 18:5310, 1999.

539. Marhin WW et al: Myc represses the growth arrest gene *gadd45*, *Oncogene* 14:2825, 1997.

540. Mitchell KO, El Deiry WS: Overexpression of c-Myc inhibits *p21WAF1/CIP1* expression and induces S-phase entry in 12-O-tetradecanoylphorbol-13-acetate (TPA)-sensitive human cancer cells, *Cell Growth Differ* 10:223, 1999.

541. Greenberg RA et al: Telomerase reverse transcriptase gene is a direct target of *c-Myc* but is not functionally equivalent in cellular transformation, *Oncogene* 18:1219, 1999.

542. Liao DJ, Dickson RB: c-myc in breast cancer, *Endocrine-Related Cancer* 7:143, 2000.

543. Eisenman RN, Thompson CB: Oncogenes with potential nuclear function: myc, myb and fos, *Cancer Surv* 5:309, 1986.

544. Croce CM: Role of chromosome translocations in human neoplasia, *Cell* 49:155, 1987.

545. Varmus H, Bishop JM: Biochemical mechanisms of oncogene activity: proteins encoded by oncogenes—introduction, *Cancer Surv* 5:153, 1986.

546. Mariani-Costantini R et al: In situ c-myc expression and genomic status of the c-myc locus in infiltrating ductal carcinomas of the breast, *Cancer Res* 48:199, 1988.

547. Adnane J et al: Proto-oncogene amplification and human breast tumor phenotype, *Oncogene* 4:1389, 1989.

548. Bonilla M et al: In vivo amplification and rearrangement of *c-myc* oncogene in human breast tumors, *J Natl Cancer Inst* 80:665, 1988.

549. Brouillet JP et al: Cathepsin D assay in primary breast cancer and lymph nodes: relationship with *c-myc, c-erb-B-2* and *int-2* oncogene amplification and node invasiveness, *Eur J Cancer* 26:437, 1990.

550. Donovan-Peluso M et al: Oncogene amplification in breast cancer, *Am J Pathol* 138:835, 1991.

551. Garcia I et al: Genetic alterations of *c-myc, c-erbB-2,* and *c-Ha-ras* protooncogenes and clinical associations in human breast carcinomas, *Cancer Res* 49:6675, 1989.

552. Guerin M et al: Overexpression of either *c-myc* or *c-erbB-2/neu* proto-oncogenes in human breast carcinomas: correlation with poor prognosis, *Oncogene Res* 3:21, 1988.

553. Nagle RB et al: Cytokeratin characterization of human prostatic carcinoma and its derived cell lines, *Cancer Res* 47:281, 1987.

554. Tsuda H et al: Alterations in copy number of *c-erbB-2* and *c-myc* proto-oncogenes in advanced stage of human breast cancer, *Acta Pathol Jpn* 41:19, 1991.

555. Varley JM et al: Alterations to either *c-erbB-2(neu)* or *c-myc* proto-oncogenes in breast carcinomas correlate with poor short-term prognosis, *Oncogene* 1:423, 1987.

556. Berns EM et al: Prognostic factors in human primary breast cancer: comparison of c-myc and HER2/neu amplification, *J Steroid Biochem Mol Biol* 43:13, 1992.

557. Berns EM et al: C-myc amplification is a better prognostic factor than HER2/neu amplification in primary breast cancer, *Cancer Res* 52:1107, 1992.

558. Spandidos DA et al: Elevated expression of the *myc* gene in human benign and malignant breast lesions compared to normal tissue, *Anticancer Res* 7:1299, 1987.

559. Whittaker JL, Walker RA, Varley JM: Differential expression of cellular oncogenes in benign and malignant human breast tissue, *Int J Cancer* 38:651, 1986.

560. Deming SL et al: C-myc amplification in breast cancer: a meta-analysis of its occurrence and prognostic relevance, *Br J Cancer* 83:1688, 2000.

561. Borg A et al: C-myc amplification is an independent prognostic factor in postmenopausal breast cancer, *Int J Cancer* 51:687, 1992.

562. Mimori K et al: Expression of ornithine decarboxylase mRNA and c-myc mRNA in breast tumours, *Int J Oncol* 12:597, 1998.

563. Pertschuk LP et al: Steroid hormone receptor immunohistochemistry and amplification of *c-myc* protooncogene: relationship to disease-free survival in breast cancer, *Cancer* 71:162, 1993.

564. Roux-Dosseto M et al: C-myc gene amplification in selected node-negative breast cancer patients correlates with high rate of early relapse, *Eur J Cancer* 28A:1600, 1992.

565. Scorilas A et al: Determination of *c-myc* amplification and overexpression in breast cancer patients: evaluation of its prognostic value against *c-erbB-2*, cathepsin-D and clinico-pathological characteristics using univariate and multivariate analysis, *Br J Cancer* 81:1385, 1999.

566. Bieche I et al: Quantitation of *MYC* gene expression in sporadic breast tumors with a real-time reverse transcription-PCR assay, *Cancer Res* 59:2759, 1999.

567. Pietilainen T et al: Expression of c-myc proteins in breast cancer as related to established prognostic factors and survival, *Anticancer Res* 15:959, 1995.

568. Mizukami Y et al: Immunohistochemical study of oncogene product *ras p21, c-myc* and growth factor EGF in breast carcinomas, *Anticancer Res* 11:1485, 1991.

569. Spaventi R et al: Immunohistochemical detection of TGF-alpha, EGF-R, c-erbB-2, c-H-ras, c-myc, estrogen and progesterone in benign and malignant human breast lesions: a concomitant expression, *In Vivo* 8:183, 1994.

570. Wang Q et al: *BRCA1* binds c-Myc and inhibits its transcriptional and transforming activity in cells, *Oncogene* 17:1939, 1998.

571. Ghosh AK et al: PTEN transcriptionally modulates *c-myc* gene expression in human breast carcinoma cells and is involved in cell growth regulation, *Gene* 235:85, 1999.

572. Hyder SM, Stancel GM, Loose-Mitchell DS: Steroid hormone-induced expression of oncogene encoded nuclear proteins, *Crit Rev Eukaryot Gene Expr* 4:55, 1994.

573. Schuchard M et al: Steroid hormone regulation of nuclear proto-oncogenes, *Endocr Rev* 14:659, 1993.

574. Dubik D, Shiu RP: Mechanism of estrogen activation of *c-myc* oncogene expression, *Oncogene* 7:1587, 1992.

575. Le RX et al: Decrease of *c-erbB-2* and *c-myc* RNA levels in tamoxifen-treated breast cancer, *Oncogene* 6:431, 1991.

576. Wong MS, Murphy LC: Differential regulation of c-myc by progestins and antiestrogens in T-47D human breast cancer cells, *J Steroid Biochem Mol Biol* 39:39, 1991.

577. Alkhalaf M, Murphy LC: Regulation of c-jun and jun-B by progestins in T-47D human breast cancer cells, *Mol Endocrinol* 6:1625, 1992.

578. Angel P, Karin M: The role of Jun, Fos and the AP-1 complex in cell-proliferation and transformation, *Biochim Biophys Acta* 1072:129, 1991.

579. Jensen EV: Studies of growth phenomenon using tritium-labeled steroids, *Proceedings of the 4th International Congress of Biochemistry* 15:119, 1958.

580. Jensen EV, DeSombre ER: Mechanism of action of the female sex hormones, *Annu Rev Biochem* 41:203, 1972.

581. Zava DT, McGuire WL: Estrogen receptor: unoccupied sites in nuclei of a breast tumor cell line, *J Biol Chem* 252:3703, 1977.

582. Edwards DP et al: Subcellular compartmentalization of estrogen receptors in human breast cancer cells, *Exp Cell Res* 127:197, 1980.

583. King WJ, Greene GL: Monoclonal antibodies localize oestrogen receptor in the nuclei of target cells, *Nature* 307:745, 1984.

584. Welshons WV, Lieberman ME, Gorski J: Nuclear localization of unoccupied oestrogen receptors, *Nature* 307:747, 1984.

585. Caruso JA, Laird DW, Batist G: Role of HSP90 in mediating cross-talk between the estrogen receptor and the Ah receptor signal transduction pathways, *Biochem Pharmacol* 58:1395, 1999.

586. Passinen S et al: The C-terminal half of Hsp90 is responsible for its cytoplasmic localization, *Eur J Biochem* 268:5337, 2001.

587. Schuh S et al: A 90,000-dalton binding protein common to both steroid receptors and the Rous sarcoma virus transforming protein, pp60v-src, *J Biol Chem* 260:14292, 1985.

588. Kousteni S et al: Nongenotropic, sex-nonspecific signaling through the estrogen or androgen receptors: dissociation from transcriptional activity, *Cell* 104:719, 2001.

589. Razandi M, Pedram A, Levin ER: Plasma membrane estrogen receptors signal to antiapoptosis in breast cancer, *Mol Endocrinol* 14:1434, 2000.

590. Gu Q, Korach KS, Moss RL: Rapid action of 17beta-estradiol on kainate-induced currents in hippocampal neurons lacking intracellular estrogen receptors, *Endocrinology* 140:660, 1999.

591. Kumar V et al: Localisation of the oestradiol-binding and putative DNA-binding domains of the human oestrogen receptor, *EMBO J* 5:2231, 1986.

592. Druege PM et al: Introduction of estrogen-responsiveness into mammalian cell lines, *Nucleic Acids Res* 14:9329, 1986.

593. Walter P et al: Cloning of the human estrogen receptor cDNA, *Proc Natl Acad Sci USA* 82:7889, 1985.

594. Migliaccio A, Rotondi A, Auricchio F: Calmodulin-stimulated phosphorylation of 17beta-estradiol receptor on tyrosine, *Proc Natl Acad Sci USA* 81:5921, 1984.

595. Migliaccio A, Rotondi A, Auricchio F: Estradiol receptor: phosphorylation on tyrosine in uterus and interaction with anti-phosphotyrosine antibody, *EMBO J* 5:2867, 1986.

596. Auricchio F et al: Regulation of hormone binding of 17B-estradiol receptor by phosphorylation-dephosphorylation of receptor on tyrosine. In Auricchio F (ed): *Sex steroid receptors*, Rome, 1985, Field Educational Italia Acta Medica.

597. Fleming H, Blumenthal R, Gurpide E: Rapid changes in specific estrogen binding elicited by cGMP or cAMP in cytosol from human endometrial cells, *Proc Natl Acad Sci USA* 80:2486, 1983.

598. Knabbe CK et al: Phorbol ester induced phosphorylation of the estrogen receptor in intact MCF-7 human breast cancer cells, *Fed Proc* 45:1899, 1986.

599. Darbon JM, Valette A, Bayard F: Phorbol esters inhibit the proliferation of MCF-7 cells: possible implication of protein kinase C, *Biochem Pharmacol* 35:2683, 1986.

600. Greene GL, Jensen EV: Monoclonal antibodies as probes for estrogen receptor detection and characterization, *J Steroid Biochem* 16:353, 1986.

601. Raam S, Vrabel DM: Evaluation of an enzyme immunoassay kit for estrogen receptor measurements, *Clin Chem* 32:1496, 1986.

602. Di Fronzo G et al: Relationship between ER-ICA and conventional steroid receptor assays in human breast cancer, *Breast Cancer Res Treat* 8:35, 1986.

603. McCarty KS Jr et al: Estrogen receptor analyses: correlation of biochemical and immunohistochemical methods using monoclonal antireceptor antibodies, *Arch Pathol Lab Med* 109:716, 1985.

604. Elliston JF et al: Ketononestrol aziridine, an agonistic estrogen receptor affinity label: study of its bioactivity and estrogen receptor covalent labeling, *Endocrinology* 121:667, 1987.

605. Monsma FJ Jr et al: Characterization of the estrogen receptor and its dynamics in MCF-7 human breast cancer cells using a covalently attaching antiestrogen, *Endocrinology* 115:143, 1984.

606. Katzenellenbogen BS et al: Structural analysis of covalently labeled estrogen receptors by limited proteolysis and monoclonal antibody reactivity, *Biochemistry* 26:2364, 1987.

607. Schwabe JW et al: The crystal structure of the estrogen receptor DNA-binding domain bound to DNA: how receptors discriminate between their response elements, *Cell* 75:567, 1993.

608. Schwabe JW, Neuhaus D, Rhodes D: Solution structure of the DNA-binding domain of the oestrogen receptor, *Nature* 348:458, 1990.

609. Shiau AK et al: The structural basis of estrogen receptor/coactivator recognition and the antagonism of this interaction by tamoxifen, *Cell* 95:927, 1998.

610. McInerney EM et al: Determinants of coactivator LXXLL motif specificity in nuclear receptor transcriptional activation, *Genes Dev* 12:3357, 1998.

611. Smith CL et al: CREB binding protein acts synergistically with steroid receptor coactivator-1 to enhance steroid receptor-dependent transcription, *Proc Natl Acad Sci USA* 93:8884, 1996.

612. Kim MY, Hsiao SJ, Kraus WL: A role for coactivators and histone acetylation in estrogen receptor alpha-mediated transcription initiation, *EMBO J* 20:6084, 2001.

613. Skipper JK et al: Identification of an isoform of the estrogen receptor messenger RNA lacking exon four and present in the brain, *Proc Natl Acad Sci USA* 90:7172, 1993.

614. Kuiper GG et al: Cloning of a novel receptor expressed in rat prostate and ovary, *Proc Natl Acad Sci USA* 93:5925, 1996.

615. Giguere V, Tremblay A, Tremblay GB: Estrogen receptor beta: re-evaluation of estrogen and antiestrogen signaling, *Steroids* 63:335, 1998.

616. Shughrue PJ, Lane MV, Merchenthaler I: Comparative distribution of estrogen receptor-alpha and -beta mRNA in the rat central nervous system, *J Comp Neurol* 388:507, 1997.

617. Mosselman S, Polman J, Dijkema R: ER beta: identification and characterization of a novel human estrogen receptor, *FEBS Lett* 392:49, 1996.

618. Pace P et al: Human estrogen receptor beta binds DNA in a manner similar to and dimerizes with estrogen receptor alpha, *J Biol Chem* 272:25832, 1997.

619. Hanstein B et al: Functional analysis of a novel estrogen receptor-beta isoform, *Mol Endocrinol* 13:129, 1999.

620. Ogawa S et al: Molecular cloning and characterization of human estrogen receptor betacx: a potential inhibitor of estrogen action in human, *Nucleic Acids Res* 26:3505, 1998.

621. Hall JM, McDonnell DP: The estrogen receptor beta-isoform (ERbeta) of the human estrogen receptor modulates ERalpha transcriptional activity and is a key regulator of the cellular response to estrogens and antiestrogens, *Endocrinology* 140:5566, 1999.

622. Palmieri C et al: Estrogen receptor beta in breast cancer, *Endocr Relat Cancer* 9:1, 2002.

623. Tora L et al: The human estrogen receptor has two independent nonacidic transcriptional activation functions, *Cell* 59:477, 1989.

624. Anzick SL et al: AIB1, a steroid receptor coactivator amplified in breast and ovarian cancer, *Science* 277:965, 1997.

625. Bautista S et al: In breast cancer, amplification of the steroid receptor coactivator gene *AIB1* is correlated with estrogen and progesterone receptor positivity, *Clin Cancer Res* 4:2925, 1998.

626. List HJ et al: Expression of the nuclear coactivator *AIB1* in normal and malignant breast tissue, *Breast Cancer Res Treat* 68:21, 2001.

627. Reiter R, Wellstein A, Riegel AT: An isoform of the coactivator *AIB1* that increases hormone and growth factor sensitivity is overexpressed in breast cancer, *J Biol Chem* 276:39736, 2001.

628. Planas-Silva MD et al: *AIB1* enhances estrogen-dependent induction of cyclin D1 expression, *Cancer Res* 61:3858, 2001.

629. Osborne CK et al: The estrogen receptor coactivator *AIB1* (*SRC3*) in combination with *HER-2* is a prognostic and predictive marker in patients with breast cancer, *Proc Am Soc Clin Oncol* 21:33a, 2002.

630. Horwitz KB, McGuire WL: Estrogen control of progesterone receptor in human breast cancer: correlation with nuclear processing of estrogen receptor, *J Biol Chem* 253:2223, 1978.

631. Chalbos D, Rochefort H: Dual effects of the progestin R5020 on proteins released by the T47D human breast cancer cells, *J Biol Chem* 259:1231, 1984.

632. Reiner GC, Katzenellenbogen BS: Characterization of estrogen and progesterone receptors and the dissociated regulation of growth and progesterone receptor stimulation by estrogen in MDA-MB-134 human breast cancer cells, *Cancer Res* 46:1124, 1986.

633. Lippman ME: Endocrine responsive cancers of man. In Williams RH (ed): *Textbook of endocrinology*, Philadelphia, 1985, WB Saunders.

634. Nardulli AM et al: Regulation of progesterone receptor messenger ribonucleic acid and protein levels in MCF-7 cells by estradiol: analysis of estrogen's effect on progesterone receptor synthesis and degradation, *Endocrinology* 122:935, 1988.

635. Read LD et al: Ligand-modulated regulation of progesterone receptor messenger ribonucleic acid and protein in human breast cancer cell lines, *Mol Endocrinol* 2:263, 1988.

636. Wei LL, Miner R: Evidence for the existence of a third progesterone receptor protein in human breast cancer cell line T47D, *Cancer Res* 54:340, 1994.

637. Beck C, Edwards D: Progesterone receptor in breast cancer. In Dickson R, Lippman ME, (eds): *Genes, oncogenes, and hormones*, Boston, 1992, Kluwer.

638. Horowitz KB: Hormone resistance in breast cancer: the role of normal and mutant steroid receptors. In Dickson R, Lippman ME (eds): *Mammary tumorigenesis and malignant progression*, Boston, 1994, Kluwer.

639. Smith DF, Toft DO: Steroid receptors and their associated proteins, *Mol Endocrinol* 7:4, 1993.

640. Tung L et al: Antagonist-occupied human progesterone B-receptors activate transcription without binding to progesterone response elements and are dominantly inhibited by A-receptors, *Mol Endocrinol* 7:1256, 1993.

641. McDonnell DP et al: Analysis of estrogen receptor function in vitro reveals three distinct classes of antiestrogens, *Mol Endocrinol* 9:659, 1995.

642. Elledge RM, McGuire WL, Osborne CK: Prognostic factors in breast cancer, *Semin Oncol* 19:244, 1992.

643. Allegra JC, Lippman ME: Estrogen receptor status and the disease-free interval in breast cancer, *Recent Results Cancer Res* 71:20, 1980.

26

Concepts and Mechanisms of Breast Cancer Metastasis

JANET E. PRICE

Chapter Outline

Once breast cancer has been diagnosed, the most important question is whether the cancer is confined to the breast or has spread to distant sites. The prognosis for recurrence and death after treatment of primary breast cancer is related to the disease stage and the presence of axillary lymph node metastases at the time of diagnosis. The general understanding of the pathogenesis of metastasis has increased considerably in the last two decades, but comparable improvements in the treatment of metastatic disease have, for the most part, not yet been realized. Most deaths of women with breast cancer result from the growth of metastases that are nonresponsive to therapy. A major obstacle to the successful treatment of metastatic disease is that the cancer cells in primary and secondary tumors are biologically heterogeneous, consisting of many different subpopulations, with a range of genetic, biochemical, immunologic, and biologic characteristics, including sensitivities to therapeutic agents.[1-5] The development of more effective therapies for metastatic breast cancer should be based on a better understanding of the mechanisms responsible for the spread of cells from the breast to distant sites, plus an appreciation of the consequences of tumor heterogeneity. This chapter discusses some of the recent findings on mechanisms of metastasis that are relevant to metastatic breast cancer.

Pathogenesis of Metastasis

To establish metastases in distant organs, cancer cells must complete a sequence of steps, each of which may be described as rate limiting (Figure 26-1). Failure to complete any of the steps will abort the process. The cells that do survive may represent selected populations of cells, and numerous experimental studies have shown that the cells recovered from metastases have enhanced metastatic capabilities compared with the original populations of cells. The metastatic potential depends on intrinsic properties of the tumor cells and their interactions with elements of the tissue environment. The essential steps in the formation of a metastasis are essentially similar for all solid tumors and consist of the following:

1. *Proliferation* of the tumor cells is supported by growth factors from the tissue environment (paracrine growth) or from the tumor cells themselves (autocrine growth). Overexpression of the tyrosine kinase receptors, such as epidermal growth factor receptor (EGFR) and *c-erbB-2*/HER2/*neu* may give the malignant cells a growth advantage, and some breast cancer cells are reported to overexpress the ligands transforming growth factor (TGF)-α and heregulin (HRG), respectively.

2. *Neovascularization* or *angiogenesis* is necessary for the continued growth of a tumor of greater than 1 to 2 mm^3. This is made possible by new blood vessel growth, promoted by angiogenic factors released by tumor cells and local stromal tissues. The balance between angiogenic promoters and inhibitors controls the establishment of a new capillary network, originating from surrounding vessels.

3. Some tumor cells show reduced or no expression of cohesive molecules, contributing to increased *motility* and therefore increasing the likelihood of detachment and movement away from the primary tumor.

4. *Invasion* from the primary tumor is a complex process involving destruction of basement membranes and connective tissues, adhesion, and motility in response to paracrine or autocrine motility factors.

5. Distant metastasis requires the entry of cancer cells into blood or lymphatic vessels, potentially leading to *dissemination* throughout the body as single cells or emboli.

6. The emboli can *arrest* in draining lymph nodes or organ capillary beds and may adhere to the endothelial cells or to exposed subendothelial basement membrane.

7. Some of the cells *extravasate*, using similar mechanisms as those for invasion of the vessels; however, extravasation is not required because some cancer cells can proliferate actively within the vessel lumen.

8. *Growth* in the new organ site, as for the original primary tumor, depends on responses to paracrine or autocrine factors and the establishment of a vascular network. Once established, a metastatic lesion can serve as the source of more metastases, that is, the phenomenon of "metastasis of metastases."

The time course of the events of metastasis can vary greatly. The survival of cells in the circulation may be relatively brief; experimental studies using various methods of labeling cancer cells that were then injected into appropriate host animals have shown that the cells can reach a potential metastasis site within minutes.[6] However, once metastases are established in a distant site, the growth rates of different metastases are highly variable. The risk of recurrence for patients with breast cancer is highest in the first 2 years after diagnosis and initial treatment, but some metastases can remain dormant for many years after apparently successful treatment.[7] The mechanisms underlying the dormancy are unknown, although recent experimental studies suggest that this may be linked to the control of angiogenesis.[8]

ANGIOGENESIS AND METASTASIS

Angiogenesis is required for the growth of primary and metastatic tumors.[9,10] The angiogenic process is mediated by factors released by malignant and normal cells in the

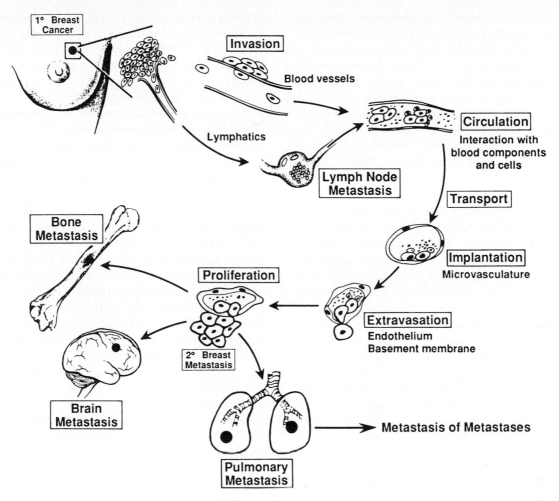

FIG. **26-1** The pathogenesis of breast cancer metastasis. The process of breast cancer metastasis is sequential and requires that metastatic cells complete all steps of the highly selective events.

microenvironment that can promote or inhibit the outgrowth of endothelial cells from established vessels. The capillary sprouts arise from the division of microvascular endothelial cells and migration of cells toward the source of the angiogenic molecules, requiring invasion and penetration of the stromal tissues. Endothelial cells undergoing sprouting express matrix-degrading proteases, including those of the matrix metalloproteinase (MMP) family and urokinase plasminogen activator (uPA). Molecules that inhibit MMP activity have been found to have antiangiogenic activity and are capable of impeding tumor growth and metastasis in preclinical models.[11] Counting the numbers and density of microscopic blood vessels in sections of breast cancer specimens has been used as a measure of angiogenesis,[12] using antibodies against endothelial markers such as factor VIII related antigen, CD34, CD105, and the integrin heterodimer $\alpha v \beta 3$ to identify the new blood vessels. Increased microvessel density is associated with a poor prognosis in most published reports.[13,14]

Breast cancer cells can release a variety of angiogenic factors, including members of the fibroblast growth factor family (FGF-1 and FGF-2), vascular endothelial growth factors (VEGFs), platelet-derived endothelial cell growth factor (PD-ECGF, also known as *thymidine phosphorylase*), interleukin (IL)-8, angiopoietins, platelet-derived growth factors (PDGFs), and TGF-α and TGF-β.[15-20] Normal cells within the tissue environment, such as endothelial cells, epithelial cells, mast cells, and leukocytes, can also release proangiogenic factors. Macrophage infiltration into invasive breast cancers can be elevated in the highly angiogenic tumors,[21] with the tumor-associated macrophages (TAMs) clustered in areas of central necrosis. TAMs can release angiogenic factors such as VEGF and tumor necrosis factor (TNF)-α, and proteolytic enzymes that activate profactors or release factors sequestered in the extracellular matrix. The appearance of necrosis in angiogenic tumors may result from the growth of the tumor cells outpacing the ingrowth of new blood vessels. Hypoxic conditions, resulting from focal ischemia, can upregulate expression of angiogenic factors, including VEGF and IL-8. Necrosis and the presence of TAMs have been shown to be indicators of aggressive phenotype of invasive breast cancers.[22]

Five members of the VEGF family have been described: types A, B, C, D, and E,[23,24] with VEGF-A most commonly being reported as an important angiogenic factor associated with poor prognosis for patients with breast cancer.[25] VEGF-A, present in four major isoforms resulting from alternate splicing, binds and activates the Flk-1/KDR-1 tyrosine kinase receptor on endothelial cells. There are some reports also of VEGF receptors on breast cancer cells, suggesting a possible autocrine mechanism.[26] VEGF-B binds to the flt-1/VEGFR-1 tyrosine kinase receptor, and in endothelial cells this has been shown to increase the expression and activity of uPA and plasminogen activator 1 (PAI-1).[27] In a study of VEGF-B levels in breast tissues, there was no significant relationship between the presence of the factor and tumor vascularity; however, there was a significant relationship with the numbers of lymph nodes with metastases.[28] VEGF-B may contribute to cancer progression by playing a role in the regulation of matrix degradation and cell adhesion of endothelial cells undergoing angiogenesis and vascular remodeling.[27] VEGF-C and VEGF-D have been associated with lymphangiogenesis, and both factors bind to the lymphatic endothelial cell receptor flt-4/VEGFR-3. Binding to the VEGFR-2 receptors requires proteolytic processing of these factors and can promote proliferation and migration of endothelial cells. VEGF-C is a growth factor for lymphatic vascular endothelium and stimulates lymphangiogenesis in chorioallantoic membrane assays. Measurements of VEGF-C RNA in tissue specimens have shown a correlation with metastasis to lymph nodes of patients with breast cancer.[29] Experimental studies demonstrated that introduction of VEGF-C into breast cancer cell lines resulted in increased intratumor lymphangiogenesis and promoted the growth and metastasis of the xenografts in immunodeficient mice.[30] VEGF-D also promotes tumor lymphangiogenesis and metastatic spread of experimental tumors via lymphatics.[31] Currently, there are relatively few reports on the expression of VEGF-D in breast cancer specimens. Kurebayashi and colleagues[29] detected VEGF-D expression only in inflammatory breast cancer (a primary specimen and an inflammatory metastasis). Evidence to date therefore suggests that VEGF-C and VEGF-D, through promotion of lymphangiogenesis, play a role in the malignant progression of breast cancer.

The significance of VEGF expression can vary depending on the histologic type of the breast cancer. A study by Lee and colleagues[32] found higher VEGF expression in invasive ductal carcinoma than in invasive lobular carcinoma. VEGF expression correlated with vessel density in the invasive ductal carcinoma specimens but not in the invasive lobular carcinomas; a different factor, or repertoire of angiogenic factors, is presumably important for promoting angiogenesis in invasive lobular carcinoma.

Angiogenesis is determined by the balance between promoters and inhibitors of new blood vessel growth. A variety of endogenous antiangiogenic molecules have been identified, including angiostatin, endostatin, thrombospondin (TSP-1), interferon-alfa and IL-12.[24] In normal tissues an inhibitory influence may predominate and the activation of an "angiogenic switch" may be required for the further growth of the cancer cells or to allow release from a dormant state. Systemic administration of angiostatin, a fragment of plasminogen, was shown to restrict the growth and metastasis of human and rodent cancers in experimental models and induce dormancy of micrometastatic foci.[8] In a transgenic mouse model of pancreatic carcinogenesis, a key component of the angiogenic switch was matrix metalloproteinase (MMP)-9, acting potentially through increased proteolytic release of VEGF-A sequestered in extracellular matrix.[33] For cultured cells isolated from patients with Li-Fraumeni syndrome the switch to an angiogenic phenotype coincided with the loss of the wild-type allele of the p53 tumor-suppressor gene, resulting in reduction of TSP-1.[34] Enforced expression of TSP-1 in the human breast cancer cell line MDA-MB-435 was found to reduce tumor growth and metastasis in immunodeficient mice, in part as a consequence of impaired angiogenesis.[35] The status of p53 may also influence angiogenesis, for example through modulation of expression of bFGF and VEGF.[36,37] The mutation status of p53 and accumulation of p53 protein in breast cancer specimens are recognized as prognostic indicators.[38] This important gene can influence many different aspects of the malignant phenotype, and one of these may be the control of angiogenesis.

INVASION

Breast cancer cell invasion through the basement membranes of ducts and lobules can result in cells entering vascular and lymphatic vessels. The penetration of basement membranes and connective tissues of the breast is mediated by the synthesis of degradative enzymes by normal and neoplastic cells in the microenvironment.[11,39] There are four major groups of proteases: (1) MMPs, collagenases, gelatinases, stromelysin; (2) cysteine proteases (cathepsin B, H, L); (3) aspartyl proteases (cathepsin D); and (4) serine proteases (i.e., plasminogen activators [uPA, tPA] and the activated product plasmin). Several inhibitory molecules have been identified, including the tissue inhibitors of metalloproteinase (TIMP-1, TIMP-2, and

TIMP-3) and plasminogen activator inhibitors (PAI-1 and PAI-2). Proteolytic activity represents a balance between the proteolytic enzymes, activators of the enzymes (e.g., the membrane type MMPs), and the inhibitory molecules. The expression of proteases is normally under the control of cytokines and growth factors such as PDGF, TGF-β, amphiregulin, EGF interferons, IL-4, and IL-6. Estrogen and progesterone can also regulate proteolytic enzyme expression and the invasive potential of breast cancer cells.[40]

Data from in vitro and experimental studies provide evidence for the role of two MMPs that degrade the collagen type IV of basement membranes, MMP-2 and MMP-9, in invasion and metastasis. Metastatic clones of heterogeneous tumors often express elevated levels of these enzymes, and the introduction of an inhibitory molecule can reduce invasive and metastatic ability. TIMP-1 can bind to and inhibit the activity of MMP-9, and TIMP-2 complexes with the latent and active forms of MMP-2. The expression levels of MMP-2, MMP-3, MMP-9, uPA, TIMP-1, and TIMP-2 were found to be elevated in breast cancer samples compared with normal tissue, and the total proteolytic activity was higher in the neoplastic samples.[41] Activated forms of MMP-2 or MMP-9 can be detected in urine and indicate organ-confined and metastatic disease of various human cancers, within and outside the urinary tract.[42] Although protease production by tumor cells is implicated in invasion, many proteases are also produced by stromal cells, in addition to the malignant epithelial cells. The net increase in protease activity in tumor tissue samples may be a function of induction of stromal cell expression of the proteases, in response to tumor-derived factors such as cytokines and extracellular matrix metalloproteinase inducer (EMMPRIN).[43,44] Immunolocalization of different components of the MMP system point to the important role of the membrane-type MMPs (MT1, MT2, and MT3-MMP) in activating MMP-2 and facilitating the invasion and clinical progression of invasive breast cancers.[45] Invasive lobular cancers were shown to express more abundant MMP-9 than invasive ductal cancers. Colocalization of MT1-MMP and MMP-2 in both types of invasive cancer was significantly associated with the presence of lymph node metastases.[46]

There is increasing recognition that the contributions of the MMP-system and uPA system to tumor progression go beyond the dissolution of barriers constraining cancer cell invasion. In addition to the degradation of extracellular matrix (ECM) and basement membranes, other actions of proteases are cleavage and activation of growth factors (e.g., latent TGF-β) and other factors that act as angiogenic factors (VEGF-C and two forms of PDGF [C and D]), which are activated or have enhanced binding to receptors after proteolytic activation.[11,47,48] Release and activation of the factors can affect the growth of the tumor, increasing local availability of growth factors to the tumor cells and to stromal cells, including the endothelial cells forming the new blood supply essential for continued tumor growth.

CELL-TO-CELL COHESION AND MOTILITY

Most tumor cells possess the cytoplasmic machinery that is necessary for active locomotion, and increased tumor cell motility is preceded by a loss of cell-to-cell cohesion. Members of the cadherin family of cell-surface glycoproteins are essential for cell-cell adhesion and maintenance of tissue integrity.[49] Cadherins are linked to the actin cytoskeleton via association with the cytoplasmic catenins α, β, and γ. β-Catenin is also involved in the Wnt-1 signaling pathway and gene transcription through interactions with the TCF-1/LEF transcription factor.[50] For many epithelial cancers the loss of contact is associated with the loss of expression of one of the cadherin family members, E-cadherin. In experimental studies the enforced expression of E-cadherin in highly malignant cells has been shown to reduce or inhibit the invasive and metastatic abilities.[51,52] Analyses of breast cancers show that loss or reduced expression of E-cadherin and catenins can correlate with a poor prognosis.[53,54] The gene is located on chromosome 16q22.1, an area of frequent loss of heterozygosity in sporadic breast cancers. Loss of E-cadherin is more common in specimens of lobular carcinoma than ductal carcinoma, which more generally show patchy expression. For the lobular types, loss of E-cadherin expression has been linked to LOH and somatic mutation in the remaining allele. No such mutations have been reported in ductal carcinomas (or cell lines derived from ductal tumors), and reduced expression is thought to be related to epigenetic changes, including promoter hypermethylation or repression by the Snail transcription factor.[49,55] In contrast, E-cadherin expression is reported to be maintained in inflammatory breast cancer, therefore showing an exception to the more general observation of loss of this molecule and poor prognosis.[56]

Tumor cell motility is an active process dependent on the release of motility-promoting factors and activation of receptors. Motility and migration of normal and malignant cells can be promoted by cytokines released by other cells in the tissue environment[57] or by the cancer cells. Autocrine motility factor (AMF) is a protein produced by malignant cells that binds to its own surface receptor and that can stimulate motility and metastatic properties in experimental systems.[58] AMF was shown to be increased in breast cancer cells exposed to heregulin β1, a ligand for two tyrosine kinase receptors commonly expressed in breast cancer that promotes invasion and migration.[59] Another factor that promotes motility is hepatocyte growth factor (HGF), also known as *scatter factor* (SF), which binds to c-met, a member of the tyrosine kinase family of cell-surface receptors. Higher expression of c-met has been reported as an independent predictor of decreased survival for women with invasive ductal breast carcinoma.[60] HGF is released by mesenchymal/stromal cells and also by epithelial cells. There are reports of coexpression of HGF and the c-met receptor in breast carcinomas, suggesting a potential autocrine mechanism of promoting motility.[61] Signaling through c-met has also been associated with enhanced survival from DNA-damaging agents and increased angiogenesis, hence contributing to survival of the metastatic cells.[62]

A recent report identified chemokine receptors as potential players in determining patterns of breast cancer metastasis. Chemokines, cytokine-like proteins, and their G protein–coupled receptors can direct the homing of hematopoietic cells, and the experimental data point to tumor cells using a similar mechanism. The chemokine receptors CXCR4 and CXCR7 were found on breast cancer tissues and cell lines. The respective ligands CXCL12/SDF-1α and CCL21/6Ckine were detected at highest levels in organs where breast cancer cells can form metastases, such as bone marrow, lymph nodes, and the lungs. Treatment with an antibody to CXCR4 blocked motility and invasion in vitro and metastasis of human breast cancer cells to lymph nodes and lungs of severe combined immunodeficient (SCID) mice.[63] Thus interfering with chemokine receptors, and blocking the cancer cell interaction with organ-derived chemokines, may be another approach for inhibiting metastasis.

CELL-TO-CELL ADHESION

Adhesion of tumor cells to other tumor cells (homotypic adhesion) or other cell types (heterotypic adhesion) is considered an essential step in the formation of metastases. Experimental studies have shown that the arrest of tumor emboli is more efficient than the arrest of single cells in capillary networks of organs such as the lungs.[64] Numerous molecules that can facilitate heterotypic adhesions and adhesion to extracellular matrix have been identified and can be classified into the general categories of cadherins, selectins, immunoglobulin-like cell adhesion molecules (CAMs), and integrins. Aberrant or dysregulated expression of many of these and other molecules, including CD44 and the 66kDa laminin receptor, have been reported in breast and other epithelial cancers.[65-72] Initial binding of tumor cells to capillary endothelial cells under flow conditions is mediated by selectin molecules, followed by more stable integrin-mediated binding and subsequent migration through the subendothelial basement membrane.[73] Experimental studies have shown increased expression of the α6β1 or αvβ3 integrins on human breast cancer cells that can metastasize in immunodeficient mice.[74,75] Interference with integrin binding, with a fragment of fibronectin or a snake venom–derived disintegrin, can diminish the growth and metastasis of the same breast cancer cells.[76,77] High expression of the αvβ3 integrin on invasive breast cancer and by endothelial cells within the tumors has directed efforts to target this molecule (e.g., with a monoclonal antibody against the integrin heterodimer) and can affect both tumor and stromal cells.[78]

LYMPHATIC METASTASIS

In the process of invasion from the primary lesion and through infiltration and expansion in the surrounding tissues, tumor cells can penetrate small lymphatic vessels. The spread of tumor cells via the lymphatics has been documented and studied for centuries. The presence of breast cancer cells in axillary lymph nodes has very high prognostic significance, yet surprisingly little is known about the mechanisms of lymphatic metastasis. In contrast to the vascular system, lymphatic capillaries lack a true basement membrane and thus may offer less resistance to penetration by tumor cells. Experimental models have shown that tumor cells can pass through gaps between lymphatic endothelial cells.[79] Recent studies have identified two related molecules, VEGF-C and VEGF-D, as mediators of interactions between tumor cells and lymphatic endothelial cells.[80] The enforced expression of either factor in experimental tumors was shown to increase lymphangiogenesis in the tumors and promote lymphatic metastasis.[30,31] Once inside the lymphatics, the tumor cells or emboli may be passively transported to arrest either in the first lymph node downstream or may bypass to more distal nodes. Cells within lymph nodes include B and T lymphocytes, macrophages, dendritic reticular cells, plasma cells, fibroblasts, and endothelial cells. Many of these can express growth factors and cytokines that can promote tumor growth, and there are few data to suggest that lymph nodes can serve as immunologic barriers, other than for eliminating small numbers of cells.[79] Experimental studies with rodent or rabbit tumors illustrated that lymph nodes can act as physical barriers to tumor cells traveling in lymphatics. However, tumor cells have also been found in venous effluent and lymphatic efferent vessels of lymph nodes with metastases. Hence, the lymph node metastases may be the source of hematogenous or further lymphatic spread.[81] Hellman[82] has proposed a "spectrum hypothesis," describing breast cancer as a spectrum of heterogeneous diseases, with increasing propensity to metastasize as tumors become more malignant through clinical evolution. His hypothesis proposes that the presence of lymph node metastases serves both as a marker of prognosis and as a source of additional metastases. The fact that lymphadenectomy does not affect overall survival may be a reflection of the systemic nature of the disease once lymph node metastasis has occurred. This has led to the use of lymphatic mapping to find the sentinel node in patients with breast cancer, similar to the techniques used in those with melanoma.[83] The sensitivity of sentinel node mapping for accurate staging has been shown to depend on the methods used to detect tumor cells within the node. Routine histopathology, immunohistochemistry, flow cytometry, and reverse transcription polymerase chain reaction (RT-PCR) are being used to detect microscopic or occult disease in the sentinel nodes. Data from such studies do not yet have sufficient follow-up to determine the prognostic significance of the microscopic disease on patient survival.[84]

HEMATOGENOUS METASTASIS

For hematogenous metastasis, tumor cells must survive transport in the circulation, arrest and form adhesions in small vessels and capillaries, and extravasate by invading through the vessel wall. The survival of a few cells may represent the selection of preexisting subpopulations of cells endowed with the properties required to form metastases. This principle has been proved in a variety of tumor types, rodent and human, from which more metastatic variants have been isolated by recovering cells that formed metastases in appropriate animal hosts (syngeneic or immunodeficient animals for human tumor studies).[64]

Death of cells within the circulation has been attributed to simple mechanical factors, most notably turbulence. Factors that contribute to the survival of cells in the circulation may include the propensity to form aggregates, either homotypic or heterotypic aggregates, with normal cells such as platelets or lymphocytes.[85,86] The ability of circulating tumor cells to deform in the microcirculation may also contribute to their ability to recirculate after initial lodgment in a capillary bed. Drugs that disrupt the cytoskeletal organization and modify the cell deformability can alter tumor cell arrest, detachment, and recirculation.[87] Components of the blood-clotting pathway may also contribute to metastatic process by trapping cells in capillaries or facilitating adherence of cells to vessel walls. Circulating tumor cells can be thromboplastic, and increased coagulability is commonly observed in patients with advanced cancers. There is good experimental evidence that fibrinolytic agents and inhibitors of platelet aggregation, such as prostacyclin, can reduce or inhibit hematogenous metastases in rodent models. However, clinical studies have yet to provide similarly convincing evidence that anticoagulant agents can effectively prevent or reduce bloodborne metastases.[88]

Once in the microcirculation, the metastatic cells interact with cells of the vascular endothelium. The interaction may begin as nonspecific lodging of the tumor cell or emboli, followed by formation of adhesions mediated by cell-surface molecules such as selectins and integrins, recognizing ligands on the endothelial cells and the subendothelial matrix.[72,89] Once bound to endothelial cells, tumor cells elicit endothelial cell retraction, resulting in the exposure of the basement membrane.[90] There is increasing evidence of phenotypic heterogeneity in capillary endothelial cells isolated from different organs and of endothelial cells populating tumors and metastases. The identification of "vascular addresses" by phage display techniques has been used to target therapy to lung metastases in experimental models.[91] Endothelial cell heterogeneity may also be a determinant of organ-specific metastasis, with tumor cells expressing a certain repertoire of cells' surface molecules being more likely to arrest and extravasate in capillaries of an organ with a particular vascular address.[92]

Extravasation of arrested tumor cells is thought to occur through mechanisms similar to those responsible for local invasion and release into the circulation. Tumor cells can penetrate the endothelial basement membrane or follow extravasating lymphocytes. Alternatively, the tumor cells can proliferate within the vessel and ultimately destroy the normal structure.[93] The invasion, survival, and growth of tumor cells in the metastatic site can be in response to factors present in the tissue or organ. Metastatic tumor cells can recognize and respond to organ-specific factors, whereas nonmetastatic counterparts fail to respond.[94,95] An example of one such factor, which differentially promoted the growth of tumor cells metastatic to lung or brain, was identified as transferrin.[96] Metastatic tumor cells were found to express more transferrin receptors than nonmetastatic cells.[97]

Recent developments in imaging technology have provided some further insights into steps of hematogenous metastasis. The basic concept of experimental in vivo videomicroscopy (IVVM) is to capture images of tumor cells within tissues and microcirculation in real time. The tumor cells being tracked need a distinguishing marker, either endogenous (e.g., melanin), a fluorescent label, or a genetically introduced marker such as green fluorescent protein. Fluorescent labeling was used to show that the rate of intravasation of cells at the site of primary implanted tumors distinguished metastatic from poorly metastatic rat mammary tumor cells, identifying this step as critical in determining the metastatic potential, at least of these tumors.[98] Chambers and colleagues[99] have included plastic microspheres with the test cell inoculum to develop an accounting technique and have shown that the survival of tumor cells within the circulation and arrest in the microcirculation is not such an inefficient process as has been previously proposed. The data from the IVVM using transplantable rodent tumors suggest that survival, arrest, and extravasation of metastatic and nonmetastatic or poorly metastatic cells in mouse liver is equally likely to occur. However, after extravasation, few of the poorly metastatic cells proliferate to form metastatic lesions; many cells persist in the tissue yet remain dormant.[99] Elimination of extravasated cells that do not become dormant may be the result of apoptosis. IVVM was used in another study to follow the fate of intravenously injected cells and showed that many of these cells underwent apoptosis in the lungs of the recipient animals within 24 to 48 hours.[100] The new imaging techniques may therefore help revise or refine the general understanding of different steps in the process of metastasis.

METASTASIS-RELATED GENES

Considering that the metastatic process should be viewed as a sequence of different events, it is not surprising that a variety of genes have been nominated as key players in determining the metastatic phenotype of breast cancer cells. Examples of breast cancer metastasis-associated genes include growth factor receptors (HER2/*neu* and EGFR), angiogenic factors, adhesion molecules such as E-cadherin, and degradative enzymes that facilitate invasion. An experimental approach used by many investigators is the identification of genes differentially expressed in metastatic versus nonmetastatic counterparts, using rodent or human tumor cells. A key point is that for optimal comparative analyses, the tumor samples should be isogenic (i.e., clones or variants of a single tumor) and vary only in the capacity for metastasis. Table 26-1 shows some examples of genes that have been implicated in the metastasis of breast cancer and for which there is experimental evidence for a potential mechanism to promote or reduce metastatic progression.

For some of these, measurements of protein in patient samples have been associated with the prognosis. An approach that has been used successfully to identify metastasis-suppressing genes is the introduction of single chromosomes into tumor cells and then the analysis of the phenotype of the resulting hybrid cells.[112] Table 26-2 identifies four genes found to have metastasis-suppressing activity in in vivo models of breast cancer. Clinical studies support the involvement of two of these in breast cancer progression (*nm23, KAI1*), with no information yet available on the other two genes. A concept emerging from studies of metastasis suppression is that of suppression of the growth and development of cells arrested in the metastatic site.[122] If so, this points to new approaches for checking the growth of metastases, which have disseminated before diagnosis and treatment of the primary tumor, by introducing agents that can reproduce the action of the suppressor gene product but with less systemic toxicity than standard antineoplastic drugs. Further information about what regulates the metastasis-associated and the metastasis-suppressor genes may identify ways to modify their expression. For example, promoter methylation can silence gene expression, and exposure of human breast cancer cells to the DNA methylation inhibitor 5-aza-2'-deoxycytidine has been reported to increase expression of *nm23* and suppress cell motility.[123]

Patterns of Metastasis

CLINICAL AND AUTOPSY FINDINGS

Clinical observations have shown that some cancers have a marked preference for metastasis in specific organs that is not necessarily related to the vascular anatomy, rate of blood flow, or the numbers of tumor cells that may arrive

TABLE 26-1 | Genes Associated with Breast Cancer Metastasis

GENE	ORIGIN	KNOWN OR PROPOSED MECHANISM	CLINICAL OBSERVATION	REFERENCES
S100A4	Upregulated in metastatic mammary tumors	Regulator of the cytoskeleton	Expression correlated with poor prognosis	101, 102
MTA-1	Differentially expressed in metastatic rat mammary tumors	Gene regulation	Gene present in node-positive breast cancers	103, 104
Osteopontin	Increased expression in metastatic clones of rat and human beast cancer	Extracellular phosphoprotein; interactions with integrins; protection from macrophagemediated killing	Elevated plasma levels associated with poor prognosis	105-107
bcl-2	Introduction into breast cancer cells conferred metastatic ability	Inhibitor of apoptosis	Expression associated with lymph node metastasis	108, 109
maspin	Reduced expression in cancer cells	Serine protease inhibitor	Reduced expression in metastatic breast cancer	110, 111

TABLE 26-2	Genes with Metastasis-Suppressing Function in Breast Cancer			
GENE	ORIGIN	KNOWN OR PROPOSED MECHANISM	CLINICAL OBSERVATIONS	REFERENCES
nm23	Differentially expressed, lost in metastatic melanoma cells	Control of cell cycle progression; protein phosphorylation; transcription	Reduced expression; absence correlated with poor prognosis	113, 114
KAI1	Chromosome hybrid studies: suppressor of prostate cancer metastasis	Tetraspanin; suggested roles in aggregation, motility, and invasion	Reduced expression in invasive breast cancers	115-117
KiSS1	Chromosome hybrid studies; suppressor of melanoma and breast cancer metastasis	Ligand for G protein–coupled receptor; inhibits invasion	—	118, 119
BRMS1	Isolated in metastasis-suppressed chromosome hybrids of breast cancer cells	Mediates gap junctional cell-cell communication; suppressed motility	—	120, 121

in the organ. In 1889 Stephen Paget[124] published an analysis of 735 autopsy records from women with breast cancer, and the nonrandom pattern of visceral metastases suggested that the process was not related to chance but rather that certain tumor cells ("seeds") had an affinity for the milieu provided by certain organs ("soils"). Studies with rodent tumors have demonstrated that the formation and anatomic locations of metastases are determined by host factors and tumor cell properties,[64] and the results have been proposed as experimental examples of Paget's seed and soil hypothesis.

The use of peritoneovenous shunts in patients with intransigent malignant ascites provided an opportunity to study some of the factors affecting metastatic spread in humans. The published studies on 29 patients with different primary tumors (the most common was ovarian carcinoma) reported that the peritoneovenous shunts gave good palliation with minimal complications. Autopsy findings from 15 patients reflected the clinical findings that the shunts did not promote widespread systemic metastasis because in only 8 of these 15 were metastases found in extraabdominal organs, whereas in the remaining 7 there was no evidence of metastasis. These results suggest that even though the tumor cells were introduced into the circulation, micrometastases formed only in some sites or did not form at all.[125,126] Thus the outcome of tumor cell dissemination is determined by both tumor cells and normal organ factors, as originally proposed by Paget.[124]

INFLUENCE OF THE ORGAN ENVIRONMENT ON METASTASIS: EXPERIMENTAL ANALYSES

Paget's hypothesis that the soil can determine whether metastases form, in combination with attributes of the metastatic cells, has been tested in various experimental rodent tumor systems and in human tumors transplanted into immunodeficient animals. Following the hematogenous distribution of radiolabeled tumor cells injected into suitable hosts has shown that cells reach the microvasculature of most organs sampled.[6,127,128] However, the proliferation of the cells occurs only in some organs. Some data from studies of metastasis-suppressor genes show that the mechanism may be growth arrest of cells in the microenvironment of the sites of metastasis, even though the growth of the primary tumor is not restricted.[122]

A model used for testing the seed and soil hypothesis was developed by Hart and Fidler, who used the B16 murine melanoma. The intravenous injection of these cells into syngeneic mice resulted in the growth of tumors in the lungs and also in fragments of ovary or lung previously grafted into the quadriceps femoris of the host mice. In contrast, no tumors formed in control grafts of kidney or at sites of surgical trauma. When radiolabeled cells were injected and the distribution patterns monitored, there were no differences between distribution to legs grafted with lung compared with the control grafts.[129] Thus the lungs (grafts or intact) provided a receptive organ for the proliferation of the few tumor cells that reached these sites.

The model of engrafting different tissues has been used recently to study aspects of organ-specific metastasis of human tumor cells, with grafts of human fetal tissue placed in SCID mice.[130,131] Injection of human prostate or lung tumors resulted in species- and tissue-specific patterns of metastasis, therefore providing systems for studying the tissue interactions involved in growth of human tumors in human tissues that may not be readily simulated with culture techniques. For example, the technique allowed analysis of mechanisms involved in the preferential homing of human prostate cancer cells to grafts of fetal bone but not to grafts of lung or intestine.[131] In vitro experiments have provided some insight into organ selectivity, by analyzing adhesion and/or growth of different tumors to cells or factors isolated from different organs. A model of human breast cancer cell interactions in tissue cultures revealed that cells isolated from primary tumors or tumor-involved lymph nodes bound preferentially to bone marrow stromal cells rather than to mammary fibroblasts, whereas epithelial cells isolated from benign or normal breast tissues revealed no preference for adhesion to the stromal cells.[132] For rodent tumors, the results of the in vitro models can provide correlates of the patterns of metastasis to different organs[94,133,134] and lead to the identification of factors found in the organs. For example, transferrin was shown to be a key lung-derived factor that promoted the growth of lung-metastatic rat mammary tumor cells.[96] In contrast, analysis of a muscle cell–conditioned medium identified adenosine as one of the active components restricting tumor cell growth, possibly accounting for the low incidence of metastasis in striated muscle.[135] The findings from these different studies provide further support for the hypothesis that elements within the organ microenvironment can modulate neoplastic proliferation and may therefore play a role in determining the distribution of metastases.[94,97]

Mechanisms of tumor growth modulation may be related to the homeostatic processes that control normal cell replication and regulate organ growth and repair. Metastatic tumor growth in areas of injury and wound repair has been documented clinically and in a number of experimental systems. One example is the promotion of mammary tumor metastases in the livers of rats following trauma to this organ, with no metastases seen in the noninjured animals.[136] In vitro assays have demonstrated that media from cultures of resorbing bones contain factors capable of modulating normal osteoblasts and also stimulating the proliferation of rodent and human breast tumor cells.[137] These results can be interpreted as the local effects of wound healing (which include neovascularization and tissue remodeling) being subverted to support the growth of cancer cells in the organ or tissue, possibly in a state of dormancy or slow proliferation since arrest in the site before the local injury.

The common sites for breast cancer metastasis, in addition to regional lymph nodes, are the lung, liver, brain, and bone, with this last site being the most commonly involved. Up to 80% of women with metastatic breast cancer may develop bone metastases.[138] Many of these are lytic lesions, and a variety of growth factors and cytokines released by cancer cells have been shown to promote the activation of osteoclasts, the cells primarily responsible for bone destruction. The destruction of bone is thought to release factors that may in turn promote the growth of cancer cells, creating a "vicious cycle."[139] Inhibitors of bone resorption, such as the bisphosphonates, can reduce the skeletal morbidity in women with advanced breast cancer.[140] The mechanism is thought to be primarily through impeding osteoclastic bone resorption. However, some experimental reports have suggested a direct inhibitory action of bisphosphonates on metastatic cells, preventing adhesion or inhibiting the activation of MMPs.[141] Analyses of clinical specimens and experimental metastatic systems have been used to delineate factors that contribute to the promotion of breast cancer metastasis in bone. An example of this is parathyroid hormone–related protein (PTHrP), which was identified as a factor responsible for hypercalcemia associated with malignancy. Clinical studies reported a high incidence of PTHrP expression in breast cancer bone metastases, with significantly lower expression in soft tissue metastases.[142] An experimental model for bone metastasis is the injection of cancer cells into the left ventricle of the heart of rodents, which can result in distribution of tumors in many organs, including bone. This model was used to demonstrate that antibodies to PTHrP reduced the extent of human breast cancer bone metastases.[143] The same model system demonstrated that TGF-β released from the matrix of resorbing bone can promote the expression of PTHrP by the cancer cells and that compromising the TGF-β receptor function in the cells reduced their potential for bone metastasis.[144] Thus interfering with components of the vicious cycle promoting bone destruction resulted in a reduction in the extent of bone metastasis. The effect of the local microenvironment may be highly significant for bone metastases. As noted previously, PTHrP expression was high in the samples of breast cancer bone metastases. However, an analysis of expression in the primary tumors did not find a correlation between PTHrP and the incidence of bone metastasis or the survival of breast cancer patients, suggesting that this measurement could not be used as a predictor of risk for bone metastasis.[145] Instead, the experimental findings may point to microenvironmental regulation of a factor that promotes osteoclast activation and bone destruction and that can enhance the growth of the breast cancer cells in the bone.

Within a tumor mass, individual cells are exposed to different microenvironments, as a function of the anatomic site, and to differences in concentrations of nutrients, oxygen growth factors, and other factors.[146] Microenvironmental factors are thought to have a major effect on the sensitivity of cancer cells to therapy, and hypoxia and low extracellular pH are two that have been studied extensively. Cells in chronically hypoxic cancers are growth inhibited and considered likely to be resistant to most anticancer drugs. Low extracellular pH can have the same effect on cell proliferation and thus compound the potential effects of chemotherapy drugs. In addition, there is increasing awareness that exposure to the stresses of hypoxia and low extracellular pH can alter gene expression in tumor cells, inducing expression of genes that can promote the survival of the cells, such as angiogenic factors or antiapoptotic factors.[147,148] Clinical observations suggest that responses of breast cancer metastases to chemotherapy are influenced by the anatomic location of the lesions, possibly related to differences in microenvironmental stresses.[149,150] Differential sensitivity to antineoplastic treatment of metastases in different locations may be a function of heterogeneity of the tumor population, with different clones metastasizing to different organs. However, the influence of the organ environment cannot be ignored. The results from experimental tumor models have demonstrated that the same tumor implanted in different organs can have different responses to a chemotherapeutic agent. For doxorubicin sensitivity this may be related to microenvironmental regulation of the *mdr* p-glycoprotein, which acts as a pump to export toxic drugs from the cells.[151] The sensitivity of mouse mammary tumor cells to different chemotherapy agents was assessed in vivo, comparing response in subcutaneous tumors with responses of cells in bone marrow, spleen, lungs, liver, and brain. The subcutaneous tumors were generally sensitive, whereas cells in liver and brain were less sensitive to alkylating agents. Sensitivity of cells in the bone marrow was variable for the different drugs tested, but the addition of an antiangiogenic combination (TNP-470/minocycline) markedly increased killing of the bone marrow metastases by cyclophosphamide.[152] Thus the microenvironment may contribute to the chemotherapy sensitivity of disseminated cancer cells, and altering an aspect of the normal stroma (in this example the vascular supply) can affect the response to chemotherapy. Understanding the impact of the microenvironment on sensitivity to different forms of therapy may identify important ways to improve the efficiency of eliminating metastatic cells.[153]

Cellular components of the tumor microenvironment also contribute to malignant progression. Growing tumors can be extensively infiltrated by lymphocytes, granulocytes, mast cells, and macrophages. Tumor-infiltrating macrophages can either destroy tumor cells or release factors that may promote the development of the tumor.[154,155] An example noted earlier is the macrophage infiltration of highly angiogenic invasive breast cancers, with potential of release of angiogenic factors by the macrophages.[21] Macrophages within mouse mammary tumors were shown to mediate the evolution of drug-resistant variants, and this effect was inhibited by oxygen radical scavengers.[156] Alternatively, highly metastatic mammary tumor cells escape such effects through reduced sensitivity to host effector

mechanisms. In some cases the highly metastatic cells are growth stimulated by the activated macrophages and were found to be more resistant to macrophage-mediated cytolysis than the poorly metastatic counterparts.[157] This may explain why highly metastatic breast cancer cells do not seem to be suppressed by host effector mechanisms. Inflammatory breast cancer is an aggressive form of locally advanced breast cancer that can be heavily infiltrated with host cells and usually has a very poor prognosis.[158]

Biologic Diversification and Heterogeneity of Metastatic Cancers

It is well established that individual cancers are composed of diverse cell populations that are heterogeneous for a variety of characteristics, including many of those once thought to be expressed homogeneously among tumor cells. The heterogeneous expression of such properties is thought to be passed on to progeny cells, at least for several generations. However, a number of factors, including microenvironmental factors, may modulate gene expression in different tumor cells. One aspect of tumor heterogeneity is the ability of one tumor cell population to influence the properties of others within the same tumor in such a way as to modify growth rates, metastatic properties, and sensitivity to chemotherapeutic agents.[1,159-162] Cellular heterogeneity is not unique to transformed cells, and normal cells and tissues can be heterogeneous for a variety of properties. However, the degree of cellular heterogeneity is often more pronounced in the malignant population than in the counterpart benign or normal tissue. Serial analysis of gene expression (SAGE) was applied to normal and malignant breast specimens, and one observation was that the normal cells showed the least variable gene expression profiles. In contrast, a high degree of diversity was found in the malignant tumor samples, although there were few genes universally upregulated in all tumors.[4]

Advances in DNA technology have introduced ways to identify the expression patterns of thousands of genes in breast cancer samples. The techniques have confirmed the high level of heterogeneity within and between different breast cancers. The characterization of 65 surgical breast cancer specimens by cDNA array analysis demonstrated many different gene profile phenotypes, including those of the normal cells within the tissue samples. This study used a hierarchical clustering method to group genes on the basis of similarities in expression patterns. Matched pairs of primary tumors and metastases from the same patient revealed overall similarities in expression of the groups of genes selected for analyses, suggesting that the molecular profile of the original tumor can be retained in the metastasis.[163] The results of another study of 117 primary invasive breast tumors from young women (<55 years) for microarray analyses were able to separate tumors into those with good versus poor prognosis profiles based on expression of groups of genes regulating cell cycle control, invasion, metastasis, and angiogenesis.[164] The challenge will be to distinguish the gene expression patterns within the heterogeneity of different tumors that are critical for the malignant progression from those that are epiphenomena of genetic instability and abnormalities in DNA repair. Advances in bioinformatics technologies will be essential to analyze the information that will obtained by using genomic and proteomic approaches to investigate breast cancer progression and prognosis.[165]

EVOLUTION OF HETEROGENEOUS NEOPLASMS

Most naturally occurring and induced neoplasms develop from the transformation and proliferation of single cells. Even in tumors in which the progeny of a single cell have diversified to heterogeneous cellular phenotypes, evidence of a clonal origin still exists. Clinical and histologic observations of tumors suggested to Foulds[166] that tumors undergo a series of changes during the course of the disease. For example, a mammary tumor that was initially diagnosed as being benign can over many months or years evolve into a malignant tumor. To explain the process of tumor evolution and progression, Nowell[167] suggested that acquired genetic variability within developing clones of tumors, combined with host selection pressures, can bring about the emergence of new clonal sublines of increased growth autonomy or malignancy. Tumor heterogeneity may be achieved because individual neoplasms display various rates of phenotypic diversification, yielding different combinations of cellular phenotypes. A benign tumor may be expected to show relatively less diversification when compared with a more malignant counterpart.[168] Studies with clonally derived populations of rodent tumors have shown that certain neoplasms had altered rates of phenotypic diversification, which may have been caused through tumor cell–tumor cell interactions that acted to stabilize the diversification within the tumor population.[3] *Phenotypic drift* and *dynamic heterogeneity* are terms used to describe changes in tumor cell properties, especially metastatic ability, which may occur more rapidly than predicated from gradual selection of diversified clones.[169,170] The more rapid changes may also be modulated by cell-cell interactions, as noted previously.[1,171,172]

One question addressed using clones of rodent and human tumors is whether metastatic variants have a growth advantage over nonmetastatic cells, such that over time the metastatic clones would constitute most cells in a tumor. One experimental approach used exploited the random integration of introduced foreign DNA molecules in the tumor cell genome as a way of generating clones with unique genetic tags, which were identified by Southern blotting. Mixed populations of tagged breast tumor cells were implanted in recipient mice and metastases recovered and analyzed to identify clones. The results from several studies were that of one or a few "growth dominant" clones emerging in both the primary and metastatic tumors.[173,174] A clinical study of clonality in breast cancer specimens used DNA ploidy analyses and immunohistochemistry for HER2/*neu* expression to assess heterogeneity. The results indicated that clonal majorities may be identified in metastases and that these clones can also be detected in the primary tumors.[175] Thus this is an example of selection of clones in metastatic tumors but not the complete dominance seen in experimental systems. This may be a function of the different ways of identifying the clones; a study of clonality of prostate tumors used *p53* mutations and found evidence of limited clonal expansion in the primary tumor yet significant clonal growth of cells with *p53* mutations in metastases.[176] However, mutations in *p53* can have significant impact on the malignant phenotype and have been linked to increased risk of relapse and metastasis in breast cancer.[38,177,177a-177c] The difference between using a "tag" that can modulate tumor cell phenotype and using an inert marker such as used in the experimental studies may be one reason for the apparent disparity in outcomes.

GENETIC AND EPIGENETIC INSTABILITY

The accumulation of genetic changes underlies malignant transformation and the progression and development of heterogeneity within tumor cell populations.[178-180] Evidence for the linkage of genetic alterations and malignant progression of tumors has come from examination of gross chromosomal alterations,[181,182] mitotic errors, and rates of spontaneous mutations in highly metastatic cells as compared with low-metastatic or nonmetastatic clones.[183] As tumors progress to the metastatic phenotype, the chromosomal alterations and karyotypic anomalies can become more complex.[184] Evidence from loss-of-heterozygosity (LOH) analyses revealed that genetic changes are relatively rare in hyperplastic breast epithelial cells; however, the incidence increases in putative premalignant lesions, with further increases in ductal carcinoma in situ (DCIS). Shared LOH profiles between synchronous DCIS and invasive breast cancers showed that the in situ neoplasms are a precursor of the invasive disease.[168] A similar conclusion was reached in studies using comparative genomic hybridization.[185]

Epigenetic modifications can also contribute to the high rates of cellular diversity found in many malignant populations. The epigenetic changes may be a function of various mechanisms, including DNA methylation,[186,187] posttranscriptional modifications, or other mechanisms that may be responsive to tumor microenvironments.[188,189] Methylation-specific polymerase chain reaction assays were used to show extensive methylation in the regulatory region of the estrogen receptor (ER)-α gene in ER-negative breast cancer specimens and cell lines. Some of the ER-positive samples also showed methylation in the promoter, resulting in phenotypic heterogeneity that may result in ER-positive tumors recurring as ER-negative tumors.[190] Heterogeneous expression of E-cadherin, the homotypic cell-cell adhesion molecule, can result from variation in methylation of the promoter region of the gene. Methylation changes were detected in samples of DCIS (i.e., an event before progression to the invasive disease). Analysis of breast cancer cells grown in culture, however, showed that the promoter methylation and E-cadherin expression can be variable, depending on conditions of growth, with methylation decreased and protein reexpression seen in cells cultured in spheroids requiring cell-cell adhesion. Thus this is an example of epigenetic plasticity, which can result in dynamic phenotypic heterogeneity, involving a gene important for the malignant progression of breast cancer.[55]

THE ORIGIN OF BIOLOGIC DIVERSITY IN METASTASES

Metastases proliferating in the same or different organs can exhibit heterogeneity in a variety of characteristics, such as capacity for further metastatic spread, hormone receptor expression, growth rates, and responses to chemotherapy.[64,191] This diversity could result from the process of tumor evolution and the influence of the organ environment.[192] Experimental studies have shown that many metastases have a clonal origin. One of these used x-irradiation of tumor cells to induce random chromosome breaks and rearrangements to generate unique karyotypic patterns, which served to identify different clones. When mixed populations were injected into mice and metastases recovered, the karyotype analyses showed that most metastases were the result of the outgrowth of single clones.[193] Analyses of breast cancer specimens have shown clonality in metastases[175,179,184]; however, some metastases develop additional genetic abnormalities, reflecting continuing diversification of the metastatic population by genetic and epigenetic mechanisms to create intralesional heterogeneity. The potential for different clonal origins of different metastases from a single primary tumor, plus the continued generation of heterogeneity in the different metastases, may contribute to differences in responses to therapy.

The Clinical Challenge of Metastatic Heterogeneity

A major obstacle to successful clinical management of established metastases may be the diversification and heterogeneity resulting from continuing evolution in response to microenvironmental signals or therapy.[194] Three areas for which tumor heterogeneity is of practical importance are the detection of disease with tumor markers or with monoclonal antibodies,[195] the design of screening procedures for novel therapies, and the use of therapies other than surgery.

HETEROGENEOUS RESPONSES TO THERAPY

There are many examples of differences in drug sensitivity among tumor cells in different human cancers, including melanoma, colon adenocarcinoma, breast carcinoma, lymphoma, and lung cancer. Of greater importance are differences in drug response between tumor cells from different metastases and from those of the primary tumor.[196] Similar to the heterogeneity in responses to chemotherapeutic agents, radiation sensitivities of cell populations in animal and human tumors are also heterogeneous.[197,198]

Although cytotoxicity or growth inhibition by a drug in vitro does not always correlate with drug sensitivity in vivo, the development of in vitro assays for tumor cell responses for the purpose of predicting the outcome of cancer therapy have been used extensively.[196,199] For these assays to be of greatest value they must use samples representative of the tumor population. The use of the tumor stem cell assay using clinical specimens was based on the rationale that drug sensitivity of the isolated cells might more accurately predict clinical response to antineoplastic agents than cells that have been maintained in tissue culture over prolonged serial passages. One consideration of the stem cell assays is that the isolation of cells from one region of a solid tumor, which could be zonally heterogeneous, coupled with low cloning efficiency of most human tumor cells may limit their use with some clinical samples. Other complications are that clonal interactions between different subpopulations of tumor cells may influence the drug sensitivities and that the cells that proliferate in such assays may not represent the highly malignant tumor populations that pose a risk for metastasis.[160,200,201]

Stimulation of the rate of formation of tumor cell variants by the restriction of subpopulation diversity may be an explanation for rapid evolution of cellular diversity within metastases.[197,202] Within the primary tumor, cell-cell interactions between different cell populations may act to impose relative phenotypic stability and thus put a check on the rate of emergence of new variants. However, in clonally derived metastases these interactions would be absent. Diversification may be unchecked, quickly converting the lesion to a heterogeneous population.[202] If a form of therapy could kill most cells in a heterogeneous tumor cell population, this could stimulate the formation of new tumor cell variants from the surviving, therapy-resistant subpopulations (iatrogenic stimulation of heterogeneity).[159] Interactions between breast cancer cells may be mediated by gap junctions, which can impose metabolic and electrical coupling between the cells. Once breast cancer cells progress from benign to malignant, gap junction coupling is lost, which may contribute to enhanced heterogeneity in the cell populations.[203] A function of the putative metastasis suppressor gene BRMS-1 is to mediate gap-junctional communication.[120]

The heterogeneous nature of responses of tumor cell populations to cytotoxic drugs or other treatment modalities, coupled with the iatrogenic stimulation of surviving tumor cell diversification, makes it unlikely that single or multiple treatment regimens will be able to kill all cells within a tumor, even if several agents are used simultaneously or sequentially. The use of repeated cycles of cytotoxic therapy with different agents followed by intervening recovery periods may result in the eventual emergence of highly resistant and increasingly malignant tumor populations. Theoretic improvements would include truncation of recovery periods to limit diversification of surviving tumor cell populations and inhibition of tumor cell diversification during recovery periods by cytostatic agents such as modulators of differentiation, hormones, growth factors, and vitamin analogs.[204]

Another approach to maximize the benefit of established chemotherapeutic drugs is to select the patients most likely to respond, based on expression of key genes in their tumors.[205] The results of numerous studies are beginning to show that some of the heterogeneously expressed genes in breast cancer may be used as predictors of response to therapy. For example, in a study of women with locally advanced breast cancer, the presence of certain mutations in the tumor-suppressor p53 gene were predictive of resistance to doxorubicin.[206] The development of agents targeting key molecules, selected on the basis of an association with poor prognosis, is also likely to improve therapeutic options and hopefully provide more target specificity. A prime example of the development of targeted therapy is the variety of different agents against the HER2/neu growth factor receptor. This receptor is expressed on normal cells but is overexpressed in a proportion of breast cancers, and high levels of expression have been associated with poor patient prognosis.[207] Clinical trials using the humanized monoclonal antibody against HER2/neu as a single agent have produced antitumor responses in 15% to 20% of women with metastatic breast cancer.[208] In combination therapy, the antibody appears to increase the efficacy of chemotherapy, resulting in higher objective response rates and prolongation of time to progression, duration of response, and overall survival.[209]

Other approaches targeting HER2/neu include gene therapy, the use of antisense, or vaccine strategies. DNA vaccines against the rodent equivalent of HER/neu have successfully inhibited the growth and metastasis of neu-expressing mammary tumors.[210] Although the HER2/neu gene product is a normal, albeit overexpressed, protein, measurable antibody and CD4-positive T-lymphocyte responses to this protein have been reported in patients with breast cancer and in those with ovarian cancer. This supports the concept that HER2 vaccine strategies may be successful in humans, using similar approaches to those used in experimental models of breast cancer.[211]

Conclusions

Metastasis of breast cancer is a highly selective process that appears to depend on both unique tumor cell phenotypes and normal host factors and should be interpreted in the context of the seed and soil hypothesis presented by Stephen Paget in 1889.[124] In breast and other cancers the contribution of regional lymph nodes and distant organ sites to the pathogenesis of metastasis has been recognized. Clinical and experimental data indicate that specific cellular mechanisms exist for tumor cell arrest and implantation, invasion, survival, and growth of metastatic cells in different organs. An important aspect of malignancy is the genetic and phenotypic instability of individual tumor cells and their ability to undergo diversification to form heterogeneous populations. Tumor diversification and heterogeneity appear to be driven by genetic and epigenetic events that can also be modulated by cell-cell interactions and elements in the tumor microenvironments. A better understanding of the molecular mechanisms regulating the process of breast cancer metastasis and of the complex interactions between the metastatic cells and the organ environment will provide a rational foundation for the design of more effective therapies for different cancers and new options for clinical management of metastatic cancer.

REFERENCES

1. Heppner GH: Cancer cell societies and tumor progression, Stem Cells 11:199, 1993.
2. Boyer CM et al: Heterogeneity of antigen expression in benign and malignant breast and ovarian epithelial cells, Int J Cancer 43:55, 1989.
3. Nicolson GL: Tumor cell instability, diversification, and progression to the metastatic phenotype: from oncogene to oncofetal expression, Cancer Res 47:1473, 1987.
4. Porter DA et al: A SAGE (serial analysis of gene expression) view of breast tumor progression, Cancer Res 61:5697, 2001.

5. Heimann R, Hellman S: Individual characterisation of the metastatic capacity of human breast carcinoma, *Eur J Cancer* 36:1631, 2000.

6. Price JE, Aukerman SL, Fidler IJ: Evidence that the process of murine melanoma metastasis is sequential and selective and contains stochastic elements, *Cancer Res* 46:5172, 1986.

7. Demicheli R et al: Time distribution of the recurrence risk for breast cancer patients undergoing mastectomy: further support about the concept of tumor dormancy, *Breast Cancer Res Treat* 41:177, 1996.

8. O'Reilly MS et al: Angiostatin induces and sustains dormancy of human primary tumors in mice, *Nat Med* 2:689, 1996.

9. Folkman J: Angiogenesis in cancer, vascular, rheumatoid and other disease, *Nat Med* 1:27, 1995.

10. Ellis LM, Fidler IJ: Angiogenesis and metastasis, *Eur J Cancer* 32A:2451, 1996.

11. Chang C, Werb Z: The many faces of metalloproteases: cell growth, invasion angiogenesis and metastasis, *Trends Cell Biol* 11:S35, 2001.

12. Weidner N, Folkman J: Tumor vascularity as a prognostic factor in cancer, *Important Adv Oncol* 26:167, 1996.

13. Weidner N et al: Tumor angiogenesis and metastasis: correlation in invasive breast carcinoma, *N Engl J Med* 324:1, 1991.

14. Gasparini G: Clinical significance of determination of surrogate markers of angiogenesis in breast cancer, *Crit Rev Oncol/Hematol* 37:97, 2001.

15. Coltrera MD et al: Expression of platelet-derived growth factor B-chain and the platelet-derived growth factor receptor β subunit in human breast tissue, *Cancer Res* 55:2703, 1995.

16. De Larco JE et al: A potential role for interleukin-8 in the metastatic phenotype of breast carcinoma cells, *Am J Pathol* 158:639, 2001.

17. De Jong JS et al: Expression of growth factors, growth inhibiting factors, and their receptors in invasive breast cancer. I. An inventory in search of autocrine and paracrine loops, *J Pathol* 184:44, 1998.

18. Brown LF et al: Vascular stroma formation in carcinoma in situ, invasive carcinoma, and metastatic carcinoma of the breast, *Clin Cancer Res* 5:1041, 1999.

19. Toi M et al: Vascular endothelial growth factor and platelet-derived endothelial cell growth factor are frequently coexpressed in highly vascularized human breast cancer, *Clin Cancer Res* 1:961, 1995.

20. Currie MJ et al: Angiopoietin-1 is inversely related to thymidine phosphorylase expression in human breast cancer, indicating a role in vascular remodeling, *Clin Cancer Res* 7:918, 2001.

21. Leek RD et al: Necrosis correlates with high vascular density and focal macrophage infiltration in invasive carcinoma of the breast, *Br J Cancer* 79:991, 1999.

22. Leek RD et al: Association of macrophage infiltration with angiogenesis and prognosis in invasive breast carcinoma, *Cancer Res* 56:4625, 1996.

23. Nicosia RF: What is the role of vascular endothelial growth factor-related molecules in tumor angiogenesis? *Am J Pathol* 153:11, 1998.

24. Hagedorn M, Bikfalvi A: Target molecules for anti-angiogenic therapy: from basic research to clinical trials, *Crit Rev Oncol/Hematol* 34:89, 2000.

25. Gasparini G, Pozza F, Harris AL: Evaluating the potential usefulness of new prognostic and predictive indicators in node-negative breast cancer patients, *J Natl Cancer Inst* 85:1206, 1993.

26. Soker S et al: Neuropilin-1 is expressed by endothelial and tumor cells as an isoform-specific receptor for vascular endothelial growth factor, *Cell* 92:735, 1998.

27. Olofsson B et al: Vascular endothelial growth factor B (VEGF-B) binds to VEGF receptor-1 and regulates plasminogen activator activity in endothelial cells, *Proc Natl Acad Sci USA* 95:11709, 1998.

28. Gunningham SP et al: VEGF-B expression in human primary breast cancers is associated with lymph node metastasis but not angiogenesis, *J Pathol* 193:325, 2001.

29. Kurebayashi J et al: Expression of vascular endothelial growth factor (VEGF) family members in breast cancer, *Jpn J Cancer Res* 90:977, 1999.

30. Skobe M et al: Induction of tumor lymphangiogenesis by VEGF-C promotes breast cancer metastasis, *Nat Med* 7:192, 2001.

31. Stacker SA et al: VEGF-D promotes the metastatic spread of tumor cells via the lymphatics, *Nat Med* 7:186, 2001.

32. Lee AHS et al: Invasive lobular and invasive ductal carcinoma of the breast show distinct patterns of vascular endothelial growth factor expression and angiogenesis, *J Pathol* 185:394, 1998.

33. Bergers G et al: Matrix metalloproteinase-9 triggers the angiogenic switch during carcinogenesis, *Nat Cell Biol* 2:737, 2000.

34. Damcron KM et al: Control of angiogenesis in fibroblasts by *p53* regulation of thrombospondin-1, *Science* 265:1582, 1994.

35. Weinstat-Saslow DL et al: Transfection of thrombospondin 1 complementary DNA into a human breast carcinoma cell line reduces primary tumor growth, metastatic potential and angiogenesis, *Cancer Res* 54:6504, 1994.

36. Ueba T et al: Transcriptional regulation of basic fibroblast growth factor gene by *p53* in human glioblastoma and hepatocellular carcinoma cells, *Proc Natl Acad Sci USA* 91:9009, 1994.

37. Koura AN et al: Regulation of genes associated with angiogenesis, growth and metastasis by specific *p53* point mutations in a murine melanoma cell line, *Oncol Rep* 4:475, 1997.

38. Silvestrini R et al: Validation of *p53* accumulation as a predictor of distant metastasis at 10 years of follow-up in 1400 node-negative breast cancers, *Clin Cancer Res* 2:2007, 1996.

39. Liotta LA, Kohn EA: The microenvironment of the tumour-host interface, *Nature* 411:375, 2001.

40. Van den Brule F et al: Genes involved in tumor invasion and metastasis are differentially modulated by estradiol and progestin in human breast cancer cells, *Int J Cancer* 52:653, 1992.

41. Garbett EA, Reed MW, Brown NJ: Proteolysis in human breast and colorectal cancer, *Br J Cancer* 81:287, 1999.

42. Moses MA et al: Increased incidence of matrix metalloproteinases in urine of cancer patients, *Cancer Res* 58:1395, 1998.

43. Heppner KJ et al: Expression of most matrix metalloproteinase family members in breast cancer represents a tumor-induced host response, *Am J Pathol* 149:273, 1996.

44. Sun J, Hemler ME: Regulation of MMP-1 and MMP-2 production through CD147/extracellular matrix metalloproteinase inducer interactions, *Cancer Res* 61:2276, 2001.

45. Ueno H et al: Expression and tissue localization of membrane-types 1, 2, and 3 matrix metalloproteinases in human invasive breast cancer, *Cancer Res* 57:2055, 1997.

46. Jones JL, Glynn P, Walker RA: Expression of MMP-2 and MMP-9, their inhibitors, and the activator MT1-MMP in primary breast carcinomas, *J Pathol* 189:161, 1999.

47. Bergsten E et al: PDGF-D is a specific, protease-activated ligand for the PDGF β-receptor, *Nat Cell Biol* 3:512, 2001.
48. Li X et al: PDGF-C is a new protease-activated ligand for the PDGF α-receptor, *Nat Cell Biol* 2:302, 2000.
49. Berx G, Van Roy F: The E-cadherin/catenin complex: an important gatekeeper in breast cancer tumorigenesis and malignant progression, *Breast Cancer Res* 3:289, 2001.
50. Gumbiner BM: Signal transduction by β-catenin, *Curr Opin Cell Biol* 7:634, 1995.
51. Meiners S et al: Role of morphogenetic factors in metastasis of mammary carcinoma cells, *Oncogene* 16:9, 1998.
52. Vleminckx K et al: Genetic manipulation of E-cadherin expression by epithelial tumor cells reveals an invasion suppressor role, *Cell* 66:107, 1991.
53. Pierceall WE et al: Frequent alterations in E-cadherin and alpha- and beta-catenin expression in human breast cancer cell lines, *Oncogene* 11:1319, 1995.
54. Bukholm IK et al: E-cadherin and α-, β- and γ-catenin protein expression in relation to metastasis in human breast carcinoma, *J Pathol* 185:262, 1998.
55. Graff JR et al: Methylation patterns of the E-cadherin 5′ CpG island are unstable and reflect the dynamic, heterogeneous loss of E-cadherin expression during metastatic progression, *J Biol Chem* 275:2727, 2000.
56. Kleer CG, van GK, Merajver SD: Persistent E-cadherin expression in inflammatory breast cancer, *Mod Pathol* 14:458, 2001.
57. Arihiro K et al: Cytokines facilitate chemotactic motility of breast carcinoma cells, *Breast Cancer* 7:221, 2000.
58. Nabi IR, Watanabe H, Raz A: Autocrine motility factor and its receptor: role in cell locomotion and metastasis, *Cancer Metastasis Rev* 11:5, 1992.
59. Talukder AH et al: Heregulin regulation of autocrine motility factor expression in human tumor cells, *Cancer Res* 60:474, 2000.
60. Ghoussoub RA et al: Expression of c-met is a strong independent prognostic factor in breast carcinoma, *Cancer* 82:1513, 1998.
61. Tuck A et al: Coexpression of hepatocyte growth factor and receptor (Met) in human breast carcinoma, *Am J Pathol* 148:225, 1996.
62. Fan S et al: Scatter factor protects epithelial and carcinoma cells against apoptosis induced by DNA-damaging agents, *Oncogene* 17:131, 1998.
63. Muller A et al: Involvement of chemokine receptors in breast cancer metastasis, *Nature* 410:50, 2001.
64. Fidler IJ: Critical factors in the biology of human cancer metastasis: twenty-eighth G.H.A. Clowes Memorial Award Lecture, *Cancer Res* 50:6130, 1990.
65. Naot D, Sionov RV, Ish-Shalom D: CD44: structure, function, and association with the malignant process, *Adv Cancer Res* 71:241, 1997.
66. Glukhova M et al: Adhesion systems in normal breast and in invasive breast carcinoma, *Am J Pathol* 146:706, 1995.
67. Cavallaro U, Christofori G: Cell adhesion in tumor invasion and metastasis: loss of the glue is not enough, *Biochim Biophys Acta* 1552:39, 2001.
68. Ruoslahti E: Fibronectin and its integrin receptors in cancer, *Adv Cancer Res* 76:1, 1999.
69. Honn KV, Tang DG: Adhesion molecules and tumor cell interaction with endothelium and subendothelial matrix, *Cancer Metastasis Rev* 11:353, 1992.
70. Castronovo V et al: Immunodetection of the metastasis-associated laminin receptor in human breast cancer cells obtained by fine-needle aspiration biopsy, *Am J Pathol* 137:1373, 1990.
71. Krause T, Turner GA: Are selectins involved in metastasis? *Clin Exp Metastasis* 17:183, 1999.
72. Cheng HC et al: Lung endothelial dipeptidyl peptidaseIV promotes adhesion and metastasis of rat breast cancer cells via tumor surface associated fibronectin, *J Biol Chem* 273:24207, 1998.
73. Haier J, Nicolson GL: Tumor cell adhesion under hydrodynamic conditions of fluid flow, *APMIS* 109:241, 2001.
74. Mukhopadhyay R, Theriault RL, Price JE: Increased levels of alpha6 integrins are associated with the metastatic phenotype of human breast cancer cells, *Clin Exp Metastasis* 17:325, 1999.
75. Felding-Habermann B et al: Integrin activation controls metastasis in human breast cancer, *Proc Natl Acad Sci USA* 98:1853, 2001.
76. Yi M, Ruoslahti E: A fibronectin fragment inhibits tumor growth, angiogenesis, and metastasis, *Proc Natl Acad Sci USA* 98:620, 2001.
77. Zhou Q et al: Contortrostatin, a dimeric disintegrin from Agkistrodon contortix, inhibits breast cancer progression, *Breast Cancer Res Treat* 61:249, 2000.
78. Gasparini G et al: Vascular integrin alpha(v)beta(3): a new prognostic indicator in breast cancer, *Clin Cancer Res* 4:2625, 1998.
79. Carr I: Lymphatic metastasis, *Cancer Metastasis Rev* 2:307, 1983.
80. Karpanen T, Alitalo K: Lymphatic vessels as targets of tumor therapy? *J Exp Med* 194:F37, 2001.
81. Fisher B: The evolution of paradigms for the management of breast cancer: a personal perspective, *Cancer Res* 52:2371, 1992.
82. Hellman S: Karnofsky memorial lecture: natural history of small breast cancers, *J Clin Oncol* 12:2229, 1994.
83. Tanis PJ et al: History of sentinel node and validation of the technique, *Breast Cancer Res* 3:109, 2001.
84. Rampaul RS et al: Pathological validation and significance of micrometastasis in sentinel nodes in primary breast cancer, *Breast Cancer Res* 3:113, 2001.
85. Fidler IJ: The relationship of embolic homogeneity, number, size and viability to the incidence of experimental metastasis, *Eur J Cancer* 9:227, 1973.
86. Liotta LA, Saidel MG, Kleinerman J: The significance of hematogenous tumor cell clumps and the metastatic process, *Cancer Res* 36:889, 1976.
87. Nicolson GL, Fidler IJ, Poste G: The effects of tertiary amine local anesthetics on the blood-borne implantation and cell surface properties of metastatic melanoma cells, *J Natl Cancer Inst* 76:511, 1986.
88. Hejna M, Raderer M, Zielinski CC: Inhibition of metastases by anticoagulants, *J Natl Cancer Inst* 91:22, 1999.
89. Kramer RH, Gonzales R, Nicolson GL: Metastatic cells adhere preferentially to extracellular matrix of endothelial cells, *Int J Cancer* 26:639, 1980.
90. Nicolson GL: Metastatic tumor cell interactions with endothelium, basement membrane and tissue, *Curr Opin Cell Biol* 1:1009, 1989.
91. Kolonin M, Pasqualini R, Arap W: Molecular addresses in blood vessels as targets for therapy, *Curr Opin Chem Biol* 5:308, 2001.

92. Belloni PN, Tressler RJ: Microvascular endothelial cell heterogeneity: interactions with leukocytes and tumor cells, Cancer Metastasis Rev 8:353, 1990.
93. Al-Mehdi AB et al: Intravascular origin of metastasis from the proliferation of endothelium-attached tumor cells: a new model for metastasis, Nat Med 6:100, 2000.
94. Rusciano D, Burger MM: Why do cancer cells metastasize into particular organs? BioEssays 14:185, 1992.
95. Herynk M, Radinsky R: The coordinated functional expression of epidermal growth factor receptor and c-met in colorectal carcinoma metastasis, In Vivo 14:587, 2000.
96. Cavanaugh PG, Nicolson GL: Lung-derived growth factor that stimulates the growth of lung-metastasizing tumor cells: identification as transferrin, J Cell Biochem 47:261, 1991.
97. Nicolson GL: Paracrine and autocrine growth mechanisms in tumor metastasis to specific sites with particular emphasis on brain and lung metastasis, Cancer Metastasis Rev 12:325, 1993.
98. Wyckoff JB et al: A critical step in metastasis: in vivo analysis of intravasation at the primary tumor, Cancer Res 60:2504, 2000.
99. Chambers AF et al: Molecular biology of breast cancer metastasis: clinical implications of experimental studies on metastatic inefficiency, Breast Cancer Res 2:400, 2000.
100. Wong CW et al: Apoptosis: an early event in metastatic inefficiency, Cancer Res 61:333, 2001.
101. Rudland PS et al: Prognostic significance of the metastasis-inducing protein S100A4 (p9Ka) in human breast cancer, Cancer Res 60:1595, 2000.
102. Platt-Higgins AM et al: Comparison of the metastasis-inducing protein S100A4 (p9Ka) with other prognostic markers in human breast cancer, Int J Cancer 89:198, 2000.
103. Nawa A et al: Tumor metastasis-associated human MTA1 gene: its deduced protein sequence, localization, and association with breast cancer cell proliferation using antisense phosphorothioate oligonucleotides, J Cell Biochem 79:202, 2000.
104. Martin MD et al: Loss of heterozygosity events impeding breast cancer metastasis contain the MTA1 gene, Cancer Res 61:3578, 2001.
105. Singhal H et al: Elevated plasma osteopontin in metastatic breast cancer associated with increased tumor burden and decreased survival, Clin Cancer Res 3:605, 1997.
106. Feng B, Rollo EE, Denhardt DT: Osteopontin (OPN) may facilitate metastasis by protecting cells from macrophage NO-mediated cytotoxicity: evidence from cell lines down-regulated for OPN expression by a targeted ribozyme, Clin Exp Metastasis 13:453, 1995.
107. Urquidi V et al: Contrasting expression of thrombospondin-1 and osteopontin correlates with absence or presence of metastatic phenotype in an isogenic model of spontaneous human breast cancer, Clin Cancer Res 8:61, 2002.
108. Sierra A et al: Bcl-2 with loss of apoptosis allows accumulation of genetic alterations: a pathway to metastatic progression in human breast cancer, Int J Cancer 89:142, 2000.
109. Del BD et al: Bcl-2 overexpression enhances the metastatic potential of a human breast cancer cell line, FASEB J 11:947, 1997.
110. Maass N et al: Decline in the expression of the serine proteinase inhibitor maspin is associated with tumor progression in ductal carcinomas of the breast, J Pathol 195:321, 2001.
111. Sheng S et al: Maspin acts at the cell membrane to inhibit invasion and motility of mammary and prostatic cancer cells, Proc Natl Acad Sci USA 93:11669, 1996.
112. Welch DR, Wei LL: Genetic and epigenetic regulation of human breast cancer progression and metastasis, Endocr Rel Cancer 5:155, 1996.
113. Hennessy C et al: Expression of the antimetastatic gene nm23 in human breast cancer: an association with good prognosis, J Natl Cancer Inst 83:281, 1991.
114. Freije JMP, MacDonald NJ, Steeg PS: Differential gene expression in tumor metastasis: nm23, Curr Top Microbiol Immunol 213:215, 1996.
115. Dong JT et al: KAI1, a metastasis suppressor gene for prostate cancer on human chromosome 11p.11.2, Science 268:884, 1995.
116. Phillips KK et al: Correlation between reduction of metastasis in the MDA-MB-435 model system and increased expression of the Kai-1 protein, Mol Carcinog 21:111, 1998.
117. Yang X et al: KAI1 protein is down-regulated during the progression of human breast cancer, Clin Cancer Res 6:3424, 2000.
118. Ohtaki T et al: Metastasis suppressor gene KiSS-1 encodes peptide ligand of a G-protein-coupled receptor, Nature 411:613, 2001.
119. Lee JH, Welch DR: Suppression of metastasis in human breast carcinoma MDA-MB-435 cells after transfection with the metastasis suppressor gene, KiSS-1, Cancer Res 57:2384, 1997.
120. Saunders MM et al: Breast cancer metastatic potential correlates with a breakdown in homospecific and heterospecific gap junctional intercellular communication, Cancer Res 61:1765, 2001.
121. Seraj MJ et al: Functional evidence for a novel human breast carcinoma metastasis suppressor, BRMS1, encoded at chromosome 11q13, Cancer Res 60:2764, 2000.
122. Welch DR, Steeg PS, Rinker-Schaeffer CW: Molecular biology of breast cancer metastasis: genetic regulation of human breast carcinoma metastasis, Breast Cancer Res 2:408, 2001.
123. Hartsough MT et al: Elevation of breast carcinoma Nm23-H1 metastasis suppressor gene expression and reduced motility by DNA methylation inhibition, Cancer Res 61:2320, 2001.
124. Paget S: The distribution of secondary growths in cancer of the breast, Lancet 1:571, 1889.
125. Tarin D et al: Clinicopathological observations on metastasis in man studied in patients treated with peritoneovenous shunts, BMJ 288:749, 1984.
126. Tarin D et al: Mechanisms of human tumor metastasis studied in patients with peritoneovenous shunts, Cancer Res 44:3584, 1984.
127. Verschraegen CF et al: Specific organ metastases of human melanoma cells injected into the arterial circulation of nude mice, Anticancer Res 11:529, 1991.
128. Price JE et al: Organ distribution of experimental metastases of a human colorectal carcinoma injected in nude mice, Clin Exp Metastasis 7:55, 1989.
129. Hart IR, Fidler IJ: Role of organ selectivity in the determination of metastatic patterns of B16 melanoma, Cancer Res 40:2281, 1980.
130. Shtivelman E, Namikawa R: Species-specific metastasis of human tumor cells in the severe combined immunodeficiency mouse engrafted with human tissue, Proc Natl Acad Sci USA 92:4661, 1995.

131. Nemeth JA et al: Severe combined immunodeficient-hu model of human prostate cancer metastasis to human bone, *Cancer Res* 59:1987, 1999.

132. Brooks B et al: Investigation of mammary epithelial cell-bone marrow stroma interactions using primary human cell culture as a model of metastasis, *Int J Cancer* 73:690, 1997.

133. Horak E, Darling DL, Tarin D: Analysis of organ-specific effects on metastatic tumor formation by studies in vitro, *J Natl Cancer Inst* 76:913, 1986.

134. Okumura Y et al: Preferential growth stimulation of metastatic rat mammary adenocarcinoma cells by organ-derived syngeneic fibroblasts in vitro, *Invasion Metastasis* 12:275, 1992.

135. Bar-Yehuda S et al: Resistance of muscle to tumor metastases: a role for a3 adenosine receptor agonists, *Neoplasia* 3:125, 2001.

136. Fisher B, Fisher ER: Experimental evidence in support of the dormant cell, *Science* 130:918, 1959.

137. Manishen WJ, Sivananthan K, Orr FW: Resorbing bone stimulates tumor cell growth: a role for the host microenvironment in bone metastasis, *Am J Pathol* 123:39, 1986.

138. Rubens RD: Bone metastases: the clinical problem, *Eur J Cancer* 34:210, 1998.

139. Chirgwin JM, Guise TA: Molecular mechanisms of tumor-bone interactions in osteolytic metastases, *Crit Rev Eukaryotic Gene Exp* 10:159, 2000.

140. Coleman RE: Management of bone metastases, *Oncologist* 5:463, 2000.

141. Boissier S et al: Bisphosphonates inhibit breast and prostate carcinoma cell invasion, an early event in the formation of bone metastases, *Cancer Res* 60:2949, 2000.

142. Powell GJ et al: Localization of parathyroid hormone-related protein in breast cancer metastases: increased incidence in bone compared with other sites, *Cancer Res* 51:3059, 1991.

143. Guise TA: Parathyroid hormone-related protein and bone metastases, *Cancer* 80S:1572, 1997.

144. Yin JJ et al: TGF-β signaling blockade inhibits PTHrP secretion by breast cancer cells and bone metastases development, *J Clin Invest* 103:197, 1999.

145. Henderson MA et al: Parathyroid hormone-related protein production by breast cancers, improved survival and reduced bone metastases, *J Natl Cancer Inst* 93:234, 2000.

146. Tannock IF: Tumor physiology and drug resistance, *Cancer Metastasis Rev* 20:123, 2001.

147. Graeber TJ et al: Hypoxia-mediated selection of cells with diminished apoptotic potential in solid tumors, *Nature* 379:88, 1996.

148. Maxwell PH et al: Hypoxia-inducible factor-1 modulates gene expression in solid tumors and influences both angiogenesis and tumor growth, *Proc Natl Acad Sci USA* 94:8104, 1997.

149. Kamby C et al: The pattern of metastases in human breast cancer: influence of systemic adjuvant therapy and impact on survival, *Acta Oncol* 27:715, 1988.

150. Pusztai L et al: Relapse after complete response to anthracycline-based combination chemotherapy in metastatic breast cancer, *Breast Cancer Res Treat* 55:1, 1999.

151. Wilmanns C et al: Modulation of doxorubicin sensitivity and level of p-glycoprotein expression in human colon carcinoma cells by ectopic and orthotopic environments in nude mice, *Int J Oncol* 3:413, 1993.

152. Holden SA et al: Host distribution and response to antitumor alkylating agents of EMT-6 tumor cells from subcutaneous tumor implants, *Cancer Chemother Pharmacol* 40:87, 1997.

153. Sausville EA: The challenge of pathway and environment-mediated drug resistance, *Cancer Metastasis Rev* 20:117, 2001.

154. Fidler IJ: Macrophages and metastasis: a biological approach to cancer therapy: presidential address, *Cancer Res* 45:4714, 1985.

155. Crowther M et al: Microenvironmental influence on macrophage regulation of angiogenesis in wounds and malignant tumors, *J Leukoc Biol* 70:478, 2001.

156. Yamashina K, Miller BE, Heppner GH: Macrophage-mediated induction of drug-resistant variants in a mouse mammary tumor cell line, *Cancer Res* 46:2396, 1986.

157. North SM, Nicolson GL: Heterogeneity in the sensitivities of 13762NF rat mammary adenocarcinoma cell clones to cytolysis mediated by extra- and intratumoral macrophages, *Cancer Res* 45:1453, 1985.

158. Ellis LM, Bland KI, Copeland EM III: Inflammatory breast cancer: advances in therapy, *Semin Surg Oncol* 4:261, 1988.

159. Poste G, Doll J, Fidler IJ: Interactions among polyclonal subpopulations affect stability of the metastatic phenotype in polyclonal populations of B16 melanoma cells, *Proc Natl Acad Sci USA* 78:6226, 1981.

160. Miller BE et al: Rates of development of methotrexate resistance in heterogeneous mouse mammary tumor cell cultures, *J Exp Ther Oncol* 1:30, 1996.

161. Jouanneau J et al: A minority of carcinoma cells producing acidic fibroblast growth factor induces a community effect for tumor progression, *Proc Natl Acad Sci USA* 91:286, 1994.

162. Martorana AM et al: Epithelial cells up-regulate matrix metalloproteinases in cell within the same mammary carcinoma that have undergone an epithelial-mesenchymal transition, *Cancer Res* 58:4970, 1998.

163. Perou CM et al: Molecular portraits of human breast tumours, *Nature* 406:747, 2000.

164. van't Veer LJ et al: Gene expression profiling predicts clinical outcome of breast cancer, *Nature* 415:530, 2002.

165. Osin P et al: Experimental pathology and breast cancer genetics: new technologies, *Recent Results Cancer Res* 152:35, 1998.

166. Foulds L: *Neoplastic development*, London, 1975, Academic Press.

167. Nowell PC: The clonal evolution of tumor cell populations, *Science* 194:23, 1976.

168. O'Connell P et al: Analysis of loss of heterozygosity in 399 premalignant breast lesions at 15 genetic loci, *J Natl Cancer Inst* 90:697, 1998.

169. Neri A, Nicolson GL: Phenotypic drift of metastatic and cell surface properties of mammary adenocarcinoma cell clones during growth in vitro, *Int J Cancer* 28:731, 1981.

170. Young SD, Hill RP: Isolation of murine tumor cell populations enriched for metastatic variants and quantification of unstable expression of the phenotype, *Clin Exp Metastasis* 4:153, 1986.

171. Miller FR, Miller BE, Heppner GH: Characterization of metastatic heterogeneity among subpopulations of a single mouse mammary tumor: heterogeneity in phenotypic stability, *Invasion Metastasis* 3:22, 1983.

172. Brodt P et al: Studies on clonal heterogeneity in two spontaneously metastasizing mammary carcinomas of recent origin, *Int J Cancer* 35:265, 1985.

173. Kerbel RS: Growth dominance of the metastatic cancer cell: cellular and molecular aspects, *Adv Cancer Res* 55:87, 1990.

174. Price JE, Bell C, Frost P: The use of a genotypic marker to demonstrate clonal dominance during the growth and

metastasis of a human breast carcinoma in nude mice, *Int J Cancer* 45:968, 1990.

175. Symmans WF et al: Breast cancer heterogeneity: evaluation of clonality in primary and metastatic lesions, *Hum Pathol* 26:210, 1994.

176. Stapleton AMF et al: Primary human prostate cancer cells harboring *p53* mutations are clonally expanded in metastases, *Clin Cancer Res* 3:1389, 1997.

177. van Slooten HJ et al: Mutations in exons 5-8 of the *p53* gene, independent of their type and location, are associated with increased apoptosis and mitosis in invasive breast carcinoma, *J Pathol* 189:504, 1999.

177a. Bland KI et al: Oncogene protein co-expression: value of Ha-*ras*, c-*myc*, c-*fos*, and p53 as prognostic discriminants for breast carcinoma, *Ann Surg* 221:706, 1995.

177b. Beenken SW et al: Molecular biomakers for breast cancer prognosis: coexpression of c-erbB-2 and p53, *Ann Surg* 233:630, 2001.

177c. Beenken S, Bland KI: Biomakers for breast cancer, *Minerva Chir (Italy)* 57:437, 2002.

178. Shen CY et al: Genome-wide search for loss of heterozygosity using laser capture microdissected tissue of breast carcinoma: an implication for mutator phenotype and breast cancer pathogenesis, *Cancer Res* 60:3884, 2000.

179. Kuukasjarvi T et al: Genetic heterogeneity and clonal evolution underlying development of asynchronous metastasis in human breast cancer, *Cancer Res* 57:1597, 1997.

180. Unger MA, Weber BL: Recent advances in breast cancer biology, *Curr Opin Oncol* 12:521, 2000.

181. Teixeira MR, Pandis N, Heim S: Cytogenetic clues to breast carcinogenesis, *Genes Chromosomes Cancer* 33:1, 2002.

182. Kittiniyom K et al: Allelic loss on chromosome band 18p11.3 occurs early and reveals heterogeneity in breast cancer progression, *Breast Cancer Res* 3:192, 2001.

183. Cifone MA, Fidler IJ: Increasing metastatic potential is associated with increasing genetic instability of clones isolated from murine neoplasms, *Proc Natl Acad Sci USA* 78:6949, 1981.

184. Pandis N et al: Cytogenetic comparison of primary tumors and lymph node metastases in breast cancer patients, *Genes Chromosomes Cancer* 22:122, 1998.

185. Buerger H et al: Genetic relation of lobular carcinoma in situ, ductal carcinoma in situ, and associated invasive carcinoma of the breast, *Mol Pathol* 53:118, 2000.

186. Bernardino J et al: DNA hypomethylation in breast cancer: an independent parameter of tumor progression? *Cancer Genet Cytogenet* 97:83, 1997.

187. Graff JR et al: E-cadherin expression is silenced by DNA hypermethylation in human breast and prostate carcinomas, *Cancer Res* 55:5195, 1995.

188. Park CC, Bissell MJ, Barcellos-Hoff MH: The influence of the microenvironment on the malignant phenotype, *Mol Med Today* 6:324, 2000.

189. Lochter A, Bissell MJ: Involvement of extracellular matrix constituents in breast cancer, *Semin Cancer Biol* 6:165, 1995.

190. Lapidus RG et al: Mapping of ER gene CpG island methylation by methylation-specific polymerase chain reaction, *Cancer Res* 58:2515, 1998.

191. Fidler IJ: Critical determinants of cancer metastasis: rationale for therapy, *Cancer Chemother Pharmacol* 43:S3, 1999.

192. Radinsky R: Modulation of tumor cell gene expression and phenotype by the organ-specific metastatic environment, *Cancer Metastasis Rev* 14:323, 1995.

193. Fidler IJ, Talmadge JE: Evidence that intravenously derived murine pulmonary metastases can originate from the expansion of a single tumor cell, *Cancer Res* 46:5167, 1986.

194. Hortobagyi GN: Developments in chemotherapy of breast cancer, *Cancer* 88:3073, 2000.

195. Kostler WJ et al: Detection of minimal residual disease in patients with cancer: a review of techniques, clinical implications, and emerging therapeutic consequences, *Cancer Detect Prev* 24:376, 2000.

196. Kern DH: Heterogeneity of drug resistance in human breast and ovarian cancers, *Cancer J Sci Am* 4:41, 1998.

197. Talmadge JE et al: The development of biological diversity and susceptibility to chemotherapy in cancer metastases, *Cancer Res* 44:3801, 1984.

198. Morstyn G et al: Heterogeneity in the radiation survival curves and biochemical properties of human lung cancer cell lines, *J Natl Cancer Inst* 73:801, 1984.

199. Cree IA et al: Correlation of the clinical response to chemotherapy in breast cancer with ex vivo chemosensitivity, *AntiCancer Drugs* 7:630, 1996.

200. Nicolson GL, Lembo TM, Welch DR: Growth of rat mammary adenocarcinoma cells in semisolid clonogenic medium not correlated with spontaneous metastatic behavior: heterogeneity in the metastatic, antigenic, enzymatic, and drug sensitivity properties of cells from different sized colonies, *Cancer Res* 48:399, 1988.

201. Price JE, Tarin D: Low incidence of tumourigenicity in agarose colonies from spontaneous murine mammary tumours, *Differentiation* 41:202, 1989.

202. Poste G et al: Evolution of tumor cell heterogeneity during progressive growth of individual lung metastases, *Proc Natl Acad Sci USA* 79:6574, 1982.

203. Nicolson GL: Breast cancer metastasis-associated genes: role in tumour progression to the metastatic state, *Biochem Soc Symp* 63:231, 1998.

204. Nicolson GL, Lotan R: Preventing diversification of malignant tumor cells during therapy, *Clin Exp Metastasis* 6:231, 1986.

205. Gasparini G, Pozza F, Harris AL: Evaluating the potential usefulness of new prognostic and predictive indicators in node-negative breast cancer patients, *J Natl Cancer Inst* 85:1206, 1993.

206. Geisler S et al: Influence of TP53 gene alterations and c-erbB-2 expression on the response to treatment with doxorubicin in locally advanced breast cancer, *Cancer Res* 61:2505, 2001.

207. Slamon DJ: Human breast cancer: correlation of relapse and survival with amplification of the HER-2/*neu* oncogene, *Science* 235:177, 1987.

208. Cook-Bruns N: Retrospective analysis of the safety of Herceptin immunotherapy in metastatic breast cancer, *Oncology* 61:58, 2001.

209. Burstein HJ et al: Clinical activity of trastuzumab and vinorelbine in women with HER2-overexpressing metastatic breast cancer, *J Clin Oncol* 19:2722, 2001.

210. Lachman LB et al: DNA vaccination against HER2/*neu* reduces breast cancer incidence and metastasis, *Cancer Gene Ther* 8:259, 2001.

211. Yip YL, Ward RL: Anti-*ErbB-2* monoclonal antibodies and *ErbB-2*-directed vaccines, *Cancer Immunol Immunother* 50:569, 2002.

CHAPTER

27

Gene Therapy of Breast Cancer

THERESA V. STRONG

DAVID T. CURIEL

Chapter Outline

Although the treatment of breast cancer has improved significantly over the past decades, locoregional recurrence and disseminated disease still represent formidable challenges for conventional therapies. The field of gene therapy is rapidly developing and has greatly expanded the opportunities for new breast cancer treatments. Defined as the introduction of genetic material for the treatment of disease, gene therapy was originally envisioned primarily for the correction of inherited genetic defects. To date, however, gene therapy has found more extensive application in the treatment of malignant disease. This comes from several realizations. First, it has been appreciated that breast cancer, like other cancers, develops through the progressive accumulation of alterations in specific genes, resulting in abnormal cell growth and invasion. These genetic abnormalities can be corrected or altered via the introduction of therapeutic genes. Second, many limitations of current gene therapy approaches pose less of a challenge in their application to the treatment of cancer. Most notably, difficulties in maintaining long-term gene expression are obviated for most approaches to gene therapy for cancer because transgene expression of a limited duration can achieve therapeutic effect. Finally, a better understanding of the molecular pathology of tumors, including the tumor microenvironment, has led to identification of new therapeutic targets that can be manipulated through gene therapy.

Based on these concepts, numerous approaches to gene therapy for breast cancer have been considered, each targeting different points in the cancer progression pathway. Given that conventional therapies for early stage breast cancer are generally effective, gene therapy approaches have focused on three clinical scenarios. One is the treatment of advanced, widely disseminated disease, for which conventional therapy is inadequate. A second potential target population is women who have responded favorably to conventional therapy but who are at high risk for recurrence. In this case, gene therapy strategies designed to eliminate micrometastatic disease with low toxicity may be considered. Finally, gene therapy has been used in patients with breast cancer in conjunction with bone marrow transplantation therapy. Depending on the application, some of the approaches evaluated to date seek to directly alter or kill the tumor cells, whereas others attempt to alter the tumor environment. This chapter reviews the basic concepts of gene therapy as they apply to the treatment of breast cancer.

Although many of these therapeutic strategies are still in preclinical development, others are under investigation in clinical trials. An updated listing of approved gene therapy trials is available in the Human Gene Transfer Clinical Trials Database through the National Institutes of Health, Office of Biotechnologies Activities (www4.od.nih.gov/oba/).

Gene Therapy Strategies

STRATEGIES TO ACCOMPLISH GENE THERAPY FOR BREAST CANCER: TARGETING THE TUMOR CELL

When gene therapy is considered for treatment of breast cancer, a critical issue is the choice of therapeutic gene. Unlike colon cancer, in which a well-defined accumulation of genetic aberrations leads to progressively more aggressive disease,[1] the genetic alterations leading to breast cancer are apparently more diverse and suggest that, at the genetic level, breast cancer is not a single disease. Molecular profiling of breast tumors[2] will likely provide a better understanding of the pathways involved. Nevertheless, a number of mutations common in breast cancer have been identified as therapeutic targets. Inherited or somatic genetic changes in tumor-suppressor genes, oncogenes, growth factor receptors, DNA repair enzymes, and/or cell signaling molecules lead to low- or high-risk carcinomas in situ, and additional changes involving genes important in invasive and angiogenesis promote metastatic spread. These tumor-specific genetic alterations can be targeted by gene therapy approaches that include *mutation compensation, molecular chemotherapy*, and *viral oncolysis*, or virotherapy (Table 27-1).

Mutation Compensation. Mutation compensation aims to correct the genetic defects that contribute to the malignant phenotype. Such correction may be accomplished by replacing the function of tumor-suppressor genes, ablating the function of a dominant oncogene, or interfering with dysregulated signal transduction pathways. For inactive tumor-suppressor genes, one logical approach is the replacement of the deficient gene. Examples of this in breast cancer include replacement of the *p53* and *BRCA1* genes[3] in deficient tumor cells, which may lead to reversion of the malignant phenotype and/or induction of apoptosis. For dominant oncogenes or dysregulated signaling proteins, it is possible to abrogate the function of the encoded proteins at many levels. Perhaps the best-studied molecule in this respect is the product of the *ERBB2 (HER2/neu)* gene, which is overexpressed in approximately 30% of breast tumors and is associated with a poor prognosis. Introduction of triplex-forming oligonucleotides that interfere with transcription of this gene has shown some effect in in vitro systems.[15] Degradation of the mRNA encoding this oncogene and interference with protein translation can be promoted through the use of specific, antisense oligonucleotides[16]; however, practical application of the technology and idiosyncrasies in the effects of specific antisense molecules have posed a challenge in this field. At the protein level, expression of intracellular antibodies against ErbB-2 promotes degradation of the protein and induces

TABLE **27-1** Gene Therapy Strategies for Breast Cancer

APPROACH	RATIONALE	REFERENCES
Mutation compensation	Targets specific gene mutations to restore normal growth or induce apoptosis	3, 4
Molecular chemotherapy	Causes local conversion of a prodrug into a toxic drug to kill tumor cells	5
Viral oncolysis	Involves tumor-specific viral replication and lysis	6-8
Genetic immunotherapy	Stimulates host immune system to recognize and eliminate tumor cells	9
Antiangiogenic	Interrupts the tumor's ability to establish a blood supply	10, 11
Bone marrow chemoprotection	Protects normal cells from high-dose chemotherapy	12
Bone marrow purging	Eliminates contaminating tumor cells for autologous bone marrow transplant	13, 14

apoptosis in ErbB-2–expressing cells.[4] Although mutation compensation is straightforward and many preclinical studies have demonstrated the utility of these strategies, significant obstacles remain for these approaches to achieve therapeutic efficacy in the clinical setting. Chief among these is the theoretical need to correct the deficit in all tumor cells to achieve a therapeutic effect. So-called "quantitative transduction" of the tumor cells is elusive, and to date no vectors for gene delivery have been able to achieve this goal. Another significant limitation stems from the accumulated genetic changes found in highly malignant cells, which may not be amenable to correction by the introduction of a single therapeutic gene.

Molecular Chemotherapy. As a method to overcome some of the practical limitations of mutation compensation, the concept of molecular chemotherapy, or "suicide" gene therapy, has also been explored. The premise of this approach is to restrict the toxic effects of a chemotherapeutic drug specifically to tumor cells by mediating conversion of a systemically delivered prodrug into a toxic metabolite within the tumor cells, as directed by an expressed transgene.[5] Molecular chemotherapy strategies may offer an advantage compared with most mutation compensation approaches in that nearby tumor cells that did not receive the transgene may also be affected by the toxin, the so-called "bystander effect." Many prodrug systems exist, but the most studied method to accomplish tumor cell killing in this way uses the thymidine kinase gene from the herpes simplex virus (HSV-tk). Expression of this gene in mammalian cells in not harmful but allows conversion of the relatively nontoxic nucleoside analog ganciclovir to a phosphorylated form that incorporates into the cellular DNA, inhibits DNA synthesis and RNA polymerase, and leads to cell death. For this and other molecular chemotherapy

approaches to be successful, transgene expression must be confined to the tumor cells; thus appropriately targeted gene delivery and expression are critical.

Viral Oncolysis. As the field of gene therapy has advanced, it has become apparent that first-generation, replication-incompetent viral vectors lack the ability to achieve quantitative transduction of tumors, limiting their therapeutic efficacy. To overcome this limitation, conditionally replicative viruses have been investigated.[6,17] These viruses are engineered such that they can replicate within genetically aberrant cancer cells, resulting in specific, intratumoral viral propagation. Replication in normal cells is absent or attenuated. The therapeutic effect may be achieved solely as a result of virus-driven tumor cell lysis or may be augmented by the addition of a therapeutic transgene, such as an immunostimulatory cytokine. These oncolytic vectors, derived from a number of different naturally occurring viruses, have shown promise in preclinical and some early clinical trials for other tumor types. Additional modifications to the vectors to enhance tumor specificity, intratumoral spread, and immune response evasion promise to further improve the potential of this approach.

STRATEGIES TO ACCOMPLISH GENE THERAPY FOR BREAST CANCER: TARGETING THE TUMOR ENVIRONMENT

Genetic Immunotherapy. A central issue in the management of women with breast cancer is the development of relatively nontoxic therapies designed to eliminate micrometastatic disease and prevent disease recurrence. *Genetic immunotherapy* refers to strategies designed to recruit the patient's immune system to identify and destroy aberrant tumor cells, by virtue of tumor-associated antigens expressed in the tumor cell.[9]

It has long been apparent that tumor cells possess some degree of immunogenicity and that furthermore, tumors employ a variety of strategies to evade detection by the host immune system. Immunotherapy seeks to stimulate the immune response to the tumor cells.

Nonspecific genetic immunotherapy uses transfer of immunomodulatory genes such as cytokines and costimulatory molecules to overcome immunologic tolerance to tumors and promote tumor rejection. This approach does not require knowledge of the tumor antigens expressed in a particular tumor. In contrast, active specific immunotherapy uses immunization with defined antigen(s) to elicit a specific antitumor immune response. Advances in the identification and characterization of tumor antigens relevant to breast cancer have expanded the possible target antigens for this approach.

Antiangiogenic Gene Therapy. The growth of tumors depends on the process of angiogenesis, which establishes the tumor blood supply. Preclinical studies suggest that interfering with the factors necessary to establish appropriate blood flow to the tumor effectively inhibit tumor growth.[10,11] Several proteins, including angiostatin, endostatin, and soluble vascular-endothelial growth factor receptor, may act to inhibit tumor cell growth when administered. Clinically, gene therapy offers some advantages compared with protein-based therapy. Long-term expression of the therapeutic gene offered by some vectors would permit a continuous, endogenous source of the protein. Furthermore, because the protein is synthesized in vivo, stability is improved compared with protein produced in vitro. In its optimal form, this approach requires a vector capable of directing long-term expression of the transgene, with the ability to regulate the level of transgene expressed.

GENE THERAPY IN CONJUNCTION WITH BONE MARROW TRANSPLANT

Gene therapy has been applied to breast cancer autologous bone marrow transplantation in two ways (see Table 27-1). One of the first applications of gene therapy for breast cancer was the transduction of normal cells in the bone marrow with a protective gene (e.g., the multidrug resistance gene) to mitigate the myelosuppressive effects of high-dose chemotherapy.[12] In a second application, viral vectors that specifically transduce and kill tumor cells have been used to purge bone marrow cells of contaminating tumor cells.[13,14]

Vectors for Gene Transfer

Once a general strategy and therapeutic gene have been determined, a second consideration for all gene therapy protocols is the choice of vector to most effectively deliver the gene. There is a vast array of choices, and these continue to expand as new vectors are characterized, modified, or synthesized to achieve more efficacious gene delivery. Gene transfer vectors generally fall into two classes—viral and nonviral, each with its advantages and disadvantages. Because the primary focus of breast cancer gene therapy is targeting and eliminating metastatic disease, the ideal gene transfer vector would possess the following attributes: (1) stability in vivo to allow intravenous delivery; (2) ability to target gene transfer to the desired cells, for example, disseminated breast tumor cells, while leaving normal cells unaltered; (3) ability to transfer large genes with the appropriate regulatory sequences; (4) ability to direct sufficiently prolonged expression of the therapeutic transgene; (5) ability to replicate autonomously or integrate at a defined chromosomal site; and (6) lack of stimulation of unwanted host immune response that might interfere with transgene expression. Nonviral gene delivery systems have advantages in that they have low toxicity and may not elicit immune responses; however, they are generally inefficient in their ability to deliver the genes, and transgene expression is transient. Viral vectors, having evolved to deliver their nucleic acids into cells, are generally much more efficient than nonviral methods but suffer from other limitations, including preexisting immune responses that may interfere with gene transduction, induction of antivector immune responses that limit the ability to repetitively dose, and potential safety concerns (including recombination with wild-type virus). Chimeric vectors combine features of different nonviral and/or viral components to achieve the desired gene delivery profile. A summary of gene therapy vectors explored for use in breast cancer therapy is found in Table 27-2. Unfortunately, none of these vectors yet meets the criteria for the ideal, and thus a major focus in the field of gene therapy has been the development of novel or modified vectors toward this end. Considerable progress has been made, including the development of vectors that target tumor cells specifically,[18-20] express their genes only in recipient tumor cells by virtue of tumor-specific promoters, evade the immune response, and replicate specifically in tumor cells.[21,22]

Conclusions

Advances in cancer treatment have significantly improved clinical outcome, but no single therapeutic intervention has yet proved effective for all breast cancers. Gene therapy offers promise to expand and complement the current arsenal of therapies that can be applied to breast cancer. In fact, gene therapy is likely to find its most useful clinical application in combination with conventional therapeutic approaches—acting to

| TABLE 27-2 | Gene Delivery Systems in Preclinical or Clinical Development for Breast Cancer |

METHOD	ADVANTAGES	DISADVANTAGES
NONVIRAL		
Liposomes	Nonimmunogenic, repeated delivery possible	Inefficient gene delivery
Naked nucleic acids	Easy to prepare, nonimmunogenic	Inefficient gene delivery
Conjugates	Targeted delivery, flexible design	Unstable, inefficient
VIRAL		
Adenovirus	Comparatively efficient gene delivery	Transient, immunogenic, preexisting antibodies
Retrovirus	Long-term expression	Risk of insertional mutagenesis, unstable in vivo, transduces dividing cells only
Poxvirus	Robust, short-term expression	Immunogenic
Adeno-associated virus	Long-term expression, nonpathogenic	Small insert size, difficult preparation
Herpes simplex virus	Efficient in vivo, large insert size	Not completely characterized
Reovirus	Specific oncolysis in cells with activated *RAS* oncogene pathway	Clinical profile not yet known
Lentivirus	Long-term expression, transduces nondividing cells	Production system not fully developed, safety
Chimeric vectors	May improve targeting, long-term expression	Not fully developed

sensitize tumor cells, increase the specificity of toxins to the tumor cells, or manipulate the immune response to promote a favorable outcome. In the coming years, the development of advanced generation gene delivery vectors should enhance the ability to target the appropriate cells and achieve optimal transgene expression, allowing gene therapy to reach its full potential and offering new hope to those with breast cancer.

ACKNOWLEDGMENT

We acknowledge support from the National Institutes of Health, 1 P50 CA89019, SPORE in Breast Cancer.

REFERENCES

1. Fearon ER, Vogelstein B: A genetic model for colorectal tumorigenesis, *Cell* 61:759, 1990.
2. van't Veer LJ et al: Gene expression profiling predicts clinical outcome of breast cancer, *Nature* 415:530, 2002.
3. Obermiller PS, Tait DL, Holt JT: Gene therapy for carcinoma of the breast: therapeutic genetic correction strategies, *Breast Cancer Res* 2:28, 2000.
4. Curiel DT: Gene therapy for carcinoma of the breast: genetic ablation strategies, *Breast Cancer Res* 2:45, 2000.
5. Vassaux G, Lemoine NR: Gene therapy for carcinoma of the breast: genetic toxins, *Breast Cancer Res* 2:22, 2000.
6. Gomez-Navarro J, Curiel DT: Conditionally replicative adenoviral vectors for cancer gene therapy, *Lancet Oncol* 1:148 2000.
7. Norman KL et al: Reovirus oncolysis of human breast cancer, *Hum Gene Ther* 13:641, 2002.
8. Toda M, Rabkin SD, Martuza RL: Treatment of human breast cancer in a brain metastatic model by G207, a replication-competent multimutated herpes simplex virus 1, *Hum Gene Ther* 9:2177, 1998.
9. Strong TV: Gene therapy for carcinoma of the breast: genetic immunotherapy, *Breast Cancer Res* 2:15, 2000.
10. Chen QR et al: Liposomes complexed to plasmids encoding angiostatin and endostatin inhibit breast cancer in nude mice, *Cancer Res* 59:3308, 1999.
11. Sauter BV et al: Adenovirus-mediated gene transfer of endostatin in vivo results in high level of transgene expression and inhibition of tumor growth and metastases, *Proc Natl Acad Sci USA* 97:4802, 2000.
12. Cowan KH et al: Paclitaxel chemotherapy after autologous stem-cell transplantation and engraftment of hematopoietic cells transduced with a retrovirus containing the multidrug resistance complementary DNA (MDR1) in metastatic breast cancer patients, *Clin Cancer Res* 5:1619, 1999.
13. Seth P et al: Adenovirus-mediated gene transfer to human breast tumor cells: an approach for cancer gene therapy and bone marrow purging, *Cancer Res* 56:1346, 1996.
14. Wu A et al: Biological purging of breast cancer cells using an attenuated replication-competent herpes simplex virus in human hematopoietic stem cell transplantation, *Cancer Res* 61:3009,2001.
15. Ebbinghaus SW et al: Triplex formation inhibits HER-2/*neu* transcription in vitro, *J Clin Invest* 92:2433, 1993.

16. Roh H et al: HER2/*neu* antisense targeting of human breast carcinoma, *Oncogene* 19:6138, 2000.

17. Ring CJ: Cytolytic viruses as potential anti-cancer agents, *J Gen Virol* 83:491, 2002.

18. Krasnykh VN, Douglas JT, van Beusechem VW: Genetic targeting of adenoviral vectors, *Mol Ther* 1:391, 2000.

19. Buchholz CJ, Stitz J, Cichutek K: Retroviral cell targeting vectors, *Curr Opin Mol Ther* 1:613, 1999.

20. Nishikawa M, Huang L: Nonviral vectors in the new millennium: delivery barriers in gene transfer, *Hum Gene Ther* 12:861, 2001.

21. Zwiebel JA: Cancer gene and oncolytic virus therapy, *Semin Oncol* 28:336, 2001.

22. Gomez-Navarro J, Curiel DT, Douglas JT: Gene therapy for cancer, *Eur J Cancer* 35:2039, 1999.

28

Angiogenesis in Breast Cancer

M. JUDAH FOLKMAN

Chapter Outline

Tumor Angiogenesis: Biologic Basis

PREVASCULAR PHASE

When a new primary tumor first arises, it is usually not vascularized. In this *prevascular* state, tumor volume is less than a few cubic millimeters. External in situ carcinomas of the skin, cervix, and oral mucous membranes, which can be observed directly, are usually thin and flat because their expansion is limited by the diffusion of nutrients and oxygen from normal vessels that lie beneath the epithelial layer. Thus a new melanoma is separated from capillary vessels in the dermis, which are already occupied by normal cells. The prevascular stage of an internal tumor, such as carcinoma in situ of the breast, can usually be seen only with microscopic examination (Figure 28-1). These tumor cells are also usually separated from host microvessels by a basement membrane. From experimental studies,[1-3] we know that these prevascular lesions exist in a steady state of tumor cell proliferation balanced by cell death. Externally located prevascular tumors may remain in this state for months to years, but we do not know about internal lesions. The onset of neovascularization, however, can be relatively sudden and is called the *angiogenic switch*.[3-6]

SWITCH TO THE ANGIOGENIC PHENOTYPE

The appearance of a thin layer of new periductal vessels may be the first evidence of neovascularization of in situ breast carcinoma (see Figure 28-1). Experimental studies of spontaneous tumors in mice, especially in transgenic mice, reveal that the angiogenic switch is a discrete event that develops during progressive stages of tumorigenesis, beginning with the premalignant stage in these mouse models (Figure 28-2).[2,3,6] The stages are similar to those in human carcinoma of the cervix, in which the onset of angiogenesis occurs during the premalignant dysplastic stage.[7] In contrast, breast cancer and other cancers are already at the in situ stage when neovascularization appears. Nevertheless, in both animal and human tumors, neovascularization usually develops before the emergence of invasive malignancy. In the 1970s, before the discovery of angiogenic proteins, increased angiogenic activity was demonstrated in breast tissue that progressed from a preoplastic to a neoplastic stage.[8,9] In human breast cancer, low-level angiogenic activity may be detected in preneoplastic lesions, such as fibrocystic disease.[10]

Increased expression of the angiogenic proteins vascular endothelial growth factor (VEGF) or basic fibroblast growth factor (bFGF)[11-15] and of the angiogenic mediators thymidine phosphorylase[16,17] and tissue factor[18] has been reported in human breast cancer. VEGF mRNA and protein levels are dramatically upregulated by human mammary fibroblasts in response to hypoxia.[19] Thus mammary stromal cells may play a role in the angiogenic phenotype in breast cancer. Also, bFGF and other angiogenic proteins can be mobilized from storage sites in the extracellular matrix in breast cancer.[20-22] Expression of VEGF in node-negative breast cancers has prognostic significance.[23] However, it should be emphasized that because the angiogenic activity of a tumor is the sum total of positive and negative regulators of angiogenesis, it would not be expected that quantification of a single angiogenic factor in tumor tissue would uniformly provide prognostic information.

The switch to the angiogenic phenotype also is understood as a shift in the net balance between positive regulators of angiogenesis (e.g., bFGF, VEGF)[24,25] and negative regulators of angiogenesis (e.g., thrombospondin-1, 16-kD prolactin, interferon-alpha, interferon-beta, platelet factor 4, angiostatin, endostatin, and others such as interleukin-12).[4,26-29] Macrophages and other host cells may contribute to the angiogenic switch in breast cancer.[30,31] However, the genetic control of these regulators is just beginning to be elucidated.[2,27,32] For example, an angiogenesis inhibitor, thrombospondin-1, may be under the control of the *p53* tumor-suppressor gene[33]; induction of wild-type *p53* in glioblastoma cells releases an angiogenesis inhibitor[34]; VEGF is in part under the control of the *VHL* suppressor gene[35] and also the *p53* suppressor gene[36]; and activation of oncogenes such as *RAS*, *RAF*, *FOS*, $SV_{40}T$ antigen, and others[27] appears to be involved in production of angiogenic factors by tumor cells.

The positive regulators of angiogenesis that are overexpressed in breast cancer must overcome a variety of negative regulators, some of which are produced by myoepithelial cells that surround ducts. These inhibitors include thrombospondin-1, bFGF soluble receptor, and tissue inhibitor and metalloproteinase-1 (TIMP-1).

Mechanisms of the Angiogenic Switch. Normal cells that have been transformed to neoplastic cells are not usually angiogenic at the outset. Experimental studies of spontaneous tumors in transgenic mice reveal that the angiogenic switch is a discrete event that develops during progressive stages of tumorigenesis, beginning with the premalignant stage in these mouse models.[3] By the time most human tumors are detected, for example, with mammography, neovascularization has usually occurred. However, most human tumors arise without angiogenic activity, exist in situ without neovascularization for months to years, and then switch to an angiogenic phenotype. Therefore the angiogenic phenotype appears after the expression of the malignant phenotype in most primary tumors. For certain

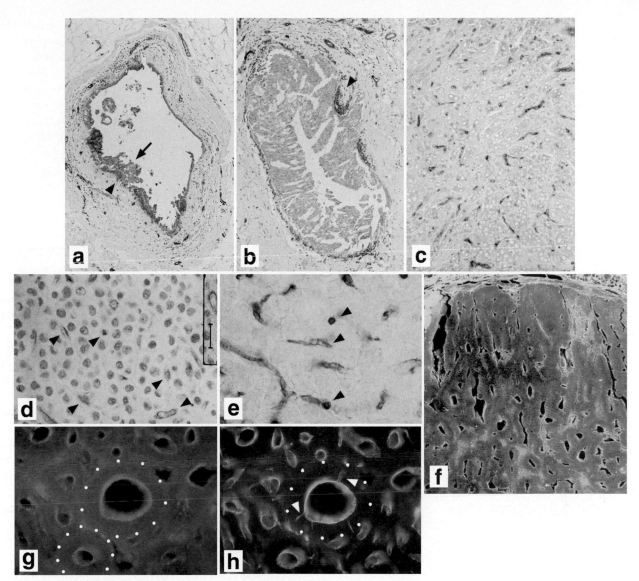

FIG. **28-1 A,** Human breast cancer. Large breast duct partially lined by duct carcinoma in situ *(arrow)* and intense angiogenesis in the immediately adjacent periductal breast stroma. Brown staining microvessels (antibody to von Willebrand factor) are indicated by the arrowhead. Note the absence of angiogenesis in the areas of breast stroma adjacent to portion of duct lined with benign duct epithelium (from Weidner and co-workers[89]). **B,** Large breast duct filled with carcinoma in situ and surrounded by new microvessels in the periductal breast stroma. Arrowhead shows invasion of microvessels through basement membrane of the duct, accompanied by invasion of tumor cells into the periductal stroma. **C,** Invasive ductal carcinoma, area of highest density of microvessels. **D,** Higher power of invasive human breast carcinoma 4-μm-thick section. Microvessels (brown stained with antibody to CD31) are indicated by arrowheads. **E,** A 50-μm-thick confocal microscopy section showing microvessels in three dimensions *(arrowheads)* surrounded by tumors cells that fill the intercapillary space. **F, G, H,** Cross sections of breast cancer in mice showing the microcylinders of tumor cells that surround each microvessel. The 100-μm thickness of these tumor microcylinders is within the range of the oxygen diffusion limit. **F,** Scanning electron microscope view of 100-μm Vibratome section of a subcutaneous MCa-IV mouse breast tumor with the skin at the top. Blood vessels appear as black holes emptied of blood and preserved in an open state by vascular perfusion of fixative. Pale necrotic regions surround perivascular rings of tumor tissue that are approximately 100 μm thick. (Original magnification 25×.) A 10-mm scale bar would equal 400 μm. *(Courtesy Donald M. McDonald, University of California, San Francisco.)* **G, H,** Large and small thin-walled blood vessels in MCa-IV mouse breast tumor labeled by vascular perfusion of green (FITC) fluorescent lectin staining (**G,** green) and CD31-immunoreactivity viewed by Cy3 fluorescence (**H,** gold). Like the lectin, CD31-immunoreactivity defines the luminal surface of the vessels but, unlike the lectin, it also labels tiny sprouts, which have no apparent lumen because they have CD31-immunoreactivity but no lectin staining. Sprouts *(white arrowheads)* about 1 μm in diameter radiate from the vessel lining into the 100-μm-thick perivascular ring of tumor tissue (outlined by white dots). Vessels preserved in open state by vascular perfusion of fixative. *(Courtesy Donald M. McDonald, University of California, San Francisco.)*

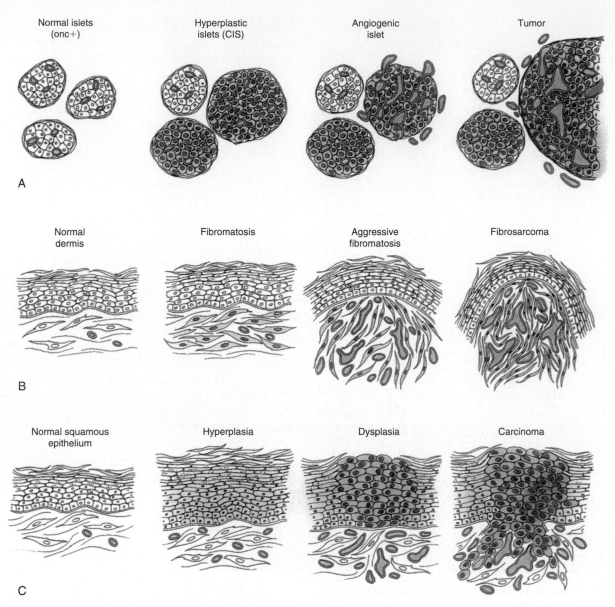

FIG. 28-2 Histologic representations of the switch to the angiogenic phenotype. **A,** Islet cell carcinoma in transgenic RIP-Tag mice.[3] **B,** Fibrosarcoma in transgenic mice.[3] **C,** Human cervical carcinoma.[3,7] *CIS,* Carcinoma in situ.

human tumors such as carcinoma of the cervix, the preneoplastic stage of dysplasia becomes neovascularized before the malignant tumor appears.[7] This sequence of events also occurs in certain spontaneously arising tumors in animals.

At least four mechanisms of the angiogenic switch have been identified in both human tumors and spontaneous tumors in mice.

Prevascular Tumors Recruit Their Own Blood Supply. This is the most common mechanism of the angiogenic switch. Approximately 95% of human cancers are carcinomas that originate as microscopic in situ lesions in an avascular epithelial layer separated by a basement membrane from underlying vasculature in the dermis or submucosa, respectively. The basement membrane is not only a physical barrier but also a molecular barrier to migrating endothelial cells. For example, tumstatin, a potent inhibitor of endothelial cell migration and proliferation, is found in collagen IV.[37] After the basement membrane has been breached by new vessel sprouts, tumor cells form multiple cell layers around each new capillary blood vessel.[38] The radius of these microcylinders is restricted to the oxygen diffusion limit for a given tumor type as originally defined by Thomlinson and Gray.[39] For example, for a human melanoma, the oxygen diffusion limit is approximately 85 microns. Beyond that distance from a capillary blood vessel, virtually all tumor cells are apoptotic (or necrotic). Within that radius, most tumor cells are viable (Figure 28-3). For a prostate carcinoma, the oxygen diffusion limit is approximately 110 microns, and it may be greater for certain tumors, such as for a chondrosarcoma or a tumor in which *p53* is mutated or absent; however, it would rarely exceed 200 microns.

Circulating Endothelial Stem Cells Participate in Tumor Angiogenesis. It is becoming clear that circulating endothelial progenitor cells derived from bone marrow can be recruited to the vascular bed of tumors and contribute to tumor growth.[40-53] VEGF is elaborated by a variety of tumor signals through both VEGFR-1 (Flt-1) and VEGFR-2 (Flt-1) on endothelial cells and can mobilize progenitor endothelial cells into the circulation, where they are recruited into the vascular bed of certain tumor types, but not others.[40,54] The current view is that microvascular endothelial cells in the vascular bed of a tumor may be recruited both from the local neighborhood and from the bone marrow. However, the *ratio* of these endothelial cells from different sources may differ by tumor type (Rafii, personal communication). Although lymphomas may recruit the majority (>90%) of their endothelial cells from the bone marrow, other tumors (e.g., breast cancer) recruit vascular endothelial cells both from the local neighborhood and to a lesser extent from the bone marrow. In contrast, in prostate cancer, most endothelial cells are recruited locally and very few are derived from bone marrow. Although the ratios of bone marrow–derived endothelium and local endothelium have not yet been elucidated for most tumors, Shahin Rafii has suggested certain possible implications. First, the

efficacy of conventional chemotherapy may eventually be shown to correlate with the percentage of bone marrow–derived endothelial cells in a tumor. Second, during conven-tional chemotherapy administered at maximum tolerated dose, the off-therapy intervals necessary to rescue bone marrow may result in a surge of progenitor endothelial cells, which could traffic to the tumor (Rafii, personal communication). Third, certain angiogenesis inhibitors may suppress the release of bone marrow–derived progenitor endothelial cells. For example, angiostatin targets progenitor endothelial cells,[55] endostatin induces apoptosis in circulating endothelial cells in tumor-bearing mice,[56] and thalidomide decreases circulating endothelial cells by tenfold in multiple myeloma.[57]

Circulating VEGF may be one of the angiogenic signals by which tumors can recruit endothelial cells from bone marrow. Subcutaneously implanted collagen gels embedded with VEGF are invaded by endothelial cells from bone marrow and from the local neighborhood.[40,54] VEGF serum concentrations closely correlate with platelet counts in cancer patients.[58] VEGF is stored, transported,[58] and released from platelets.[59] Furthermore, it has been reported that platelet counts have prognostic significance for cancer patients—higher platelet counts correlate with a worse prognosis.[60-62] Therefore it is possible that for those types of tumors that recruit bone marrow–derived endothelial cells, communication from tumor to bone marrow may be mediated in part by the VEGF in circulating platelets. According to Pinedo and colleagues,[61] "these results do not at this time have a direct impact on clinical cancer therapy." However, he emphasizes that "oncologists should be aware of a potential role for

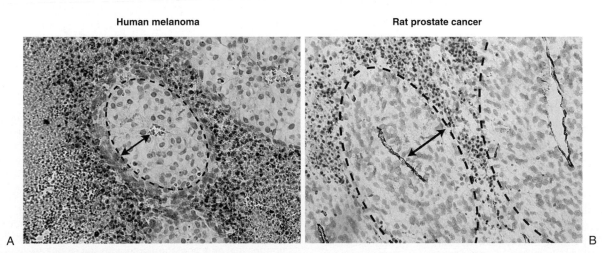

Human melanoma **Rat prostate cancer**

FIG. **28-3** **A,** A cuff of live tumor cells around a microvessel in a human melanoma growing in a SCID mouse has an average radius of 85 microns. The appearance of an ellipsoid is due to the way the section is cut. **B,** A cuff of rat prostate cancer cells around a microvessel has an average radius of 110 microns. *(From Folkman J, Kalluri R: Tumor angiogenesis. In Kufe DW et al [eds]: Cancer medicine, ed 6, Hamilton, Ontario, 2003, Decker.)*

platelets in cancer growth" and in tumor angiogenesis. "For example, bone marrow–supportive agents, currently used in high-dose chemotherapy, contribute to platelet production and thereby may influence response to therapy."[60]

Nonendothelial Host Cells May Contribute to the Angiogenic Switch by Amplifying Tumor Angiogenesis. In addition to recruiting vascular endothelium from the host, certain tumors may also attract mast cells,[63] macrophages,[64] and inflammatory cells.[65,66] These cells can amplify tumor angiogenesis by releasing pro-angiogenic molecules such as bFGF[63,67] or by releasing metalloproteinases, which can mobilize VEGF and other angiogenic proteins.[68] Tumor angiogenesis and tumor growth are significantly diminished in mice deficient in metalloproteinase-9.[65] Certain tumor cells may also trigger host stromal cells in the tumor bed to overexpress the angiogenic protein VEGF.[69] This is a novel mechanism of amplification of the angiogenic phenotype once it has been initiated.

Vessel Cooption. In certain metastases (e.g., in the mouse brain), tumor cells exit from microvessels in the target organ, encircle these vessels, cause the endothelial cells to undergo apoptosis, and finally induce neovascular sprouts from neighboring vessels. This process, called *cooption,* may represent an intermediate or alternative step in the switch to the angiogenic phenotype.[70,71]

In summary, the hypothesis that all malignancies are angiogenesis dependent and that antiangiogenic therapy may control tumor growth appears to be true for all of these mechanisms of angiogenic switching.

Persistence of Nonangiogenic Tumor Cells in the Vascularized Tumor. After a nonangiogenic microscopic in situ carcinoma has become neovascularized, the tumor still contains a significant proportion of tumor cells that have not switched.[72] Vascularized human primary tumors appear to contain a mixture of *angiogenic* and *nonangiogenic* tumor cells. The nonangiogenic tumor cells can be isolated from a human tumor removed at surgery by implanting numerous tiny pieces (1 mm³) of tumor into the subcutaneous dorsum of immunodeficient SCID mice or by implanting cultured human tumor cells.[72] Although a few tumors grow to a palpable and visible size (100 mm³ to >1000 mm³) within a few weeks and a few others appear after several months, most human tumor transplants remain invisible in the majority of mice, a phenomenon called *no take.* However, upon opening the skin of these mice, one invariably finds a tiny (<0.5 to 1 mm³) whitish avascular or poorly vascularized tumor that is transplantable, contains proliferating and apoptotic tumor cells, but does not expand or metastasize. A few of these nonangiogenic dormant

tumors have spontaneously become angiogenic after 1 month or more, depending on the tumor type, and have then grown. In contrast, others (e.g., osteosarcoma) have remained nonangiogenic and dormant up to 3 years after being transplanted to new mice every 8 months[72,73] (Figure 28-4). Some tumor types that remain nonangiogenic can be rapidly switched to the angiogenic phenotype through transfection with the *ras* oncogene, which significantly increases tumor cell production of VEGF and decreases thrombosponsin-1 production.[73] Furthermore, nonangiogenic tumor cells can be labeled with green fluorescent protein and mixed 1:1 with angiogenic tumor cells that are not labeled.[73] The resulting large neovascularized tumor that grows rapidly contains tiny (<0.5 mm) green nonangiogenic colonies dispersed throughout. When the nonangiogenic green tumor cells are mixed with a decreasing fraction of angiogenic tumor cells, there is a long latent period of 1 month or more before neovascularized tumors arise. The latent period appears to be the time required for the angiogenic tumor cells to accumulate to a threshold population sufficient to recruit new blood vessels for the whole tumor. Once neovascularization has occurred, spontaneous metastases may appear in the lung (depending on the tumor type). Nonangiogenic tumor cells form microscopic nonangiogenic metastases

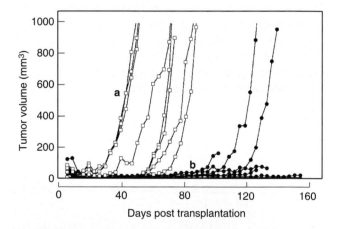

FIG. 28-4 Tumor growth curves of subcutaneous xenotransplants of human liposarcoma in severe combined immunodeficient (SCID mice). Tumor cells were transplanted into groups of 28 mice. A majority of the tumors remained as nonangiogenic in situ tumors of less than 1 mm³ beyond 150 days. Some tumors switched to the angiogenic phenotype by approximately 30 days, whereas others did not become angiogenic until 100 days or more. Once the tumors were angiogenic, the growth rates of the angiogenic tumors were similar to one another. This experiment reveals that human tumors that are angiogenic contain subclones of nonangiogenic tumor cells mixed with angiogenic tumor cells. *(From Folkman J, Kalluri R: Tumor angiogenesis. In Kufe DW et al [eds]: Cancer medicine, ed 6, Hamiltan, Ontario, 2003, Decker.)*

(Udagawa and co-workers, personal communication). These studies indicate that a nonangiogenic, dormant primary tumor may not shed tumor cells into the circulation. Once it switches to the angiogenic phenotype, it may then shed both angiogenic and nonangiogenic tumor cells into the circulation. The nonangiogenic tumor cells may be the source of microscopic metastases, which are capable of remaining dormant for prolonged periods. It has also been reported that in some instances, tumor cells may remain dormant as solitary cells.[74,75]

ONSET OF NEOVASCULARIZATION PERMITS EXPANSION OF TUMOR MASS, INVASION, AND METASTASIS

Expansion of Tumor Mass. As new capillaries are induced to sprout from preexisting capillaries and venules, tumor cells grow around them. Three or more concentric layers of tumor cells may encircle a single capillary tube. The replication of new capillaries, each supporting a microcylinder of tumor cells, permits rapid expansion of tumor mass. A segment of capillary tube formed by a single endothelial cell can support 5 to 50 tumor cells, based on the finding that a gram of tumor contains approximately 20 million endothelial cells and 10^8 to 10^9 tumor cells.[76,77] A large breast carcinoma of 1 cm^3 or greater may appear white or pale on gross examination and thus is often assumed to be avascular. However, microscopic examination reveals a fine vascular network interspersed with tumor cells. The microvessels are often difficult to see on a routine 4-µm-thick paraffin section, because their lumina are compressed. However, if endothelial cells are highlighted with antibody to von Willebrand factor or to CD34, the microvessels are more readily visualized. Furthermore, if the thickness of the histologic section is increased to 50 µm, it is possible to see microvessels projecting in three dimensions, and each vessel is surrounded by a microcylinder of three to four layers of tumor cells (Tedrow, unpublished data).

The stimulation of tumor cell growth after the onset of neovascularization is usually ascribed to perfusion of the tumor cells by new blood flow, which delivers oxygen and nutrients and removes catabolites. A paracrine effect of endothelial cells on tumor cell growth may be equally important.[27,32,78,79] In vitro studies reveal that tumor cells grow preferentially around capillary tubes despite the absence of flow.[80] Endothelial cells also produce growth and survival factors such as insulin-like growth factor-I (IGF-I), bFGF, platelet-derived growth factor (PDGF-BB), heparin-binding epithelial growth factor (HB-EGF), and granulocyte-macrophage colony-stimulating factor. Because a neovascularized tumor is flooded with growth factors

and survival factors, complete blockade of neovascularization by an angiogenesis inhibitor could result in disappearance of growth factors, survival factors, or both. In animal[81-84] and human tumors,[85] the induction of angiogenesis correlates with a significant decrease in apoptosis (by as much as sevenfold in mice). Nevertheless, in these tumors the proliferation rate of tumor cells remains equivalently high in the prevascular and in the vascularized tumor (up to 40% by bromo-deoxy-uridine [BrdU]). This pattern is observed in a variety of tumor types. It indicates that tumor expansion after neovascularization may depend mainly on a decrease in apoptosis.[35,81] Analogous systems are found in *MYC*-dependent lymphoma cells or in fibroblasts with dysregulated *MYC*-expression. Both cell types grow in the presence of IGF-I or IGF-II, respectively, but die when these factors are withdrawn.[86]

Although the absence of angiogenesis prevents expansion of tumor mass beyond a microscopic size of a few millimeters, the presence of angiogenesis is necessary but not sufficient for expansion of tumor mass.[87] Some benign tumors, such as adrenal adenoma, may lack the proliferative capacity to match their high angiogenic activity. Conversely, the rate of expansion of a tumor mass can be regulated independently of tumor cell proliferation. Some human tumors (e.g., prostate and breast cancer) grow slowly for years and then seem to shift to a rapid rate of expansion of tumor mass. Neglected breast cancers that have attained a large size may slow their growth, possibly from diminished angiogenic activity. Experimental evidence for this idea comes from murine fibrosarcoma cells transfected with the angiogenesis inhibitor angiostatin.[82,83,88] Inoculation of mice with transfected cells that express increasing levels of angiostatin yields tumors that grow slowly (i.e., 77% inhibition of tumor growth compared with nontransfected tumor cells in the same period). Furthermore, because it is now clear that tumor burden can inhibit angiogenesis, the slowing of certain tumors as they increase in size could be attributable in part to angiogenic mechanisms.[82-84]

Invasion. Tumor invasion may be facilitated by neovascularization. Although microinvasion may be observed in a carcinoma in situ of the breast before it has become neovascularized[89] (i.e., a thin file of tumor cells breaches the basic membrane of a duct filled with tumor), after neovascularization, invasion into adjacent connective tissue occurs along a broad front and tumor cords follow the path of newly generated blood vessels.[80] Microvascular endothelial cells under the stimulus of angiogenic proteins (e.g., bFGF, VPF/VEGF) increase their expression of proteolytic enzymes (e.g., collagenase IV),[90-94] which contribute to the invasiveness of endothelial cells and tumor cells. The ability of growing capillaries to liquefy extracellular matrix is clearly illustrated by the following experiment.[95,96] India ink (containing carbon particles of approximately 200 angstroms) is injected into a rabbit cornea so that the ink is trapped in a square corneal pocket, like a tattoo, between a tumor implant and the vascular bed at the limbal edge of the cornea. As new blood vessels are attracted into the cornea by the tumor, they first encounter the India ink. India ink is dispersed only from the inferior border of the pocket, coincident with dissolution of the corneal matrix by the neovascular front. The superior border of the India ink, contiguous to the avascular tumor, remains intact. Only after the tumor has become neovascularized is it capable of invading the corneal pocket and dispersing all of the India ink. In the absence of neovascularization, India ink remains sharply demarcated in the corneal pocket.[95] This result suggests that the proteolytic activity produced by proliferating capillary blood vessels may enhance invasion of endothelial cells into extracellular matrix but may also contribute to the invasiveness of tumor cells. Therefore antiangiogenic therapy could inhibit tumor invasion. Conversely, certain protease inhibitors are antiangiogenic.[96,97] However, some protease inhibitors may also decrease the enzymatic release of angiogenesis inhibitors (e.g., angiostatin, endostatin, tumstatin). When human skin grafted to immunodeficient mice was inoculated with human breast cancer cells, the resulting tumors became vascularized by human blood vessels. When the animals were injected with antibody against alpha$_v\beta_3$ integrin on the human endothelial cells, angiogenesis was inhibited, but so was tumor invasiveness, despite the fact that the tumor cells lacked the alpha$_v\beta_3$ receptor.[98,99]

Metastasis. Experimental and clinical evidence suggest that the process of metastasis is also angiogenesis dependent.[24,100] For a tumor cell to metastasize successfully, it must breach several barriers and be able to respond to specific growth factors.[101,102] Tumor cells must gain access to the vasculature in the primary tumor, survive the circulation, arrest in the microvasculature of the target organ,[103] exit from this vasculature,[104] grow in the target organ, and induce angiogenesis.[96,105] Thus angiogenesis appears to be necessary at both the beginning and end of the metastatic cascade.

In experimental animals, tumor cells are generally found in the circulation only after a primary tumor has become vascularized.[90,106] The number of cells shed from the primary tumor correlates with the density of vessels in the primary tumor and with the number of lung metastases observed subsequently. Tumor cells can enter the circulation by penetrating through proliferating capillaries whose basement membranes are fragmented and leaky.[106,107] Increasing tumor angiogenesis has also been correlated with increased tumor cell shedding into the circulation in human tumors.[108] Furthermore, angiogenic factors from tumors (bFGF and VEGF) induce plasminogen activator and collagenases in proliferating endothelial cells and contribute to the degradation of basement membranes.[92,93,109] Other evidence that metastasis is angiogenesis dependent is based on the suppression of metastatic growth in mice treated with endothelial-specific angiogenesis inhibitors, such as angiostatin or endostatin. The metastases remain dormant at a microscopic size. Dormancy occurs despite the fact that the angiogenesis inhibitors have no inhibitory effect on the tumor cells in vitro. In these animals, microscopic dormant metastases are harmless, and the mice appear perfectly healthy for as long as the inhibitor is administered (up to 2 to 10 months in current studies).[83] In another animal tumor model, lung metastases remain nonangiogenic and avascular, even after the original primary tumor has been removed. These mice are healthy for as long as they have been observed (up to 1 year at the time of this writing), or almost half their normal life span (O'Reilly, unpublished data). The dormant, nonangiogenic metastases can be induced to grow at any time through local trauma to the chest or systemic administration of transforming growth factor-β (TGF-β) (O'Reilly and co-workers, unpublished data). Correlative clinical data also suggest that metastatic potential may depend on the intensity of angiogenesis. Neovascularization can be quantified in human tumors by staining histologic sections with an antibody to von Willebrand factor, an endothelial cell marker. This method also reveals a significant direct correlation between the highest density of microvessels in a histologic section of invasive breast cancer and the occurrence of future metastases.[89] In other tumor types, microvessel counts also correlate with metastatic risk and clinical outcome (see the section on clinical applications of angiogenesis research).

Angiogenesis Progression. Rak and colleagues[27,32,110] proposed the term *angiogenic progression* in a hypothesis that states that "a stepwise accumulation of genetic alterations during tumor progression is likely to be paralleled by a stepwise increase in angiogenic competence of tumor cells." Angiogenesis and neoplastic progression have also been linked in animal tumors.[111] For example, a primary breast cancer may produce one angiogenic protein, for example, VEGF, but subsequent metastases may produce up to six angiogenic proteins.[112] In the advanced stages of breast cancer or other malignancies, the clinical picture is one of new metastases that parasitize the circulation and that appear ever more frequently at decreasing intervals.

Angiogenesis in Breast Cancer Correlates with Tumor Aggressiveness

QUANTIFICATION OF INTRATUMORAL MICROVESSEL DENSITY

Weidner and associates[89] first reported that quantification of microvessel density in breast cancer was an independent prognostic indicator of metastatic risk and mortality. Microvessels were highlighted in histologic sections by staining with an antibody to von Willebrand factor. In subsequent studies, other endothelial markers have been used, such as CD31.[113] Without such endothelial markers, microvessels are often difficult to visualize in the standard histologic section, which is cut at 4-μm thickness. This is in part because of the closure of some vessels by compressive interstitial pressures.

Weidner and colleagues also found that microvessels were not homogeneously distributed but that there were areas of increased microvessel density. Quantification of the number of vessels in these areas gave the best predictive values for overall survival. The method that Weidner described for preparing the histologic sections and for counting microvessels has previously been described in detail.[96] However, the critical steps are as follows: Paraffin blocks are selected that contain the invasive components of breast cancer specimens by observing corresponding sections stained with hematoxylin and eosin. Areas of highest microvessel density (vascular hotspots) are selected by scanning a tumor section at low magnification (10 to 100×). A generous section through the middle of the tumor (which includes the tumor periphery) is selected for microvessel analysis. A low-background staining and highly specific and intense labeling of endothelial cells are required. Areas of highest microvessel density (vascular hotspots) are encountered predominantly at the peripheral tumor margin. A higher magnification (approximately 200×) is then used to count individual stained microvessels. Weidner and co-workers[89] suggested a field size of 0.74 mm², although other magnifications have been reported. Focusing on a smaller area, corresponding to a higher magnification (400×), improves the detail of the image, allowing the identification of more single endothelial cell sprouts. However, areas smaller than approximately 0.15 mm² (e.g., >400×) or areas significantly larger than 0.74 mm² (e.g., <200×) may decrease the correlation of microvessel density with clinical outcome. When microvessels are counted in a field, it is not necessary to identify a lumen or red cells in a vessel, nor is a cutoff caliber size used. Both single cell sprouts and larger vessels are included in the counts. Even if distinct clusters give the impression of being part of one larger vessel transected by the plane of the tissue section more than once, they are counted as separate microvessels. Averaging counts of all the vessels in a section does not correlate with clinical outcome, but quantification of hotspots does.[114] In more than 3200 cases worldwide of breast cancer assessed for angiogenic activity, 80% of the studies that included multivariant analysis found that angiogenesis is a significant prognostic indicator of overall survival.[115] Intratumoral microvessel density is a prognostic indicator in patients who are lymph node negative, and this may be an important use for this method. A similar method has been successful in the majority of reports for a variety of other tumors from many centers worldwide. A summary of reports on microvessel density as a prognostic indicator in breast cancer is presented in Tables 28-1 and 28-2. Gasparini[115] and Weidner and Folkman[96] review these studies.

BIOLOGIC BASIS OF THE CORRELATION OF INTRATUMORAL MICROVESSEL DENSITY WITH CLINICAL OUTCOME

Most studies since Weidner's report[89] in 1991 reveal that the higher the microvessel count in areas of highest vessel density, the lower the overall survival. The decreased survival is generally related to increased metastatic risk. Possible biologic explanations for this correlation include the following:

1. Increasing microvessel density provides an increased vascular surface area for cells to escape from the primary tumor into the main circulation.
2. Because of the clonal origin of metastases, a primary tumor containing a high proportion of angiogenic malignant cells is more likely to generate metastases that are already angiogenic when they arrive at the target tissue.[105,147,148]
3. Some tumor cells produce multiple angiogenic factors compared with others and thus have a higher probability of rapid tumor growth.[112]
4. Certain angiogenic factors such as bFGF and VEGF also upregulate production of metalloproteinases by endothelial cells and increase the possibility that tumor cells enter the circulation.[27]
5. Endothelial cells in the vascular bed of a tumor release cytokines that can facilitate metastasis. For example, interleukin-6, produced by endothelial cells, is a motility factor for breast cancer cells and may facilitate their escape from a vascularized tumor into the circulation.[148-150]
6. There are also confounding biologic factors that could explain some reports that find no prognostic value for microvessel density. For example,

TABLE 28-1 | Journal Reports of a Positive Association between Tumor Angiogenesis and Tumor Aggressiveness

AUTHORS	NO. OF PATIENTS	NO. OF NODE-NEGATIVE PATIENTS	TUMOR ANGIOGENESIS: POSITIVE ASSOCIATIONS	COMMENTS
Weidner[89]	49	—	Lymph node metastases and distant metastases	1st study of iMVD
Bosari[116]	180	151	LN mets LVI	1st confirmation
Horak[113]	103	64	LN mets, HG, TS, OS	1st use of CD31 for iMVD
Weidner[117]	165	83	RFS, OS, LN mets, TS, HG	1st study of RFS and OS in ANN and ANP patients
Visscher[118]	58	28	RFS	1st image analysis of iMVD
Toi[119]	125	57	LN mets, RFS epidermal growth factor receptor, CERBB2	
Gasparini[120]	254	0	RFS, OS, D mets age, menopause, HG	
Obermair[121]	64	32	LN mets, HG	
Gasparini[122]	165	—	RFS, OS	Analysis of p53
Fox[123]	109	109	RFS, OS	Chalkley point eyepiece graticule used
Obermair[124]	106	—	RFS	
Toi[125]	328	130	RFS	
Gasparini[126]	191	0	RFS, OS	
Inada[127]	110	110	RFS	
Charpin[128]	133	—	Nottingham prognostic index	
Barbareschi[129,130]	191	0	RFS, OS, ER	
Bevilacqua[131]	211	211	RFS	
Ogawa[132]	155	91	RFS, OS, LVI, ER	
Obermair[133]	230	—	RFS	
Chu[134]	81	—		
Heimann[135]	167	167	OS	First to show that "the prognostic usefulness of microvessel density is maintained after more than 15 years of follow-up"
Ravazoula[136]	106	86	Predicts hematogenous metastases	3- to 10-yr follow-up
Karaiossifidi[137]	52	52	Early relapse	
Kato[138]	109		AMC or HMC "Univariate analysis showed that AMC or HMC was a statistically significant predictor of overall survival in all patients (p = .0086 and p = .0307 respectively)" p 49	
Bertin[139]	33		"Microvessel count correlates with desmoplastic-rich stroma"	

Data from Weidner N, Folkman J: Tumor vascularity as a prognostic factor in cancer. In DeVita VT, Hellman S, Rosenberg SA (eds): *Important advances in oncology*, Philadelphia, 1996, Lippincott-Raven; and Gasparini G: *Eur J Cancer* 32A:2485, 1996.

AMC, Average microvessel count per square millimeter; *ANN*, axillary node negative; *ANP*, axillary node positive; *D mets*, distant metastases; *ER*, estrogen receptor; *HG*, histograde; *HMC*, highest microvessel count per square millimeter; *iMVD*, intratumoral microvessel density; *LN*, lymph node; *LVI*, lymphatic vascular invasion; *mets*, metastases; *OS*, overall survival; *RFS*, relapse-free survival; *TS*, tumor size.

For additional reports which compare intensity of tumor vascularization to parameters of breast cancer other than relapse or survival, see references 214, 215, 216, 217, 218, and 219.

TABLE 28-2	Journal Reports of a Negative Association between Tumor Angiogenesis and Tumor Aggressiveness

AUTHORS	NO. OF PATIENTS	NO. OF NODE-NEGATIVE PATIENTS	TUMOR ANGIOGENESIS: POSITIVE ASSOCIATIONS	COMMENTS
Hall[140]	87	50	No analysis of RFS or OS	Different counting method than Weidner[89]; short follow-up Only 6% relapse in ANN
Van Hoef[141]	93	0	HG ($p = .27$)	MV counts seem too high for area given
Milliaris[142]	42	—	No analysis of RFS or OS	
Axelsson[143]	220	110		Series limited to ductal carcinoma; patients are specially selected
Siitonen[144]	77	77	RFS, OS not analyzed	
Goulding[145]	165	Not stated	No correlation with RFS or OS	
Costello[146]	87	87	No correlation with RFS or OS	Area of field = 0.22 mm^2

ANN, Axillary node negative; *HG,* histograde; *OS,* overall survival; *RFS,* relapse-free survival.

mouse experiments reveal that tumor burden can influence angiogenesis at a remote site (see later discussion).[82-84]

MICROVESSEL DENSITY MAY NOT BE USEFUL FOR PREDICTING EFFICACY OF THERAPY

Although microvessel density is a useful prognostic indicator of metastatic risk in many tumors, it may not be a good indicator of therapeutic efficacy for several reasons. In normal tissues, the degree of vascularization and oxygen/nutrient demand are tightly coupled. In tumors, however, the degree of vascularization and tumor growth are loosely coupled, or even uncoupled. This may be because in tumor cells, expression of angiogenic factors, such as VEGF, are no longer regulated by oxygen concentration. During tumor regression under antiangiogenic therapy, microvessel density may decrease if capillary dropout exceeds tumor cell dropout (autolysis), increase if tumor cell dropout exceeds capillary dropout, or remain the same if disappearance of capillaries and tumor cells parallel each other. Mice bearing human osteosarcomas were treated with endostatin until there was more than a 50% inhibition of tumor growth[151] (Figure 28-5). Despite the fact that this drug inhibited growth of both treated tumors depicted, the intensity of vascularization after treatment differed significantly between the tumors. Microvascular density was quantified over the entire histologic section rather than over vascular hotspots to avoid the effects of heterogeneity of vascularization in the tissue sample. Microvascular density dropped sharply in one treated tumor but rose slightly in the second, yet both tumors

were equivalently reduced in size by the treatment relative to control. Thus detection of a decrease in microvessel density during treatment with an angiogenesis inhibitor suggests that the agent is active. However, the absence of a drop in microvessel density does not indicate that the agent is ineffective.[152] Understanding this distinction between the usefulness of microvessel density as a prognostic indicator of future metastatic risk or mortality in contrast to its problematic status as a predictor of therapeutic efficacy is important in the design of clinical trials of angiogenesis inhibitors. Biopsies of tumors or lymph nodes for microvessel density, before or after antiangiogenic therapy, may not be useful. Furthermore, selecting patients for such clinical trials on the basis of whether their tumor is highly vascularized also appears to be unnecessary. In fact, experimental studies show that a given dose of an angiogenesis inhibitor is more effective in poorly vascularized tumors. Highly vascularized tumors require larger doses.[153]

Dormant Breast Cancer

It is not uncommon for a patient with node-negative breast cancer to remain asymptomatic for 10 to 12 years and then experience the sudden appearance of metastases. This phenomenon, called *tumor dormancy,* can be defined as microscopic disease in which there is no expansion of tumor mass.[154] There has been no satisfactory explanation for this long-term dormancy, nor is it clear where the tumor cells resided or whether they

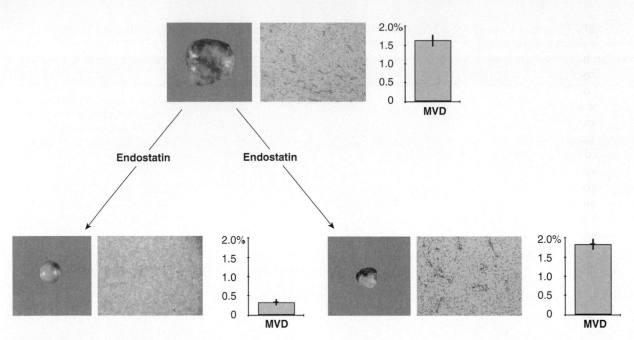

FIG. **28-5** Human osteosarcomas growing in immunodeficient mice were treated with endostatin. Endostatin significantly inhibited tumor growth. Despite the fact that endostatin inhibited both treated tumors depicted here, the intensity of vascularization after treatment differed significantly between the tumors. Microvascular density *(MVD)* was quantified over the entire histologic section rather than over vascular hotspots to avoid the effects of heterogeneity of vascularization in the tissue sample. Sections were scored by imaging as many microscopic fields at 200× as necessary to cover the entire section. Microvascular density dropped sharply in one treated tumor but rose slightly in the second, yet both tumors were equivalently reduced in size by the treatment relative to control. *(Modified from Hlatky L, Hahnfeldt P, Folkman J: J Natl Cancer Inst 94:883, 2002.)*

were proliferating or quiescent. Different explanations include the following: (1) The tumor cells could be in a prolonged G_0 state, removed from the cell cycle,[155] (2) the cells could be immunologically suppressed,[156-158] (3) tumor cells could be dormant because of hormone withdrawal,[159] (4) tumor cells could be proliferating continuously but take years to produce a tumor of the size that can be detected clinically, or (5) expansion of microscopic metastases could be constrained throughout the dormant period but undergo a sudden change from a resting microtumor to an enlarging tumor mass within a year or less of the time of first clinical detection. The results reported by Demichelli and co-workers[160,161] best fit this model. They show that the mean rate of growth of the metastatic tumor, once it has grown beyond the dormant stage and has been detected clinically, is similar from one patient to another and is independent of the length of the dormant period. This model of tumor dormancy most closely resembles experimental models of blocked angiogenesis. Holmgren and colleagues[81] proposed a new concept of tumor dormancy based on murine lung metastases that are held dormant at a microscopic size for as long as their angiogenesis is completely blocked by administration of angiostatin. In these animals, proliferating tumor cells are balanced by apoptotic tumor cells. A provocative finding is that inhibition of angiogenesis significantly increases tumor cell apoptosis but has no effect on the high rate of tumor cell proliferation. Subsequent reports confirm that angiogenesis and apoptosis are inversely correlated, whereas tumor cell proliferation is independent of angiogenesis.[82,83,162]

Influence of Tumor Burden on Angiogenesis at Remote Sites: Implications for Breast Cancer

Patients with locally advanced breast cancer who have no detectable metastases may often develop rapid growth of metastases after removal of the large breast tumor.[163] A possible explanation for this observation is that tumor burden can suppress tumor growth.[164] A suggested mechanism for this phenomenon comes from the recent discovery that increasing mass of a primary tumor inhibits angiogenesis at remote sites and that this process is mediated by angiostatin.[81,84,163]

The inhibition of metastatic growth by a primary tumor may be only one pattern of a group of common patterns of presentation of metastases, some of which

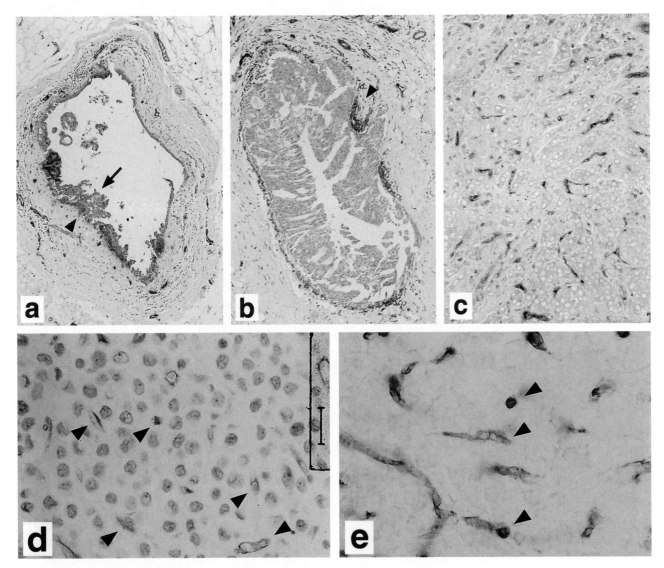

COLOR PLATE **1** **A,** Human breast cancer. Large breast duct partially lined by duct carcinoma in situ *(arrow)* and intense angiogenesis in the immediately adjacent periductal breast stroma. Brown staining microvessels (antibody to von Willebrand factor) are indicated by the arrowhead. Note the absence of angiogenesis in the areas of breast stroma adjacent to portion of duct lined with benign duct epithelium (from Weidner and co-workers[89]). **B,** Large breast duct filled with carcinoma in situ and surrounded by new microvessels in the periductal breast stroma. Arrowheads show invasion of microvessels through basement membrane of the duct, accompanied by invasion of tumor cells into the periductal stroma. **C,** Invasive ductal carcinoma, area of highest density of microvessels. **D,** Higher power of invasive human breast carcinoma 4-μm-thick section. Microvessels (brown stained with antibody to CD31) are indicated by arrowheads. **E,** A 50-μm-thick confocal microscopy section showing microvessels in three dimensions *(arrowheads)* surrounded by tumors cells that fill the intercapillary space.

Continued

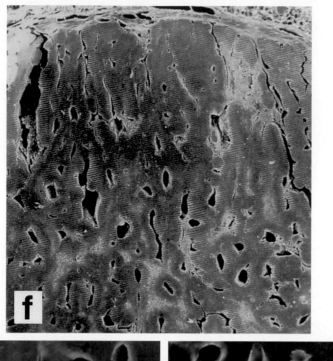

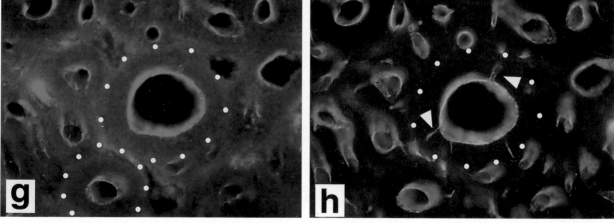

COLOR PLATE **1 cont'd F, G, H,** Cross sections of breast cancer in mice showing the microcylinders of tumor cells that surround each microvessel. The 100-μm thickness of these tumor microcylinders is within the range of the oxygen diffusion limit. **F,** Scanning electron microscope view of 100-μm Vibratome section of a subcutaneous MCa-IV mouse breast tumor with the skin at the top. Blood vessels appear as black holes emptied of blood and preserved in an open state by vascular perfusion of fixative. Pale necrotic regions surround perivascular rings of tumor tissue that are approximately 100 μm thick. (Original magnification 25×.) A 10-mm scale bar would equal 400 μm. *(Courtesy Donald M. McDonald, University of California, San Francisco.)* **G, H,** Large and small thin-walled blood vessels in MCa-IV mouse breast tumor labeled by vascular perfusion of green (FITC) fluorescent lectin staining (**G,** green) and CD31-immunoreactivity viewed by Cy3 fluorescence (**H,** gold). Like the lectin, CD31-immunoreactivity defines the luminal surface of the vessels but, unlike the lectin, it also labels tiny sprouts, which have no apparent lumen because they have CD31-immunoreactivity but no lectin staining. Sprouts *(white arrowheads)* about 1 μm in diameter radiate from the vessel lining into the 100-μm-thick perivascular ring of tumor tissue (outlined by white dots). Vessels preserved in open state by vascular perfusion of fixative. *(Courtesy Donald M. McDonald, University of California, San Francisco.)*

are observed in patients with breast cancer. Four common patterns and a rare pattern of metastatic presentation have been proposed.[163]

The first pattern, in which metastases grow after removal of the primary tumor, is analogous to a mouse model of Lewis lung carcinoma in which lung metastases remain microscopic while a primary tumor is present (and generating angiostatin) but grow rapidly within 5 days after the primary tumor is removed.[81 84,163]

The second pattern, in which metastases grow concomitantly with the primary tumor, is analogous to a mouse model of a subclone of Lewis lung carcinoma in which the primary tumor does not suppress its lung metastases and does not generate detectable levels of angiostatin in the circulation.[84]

The third pattern, known to oncologists as the *occult primary*,[1] could be based on metastatic cells that outgrow the primary tumor and suppress its angiogenesis. This is speculation, and there are no animal models, with the possible exception of one report, in which metastatic cells were seeded in the lungs, followed later by implantation of a subcutaneous tumor, whose growth was inhibited.[165]

The fourth pattern, in which metastases remain dormant for years following removal of the primary tumor, is observed in breast cancer, colon cancer, Ewing's sarcoma, and many other tumor types. Again, the mechanism of this prolonged dormancy is unknown. However, recent reports indicate that once metastases become clinically detectable, they display a similar rate of growth that is independent of the number of years of dormancy.[160,161] This observation is consistent with a model of microscopic dormant metastases that do not expand until sometime within a year of becoming clinically detectable.[160,161] It can be speculated that these metastases originated from cells that were not angiogenic but underwent the switch to the angiogenic phenotype before becoming clinically detectable. No animal model has been reported. However, in our laboratory, O'Reilly has demonstrated a B16 melanoma in C57Bl/6 mice in which dormant, nonangiogenic lung metastases of less than 0.1 to 0.2 mm diameter are found as late as 6 months after removal of the primary tumor in otherwise healthy mice. This is one fourth the normal life span of these animals (O'Reilly, personal communication). A study of nonangiogenic tumor cells that escape from the primary tumor and the mechanism by which their metastases switch to the angiogenic phenotype may be a fruitful area of research.

A fifth pattern of metastatic presentation is occasionally observed, for example, when removal of a renal cell carcinoma is followed by regression of lung metastases. One can speculate that the metastases may have been dependent on high production of circulating angiogenic factors[166] (and possibly other growth factors) from the primary tumor. In renal cell carcinomas, high tumor levels of bFGF correlate with high mortality.[166] In fact, we found that 10% of a group of patients with a wide spectrum of malignancies had abnormally elevated levels of the angiogenic polypeptide bFGF in their serum and 37% of 950 patients had abnormally elevated levels of bFGF in urine.[167]

The clinical presentations of metastases are discussed here in terms of angiogenic mechanisms, because this approach offers a plausible unifying explanation for the different patterns that oncologists see in their cancer patients. The similarity of animal models to human patterns of metastasis presentation does not prove that angiogenic control of metastatic growth is responsible for the behavior of metastases in cancer patients. These mechanisms have yet to be demonstrated in human cancer. However, clinicians who are aware of them may be able to uncover evidence that supports or rejects the hypothesis.

Principles of Antiangiogenic Therapy in the Clinic: Guidelines for Designs of Clinical Protocols

Certain guidelines are emerging from laboratory and clinical experience that may be helpful in the design of protocols for antiangiogenic therapy in breast cancer, as well as in other types of cancer.

OBJECTIVE

A goal of antiangiogenic therapy is to regress a focus of proliferating microvessels, that is, to restore a local area of migrating and proliferating endothelial cells to their normal resting state. When used in cancer therapy, antiangiogenic therapy differs from cytotoxic chemotherapy, in which the objective is to kill as many tumor cells as possible in the shortest possible time with the maximum tolerated dose. Antiangiogenic therapy is usually administered for prolonged periods, without interruption, at the highest effective dosage that does not cause toxicity. It is neither necessary nor efficacious to discontinue an angiogenesis inhibitor at intervals, as is done for cytotoxic therapy. For example, infants with life-threatening hemangiomas have been treated daily for 9 months to 1 year with interferon-alpha. Low-dose daily interferon-alpha (3 million U/m^2/day for children or 3 million U/day for adults), which inhibits production by tumors of the pro-angiogenic protein bFGF, has been administered for 8 months to 1 year to patients with recurrent high-grade giant cell tumors of the mandible and maxilla and has resulted in complete regression that has remained durable for up to 6 years' follow-up.[168,169] Stable disease can also be a goal of antiangiogenic therapy. In current clinical trials of endostatin, some patients with metastatic disease who self-inject the drug subcutaneously every day have had stable disease for up to a year at the time of this writing. Tumor growth is arrested. The patients regain weight, strength, and hair. There has been virtually no toxicity. *Tumor arrest* may be a better term than *stable disease* for this condition, because stable disease induced by conventional cytotoxic chemotherapy is often limited by eventual acquired drug resistance, is associated with the side effects of chemotherapy, and connotes probable failure of conventional cytotoxic chemotherapy.

DIRECT AND INDIRECT ANGIOGENESIS INHIBITORS

In designing a clinical trial for antiangiogenic therapy of cancer, especially breast cancer, it is helpful to understand that angiogenesis inhibitors can be either direct or indirect (Figure 28-6).

Direct angiogenesis inhibitors such as vitaxin,[170] angiostatin,[84,171,172] endostatin,[82,173] 2-methoxyestradiol, combretastatin, NM-3, thrombospondin, ultralow-dose continuous paclitaxel,[174] and others prevent vascular endothelial cells from proliferating, migrating, or increasing their survival in response to a spectrum

Types of Angiogenesis Inhibitors

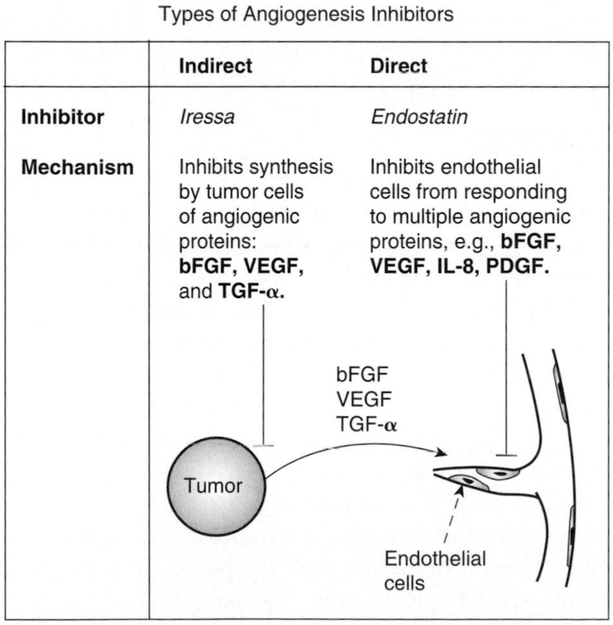

FIG. **28-6** Direct angiogenesis inhibitors are less likely to induce acquired drug resistance because they inhibit endothelial cells in the tumor bed from responding to a wide spectrum of pro-angiogenic proteins from tumor or from stroma. In contrast, indirect angiogenesis inhibitors block an oncogene expressed by the tumor, or a tumor cell product, or the receptor for that product. This permits the emergence of mutants producing pro-angiogenic proteins that might not be antagonized by the indirect angiogenesis inhibitor. (See text for abbreviations.) *(From Folkman J, Kalluri R: Tumor angiogenesis. In Kufe DW et al [eds]: Cancer medicine, ed 6, Hamilton, Ontario, 2003, Decker.)*

of pro-angiogenic proteins, including VEGF, bFGF, interluekin-8, PDGF, and platelet-derived endothelial cell growth factor (PD-ECGF). Direct angiogenesis inhibitors are the least likely to induce acquired drug resistance, because they target genetically stable endothelial cells rather than unstable mutating tumor cells.[175] Tumors in mice treated with antiangiogenic therapy did not develop drug resistance.[176]

Indirect angiogenesis inhibitors generally inhibit expression of a tumor cell product, neutralize the tumor product itself, or block its receptor on endothelial cells. Examples include (1) EGF tyrosine kinase inhibitors, which block production of the pro-angiogenic proteins, VEGF, bFGF, and TGF-α (e.g., gefitinib [Iressa], erlotinib HCl [Tarceva], cetuximab [Erbitux]); (2) an antibody that neutralizes VEGF (e.g., bevacizumab; note that in references 176a and 176b bevacizumab [Avastin] was inadvertently tabulated as a "direct" angiogenesis inhibitor, but it is an "indirect" angiogenesis inhibitor); or (3) inhibitors of VEGF receptors on endothelium (e.g., PTK787, ZD6474, SU11248). For indirect angiogenesis inhibitors, it may be important to know in advance if the tumor is producing one or more of the angiogenic proteins that are counteracted by the angiogenesis inhibitor[112] (Figure 28-7).

Therefore it may be valuable to stratify patients who are receiving an indirect angiogenesis inhibitor, analogous to the selection of patients who receive trastuzumab (Herceptin) or tamoxifen. Also, indirect angiogenesis inhibitors are susceptible to acquired drug resistance as the tumor cells undergo mutation and produce angiogenic proteins not covered by the indirect angiogenesis inhibitor. Drug resistance is less likely to occur with the use of direct angiogenesis inhibitors, because they prevent endothelial cells from responding to a wide range of pro-angiogenic factors.

LOW TOXICITY

Most angiogenesis inhibitors are not toxic to highly replicating cell populations such as in the gut, bone marrow, bladder, or skin. In fact, the more *selective* an angiogenesis inhibitor is for endothelial cells, the less likely it is to cause diarrhea, bone marrow suppression, and hair loss. Delayed wound healing and contraception[177] are two side effects common to some angiogenesis inhibitors. Of course, there may be side effects unrelated to the antiendothelial activity of these inhibitors. For example, when TNP-470 is administered at levels higher than its effective dosage, side effects may develop in the central nervous system, and this was also observed in preclinical animal studies. This toxicity has now been eliminated in tumor-bearing mice through a modification of TNP-470 in which the drug is conjugated to a polymer, hydroxypropyl methacrylamide, so that it no longer enters the cerebrospinal fluid (Satchi-Fainaro, personal communication).

Production of pro-angiogenic proteins by human tumors

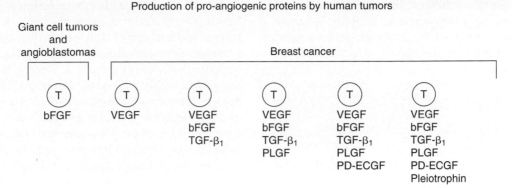

FIG. **28-7** High-grade giant cell tumors and angioblastomas produce mainly bFGF as their angiogenic stimulator. In contrast breast cancers produce a spectrum of different angiogenic proteins. (See text for abbreviations.) *(From Relf M et al: Cancer Res 57:963, 1997.)*

In contrast, angiostatin[83,84] and endostatin[82] are *specific* inhibitors of endothelial proliferation and have no effect on a wide spectrum of other cell types tested up to the time of this writing. Nor do they have any effect on resting, nonproliferating endothelial cells. No toxicity of any kind from these inhibitors has been detected in animals to date, and these drugs are both very safe in phase I/II clinical trials so far.

CONTINUOUS VERSUS BOLUS DOSING

Experimental studies in tumor-bearing animals have shown that continuous dosing of an angiogenesis inhibitor is approximately tenfold more effective than bolus dosing.[178] For example, continuous administration of endostatin by a microosmotic Alzet pump implanted into the peritoneal cavity caused regression of human tumors in mice, whereas the same amount of endostatin given as an intraperitoneal dose as a bolus every 24 hours did not regress the same tumor (Figure 28-8). These experiments indicate that if endothelial cells in a tumor bed are constantly exposed to pro-angiogenic proteins issuing from adjacent tumor cells, then to counter this stimulation with antiangiogenic therapy requires the continual presence

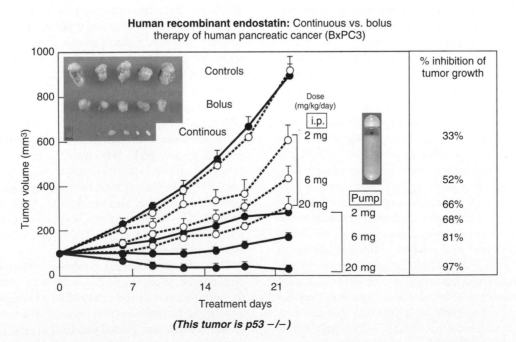

Human recombinant endostatin: Continuous vs. bolus therapy of human pancreatic cancer (BxPC3)

(This tumor is p53 −/−)

FIG. **28-8** Demonstration in tumor-bearing mice that continuous infusion of endostatin is approximately 10 times more effective than single daily bolus injection. Continuous infusion leads to tumor regression, whereas bolus injection of the same dose does not. *(From Folkman J, Kalluri R: Tumor angiogenesis. In Kufe DW et al [eds]: Cancer medicine, ed 6, Hamilton, Ontario, 2003, Decker.)*

of an angiogenesis inhibitor (or inhibitors) in the lumen. In a sense, the angiogenesis inhibitor is *titrated* against the total amount of pro-angiogenic activity from a tumor during the therapeutic attack against the tumor.

Common Misperceptions about Antiangiogenic Therapy

Certain common misperceptions about the mechanisms of angiogenesis and about antiangiogenic therapy may be problematic in the design of protocols for clinical trials. For example, it is often assumed that tumors that are avascular or poorly vascularized cannot be treated with an angiogenesis inhibitor.[4] This assumption originates from observations of gross specimens of tumors, some of which appear to be highly vascularized, whereas others are pale or white and appear not to be vascularized. In fact, the gross appearance of a tumor, whether it is observed before or after it has been removed from the patient, does not accurately reflect the intensity of neovascularization at the microscopic level. Virtually all tumors that are of clinically detectable size (>2 to 3 mm) are neovascularized. In principle, they are treatable with an angiogenesis inhibitor, although some tumors may be greater producers of angiogenic activity than others and require higher dosages of an angiogenesis inhibitor. In experimental animals, poorly vascularized, more slowly growing bladder cancers responded to a given dose of angiogenesis inhibitors with greater efficacy than did highly vascularized, rapidly growing tumors. Furthermore, antiangiogenic therapy may also be used to maintain the dormancy of microscopic metastases that are not neovascularized.[83]

Another common misperception is that large, established tumors cannot be treated with an angiogenesis inhibitor, presumably because the vessels would no longer be growing or would be mature. Even in large tumors, endothelial cells in the new microvessels in a tumor bed have a high turnover rate compared with endothelial cells in quiescent microvessels outside the tumor.[179] Most tumor microvessels consist of thin-walled capillary tubes with or without pericytes but with little or no smooth muscle. After an angiogenic stimulus is removed from the rabbit cornea, neovessels involute and disappear within 1 to 2 weeks. However, the preexisting or established vessels in the sclera at the limbal edge of the cornea remain intact. These vessels may be equivalent to the arterial and venous feeder vessels of a tumor. It is not yet known whether some tumors may produce a combination of pro-angiogenic proteins that can produce mature, stabilized microvessels, which may not be as susceptible to certain angiogenesis inhibitors.

It is often assumed that only malignant tumors are treatable with antiangiogenic therapy. However, both benign and malignant tumors can be angiogenic. For example, a prostate gland enlarged by benign prostatic hypertrophy is neovascularized. Adrenal adenomas are benign but highly angiogenic tumors. Also, in children, benign hemangiomas and a benign giant cell tumor of the mandible have regressed completely with interferon-α therapy. One can speculate that certain slow-growing benign tumors, such as fibromas and neurofibromas, may be candidates for antiangiogenic therapy, especially because this form of therapy does not depend on a large pool of proliferating tumor cells.

Another common misperception is that antiangiogenic therapy should not be used before chemotherapy because an angiogenesis inhibitor closes blood vessels and thus reduces access to a chemotherapeutic drug. Just the opposite is true. First, Teicher and colleagues[180] have shown that antiangiogenic therapy increases flow and oxygen delivery as well as drug delivery to a tumor. Second, O'Reilly and associates[82,83] and Holmgren and co-workers[81] reported that during inhibition of angiogenesis by either angiostatin or endostatin, apoptosis of tumor cells increased threefold to sevenfold but tumor cell proliferation remained high. These data argue that after a bulky tumor is reduced to a small tumor of microscopic size by antiangiogenic therapy, the residual tumor population should remain sensitive to cytotoxic chemotherapy. The mechanism by which antiangiogenic therapy would increase drug delivery and blood flow to a tumor as reported by Teicher is not clear but may be based on the lowering of interstitial pressure[181] as a tumor becomes unpacked by capillary dropout.

It is important to distinguish antiangiogenic from antivascular therapy.[182] Antivascular therapy, for example, with combretastatin, which can bring about rapid regression of large bulky tumors, depends on occlusion of tumor vasculature, in part by desquamation of endothelial cells into the lumen.

Some scientists have assumed that the efficacy of antiangiogenic therapy would be limited by tumor cells that are p53 deficient[182a] and/or hypoxic.[182b] However, there is considerable evidence to the contrary.[182c,182d] In fact, at least two angiogenesis inhibitors, 2-methoxyestradiol and endostatin, have been demonstrated to downregulate expression of hypoxia inducible factor-1α (HIF 1α), thus overriding tumor cell response to hypoxia.[182d]

There is also confusion about whether radiotherapy can be used in combination with antiangiogenic therapy because of the notion that antiangiogenic therapy might decrease oxygen delivery to a tumor and lead to radioresistance. However, Teicher and colleagues[183] have reported that antiangiogenic therapy potentiates radiotherapy and increases tumor oxygenation in tumor-bearing animals, at least during the initial stages of antiangiogenic therapy.

It has been assumed that leukemia, called the *liquid tumor*, would not be dependent on angiogenesis. In fact, it has been reported that the bone marrow in human leukemia is highly angiogenic,[184] with up to a sevenfold increase in microvessel density in acute lymphoblastic leukemia of children compared with nonleukemic bone marrows ($p < .0001$). Confocal microscopy reveals that leukemic tumor cells in the marrow are configured as microcylinders around capillary vessels, not unlike the configuration of microcylinders of tumor cells around new microvessels in solid tumors, for example, in breast cancer (see Figure 28-1).

Certain Conventional Anticancer Drugs May Also Inhibit Angiogenesis

Steiner[185] first showed in 1992 that of 17 cytotoxic drugs tested in the chick embryo, only adriamycin and its analogs or etoposide specifically inhibited angiogenesis. Mitoxantrone inhibited angiogenesis to a lesser extent. It has been demonstrated that paclitaxel (Taxol) inhibits angiogenesis in animals below the cytotoxic dose.[186] Of interest is that although Taxol is usually administered for metastatic breast cancer once every 3 weeks for approximately six to seven such cycles, scattered reports exist of patients treated for 20 cycles or more who have stable disease. Drug resistance does not appear to have developed in these patients. A possible explanation is that the tumor compartment may have become drug resistant but the endothelial cell compartment has not.

Vascular endothelial cells in the tumor bed are the first to be exposed to chemotherapy. However, conventional cytotoxic chemotherapy is usually administered at a maximum tolerated dose, followed by treatment-free intervals to allow recovery of bone marrow and gastrointestinal tract cells. Therefore, during treatment-free intervals, endothelial are untreated.[187] Browder and co-workers[187] showed that by administering cyclophosphamide at more frequent intervals and at lower dosages, apoptosis of endothelial cells in the tumor bed *preceded* tumor cell apoptosis by 4 to 5 days. Browder and co-workers used the term *antiangiogenic chemotherapy*. At these close intervals, the cytotoxic drug was converted to an angiogenesis inhibitor. It was effective even when the tumor was made completely resistant to cyclophosphamide. Klement and colleagues[188] confirmed this result with a different cytotoxic agent, and in

an accompanying editorial, Hanahan, Bergers, and Bergsland[189] provided the term *metronomic therapy*. The two terms do not have precisely the same meaning. *Antiangiogenic chemotherapy* signifies that the target of the chemotherapy is microvascular endothelium in the tumor bed. *Metronomic therapy* indicates that the schedule of administration is at regular intervals. A recent in vitro study showed that ultralow picomolar concentrations of paclitaxel, administered continuously, inhibited endothelial cell proliferation[174] (Table 28-3).

This study suggests the possibility that prolonged ultralow dosages of paclitaxel, or even sustained-release subcutaneous dosing of paclitaxel, could be used in cancer patients whose tumor had become resistant to dosing every 3 weeks or weekly.

These results might also help explain why some patients who receive long-term maintenance or even palliative chemotherapy have stable disease beyond the time that the tumor would have been expected to develop drug resistance. Patients with slow-growing cancers who are on antiangiogenic scheduling of chemotherapy involving continuous infusion 5-fluorouracil,[190-192] weekly paclitaxel,[193,194] or daily oral etoposide[195-197] have shown an improved outcome, despite the fact that in some of these patients the tumors had already become drug resistant to conventional chemotherapy.

Tamoxifen inhibits growth of human microvascular endothelial cells and induces apoptosis in these cells in vitro. It also inhibits angiogenesis in the chick embryo in vivo.[198-200] Thus it is possible that some part of the antitumor effect of tamoxifen is related to its antiangiogenic activity, however weak this activity may be relative to other angiogenesis inhibitors.

TABLE 28-3 Inhibition of Human Microvascular Endothelial Cell (HMVEC) Proliferation by Chemotherapeutics

COMPOUNDS	IC_{50} (pM)
Paclitaxel	0.1
5-Fluorouracil	5,000
Camptothecin	10,000
Doxorubicin	100,000
Cisplatin	5,000,000

Modified from Wang J et al: *Anticancer Drugs* 14:13, 2003. HMVEC were grown in 96-well plate with EGM2 medium containing growth factors and fetal bovine serum (FBS). The cells were incubated with compounds at various concentrations for 3 days before MTS reagents were used to quantify the live cells. The IC_{50} (concentration to achieve 50% of maximum inhibition) was the average of three independent experiments.[174]

Drugs Discovered to Be Angiogenesis Inhibitors after They Were Approved for Another Use

Celecoxcib,[201] a cyclooxygenase-2 inhibitor used in the management of arthritis; rosiglitazone, a PPAR-gamma ligand used in type 2 late-onset diabetes[202]; and zolendrenate,[203] a bisphosphonate used to treat osteoporosis have recently been reported to inhibit angiogenesis. Celecoxib is already being studied in a clinical trial in combination with thalidomide and low-dose cyclophosphamide.[203a] Celecoxib also mobilizes endostatin from platelets and increases the blood level of endostatin.[204,205] In the future, it is possible that celecoxib, rosiglitazone, and zoledronate may be administered chronically in cancer, as they now are administered for nonneoplastic diseases. One can also speculate that these types of relatively nontoxic drugs could be used as a platform of antiangiogenic therapy to which other agents could be added.

Conclusions and Future Directions

This review of the role of angiogenesis in breast cancer is based on principles of the angiogenic process that have been elucidated in the laboratory and are being translated to clinical application, not only in breast cancer but also in other neoplastic and nonneoplastic diseases. Angiogenesis research[206,207] is 30 years old and can be divided into three periods of development: The 1970s were devoted mainly to the development of methods to study blood vessel growth in vitro and in vivo. The 1980s saw the discovery of molecules that mediate angiogenesis, including inducers and inhibitors of angiogenesis. Proof of principle demonstrated that tumor growth is angiogenesis dependent. In the 1990s, a first generation of angiogenesis inhibitors entered clinical trial. These new molecules could inhibit tumor angiogenesis, but not completely; they could slow tumor growth in animals but could not induce tumor regression. By the mid-1990s came the discovery of a second generation of angiogenesis inhibitors, angiostatin and endostatin, capable for the first time of turning off tumor angiogenesis completely or nearly completely. These proteins are internal fragments of larger proteins, which themselves do not inhibit angiogenesis. They could induce regression of tumors in animals, maintain tumor dormancy, and when combined, eradicate tumors. Also, by the mid-1990s genetic proofs that tumors are angiogenesis dependent were reported.[40,54,208-210]

The discovery of this second generation of powerful endogenous angiogenesis inhibitors led immediately to novel concepts (and proofs for many of them) that were not even imagined 10 years ago, including the demonstration that (1) tumor mass controls tumor growth by regulation of angiogenesis, even at remote sites; (2) angiogenesis correlates inversely with tumor cell apoptosis but is independent of proliferation; (3) four common clinical patterns of metastasis presentation are governed by angiogenic mechanisms; (4) the endothelial cell population and the tumor cell population in a tumor require different therapeutic approaches with different schedules; (5) human leukemia is angiogenic[184]; (6) a tumor that has become resistant to a cytotoxic drug by virtue of a dose schedule that is optimally effective for the tumor cell compartment may possibly be converted to a drug-sensitive tumor by changing the dose schedule so that it is optimal for the endothelial compartment; (7) antiangiogenic therapy is a strategy to bypass drug resistance; and (8) continuous administration of an angiogenesis inhibitor is more effective against experimental tumors than bolus administration.

The development of a method to quantify tumor vascularization in histologic sections of breast cancer by microvessel density has led to the recognition that tumor angiogenesis may be an independent prognostic indicator in node-negative breast cancer, as well as in other tumors. However, microvascular density has not turned out to be useful for determining efficacy of antiangiogenic therapy. There is a need for surrogate markers in the blood or urine that would correlate with efficacy of antiangiogenic therapy. It remains to be seen whether quantification of circulating endothelial cells will correlate with tumor response to antiangiogenic therapy.

If recently discovered potent angiogenesis inhibitors (e.g., angiostatin, endostatin, inhibitors of $\alpha_v\beta_3$, and others) show efficacy in the clinic similar to their antitumor activity in experimental animals, then it is conceivable that it may not be necessary to continue antiangiogenic therapy for life but rather for more limited periods.

Furthermore, if the absence of drug resistance continues to be a prominent feature of antiangiogenic therapy in the clinic, it should be possible for a patient who has discontinued antiangiogenic therapy to resume it in the event of tumor recurrence. If such a scenario becomes reality, there will be an increasing need for molecular diagnostic methods to detect tumor recurrence before the tumor mass is large enough to be located with conventional imaging methods. We can ask whether it will eventually be possible to guide the dose and schedule of antiangiogenic therapy in prostate cancer, for example, by following the serum prostate-specific antigen or by detecting serum markers of neovascularization.[211] Beyond this, could breast cancer recurrences be treated similarly, once a molecular marker has been developed for breast cancer that is as efficient as prostate-specific antigen is for prostate cancer?

As our understanding of the genetic background of the angiogenic phenotype increases, it may become possible to turn off tumor angiogenesis with gene therapy.[212,213] Regardless of whether gene therapy can be successfully used to turn off angiogenesis, the administration of exogenous angiogenesis inhibitors may facilitate the application of gene therapy directed against the tumor cell population. It is precisely because antiangiogenic therapy can hold a tumor at a microscopic dormant size while permitting continual proliferation of tumor cells that we are beginning to think that eventually antiangiogenic therapy may become a platform for low-dose (metronomic) chemotherapy, radiotherapy, immunotherapy, gene therapy, and in selected cases, conventional chemotherapy.

Acknowledgments

Supported by The Breast Cancer Foundation and grants from the National Institutes of Health P01 CA45548; R37 CA 37395; and RO1 CA64481, and a grant to Children's Hospital from EntreMed, Inc., Rockville, MD.

References

1. Gimbrone MA Jr et al: Tumor dormancy in vivo by prevention of neovascularization, *J Exp Med* 136:261, 1972.
2. Hanahan D et al: Transgenic mouse models of tumor angiogenesis: the angiogenic switch, its molecular controls, and prospects for preclinical therapeutic models, *Eur J Cancer* 32A:2386, 1996.
3. Hanahan D, Folkman J: Patterns and emerging mechanisms of the angiogenic switch during tumorigenesis, *Cell* 86:353, 1996.
4. Folkman J: Antiangiogenic therapy. In DeVita VT Jr, Hellman S, Rosenberg SA (eds): *Cancer: principles & practice of oncology*, ed 5, Philadelphia, 1997, Lippincott-Raven.
5. Folkman J et al: Induction of angiogenesis during the transition from hyperplasia to neoplasia, *Nature* 339:58, 1989.
6. Kandel J et al: Neovascularization is associated with a switch to the export of bFGF in the multistep development of fibrosarcoma, *Cell* 66:1095, 1991.
7. Smith-McCune KK, Weidner N: Demonstration and characterization of the angiogenic properties of cervical dysplasia, *Cancer Res* 54:800, 1994.
8. Brem SS, Jensen HM, Gullino PM: Angiogenesis as a marker of preneoplastic lesions of the human breast, *Cancer* 41:239, 1978.
9. Gimbrone MA Jr, Gullino PM: Neovascularization induced by intraocular xenografts of preneoplastic and neoplastic mammary tissues, *J Natl Cancer Inst* 56:305, 1976.
10. Guinebretiere JM et al: Angiogenesis and risk of breast cancer in women with fibrocystic disease, *J Natl Cancer Inst* 86:635, 1994.
11. Anan K et al: Vascular endothelial growth factor and platelet-derived growth factor are potential angiogenic and metastatic factors in human breast cancer, *Surgery* 119:333, 1996.
12. Brown LF et al: Expression of vascular permeability factor (vascular endothelial growth factor) and its receptors in breast cancer, *Hum Pathol* 26:86, 1995.
13. Chaudhury TK, Lerner MP, Nordquist RE: Angiogenesis by human melanoma and breast cancer cells, *Cancer Lett* 11:43, 1980.
14. McLeskey SW et al: Fibroblast growth factor overexpressing breast carcinoma cells as models of angiogenesis and metastasis, *Breast Cancer Res Treat* 39:103, 1996.
15. Yoshiji H et al: Expression of vascular endothelial growth factor, its receptor, and other angiogenic factors in human breast cancer, *Cancer Res* 56:2013, 1996.
16. Fox SB et al: The angiogenic factor platelet-derived endothelial cell growth factor/thymidine phosphorylase is up-regulated in breast cancer epithelium and endothelium, *Br J Cancer* 73:275, 1996.
17. Toi M et al: Expression of platelet-derived endothelial cell growth factor/thymidine phosphorylase in human breast cancer, *Int J Cancer* 64:79, 1995.
18. Contrino J et al: In situ detection of tissue factor in vascular endothelial cells: correlation with the malignant phenotype of human breast disease, *Nature Med* 2:167, 1996.
19. Hlatky L et al: Mammary fibroblasts may influence breast tumor angiogenesis via hypoxia-induced vascular endothelial growth factor up-regulation and protein expression, *Cancer Res* 54:6083, 1994.
20. Briozzo P et al: MCF7 mammary cancer cells respond to bFGF and internalize it following its release from extracellular matrix: a permissive role of cathepsin D, *Exp Cell Res* 194:252, 1991.
21. Herron GS et al: Secretion of metalloproteinases by stimulated capillary endothelial cells. I. Production of procollagenase and prostromelysin exceeds expression of proteolytic activity, *J Biol Chem* 261:2810, 1986.
22. Hildenbrand R et al: Urokinase plasminogen activator induces angiogenesis and tumor vessel invasion in breast cancer, *Pathol Res Pract* 191:403, 1995.
23. Gasparini G et al: Prognostic significance of vascular endothelial growth factor protein in node-negative breast carcinoma, *J Natl Cancer Inst* 89:139, 1997.
24. Dickson RB, Lippman ME: Molecular determinants of growth, angiogenesis, and metastases in breast cancer, *Semin Oncol* 19:286, 1992.
25. Riegel AT, Wellstein A: The potential role of the heparin-binding growth factor pleiotrophin in breast cancer, *Breast Cancer Res Treat* 31:309, 1994.
26. Folkman J: Clinical applications of research on angiogenesis, *N Engl J Med* 333:1757, 1995.
27. Rak J, Filmus J, Kerbel RS: Reciprocal paracrine interactions between tumor cells and endothelial cells: the `angiogenesis progression' hypothesis, *Eur J Cancer* 32A:2438, 1996.
28. Voest EE et al: Inhibition of angiogenesis in vivo by interleukin 12, *J Natl Cancer Inst* 87:581, 1995.
29. Dong Z et al: Macrophage-derived metalloelastase is responsible for generation of angiostatin in Lewis lung carcinoma, *Cell* 88:801, 1997.
30. Kerbel R, Folkman J: Clinical translation of angiogenesis inhibitors, *Nat Rev Cancer* 2:727, 2002.

31. Lewis CE et al: Cytokine regulation of angiogenesis in breast cancer: the role of tumor-associated macrophages, *J Leukoc Biol* 57:747, 1995.

32. Rak J et al: Oncogenes as inducers of tumor angiogenesis, *Cancer Metastasis Rev* 14:263, 1995.

33. Dameron KM et al: Control of angiogenesis in fibroblasts by p53 regulation of thrombospondin-1, *Science* 265:1582, 1994.

34. Van Meir EG et al: Release of an inhibitor of angiogenesis upon induction of wild type p53 expression in glioblastoma cells, *Nat Genet* 8:171, 1994.

35. Wizigmann-Voos S et al: Up regulation of vascular endothelial growth factor and its receptors in von Hippel-Lindau disease-associated and sporadic hemangioblastomas, *Cancer Res* 55:1358, 1995.

36. Mukhopadhyay D, Tsiokas L, Sukhatme VP: Wild-type p53 and v-src exert opposing influences on human vascular endothelial growth factor gene expression, *Cancer Res* 55:6161, 1995.

37. Maeshima Y et al: Identification of the anti-angiogenic site within vascular basement membrane-derived tumstatin, *J Biol Chem* 276:15240, 2001.

38. Weidner N: Tumoural vascularity as a prognostic factor in cancer patients: the evidence continues to grow, *J Pathol* 184:119, 1998.

39. Thomlinson R, Gray L: The histological structure of some human lung cancers and the possible implications for radiotherapy, *Br J Cancer* 9:539, 1955.

40. Lyden D et al: Impaired recruitment of bone-marrow-derived endothelial and hematopoietic precursor cells blocks tumor angiogenesis and growth, *Nat Med* 7:1194, 2001.

41. Asahara T et al: Isolation of putative progenitor endothelial cells for angiogenesis, *Science* 275:964, 1997.

42. Shi Q et al: Evidence for circulating bone marrow-derived endothelial cells, *Blood* 92:362, 1998.

43. Hatzopoulos AK et al: Isolation and characterization of endothelial progenitor cells from mouse embryos, *Development* 125:1457, 1998.

44. Asahara T et al: VEGF contributes to postnatal neovascularization by mobilizing bone marrow-derived endothelial progenitor cells, *EMBO J* 18:3964, 1999.

45. Murohara T et al: Transplanted cord blood-derived endothelial precursor cells augment postnatal neovascularization, *J Clin Invest* 105:1527, 2000.

46. Rafii S: Circulating endothelial precursors: mystery, reality, and promise, *J Clin Invest* 105:17, 2000.

47. Peichev M et al: Expression of VEGFR-2 and AC133 by circulating human CD34(+) cells identifies a population of functional endothelial precursors, *Blood* 95:952, 2000.

48. Gehling UM et al: In vitro differentiation of endothelial cells from AC133-positive progenitor cells, *Blood* 95:3106, 2000.

49. Hattori K et al: Vascular endothelial growth factor and angiopoietin-1 stimulate postnatal hematopoiesis by recruitment of vasculogenic and hematopoietic stem cells, *J Exp Med* 193:1005, 2001.

50. Hattori K et al: Plasma elevation of stromal cell-derived factor-1 induces mobilization of mature and immature hematopoietic progenitor and stem cells, *Blood* 97:3354, 2001.

51. Hattori K et al: Placental growth factor reconstitutes hematopoiesis by recruiting VEGFR1(+) stem cells from bone-marrow microenvironment, *Nat Med* 8:841, 2002.

52. Heissig B et al: Recruitment of stem and progenitor cells from the bone marrow niche requires MMP-9 mediated release of kit-ligand, *Cell* 109:625, 2002.

53. Reyes M et al: Origin of endothelial progenitors in human postnatal bone marrow, *J Clin Invest* 109:337, 2002.

54. Lyden D et al: Id1 and Id3 are required for neurogenesis, angiogenesis and vascularization of tumour xenografts, *Nature* 401:670, 1999.

55. Ito H et al: Endothelial progenitor cells as putative targets for angiostatin, *Cancer Res* 59:5875, 1999.

56. Monestiroli S et al: Kinetics and viability of circulating endothelial cells as surrogate angiogenesis marker in an animal model of human lymphoma, *Cancer Res* 61:4341, 2001.

57. Bertolini F et al: Thalidomide in multiple myeloma, myelodysplastic syndromes and histiocytosis: analysis of clinical results and of surrogate angiogenesis markers, *Ann Oncol* 12:987, 2001.

58. Verheul HM et al: Platelet: transporter of vascular endothelial growth factor, *Clin Cancer Res* 3:2187, 1997.

59. Mohle R et al: Constitutive production and thrombin-induced release of vascular endothelial growth factor by human megakaryocytes and platelets, *Proc Natl Acad Sci USA* 94:663, 1997.

60. Verheul HM, Pinedo HM: Tumor growth: a putative role for platelets? *Oncologist* 3:II, 1998.

61. Pinedo HM et al: Involvement of platelets in tumour angiogenesis? *Lancet* 352:1775, 1998.

62. Verheul HM et al: Vascular endothelial growth factor-stimulated endothelial cells promote adhesion and activation of platelets, *Blood* 96:4216, 2000.

63. Folkman J: The role of angiogenesis in tumor growth, *Semin Cancer Biol* 3:65, 1992.

64. Polverini PJ, Leibovich SJ: Induction of neovascularization in vivo and endothelial proliferation in vitro by tumor-associated macrophages, *Lab Invest* 51:635, 1984.

65. Bergers G et al: Matrix metalloproteinase-9 triggers the angiogenic switch during carcinogenesis, *Nat Cell Biol* 2:737, 2000.

66. Coussens LM et al: MMP-9 supplied by bone marrow-derived cells contributes to skin carcinogenesis, *Cell* 103:481, 2000.

67. Schulze-Osthoff K et al: In situ detection of basic fibroblast growth factor by highly specific antibodies, *Am J Pathol* 137:85, 1990.

68. Fang J et al: Matrix metalloproteinase-2 is required for the switch to the angiogenic phenotype in a tumor model, *Proc Natl Acad Sci USA* 97:3884, 2000.

69. Fukumura D et al: Tumor induction of VEGF promoter activity in stromal cells, *Cell* 94:715, 1998.

70. Holash J et al: Vessel cooption, regression, and growth in tumors mediated by angiopoietins and VEGF, *Science* 284:1994, 1999.

71. Kim ES et al: Potent VEGF blockade causes regression of coopted vessels in a model of neuroblastoma, *Proc Natl Acad Sci USA* 99:11399, 2002.

72. Achilles EG et al: Heterogeneity of angiogenic activity in a human liposarcoma: a proposed mechanism for "no take" of human tumors in mice, *J Natl Cancer Inst* 93:1075, 2001.

73. Udagawa T et al: Persistence of microscopic human cancers in mice: alterations in the angiogenic balance accompanies loss of tumor dormancy, *FASEB J* 16:1361, 2002.

74. Luzzi KJ et al: Multistep nature of metastatic inefficiency: dormancy of solitary cells after successful extravasation and limited survival of early micrometastases, *Am J Pathol* 153:865, 1998.

75. Cameron MD et al: Temporal progression of metastasis in lung: cell survival, dormancy, and location dependence of metastatic inefficiency, *Cancer Res* 60:2541, 2000.

76. Folkman J: Tumor angiogenesis and tissue factor, *Nature Med* 2:167, 1996.

77. Folkman J: The influence of angiogenesis research on management of patients with breast cancer, *Breast Cancer Res Treat* 36:109, 1995.

78. Hamada J et al: Separable growth and migration factors for large-cell lymphoma cells secreted by microvascular endothelial cells derived from target organs for metastasis, *Br J Cancer* 66:349, 1992.

79. Hamada J et al: A paracrine migration-stimulating factor for metastatic tumor cells secreted by mouse hepatic sinusoidal endothelial cells: identification as complement component C3b, *Cancer Res* 53:4418, 1993.

80. Nicosia RF, Tchao R, Leighton J: Interactions between newly formed endothelial channels and carcinoma cells in plasma clot culture, *Clin Exp Metastasis* 4:91, 1986.

81. Holmgren L, O'Reilly MS, Folkman J: Dormancy of micrometastases: balanced proliferation and apoptosis in the presence of angiogenesis suppression, *Nat Med* 1:149, 1995.

82. O'Reilly MS et al: Endostatin: an endogenous inhibitor of angiogenesis and tumor growth, *Cell* 88:277, 1997.

83. O'Reilly MS et al: Angiostatin induces and sustains dormancy of human primary tumors in mice, *Nature Med* 2:689, 1996.

84. O'Reilly MS et al: Angiostatin: a novel angiogenesis inhibitor that mediates the suppression of metastases by a Lewis lung carcinoma, *Cell* 79:315, 1994.

85. Lu C, Tanigawa N: Spontaneous apoptosis is inversely related to intratumoral microvessel density in gastric carcinoma, *Cancer Res* 57:221, 1997.

86. Evans GI: Old cells never die, they just apoptose, *Trends Cell Biol* 4:191, 1994.

87. Ribatti D et al: Angiogenesis induced by B-cell non-Hodgkin's lymphomas: lack of correlation with tumor malignancy and immunologic phenotype, *Anticancer Res* 10:401, 1990.

88. Cao Y et al: Expression of angiostatin cDNA in a murine fibrosarcoma suppresses primary tumor growth and produces long-term dormancy of metastases, *J Clin Invest* 101:1055, 1998.

89. Weidner N et al: Tumor angiogenesis correlates with metastasis in invasive breast carcinoma, *N Engl J Med* 324:1, 1991.

90. Liotta LA, Steeg PS, Stetler-Stevenson WG: Cancer metastasis and angiogenesis: an imbalance of positive and negative regulation, *Cell* 64:327, 1991.

91. Mignatti P et al: In vitro angiogenesis on the human amniotic membrane: requirement for basic fibroblast growth factor-induced proteinases, *J Cell Biol* 108:671, 1989.

92. Moscatelli D, Gross JL, Rifkin DB: Angiogenic factors stimulate plasminogen activator and collagenase production by capillary endothelial cells, *J Cell Biol* 91:201a, 1981 (abstract).

93. Nagy JA et al: Pathogenesis of tumor stroma generation: a critical role of leaky blood vessels and fibrin deposition, *Biochim Biophys Acta* 948:305, 1989.

94. Ray JM, Stetler-Stevenson WF: The role of matrix metalloproteases and their inhibitors in tumor invasion, metastasis and angiogenesis, *Eur Respir J* 7:2062, 1994.

95. Smolin G, Hyndiuk RA: Lymphatic drainage from vascularized rabbit cornea, *Am J Ophthalmol* 72:147, 1971.

96. Weidner N, Folkman J: Tumor vascularity as a prognostic factor in cancer. In DeVita VT Jr, Hellman S, Rosenberg SA (eds): *Important advances in oncology*, Philadelphia, 1996, Lippincott-Raven.

97. Wojtowicz S et al: Phase I of batimastat (BB-94), a novel matrix metalloproteinase inhibitor in patients with advanced cancer, *J Immunother* 16:249, 1994 (abstract).

98. Brooks PC et al: Integrin $\alpha v\beta 3$ antagonists promote tumor regression by inducing apoptosis of angiogenic blood vessels, *Cell* 79:1157, 1994.

99. Brooks PC et al: Anti-integrin $\alpha v\beta 3$ blocks human breast cancer growth and angiogenesis in human skin, *J Clin Invest* 96:1815, 1995.

100. Ellis LM, Fidler IJ: Angiogenesis and breast cancer metastasis, *Lancet* 346:388, 1995.

101. Fidler IJ, Gersten DM, Hart OR: The biology of cancer invasion and metastasis, *Adv Cancer Res* 28:149, 1978.

102. Nicolson GL: Cancer metastasis, *Sci Am* 240:66, 1979.

103. Netland PA, Zetter BR: Organ-specific adhesion of metastatic tumor cells in vitro, *Science* 224:1113, 1984.

104. Boxberger HJ et al: An in vitro model study of BSp73 rat tumor cell invasion into endothelial monolayer, *Anticancer Res* 9:1777, 1989.

105. Weinstat-Saslow D, Steeg PS: Angiogenesis and colonization in the tumor metastatic process: basic and applied advances, *FASEB J* 8:401, 1994.

106. Liotta LA et al: Metastatic potential correlates with enzymatic degradation of basement membrane collagen, *Nature* 284:67, 1980.

107. Dvorak HF et al: Identification and characterization of the blood vessels of solid tumors that are leaky to circulating macromolecules, *Am J Pathol* 133:95, 1988.

108. McCulloch P, Choy A, Martin L: Association between tumor angiogenesis and tumor cell shedding into effluent venous blood during breast cancer surgery, *Lancet* 346:1334, 1995.

109. Kalebic T et al: Basement membrane collagen: degradation by migrating endothelial cells, *Science* 221:281, 1983.

110. Rak JW et al: Progressive loss of sensitivity to endothelium-derived growth inhibitors expressed by human melanoma cells during disease progression, *J Cell Physiol* 159:245, 1994.

111. Ziche M, Gullino PM: Angiogenesis and neoplastic progression in vitro, *J Natl Cancer Inst* 69:483, 1982.

112. Relf M et al: Expression of the angiogenic factors vascular endothelial growth factor, acidic and basic fibroblast growth factor, tumor growth factor beta-1, platelet-derived endothelial cell growth factor, placenta growth factor, and pleiotrophin in human primary breast cancer and its relation to angiogenesis, *Cancer Res* 57:963, 1997.

113. Horak ER et al: Angiogenesis, assessed by platelet/endothelial cell adhesion molecule antibodies, as indicator of node metastases and survival in breast cancer, *Lancet* 340:1120, 1992.

114. Vermeulen PB et al: Quantification of angiogenesis in solid human tumours: an international consensus on the methodology and criteria of evaluation, *Eur J Cancer* 32A:2474, 1996.

115. Gasparini G: Clinical significance of the determination of angiogenesis in human breast cancer: update of the biological background and overview of the Vicenza studies, *Eur J Cancer* 32A:2485, 1996.

116. Bosari S et al: Microvessel quantitation and prognosis in invasive breast carcinoma, *Hum Pathol* 23:755, 1992.

117. Weidner N et al: Tumor angiogenesis: a new significant and independent prognostic indicator in early-stage breast cancer, *J Natl Cancer Inst* 84:1875, 1992.

118. Visscher DW et al: Prognostic significance of image morphometric microvessel enumeration in breast cancer, *Anal Quant Cytol Histol* 15:88, 1993.

119. Toi M, Kashitani J, Tominaga T: Tumor angiogenesis is an independent prognostic indicator of primary breast carcinoma, *Int J Cancer* 55:371, 1993.

120. Gasparini G et al: Tumor microvessel density, p53 expression, tumor size and peritumoral lymphatic vessel invasion are relevant prognostic markers in node-negative breast carcinoma, *J Clin Oncol* 12:454, 1994.

121. Obermair A et al: Influence of tumoral microvessel density on the recurrence-free survival in human breast cancer: preliminary results, *Onkologie* 17:44, 1994.

122. Gasparini G et al: Prognostic value of p53 expression in early-stage breast carcinoma compared with tumor angiogenesis, epidermal growth factor receptor c-erbB2, cathepsin D, DNA ploidy, parameters of cell kinetics and conventional features, *Int J Oncol* 4:155, 1994.

123. Fox SB et al: Tumor angiogenesis in node-negative breast carcinomas: relationship with epidermal growth factor receptor, estrogen receptor, and survival, *Breast Cancer Res Treat* 29:109, 1994.

124. Obermair A et al: Tumor vascular density in breast tumors and their effect on recurrence-free survival, *Chirurg* 65:611, 1994.

125. Toi M et al: Tumor angiogenesis in breast cancer: its importance as a prognostic indicator and the association with vascular endothelial growth factor expression, *Breast Cancer Res Treat* 36:193, 1995.

126. Gasparini G et al: Tumor angiogenesis predicts clinical outcome of node-positive breast cancer patients treated with adjuvant hormone therapy or chemotherapy, *Cancer J Sci Am* 1:131, 1995.

127. Inada K et al: Significance of tumor angiogenesis as an independent prognostic factor in axillary node-negative breast cancer, *Gan To Kagaku Ryoho* 22:59, 1995.

128. Charpin C et al: CD31 quantitative immunocytochemical assays in breast carcinomas: correlation with current prognostic factors, *Am J Clin Pathol* 103:443, 1995.

129. Barbareschi M et al: Microvessel density quantification in breast carcinomas: assessment by light microscopy vs a computer-aided image analysis system, *Appl Immunohistochem* 3:75, 1995.

130. Barbareschi M et al: Novel methods for the determination of the angiogenic activity of human tumors, *Breast Cancer Res Treat* 36:181, 1995.

131. Bevilacqua P et al: Prognostic value of intratumoral microvessel density, a measure of tumor angiogenesis, in node-negative breast carcinoma—results of a multiparametric study, *Breast Cancer Res Treat* 36:205, 1995.

132. Ogawa Y et al: Microvessel quantitation in invasive breast cancer by staining for factor VIII-related antigen, *Br J Cancer* 71:1297, 1995.

133. Obermair A et al: Microvessel density and vessel invasion in lymph-node–negative breast cancer: effect on recurrence-free survival, *Int J Cancer* 62:126, 1995.

134. Chu JS et al: Correlation between tumor angiogenesis and metastasis in breast cancer, *J Formos Med Assoc* 94:373, 1995.

135. Heimann R et al: Angiogenesis as a predictor of long-term survival for patients with node-negative breast cancer, *J Natl Cancer Inst* 88:1764, 1996.

136. Ravazoula P et al: Angiogenesis and metastatic potential in breast carcinoma, *The Breast* 5:418, 1996.

137. Karaiossifidi H et al: Tumor angiogenesis in node-negative breast cancer: relationship with relapse free survival, *Anticancer Res* 16:4001, 1996.

138. Kato T et al: Clinicopathologic study of angiogenesis in Japanese patients with breast cancer, *World J Surg* 21:49,1997.

139. Bertin N et al: Thrombospondin-1 and -2 messenger RNA expression in normal, benign, and neoplastic human breast tissues: Correlation with prognostic factors, tumor angiogenesis, and fibroblast desmoplasia, *Cancer Res* 57:396, 1997.

140. Hall NR et al: Is the relationship between angiogenesis and metastasis in breast cancer real? *Surg Oncol* 1:223, 1992.

141. Van Hoef ME et al: Assessment of tumor vascularity as a prognostic factor in lymph node-negative invasive breast cancer, *Eur J Cancer* 29A:1141, 1993.

142. Miliaras D, Kamas A, Kalekou H: Angiogenesis in invasive breast carcinoma: is it associated with parameters of prognostic significance? *Histopathology* 26:165, 1995.

143. Axelsson K et al: Tumor angiogenesis as a prognostic assay for invasive ductal breast carcinoma, *J Natl Cancer Inst* 87:997, 1995.

144. Siitonen SM et al: Comparison of different immunohistochemical methods in the assessment of angiogenesis: lack of prognostic value in a group of 77 selected node-negative breast carcinomas, *Mod Pathol* 8:745, 1995.

145. Goulding H et al: Assessment of angiogenesis in breast carcinoma: an important factor in prognosis? *Hum Pathol* 26:1196, 1995.

146. Costello P et al: Prognostic significance of microvessel density in lymph node negative breast carcinoma, *Hum Pathol* 26:1181, 1995.

147. Kerbel RS et al: Clonal dominance of primary tumors by metastatic cells: genetic analysis and biological implications, *Cancer Surv* 7:597, 1988.

148. Tamm I et al: Cell-adhesion–disrupting action of interleukin 6 in human ductal breast carcinoma cells, *Proc Natl Acad Sci USA* 91:3329, 1994.

149. Chiu JJ, Sgagias MK, Cowan KH: Interleukin 6 acts as a paracrine growth factor in human mammary carcinoma cell lines, *Clin Cancer Res* 2:215, 1996.

150. Motro B et al: Pattern of interleukin 6 gene expression in vivo suggests a role for this cytokine in angiogenesis, *Proc Natl Acad Sci USA* 87:3092, 1990.

151. Folkman J: Angiogenesis-dependent diseases, *Semin Oncol* 28:536, 2001.

152. Hlatky L, Hahnfeldt P, Folkman J: Clinical application of antiangiogenic therapy: microvessel density, what it does and doesn't tell us, *J Natl Cancer Inst* 94:883, 2002.

153. Beecken WD et al: Effect of anti-angiogenic therapy on slowly growing, poorly vascularized tumours in mice, *J Natl Cancer Inst* 93:382, 2001.

154. Folkman J: New perspectives in clinical oncology from angiogenesis research, *Eur J Cancer* 32A:2534, 1996.

155. Meltzer A: Dormancy and breast cancer, *J Surg Oncol* 43:181, 1990.

156. Vitetta ES, Uhr JW: Monoclonal antibodies as agonists: an expanded role for their use in cancer therapy, *Cancer Res* 54:5301, 1994.

157. Wheelock EF, Weinhold KJ, Levich J: The tumor dormant state, *Adv Cancer Res* 34:107, 1981.

158. Yanai S et al: Antitumor activity of a medium-chain triglyceride solution of the angiogenesis inhibitor TNP-470

(AGM-1470) when administered via the hepatic artery to rats bearing Walker 256 sarcoma of the liver, *J Pharmacol Exp Ther* 271:1267, 1994.

159. Noble RL, Hoover L: A classification of transplantable tumors in Nb rats controlled by estrogen from dormancy to autonomy, *Nature Med* 35:2935, 1975.

160. Demicheli R et al: Time distribution of the recurrence risk for breast cancer patients undergoing mastectomy: further support about the concept of tumor dormancy, *Breast Cancer Res Treat* 41:177, 1996.

161. Demicheli R et al: Local recurrences following mastectomy: support for the concept of tumor dormancy, *J Natl Cancer Inst* 86:45, 1994.

162. Wu J: Apoptosis and angiogenesis: two promising tumor markers in breast cancer, *Anticancer Res* 16:2233, 1996.

163. Folkman J: Angiogenesis in cancer, vascular, rheumatoid and other disease, *Nature Med* 1:27, 1995.

164. Prehn RT: The inhibition of tumor growth by tumor mass, *Cancer Res* 51:2, 1991.

165. Yuhas JM, Pazmino NH: Inhibition of subcutaneously growing line 1 carcinomas due to metastatic spread, *Cancer Res* 34:2005, 1974.

166. Nanus DM et al: Expression of basic fibroblast growth factor in primary human renal tumors: correlation with poor survival, *J Natl Cancer Inst* 85:1597, 1993.

167. Nguyen M et al: Elevated levels of an angiogenic peptide, basic fibroblast growth factor, in the urine of patients with a wide spectrum of cancers, *J Natl Cancer Inst* 86:356, 1994.

168. Kaban LB et al: Antiangiogenic therapy of a recurrent giant cell tumor of the mandible with interferon alfa-2a, *Pediatrics* 103:1145, 1999.

169. Kaban LB et al: Antiangiogenic therapy with interferon alpha for giant cell lesions of the jaws, *J Oral Maxillofac Surg* 60:1101, 2002.

170. Gutheil JC et al: Targeted antiangiogenic therapy for cancer using Vitaxin: a humanized monoclonal antibody to the integrin alphavbeta3, *Clin Cancer Res* 6:3056, 2002.

171. Moser TL et al: Angiostatin binds ATP synthase on the surface of human endothelial cells, *Proc Natl Acad Sci USA* 96:2811, 1999.

172. Troyanovsky B et al: Angiomotin: an angiostatin binding protein that regulates endothelial cell migration and tube formation, *J Cell Biol* 152:1247, 2001.

173. Dixelius J: Endostatin-induced tyrosine kinase signaling through the Shb adapter protein regulates endothelial cell apoptosis, *Blood* 95:4304, 2000.

174. Wang J et al: Paclitaxel at ultra low concentrations inhibits angiogenesis without affecting cellular microtubule assembly, *Anticancer Drugs* 14:13, 2003.

175. Kerbel RS: Inhibition of tumor angiogenesis as a strategy to circumvent acquired resistance to anticancer therapeutic agents, *Bioessays* 13:31, 1991.

176. Boehm T et al: Antiangiogenic therapy of experimental cancer does not induce drug resistance, *Nature* 390:404, 1997.

176a. Kerbel R, Folkman J: Clinical translation of angiogenesis inhibitors, *Nat Rev Cancer* 2:727,2002.

176b. Folkman J, Kalluri R: Tumor angiogenesis. In Kufe DW et al (eds): *Cancer medicine*, ed 6, Hamilton, Ontario, 2003, Decker.

177. Klauber N et al: Critical components of the female reproductive pathway are suppressed by the angiogenesis inhibitor AGM-1470, *Nature Med* 3:443, 1997.

178. Kisker O et al: Continuous administration of endostatin by intraperitoneally implanted osmotic pump improves the efficacy and potency of therapy in a mouse xenograft tumor model, *Cancer Res* 61:7669, 2001.

179. Denekamp J: Vascular attack as a therapeutic strategy for cancer, *Cancer Metastasis Rev* 3:267, 1990.

180. Teicher BA et al: Antiangiogenic treatment (TNP-470/Minocycline) increases tissue levels of anticancer drugs in mice bearing Lewis lung carcinoma, *Oncol Res* 27:237, 1995.

181. Jain R: Barriers to drug delivery in solid tumors, *Sci Am* 271:58, 1994.

182. Huang X et al: Tumor infarction in mice by antibody-directed targeting of tissue factor to tumor vasculature, *Science* 275:547, 1997.

182a. Yu JL et al: Effect of p53 status on tumor response to antiangiogenic therapy, *Science* 295:1526, 2002.

182b. Pennacchietti S et al: Hypoxia promotes invasive growth by transcriptional activation of the met protooncogene, *Cancer Cell* 3:347, 2003.

182c. Browder T et al: Antiangiogenic therapy and p53, *Science* 297:471a, 2002.

182d. Kieran MW, Folkman J, Heymach J: Angiogenesis inhibitors and hypoxia, *Nat Med*, 2002 (in press).

183. Teicher BA et al: Antiangiogenic agents can increase tumor oxygenation and response to radiation therapy, *Radiat Oncol Invest* 2:269, 1995.

184. Perez-Atayde AR et al: Spectrum of tumor angiogenesis in the bone marrow of children with acute lymphoblastic leukemia, *Am J Pathol* 150:815, 1997.

185. Steiner R: Angiostatic activity of anticancer agents in the chick embryo chorioallantoic membrane (CHE-CAM) assay. In Steiner R, Weisz P, Langer R (eds): *Angiogenesis: key principles-science-technology-medicine*, Basel, Switzerland, 1992, Birkhauser Verlag.

186. Belotti D et al: The microtubule-affecting drug paclitaxel has antiangiogenic activity, *Clin Cancer Res* 2:1843, 1996.

187. Browder T et al: Antiangiogenic scheduling of chemotherapy improves efficacy against experimental drug-resistant cancer, *Cancer Res* 60:1878, 2000.

188. Klement G et al: Continuous low-dose therapy with vinblastine and VEGF receptor-2 antibody induces sustained tumor regression without overt toxicity, *J Clin Invest* 105:R15, 2000.

189. Hanahan D, Bergers G, Bergsland E: Less is more, regularly: metronomic dosing of cytotoxic drugs can target tumor angiogenesis in mice, *J Clin Invest* 105:1045, 2000.

190. Efficacy of intravenous continuous infusion of fluorouracil compared with bolus administration in advanced colorectal cancer: Meta-analysis Group In Cancer, *J Clin Oncol* 16:301, 1998.

191. Gabra H et al: Weekly doxorubicin and continuous infusional 5-fluorouracil for advanced breast cancer, *Br J Cancer* 74:2008, 1996.

192. Hansen RM et al: Phase III study of bolus versus infusion fluorouracil with or without cisplatin in advanced colorectal cancer, *J Natl Cancer Inst* 88:668, 1996.

193. Abu-Rustum NR et al: Salvage weekly paclitaxel in recurrent ovarian cancer, *Semin Oncol* 24:S15, 1997.

194. Loffler TM et al: Schedule- and dose-intensified paclitaxel as weekly 1-hour infusion in pretreated solid tumors: results of a phase I/II trial, *Semin Oncol* 23:32, 1996.

195. Kakolyris S et al: Treatment of non-small-cell lung cancer with prolonged oral etoposide, *Am J Clin Oncol* 21:505, 1998.

196. Chamberlain MC: Recurrent supratentorial malignant gliomas in children: long-term salvage therapy with oral etoposide, *Arch Neurol* 54:554, 1997.
197. Neskovic-Konstantinovic ZB et al: Daily oral etoposide in metastatic breast cancer, *Anticancer Drugs* 7:543, 1996.
198. Gagliardi A, Collins DC: Inhibition of angiogenesis by antiestrogens, *Cancer Res* 53:533, 1993.
199. Gagliardi AR, Hennig B, Collins DC: Antiestrogens inhibit endothelial cell growth stimulated by angiogenic growth factors, *Anticancer Res* 16:1101, 1996.
200. Munn RK et al: Tamoxifen induces apoptosis in human microvascular endothelial cells, *Proc Am Assoc Cancer Res* 38:266, 1997 (abstract 1784).
201. Kishi K et al: Preferential enhancement of tumor radioresponse by a cyclooxygenase-2 inhibitor, *Cancer Res* 60:1326, 2000.
202. Panigrahy D et al: PPARgamma ligands inhibit primary tumor growth and metastasis by inhibiting angiogenesis, *J Clin Invest* 110:923, 2002.
203. Wood J et al: Novel antiangiogenic effects of the bisphosphonate compound zoledronic acid, *J Pharmacol Exp Ther* 302:1055, 2002.
203a. Kieran M et al: 4-drug anti-angiogenic chemotherapy: results from a phase I feasibility trial of oral thalidomide, celecoxib, etoposide and cyclophosphamide in patients with recurrent or progressive cancer, *Proc Am Assoc Cancer Res* 44:1363, 2003 (abstract 173).
204. Ma L et al: Platelets modulate gastric ulcer healing: role of endostatin and vascular endothelial growth factor release, *Proc Natl Acad Sci USA* 98:6470, 2001.
205. Ma L, del Soldato P, Wallace JL: Divergent effects of new cyclooxygenase inhibitors on gastric ulcer healing: shifting the angiogenic balance, *Proc Natl Acad Sci USA* 99:13243, 2002.
206. Folkman J: Tumor angiogenesis: therapeutic implications, *N Engl J Med* 285:1182, 1971.
207. Folkman J: Anti-angiogenesis: new concept for therapy of solid tumors, *Ann Surg* 175:409, 1972.
208. Arbiser JL et al: Oncogenic H-ras stimulates tumor angiogenesis by two distinct pathways, *Proc Natl Acad Sci USA* 94:861, 1997.
209. Streit M et al: Thrombospondin-2: a potent endogenous inhibitor of tumor growth and angiogenesis, *Proc Natl Acad Sci USA* 96:14888, 1999.
210. Chin L et al: Essential role for oncogenic Ras in tumour maintenance, *Nature* 400:468, 1999.
211. Nguyen M et al: Vascular expression of E-selectin is increased in estrogen-receptor-negative breast cancer, *Am J Pathol* 150:1307, 1997.
212. Harris AL et al: Gene therapy through signal transduction pathways and angiogenic growth factors as therapeutic targets in breast cancer, *Cancer* 74:1021, 1994.
213. Harris AL et al: Breast cancer angiogenesis: therapy target and prognostic factor, *Eur J Cancer* 31A:831, 1995.
214. Aranda FI, Laforga JB: Microvessel quantitation in breast ductal invasive carcinoma: correlation with proliferative activity, hormonal receptors and lymph node metastases, *Pathol Res Pract* 192:124, 1996.
215. Gasparini G et al: Determination of angiogenesis adds information to estrogen receptor status in predicting the efficacy of adjuvant tamoxifen in node-positive breast cancer patients, *Clin Cancer Res* 2:1191, 1996.
216. Hayes DF: Angiogenesis and breast cancer, *Hematol Oncol Clin North Am* 8:51, 1994.
217. Macaulay VM et al: Breast cancer angiogenesis and tamoxifen resistance, *Endocr Relat Cancer* 2:97, 1995.
218. Runkel S, Wayss K, Melchert F: Angiogenesis of human breast cancers: neovascularization in xenotransplants and oxygenation in situ in patients, *Gynakol Geburtschifliche Rundsch* 35:68, 1995.
219. Salven P et al: Endothelial Tie growth factor receptor provides antigen marker for assessment of breast cancer angiogenesis, *Br J Cancer* 74:69, 1996.

CHAPTER

29

Immunology and the Role of Immunotherapy in Breast Cancer

PETER S. GOEDEGEBUURE

TOBY J. DUNN

TIMOTHY J. EBERLEIN

Chapter Outline

Other chapters in this book have emphasized the indication and specific uses of the traditional modalities of treatment of breast cancer, such as breast conservation, the importance of surgical margins, indications for mastectomy, indications for radiation therapy, and indications and regimens of chemotherapy and hormone therapy. However, the fact remains that patients who have recurrent metastatic breast cancer usually succumb to the disease. Thus alternative systemic therapies for the treatment of breast cancer need to be developed.

Immunotherapy for tumor was first used more than a century ago by William Coley, who used extracts of pyogenic bacteria to treat tumors.[1] The concept of immune-surveillance was first suggested by Ehrlich in 1909, but it was not until 1959 that Thomas postulated that the outgrowth of tumors was immunologically controlled. The theory of immune-surveillance was formally introduced by Burnet in 1967.[2]

This hypothesis holds that the immune system functions to detect and remove malignant cells as they arise, thereby preventing the growth of clinically apparent cancers in most individuals. Thus a patient with a clinically detectable breast malignancy would represent a failure of the immune system. The theory of immune-surveillance has become more widely accepted because of recent experimental evidence.

A direct role for lymphocytes and interferon-γ (IFN-γ) in tumor suppression was demonstrated by Schreiber and colleagues, who used mice deficient for lymphocytes and/or IFN-γ.[3] At the age of 18 months, 50% of the lymphocyte-deficient mice had developed tumors of gastrointestinal origin, whereas 80% of mice deficient for both lymphocytes and IFN-γ developed primarily breast and colon cancers. In contrast, wild-type control animals had no evidence of tumors.

Recent advances in cellular and molecular biology have elucidated the complexity of oncogenesis and cancer progression. Advances in cellular and molecular biology have led to an improved understanding of the interaction between malignant cells and the immune system.[4] Collectively, the new knowledge has caused a resurgence of interest in the immunology of cancer and in cancer immunotherapy.

Traditionally, breast cancer has not been considered an immunologically responsive tumor, in contrast to other human solid malignancies such as melanoma and renal cell cancer. Other than the monoclonal antibody trastuzumab (Herceptin) directed against the *HER2/neu* receptor,[5] there are currently no immunologic-based therapies approved by the U.S. Food and Drug Administration (FDA) for treatment of breast cancer. However, other immunologic-based therapies are under extensive preclinical and clinical evaluation and have the potential to provide clinicians with another modality of treatment for patients with breast cancer.

This chapter provides a summary of the basic and clinical science that defines the current status of tumor immunology and the prospects for successful immunotherapy of breast cancer. By the end of this chapter, it is hoped that the reader will appreciate the importance of the immune response in breast cancer and recognize the potential application of immune strategies for the treatment of breast cancer, either as a single modality or in combination with other, more established therapies.

Basics of Tumor Immunology

IMMUNE EFFECTOR CELLS

A number of immune effector cells have the ability to eradicate tumor cells directly or indirectly (Table 29-1). Innate immune cells, including macrophages, natural killer (NK) cells, and neutrophils, characteristically do not need sensitization to respond to an immunogen. Macrophages and neutrophils are generally not cytotoxic to tumor cells unless activated by bacterial products. Macrophages may exert direct antitumor activity through secretion of tumor necrosis factor or oxyradicals such as nitric oxide. More important perhaps is the ability of macrophages and neutrophils to phagocytose and destroy antibody-coated tumor cells. In addition, macrophages can present tumor antigens to T cells.

NK cells are a distinct population of lymphocytes that can efficiently lyse tumor cells. NK cells express receptors that recognize specific major histocompatibility complex (MHC) alleles. Binding of the receptor to MHC molecules blocks the lytic machinery of the NK cell. Thus, as long as the MHC expression on tumor cells is intact, the NK cells will not lyse the tumor cells. Loss of expression of one or

TABLE 29-1   Immune Effector Cells Against Tumor

EFFECTOR CELLS	MAIN FUNCTIONS
Macrophage	Phagocytosis, direct tumor cell lysis, ADCC, antigen presentation, cytokine secretion
Dendritic cell	Antigen presentation; stimulation of T, B, and NK cells; cytokine and chemokine secretion
NK cell	Direct tumor cell lysis, ADCC, cytokine (e.g., IFN-γ) secretion
Neutrophil	Direct tumor cell lysis, cytokine secretion
T lymphocyte	Antigen-specific tumor cell lysis, cytokine secretion
B lymphocyte	Antigen-specific antibody formation, cytokine secretion

ADCC, Antibody-dependent cellular cytotoxicity.

more alleles may remove the "brake" and make tumor cells more susceptible to tumor lysis.[6]

The innate immune system often works synergistically with the acquired or adaptive immune system. Of the two arms of the immune system, acquired immunity consisting of the B- and T-lymphocyte response may be the most potent against solid tumors. Whereas innate immunity is mediated by nonspecific effector cells, acquired immunity is mediated by specific effector cells that recognize tumor antigens. Truly tumor-specific antigens have been discovered that are either unique or shared by other tumors; these can be recognized by antibodies or T cells through specific receptors.

The role of B cells and antibodies in antitumor responses is poorly understood. Tumor-specific antibodies are often present in the serum of patients without correlation to clinical status. Possible mechanisms of tumor cell lysis involve complex formation between antibody and tumor cells, followed by opsonization by macrophages (phagocytosis). The presence of complement may enhance this process. Alternatively, the Fc part of the antibody may be bound by Fc-receptor positive effector cells, such as NK cells, macrophages, and neutrophils. Ligation of the Fc receptor triggers the lytic machinery, which leads to tumor cell lysis. This process is called *antibody-dependent cellular cytotoxicity* (ADCC).

T cells, in contrast to antibodies, may directly lyse tumor cells and are considered more essential for rejection of solid tumors than B cells. "Spontaneous" regression of solid tumors has sporadically been observed and is thought to be mediated by tumor-specific T cells. T-cell–mediated lysis is dependent on activation of the lytic machinery after recognition of tumor antigens by an antigen-specific receptor, known as the *T-cell receptor* (TcR). The TcR is expressed on every T cell and is encoded by genetically uniquely rearranged gene fragments, yielding a large repertoire of TcR molecules with a different antigen specificity.[7] The TcR molecule is designed to bind to molecules of the MHC; CD8+ T cells bind to MHC class I molecules, which are expressed on all nucleated cells, and CD4+ T cells generally bind to MHC class II molecules, which are expressed predominantly on cells of the immune system. Whereas CD8 T cells are primarily cytotoxic, CD4 T cells primarily secrete cytokines that support or inhibit the function of other cells, including immune effector cells (Figure 29-1).

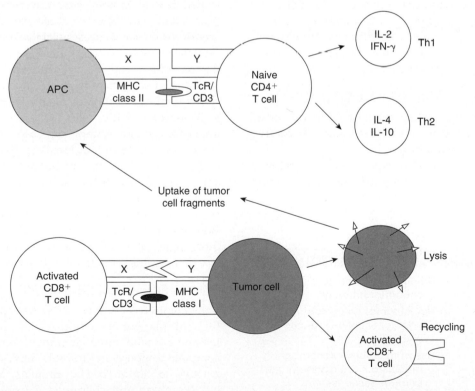

FIG. 29-1 Schematic overview of CD4 and CD8 T-cell activation. Major histocompatibility complex *(MHC)* class I-peptide complex is recognized by the T-cell receptor *(TcR)* on CD8 T cells. When costimulatory signals are provided through costimulatory molecules, represented by the X-Y interaction, the CD8 T cell is activated and the tumor cell is lysed. The CD8 T cell recycles, and tumor cell fragments can be taken up by antigen-presenting cells *(APCs),* such as dendritic cells. The APCs process antigen and present antigenic peptides by MHC class II to CD4 T cells. When costimulation is provided, CD4 T cells are activated and differentiate into Th1 or Th2 effector cells.

T-cell activation is a two-signal process. In addition to the TcR binding to the MHC-peptide complex, a second, costimulatory signal is required. This signal is provided through interaction of certain ligands on the antigen-presenting cell and their receptors on the T cell. When properly activated, T cells undergo cell division (clonal expansion) and become functionally active. Expansion of T cells is also dependent on the availability of growth factors, such as interleukin (IL)-2. Most CD8+ T cells do not produce sufficient amounts of IL-2 to sustain proliferation and are dependent on CD4+ T cells for their IL-2, in particular the CD4+ T helper (Th) 1 cells. Because most tumor cells do not express MHC class II, CD4+ T cells are dependent on presentation of tumor antigen by professional antigen-presenting cells, such as dendritic cells and macrophages. B cells, on the other hand, are dependent on IL-4 produced by CD4+ Th2 cells.

Generally, an immune response is characterized by stimulation of an innate immune response as a first line of defense, followed by an acquired immune response and induction of immunologic memory. Dendritic cells are thought to bridge innate and acquired immune responses. As such, each immune response involves multiple different subsets of immune cells, each secreting a unique panel of cytokines, which makes an immune response a complex process. Induction of an antitumor immune response in a cancer patient is more complex because the tumor cells managed to coexist in often immunologically competent hosts. Nonetheless, progress has been made over the years.

EARLY STAGES OF IMMUNE INTERVENTION

Several types of immunotherapy exist: (1) active, either nonspecific or specific; (2) adoptive; and (3) passive immunotherapy (Table 29-2).

As mentioned, the first attempts to boost a patient's immune system to reject a tumor involved injecting

TABLE 29-2 | Strategies of Immunotherapy

STRATEGY	CHARACTERIZATION
Active immunization	Stimulation of the host's antitumor immunity
Specific	Use of tumor antigen to activate adaptive immune response
Nonspecific	Use of microbial or chemical modulators to activate innate immune response
Adoptive immunotherapy	Transfer of immune cells or factors (e.g., cytokines, chemokines)
Passive immunotherapy	Transfer of tumor-specific antibodies

killed bacteria. This strategy emphasized nonspecific activation of immune responses. Some of the most common bacterial vaccines tested in an adjuvant setting in breast cancer include *Bacillus Calmette-Guerin* (BCG), *Corynebacterium parvum* (*C. parvum*), and *Pseudomonas*-based vaccines. However, none of these vaccines by themselves or in combination with chemotherapy or hormone therapy significantly increased disease-free survival.[8-10] These trials were performed in the late 1970s and throughout most of the 1980s.

An alternative strategy pioneered by Dr. S. Rosenberg and colleagues at the National Cancer Institute (NCI) involved the adoptive transfer of activated lymphocytes into cancer patients. Initially, the lymphocytes were obtained from peripheral blood and activated with high-dose IL-2 to generate so-called lymphokine-activated killer (LAK) cells.[11] Later, T cells were extracted from the patient's tumor, the so-called tumor-infiltrating lymphocytes.[12] Other investigators attempted to treat patients with a lysate of either the patient's tumor cells[13] or from histologically matched allogeneic tumor cell lines.[14,15]

Even though these strategies were based on the supposition that tumor-specific T cells exist and circulate in cancer patients, and tumor antigens are shared among tumors, very few tumor antigens had been identified. Most of these came from serologic identification in a process called *autologous typing*, established by L. Old and colleagues[16] in the 1970s. The demonstration and characterization of tumor-specific antibodies led to attempts to attach antibodies to tumor cells with the Fc portion being available for crosslinking to Fc-positive killer cells (ADCC). This transfer of antibodies was an example of passive immunotherapy.

Unequivocal proof for the existence of antigens specifically expressed in tumors but not in normal tissues was obtained in 1991.[17] In subsequent years, numerous tumor antigens were identified both for T cells and B cells, primarily through the screening of cDNA expression libraries made from tumors (Table 29-3, discussed in more detail later). Consequently, active specific immunization became more frequently used.

TUMOR ESCAPE MECHANISMS

The promise of immune-based therapies is embodied by multiple human clinical trials in patients with melanoma who have demonstrated the occasional complete response and durable remission using T cells reactive to tumor-specific antigens, as demonstrated by Rosenberg and colleagues.[18] Complete responses, however, are the exception rather than the rule. With the availability of both innate and acquired immunity, one wonders why these systems have failed in cancer patients despite the expression of specific tumor antigens. Clearly, tumors must develop mechanisms

TABLE 29-3 | Examples of Tumor Antigens Recognized by T or B Cells

I. CLASS I—RESTRICTED ANTIGENS RECOGNIZED BY CD8 T CELLS

Shared*	Melanoma	MAGE-1, NY-ESO-1
	Breast cancer	*HER2/neu*, MUC1, mammaglobin
	Colon cancer	CEA
Unique	Melanoma	MUM-1, CDK4, β-catenin
	Renal carcinoma	HLA-A2
	Bladder carcinoma	KIA0205

II. CLASS II—RESTRICTED ANTIGENS RECOGNIZED BY CD4 T CELLS

Shared	Melanoma	MAGE-1, NY-ESO-1
	Breast cancer	*HER2/neu*
Unique	Melanoma	CDC27, LDFP

III. ANTIGENS RECOGNIZED BY ANTIBODIES

Shared	Melanoma	MAGE-1, NY-ESO-1
	Breast cancer	*HER2/neu*, MUC1, mammaglobin
	Colon cancer	CEA

CDK4, cyclin-dependent kinase 4; *CEA*, carcinoembryonic antigen; *LDFP*, low-density-lipid receptor fusion protein; *MUM-1*, melanoma-ubiquitous mutated-1.
*Shared antigens include those shared among tumors of the same histologic type, as well as antigens shared by various types of cancers.

TABLE 29-4 | Tumor Escape Mechanisms

MECHANISM	CHARACTERISTICS
Tumor related	No expression of tumor antigens
	Dysfunctional processing of tumor antigens
	Decreased expression of MHC molecules
	Decreased expression of costimulatory molecules
	Secretion of immunosuppressive factors
	Induction of T-cell apoptosis
	Induction of T-cell tolerance
Host related	Inherited or acquired immunodeficiency
	Treatment-related immunosuppression
	Age-related immunosuppression
	Defective antigen presentation by immune effector cells
	No access to tumor cells

MHC, Major histocompatibility complex.

by which to evade an effective immune response. Extensive research during the last decade has elucidated several escape mechanisms that permit tumor cells to avoid elimination by immune effector cells.

Elimination of tumor cells by T cells has failed in cancer patients because of host-related issues, tumor-related issues, or both[19,20] (Table 29-4). The tumor cells may not, for example, be immunosensitive because they lack antigens that induce a T-cell response. With the exception of malignant melanoma, most solid tumor cells do not induce a strong T-cell response in vitro. Circumstantial evidence suggests that lack of expression of dominant tumor antigens is an important factor. In addition, the expression of certain or all MHC alleles on the tumor cells may be lower or completely lacking, resulting in decreased antigen presentation. Loss of expression has been positively correlated with tumor aggressiveness and metastatic potential. Furthermore, the tumor cells may not be able to process or present tumor antigen effectively. Finally, tumor cells may also be resistant to tumoricidal effector mechanisms such as induction of apoptosis through the apoptosis-inducing molecule Fas.

Different from immunosensitivity is immunogenicity. For example, tumor cells may express tumor antigens but still not induce an immune response because the tumor cells lack the expression of costimulatory molecules. Furthermore, tumor cells may produce immunosuppressive factors that inhibit T-cell function or induce signaling defects in T cells, transforming growth factor (TGF)-β and IL-10 secretion by tumor cells has been shown to inhibit T-cell activation. Soluble MUC1 secreted by multiple human epithelial cancers, including breast cancer, has been shown to induce immune suppression by blocking T-cell activation, presumably through interference with costimulation.[21] In addition, tumor cells may secrete soluble factors that downregulate T-cell molecules involved in signal transduction.[19]

As another example of a lack of immunogenicity, the antigen may be shed (e.g., CA 125 in ovarian cancer and CEA in colon cancer), or it may induce T-cell tolerance. Tolerance induction may be related to the low avidity of the interaction between T cell and tumor cell. Finally, the tumor cells may induce apoptosis in activated T cells. Apoptosis, or programmed cell death, is a special type of physiologic death and is distinct from nonphysiologic accidental cell death or necrosis. In some models, tumor cells have been demonstrated to produce cell surface or soluble Fas ligand, which can bind to the Fas receptor expressed on activated T cells and thereby induce apoptosis in T cells.[20]

Host-related factors that induce tumor escape include (1) immunodeficiency (either inherited or acquired) that may increase the incidence of tumors; (2) immunosuppression induced by radiation treatment, chemotherapeutic drugs, or chemical or physical carcinogens; (3) tumor progression that may outpace tumor regression; (4) deficient presentation of tumor antigens by antigen-presenting cells, as was demonstrated for the breast cancer antigens MUC1[22] and *HER2/neu*; (5) lack of access of effector cells to the tumor; or (6) expression of immunodominant antigens on parental tumor that prevents stimulation with other tumor antigens.

The last mentioned mechanism is an intriguing phenomenon that was described in the 1980s but has so far not been explained. There appears to be a hierarchy in the immune response to various tumor antigens because the host fails to recognize all antigens simultaneously. The expression of an immunodominant antigen would prohibit the immune system from responding to antigen-negative tumor cells. A less clear failure of the host to mount an antitumor immune response is related to age. Over time, there may be a decrease in effectiveness of the immune response.

How to Overcome Tumor Escape Mechanisms

With the results of the first controlled clinical studies showing disappointing results, investigators rethought their strategies. The large number of possible escape mechanisms seen in tumors demanded a more sophisticated approach than was currently used. Several developments in the early to mid-1990s permitted the design of more sophisticated vaccines. The main aspects that investigators focused on were (1) optimization of the cytokine environment for T cells, (2) provision of adequate costimulation of T cells, and (3) identification of tumor-associated antigens encoding T-cell epitopes. More recently, there is a renewed interest in understanding immune mechanisms of tumor tolerance.

CYTOKINE ENVIRONMENT

The simplest way to ensure the local presence of a particular cytokine is to inject the cytokine locally, in or near the tumor. This limits application to mostly primary tumors that are fairly easily accessible. In addition, it is difficult to maintain a certain concentration of the cytokine in situ.

To ensure that a particular cytokine is secreted continuously at the tumor site, investigators explored the use of various delivery systems that would permit a direct targeting of the tumor environment. Vaccines consisting of replicating or nonreplicating tumor cells genetically engineered to express a cytokine showed promise in murine models, including breast cancer models.[23]

In addition to secretion of stimulatory cytokine, the availability of additional tumor antigen may promote antitumor responses. Comparisons between interleukins and proinflammatory cytokines such as IFN-γ, granulocyte-macrophage colony-stimulating factor (GM-CSF), and tumor necrosis factor (TNF)-α suggest that multiple cytokines induced potent antitumor immune responses and protected mice from subsequent tumor challenge.[23] Evaluation of the underlying mechanism reveals that the cytokine secreted by the engineered tumor cells usually induced an inflammatory response followed by an influx of nonspecific immune cells. Although each cytokine evokes a unique response, common factors in the cascade of events that lead to successful tumor eradication are the influx of granulocytes, primarily neutrophils, followed by an influx and activation of CD8 T cells.[24] Initial tumor lysis is mediated by granulocytes; this lysis leads to mobilization of antigen-presenting cells and, subsequently, of CD8 T cells. Depletion of T cells or granulocytes, as well as blocking the release of secondary cytokines, impairs the antitumor response. Therefore crosstalk between nonspecific and specific immune cells appears essential.

COSTIMULATION: ROLE OF B7

The finding that B7, later defined as B7.1 (CD80), and B7.2 (CD86) are ligands for CD28 on the T cells[25] provides a strong stimulus in vaccine design. The CD28-B7 interaction provides a costimulatory signal for naïve resting T cells. Without the costimulatory signal, T cells are induced into a state of unresponsiveness, so-called anergy. T-cell activation is dependent on two signals, one through crosslinking of the TcR and the other through costimulatory molecules. Of the costimulatory molecules, CD28 is critical for initiation of T-cell stimulation and subsequent IL-2 production and proliferation. Successful T-cell activation is dependent on reaching a threshold of crosslinked TcR molecules. The threshold number is significantly reduced when a costimulatory signal is provided, thereby making T cells more sensitive to antigenic stimulation.[26]

Expression of B7.1 and B7.2 is generally limited to professional antigen-presenting cells: macrophages, dendritic cells, and activated B cells. Most epithelial cells, and epithelial tumors, do not express B7.1 or B7.2, which could explain why tumor cells fail to elicit effective antitumor T-cell responses. Transfer of B7.1 or B7.2 into a variety of moderately immunogenic murine tumors, including breast carcinomas, followed by immunization has led to tumor rejection.[27,28] However, immunogenicity of poorly immunogenic tumors is not altered after B7.1 coexpression.[28,29]

COSTIMULATION: ROLE OF CTLA-4

Shortly after the identification of B7.1 and B7.2 as ligands for CD28, it was found that a second receptor expressed on T cells could bind B7 molecules.[25]

This receptor, named cytotoxic T lymphocyte antigen-4 (CTLA-4, CD152), is expressed on activated T cells, and crosslinking of the receptor leads to inhibition of proliferation. CTLA-4 is homologous to CD28 but has a 50- to 2000-fold higher binding affinity for the B7 molecules than CD28. Blockade of CTLA-4 with intact antibody or Fab fragments enhances T-cell proliferation. This feature has been exploited in murine tumor models with the idea that blockade of CTLA-4 might enhance T-cell responses to tumor.

Administration of the anti-CTLA-4 antibody has indeed shown a dramatic improvement of antitumor immunity and has led to rejection of preestablished tumors.[30,31] However, CTLA-4 blockade by itself is not effective against poorly immunogenic tumors such as the experimental mammary tumor SM1.[32] When combined with a vaccination strategy such as irradiated or cytokine gene-transformed tumor cells, however, poorly immunogenic tumors can also be rejected, including the SM1.[32]

COSTIMULATION: USE OF DENDRITIC CELLS

Of all professional antigen-presenting cells such as macrophages, activated B cells, and dendritic cells, the dendritic cells are primarily responsible for induction of primary immune responses mediated by T and B lymphocytes and establishment of immunologic memory.[33] The discovery of conditions for in vitro culture and expansion of dendritic cells from both mice and humans[34,35] opens new avenues for vaccine design. Key for in vitro generation of dendritic cells is the addition of GM-CSF. Since then, a large body of literature has accumulated on the origin and differentiation pathways of dendritic cells, as well as on their potential use as antigen-presenting cells for induction of antitumor immune responses (reviewed in reference 36).

Currently, the three main subsets of human dendritic cells are derived from CD34+ progenitor cells. CD34+ myeloid progenitor cells differentiate into monocytes (dendritic cell precursors) that give rise to immature interstitial dendritic cells in the presence of GM-CSF and IL-4. CD34+ myeloid progenitor cells can also differentiate into nonmonocytic cells that further differentiate into Langerhans dendritic cells in the presence of GM-CSF, IL-4, and TGF-β. Finally, CD34+ lymphoid progenitor cells can give rise to lymphoid dendritic cells in the presence of IL-3.

Immature dendritic cells have a high phagocytic capacity that is greatly reduced upon maturation. Following antigen uptake, immature dendritic cells migrate to lymphoid organs and undergo maturation. In lymphoid organs, T cells (both CD4 and CD8) and B cells are stimulated. In addition, dendritic cells can secrete cytokines after antigen uptake, which stimulate innate immune cells such as eosinophils, macrophages, and NK cells. As such, dendritic cells are of great importance for induction of both innate and adaptive immune responses. Within adaptive immunity, dendritic cells are essential for both cellular as well as humoral responses.

It has recently become evident that in addition to the existence of distinct dendritic cell subsets that exhibit distinct functions, dendritic cell functions can be altered by cytokines. For example, dendritic cells that normally induce Th1 responses can switch to inducing Th2 (or regulatory T cells (T_{reg}), as discussed later) responses in the presence of antiinflammatory cytokines, such as IL-10 or TGF-β, or with steroids or prostaglandin E_2. A dominant Th2 response would promote a humoral response but inhibit a cellular immune response. Therefore soluble factors that skew dendritic cell function can negatively affect the antitumor immune response.

IDENTIFICATION OF TUMOR ANTIGENS

The third major improvement in the early to mid-1990s was the development of techniques to identify T- and B-cell epitopes uniquely expressed on tumor cells. Boon and colleagues[17] popularized T-cell screening of a cDNA expression library made of mRNA from tumor cells. The expression library was made in cells with the same human leukocyte antigen (HLA) allele as the restriction element for the tumor-specific T-cell clones used for screening so that reconstitution of the HLA-antigen complex conferred recognition by the T-cell clone. Recognition was evaluated by release of cytokines or cytolytic activity.

This technique has been adopted by others with or without modifications and has led to the identification of more than 50 antigens already, most of which are identified in malignant melanoma[37,38] (see Table 29-3). In addition to this genetic approach, a more biochemical approach was successfully used in which antigenic peptides are eluted from cell-surface HLA molecules on tumor cells. The peptide pool is fractionated by reverse-phase high-performance liquid chromatography (HPLC) and individual fractions are screened with tumor-specific T-cell clones in a reconstitution assay similar to that previously described by pulsing each fraction onto target cells.[37-39]

A third technique that is commonly used is the serologic identification of antigens by recombinant expression cloning, known as *SEREX*.[40] This method is based on the screening of a cDNA expression library from tumor-derived mRNA, similar to the method used by Boon and colleagues. However, the expression library is screened with serum antibodies from the patient bearing the original tumor. The presence of tumor-specific antibodies in serum of cancer patients was clearly demonstrated by Old and colleagues in the 1970s.[16] The implementation of molecular cloning techniques leading to SEREX dates from 1995.[40] Since then, more than 2000 antigens have been identified with the aid of SEREX on a variety of tumors, including melanoma, breast,[41,42] lung, colon, renal, and testis cancers, but also nonsolid tumors such as Hodgkin's lymphomas. An advantage of SEREX over other techniques is that by identifying immunogenic proteins uniquely expressed in tumors, T-cell epitopes may subsequently be identified as well. Selecting for high-titer IgG antibodies in the serum during the screening process increases the likelihood that the identified immunogenic protein also contains T-cell epitopes. This has proved correct for a number of molecules, including the breast cancer antigens *HER2/neu* and NY-ESO.[43]

Mechanisms of Immune Tolerance to Tumor

Although clear evidence of existing antitumor immune responses can be obtained in most cancer patients, the response is not effective. In addition to the possibilities listed in Table 29-4, several mechanisms for immune evasion of tumor have recently become clear. For dendritic cell precursors to undergo differentiation into mature dendritic cells capable of stimulating T cells, distress signals are required. Tumor cells that initially grow and behave as healthy cells do not induce those signals. Thus even though dendritic cells may capture and present tumor antigen, the lack of distress signals results in the inability to undergo maturation and provide costimulation to T cells. When these dendritic cells encounter T cells, either T-cell anergy or deletion is induced.[4,44]

Strategies such as treatment with BCG may induce "danger" signals, but clinical testing has taught us that repeated injection of BCG does not cure cancer.[8] More detailed knowledge on various forms of stress-induced and lymphocyte-induced tumor cell death is required to better understand the distress signals that lead to maturation of dendritic cells.

Recent studies demonstrated an additional escape mechanism in which tumor cells either did not reach draining lymph nodes[45] or tumor cells reaching lymph nodes were physically separated from T cells.[46] In both cases, immune effector cells were not induced and the tumor cells were ignored.

Even when immune effector cells are induced, the presence of suppressor cells may block effector function.

Three types of lymphocytes have recently been identified that could potentially interfere with the host's ability to mount an effective antitumor response. NKT cells, CD4+CD25+ regulatory T cells (T_{reg}), and CD8$\alpha\alpha$+$\gamma\delta$T cells, are regulatory or suppressor T cells that maintain self-tolerance by suppressing autoreactive CD4 and CD8 T cells.[4] Lack of these regulatory lymphocytes has been shown to be associated with autoimmune disease. Consequently, this implies that removal of regulatory cells would promote antitumor responses.

This assumption has been recently proved correct in animal models in which antibody-mediated depletion of T_{reg}[47,48] or $\gamma\delta$T cells,[49] adoptive transfer of purified NKT cells,[50] or depletion of NKT cells[51] improved antitumor efficacy in murine tumor models. In addition, a recent study demonstrated an increased prevalence of T_{reg} in the blood and tumor microenvironment of breast cancer and pancreas cancer patients compared with the prevalence of T_{reg} in the blood of normal donors.[52] Similar observations were made in patients with lung and ovarian cancer.[53]

Clinical Evaluation

Although the previously mentioned topics drastically improved our understanding of basic immune responses and permitted the design of new generations of vaccines, clinical translation has been difficult. When tested in animal models, mostly mouse models, the majority of vaccines induced tumor rejection as well as protection against a rechallenge with the same tumor cells.

However, when testing vaccines clinically, one should realize the following: Most vaccines used in animal models are used as prophylactic vaccines or used to treat early tumors established less than a week. Very few reports exist on successful treatment of preexisting and established tumors in mice. Moreover, most of the tumors used are transplantable tumors to which the animals have not been exposed previously and thus the immune system has not been tolerized to the tumor. If tumors are given time to adapt to their environment under pressure of a competent immune system, as is the case with human tumors, successful immunologic intervention becomes much more difficult.

To date, a few transgenic mouse models have been generated in which a tumor antigen such as erbB2 or MUC1 is expressed as a transgene (reviewed in reference 54). These models have the advantage that spontaneous tumors reproducibly develop in a fashion similar to human cancers. At the same time, the presence of the transgene has induced T- and B-cell tolerance to the tumor antigen that needs to be overcome by immunologic intervention. Therefore use of vaccines in patients with metastatic disease might be predicted to fail. Testing of prophylactic vaccines in humans for most tumors requires many years of following patients.

An additional problem is that investigators currently do not know how to accurately measure anticancer activity of a vaccine. Measuring distinct T-cell responses in vitro, such as the ability to lyse tumor cells, has not proved predictive of clinical responses. In the absence of a surrogate marker for antitumor activity, the question becomes how to evaluate efficacy. Relying on criteria used for evaluation of chemotherapeutic drugs may not be accurate either because the kinetics of a response to chemotherapy most likely is not the same as a response to immunotherapy. In fact, immunotherapy of preexisting tumors generally does not lead to a rapid regression. Therefore the only valid end point to date is clinical outcome, and this usually requires several years to obtain.

Antibody Therapy in Breast Cancer

The human proto-oncogene *HER2/neu* encodes a transmembrane growth-factor receptor related to the epidermal growth-factor receptor that has been specifically targeted in the treatment of breast cancer. *HER2/neu* gene amplification and subsequent overexpression of the wild-type protein occurs in 25% to 30% of human breast carcinomas.[55] In breast cancer, *HER2/neu* overexpression is an independent predictor of both relapse-free and overall survival. The *HER2/neu* receptor is not merely a marker of a more malignant phenotype but also plays an integral role in the biology and pathogenesis of breast cancer. Early studies demonstrated that *HER2/neu* overexpression alone could induce malignant transformation,[56] and additional studies have implicated overexpression of *HER2/neu* in the progression of metastatic disease and resistance to therapy.[57]

Characterization of the receptor and development of antireceptor antibodies have led to a novel approach to the treatment of breast cancer. Trastuzumab (Herceptin) is a recombinant humanized monoclonal antibody directed against the *HER2/neu* receptor.[58] Although the mechanism of its antitumor activity is not entirely clear, monoclonal antibody against *HER2/neu* appears to produce apoptosis in tumor cells overexpressing the protein. It is currently approved for use as a single agent for those patients with metastatic breast cancer whose tumors overexpress the *HER2/neu* protein and who have received one or more chemotherapy regimens for metastatic disease. It is also approved for use as a first-line therapy in combination with paclitaxel for the treatment of *HER2/neu* overexpressing metastatic breast cancer. It remains the only FDA-approved immunologic-based therapy for the treatment of breast cancer.

Current Clinical Trials

Ongoing clinical trials do not yet reflect the latest preclinical discoveries. Of 64 current clinical trials for immune-based treatment of breast cancer, 30 protocols include treatment with tumor-specific antibodies (Table 29-5). Of these, the majority involves the anti-*HER2/neu* antibody trastuzumab (Herceptin). The vaccines (9 out of 64) contain tumor antigens in the form of a peptide, protein, RNA, or tumor cell for induction of specific T- and/or B-cell responses. Treatments involving bone marrow/stem cell transplantation comprise 25% of the 64 protocols; 11 out of 16 are combined with chemotherapy. Of the eight protocols that involve cytokines and biologic-response modifiers, seven are combined with chemotherapy. The cytokine most commonly used in this group is G-CSF. Gene therapy is not (yet) being tested for breast cancer, although two protocols, one vaccine and one bone marrow–transplantation protocol, involve gene-modified cells. Only one trial involves treatment with a nonspecific vaccine (*Corynebacterium granulosum*).

Summary

- Breast cancers express antigens recognized by T and B lymphocytes.
- Objective clinical responses have been observed after immune-based therapy.
- Immunotherapy may be successful as an adjuvant therapy to prevent metastatic and recurrent disease.
- Future directions of investigations may include combinations of various immune-based strategies such as immunization combined with inhibition/depletion of suppressor cells.

TABLE 29-5 Ongoing Clinical Trials Involving Immune Therapy

TREATMENT	NUMBER OF TRIALS
Vaccines	9
Antibody therapy	30
Bone marrow/stem cell therapy	16
Cytokines/biologic-response modifiers	8
Nonspecific vaccines	1

From http://cancernet.nci.nih.gov/clinical_trials/.

- Future directions may also include combination therapy such as immunotherapy (e.g., trastuzumab) and chemotherapy.

REFERENCES

1. Coley WB: The treatment of malignant tumors by repeated inoculation of erysipelas: with a report of ten original cases, *Am J Med Sci* 105:487, 1893.
2. Burnet FM: Immunological aspects of malignant disease, *Lancet* 1:1171, 1967.
3. Shankaran V et al: IFNγ and lymphocytes prevent primary tumour development and shape tumour immunogenicity, *Nature* 410:1107, 2001.
4. Smyth MJ, Godfrey DI, Trapani JA: A fresh look at tumor immunosurveillance and immunotherapy, *Nature Immunol* 2:293, 2001.
5. McNeil C: Herceptin raises its sight beyond advanced breast cancer, *J Natl Cancer Inst* 90:882, 1998.
6. Moretta A et al: Natural cytotoxicity receptors that trigger human NK-cell-mediated cytolysis, *Immunol Today* 21:228, 2000.
7. Davis MM, Bjorkman PJ: T-cell antigen receptor genes and T-cell recognition, *Nature* 334:395, 1988.
8. Hubay CA et al: Adjuvant endocrine therapy, cytotoxic chemotherapy and immunotherapy in stage II breast cancer: 6-year result, *J Steroid Biochem* 23:1147, 1985.
9. Hortobagyi GN et al: Combined antiestrogen and cytotoxic therapy with pseudomonas vaccine immunotherapy for metastatic breast cancer: a prospective, randomized trial, *Cancer* 60:2596, 1987.
10. Fischer B et al: Evaluation of the worth of *Corynebacterium parvum* in conjunction with chemotherapy as adjuvant treatment for primary breast cancer: eight-year results from the National Surgical Adjuvant Breast and Bowel Project B-10, *Cancer* 66:220, 1990.
11. Rosenberg SA et al: A progress report on the treatment of 157 patients with advanced cancer using lymphokine-activated killer cells and interleukin-2 or high-dose interleukin-2 alone, *N Engl J Med* 316:889, 1987.
12. Rosenberg SA et al: Use of tumor-infiltrating lymphocytes and interleukin-2 in the immunotherapy of patients with metastatic melanoma, *N Engl J Med* 319:1676, 1988.
13. Berd D et al: Treatment of metastatic melanoma with an autologous tumor-cell vaccine: clinical and immunologic results in 64 patients, *J Clin Oncol* 8:1858, 1990.
14. Mitchell MS et al: Active specific immunotherapy for melanoma: phase I trial of allogeneic lysates and a novel adjuvant, *Cancer Res* 48:5883, 1988.
15. Bystryn J-C et al: Immunogenicity of a polyvalent melanoma antigen vaccine in humans, *Cancer* 61:1065, 1988.
16. Old LJ: Cancer immunology: the search for specificity—G.H.A. Clowes memorial lecture, *Cancer Res* 41:361, 1981.
17. Van der Bruggen P et al: A gene encoding an antigen recognized by cytolytic T lymphocytes on a human melanoma, *Science* 254:1643, 1991.
18. Rosenberg SA: Development of cancer immunotherapies based on identification of the genes encoding cancer regression antigens, *J Natl Cancer Inst* 88:1635, 1996.
19. Finke J et al: Where have all the T cells gone? Mechanisms of immune evasion by tumors, *Immunol Today* 20:158, 1999.
20. Ferrone S et al: How much longer will tumour cells fool the immune system? *Immunol Today* 21:70, 2000.
21. Chan AK et al: Soluble MUC1 secreted by human epithelial cancer cells mediates immune suppression by blocking T-cell activation, *Int J Cancer* 82:721, 1999.
22. Hiltbold EM et al: The mechanism of unresponsiveness to circulating tumor antigen MUC1 is a block in intracellular sorting and processing by dendritic cells, *J Immunol* 165:3730, 2000.
23. Allione A et al: Immunizing and curative potential of replicating and nonreplicating murine mammary adeno-carcinoma cells engineered with interleukin (IL)-2, IL-4, IL-6, IL-7, IL-10, tumor necrosis factor α, granulocyte-macrophage colony-stimulating factor, and γ-interferon gene or admixed with conventional adjuvants, *Cancer Res* 54:6022, 1994.
24. Musiani P et al: Role of neutrophils and lymphocytes in inhibition of a mouse mammary adenocarcinoma engineered to release IL-2, IL-4, IL-7, IL-10, IFN-α, IFN-γ, and TNF-α, *Lab Invest* 74:146, 1996.
25. Linsley PS et al: Human B7-1 (CD80) and B7-2 (CD86) bind with similar avidities but distinct kinetics to CD28 and CTLA-4 receptors, *Immunity* 1:793, 1994.
26. Viola A, Lanzavecchia A: T-cell activation determined by T-cell receptor number and tunable thresholds, *Science* 273:104, 1996.
27. Townsend SE, Allison JP: Tumor rejection after direct costimulation of CD8+ T cells by B7-transfected melanoma cells, *Science* 259:368, 1993.
28. Ostrand-Rosenberg S: Tumor immunotherapy: the tumor cell as an antigen-presenting cell, *Current Biol* 6:722, 1994.
29. Hurwitz AA et al: Enhancement of the antitumor immune response using a combination of interferon-γ and B7 expression in an experimental mammary carcinoma, *Int J Cancer* 77:107, 1998.
30. Leach DR, Krummel MF, Allison JP: Enhancement of anti-tumor immunity by CTLA-4 blockade, *Science* 271:1734, 1996.
31. Chambers CA et al: CTLA-4-mediated inhibition in regulation of T-cell responses: mechanisms and manipulation in tumor immunotherapy, *Annu Rev Immunol* 19:565, 2001.
32. Hurwitz AA et al: CTLA-4 blockade synergizes with tumor-derived granulocyte-macrophage colony-stimulating factor for treatment of an experimental mammary carcinoma, *Proc Natl Acad Sci USA* 95:10067, 1998.
33. Bancherau J, Steinman RM: Dendritic cells and the control of immunity, *Nature* 392:245, 1998.
34. Inaba K et al: Generation of large numbers of dendritic cells from mouse bone marrow cultures supplemented with granulocyte/macrophage colony-stimulating factor, *J Exp Med* 17:1693, 1992.
35. Romani N et al: Proliferating dendritic cell progenitors in human blood, *J Exp Med* 180:83, 1994.
36. Bancherau J et al: Immunobiology of dendritic cells, *Annu Rev Immunol* 18:767, 2000.
37. Wang R-F: Human tumor antigens: implications for cancer vaccine development, *J Mol Med* 77:640, 1999.
38. Cox AL et al: Identification of a peptide recognized by five melanoma-specific human cytotoxic T-cell lines, *Science* 264:716, 1994.
39. Tanaka Y et al: Mammaglobin-A is a tumor-associated antigen in human breast carcinoma, *Surgery* 133:74, 2003.
40. Sahin U et al: Human neoplasms elicit multiple specific immune responses in the autologous host, *Proc Natl Acad Sci USA* 92:11810, 1995.

41. Obata Y et al: Identification of cancer antigens in breast cancer by the SEREX expression cloning method, *Breast Cancer* 6:305, 1999.

42. Jager D et al: Identification of a tissue-specific putative transcription factor in breast tissue by serological screening of a breast cancer library, *Cancer Res* 61:2055, 2001.

43. Jager E et al: Simultaneous humoral and cellular immune response against cancer-testis antigen NY-ESO-1: definition of human histocompatibility leukocyte antigen (HLA)-A2-binding peptide epitopes, *J Exp Med* 187:265, 1998.

44. Pardoll D: T cells and tumours, *Nature* 411:1010, 2001.

45. Ochsenbein AF et al: Immune surveillance against a solid tumor fails because of immunological ignorance, *Proc Natl Acad Sci USA* 96:2233, 1999.

46. Ochsenbein AF et al: Roles of tumour localization, second signals, and cross priming in cytotoxic T-cell induction, *Nature* 411:1058, 2001.

47. Onizuka S et al: Tumor rejection by in vivo administration of anti-CD25 (interleukin-2 receptor α) monoclonal antibody, *Cancer Res* 59:3128, 1999.

48. Sutmuller RP et al: Synergism of cytotoxic T lymphocyte-associated antigen 4 blockade and depletion of CD25+ regulatory T cells in antitumor therapy reveals alternative pathways for suppression of autoreactive cytotoxic T lymphocyte responses, *J Exp Med* 194:823, 2001.

49. Seo N et al: Depletion of IL-10- and TGF-β-producing regulatory γδT cells by administering a daunomycin-conjugated specific monoclonal antibody in early tumor lesions augments the activity of CTLs and NK cells, *J Immunol* 163:242, 1999.

50. Moodycliffe AM et al: Immune suppression and skin cancer development: regulation by NKT cells, *Nature Immunol* 1:521, 2000.

51. Terabe M et al: NKT cell-mediated repression of tumor immunosurveillance by IL-13 and the IL-4R-STAT6 pathway, *Nature Immunol* 1:515, 2000.

52. Liyanage UK et al: Prevalence of regulatory T cells is increased in peripheral blood and tumor microenvironment of patients with pancreas or breast carcinoma, *J Immunol* 169:2756, 2002.

53. Woo EY et al: Regulatory CD4+CD25+ T cells in tumors from patients with early-stage non-small cell lung cancer and late-stage ovarian cancer, *Cancer Res* 61:4766, 2001.

54. Gendler SJ, Mukherjee P: Spontaneous adenocarcinoma mouse models for immunotherapy, *Trends in Molec Med* 7:471, 2001.

55. Slamon DJ et al: Studies of the HER2/neu proto-oncogene in human breast and ovarian cancer, *Science* 244:707, 1989.

56. Di Fiore PP et al: ErbB-2 is a potent oncogene when overexpressed in NIH/3T3 cells, *Science* 237:178, 1987.

57. Braun S et al: ErbB-2 overexpression on occult metastatic cells in bone marrow predicts poor clinical outcome of stage I-III breast cancer patients, *Cancer Res* 61:1890, 2001.

58. Carter P et al: Humanization of an anti-p185[Her2] antibody for human cancer therapy, *Proc Natl Acad Sci USA* 89:4285, 1992.

XI

SCREENING AND DIAGNOSIS OF BREAST DISEASE

30

Examination Techniques: Roles of the Physician and Patient in Evaluating Breast Diseases

FRANCIS E. ROSATO

ERNEST L. ROSATO

Chapter Outline

- Presentation of Breast Cancer
- History
- Physical Examination
  Technique of Self-Examination

- Diagnostic Tests
  Noninvasive Tests
  Invasive Tests

Breast cancer has reached epidemiologic proportions, with approximately 10% of women who live to age 70 developing some form of the disease. Early diagnosis has been stressed with the hope of producing better outcomes. To promote earlier diagnosis there has been extensive education on breast self-examination. This has been urged by the American Cancer Society as a technique that should have positive impact on preventing breast cancer. Its efficacy has been supported in many studies, yet there has been no definitive evidence that breast self-examination has an ultimate effect on survival.[1] Screening mammography has great potential particularly in the detection of nonpalpable lesions. However, a controversy has surfaced between Canadian and American studies as to its true efficacy.[2] The Canadian study failed to show an effective impact on breast cancer mortality, whereas American studies have indicated as much as a 25% reduction in breast cancer mortality with the use of screening mammography combined with physical examination. The fact remains that if the detection of subclinical lesions is of importance, it should be reflected in a decrease in the age-adjusted mortality rate. However, this is not yet evident.[3] It is good to remember that timely diagnosis is even more difficult in women younger than age 50. Although only one third of cancers occur in this age group, two thirds of medical-legal suits related to delay in diagnosis are in the age group younger than 50 years.[4]

Presentation of Breast Cancer

According to the American College of Surgeons' recent survey of more than 17,000 cases, conducted by the Commission on Cancer, there are a variety of ways in which breast cancer comes to the forefront.[5] The most frequent mode of diagnosis is through a self-discovered mass (42%), whereas physician-discovered masses account for 24%. The American College of Surgeons' survey also shows the increasingly significant role of screening mammography in the diagnosis of breast cancer (36%), second only to self-discovered lumps. At our institution, approximately 50% of all breast biopsies are performed for lesions not detectable by any method other than mammography and require a needle-localizing technique.

Abnormalities discovered by physicians accounted for only 24% of lesions diagnosed. This statistic emphasizes the need for training in breast examination, especially by those in the primary care fields.[6-8]

Abnormalities to be noted by either the doctor or the patient include skin retraction, nipple erosion, nipple discharge, peau d'orange or edema of the breast skin, heat and redness as would be seen in an inflammatory reaction, and the presence of axillary or supraclavicular adenopathy in the absence of a breast mass—so-called occult breast cancer.[9] One can hope and even predict that with continued increased publicity, particularly as well-known national figures share their experience with this disease, there should be less delay in diagnosis. The availability of breast conservation and better physician training should help as well.

History

It is important to detail how a breast mass was discovered and how long it has been present. When a breast cancer has been present for a long time, if it has not metastasized, it usually can be viewed as favorable, even if it is locally advanced. Presumably, active immunity is confining the lesion. The symptom of pain usually is more often associated with lumpy breast syndrome than with cancer. In one series, only 0.4% of people who presented with breast pain alone will eventuate with a diagnosis of cancer.[10]

Changes in the size of a mass are likewise important to detail. Lesions that grow inexorably are more likely to be cancer than lesions that wax and wane with menstrual cycle, which usually indicates lumpy breast syndrome.

A history of nipple discharge can also be indicative of cancer. To be significant, however, the discharge should be spontaneous and not a result of forcible manual compression. The discharge is also significant if it is unilateral, is localized to a single duct, and occurs in an older patient. Discharges associated with cancer can be clear, bloody, or serous. A benign cause for discharge is indicated by bilaterality, multiductal origin, and a discharge that is usually milky, green, or greenish blue.[11] Again, when nipple discharge occurs, particularly of the type indicative of cancer and associated with a mass, 11% of such patients ultimately are proved to have breast cancer.[12] On the other hand, if nipple discharge is the sole finding and unassociated with masses or other abnormalities, less than 1% of the patients eventuate with the diagnosis of cancer.[13]

The history of cancer in a first-degree relative (mother, sister, or maternal aunt) increases the risk threefold. This factor is true only for a family history on the maternal side. Paternal history is usually not accepted as carrying a risk factor. If the first-degree relative develops bilateral breast cancer before menopause, the risk goes up sixfold to sevenfold, making prophylactic mastectomy a viable consideration in such individuals.[14] A history of breast cancer certainly requires increased vigilance in monitoring possible lesions in the remaining breast. It is estimated that approximately 15% of women with unilateral breast cancer will develop cancer in the remaining contralateral breast in their lifetime. In those who develop their first breast cancer at an early age, this percentage is even higher, and continued, close surveillance of the contralateral breast is required.[15]

The critical and oft-debated role of estrogen use is an important consideration. The use of an estrogen supplement in the postmenopausal state is under particular scrutiny. In an excellent review article, the risk of breast cancer was in fact significantly greater in those who were using estrogen alone and in those who were using combinations of estrogen and progesterone than in a similar postmenopausal group who were not undergoing hormonal replacement therapy. It is important to remember, however, that the increase is still slight. Other studies contest these findings, and in any event, one must weigh the risk against the benefits of postmenopausal estrogen replacement, particularly in terms of guarding against heart disease, stroke, osteoporosis, and even, as some suggest, colon cancer.[16] In a setting other than postmenopausal replacement, the question of the safety of estrogen as an oral contraceptive is likewise often discussed. The weight of literature suggests that the dosages used in oral contraceptives do not increase the risk of breast cancer.[17]

A history of alcohol intake is important because several recent studies support the notion that alcohol intake above a certain level may be associated with an increase in breast cancer incidence. With the consumption of as little as three to nine drinks per week, the incidence of breast cancer in one study was reported to be 1.3 times the normal rate. Consumption of more than 15 g of alcohol daily was associated with a risk factor of 1.6.[18]

Physical Examination

The American Cancer Society has outlined recommendations for the frequency of physical examinations by a physician: for women younger than 40 years, one examination every 3 years, and in women older than 40 years, one examination every year.

The technique of examination of the breast should include inspection and palpation of the entire breast and lymph node–bearing areas. The physician, standing in front of the patient, should first inspect the breasts with the patient's arms by her sides (Figure 30-1, *A*), with her arms straight up in the air (Figure 30-1, *B*), and with her hands on her hips with and without pectoral contraction (pressing in on the hips) (Figure 30-1, *C*). The general shape, size, and symmetry of the breasts should be noted, as well as any edema (peau d'orange), erythema, nipple inversion or change, and skin retraction. With the arms extended forward, the patient should then be asked to lean forward, once again to check for retraction. The node-bearing areas include the

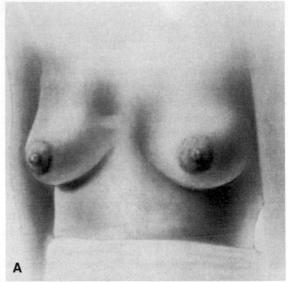

A

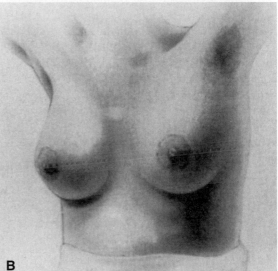

B

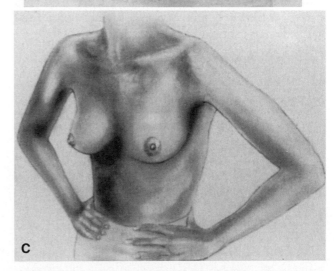

C

FIG. **30-1** Technique of inspection of the breast. Standing in front of the patient, the physician should inspect the patient with the patient's arms at the sides **(A)**, arms straight up in the air **(B)**, and hands on hips **(C)**.

cervical area (Figure 30-2, *A*), the supraclavicular and infraclavicular areas (Figure 30-2, *B*), and the axilla (Figure 30-2, *C*). Each of these regions should be palpated carefully and any adenopathy noted. Any node that is firm and larger than 5 mm in diameter should be suspect. The examination of the patient in the supine position (Figure 30-3) allows the breast to be flattened along the chest wall and thus facilitates palpation. The examiner should gently palpate the breast, making certain to examine the entire breast from the sternum to the clavicle, posteriorly to the latissimus, and inferiorly to the rectus sheath. Particular care should be given to following the extension of breast tissue into the axilla, the so-called axillary tail of Spence. Baby powder may aid the examining fingers to glide over the breast without friction from the patient's skin. The examination is performed with the palmar fingers flat, never grasping or pinching. The breast can also be molded or cupped in the examiner's hand, once again to check for retraction. The nipple/areola complex should be inspected carefully for subtle changes in the epithelium, retroareolar masses, and nipple discharge.

An accurate record of any significant physical findings should be documented carefully. Many physicians use a written description incorporated in the progress notes. A diagram or photograph may be more objective and accurate in relating the findings. Photographs may be useful in following the progression or regression of advanced lesions that have skin changes that are difficult to describe. Diagrams (Figure 30-4, *A* and *B*) are useful to record the location of a mass or nodularity. We prefer to localize masses or other abnormalities by superimposing the radials of a clock on the breast and detailing location along a specific radial in centimeters from the areolar margin (Figure 30-4, *C*). The size, shape, consistency, mobility, and delineation of any palpable mass should be noted.

TECHNIQUE OF SELF-EXAMINATION

Breast self-examination is a three-step method: (1) inspection in front of a mirror with the arms by the sides, straight up in the air overhead, and on the hips, looking for changes in contour, skin color or texture, and nipple changes; (2) palpation in the shower; and (3) palpation in the supine position on a couch or a bed.

Palpation can be performed in several directions: horizontal or vertical (Figure 30-5, *A* and *B*), radial (Figure 30-5, *C* and *D*), or circular (Figure 30-5, *E* and *F*). A study designed to evaluate the relative effectiveness of these three patterns determined that the vertical pattern was the most thorough in examining breast tissue. Patients also need to be taught to discern a lump from "lumpiness."

Patients should start breast self-examination in their late twenties to early thirties and continue for the rest

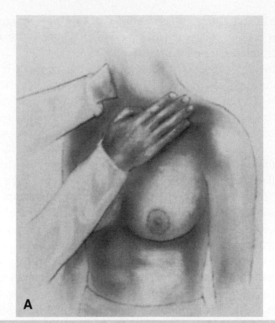

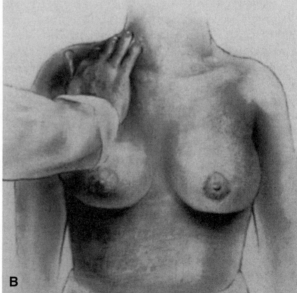

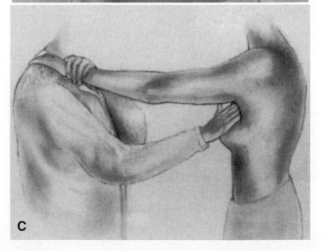

FIG. **30-2** Technique of palpating the cervical area **(A)**, supraclavicular and infraclavicular areas **(B)**, and axilla **(C)**.

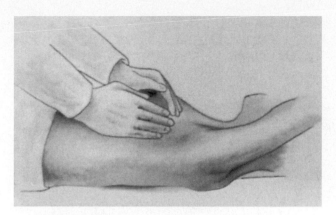

F I G. **30-3** Palpation of the breast with the patient in the supine position.

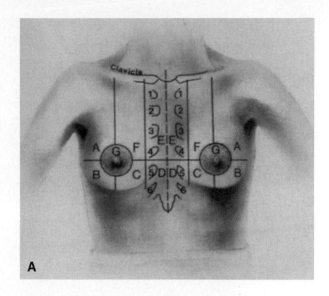

A

of their lives. The self-examination is best performed 5 to 10 days after the onset of menses. Postmenopausal women should be instructed to do the examination on the same day of every month.

Despite all of the publicity about breast cancer and education about breast self-examination, only one fourth of women routinely perform breast self-examination. There is a need to disseminate information to increase the participation of patients. There does seem to be a positive effect on survival for tumors discovered by breast self-examination. Most probably, this is related to the fact that the disease is discovered at an earlier stage in patients performing routine examination.[19,20]

Diagnostic Tests

Having completed the history and physical examination, several noninvasive and invasive tests are available for further evaluation of any suspected disease.

NONINVASIVE TESTS

Mammography. Mammography using a low-dose film/screen technique delivers a dose as low as 0.1 rad per study.[21,22] By comparison, a chest x-ray study delivers 0.025 rad per study. Based on the observation that women exposed to large doses of radiation could develop breast cancers, investigators speculated as to the risk associated with mammography. There have been no cases reported of breast cancer developing as a consequence of screening mammography, and the benefit of detecting a small cancer, which is often curable with current therapeutic modalities, far outweighs any theoretical risk.[23,24] According to Feig[24]:

This risk estimate of 3.5 cancers per million women per year per rad means that if one million women aged 30 or older each received a mean breast dose of one rad there would, after a

BREAST DIAGRAM

PATIENT :_____   DATE :_____

AGE :_____   MED REC NO :_____

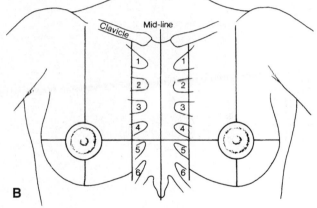

B

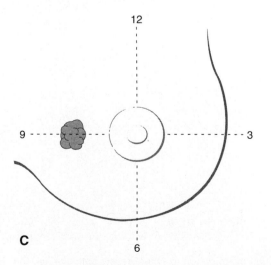

C

F I G. **30-4 A** and **B,** Diagrams of the breast to record location of a mass or nodulation. **C,** Mass noted along 9 o'clock radial right breast 3 cm from areolar edge.

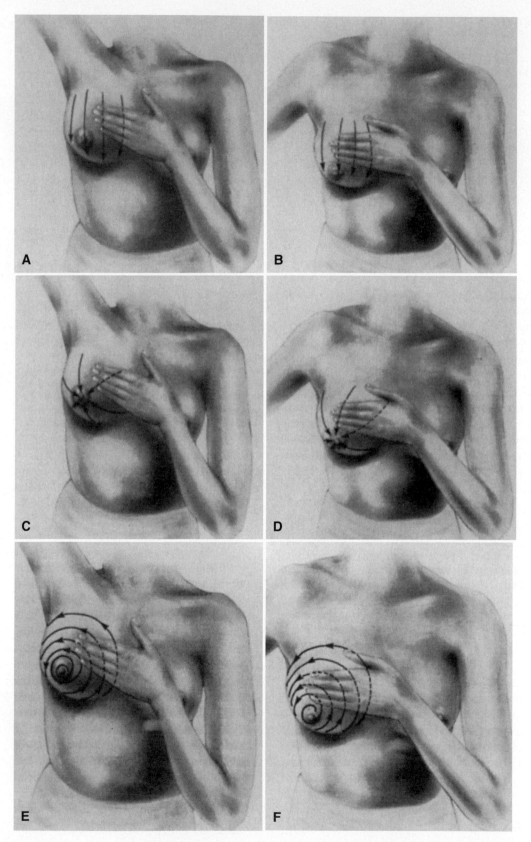

FIG. **30-5** Self-examination of the breast; palpation in the vertical or horizontal (**A** and **B**), radial (**C** and **D**), and circular directions (**E** and **F**).

minimal latent period of ten years, be an excess incidence of 3.5 cancers each year in the population. Examination with current low-dose technique (mean breast dose of 0.3 rad for a two view study) would carry a hypothetical risk of about one excess cancer case per year per million women examined. If there were a 50% breast cancer mortality, the hypothetical risk would be one excess death per two million women examined. This level of risk (hypothetical), one death per two million women per year, is extremely small and can be equated with the following: 200 miles travelled by air, 30 miles travelled by car, smoking one half of one cigarette, 3/4 of a minute of mountain climbing, and ten minutes of being a man aged 60.

Despite the fact that most physicians agree that mammography is an effective screening tool, only 8% to 15% of asymptomatic women have this study as part of a routine annual evaluation. In fact, only 15% to 20% of women older than 50 have ever had a mammogram.[25] Data from the Health Insurance Plan and Breast Cancer Detection Demonstration Project studies suggest that mammography (with physical examination) was effective in diagnosing nonpalpable lesions, with a survival advantage resulting from the earlier stage at detection.[25-27]

There are indications for mammography in both a screening and diagnostic setting. Patients with tumors or areas of asymmetry, nipple discharge, skin retraction, or axillary adenopathy should be evaluated with mammography. The study is not very useful in the teenage group because of the density of the breast but is indicated if a malignant process is suspected. The false-negative rate is about 10% to 15%. Therefore the physician must be vigilant while performing the physical examination and not make a therapeutic decision based entirely on a negative mammogram.

All patients with a personal history of lobular neoplasia or carcinoma of the breast, a family history of carcinoma of the breast, intraductal papillomatosis, or gross cystic disease should receive a mammogram at regular intervals. In addition, the American Cancer Society and American College of Radiology have outlined recommendations regarding screening mammography for asymptomatic women: For women 40 to 49 years of age, studies should be obtained every 12 to 24 months; for those older than 50, annual mammography is recommended. The National Institutes of Health recommends that these guidelines be applied to women younger than 50 years who are in high-risk groups (i.e., those with personal or family histories of breast carcinoma).

Mammographic abnormalities that warrant further evaluation include masses, microcalcifications,[28] stellate densities or architectural distortion, and a "changing mammogram."[29] Biopsy specimens of these suspicious findings reveal carcinoma in 20% to 30% of cases, depending on the institution.[30-32]

Ultrasound. Ultrasound has been used since the early 1950s. It is most helpful and accurate[33,34] in the evaluation of the dense breast and in differentiating between cystic and solid masses.[35] Unfortunately, masses that are smaller than 5 to 10 mm may not be visualized, and masses in fatty breasts are also difficult to visualize. Its advantages are that there is no radiation, and it is essentially painless. Thermography and transillumination, previously evaluated, are not effective and no longer in use.

Computed Tomography and Magnetic Resonance Imaging Scans. The use of computed tomography (CT) and magnetic resonance imaging (MRI) scanning for the evaluation of breast disease is now being investigated. These techniques may play a role in evaluating the axilla, mediastinum, and supraclavicular areas for adenopathy and may aid in clinical staging of malignant processes.[36]

Recent publications claim that MRI can correctly identify residual or primary cancer and accurately predict the extent of cancer in nearly all patients undergoing this study. It was hoped by some that it could be a valuable tool in giving the most precise preoperative information as to extent of disease in patients with a known diagnosis of breast cancer.[37] At our own institution, we found MRI with gadolinium to be particularly helpful in resolving the nature of a suspected breast mass, which is still of uncertain nature after both mammography and ultrasound and, in addition, have found it to be of help in individuals presenting with axillary metastases and negative breast imaging studies, in which MRI has been the only modality to identify the primary lesion in what would otherwise be considered "occult breast cancer."

INVASIVE TESTS

Aspiration Cytology. Aspiration cytology involves the use of a fine needle (20 gauge or smaller) with a syringe to aspirate cells from a suspicious area, smearing cells on a glass slide, fixing them immediately to prevent air drying, and then staining for cytologic evaluation. If specimens are obtained correctly, this procedure is extremely accurate (see Chapter 37 for a comprehensive review of fine needle aspiration cytopathology techniques and results). However, specific histologic diagnosis may be impossible because of the inability to maintain architectural patterns with aspiration. Stereotactic techniques for sampling nonpalpable lesions have been described and are commonly used in the United States.[38-40] A limitation to this technique is the inability to determine accurately estrogen and progesterone receptors on a specimen of such small size. Methods of determining receptor status on these specimens are being developed but are not uniformly available in surgical pathology laboratories.[41,42]

There has been a growing interest in the noninvasive variant for breast cytology, which uses a suction device, placed over the nipple areolar complex, to obtain fluid for cytopathologic evaluation. In addition, such aspirated breast fluid can be analyzed for tumor markers. Prostate-specific antigen, in particular, has been of early interest because it correlates better with the diagnosis in those with breast cancer, and in those at increased risk, it helps quantitate the level of that risk.[43]

Core Needle Biopsy. Needle biopsies using large-bore needles are often performed. They are more invasive than needle aspiration. They are more accurate and can be used for receptor determinations. These biopsies can also be done stereotactically or with ultrasound guidance.[44]

Open Biopsy

Excisional Biopsy. Excisional biopsy refers to removal of all gross evidence of disease, usually with a small rim of normal breast tissue. It is important to plan all incisions carefully in case there is a need for subsequent surgical procedures should the lesion be malignant. Generally, it is preferable to use a circumareolar (incision G) or curvilinear incision (incision A through I) along Langer's lines (Figure 30-6). Most biopsies can be performed with local anesthesia, usually with intravenous sedation, on an outpatient basis with good patient acceptance and comfort. Frozen section may be performed, and a portion of

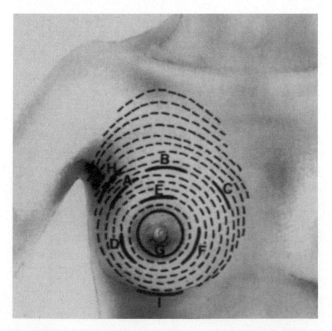

F I G. **30-6** Excisional biopsy using a circumareolar *(G)* or curvilinear *(A to I)* incision parallel to Langer's lines.

the specimen can then be preserved for estrogen and progesterone receptor tests.

Incisional Biopsy. For larger lesions not amenable to excisional biopsy, an incisional biopsy should be performed. This can also be performed under local anesthesia and on an outpatient basis without discomfort for the patient. Similar considerations for subsequent surgical procedures should be made when planning the incision. Usually 1 ml of tumor is required for receptor determination.

Needle-Guided Biopsy. Screening mammography is responsible for locating many suspicious lesions before they are clinically apparent. The technique of needle localization was developed to permit biopsies to be performed by precisely removing the lesion without sacrificing normal surrounding breast tissue. The patient is taken to the mammography unit, where, based on the original films, a needle is introduced into the breast and directed toward the lesion. Repeat mammography is then performed with the needle secured to confirm the proximity of the needle to the suspicious area. The needle can be left in place or replaced with a variety of hook wires,[31,32,45-47] and the patient is sent to the operating room.

The surgeon then performs a biopsy of the area localized by the needle. The specimen should then be radiographed to confirm the presence of the abnormality. If the specimen does not contain the lesion, additional pieces of tissue should be submitted until the lesion has been removed (see Chapter 38). In our experience, 26% of needle-guided biopsies performed for microcalcifications proved to contain cancerous specimens, whereas 13% performed for nonpalpable soft tissue densities were found to contain cancerous specimens. Most cases (76%) were stage I.

Ultrasound-Guided Biopsy. For lesions that are nonpalpable but are visualized on ultrasound evaluation, ultrasound-guided biopsy may be used intraoperatively for localization. With the patient in the supine position, the breast is scanned using a handheld transducer. The skin overlying the lesion is marked with a marking pencil; the biopsy is then performed in the standard fashion. Covered by a sterile sheath, the transducer can also be used in the operating room to aid the surgeon in locating the lesion and to confirm that the area has been excised by rescanning the area after the specimen has been removed. Cyst aspiration can also be performed under ultrasound guidance.[35]

Nipple Discharge Smear. After eliciting nipple discharge, the secretions can be smeared on a glass slide, fixed, and submitted for cytologic evaluation. Reportedly, cytology has a false-negative rate of 18% and a false-positive rate of 2.5%, so care must be exercised in interpreting these results.[11]

Nipple Biopsy. Changes in the epithelium of the nipple, often associated with itching or nipple discharge, often warrant nipple biopsy. A wedge of the nipple/areola complex can be excised under local anesthesia, with the edges reapproximated with minimal deformity.

Galactography. Injection of contrast into one of the ducts through the orifice at the areola may demonstrate ductal ectasia, obstruction, or a filling defect. This test is rarely used because it is time consuming and often painful and also requires a repeat mammogram after the injection.

Breast ductoscopy is in the earliest stages of development. This allows direct visualization of the duct epithelium and biopsy or brush cytology when indicated. It is too soon to tell if it will have a future role.

Pneumocystography. Pneumocystography, or injection of air into a cyst cavity after aspiration of the cyst, is another test that is rarely, if ever, used.

REFERENCES

1. Harris JR et al: Breast cancer, *N Engl J Med* 327:319, 1992.
2. Courteau JP, Bouchard F: Canadian National Breast Screening Study, *Can Med Assoc J* 148:875, 1993.
3. Mittra I: Breast screening: the case for physical examination without mammography, *Lancet* 343:342, 1994.
4. Lannin DR et al: Difficulties in diagnosis of carcinoma of the breast in patients less than fifty years of age, *Surg Gynecol Obstet* 177:457, 1993.
5. Osteen RT et al: Breast cancer survey, *J Am Coll Surg* 178:213, 1994.
6. Campbell HS et al: Improving physicians' and nurses' clinical breast examination: a randomized controlled trial, *Am J Prev Med* 7:1, 1991.
7. Pilgrim C et al: Improving clinical breast examination training in a medical school: a randomized controlled trial, *J Gen Intern Med* 8:685, 1993.
8. Wiecha JM, Gann P: Provider confidence in breast examination, *Fam Pract Res J* 13:37, 1993.
9. Bays JK: Physical and mammographic diagnosis of breast cancer and initial workup, *J Am Med Wom Assoc* 47:158, 1992.
10. Gadd NA, Souba WW: Evaluation and treatment of benign breast disorders. In Bland KI, Copeland EM (eds): *The breast: comprehensive management of benign and malignant diseases,* ed 2, Philadelphia, 1998, WB Saunders.
11. Leis HP: Management of nipple discharge, *World J Surg* 13:736, 1989.
12. Morrow M: Nipple discharge. In Harris JR et al (eds): *Breast diseases,* ed 2, Philadelphia, 1991, JB Lippincott.
13. Chaudary MA et al: Nipple discharge: the diagnostic value of testing for occult blood, *Ann Surg* 196:651, 1982.
14. Sattin RW et al, and the Cancer and Steroid Hormone Study: Family history and the risk of breast cancer, *JAMA* 253:1908, 1985.
15. Wanebo HJ et al: Bilateral breast cancer: risk reduction by contralateral biopsy, *Ann Surg* 201:667, 1985.
16. Colditz GA et al: The use of estrogens and progestins and the risk of breast cancer in postmenopausal women, *N Engl J Med* 332:1589, 1995.
17. Cancer and Steroid Hormone Study of the Centers for Disease Control and the National Institute of Child Health and Human Development, *N Engl J Med* 315:405, 1986.
18. Willett WC et al: Moderate alcohol consumption and the risk of breast cancer, *N Engl J Med* 316:1174, 1987.
19. Foster RS et al: Breast self-examination practices and breast cancer stage, *N Engl J Med* 299:265, 1978.
20. Foster RS, Costanza MC: Breast self-examination practices and breast cancer survival, *Cancer* 53:999, 1984.
21. Dodd GD: Mammography, state of the art, *Cancer* 39:2796, 1977.
22. National Council on Radiation Precaution and Measurements: *Mammography: a user's guide,* Bethesda, MD, 1986.
23. Feig SA: Assessment of the hypothetical risk from mammography and evaluation of the potential benefit, *Radiol Clin North Am* 21:173, 1983.
24. Feig SA: Radiation risk from mammography: Is it clinically significant? *AJR Am J Roentgenol* 143:469, 1984.
25. Howard J: Using mammography for cancer control: an unrealized potential, *Cancer* 37:33, 1987.
26. Baker LH: Breast cancer detection demonstration project: a five year summary report, *Cancer* 32:194, 1982.
27. Strax P, Venet L, Shapiro S: Value of mammography in reduction of mortality from breast cancer in mass screening, *AJR Am J Roentgenol* 117:686, 1973.
28. Sickles EA: Breast calcifications: mammographic evaluation, *Radiology* 160:289, 1986.
29. Wilhelm MC: The changing mammogram: a primary indication for needle localization biopsy, *Arch Surg* 121:1311, 1986.
30. Landercasper J et al: Needle localization and biopsy of nonpalpable lesions of the breast, *Surg Gynecol Obstet* 162:399, 1987.
31. Marrujo G, Jolly PC, Hall MH: Nonpalpable breast cancer: needle-localized biopsy for diagnosis and considerations for treatment, *Am J Surg* 151:599, 1986.
32. Rosenberg AL et al: Clinically occult breast lesions: localization and significance, *Radiology* 162:167, 1987.
33. Cole-Beuglet C et al: Ultrasound mammography: a comparison with radiographic mammography, *Radiology* 139:693, 1981.
34. Piccoli CW: Current utilization and future techniques of breast ultrasound, *Curr Opin Radiol* 4:39, 1992.
35. Pearce RB: Ultrasound, a useful adjunct to breast mammography, *Diagn Imaging* 114, 1986.
36. Boetes C et al: Breast tumors: comparative accuracy of MR imaging relative to mammography and ultrasound for demonstrating extent, *Radiology* 197:743, 1995.
37. Esserman L et al: Utility of magnetic resonance imaging in the management of breast cancer: evidence for improved preoperative staging, *J Clin Oncol* 17:110, 1999.
38. Gent HJ: Stereotaxic needle localization and cytological diagnosis of occult breast lesions, *Ann Surg* 204:580, 1986.
39. Nordenstrom B, Azjicek J: Stereotaxic needle biopsy and preoperative indications of nonpalpable mammary lesions, *Acta Cytol* 21:350, 1977.
40. Svane G: Stereotaxic needle biopsy of nonpalpable breast lesions: a clinical and radiological followup, *Acta Radiol (Diagn)* 24:385, 1983.

41. Silversward C, Humla SA: Estrogen receptor analysis on needle aspirates from human mammary cancer, *Acta Cytol* 24:54, 1980.

42. Silversward C et al: Estrogen receptors: analysis on fine needle aspirates and on histologic biopsies from human breast cancer, *Eur J Cancer* 16:1351, 1980.

43. Sauter E et al: Prostate-specific antigen levels in nipple aspirate fluid correlate with breast cancer risk, *Cancer Epidemiol Biomarkers Prev* 5:967, 1996.

44. Parker SH et al: Percutaneous large bore breast biopsy: a multi-institutional study, *Radiology* 193:359, 1994.

45. Herman G et al: Percutaneous localization of nonpalpable breast lesions, *Dis Breast* 9:4, 1983.

46. Kalisher L: An improved needle for localization of nonpalpable breast lesions, *Radiology* 128:815, 1978.

47. Kopans DB et al: A modified needle-hookwire to simplify preoperative localization of occult breast lesions, *Radiology* 134:781, 1980.

CHAPTER

31

Breast Imaging

LAWRENCE W. BASSETT

MARK SHIROISHI

Chapter Outline

Breast imaging includes all of the diagnostic imaging methods used to detect and diagnose diseases of the breast. The most commonly used breast imaging procedure is *mammography,* defined as an x-ray examination of the breasts. Since the first report on mammography in the United States in the 1930s, mammography has undergone striking technological improvements that have improved its sensitivity and accuracy.[1] Quality assurance procedures have also improved mammography in the United States.[2] In addition, standardized reporting has been developed to improve the communication of the results of mammography and appropriate management recommendations.[3]

The two major types of mammography are screening mammography and diagnostic mammography. *Screening mammography* is used to detect unexpected breast cancer in asymptomatic women. *Diagnostic mammography* is used to evaluate the breasts of patients with symptoms, such as a lump or nipple discharge. Mammography is also used to guide interventional procedures of the breast, including prebiopsy needle localization, needle aspiration, core needle biopsy (CNB), and ductography.[4-8]

Ultrasonography, the use of sonic energy to produce an image of the breast, is the next most commonly used modality for diagnostic imaging of the breast. In the past, the use of ultrasonography has primarily been restricted to differentiating benign from solid masses.[9] However, ultrasonography is increasingly being used to guide fine-needle aspiration, CNB, and prebiopsy needle localization of suspicious-looking solid masses.[4,10] In addition, criteria for the differentiation of benign and malignant solid masses by high-resolution ultrasonography are under investigation.[11]

Other modalities with potential usefulness in the diagnosis of breast diseases include digital mammography, magnetic resonance imaging (MRI), and radionuclide imaging. Diagnostic imaging also has a role in identifying or documenting metastases to other organs in appropriate patients with breast cancer.

Mammography

SCREENING MAMMOGRAPHY: GUIDELINES AND CONTROVERSIES

Breast cancer is the most common noncutaneous malignancy in women and, in recent years, has accounted for 30% of new cancer cases in American women.[12] Each year, approximately 185,000 new cases of breast cancer are diagnosed and about 45,000 women will die of this disease.[13] The risk of developing breast cancer increases with age, with women older than age 40 being at greatest risk. Although multiple risk factors have been identified, three fourths of women who develop the disease

have no special risk factors other than increasing age.[14] The benefit of screening mammography for women older than 50 years is universally accepted.[15,16] Breast cancer death rates from 1989 to 1998 have fallen in every age and racial group of women, and this is largely attributable to mammographic screening.[17]

In randomized controlled trials, noncompliance in the study group and contamination in the control group are necessary tradeoffs to avoid self-selection and length-bias sampling. However, this results in dilution of the data and an underestimation of the real benefit of screening. In 2001 Tabar and colleagues[18] reported that for women aged 40 to 69, a 63% reduction in breast carcinoma mortality was found among women who *actually underwent* screening mammography, far greater than that previously noted by others.[19,20] Even after correcting for possible selection bias, a 50% mortality reduction was found. In these screened women, cancers were detected at a considerably earlier stage compared with those who did not undergo screening. Therefore screening mammography has the potential to reduce breast cancer mortality by at least 50% and perhaps even more.

Recently, it has been proposed that reductions in breast cancer mortality after the introduction of screening are primarily related to improvements in therapeutic modalities.[21,22] It has been suggested that only one third of the recent reduction in breast cancer mortality in the United Kingdom is due to screening mammography, with the balance attributable to advances in therapy.[19] However, Tabar and colleagues[18] counter that if this were true, then a similar decrease in mortality should be seen in those who did not undergo screening mammography. This was not seen, and Tabar and co-workers go on to claim that up to 70% of the mortality reduction seen was due to screening. Regardless of the exact percentage of contribution, there is no question that screening mammography leads to the detection of smaller cancers and decreased mortality.

SCREENING FOR WOMEN 40 TO 49 YEARS OLD

In 1989 consensus guidelines put forth by the American Cancer Society, the National Cancer Institute (NCI), and 11 other major medical organizations recommended mammographic screening every 1 to 2 years for women aged 40 to 49 and yearly for those older than 50.

Since 1975 some have questioned the efficacy of screening for women 40 to 49 years.[23] Although breast cancer is the leading cause of death for these younger women, it has been argued that screening should begin at age 50 because only 16% of all breast cancers occur in women younger than 50.[24] However, almost 20% of all deaths attributed to breast cancer and 34% of all expected years of life lost to breast cancer involve women 40 to 49 years.[25] Cancers occurring in this younger population of women tend to be faster growing, and the breasts tend to be denser, making tumor detection, especially detection of noncalcified ones, difficult.[26]

The Health Insurance Plan (HIP) study was the first randomized controlled trial to provide scientific evidence of the potential of screening mammography to reduce mortality. Among women 50 years and older, a decreased breast cancer mortality was evident by 4 years after entry. For women 40 to 49 years, a decreased mortality was seen 7 years after entry. At 18 years of follow-up, a mortality reduction of nearly 25% was found in each group.[25,27]

Although the HIP study seems to demonstrate the benefit of screening for women 40 to 49 years old, there may be reason to question the validity of its results.[28] First, a longer period of follow-up was necessary to detect a mortality reduction in women 40 to 49 years, implying that some of the benefit of screening may have occurred when these women were in their fifties. On the other hand, there are several explanations why a delayed demonstration of mortality reduction occurred in these women.[29] First, breast cancer incidence and mortality rates are lower in women 40 to 49 years than in women 50 and older. Second, the sensitivity of mammography appears to be lower in younger women. Third, the higher rates of ductal carcinoma in situ (DCIS) in women aged 40 to 49 and the slow progression of it to invasive carcinoma require a longer time to manifest a mortality difference. Another frequent criticism of the HIP study involved the use of both physical examination and mammography, thus making it difficult to determine the relative contribution of each to mortality reduction.[28] Since the HIP trial, there have been six (or seven if the Swedish Two-County trial is counted as two separate studies) other randomized controlled trials (Table 31-1) that included women aged 40 to 49 years, with four demonstrating mortality reductions of 22% to 44%.[30] Although the Stockholm trial resulted in a relative risk of 1.08 for women 40 to 49 years at 11.4 years of follow-up, it should be noted that it used only one-view mammography, had a 28-month screening interval, and had only two screening rounds. The Canadian National Breast Screening Study-1 (NBSS-1) showed a relative risk of 1.14 at 10.5 years of follow-up; however, many questionable aspects of its design have made its data interpretation difficult, as is discussed in detail later in this chapter.

None of randomized controlled trials alone included enough women of this age group to provide statistical significance. Despite this, the aforementioned results suggest a likely benefit of mammographic screening for younger women if proper mammographic technique is used and screening intervals are appropriate.[31] With the exception of the NBSS-1, all of these studies were designed to include a wide range of ages and have been retrospectively stratified and analyzed by age subgroups. Major deficiencies limiting mortality reduction are readily apparent in each of these studies, particularly in the 40- to 49-year-old group.[32,33] These included biennial rather than annual screening (tumor growth rates are faster in younger women), use of single-view mammography, insufficient recall rates, excessively high thresholds for recommending biopsy, poor-quality mammography, inappropriately short follow-up intervals, noncompliance of some study group women, and control group contamination (obtaining mammography outside of study).

In 1992 the NBSS-1 seemed to demonstrate that, at 7 years of follow-up, there was no benefit for screening in women aged 40 to 49.[34] In 1993 Elwood, Cox, and Richardson[35] performed the first meta-analysis of these

| TABLE 31-1 | Selected Details of Randomized Controlled Trials of Breast Cancer Screening in Women 40 to 49 Years Old |

RANDOMIZED CONTROLLED TRIAL	START DATE	SCREENING MODALITY*	SCREENING INTERVAL (mo)	NO. OF ROUNDS	RELATIVE RISK (95% CI)	FOLLOW-UP (yr)
Health Insurance Plan	1963	2-view MM + CBE	12	4	$0.77^{0.53\text{-}1.1}$	18
Malmo	1976	2/1-view MM	18-24	6	$0.64^{0.45\text{-}0.8}$	10-15.5†
Swedish Two-County	1977	1-view MM	24	5-6	$0.87^{0.54\text{-}1.4}$	13
Edinburgh	1979	2/1-view MM + CBE	24	4	$0.78^{0.46\text{-}1.3}$	10-14‡
Canada: NBSS-1§	1980	2-view MM + CBE	12	5	$1.14^{0.83\text{-}1.5}$	10.5
Stockholm	1981	1-view MM	28	2	$1.08^{0.54\text{-}2.1}$	11.4
Gothenburg	1982	2/1-view MM	18	5	$0.56^{0.32\text{-}0.9}$	11

Modified from Sirovich BE, Sox, HC Jr: *Surg Clin North Am* 79:961, 1999.

CBE, Clinical breast examination; *CI*, confidence interval; *NBSS*, National Breast Screening Study.

*1-view MM, One-view mammography; 2-view MM, two-view mammography; 2/1-view, two views performed on the first screen, with one view on subsequent examinations.

†The Malmo trial consisted of two cohorts with follow-up periods of 10 and 15.5 years at the time of the 1997 publication.

‡The Edinburgh trial contained three cohorts with follow-up periods of 10, 12, and 14 years at the time of the 1997 publication.

§Study design consisted of randomization of volunteers after clinical breast examination.

trials and found no benefit for women 40 to 49 years. However, when this study was published, follow-up was inadequate and evidence of benefit was just beginning to emerge. In addition to the use of old data, the lack of statistical power was largely ignored in this analysis.[28,36] Although the American Cancer Society resisted making any changes to screening recommendations pending further study, these findings set the stage for the NCI to recommend against screening for this age group.[15,37]

In 1993 a meta-analysis of the major randomized controlled trials published by the NCI's International Workshop on Screening for Breast Cancer concluded that there was no benefit from screening for women aged 40 to 49 after 5 to 7 years of follow-up and only marginal benefit 10 to 12 years after entry.[15] Although more recent follow-up data from six of the eight trials and inferential data from nonrandomized controlled trials were available, these were either not included or discounted.[29,36]

The Canadian NBSS-1 trial was the only trial specifically designed to study screening in women aged 40 to 49. However, advocates of screening assert that it contained several design flaws that made its data difficult to compare with those of the other seven randomized controlled trials.[29] First, selection bias was likely given the completely volunteer nature of their study and control groups. This is in contrast to the inclusion of all women in a defined population from the other trials. Second, there were higher-than-expected rates of breast cancers in both the study and control groups of the NBSS-1.[34] The observed to expected cancers in the first year of screening was 3.2 in the study group and 2.6 in the control group. Third, the NBSS-1 was unique in that it prescreened both study and control patients with a physical examination before randomization. This led to the randomization of more advanced breast cancers in both the study and control group. Furthermore, assignment bias seems likely given the fact that the rate of advanced cancers (four or more positive nodes) was 3.8 times higher in the study group than in the control group.[34] In addition, several experts, some of whom were consultants to the study, complained that the mammographic technique used in the Canadian study was unsatisfactory.[38] In fact, several consultants refused to continue to participate because of concerns about image quality. During the first 5 years of the 8-year study, mediolateral oblique projections were not used. In Vancouver, where NBSS screening began in 1983, a 1972 mammography machine was used until 1987. External radiologic review from 1980 to 1985 found that 49% to 75% of mammograms were considered satisfactory.[39]

Since 1993, multiple meta-analyses of the eight randomized controlled trials have been performed, each demonstrating further effectiveness of screening mammography for women 40 to 49 years. Excluding data from the NBSS-1 trial, Smart and co-workers,[29]

in 1995, demonstrated a statistically significant 23% mortality reduction for women aged 40 to 49 years.

One area of contention surrounding interpretation of data from the trials of screening mammography involves the exact definition of each age group. Two alternatives are at odds with each other: age at entry versus age at diagnosis.[28] Age at entry appears to be the appropriate measure because more cancers are diagnosed at an earlier age with screening. Thus, if age at diagnosis is used as a basis for subgroup assignment, relatively more cases of cancer will be seen in the screening group for the youngest women and therefore more will be at risk for death related to breast cancer.[40] For women 40 to 49 years, how much of the reduction in mortality was due to cancers detected after age 50? According to Tabar, Duffy, and Chen,[41] for women aged 40 to 49 in the Swedish Two-County Trial, 64% of all breast cancer diagnoses and 67% of all cancer deaths occurred before they reached age 50.

In 1996 results of a nonrandomized, population-based study in Uppsala, Sweden, supported the screening of women younger than 50.[40] Although actual mortality rate reduction data were not used, this program found 7-year survival rates of 92% and 87% for cancers detected both at screening and between screening in women younger than 50 and those older than 50, respectively. This can be compared with the 7-year survival rate for breast cancer patients in the general Swedish population of 70%.

As previously mentioned, there has been no single randomized controlled trial that has included enough women between 40 and 49 years to definitively demonstrate a benefit from mammographic screening.[31] Feig[28] has postulated that the Uppsala program could have provided proof of benefit of screening if it had been conducted as a randomized controlled trial. However, this would have required the inclusion of many more women.

The Breast Cancer Detection Demonstration Project (BCDDP) was the largest mammographic screening study of women aged 40 to 49. Although it was not a randomized controlled trial either, it demonstrated results consistent with the Uppsala findings. No difference in survival rates for cancers detected at screening only was found for women 40 to 49 years compared with women 50 to 59 and 60 to 69 years. At 14-year follow-up, survival rates of 85%, 83%, and 84% were found for women aged 40 to 49, 50 to 59, and 60 to 69 years, respectively.[28,42]

In 1996 a meta-analysis of randomized trials presented in Falun, Sweden, demonstrated a 24% decrease in mortality rate from screening in women aged 40 to 49 years.[43] It has been estimated that the actual mortality decrease can be as high as 35% if two-view mammography, double reading, and state-of-the-art technique are used.[32]

In 1997 a meta-analysis of the eight randomized controlled trials presented at the National Institutes of Health (NIH) Consensus Development Conference showed a statistically significant 18% mortality reduction at 10.5 to 18 years of follow-up.[44] When the five Swedish trials alone were examined with follow-up data, a statistically significant 29% mortality reduction was evident. However, despite these findings, the panel concluded that there was insufficient evidence to support a recommendation for universal screening mammograms in women 40 to 49 years. This was based largely on their finding that some studies found lower mortality from breast cancer in screened women after 10 years while others did not. In addition, the committee cited potential harm from false-negative and false-positive readings, potential for adverse psychosocial consequences from abnormal mammograms, and potential risk from radiation exposure.[45] Responding to pressure from the Senate subcommittee overseeing its funding, the NCI reversed the NIH's initial recommendations and supported screening mammography every 1 to 2 years for younger women at average risk.[30,46] The more frequent occurrence of interval cancers among women younger than 50 has led some to advocate semiannual screening of this population.[40,47]

Public perception of the mammographic debate differs from that seen in academia. A recent survey of women found that most favored beginning mammographic screening *before* the age of 40 and only 5% believed that a first mammogram should be obtained at age 50 or older.[48] Many believed that cost and not a question of benefit was the central issue in this controversy.

In 1999 the 16-year follow-up of the UK Trial of Early Detection of Breast Cancer demonstrated a 27% decreased breast cancer mortality in women aged 45 to 64 years, with no evidence of less benefit in women aged 45 to 46 years at the start of screening.[49] These data supported evidence from the Edinburgh randomized trials, which, at 14-years of follow-up, showed a mortality reduction of 21% as a result of screening mammography for women 45 to 49 years.[50] In 2000 a Japanese study demonstrated the superior effectiveness of screening mammography to detect a high proportion of stage I cancers and absence of nodal involvement in younger women.[51]

Current screening guidelines vary by location.[30] Most European nations continue to screen only women older than age 50. However, in the United States, there is considerable overlap and disagreement among various organizations (Table 31-2). Undoubtedly, controversy over the efficacy of mammographic screening will remain, and likewise, screening guidelines will be altered.

By 2015, the American Cancer Society has proposed goals that include a 50% reduction in cancer mortality and a 25% reduction in cancer incidence.[52] If 90% of

---

TABLE 31-2 Breast Cancer Screening Guidelines of Selected Professional Groups

ORGANIZATION OR COUNTRY	AGES 40-49	AGES 50-69	UPPER AGE LIMIT
American Cancer Society	MM yearly CBE yearly BSE monthly	MM yearly CBE yearly BSE monthly	No upper age limit; consider health status and comorbidity
American College of Physicians	MM based on individual informed decision CBE yearly	MM every 1-2 yr CBE yearly	No upper limit specified
National Cancer Institute	MM every 1-2 yr CBE yearly BSE monthly	MM every 1-2 yr CBE yearly BSE monthly	Continue screening unless otherwise indicated by health status
U.S. Preventive Services Task Force (USPSTF)*	MM—(C) CBE—(C) BSE—(C)	MM every 1-2 yr—(A) CBE—(C) BSE—(C)	MM/CBE—(C); however, may be reasonable to screen women with a reasonable life expectancy
Canada	MM yearly—1 province CBE yearly—1 province	MM every 2 yr—4 provinces CBE every 2 yr—4 provinces	Through age 69
Sweden	MM every 18 mo—50% of counties	MM every 2 yr—all counties	Through age 74
United Kingdom	—	MM every 3 yr	Through age 64

Modified from Sirovich BE, Sox HC Jr: *Surg Clin North Am* 79:961, 1999.

BSE, Breast self-examination; *CBE,* clinical breast examination; *MM,* mammography.

*The strength of the USPSTF recommendations is abbreviated with the letter of the rating in parentheses.

A: There is good evidence to support the recommendation that the condition be specifically considered in a periodic health examination.

B: There is fair evidence to support the recommendation that the condition be specifically considered in a periodic health examination.

C: There is insufficient evidence to recommend for or against the inclusion of the condition in a periodic health examination, but recommendations may be made on other grounds.

women older than age 40 are screened, it is theorized that these goals can be achieved for breast cancer as early as 2008.[53] It is imperative that a national initiative to screen women of all socioeconomic groups become a public health priority.

PERFORMING THE EXAMINATION

To have the greatest possible impact, screening mammography must be widely used. Therefore screening should be done as efficiently as possible and at the lowest possible cost. For example, it has been recommended that mammography screening be done in high-volume settings where the radiologic technologist performs as many examinations as can be done properly each day and the interpreting physician batch-reads the films later in the day.[54,55] The U.S. General Accounting Office has studied costs and quality in mammography and concluded that high-volume performance sites are more likely to provide higher-quality examinations at lower cost.[56]

For screening mammography, two views of the breast are performed: the mediolateral oblique (MLO) and the craniocaudal (CC). The MLO view is the most effective single view because it includes the greatest amount of breast tissue and is the only whole-breast view to include the all of the upper outer quadrant and axillary tail (Figures 31-1 and 31-2).[57] Compared with the MLO view, the CC view provides better visualization of the medial aspect of the breast and better image detail because greater compression of the breast is usually possible (Figures 31-3 and 31-4).[58]

The importance of proper breast compression during mammography cannot be overemphasized. The compression device (1) holds the breast still and thereby prevents motion unsharpness, (2) brings objects closer to the film and reduces blur, (3) separates overlapping tissues that might obscure underlying lesions, and (4) decreases the radiation dose of mammography by making the breast less thick (Figure 31-5). Although breast compression may be uncomfortable, if properly performed it is rarely painful.[59] Few women avoid mammograms because of the discomfort of compression.[60]

DIAGNOSTIC MAMMOGRAPHY

Diagnostic mammography, also called *consultative* or *problem-solving mammography*, is indicated when there are clinical findings such as a palpable lump or abnormal results on a screening examination that require additional imaging. The diagnostic examination is usually tailored to the clinical findings on the individual patient or a specific screening abnormality.[54] The radiologist is

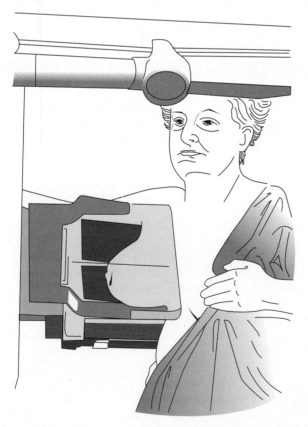

FIG. **31-1** Positioning of a woman for mediolateral oblique view.

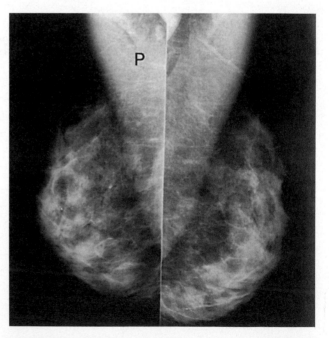

FIG. **31-2** Properly performed right and left mediolateral oblique mammograms. Note the large amount of pectoral muscle *(P)* shown, which ensures that a large amount of the breast tissue and axilla are included in the image. The breasts should be viewed back-to-back as shown here to identify asymmetries in fibroglandular tissue distribution.

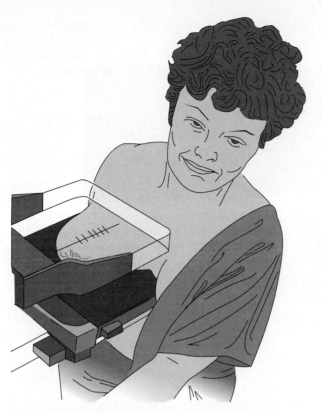

FIG. **31-3** Positioning of woman for craniocaudal view.

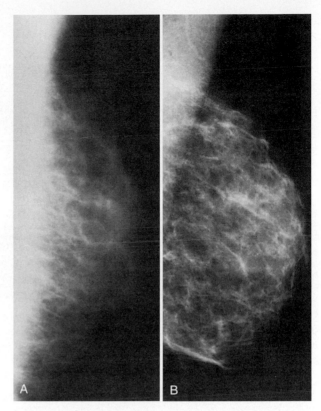

FIG. **31-5** Importance of compression is shown in these inadequately compressed (A) and properly compressed (B) films of the same breast. Compression prevents blurring by holding structures still and bringing them closer to the film, and it evens out the thickness of the breast so that details can be seen in both the thicker tissues near the chest wall and the thinner superficial tissues.

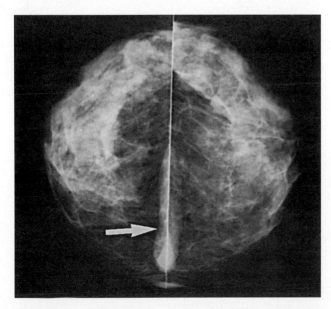

FIG. **31-4** Properly performed right and left craniocaudal mammograms. When placed on the viewbox, the lateral aspect of the breasts is placed at the top, and the breasts are viewed back-to-back as shown here. Note pectoral muscle *(arrow)* visualized near the chest wall at the medial aspects of the breasts.

usually on site during the performance of diagnostic mammography.

Performing the Examination. If the standard MLO and CC views have not been done as part of a recent screening examination, the diagnostic examination should also begin with these two views. If there is a palpable mass, the referring health care provider should communicate the presence and location of the mass to the mammography facility at the time the examination is scheduled. The mammography facility usually confirms the clinical findings with the patient at the time of her examination.

The radiologic technologist or the radiologist palpates the mass and places a radiopaque BB (lead marker) directly over it before the mammograms are performed. The palpation of a reported lump by the radiologic technologist or radiologist is termed a *correlative breast examination* and should not be considered a substitute for a complete clinical breast examination by the patient's referring health care provider. On the mammograms,

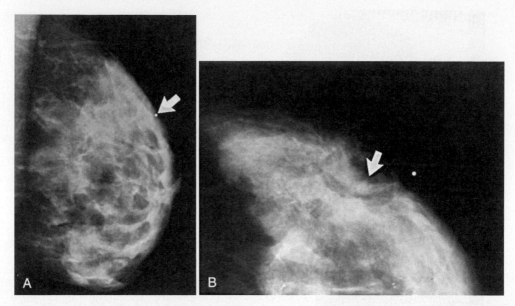

FIG. **31-6** Mammograms of a 45-year-old woman with a palpable mass. **A,** Mediolateral oblique view. Radiopaque lead "BB" *(arrow)* was placed directly over the palpable mass just before the mammograms were performed. **B,** Close-up of craniocaudal view shows a subtle architectural distortion *(arrow)* posterior to the BB.

the BB will indicate the exact location of any palpable findings (Figure 31-6).

In addition to the MLO and CC views, the diagnostic examination may include a variety of additional mammographic views that are intended to better localize or define the nature of abnormalities.[61-65] The most commonly used additional views are the 90-degree lateral and spot compression views. The 90-degree lateral view is used along with the CC view to triangulate the exact location of an abnormality. Spot compression can be done in any projection. It involves the use of a small compression device placed directly over an abnormal area (Figures 31-7 and 31-8). The smaller compression device allows for greater compression over the area of interest and displaces overlying tissues that could obscure the lesion. Magnification technique is often combined with spot compression to better resolve the margins of masses and calcifications. Ultrasonography is also commonly used during diagnostic examinations.

Mammography before Biopsy of a Suspicious Palpable Mass. For women older than age 30, diagnostic mammography should be performed even when a biopsy is planned for a palpable breast lump. The purpose of mammography before the scheduled biopsy is to (1) better define the nature of the palpable abnormality (see Figure 31-6), (2) detect unexpected lesions in the ipsilateral or contralateral breast (see Figure 31-8), and

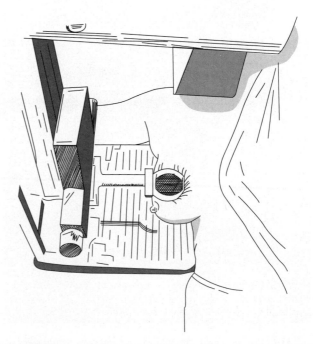

FIG. **31-7** Positioning of the breast for spot compression views. The small spot compression device achieves greater compression over a localized area of interest and displaces adjacent breast tissue away from the area.

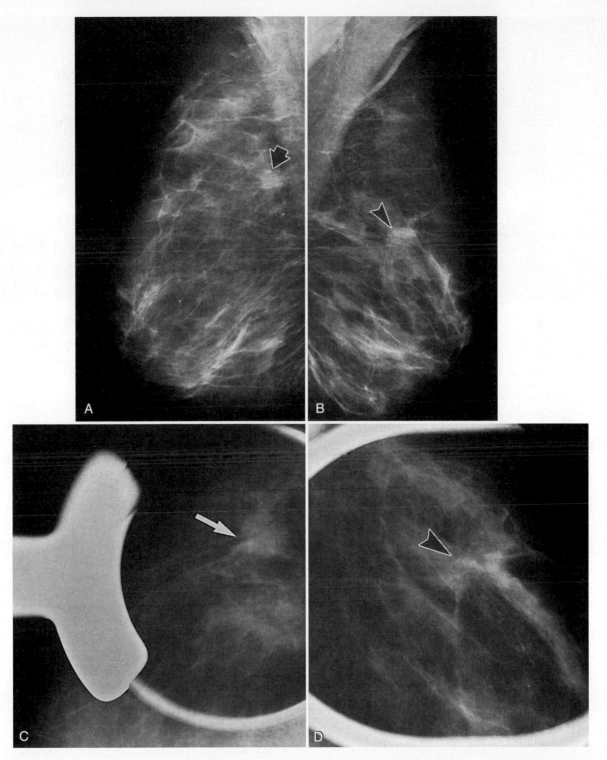

FIG. **31-8** Bilateral carcinomas in a woman with a palpable mass in the right breast. Right **(A)** and left **(B)** mediolateral oblique views show a suspicious mass in the right breast *(arrow)* at the site of the palpable abnormality and an unexpected nonpalpable abnormality in the left breast *(arrowhead)*. **C** and **D,** Spot compression magnification views reveal that the right breast mass *(arrow)* has an irregular shape with spiculations and that the left breast lesion *(arrowhead)* is associated with architectural distortion.

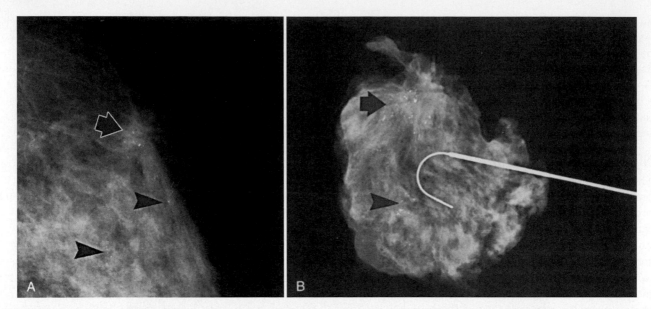

FIG. **31-9** Invasive cancer with extensive intraductal carcinoma component in a woman with a palpable mass. **A,** Close-up of upper breast revealed a spiculated mass *(arrow)* at the site of the palpable mass. The mass contained multiple calcifications of varying size and shape. Additional clusters of calcifications *(arrowheads)* were identified extending into the tissue adjacent to the mass. **B,** Specimen radiograph verifies excision of the spiculated mass *(arrow)* and several clusters of calcifications *(arrowhead)* outside of the mass. Pathologic examination revealed invasive ductal carcinoma with extensive intraductal component.

(3) identify an extensive intraductal component of a palpable invasive carcinoma (Figure 31-9).

STANDARDIZED TERMINOLOGY FOR MAMMOGRAPHY REPORTS

The American College of Radiology Breast Imaging Reporting and Data System (BI-RADS) was devised to standardize mammographic terminology, reduce confusing interpretations, and facilitate outcome monitoring.[3,66] BI-RADS uses a standardized lexicon to facilitate the uniformity of mammography reports from different radiology facilities.

The standardized mammography report also includes an overall assessment of the probability of malignancy that is incorporated in an impression at the end of every report. The inclusion of a "Final Assessment" is required by the federal Mammography Quality Standards Act (MQSA). There are six assessment categories, each associated with a management recommendation. BI-RADS category "0"—"Incomplete Assessment" identifies cases in which additional imaging is needed before a final assessment can be made. Once the additional imaging is accomplished, the case is assigned one of the five Final Assessment categories (Table 31-3). The inclusion of the Final Assessment in the "Impression" section of every mammography report prevents equivocation by the interpreter or misunderstanding by the referring health care provider regarding the significance of the findings

TABLE **31-3** | Mammography Final Assessment Categories

CATEGORY	ASSESSMENT	DESCRIPTION, RECOMMENDATION
1	Negative	There is nothing to comment on. Routine screening.
2	Benign finding	A definitely benign finding. Routine screening.
3	Probably benign finding	Very high probability of benignity. Short-term follow-up recommended to establish stability.
4	Suspicious-looking abnormality	Not characteristic but has reasonable probability of malignancy. Biopsy should be considered.
5	Highly suggestive of malignancy	Very high probability of malignancy. Appropriate action should be taken.
6	Known cancer	Appropriate action.

Modified from the American College of Radiology Breast Imaging Reporting and Data System (BI-RADS).

and the management recommendation. The Final Assessment also facilitates the follow-up and tracking of patients, because each Final Assessment category is associated with one specific follow-up recommendation. A new sixth category has been added for cases in which a biopsy has already proved cancer, but additional evaluation is being performed. An example would be imaging to evaluate a response to induction chemotherapy.

NORMAL MAMMOGRAPHIC FINDINGS

There is a wide range of appearances of the normal breast on mammography in regard to size, shape, and breast tissue composition. Breast tissue composition can range from almost all fat to extremely dense fibroglandular tissue, and this composition directly relates to the sensitivity of mammography. Because breast cancers are radiodense, radiolucent fat (dark gray to black on mammograms) provides an excellent background on which to detect small cancers, but dense fibroglandular tissue (white on mammograms) can obscure breast cancers.

In the BI-RADS system, the breast tissue composition is divided into four categories (Figure 31-10): (1) The breast is almost entirely fat; (2) there are scattered islands of fibroglandular densities that could obscure lesions on mammography; (3) the breast tissue is heterogeneously dense, which may lower the sensitivity of mammography; and (4) the breast tissue is extremely dense, which lowers the sensitivity of mammography.[3] Because young women tend to have more fibroglandular tissue, their breasts are usually more radiopaque than those of older women. However, it is important to understand that there is a wide variation in breast tissue density among women of the same age: Some young women have almost completely fatty breasts, and some older women have extremely dense breasts.

During pregnancy the breasts increase in density. An increase in density has also been associated with exogenous hormone therapy in some postmenopausal women.[67]

ABNORMAL MAMMOGRAPHIC FINDINGS

Masses and calcifications are the most common abnormalities encountered on mammograms, and the radiographic features of these abnormalities are important clues to their etiology. In the standardized mammography report, the descriptors used for masses and calcifications indicate the likelihood of malignancy. Other significant findings include new or evolving lesions, bilaterally asymmetric distribution of the fibroglandular tissue, architectural distortion, skin thickening or retraction, nipple retraction, and axillary node enlargement.

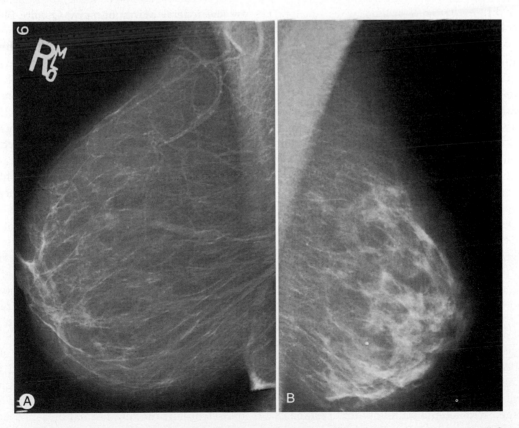

FIG. 31-10 Four categories of mammographic breast tissue composition. A, The breast tissue is almost all fatty. B, There are scattered islands of fibroglandular tissue that could obscure a lesion on mammography.

Continued

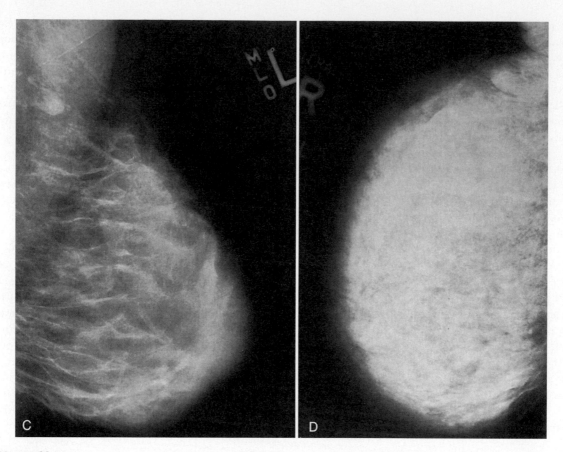

FIG **31-10, cont'd C,** The breast is heterogeneously dense. This may lower the sensitivity of mammography. **D,** The breast is extremely dense, which lowers the sensitivity of mammography.

Masses. A *mass* can be defined as a space-occupying lesion that is seen on at least two mammographic projections. Masses are described by their shape, margins, and density. The *shape* can be round, oval, lobulated, or irregular (Figure 31-11). Oval and round masses are usually benign. An irregular shape suggests a greater likelihood of malignancy.

The *margins* of masses are also an important indicator of the likelihood of malignancy.[68] Margins can be described as circumscribed, microlobulated (multiple tiny lobulations), obscured (partially hidden by adjacent tissue), indistinct, or spiculated (Figure 31-12). *Circumscribed* margins favor a benign etiology, with the likelihood of malignancy being very low, probably less than 2%.[69-71] Ultrasonography is used to establish whether a solitary circumscribed mass is cystic or solid. If it is cystic, no further workup is needed. If it is solid, magnification mammography may be required to confirm that all of the margins of a solid mass are truly circumscribed. A solitary circumscribed solid mass is usually managed with a 6-month follow-up to establish that it is stable (not growing). If it is stable, continued mammographic surveillance is recommended for at

least 2 years.[72,73] The presence of multiple circumscribed masses is even stronger evidence of benignity, suggesting cysts, fibroadenomas, or benign intramammary lymph nodes,[65] and follow-up in 1 year is usually sufficient.

Microlobulated margins increase the likelihood of malignancy.[70] If the mass is directly adjacent to fibroglandular tissue of similar density, the margin may be *obscured,* in which case spot compression is used in an attempt to show the margins of the mass more completely.[62] The finding of *indistinct* margins suggests a possibility of malignancy. A mass with *spiculated* margins has lines radiating from its border and is highly suggestive of malignancy. An area of spiculation without any associated mass is called an *architectural distortion.*

The *density* of a mass also provides a clue as to its etiology. In general, benign masses tend to be lower in density than malignant masses. Malignant masses tend to have high radiodensity compared with benign masses or surrounding normal breast tissue. However, the density of a mass is not always a reliable sign as to whether it is benign or malignant.[74]

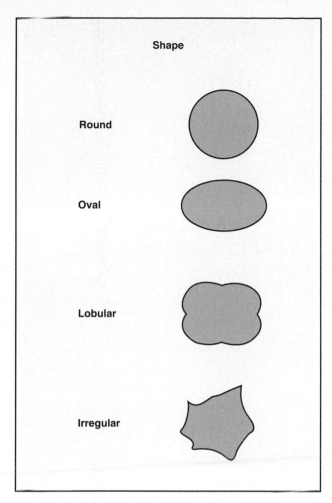

Shape

Round

Oval

Lobular

Irregular

FIG. **31-11** Standardized terminology for the shape of masses.

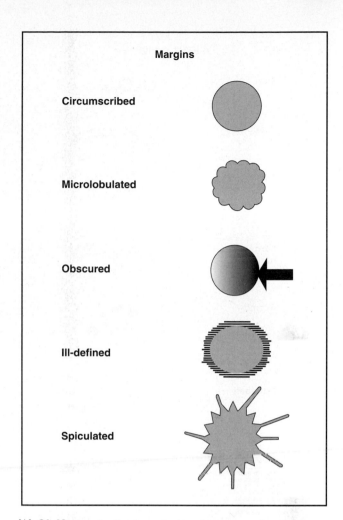

Margins

Circumscribed

Microlobulated

Obscured

Ill-defined

Spiculated

FIG. **31-12** Standardized terminology for the margins of masses.

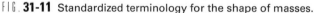

A variety of findings associated with masses may provide additional clues to their etiology. For example, calcifications in a mass often provide definitive information. The calcifications of fibroadenomas tend to be large and dense; these calcifications may be in the center or on the rim of the fibroadenoma. Fine, granular calcifications may be found in benign or malignant masses. Other findings that may be associated with a mass include skin retraction, nipple retraction, and skin thickening.

Calcifications. Calcium is a silver-white, bivalent, metallic element of the alkaline-earth group. Calcification is the deposition of calcium salts in tissues. In the breast, calcification usually occurs in the form of calcium hydroxyapatite or tricalcium phosphate.[75] In standardized terminology, calcifications are divided into three general groups: those that are typically benign, those that are indeterminate, and those that have a higher probability of malignancy. Typically, *benign* calcifications can be identified by their mammographic features and include skin, vascular, coarse, large

rodlike, round, eggshell, and milk of calcium types (Figure 31-13). *Intermediate* calcifications and those having a *higher probability of malignancy* can be described as amorphous or indistinct; pleomorphic or heterogeneous; or fine, linear, and branching (casting) (Figure 31-14).

Calcifications are also characterized by their distribution: *Grouped* or *clustered* calcifications include more than five calcifications in a small area (<2 cm³) and can be benign or malignant. *Linear* calcifications are distributed in a line that may have small branch points. *Segmental* calcifications are distributed in a duct and its branches. *Regional* calcifications occur in a larger volume of breast tissue and not necessarily in a ductal distribution. *Diffuse/scattered* calcifications are distributed randomly throughout the breast and are almost always benign.

BENIGN MASSES

Fibroadenomas are the most common masses in women younger than 30 years. Mammographically, fibroadenomas appear as round, oval, or lobulated masses with

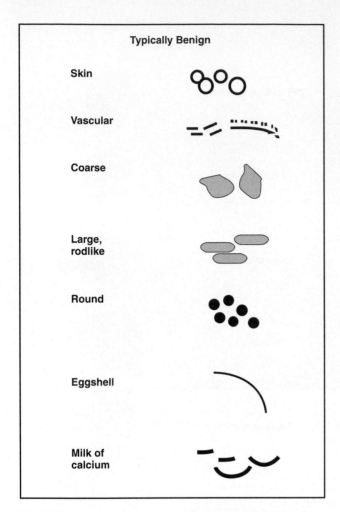

FIG. **31-13** Morphology of typically benign calcifications.

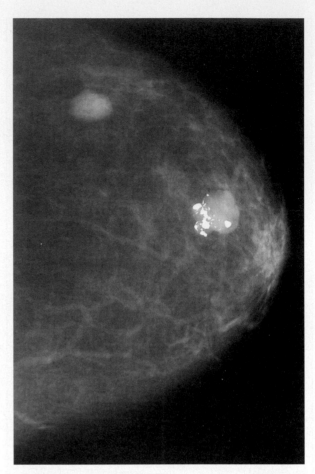

FIG. **31-15** Fibroadenoma. Craniocaudal mammogram reveals a lobular, circumscribed mass with typically benign coarse calcifications of fibroadenoma. The oval circumscribed mass proved to be a fibroadenoma based on core needle biopsy.

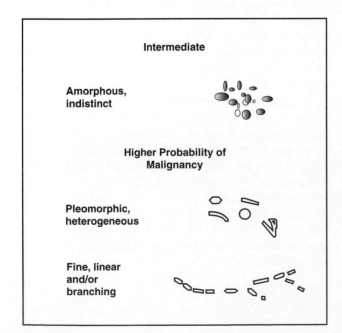

FIG. **31-14** Morphology of indeterminate calcifications and calcification with a higher probability of malignancy.

circumscribed margins (Figures 31-15 to 31-17). They may be solitary or multiple. In older women, they tend to develop characteristic coarse calcifications (see Figure 31-17).

Cysts are round to oval, circumscribed masses that can be solitary or multiple (Figure 31-18, *A*). They are most commonly seen in women aged 40 to 50. The fluid within cysts can be demonstrated with ultrasonography (Figure 31-18, *B*). If characteristic findings of cysts are present, the ultrasonographic diagnosis approaches 100%, thus eliminating the need for aspiration or biopsy.[76] Cysts tend to fluctuate in size over serial mammographic examinations, usually decreasing in size over time.[77]

Intramammary lymph nodes are commonly discovered on mammograms.[78] Intramammary nodes are usually found in the upper outer quadrant of the breast, near the axilla, and can be solitary or multiple. The indentation of the hilum may result in a reniform, or kidney, shape. A central radiolucency, representing fat within the hilum

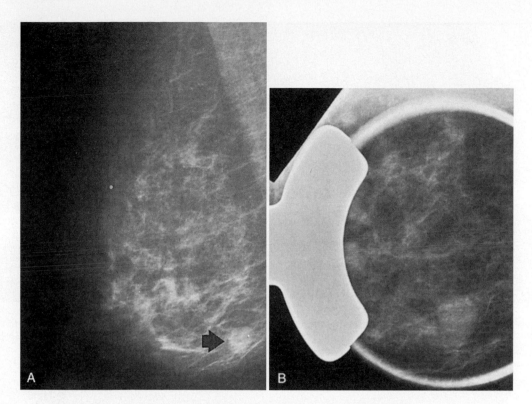

F I G. **31-16** Fibroadenoma **A,** Mediolateral oblique mammogram shows a round to oval mass *(arrow)* in the inferior aspect of the breast with a solitary calcification. **B,** Spot compression and magnification views show that the margins of the mass are circumscribed. Core biopsy revealed fibroadenoma.

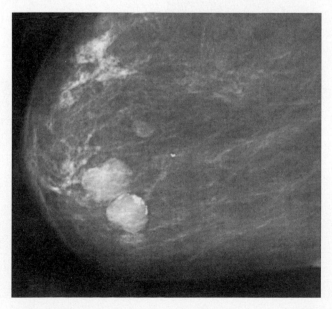

F I G. **31-17** Multiple fibroadenomas. There are several lobulated, circumscribed masses. One of the masses shows the typically benign coarse, rim calcifications of a fibroadenoma.

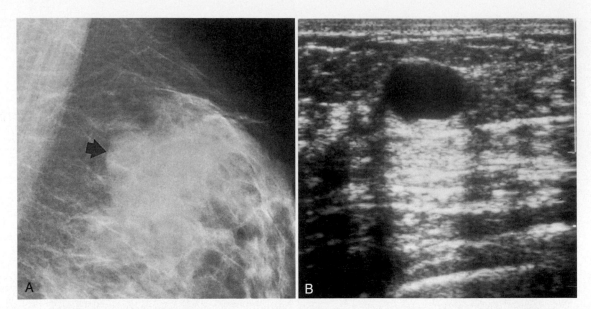

FIG. **31-18** Cyst. **A,** Close-up of a mediolateral oblique mammogram shows a mass with circumscribed posterior margins *(arrow)* and obscured anterior margins. **B,** Ultrasonography revealed that the mass has a circumscribed border, anechoic interior (no interior echoes), and enhancement of echoes posterior to the mass.

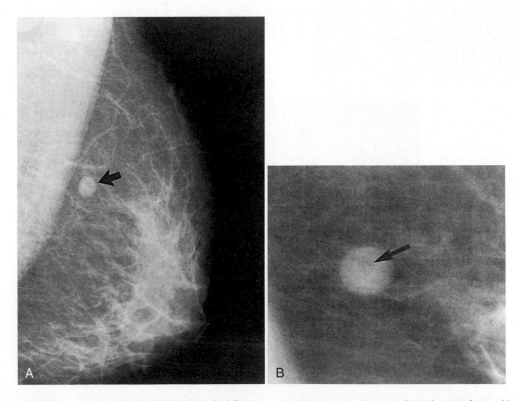

FIG. **31-19** Intramammary lymph node. **A,** Mediolateral oblique mammogram reveals a small oval mass *(arrow)* in the posterosuperior aspect of the breast. **B,** Spot compression-magnification view shows a central radiolucency *(arrow),* which is characteristic of an intramammary lymph node.

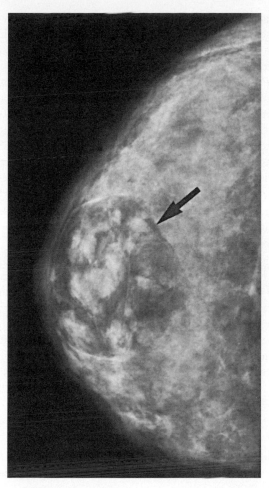

FIG. **31-20** Lipofibroadenoma. Craniocaudal mammogram shows a mass *(arrow)* composed of radiolucent fat and soft tissue densities.

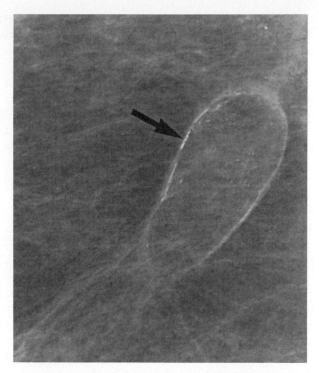

FIG. **31-21** Fat necrosis. Close-up of mammogram 2 years after biopsy shows typical lipid-filled cyst with calcification of fibrous capsule *(arrow)*.

necrosis is usually a round to oval, radiolucent lipid cyst (Figures 31-21 and 31-22). Often the wall of the cyst calcifies (see later discussion). Occasionally the fibrosis associated with posttraumatic fat necrosis results in an irregular, spiculated scar that can mimic malignancy (see Figure 31-22).

of the node, is a characteristic feature (Figure 31-19). On ultrasonography, lymph nodes may have a highly echogenic center—a pathognomonic sign for intramammary lymph nodes.

Lipofibroadenoma, sometimes called a *hamartoma of the breast,* is another benign breast mass with characteristic radiographic features.[79] The mass contains a combination of fatty and soft tissue densities surrounded by a fibrous capsule (Figure 31-20). The proportion of fatty and parenchymal tissue components can vary; thus the lesion may be relatively radiolucent or radiodense.

Lipomas have a typical mammographic appearance. The lipoma is radiolucent and surrounded by a visible, thin fibrous capsule. Lipomas are always benign and usually found incidentally on mammography, although they occasionally may be palpable. In the fatty breast it may be difficult to determine whether a finding is a lipoma or normal fatty tissue.

Posttraumatic fat necrosis may manifest as a mass, calcifications, or both.[80] The mass associated with fat

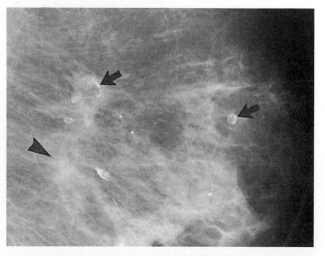

FIG. **31-22** Fat necrosis. Multiple calcifying lipid cysts *(arrows)* and fibrosis *(arrowhead)* at the site of previous lumpectomy.

Postsurgical hematomas are usually round to oval and dense (Figure 31-23, *A*). They may rapidly increase in size immediately after surgery, but they resolve slowly. Although ultrasonography may show an anechoic interior in the early stages of development, the hematoma will later show a mixture of cystic and solid components (Figure 31-23, *B*).

Postsurgical scars may show an irregular shape and spiculated margins, a mammographic appearance similar to that of invasive carcinomas (Figure 31-24). Adjacent skin thickening and retraction also mimic the findings of an advanced breast cancer. Hence, a knowledge of previous surgeries and their location is extremely important when interpreting mammograms.

Baseline mammograms are usually performed 6 months to 1 year after surgery.[81] Unlike carcinomas, scars tend to decrease in size over interval examinations, change their shape and appearance on mammograms taken in different projections, and be nonpalpable or barely palpable despite a relatively large size on mammograms.

Radial scars are benign lesions that are said to occur in approximately 1 in 1000 screening mammograms.[82]

These scars, which occur in the absence of previous surgery, are a subject of controversy among pathologists, with nine different names having been given to them (e.g., *infiltrating epitheliosis, benign sclerosing ductal proliferation*). *Radial scar* best describes the mammographic appearances: relatively long spicules emanating from a center that may be radiolucent (Figure 31-25). Calcifications may or may not be present.

It is important to differentiate radial scar from invasive carcinoma, which is also characterized by spiculations. Unlike carcinoma, radial scar is neither palpable nor associated with skin thickening or retraction. Although the radiolucent center of radial scars is an important clue to the correct diagnosis, excisional biopsy is needed to rule out malignancy with certainty.[83]

BENIGN CALCIFICATIONS

Skin (dermal) calcifications are secondary to dermatitis or residue from deodorants. They are usually located near the skin on at least one of the mammographic views.[84] The calcifications are usually low in density, often with a central radiolucency.[65] If the dermal origin of the calcifications is not certain, maneuvers are

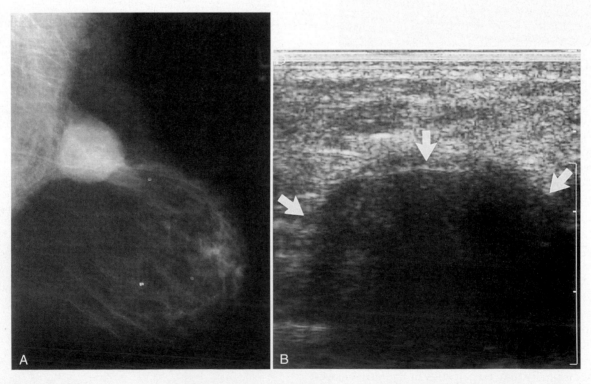

FIG. 31-23 Postsurgical hematoma. A 45-year-old woman had a biopsy of a palpable mass. Pathologic examination revealed that the mass was a fibroadenoma. However, 2 weeks later the patient noticed a new palpable mass at the site of surgery. **A,** Mediolateral mammogram reveals a round mass at the surgical site. **B,** Ultrasonography reveals a large, oval mass *(arrows)* with no interior echoes near the chest wall. The diagnosis was postsurgical hematoma. The mass completely resolved in 3 months.

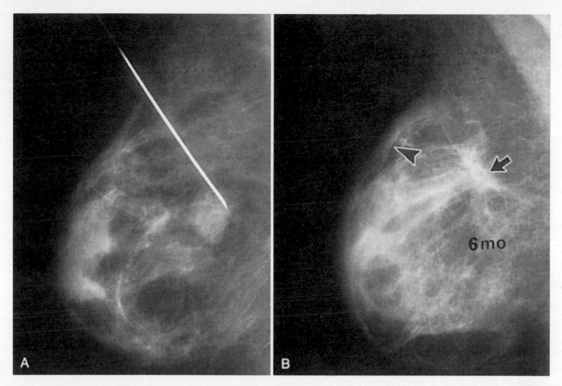

FIG. **31-24** Postsurgical scar. A 50-year-old woman had an ill-defined mass detected with screening mammography. An excisional biopsy preceded by needle localization was scheduled. **A,** Mediolateral mammogram during localization procedure shows the tip of the needle positioned immediately posterior to the mass. Biopsy revealed invasive carcinoma. **B,** Mediolateral mammogram 6 months after surgery shows a spiculated mass *(arrow)* and skin thickening *(arrowhead)* at the surgical site.

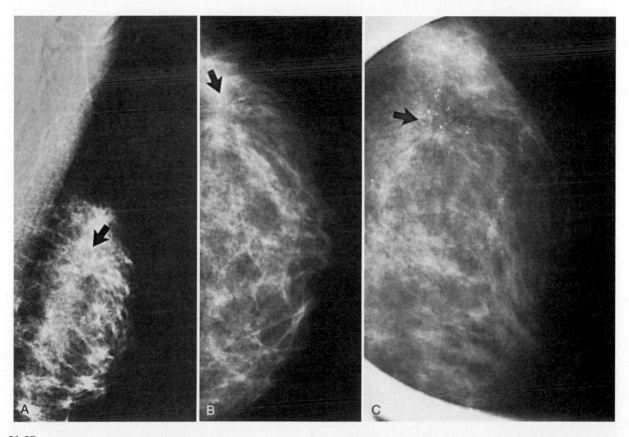

FIG. **31-25** Radial scar. A 55-year-old woman had a screening mammogram. The left mediolateral oblique **(A)** and craniocaudal **(B)** views show an architectural distortion *(arrows)* in the upper outer quadrant. **C,** Spot compression-magnification view over the abnormality reveals multiple spicules emanating from a radiolucent center *(arrow).* There are numerous punctate calcifications. Biopsy revealed radial scar.

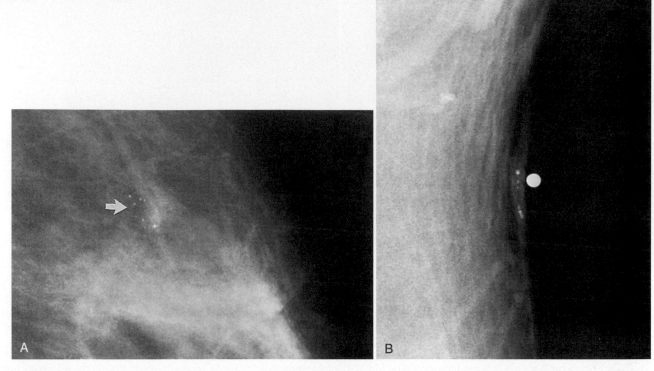

F I G. **31-26** Skin calcifications. Multiple punctate calcifications had been identified in the left breast on the screening mammograms of a 44-year-old woman. Because the calcifications were close to the skin on both mediolateral oblique (MLO) and craniocaudal views, it was possible that the calcifications were in the skin. A radiopaque BB was placed on the skin overlying the calcifications, and an x-ray projection tangential to the BB was performed. **A,** Close-up from original MLO view shows clustered, low-density calcifications *(arrow).* **B,** Close-up of tangential view shows the calcifications in the skin directly under the radiopaque BB. Because dermal calcifications are benign, nothing further was done.

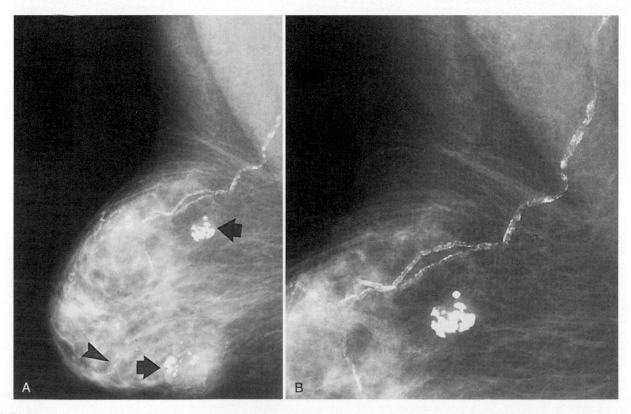

F I G. **31-27** Typically benign calcifications. **A,** Right mediolateral oblique view shows prominent vascular calcifications, calcification in two degenerating fibroadenomas *(arrows)* and benign secretory calcifications *(arrowhead).* **B,** Close-up shows typical "railroad track" vascular calcifications and "popcorn" calcifications of fibroadenoma.

performed to direct the x-ray beam tangential to the portion of the skin containing the calcifications (Figure 31-26). The tangential view can prove that calcifications are in the skin, eliminating the need for a biopsy.

Vascular calcifications are characterized by linear, parallel calcifications, referred to as a *railroad track* configuration (Figure 31-27). The calcifications are said to be more common in women with diabetes, but in fact, they are commonly seen in women with no history of diabetes.[85]

Fibroadenoma calcifications are usually coarse. The cacifications are usually centrally placed, are arranged in "popcorn" configuration (see Figure 31-27), or may be positioned on the rim of the fibroadenoma (see Figure 31-17). However, when calcifications occur within the ducts of the fibroadenoma, they may be indistinguishable from those of malignancy and a biopsy may be necessary.

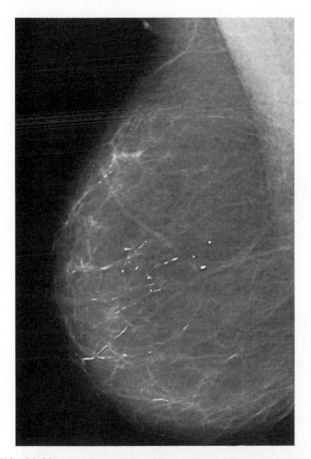

FIG. **31-28** Typically benign calcifications. Secretory calcifications of duct ectasia. Unlike the calcifications of ductal carcinoma in situ, these calcifications are solid, rodlike, and relatively well separated and rarely show branching.

Secretory calcifications, or the calcifications of duct ectasia, involve the intermediate and larger ducts of the breast. Most women with this condition are asymptomatic. Although the exact cause of duct ectasia is uncertain, the calcifications are quite characteristic. The calcifications are usually thick and solid, representing calcium deposits in the benign secretions within dilated ducts (Figures 31-27 and 31-28). They are often bilateral and in the subareolar location. A unilateral, segmental distribution of duct ectasia manifesting as calcification may be confused with comedo carcinoma, because both may show linear and branching configurations. Unlike comedo carcinoma, the calcifications of duct ectasia are solid, smooth, continuous rods, often more than 1 mm in diameter and more widely spaced than comedo carcinoma calcifications. In addition, the calcifications of duct ectasia usually do not branch.[86]

Posttraumatic fat necrosis calcifications usually develop within the fibrous walls of developing lipid cysts. In the early stages of development, they may be confused with malignant calcifications, but with time, they take on a characteristic egg-shell configuration around the lipid-filled cysts (see Figures 31-21 and 31-22).[80,87] These lesions are commonly found at the location of a previous biopsy, providing a further clue to their etiology.

Milk of calcium is free-floating calcium within cysts, usually tiny cysts. The mammographic features of this condition are pathognomonic; similar to the sediment at the bottom of a cup of tea, they change their appearance with different radiographic projections.[88] These gravity-dependent calcifications appear as amorphous and round or ovoid smudges on craniocaudal projections (Figure 31-29, *A*). However, they are sharp and linear to crescent-shaped on 90-degree lateral views (Figure 31-29, *B*). Milk of calcium does not require a biopsy, but carcinoma may arise nearby, in which case the calcifications should be inspected carefully to rule out coexistent carcinoma.

MALIGNANT MASSES

The most common malignant breast mass is invasive breast carcinoma. The mass of invasive carcinoma is typically irregular in shape, indistinct or spiculated on its margin, and high in radiographic density compared with normal parenchymal tissue (Figure 31-30). The mass may contain pleomorphic calcifications. Less commonly, the mass is circumscribed. There are several subtypes of invasive cancer, with the different histologic types differing in prognoses.[89]

Invasive Ductal Carcinoma, Not Otherwise Specified. The most common carcinoma, the not otherwise specified (NOS) type, usually presents as a mass.

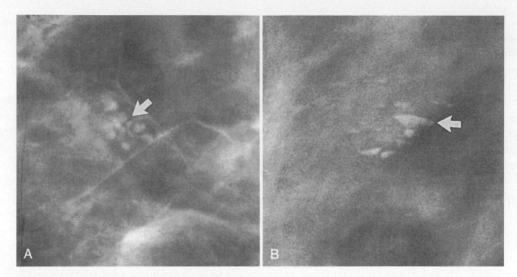

FIG. **31-29** Typically benign calcifications. Milk of calcium detected on the screening mammograms of a 41-year-old woman. **A,** Close-up of craniocaudal view shows a cluster of amorphous, round calcifications *(arrow)*. **B,** Close-up of 90-degree lateral view demonstrates layering of the gravity-dependent calcifications *(arrow)*.

Most of these masses have the irregular shape, indistinct or spiculated margins, and high radiographic density characteristic of malignancy (Figures 31-30 to 31-32). Although most NOS-type carcinomas have indistinct or spiculated margins, occasionally they have partially circumscribed margins (Figure 31-33).

Spot compression-magnification films usually reveal indistinct margins at some portion of the boundary of an otherwise circumscribed carcinoma. Approximately 40% of invasive ductal carcinomas of the NOS type are associated with malignant calcifications (see Figure 31-30, *B*).

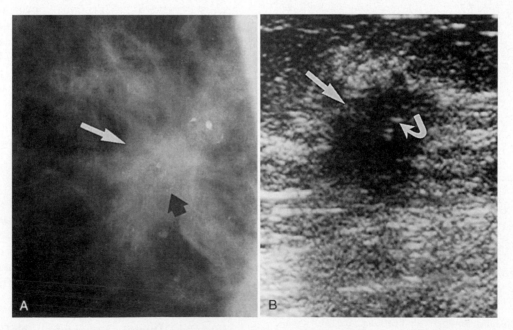

FIG. **31-30** Typical invasive carcinoma. **A,** Close-up of mammogram showing typical invasive carcinoma mass, manifested by irregular shape, spiculated margins *(white arrow)*, high radiographic density, and numerous calcifications of varying size and shape *(black arrow)*. **B,** Ultrasonography shows that the mass *(straight arrow)* has an irregular shape, ill-defined margins, and low-level heterogeneous echoes within it. The bright echoes *(curved arrow)* within the mass represent calcifications.

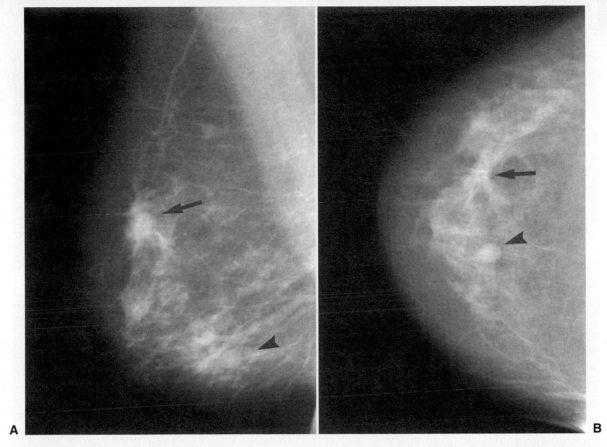

FIG. **31-31** Invasive ductal carcinoma, not otherwise specified (NOS) and a cyst in a 54-year-old asymptomatic woman referred for screening mammograms. **A** and **B,** Right mediolateral and craniocaudal views show an irregular, spiculated mass *(arrows)* and an oval, circumscribed mass *(arrowheads).* On ultrasonography the circumscribed mass proved to be a cyst. At biopsy the irregular mass proved to be invasive ductal carcinoma.

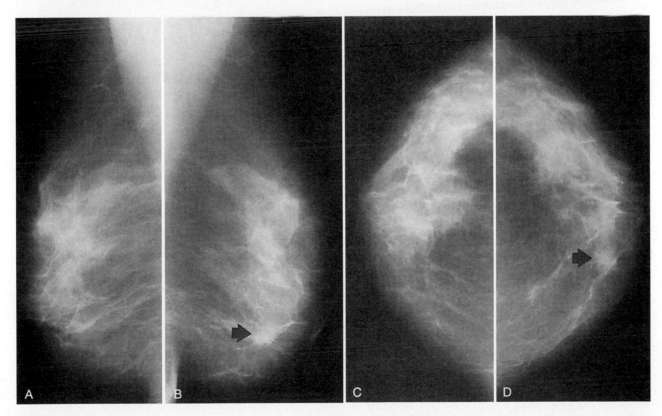

FIG. **31-32** Invasive ductal carcinoma, not otherwise specified (NOS). A 47-year-old woman had bilateral screening mammograms. Right **(A)** and left **(B)** mediolateral oblique views and right **(C)** and left **(D)** craniocaudal views show a 1.5-cm round, spiculated mass *(arrows),* approximately the same density as the surrounding fibroglandular tissue, in the lower inner quadrant of the left breast.

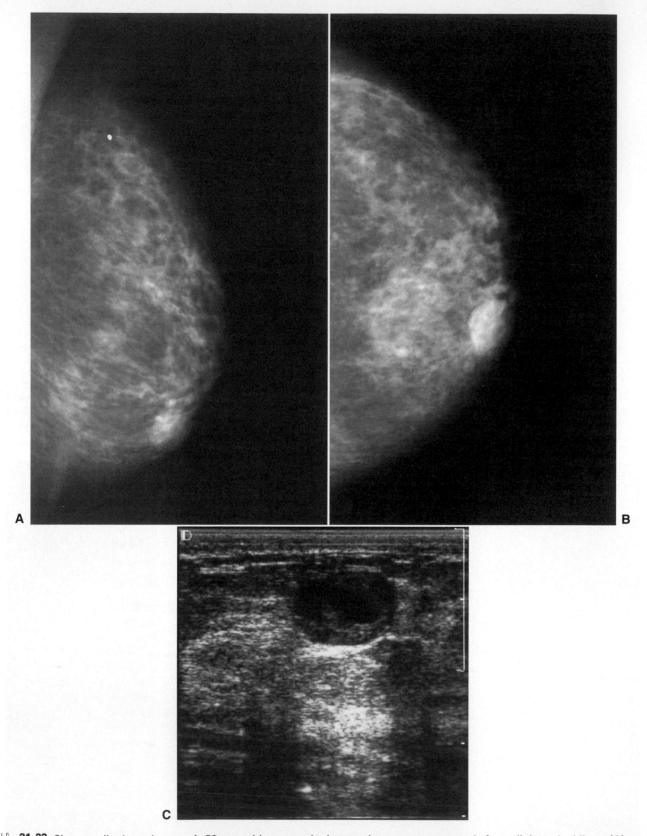

FIG. **31-33** Circumscribed carcinoma. A 58-year-old woman had screening mammograms. Left mediolateral oblique **(A)** and craniocaudal **(B)** views show a 2-cm lobulated, circumscribed subareolar mass. **C,** Ultrasonography revealed a complex mass, consisting of both cystic and solid components. Open biopsy revealed invasive ductal carcinoma, not otherwise specified.

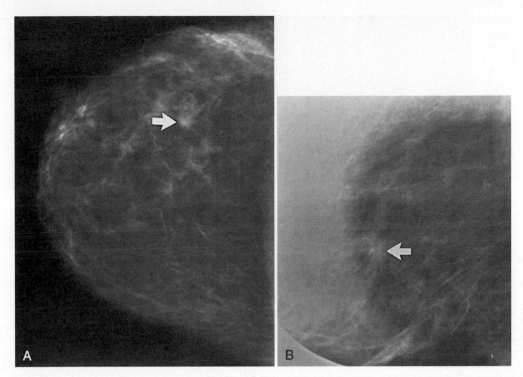

FIG. **31-34** Tubular carcinoma. A 48-year-old woman had screening mammograms. **A,** Right craniocaudal view shows irregular density *(arrow)* in the outer hemisphere. **B,** Spot compression-magnification view in mediolateral projection confirms the presence of a small spiculated mass *(arrow).* Biopsy revealed tubular carcinoma.

Tubular Carcinomas. Tubular carcinomas grow very slowly and are usually small when they are first detected on mammographic screening. They have an excellent prognosis relative to the NOS-type cancers. Other than a characteristically small size, they have the mammographic features of the usual NOS type of invasive breast carcinoma: irregular shape, spiculated margins, and high radiographic density (Figure 31-34).[90]

Medullary Carcinomas. Medullary carcinomas are often oval or lobulated in shape and frequently have circumscribed margins (Figure 31-35).[91] In addition to their benign-appearing mammographic features, the clinical findings may also mimic a benign lesion and they have a tendency to occur in younger women. This combination of features results in delayed diagnosis of many medullary carcinomas. Necrosis, cavitation, and bleeding may result in a rapid increase in lesion size; the presence of fluid within the tumor can be identified with ultrasonography (Figure 31-36).

Colloid Carcinomas. Also called *mucinous carcinomas,* colloid carcinomas often show relatively circumscribed

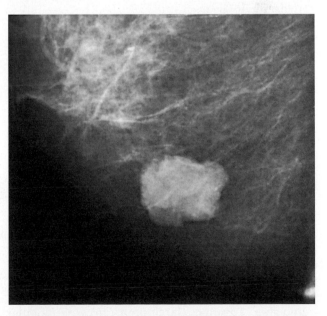

FIG. **31-35** Medullary carcinoma. A 39-year-old woman felt a mass in her right breast. On palpation the mass was freely movable. Close-up of mediolateral oblique mammogram reveals a lobular mass with circumscribed margins. Biopsy revealed medullary carcinoma.

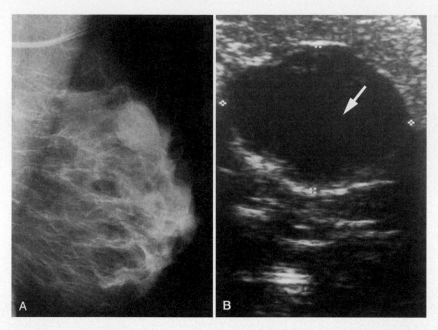

FIG. **31-36** Medullary carcinoma. A 41-year-old woman felt a movable mass in the upper outer quadrant of her left breast. A diagnostic mammogram was ordered. **A,** Left mediolateral oblique view shows an oval mass under the radiopaque BB, which was placed over the palpable mass. **B,** Ultrasonography reveals a lobulated mass with a thick wall surrounding an anechoic fluid-filled center *(arrow)*. Biopsy revealed medullary carcinoma with central hemorrhagic necrosis.

margins, but portions of the margin are usually microlobulated or indistinct (Figure 31-37). Because of their compressibility, colloid carcinomas commonly may have radiographic density similar to that of normal fibroglandular tissue.

Invasive Papillary Carcinoma. Invasive papillary carcinoma, a rare invasive cancer, may appear as a solitary, circumscribed nodule or as a multinodular pattern.[92]

Intracystic Carcinoma. Adenocarcinoma arising from the wall of a cyst is a rare lesion.[93] If the tumor is totally intracystic, the cancer is noninvasive and the prognosis is excellent. The most common histologic type is papillary adenocarcinoma. The mass is often large and circumscribed on mammography. Ultrasonography may show both fluid and solid components. The solid portions often surround the central fluid-filled portion, or the solid components may project from a portion of the wall of the cyst into the center of the fluid.

Invasive Lobular Carcinoma. Invasive lobular carcinoma can appear as a mass with an irregular shape and spiculated or ill-defined margins on mammograms (Figure 31-8). However, it is not uncommon for mammograms of invasive lobular carcinoma to show only a poorly defined asymmetric density (see Figure 31-38), an architectural distortion (Figure 31-39), or no recognizable abnormal findings.[94] Because they are often difficult to appreciate on mammography or palpation, even when relatively advanced in size, invasive lobular carcinomas are sometimes referred to as "sneaky" cancers.[95,96] They also have a higher rate of bilaterality than other carcinomas (see Figure 31-8).

Breast Metastases from Extramammary Malignancies. Metastatic foci to the breast from extramammary sites are uncommon. Metastases to the breast can originate from a variety of primary sites.[97] The patient invariably has a known history of the extramammary malignancy before the mammographic examination. Metastatic melanoma is the largest reported source of metastases to the breast. The metastatic lesions usually have a round shape and indistinct margins (Figure 31-40). Most metastatic foci to the breast are solitary lesions, although multiple masses may be seen occasionally (Figure 31-41).[98]

MALIGNANT CALCIFICATIONS

Calcifications associated with breast cancer are dystrophic; they are deposited in abnormal tissue, not as a result of elevated levels of calcium or phosphate in the blood. Malignant calcifications may occur with or without the presence of a mass, and they are typically

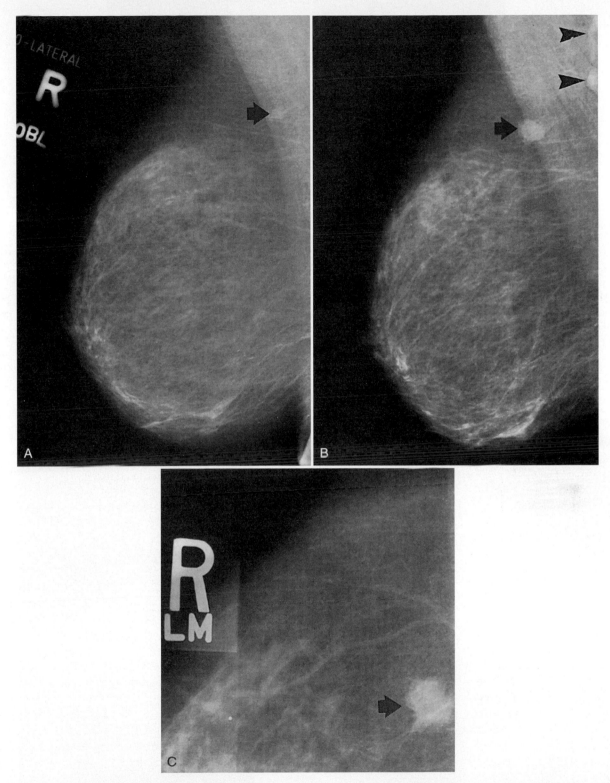

FIG. **31-37** Colloid (mucinous) carcinoma. A 45-year-old woman had annual screening mammograms that revealed an evolving density. **A,** Initial right mediolateral oblique (MLO) view was considered normal. A density *(arrow)* in the axilla was assumed to be a benign lymph node. **B,** Right MLO view 2 years later reveals that the density has increased in size. The lymph nodes *(arrowheads)* in the axilla have benign mammographic features and are now seen because of better mammographic positioning. **C,** Lateral medial spot compression-magnification view reveals a mass *(arrow)* with an irregular shape and indistinct posterior margins. Biopsy revealed colloid carcinoma.

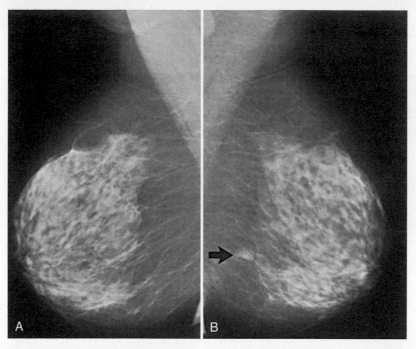

FIG. **31-38** Invasive lobular carcinoma. A 45-year-old woman had had annual screening mammograms since the age of 40. On the most recent examination, comparison of the right **(A)** and left **(B)** mediolateral oblique views showed in the left breast an asymmetric density *(arrow)* that was not present on previous examinations. Biopsy revealed invasive lobular carcinoma.

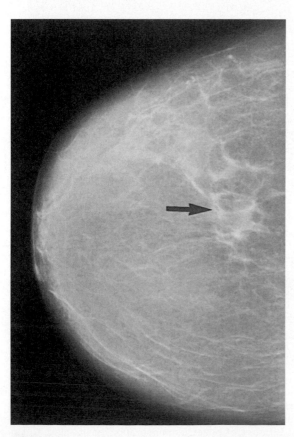

FIG. **31-39** Invasive lobular carcinoma. Left craniocaudal view from screening mammograms reveals an architectural distortion *(arrow)* in the right breast. Palpation of the area failed to reveal any abnormality. Core needle biopsy revealed invasive lobular carcinoma.

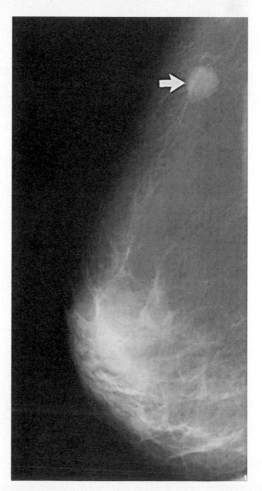

FIG. **31-40** Lung carcinoma metastatic to the breast. A 54-year-old woman with a known history of lung carcinoma noticed a mass *(arrow)* in the superior aspect of her right breast. Mammograms revealed a solitary, round, ill-defined mass at the site of the palpable abnormality. Biopsy revealed metastatic carcinoma.

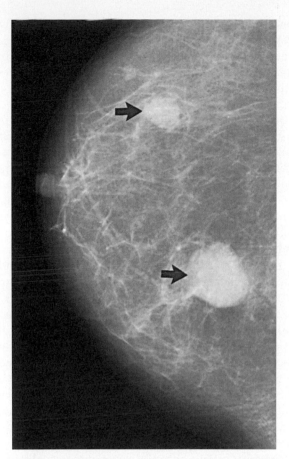

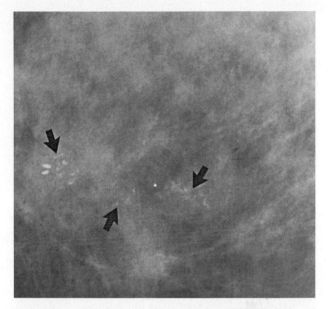

FIG. **31-42** Noncomedo ductal carcinoma in situ. A 48-year-old woman had multiple calcifications detected on screening mammography. Close-up of the calcifications reveals three groups of numerous clustered calcifications *(arrows)* that vary in size and shape. Biopsy following needle wire localization revealed noncomedo carcinoma.

FIG. **31-41** Lymphoma metastatic to the breast. A 48-year-old woman with lymphoma noticed a mass in the right breast. Right craniocaudal views show two ill-defined masses *(arrows)*. Ultrasonography revealed that the masses were solid. Fine-needle aspiration confirmed the diagnosis of metastatic lymphoma.

grouped or clustered; pleomorphic (varying in size and shape) (Figures 31-42 and 31-43); fine, linear, and branching (Figures 31-44 and 31-45) and numerous. The greater the number of calcifications in a cluster, the greater the likelihood of malignancy, with a group containing fewer than five calcifications being unlikely to represent malignancy.[99] The distribution of the calcifications can be linear, linear and branching, or segmental.

Ductal Carcinoma in Situ. DCIS, or intraductal carcinoma, is a precursor to invasive breast cancer, which on microscopic examination does not yet show clear evidence of stromal invasion.[100-102] Before the widespread use of mammography, DCIS represented less than 5% of newly detected breast cancers.[103] Today, DCIS makes up approximately 30% of newly detected breast cancers, with most DCIS cases being detected with screening mammography. Approximately 75% of DCIS cases are detected because of mammographically visible calcifications.

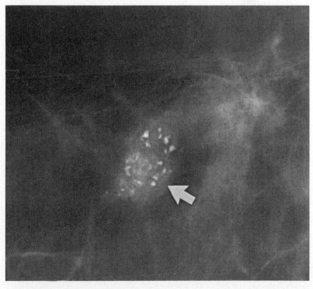

FIG. **31-43** Noncomedo carcinoma. Suspicious calcifications were detected on the screening mammograms of a 60-year-old woman. Close-up of calcifications reveals that the calcifications are numerous, clustered, pleomorphic (varying in size and shape), and associated with a soft tissue density *(arrow)*. Biopsy revealed noncomedo ductal carcinoma in situ with surrounding inflammatory response.

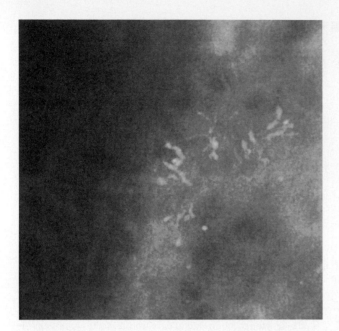

FIG. **31-44** Comedo ductal carcinoma in situ. Fine, linear, and branching calcifications of comedo carcinoma.

A major breakthrough in knowledge about DCIS occurred when Holland and co-workers[104,105] described their mastectomy specimen findings. They concluded that DCIS typically is distributed within a single lobe of a duct system without intervening areas of normal tissue. This observation was contrary to the then-popular concept of a multifocal origin of breast cancer and was more consistent with the fact that breast cancer recurrences are usually in the region of the original tumor.[86,106] DCIS includes a spectrum of lesions, and individual cases do not have the same propensity for eventual invasion and metastasis.

Several classification systems have been developed based on the extent of the lesion, clinical findings, and histologic features. The most commonly used classification system divides DCIS into two major types: the more aggressive comedo carcinoma and the more indolent noncomedo carcinoma. In excised specimens containing comedo carcinoma, the involved ducts typically extrude a thick material resembling a comedone. Today, aggressive malignant cytologic features, such as the degree of nuclear atypia, are considered more important than the presence of central lumen necrosis in the histologic diagnosis of comedo carcinoma.[100] In fact, DCIS is often intermediate in the degree of malignant cytologic features or intermixed, and the prognosis depends on the prevalent nuclear grade. Micropapillary and cribriform DCIS are the most common histologic subtypes of noncomedo DCIS. The visible calcifications of comedo carcinoma closely match the actual extent of the lesion, but noncomedo carcinoma may be considerably more extensive than suggested by its calcifications.

The calcifications of comedo carcinoma usually occur in the central debris of ducts involved by tumor cells

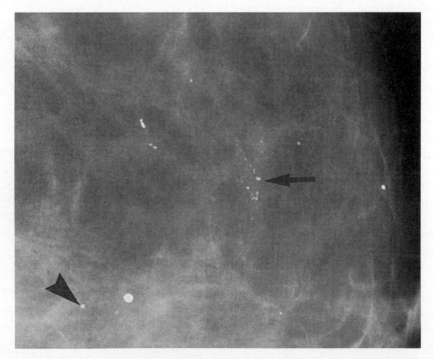

FIG. **31-45** Comedo ductal carcinoma in situ. The cluster of calcifications *(arrow)* is composed of multiple fine, granular calcifications (compare with the solid, rodlike calcifications of duct ectasia in Figure 31-30) and the benign punctuate calcification below *(arrowhead).*

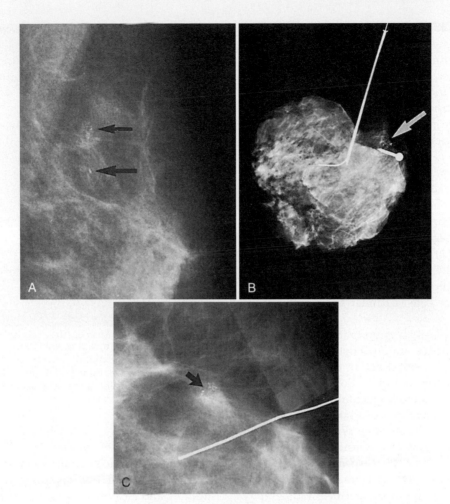

FIG. **31-46** Residual noncomedo ductal carcinoma in situ (DCIS) following lumpectomy. **A,** The barely visible calcifications *(arrows)* are numerous, tiny, and pleomorphic. **B,** Specimen radiography following wire localization verifies the presence of calcifications at the edge of the excised tissue. Histologic examination revealed micropapillary DCIS with clear margins. **C,** Preradiotherapy magnification mammograms of the surgical site revealed residual calcifications *(arrow)* in the breast. (The radiopaque wire was placed on the surface of the breast to mark the surgical site.) Reexcision following wire localization revealed micropapillary DCIS.

undergoing necrosis. As a result, the morphology of the calcifications of comedo carcinoma is typically fine, linear, and branching, suggesting casting of the duct system[107,108] (see Figures 31-44 and 31-45). The calcifications of noncomedo carcinoma represent dystrophic laminated calcifications in intraductal cellular debris or calcified secretions in the cribriform spaces of noncomedo DCIS. These granular calcifications are fine particles characterized by variable size and shape (Figures 31-42, 31-43, and 31-46). However, radiographic features are not always reliable in differentiating between comedo and noncomedo carcinoma.[109]

In slightly more than 10% of DCIS cases, a soft tissue mass can also be seen on mammograms (see Figure 31-43). This soft tissue mass is a manifestation of a solid mass of tumor cells or associated inflammation, edema, and fibrosis at the periphery of involved

ducts.[110] Table 31-4 shows the approximate frequency of the most common radiographic manifestations of DCIS. Less common manifestations of DCIS include asymmetry; dilated retroareolar ducts; an ill-defined, rounded tumor; architectural distortion; and a developing density.

TABLE **31-4** Mammographic Manifestations of Ductal Carcinoma In Situ

MAMMOGRAPHIC FINDING	FREQUENCY (%)
Calcifications alone	75
Calcifications plus soft tissue density	10
Soft tissue abnormality alone	10
No mammography findings	5

Invasive Cancer with Extensive Intraductal Component. Invasive tumors are classified as having an extensive intraductal component (EIC positive) if they are predominately intraductal with small areas of invasion or predominantly invasive with one of the following conditions: (1) DCIS fills nonobliterated ducts within the invasive cancer, or (2) there is DCIS in the tissue adjacent to the invasive tumor[105] (see Figure 31-9).

The significance of the EIC-positive designation is the greater incidence of local recurrence of breast cancer after surgical excision and radiotherapy. One study reported the incidence of recurrence for EIC-positive cases to be approximately 25% at 5 years compared with 6% for EIC-negative cases.[111] This report verifies observations of others that the presence of EIC in DCIS is a marker for widespread residual tumor after excision.[103,104,112-115] If all of the EIC is successfully removed, the local recurrence rate is similar to that of tumors without EIC.

Mammography plays an important role in the management of EIC-positive tumors. First, mammographic wire localization is essential before the surgical excision. If the purpose of the localization procedure is to excise all of the lesion for segmental resection before radiotherapy and not just to take a sample for diagnostic purposes, multiple localization wires may be used to bracket the full extent of the lesion.[116] At the time of surgical excision of DCIS, a specimen radiograph should always be performed (see Figure 31-46). However, it should be borne in mind that specimen radiography is not an adequate tool to ensure that malignant calcifications have been completely removed.[117]

Traditionally, it is the pathologist's responsibility to determine whether the margins of a resected tissue are free of tumor. However, the complex branching of the breast ductal system may lead to errors regarding whether the intraductal tumor has been completely removed (Figures 31-46 and 31-47). Therefore it is important that in cases with extensive DCIS manifested by calcifications, mammography be performed after surgery and before radiotherapy to look for residual malignant calcifications.[116,118]

To minimize the discomfort associated with mammographic compression, the pretherapy mammograms are delayed until just before radiotherapy, usually 3 to 5 weeks after surgery. At our institution, postsurgical preradiotherapy examination is performed with a wire over the surgical site. In addition to standard views, microfocus magnification views are performed over the scar (see Figure 31-46, *C*). If the preradiotherapy mammograms disclose residual calcifications, a reexcision is performed after mammographically guided wire localization (see Figure 31-47). Most reexcisions performed for residual calcifications at the lumpectomy site reveal residual carcinoma.[119]

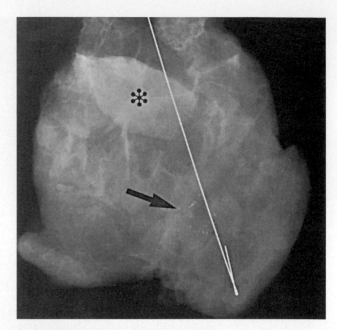

FIG. **31-47** Specimen radiograph following wire localization of residual calcifications *(arrow)* of comedo carcinoma. Preradiotherapy mammograms had demonstrated these calcifications adjacent to the postsurgical hematoma.*

If only a few calcifications remain, reexcision is not always performed, but it is still important to know the number and location of these calcifications so that they are not mistaken for recurrent tumor on follow-up mammograms.

INDIRECT SIGNS OF BREAST CANCER

Mammographic evidence of malignancy can be divided into primary, secondary, and indirect signs. *Primary signs* include a mass and calcifications. *Secondary signs,* such as skin thickening and retraction, are usually evident on clinical breast examination. When seen on mammograms, they are usually associated with an advanced cancer. *Indirect,* or *subtle, signs* are associated with nonpalpable breast cancers and include a neodensity or evolving density, architectural distortion, and bilaterally asymmetric tissue density. These indirect signs have been reported to be the only evidence of malignancy in up to 20% of mammographically detected cancers.[120]

Evolving Density. Because the breasts of postmenopausal women are expected to undergo involution, the appearance of a new or growing density should be considered a possible sign of breast cancer in this age group.[121] By definition, detection of a neodensity requires access to previous mammograms (Figure 31-48).[122] An "evolving density" is one that was present at least in retrospect on a previous examination

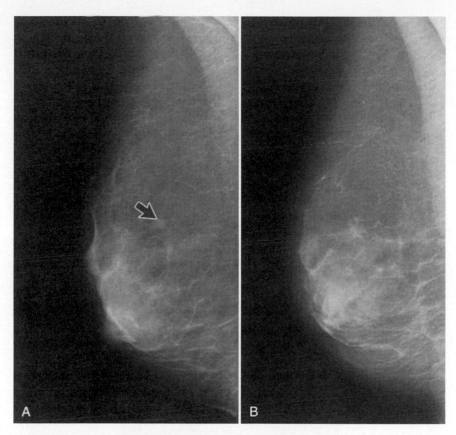

FIG. **31-48** Neodensity. Right mediolateral oblique screening mammogram **(A)** of a 45-year-old woman revealed a small density *(arrow)*, which was not present on screening mammograms performed 1 year earlier **(B)**. Biopsy revealed mucinous carcinoma.

but that was smaller and perhaps not recognized as being significant (see Figure 31-37). If a new or evolving density has mammographic features that could represent a cyst, sonography or needle aspiration should be done. If the existence of a simple cyst is proved by either method and the cyst matches the site of the mammographic abnormality, no further workup is necessary.

Tissue densities caused by hormone replacement therapy can usually be differentiated from neodensities associated with breast cancer. The densities caused by exogenous hormone therapy are usually present bilaterally and in several areas of the same breast. If there is a solitary neodensity in a woman receiving hormone replacement therapy, it may be difficult to rule out breast cancer. In this situation, it may be useful to stop hormone replacement therapy for 2 to 3 months. If the neodensity persists, a biopsy should be considered.

Architectural Distortion. An architectural distortion may be the earliest sign of breast carcinoma (see Figure 31-39). Architectural distortions can also be associated with surgical scars (see Figure 31-24) and radial scars (see Figure 31-25). Because postsurgical scarring can also result in distortions of the parenchyma, it is important to be aware of the location of any previous surgeries.[123] Some radiologists find it useful before performing mammograms for the radiologic technologist to place a wire directly over surgical scars to mark the exact site of the scar.[81]

Asymmetric Density. *Asymmetric density* refers to a relative increase in the volume of fibroglandular tissue in one breast compared with the corresponding area in the contralateral breast. Because asymmetric breast tissue usually is a normal variation, the asymmetry should not be considered significant unless it is associated with suspect clinical or mammographic features. If there is a question regarding the nature of a localized region of asymmetric breast tissue, spot compression views can be used to determine whether the area of increased density is normally compressible.

Magnification views might also disclose an underlying mass, clustered calcifications, or an architectural distortion associated with an asymmetric density,

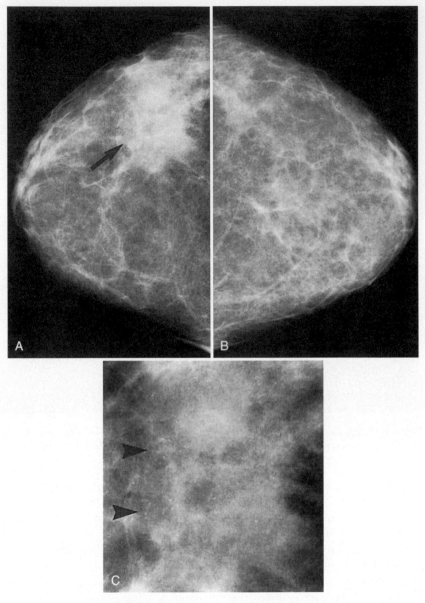

FIG. 31-49 Asymmetric density. **A** and **B,** Craniocaudal mammograms from the screening examination of a 48-year-old woman revealed an asymmetric density *(arrow)* in the right breast. **C,** Magnification mammogram revealed multiple calcifications *(arrowheads)* associated with the asymmetric density. Biopsy revealed invasive ductal carcinoma, not otherwise specified.

findings that would justify a biopsy (Figure 31-49). Ultrasonography is generally not useful for evaluating an area of asymmetric density.[124] Asymmetric breast tissue in the axilla is a common normal variant that should not be mistaken for a significant asymmetric density.[125]

Abnormal Axillary Nodes. Axillary nodes are commonly seen on the MLO view. Normal nodes tend to be oval or kidney-shaped with a central radiolucency (hilar fat) (Figure 31-50). Abnormal nodes are more likely to be round, dense in the center, and larger than 2 cm (Figure 31-51).[126] However, small nodes, even with central radiolucency, can harbor early metastases.

Thus mammography cannot be considered a substitute for axillary node dissection.

SPECIAL SITUATIONS

Inflammatory Carcinoma. Inflammatory carcinoma is a clinical diagnosis based on the findings of an inflamed breast, which may feel hot and heavy to the patient. Inflammatory carcinoma is associated with diffuse skin thickening on mammography and overall increased breast density. The differentiation of mastitis from carcinoma with lymphangitic spread (inflammatory carcinoma) may be difficult. In both conditions, the primary lesion may be completely

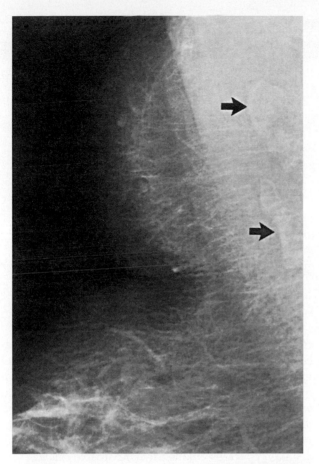

FIG. **31-50** Normal axillary nodes. Close-up of mediolateral oblique mammogram shows normal axillary nodes *(arrows)* with oval shapes and radiolucent fatty centers.

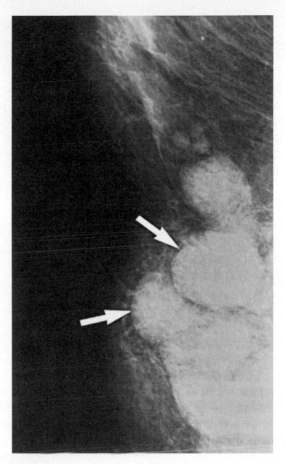

FIG. **31-51** Abnormal lymph nodes. Close-up of mediolateral oblique mammogram shows large, round, dense axillary lymph nodes *(arrows)*. Biopsy revealed metastatic adenocarcinoma from an unknown primary.

obscured by edema. In this situation, abscess may be excluded mammographically only if typical branching malignant calcifications are present. In general, the diagnosis of inflammatory carcinoma is made clinically unless the mammogram reveals an obvious malignancy.

Generalized skin thickening may also be associated with an abscess, progressive systemic sclerosis, obstruction of the superior vena cava, pemphigus, nephrotic syndrome, congestive heart failure, lymphoma, lymphatic extension from contralateral breast carcinoma, or changes secondary to radiotherapy.

Paget's Disease. Paget's disease of the nipple and areola is an uncommon condition in which malignant cells from intraductal or invasive ductal carcinoma migrate to the nipple skin, resulting in a clinical presentation of a chronic, moist, scaly, or erythematous eruption, with symptoms of itching, burning, oozing, or bleeding. These clinicopathologic changes in the nipple are pathognomonic of the early clinical presentation of breast carcinoma. A palpable or mammographically

visible mass may or may not be present. The prognosis of a woman with Paget's disease of the nipple depends on the nature of the underlying carcinoma. Usually the underlying tumor is intraductal, and the patient has an excellent prognosis. Subareolar calcifications of DCIS are sometimes present.

POSITIVE PREDICTIVE VALUE OF MAMMOGRAPHY FOR BREAST CANCER

The *positive predictive value* (PPV) is here defined as the number of cancers found at biopsy divided by the number of biopsies performed. This statistic is also known as the *true-positive biopsy rate* (or *yield*). In the literature, the true-positive biopsy rates for mammographically detected abnormalities are reported at from 10% to 40%.[6,69,70,127-129] In the past, rates as low as 10% were considered appropriate to maximize the number of early cancers detected by screening mammography.[130] However, concern over excessive numbers of false-positive mammograms leading to unnecessary investigations and surgical interventions has kept many

TABLE 31-5	Comparison of Palpable and Nonpalpable Carcinomas in 372 Biopsies		
FEATURE	**PALPABLE (%)**	**NONPALPABLE (%)**	**p VALUES***
Number of cases	143 (38)	229 (62)	—
Number of cancers	48 (34)	72 (31)	.669
Average size of cancer masses [SD]	3.7 cm [3.0]	2.0 cm[†] [1.3]	.239
Median size of malignant masses	2.8 cm	1.5 cm[†]	.183
Cancers with positive axillary nodes	16 (33)	11 (15)	.020
Cancers with distant metastases	5 (10)	0 (0)	—
Noninvasive, ≤1 cm invasive cancers with negative axillary nodes	6 (13)	34 (47)	<.001
Invasive cancers ≤1 cm with negative axillary nodes	4 (8)	11 (15)	.259

Modified from Bassett LW et al: *AJR Am J Roentgenol* 157:21, 1991.
*<.05 (is statistically significant).
†Only 38 of the nonpalpable lesions had a measurable tumor mass; the other 34 were manifested only by calcifications. Therefore the actual average size of nonpalpable cancers was much smaller than 2 cm.

referring physicians from ordering mammography screening.[131] Furthermore, the biopsies performed after screening can become the major cost associated with breast cancer screening with mammography.[132] Radiologists are being encouraged to audit their own practices to determine their true-positive rates, false-negative biopsy rates, and other measures of effectiveness.[133-135]

It is important to be aware of the true positive biopsy rates (sensitivity) for nonpalpable and palpable lesions and the radiologic differences evident for these abnormalities. The results of my (LWB) medical practice audit is consistent with that of others in the literature.[136] The results of 372 biopsies in 346 patients over a 9-year period were reviewed. All of these biopsies were performed by an experienced breast surgeon. Palpable versus nonpalpable lesions were compared for PPV, size of the cancers at time of biopsy, status of the axillary lymph nodes, and presence or absence of distant metastases at the time of biopsy (Table 31-5). Of the 372 biopsies, 143 (38%) were done because of a palpable mass and 229 (62%) because of nonpalpable, mammographically detected abnormalities. Of the 143 biopsies done because of a palpable mass, 48 yielded a primary breast malignancy, for a PPV of 34%. Of the 229 biopsies done because of nonpalpable, mammographically detected abnormalities, 72 revealed a primary breast carcinoma, for a PPV of 31%.

In this review, the histopathologic diagnoses of the nonpalpable carcinomas included 39 invasive ductal carcinomas, 23 noninvasive ductal carcinomas (DCIS), 5 colloid carcinomas, 4 invasive lobular carcinomas, and 1 invasive tubular carcinoma. There was not a significant difference in the PPVs of carcinomas detected for biopsies of palpable versus nonpalpable lesions.

However, mammography detected much smaller cancers overall, and there was a statistically significant greater percentage of cancers detected only with mammography that were noninvasive or invasive and that were 1 cm or smaller with negative axillary lymph nodes (p <.001). There were also fewer carcinomas with positive axillary lymph nodes overall (p = .02) and no distant metastases among the nonpalpable cancers.

Several strategies have been used to reduce the number of avoidable biopsies performed because of false-positive results on screening mammograms. One strategy is to do a complete workup for abnormalities found on screening mammograms, including the appropriate use of magnification mammography and spot compression applied over a suspect area.

Another strategy, the use of sonography for the evaluation of masses, eliminates the need for biopsies of most cysts and may in the future eliminate many other unnecessary biopsies. Although these methods have resulted in a higher PPV for the biopsy of nonpalpable masses, they have been less successful in reducing the number of biopsies for benign calcifications. The true-positive biopsy rates for specific mammographic findings in my (LWB) practice are shown in Table 31-6.

Imaging-Guided Interventional Procedures

A variety of interventional procedures are guided by imaging. The most common of these is prebiopsy needle localization of nonpalpable lesions before excisional biopsy. Fine-needle aspiration cytology (FNAC) and CNB of the breast can also be performed under imaging guidance. In addition, ductography has been used in many practices for the purpose of

| TABLE 31-6 | Positive Predictive Value (PPV) for Specific Mammographic Findings in 229 Biopsies of Nonpalpable Lesions |

FINDING	NUMBER (% OF TOTAL)*	MALIGNANT (PPV)†
Calcifications only	143 (62)	34 (24%)
Mass only	42 (18)	20 (48%)
Mass with calcifications	11 (5)	8 (73%)
Architectural distortion	7 (3)	4 (57%)
Asymmetric density	4 (2)	1 (25%)
Neodensity	22 (10)	5 (23%)
TOTAL	229	72

*Percentage of total cases with this mammographic feature.
†Percentage of total cases with this mammographic feature that proved malignant.

determining the cause of unilateral bloody or serous nipple discharge.

PREBIOPSY NEEDLE LOCALIZATION

Imaging-guided needle localization is indicated before the surgical excision of any nonpalpable mammographic lesion. The purpose of needle localization is to ensure removal of a clinically occult lesion with the smallest possible breast deformity. Some variations on the needle localization method include (1) a direct needle approach in which the tip of a hypodermic needle is inserted as close as possible to the mammographic abnormality and left in place when the patient goes to surgery (see Figure 31-24, A);[137] (2) a "spot" method in which methylene blue dye is injected into the breast tissue through a needle positioned near the mammographic abnormality;[138] and (3) a needle-wire method wherein a malleable wire with a barbed or round end is positioned at the site of the abnormality[139-141] (see Figures 31-46, B, and 31-47). The needle-wire method is most commonly used today.

The prebiopsy localization procedure begins with an evaluation of the abnormality that should include imaging in two orthogonal projections, usually craniocaudal and 90-degree lateral views. Based on the initial films, the location of the lesion and the most appropriate approach to the lesion are determined. A mammogram is performed, with compression sustained while the film is being processed. Using the first film as a guide, the physician determines the location of the lesion relative to a radiopaque alphanumeric grid or holes in the compression device.

The needle is introduced through the skin and advanced to the approximate depth of the lesion. A second mammogram is performed to determine whether the needle is close enough to the lesion. If the needle placement is satisfactory, the modified compression plate is released. An orthogonal view is performed to evaluate the depth of the needle tip relative to the lesion. If the needle tip is too proximal or distal, the depth of the needle tip is adjusted. Once the needle tip is in the desired location, the wire is advanced through the needle until it is firmly in place. In my (LWB) practice, the tip of the wire is positioned slightly posterior and distal to the lesion. The patient is sent to surgery either with the needle removed and a barbed-tip hookwire identifying the site of the lesion or with the needle anchored in place with a J-wire.

Specimen Radiography. Immediately after the surgeon has excised the biopsy specimen, radiographs of the specimen should be performed to verify that the nonpalpable lesion has been removed (see Figure 31-46, B).[142-144] In addition, specimen radiography can help the pathologist focus the histologic examination on the suspect area.

Immediately after inspection of the specimen radiograph and before the specimen is sent to pathology, a pin or 25-gauge needle is inserted into the specimen at the exact site of the lesion. A second specimen radiograph with the pin or needle in place at the site of the lesion is sent to the pathologist along with the specimen. Methods for improving the quality of specimen radiographs include compression of the specimen and magnification mammography.[145] If the suspect lesion is not identified in the specimen radiograph, removal of more tissue is usually indicated.

Lesions containing microcalcifications deserve special consideration. The importance of mentioning the presence of the calcifications in the pathology report should be communicated to pathologists interpreting the breast biopsy. There are two reasons why microcalcifications present in the specimen radiograph might not be mentioned in the pathology report. First, the calcifications might not be seen by the pathologist because they are not in the sectioned tissue. Reevaluation of other sections of the remaining tissue by the pathologist is warranted. Second, calcium oxalate calcifications might not be seen easily with hematoxylin and eosin staining, although they can be appreciated with polarized light.[146] If additional sections and polarized light fail to show calcifications in the histologic sections, radiography of the histologic paraffin blocks may disclose the location of the missing calcifications.[147] Additional sectioning can then be performed. Calcifications may also be lost during the preparation of the specimen; however, a review of the tissue specimens or the paraffin blocks should reveal some remaining calcifications.[148]

IMAGING-GUIDED NEEDLE BIOPSY

It is estimated that some 500,000 to 1 million breast biopsies are performed each year in the United States.[69]

This statistic translates to somewhere between 400,000 to 700,000 benign breast biopsies. In addition to tremendous costs, false-positive biopsies lead to unnecessary morbidity and are a barrier to women participating in breast cancer screening projects.[131] Imaging-guided needle biopsy offers an attractive alternative to surgical biopsy for mammographically detected abnormalities. Needle biopsy is generally less expensive than surgery, results in less morbidity, and leaves no scar. But is it accurate enough to replace surgery? In Europe, *FNAC* has reduced the costs of screening programs by greatly reducing the number of excisional biopsies performed.[149] Although FNAC has been less successful in the United States, CNB of the breast is gaining acceptance in many practices.

Needle biopsy of occult lesions can be guided with stereotactic mammography or ultrasonography. The modality chosen to guide the needle biopsy depends on (1) which technique best depicts the abnormality, (2) the location of the lesion within the breast, and (3) the operator's preferences. Stereotaxis uses the principle of triangulation to ascertain the exact location of an abnormality based on the shift in its position observed on two images taken at different angles off of the midline.[150] Stereotactic equipment includes add-on devices that are mounted on mammography units and dedicated stereotactic biopsy tables. With the add-on devices, the patient usually sits up during the procedure. Following the needle biopsy, the add-on stereotactic device is removed and the mammography unit can be used for screening and diagnostic examinations. With use of the dedicated stereotactic tables, the patient lies prone during the procedure with the breast suspended through an opening in the table. The dedicated tables are more expensive and can be used only for biopsy or localization procedures.

FINE-NEEDLE ASPIRATION CYTOLOGY

FNAC of nonpalpable breast lesions has been very successful in some practices in the United States and Canada,[4,151,152] yet the method has not gained wide acceptance in these countries. Obstacles to the use of FNAC for mammographically detected abnormalities have included inadequate numbers of skilled cytopathologists to promote and validate the procedure, the variability in reported accuracy from one institution to another, the high rates of insufficient samples, the requirement for extremely accurate needle placement, and the medicolegal environment.[153,154] Even if adequate specimens are obtained with FNAC, a definitive diagnosis is not always possible and it cannot differentiate in situ carcinoma from invasive breast carcinoma.

In some practices, a high rate of insufficient specimens has been the major limitation to the use of FNAC for nonpalpable lesions, with insufficient rates as high as 54% reported.[155-158] Methods that can improve the results of FNAC for nonpalpable lesions include (1) more vigorous sampling of lesions, (2) on-site evaluation of specimens by a cytopathologist or a cytotechnologist, (3) exclusive use of stereotactic or ultrasonographic guidance for nonpalpable lesions, (4) a stereotactic equipment calibration program to ensure accurate targeting of lesions, and (5) verification of initial needle placement with stereotactic images before the lesion is sampled.[153] Unfortunately, some of these methods also increase the cost of performing FNAC.

CORE NEEDLE BIOPSY

Several investigators believe that CNB of the breast is superior to FNAC because (1) the interpretation can be rendered by pathologists who do not have special training in cytopathology, (2) insufficient specimens are unusual, (3) CNB can usually differentiate in situ from invasive carcinoma, and (4) CNB can more completely characterize lesions.[8,159] CNB of the breast can be guided with stereotactic mammography or ultrasonography.

Vacuum-Assisted Devices. Limitations of traditional automated Tru-Cut (ATC) CNB include cases with insufficient samples to make a definitive diagnosis and problem histologies, such as a typical ductal hyperplasia and radial scar, for which excisional biopsy is needed to rule out associated malignancy.[160-163] Vacuum-assisted devices (VADs) have been developed to improve tissue sampling by obtaining larger and more intact samples with only one insertion of the biopsy needle.[164] The most important contribution of VADs has been in the evaluation of calcifications, in which cases of sampling errors or indeterminate pathology results are problematic. VAD tissue acquisition devices are available in 14- and 11-gauge sizes. Comparisons with ATC show improvements in most aspects, including few insufficient samples and discordant pathology. However, larger sample size has not reduced the incidence of carcinoma in situ found at excisional biopsy following a core biopsy diagnosis of atypical ductal hyperplasia (ADH).[165] VADs have recently been made available for ultrasound-guided biopsy. The exact benefits of ultrasound-guided biopsy remain to be determined.

Indications for Core Biopsy. Whereas there is general agreement that CNB is indicated when mammographic findings are suspect for malignancy (BI-RADS category 4), there are differences of opinion about the use of CNB for abnormalities that are probably benign (category 3) and highly suggestive of malignancy (category 5). Some investigators have asserted that probably benign lesions are good candidates for CNB, because needle biopsy of these lesions might uncover breast cancers when they are smaller and patients thus have a better prognosis.[166] However, the expected yield of breast cancers from cases with probably benign findings is very low.[71,73] One report suggests that subjecting the large number of women with probably benign findings to needle biopsy would undermine efforts to reduce the costs of screening mammography and could actually increase the overall costs of screening.[167] In my (LWB) practice, CNB for probably benign findings are limited to women who are too anxious to wait for a follow-up examination to confirm benignity. Only 2% of CNBs have been performed for probably benign findings, and none of these have revealed carcinoma.

Some investigators believe that CNB is inappropriate for lesions that are highly suggestive of malignancy. An example is an irregular, spiculated, dense mass. Because malignancy is almost certain with such as a mass, the surgeon may choose to discuss treatment options with the patient based on the imaging findings and proceed directly to one-stage surgery. The one-stage procedure for nonpalpable lesions that are highly suggestive of malignancy includes excision of the lesion, frozen section to confirm the diagnosis of malignancy, and definitive surgery once the frozen section is shown to be positive for cancer.

The one-stage operation reduces costs by eliminating a separate biopsy for tissue diagnosis.[168] Nevertheless, some surgeons routinely perform a two-stage procedure for lesions that are mammographically highly suggestive of malignancy. After a separate biopsy to confirm the diagnosis, these surgeons discuss options for treatment with the patient and schedule definitive surgery. CNB is cost effective for lesions that are highly suggestive of malignancy only if a two-stage procedure is planned.

Analysis of Data and Management of CNB Cases.
It is important that physicians performing CNB collect and analyze their results to evaluate the effectiveness of the procedure. This means determining the number of true-positive, false-positive, true-negative, and false-negative biopsy results. A true-positive CNB result is one that is correctly interpreted to be intraductal or invasive carcinoma and confirmed as one or the other at subsequent surgery. A false-positive CNB result is one that is incorrectly interpreted as showing carcinoma, and carcinoma is not found at excisional biopsy. Long-term follow-up is usually required to verify true-negative results, but the exact length of follow-up required to verify a true-negative result is not yet standardized. Some investigators define long-term follow-up as 1 year, whereas others define it as 2 years.

High-risk lesions, such as lobular carcinoma in situ (LCIS) and ADH, are considered benign for statistical and medical audit purposes.[123,136] However, many physicians recommend open biopsy after a CNB diagnosis of LCIS or ADH.[169] If ADH is diagnosed based on CNB results, an excisional biopsy is recommended because of the difficulty in differentiating ADH from intraductal carcinoma on the basis of CNB.[170] In reported series, 50% of cases originally interpreted as ADH based on CNB results have turned out to be intraductal carcinoma at excisional biopsy.[170,171]

There are some contraindications to CNB. Certain mammographic findings indicate a condition best managed with complete excision. For example, if calcifications are few in number and not tightly clustered, CNB sampling errors are highly likely to occur. There are also limitations related to the location of the lesion or the size of the breast. A lesion very close to the skin or located in a very small breast may not be suitable for CNB because of the required throw of the needle. It may not be possible to visualize lesions adjacent to the chest wall on a stereotactic biopsy unit. If these lesions are not depicted on ultrasonography, they require excisional biopsy.

DUCTOGRAPHY (GALACTOGRAPHY)

Ductography is the injection of contrast medium into the lactiferous ducts in an attempt to preoperatively determine the nature, location, and extent of lesions causing serous or bloody discharge. A serous or bloody discharge from the nipple may be caused by an intraductal papilloma (Figure 31-52), "fibrocystic changes,"

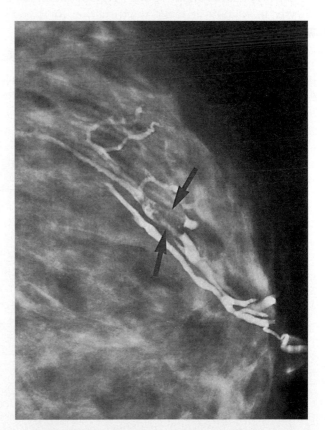

FIG. **31-52** Ductogram demonstrating solitary papilloma. A 50-year-old woman presented with bloody discharge from the left nipple. A ductogram revealed a filling defect *(arrows)* in the discharging duct system. Surgery revealed a benign solitary papilloma at the site of the defect.

duct ectasia, or carcinoma. Although bloody nipple discharge is usually associated with benign conditions, approximately 15% of these cases are secondary to carcinoma.[172] Ductography is not useful in cases of discharge from multiple orifices or discharge of milky or greenish color.

During the procedure, the duct that is discharging is cannulated and a small volume of water-soluble contrast material is injected. Mammograms are then taken in two projections, preferably with magnification mammography technique. When a filling defect is demonstrated, the ductogram may be repeated shortly before surgery using a mixture of methylene blue dye and contrast material. The blue dye identifies the abnormal duct, and the contrast medium verifies that the duct contains the filling defect.[173]

Ductography is effective in showing the cause of the discharge in almost all cases. Only half of the carcinomas demonstrated by filling defects on ductography are evident on conventional mammograms, and cytologic analysis is even more unreliable in identifying malignant cells in the fluid from these cancers.[172]

Some surgeons believe that preoperative ductography allows them to do less radical surgery for serous or bloody nipple discharge.[174] Other surgeons prefer to go directly to solitary or major duct excision for bloody nipple discharge.

ULTRASONOGRAPHY

In the early 1950s the breast was one of the first organs to be examined with ultrasonography.[175] Later, a number of ultrasonographers developed equipment especially for breast imaging.[176,177] After encouraging results, some ultrasonographers advocated the method for breast cancer screening, suggesting it was as effective as mammography.[176-179] Subsequent investigators could not reproduce these results and found that ultrasonography was inferior to mammography for the detection of early breast cancer masses.[180,181] In addition, ultrasonography could not reliably detect microcalcifications, the hallmark of intraductal carcinoma. Nonetheless, ultrasonography was very accurate in the diagnosis of cysts, eliminating the need for about 20% of the biopsies that had been performed in the past (see Figure 31-18, B).[76]

Ultrasound was eventually recognized to be an important adjunct to mammography, but its role was primarily limited to determining whether nonpalpable masses were cystic or solid.[9,182,183] With the evolution of ultrasonographic technology, including the introduction of higher-resolution transducers and imagng protocols tailored for the breast, there has been a renewed interest in expanding the role of ultrasonography for the evaluation of breast diseases. Ultrasonography is an excellent method for guiding some interventional procedures (Figure 31-53).[4,184,185] Although ultrasonography is not recommended for breast cancer screening, there are reliable ultrasonographic criteria that can differentiate benign from malignant solid masses.[11] In some practices, it is used to identify occult multicentric or bilateral disease in women with a mammographically or clinically evident

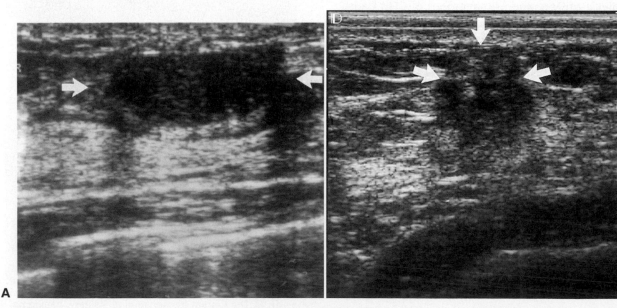

A   B

FIG. 31-53 Ultrasonography of fibroadenoma versus carcinoma. A, The fibroadenoma (arrows) has an oval shape with width greater than height, circumscribed margins, and homogeneous low-level echoes. B, The invasive carcinoma (arrows) has an irregular shape, ill-defined margins, and heterogeneous echogenicity.

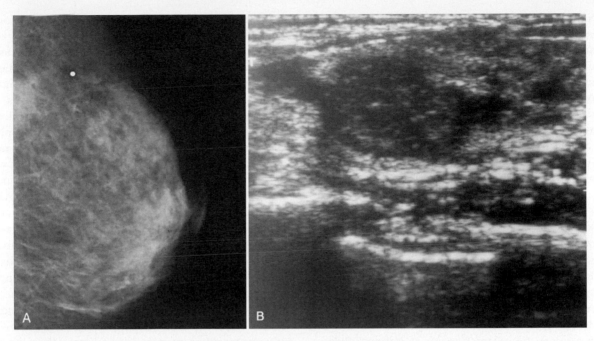

FIG. **31-54** Ultrasonography of carcinoma. A 60-year-old woman felt a firm mass in her left breast. **A,** Mammogram shows a poorly defined density posterior to radiopaque BB placed at the site of the palpable mass. **B,** Ultrasonography shows a lobulated, partially ill-defined mass with heterogeneous low-level echoes. Biopsy revealed invasive ductal carcinoma.

breast carcinoma.[185] These newer roles for ultrasonography have not yet been widely accepted.[186]

Criteria for differentiating benign from malignant solid masses with ultrasonography are of special interest. Ultrasonographic features suggesting benignity include the absence of malignant findings; ellipsoid shape (a length along the plane of the breast that is greater than the height of the mass); thin, echogenic pseudocapsule (circumscribed margins); hyperechogenicity (bright ultrasound echoes); homogeneous internal echoes; and enhanced echoes distal to the mass (see Figure 31-53, *A*).[11] Features suggesting malignancy include an irregular shape, indistinct margins, spiculation, microlobulation, a height that is greater than the width of the lesion in the plane of the breast (Figure 31-53, *B*), hypoechogenicity, and shadowing (attenuation of echoes distal to the mass) (Figures 31-54 and 31-55). Ultrasonography can also be used to evaluate the integrity of silicone breast implants.[187] However, it is not as accurate as MRI for detecting implant ruptures.[188]

OTHER BREAST IMAGING TECHNOLOGIES

Digital Mammography. Digital mammography is a type of mammography that records the radiographic image electronically in a digital format rather than directly on film. The image is kept in a digital format in a computer and can either be displayed on a florescent monitor or be transferred to a hard copy (film). It is hoped that digital mammography will eventually solve

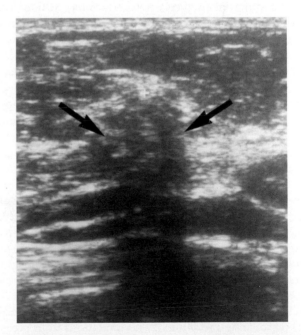

FIG. **31-55** Ultrasonography of carcinoma. A 46-year-old woman noted a mass in her left breast. Mammograms were negative. Ultrasonography showed an irregular, poorly defined mass *(arrows)* with low-level internal echoes. Note the marked posterior echo attenuation ("posterior shadowing"). Biopsy revealed invasive ductal carcinoma.

many of the problems inherent in film mammography, such as limited contrast, film storage, and lost films.[78]

Potential advantages of digital studies are the ability to do image manipulation on the display monitor, to use computer-aided diagnosis, and to transmit the images over long distances (teleradiography).[189] *Computer-aided diagnosis* refers to the use of a computer to assist in interpretation by scanning images for abnormalities or using artificial intelligence to determine the probability of malignancy.[190-192] The ability of teleradiography to send digital images over long distances opens the possibilities for greater access to previous studies and consultations with experts.[193]

Magnetic Resonance Imaging. The first reports on MRI for the evaluation of breast cancer in the mid-1980s were focused on breast tissue characterization using T_1- and T_2-weighted images.[194] These early investigations were disappointing. Heywang and co-workers[195] and Heywang-Kobrunner[196] first applied the use of magnetic resonance contrast agents to improve differentiation of benign from malignant lesions. The results were encouraging; most malignant tumors showed enhancement, and most benign tumors did not. Several other investigators have confirmed the value of contrast-enhanced MRI.[197,198] Clinical investigations show a range of sensitivities, from 88% to 100%.[199,200] However, the specificity of MRI may be relatively low, because many benign lesions show contrast enhancement.[196,197,201]

Two different methods for performing MRI of the breast for the assessment of breast tumors with gadolinium enhancement are emerging: (1) two-dimensional, medium-resolution imaging during gadolinium enhancement and (2) three-dimensional, high-resolution imaging after gadolinium enhancement. Proponents of the two-dimensional approach believe that the most useful information concerning breast lesions is the time course of gadolinium enhancement; malignant tumors enhance more rapidly and more intensely than benign tumors. Yet some investigators have shown an overlap in the enhancement patterns of malignant and benign breast tumors. Those advocating three-dimensional, high-resolution imaging believe it to be more effective because whole-breast images are obtained, allowing for the detection of multicentric lesions (Figure 31-56). Furthermore, with three-dimensional, whole-breast imaging, it is not necessary to know the site of the abnormality before beginning the examination.

The potential advantages of MRI of the breast include (1) no ionizing radiation; (2) no limitations from breast density; (3) ability to localize lesions seen on only one mammographic projection; (4) better characterization of lesions as benign or malignant; (5) improved evaluation of the extent of tumors, including multiple foci; and (6) surveillance of the postlumpectomy breast, which can be difficult to evaluate mammographically.

There are also a number of disadvantages associated with MRI: (1) cost; (2) unreliable depiction of microcalcifications; (3) lack of standardization of magnetic resonance sequences and methodologies used to image breast tumors; (4) inability to complete an MRI scan in some patients because of claustrophobia or indwelling metal devices, such as pacemakers and aneurysm clips.

Radionuclide Imaging. Another area of active investigation involves radionuclide scanning of the breast after the injection of radionuclide-labeled substances that concentrate in breast tumors. For example, tumor uptake has been identified on positron emission tomography after the injection of fluorine-18 2-deoxy-2-fluoro-D-glucose.[202] This agent also accumulates in axillary nodes, thus potentially indicating nodal status without surgery being necessary. Other investigators are scanning the breasts after the injection of technetium ^{99m}Tc-sestamibi (2-methoxy isobutyl isonitrile)[203,204] (Figure 31-57). Sestamibi has been reported to have a high sensitivity and high negative predictive value for breast carcinoma. The high negative predictive value of this agent could make it an important adjunct to mammography by potentially reducing the number of biopsies done for benign findings. Additional studies are needed to determine cost-effectiveness and sensitivity and specificity in actual clinical populations.

STAGING AND FOLLOW-UP OF WOMEN WITH BREAST CANCER

Follow-up of the Conservatively Treated Breast. Follow-up evaluation after initial treatment with breast conservation surgery, with or without adjuvant systemic therapy, consists of a mammogram before starting radiation therapy.[205] The preradiotherapy mammogram is most useful for women with extensive in situ (intraductal) carcinoma or the invasive carcinoma that coexists with an EIC; these pathologic variants are often detectable by visible calcifications mammographically (see Figures 31-46 and 31-47).[107] Preoperative mammography and specimen radiography performed at the time of surgery are essential to document that calcifications were present and that calcifications were indeed removed. However, specimen radiography is not reliable in determining whether all of the tumor was removed.[117]

It has been recommended that mammograms be done at 6-month intervals for 2 years after lumpectomy and radiotherapy and annually thereafter.[81,206] On mammograms, recurrent carcinoma can be manifested by a

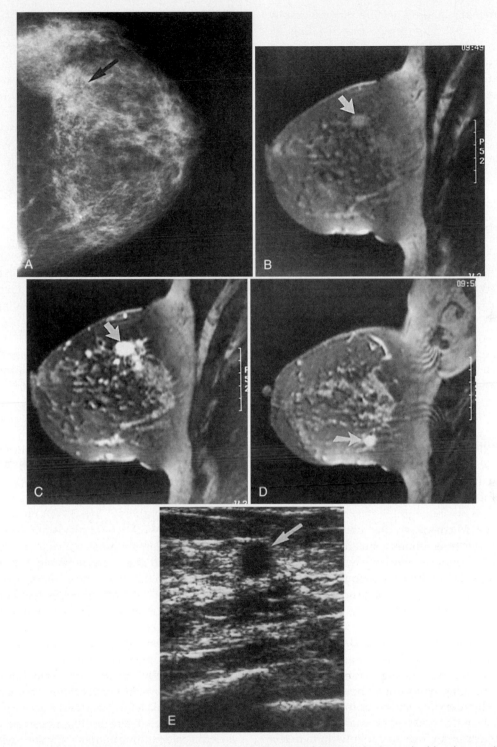

FIG. **31-56** Magnetic resonance imaging (MRI) of the breast. A 45-year-old woman had a palpable abnormality in the upper outer quadrant of her left breast. **A,** Left craniocaudal view shows an architectural distortion *(arrow)* at the site of the palpable abnormality. Precontrast **(B)** and postcontrast **(C)** sagittal T_1-weighted fat saturation three-dimensional, high-resolution MRI images show intense enhancement of the abnormal area *(arrow)* on postcontrast images. **D,** Postcontrast sagittal MRI images reveal a second lesion *(arrow),* inferior and medial to the first lesion, with intense contrast enhancement. **E,** Ultrasonography confirmed the presence of the second lesion *(arrow),* which had irregular margins. Fine-needle aspiration of the palpable abnormality and ultrasound-guided core needle biopsy of the nonpalpable lesion revealed multicentric invasive ductal carcinoma.

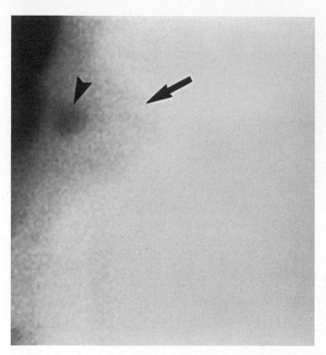

FIG. **31-57** Sestamibi radionuclide imaging of the breast *(arrow)* reveals intense radionuclide uptake at the site of a breast carcinoma *(arrowhead). (Courtesy Iraj Khalkhali, M.D., Los Angeles, CA.)*

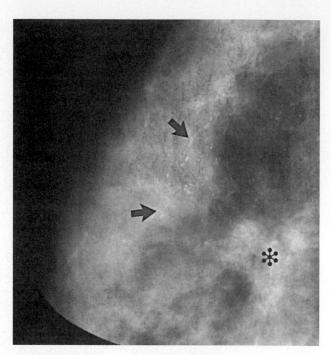

FIG. **31-58** Recurrent breast carcinoma. Close-up of mammogram performed 3 years after lumpectomy shows calcifications *(arrows)* near the intramammary surgical scar.*

mass or calcifications (Figure 31-58). The importance of 6-month interval mammography is not universally accepted. More clinical investigation is needed to determine whether annual mammography would suffice.[207]

Follow-up after Mastectomy. For patients who are treated with mastectomy, routine imaging follow-up involves annual mammography of the contralateral breast. Mammography of the mastectomy site is not believed to have clinical utility because it does not increase the detection of locally recurrent disease.[208]

Evaluation for Metastases from Breast Cancer. The most common sites for distant metastases from breast carcinoma are the skeleton, lung, liver, and brain.[209,210] Several imaging examinations are available that can potentially identify metastases to these organs. Surveys of patients with breast cancer indicate that most of these patients prefer an intensive follow-up to detect asymptomatic disease, including metastases.[211] Surveys of physicians who care for breast cancer patients indicate that most of these physicians also favor intensive surveillance programs of breast cancer patients who are asymptomatic.[212] However, for purposes of cost-effectiveness, there should be a reasonable anticipated yield and an expected effect on patient management and outcome when imaging examinations are ordered on asymptomatic breast cancer patients.

Several large, population-based studies have revealed that metastatic workups for stage I or II breast cancer are not cost effective because of the low yield of the examination and the lack of a proven effect on management or survival.[213-215] My (LWB) current policy is to limit imaging workups for metastatic disease to women with stage III carcinoma, in which (1) the tumor is larger than 5 cm and there are movable ipsilateral positive axillary nodes, (2) the invasive tumor is associated with positive ipsilateral axillary nodes fixed one to another or to other structures, or (3) the tumor has direct extension to the chest wall or skin.[213] These women receive a bone scan, chest radiographs, and if liver function tests are abnormal, imaging of the liver.

Skeletal Metastases. Radionuclide scanning is more effective than conventional radiography for the detection of skeletal metastases because radionuclide scans have higher sensitivity and can survey the entire skeleton in one examination (Figure 31-59).[216] Despite the low yield of bone scans in asymptomatic women with stage I or II breast carcinoma, many clinicians have continued to recommend *baseline* bone scans on the basis that they could be useful for comparison with subsequent scans performed if symptoms develop or abnormal results are later obtained on a routine scan.[217] Routine baseline bone scans are unlikely to be useful in patients with stage I or II disease in view of (1) the small number of patients who will later have positive scans

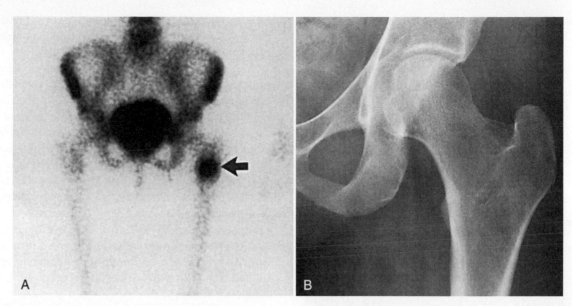

FIG. **31-59** High sensitivity of radionuclide scans. Radionuclide scan was performed in a woman with diagnosed stage III breast carcinoma. **A,** ^{99m}Tc radionuclide bone scan shows abnormal area of intense radionuclide uptake *(arrow)* in the proximal left femur. Additional intense radionuclide activity in the bladder and iliac wings is normal. **B,** Radiograph shows no evidence of a lesion in the femur. Needle biopsy confirmed metastasis.

and (2) evidence from long-term clinical trials indicating that earlier detection of metastases does not reduce overall mortality.[218-221] Furthermore, several studies have reported the problem of false-positive bone scans when screening for metastases in asymptomatic patients.[221]

In my (LWB) practice, ^{99m}Tc-diphosphonate whole-body radionuclide scans are performed on symptomatic patients or asymptomatic patients with stage III disease. Although bone scans are sensitive for the detection of metastases, many benign conditions can result in abnormal scan results. Correlation of clinical, radionuclide, and radiographic findings is important when imaging studies are performed. Therefore, unless the findings from the bone scan are definitive for metastases, radiographs of symptomatic regions or localized areas of abnormal isotope accumulation should be performed. Breast metastases to the skeleton may show unusual radiographic manifestations, and it is important to be aware of these findings to avoid an incorrect diagnosis (Figures 31-60 to 31-64). MRI can be useful when the findings of radionuclide scans and radiographs are discordant or indeterminate (Figure 31-65).[222]

Lung Metastases. Because of its relatively low cost compared with the other imaging modalities, conventional chest radiography is the most reasonable approach to (1) detect unsuspected disease, (2) serve as a baseline for monitoring, and (3) be used for routine

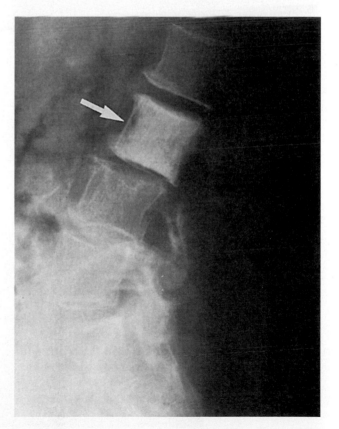

FIG. **31-60** Blastic metastasis *(arrow)* to spine from breast carcinoma. "Ivory vertebrae" can also be seen in Paget's disease, lymphoma, and hemangioma.

follow-up.[223] Signs of metastatic breast carcinoma include pulmonary nodules, adenopathy, lymphangitic spread, and pleural masses or effusions (Figures 31-66 and 31-67). High-resolution computed tomography (CT) is the method of choice to evaluate equivocal findings on chest radiography and to identify additional nodules in cases of positive results (see Figure 31-67).[224]

Investigators have questioned the use of routine chest radiography to detect intrathoracic metastases in asymptomatic breast cancer patients, especially those with stage I disease, despite the relatively low cost of chest radiography. One problem is the low yield of routine chest radiographs in patients with stage I disease, reported at less than 0.5% in asymptomatic women who had routine chest radiographs after the diagnosis of stage I breast carcinoma.[218] Another problem is that false-positive results from chest radiographs can lead to expensive diagnostic workups.[225,226] Two large, randomized controlled studies failed to show a significant outcome benefit when routine chest radiography was used to detect metastases earlier in women with various stages of carcinoma.[214,218]

Liver Metastases. Both radionuclide scanning and ultrasonography have been used to detect liver metastases. Although liver metastases are not as common as lung or bone metastases, they are associated with a worse prognosis.[210] To be detected reliably with [99mTc]-sulfur colloid liver scans, metastases generally must be larger than 2 cm.[227] Ultrasonography can also identify liver metastases 2 cm or larger, and it is often used to localize these lesions for biopsy or FNAC.[228,229]

As with screening for bone and lung metastases, the yield of screening for liver metastases with radionuclide scans or ultrasonography is low. In one retrospective

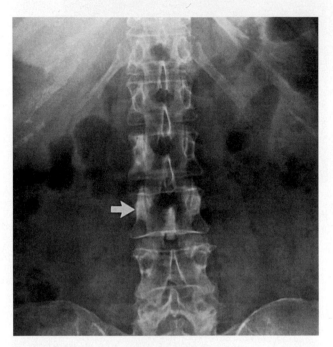

FIG. **31-61** Breast cancer blastic metastasis *(arrow)* to pedicle of L3.

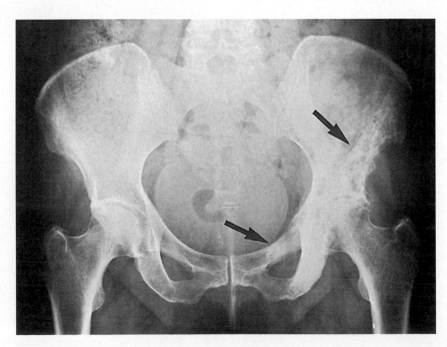

FIG. **31-62** Mixed lytic and blastic metastases *(arrows)* to the left pelvis in a woman with breast cancer who was complaining of pain in the left hip.

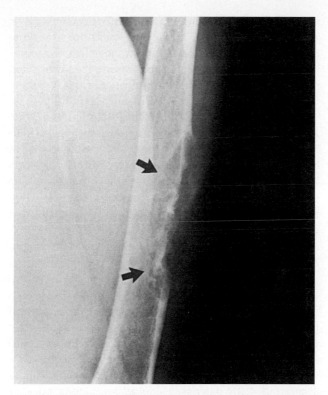

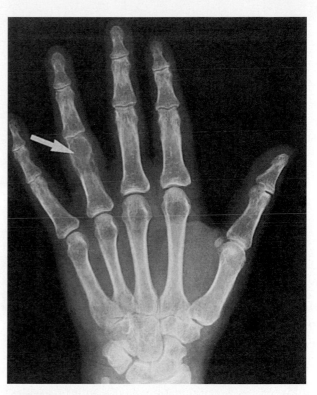

FIG. **31-63** Lytic expansile cortical metastasis *(arrow)* in the femur of a woman with breast cancer. Metastases usually involve the medullary canal, and this is an unusual finding that can occur with breast cancer.

FIG. **31-64** Lytic breast cancer metastasis *(arrow)* to proximal phalanx of hand. It is unusual for metastases to occur in the hands or feet, locations that suggest breast, lung, or renal carcinoma.

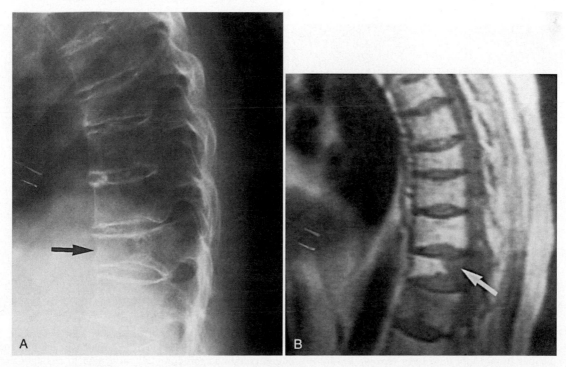

FIG. **31-65** Magnetic resonance imaging (MRI) of metastases. A 70-year-old woman with breast cancer complained of back pain. **A,** Lateral radiograph of the thoracic spine reveals a compressed vertebra *(arrow)*, which could be due to osteoporosis or metastasis. **B,** Sagittal T$_1$-weighted MRI reveals loss of normal high signal intensity of the bone marrow in the posterior aspect of the compressed vertebra *(arrow)*, which is indicative of a metastatic lesion.

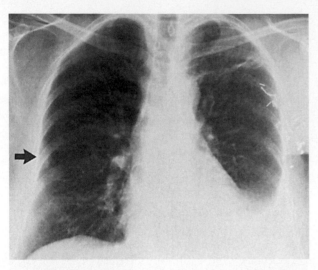

FIG. **31-66** Chest radiograph of a woman with metastatic breast carcinoma shows metallic clips from previous left axillary node dissection, scarring of the left upper lobe, malignant left pleural effusion, and right pleural metastasis (arrow).

scans were eventually determined to be falsely positive. Another study showed that the yield for detecting metastases using radionuclide scans or ultrasonography was less than 0.5%.[218] Large, randomized controlled studies have also failed to show a benefit from screening with ultrasonography for liver metastases.[214,215]

CT and MRI are more sensitive than radionuclide imaging or ultrasonography in the detection of liver metastases.[231] CT scans of the liver should be done both before and after intravenous contrast injection because some breast metastases may show up on one of these examinations but not the other (Figures 31-68 and 31-69). There is no evidence in the literature that routine imaging of the liver with either CT or MRI has clinical utility in asymptomatic patients with breast carcinoma.

Brain Metastases. Breast cancer is second only to lung carcinoma as a cause of intracerebral and orbital metastases, but few patients have brain metastases at the time of breast cancer diagnosis, especially when the tumor is detected at stage I or II.[232,233] In CT examinations, brain metastases may be nodular or ring-shaped, single or multiple. Brain metastases are usually associated with extensive edema and show varying amounts of enhancement with intravenous contrast agents.[234] One review of breast cancer patients at all stages who were undergoing radionuclide brain

study of 234 asymptomatic patients with breast carcinoma at various stages, preoperative radionuclide liver scanning identified metastases in only 1% of the patients.[230] Furthermore, in that study, 8 of 11 positive

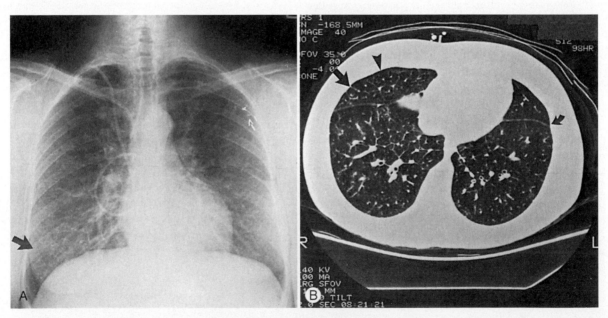

FIG. **31-67** A 52-year-old woman with a history of breast cancer came to her physician complaining of increasing dyspnea. **A,** A chest radiograph in the hospital revealed changes from previous axillary node dissection and mild reticulation of the lungs, most conspicuous in the right lung base (arrow). **B,** High-resolution computed tomography, performed to evaluate for possible lymphangitic spread of breast cancer, shows prominence of the interlobular septae (small arrow) and centrilobular interstitium (arrowhead). There is also subtle beading of the interfissural surfaces (arrow). These changes were considered diagnostic for lymphangitic carcinomatosis.

the detection of brain metastases.[237] Despite these improvements in the sensitivity of imaging modalities for the detection of cerebral metastases, there are no studies suggesting any usefulness in routine imaging with any modality for the detection of cerebral metastases in asymptomatic women with breast carcinoma.

Quality-of-Life Issues. One large, randomized controlled study investigated quality-of-life issues related to surveillance for metastatic disease in breast cancer patients.[215] The results suggested that type of follow-up (i.e., intensive surveillance versus routine clinical management) does not affect various dimensions of health-related quality of life. These dimensions include overall health and quality-of-life perception, emotional well-being, body image, social functioning, symptoms, and satisfaction with health care. These parameters were almost identical between intensive and clinical only surveillance groups. No comparison differences in any of the dimensions of quality-of-life issues were statistically significant between the two groups. Nonetheless, more than 70% of the breast cancer subjects said they wanted to be seen frequently by a physician and undergo diagnostic tests even if they were free of symptoms. This preference for intensive surveillance was not affected by whether the patient had been assigned to the intensive or minimalist follow-up regimen. Education of both physicians and patients seems to be an issue of extreme importance to provide cost-effective follow-up management of patients with breast cancer.

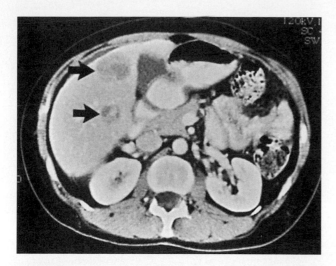

FIG. **31-68** A 40-year-old woman with diagnosed stage III breast carcinoma had abnormal liver function tests. Intravenous contrast-enhanced computed tomography image of the liver shows two hypodense lesions *(arrows)* from metastatic breast carcinoma.

scanning and CT scanning found that imaging studies failed to identify brain metastases in the absence of neurologic symptoms.[235]

Because of its greater sensitivity, MRI has largely replaced CT scanning for the detection and evaluation of brain lesions.[236] Contrast-enhanced MRI further increases the number of suspected cerebral metastases that can be detected.[232] Contrast-enhanced MRI has also proved superior to double-dose delayed CT for

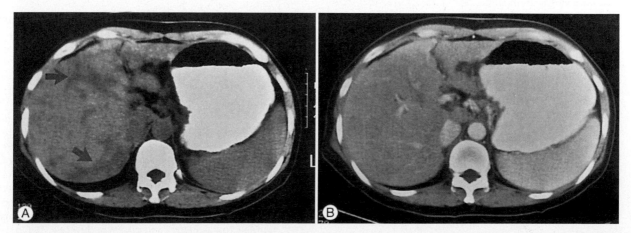

FIG. **31-69** A 53-year-old woman with stage III breast carcinoma had abnormal liver function tests. **A,** Precontrast computed tomography (CT) scan of the liver shows inhomogeneous hypodense zones *(arrows)* caused by metastatic breast carcinoma. **B,** Intravenous contrast-enhanced CT scan of same patient. The vascular metastases were masked by the contrast agent.

REFERENCES

1. Bassett LW, Gold RH, Kimme-Smith C: History of the technical development of mammography in syllabus. In Haus AG, Yaffe MJ (eds): *RSNA categorical course in physics,* Oak Brook, IL, 1994, Radiological Society of North America.

2. Hendrick RE: Quality assurance in mammography: accreditation, legislation, and compliance with quality assurance standards, *Radiol Clin North Am* 30:243, 1992.

3. American College of Radiology (ACR): *Breast imaging reporting and data system (BI-RADS™),* Reston, VA, 1993, ACR.

4. Fornage BD, Coan JD, David CL: Ultrasound-guided needle biopsy of the breast and other interventional procedures, *Radiol Clin North Am* 30:167, 1992.

5. Homer MJ: Localization of nonpalpable breast lesions: technical aspects and analysis of 80 cases, *AJR Am J Roentgenol* 140:807, 1983.

6. Homer MJ, Smith TH, Safaii H: Prebiopsy needle localization, *Radiol Clin North Am* 30:139, 1992.

7. Jackson VP, Bassett LW: Stereotactic fine-needle aspiration biopsy for nonpalpable breast lesions, *AJR Am J Roentgenol* 154:1196, 1990.

8. Parker SH et al: Stereotactic breast biopsy with a biopsy gun, *Radiology* 176:741, 1990.

9. Bassett LW et al: Automated and hand-held breast ultrasound: effect on patient management, *Radiology* 165:103, 1987.

10. Fornage BD: Percutaneous biopsies of the breast: state-of-the-art, *Cardiovasc Intervent Radiol* 14:29, 1991.

11. Stavros AT et al: Solid breast nodules: use of sonography to distinguish between benign and malignant lesions, *Radiology* 196:123, 1995.

12. Shen Y, Zelen M: Screening sensitivity and sojourn time from breast cancer early detection clinical trials: mammograms and physical examinations, *J Clin Oncol* 19:3490, 2001.

13. Parker SL et al: Cancer statistics, 1996, *CA Cancer J Clin* 65:5, 1996.

14. Seidman H, Stellman SD, Mushinski MH: A different perspective on breast cancer risk factors: some implications for the nonattributable risk, *CA Cancer J Clin* 32:301, 1982.

15. Fletcher SW et al: Report of the International Workshop on Screening for Breast Cancer, *J Natl Cancer Inst* 85:1644, 1993.

16. Tabár L et al: Reduction in mortality from breast cancer after mass screening with mammography: randomised trial from the Breast Cancer Screening Working Group of the Swedish National Board of Health and Welfare, *Lancet* 1:829, 1985.

17. Howe HL et al: Annual report to the nation on the status of cancer (1973 through 1998), featuring cancers with recent increasing trends, *J Natl Cancer Inst* 93:824, 2001.

18. Tabar L et al: Beyond randomized controlled trials: organized mammographic screening substantially reduces breast carcinoma mortality, *Cancer* 91:1724, 2001.

19. Blanks RG et al: Effect of NHS breast screening programme on mortality fro.n breast cancer in England and Wales, 1990-8: comparison of observed with predicted mortality, *BMJ* 321:665, 2000.

20. Fracheboud J et al: Interval cancers in the Dutch breast cancer screening programme, *Br J Cancer* 81:912, 1999.

21. Baum M: Screening mammography re-evaluated, *Lancet* 355:751, 2000.

22. Peto R et al: UK and USA breast cancer deaths down 25% in year 2000 at ages 20-69 years, *Lancet* 355:1822, 2000.

23. Feig SA: Mammography screening: published guidelines and actual practice, *Recent Results Cancer Res* 105:78, 1987.

24. Feig SA: Screening guidelines and controversies. In Bassett LW et al (eds): *Diagnosis of diseases of the breast,* Philadelphia, 1997, WB Saunders.

25. Shapiro S et al: *Periodic screening for breast cancer: the Health Insurance Plan project and its sequelae, 1963-1986,* Baltimore, 1988, Johns Hopkins University Press.

26. Feig SA et al: Analysis of clinically occult and mammographically occult breast tumors, *AJR Am J Roentgenol* 128:403, 1977.

27. Shapiro S et al: Ten- to fourteen-year effect of screening on breast cancer mortality, *J Natl Cancer Inst* 69:349, 1982.

28. Feig SA: Methods to identify benefit from mammographic screening of women aged 40-69 years, *Radiology* 201:309, 1996.

29. Smart CR et al: Benefit of mammography screening in women ages 40-49 years, *Cancer* 75:1619, 1995.

30. Sirovich BE, Sox HC: Breast cancer screening, *Surg Clin North Am* 79:961, 1999.

31. Kopans DB, Halpern E, Hulka CA: Statistical power in breast cancer screening trials and mortality reduction among women 40-49 years of age with particular emphasis on the National Breast Screening Study of Canada, *Cancer* 74:1196, 1994.

32. Feig SA: Estimation of currently attainable benefit from mammographic screening of women aged 40-49 years, *Cancer* 75:2412, 1995.

33. Moskowitz M: Retrospective reviews of breast cancer screening: what do we really learn from them? *Radiology* 199:615, 1996.

34. Miller AB et al: Canadian National Breast Screening Study. 1. Breast cancer detection and death rates among women aged 40-49 years, *Can Med Assoc J* 147:1459, 1992.

35. Elwood JM, Cox B, Richardson AK: The effectiveness of breast cancer screening by mammography in younger women, *Online J Curr Clin Trials* Doc No 32, 1993.

36. Sickles EA, Kopans DB: Deficiencies in the analysis of breast cancer screening data, *J Natl Cancer Inst* 85:1621, 1993.

37. Volkers N: NCI replaces guidelines with statement of evidence, *J Natl Cancer Inst* 86:14, 1994.

38. Burhenne LJW, Burhenne HJ: The Canadian National Breast Screening Study: a Canadian critique, *AJR Am J Roentgenol* 161:761, 1993.

39. Baines CJ et al: Canadian National Breast Screening Study: assessment of technical quality by external review, *AJR Am J Roentgenol* 155:743, 1990.

40. Thurfjell EL, Lindgren JAA: Breast cancer survival rates with mammographic screening: similar favorable survival rates for women younger and those older than 50 years, *Radiology* 201:421, 1996.

41. Tabar L, Duffy SW, Chen HH: Re: quantitative interpretation of age-specific mortality reductions from the Swedish Breast Cancer Screening Trials, *J Natl Cancer Inst* 88:52, 1996.

42. Smart CR: Highlights of the evidence of benefit for women aged 40-49 years from the 14-year follow-up of the Breast Cancer Detection Demonstration Project, *Cancer* 74:296, 1994.

43. Swedish Cancer Society and the Swedish National Board of Health and Welfare: Breast-cancer screening with mammography in women aged 40-49 years, *Int J Cancer* 68:693, 1996.

44. Hendrick RE et al: Benefit of screening mammography in women aged 40-49: a new meta-analysis of randomized controlled trials, *J Natl Cancer Inst Monogr* 22:87, 1997.

45. National Institutes of Health Consensus Development Panel: National Institutes of Health Consensus Development Conference Statement: breast cancer screening for women ages 40-49, *J Natl Cancer Inst Monogr* 89:1015, 1997.

46. National Cancer Advisory Board: *Mammography recommendations for women 40-49*, Bethesda, MD, 1997, National Cancer Institute.

47. Feig SA: Determination of mammographic screening intervals with surrogate measures for women aged 40-49 years, *Radiology* 193:311, 1994.

48. Woloshin S et al: Women's understanding of the mammography screening debate, *Arch Intern Med* 160:1434, 2000.

49. UK Trial of Early Detection of Breast Cancer Group: 16-year mortality from breast cancer in the UK trial of Early Detection of Breast Cancer, *Lancet* 353:1909, 1999.

50. Alexander FE, Anderson TJ, Brown HK: 14 years of follow-up from the Edinburgh randomised trial of breast-cancer screening, *Lancet* 353:1903, 1999.

51. Morimoto T et al: Breast cancer screening by mammography in women aged under 50 years in Japan, *Anticancer Res* 20:3689, 2000.

52. Byers T et al: The American Cancer Society Challenge Goals: how far can cancer rates decline in the U.S. by the year 2015? *Cancer* 86:715, 1999.

53. Cady B, Michaelson JS: The life-sparing potential of mammographic screening, *Cancer* 91:1699, 2001.

54. American College of Radiology (ACR): *Standards for the performance of diagnostic mammography and problem-solving breast evaluation [Adopted by the ACR Council 1994] in ACR Digest of Official Actions*, Reston, VA, 1994, ACR.

55. Sickles EA et al: Mammographic screening: how to operate successfully at low cost, *Radiology* 160:95, 1986.

56. General Accounting Office: *Screening mammography: low cost services do not compromise quality*, Washington, DC, 1990, General Accounting Office.

57. Bassett LW, Gold RH: Breast radiography using the oblique projection, *Radiology* 149:585, 1983.

58. Helvie MA et al: Breast thickness on routine mammograms: effect on image quality and radiation dose, *AJR Am J Roentgenol* 163:1371, 1994.

59. Jackson VP, Lex AM, Smith DJ: Patient discomfort during screen-film mammography, *Radiology* 168:421, 1988.

60. Stomper PC et al: Is mammography painful: a multicenter patient study, *Arch Intern Med* 148:521, 1988.

61. American College of Radiology Committee on Quality Assurance in Mammography: *Mammography quality control*, Reston, VA, 1992, ACR.

62. Berkowitz JE, Gatewood MB, Gayler BW: Equivocal mammographic findings: evaluation with spot compression, *Radiology* 171:369, 1989.

63. Faulk RM, Sickles EA: Efficacy of spot compression-magnification and tangential views in mammographic evaluation of palpable breast masses, *Radiology* 185:87, 1992.

64. Feig SA: Importance of supplementary mammographic views to diagnostic accuracy, *AJR Am J Roentgenol* 151:40, 1988.

65. Feig SA: Breast masses: mammographic and sonographic evaluation, *Radiol Clin North Am* 30:67, 1992.

66. D'Orsi CJ, Kopans DB: Mammographic feature analysis, *Semin Roentgenol* 28:204, 1993.

67. McNicholas MM et al: Pain and increased mammographic density in postmenopausal women, *AJR Am J Roentgenol* 163:311, 1994.

68. Gold RH, Montgomery CK, Rambo ON: Significance of margination of benign and malignant infiltrative mammary lesions: roentgenologic-pathologic correlation, *AJR Am J Roentgenol* 118:881, 1973.

69. Hall FM et al: Nonpalpable breast lesions: recommendations for biopsy based on suspicion of carcinoma at mammography, *Radiology* 167:353, 1988.

70. Moskowitz M: The predictive value of certain mammographic signs in screening for breast cancer, *Cancer* 51:1007, 1983.

71. Sickles EA: Nonpalpable, circumscribed, noncalcified solid breast masses: likelihood of malignancy based on lesion size and age of patient, *Radiology* 192:439, 1994.

72. Brenner RJ, Sickles EA: Acceptability of periodic follow-up as an alternative to biopsy for mammographically detected lesions interpreted as probably benign, *Radiology* 171:645, 1989.

73. Sickles EA: Periodic mammographic follow-up of probably benign lesions: results in 3,184 consecutive cases, *Radiology* 179:463, 1991.

74. Jackson VP et al: Diagnostic importance of radiographic density of noncalcified breast masses: analysis of 91 lesions, *AJR Am J Roentgenol* 157:25, 1991.

75. Lanyi M: Pathogenesis, pathophysiology, and composition of breast calcifications. In *Diagnosis and differential diagnosis of breast calcifications*, New York, 1986, Springer-Verlag.

76. Hilton SV et al: Real-time breast sonography: application in 300 consecutive patients, *AJR Am J Roentgenol* 147:479, 1986.

77. Brenner RJ et al: Spontaneous regression of interval benign cysts of the breast, *Radiology* 193:365, 1994.

78. Feig SA, Yaffe M: Digital imaging systems. In Basset LW et al (eds): *Diagnosis of diseases of the breast*, Philadelphia, 1996, WB Saunders.

79. Crothers JG et al: Fibroadenolipoma of the breast, *Br J Radiol* 48:191, 1985.

80. Bassett LW, Gold RH, Mirra JM: Nonneoplastic breast calcifications in lipid cysts: development after excision and primary irradiation, *AJR Am J Roentgenol* 138:335, 1981.

81. Mendelson EB: Evaluation of the postoperative breast, *Radiol Clin North Am* 30:107, 1992.

82. Tabár L, Dean PB: Stellate lesions. In *Teaching atlas of mammography*, New York, 1985, Thieme Stratton.

83. Orel SG et al: Radial scar with microcalcifications: radiologic-pathologic correlation, *Radiology* 183:479, 1992.

84. Kopans DB, Meyer JE, Grabbe J: Dermal deposits mistaken for breast calcifications, *Radiology* 149:592, 1983.

85. Sickles EA, Galvin HB: Breast arterial calcifications in association with diabetes mellitus: too weak a correlation to have clinical utility, *Radiology* 171:577, 1989.

86. Bassett LW: Mammographic analysis of calcifications, *Radiol Clin North Am* 30:93, 1992.

87. Bassett LW, Gold RH, Cove HC: Mammographic spectrum of traumatic fat necrosis: the fallibility of "pathognomonic" signs of carcinoma, *AJR Am J Roentgenol* 130:119, 1978.

88. Sickles EA, Abele JS: Milk of calcium within tiny benign breast cysts, *Radiology* 141:655, 1981.

89. World Health Organization: *Histological typing of breast tumors*, vol 2, Geneva, 1981, World Health Organization.

90. Leibman AJ, Lewis M, Kruse B: Tubular carcinoma of the breast, *AJR Am J Roentgenol* 160:263, 1993.

91. Meyer JE et al: Medullary carcinoma of the breast: mammographic and US appearance, *Radiology* 170:79, 1989.

92. Mitnick JS et al: Invasive papillary carcinoma of the breast: mammographic appearance, *Radiology* 177:803, 1990.

93. Czernobilsky B: Intracystic carcinoma of the female breast, *Surg Gynecol Obstet* 124:93, 1967.

94. Helvie MA et al: Invasive lobular carcinoma: imaging features and clinical detection, *Invest Radiol* 28:202, 1993.

95. Hilleran DJ et al: Invasive lobular carcinoma: mammographic findings in a 10-year experience, *Radiology* 178:149, 1991.

96. Sickles EA: The subtle and atypical mammographic features of invasive lobular carcinoma, *Radiology* 178:25, 1991.

97. Toombs BD, Kalisher L: Metastatic disease to the breast: clinical, pathologic, and radiographic features, *AJR Am J Roentgenol* 129:673, 1977.

98. Bohman LG et al: Breast metastases from extramammary malignancies, *Radiology* 144:309, 1982.

99. Powell RW, McSweeney MB, Wilson C: X-ray calcifications as the only basis for breast biopsy, *Ann Surg* 197:555, 1983.

100. Page DL, Anderson TJ (eds): *Diagnostic histopathology of the breast,* Edinburgh, 1987, Churchill Livingstone.

101. Betsill WL et al: Intraductal carcinoma: long-term follow-up after treatment by biopsy alone, *JAMA* 239:1863, 1978.

102. Page DL et al: Intraductal carcinoma of the breast: follow-up after biopsy only, *Cancer* 49:751, 1982.

103. Lagios MD: Duct carcinoma in situ, *Surg Clin North Am* 70:853, 1990.

104. Holland R et al: The presence of an extensive intraductal component following a limited resection correlates with prominent residual disease in the remainder of the breast, *J Clin Oncol* 8:113, 1990.

105. Holland R et al: Clinical practice: extent distribution, and mammographic/histological correlations of breast ductal carcinoma in situ, *Lancet* 335:519, 1990.

106. Paulus DD: Conservative treatment of breast cancer: mammography in patient selection and follow-up, *AJR Am J Roentgenol* 143:483, 1984.

107. Dershaw DD: Mammography in patients with breast cancer treated by breast conservation (lumpectomy with or without radiation), *AJR Am J Roentgenol* 164:309, 1995.

108. Dershaw DD, Abramson A, Kinne DW: Ductal carcinoma in situ: mammographic findings and clinical implications, *Radiology* 170:411, 1989.

109. Stomper PC, Connolly JL: Ductal carcinoma in situ of the breast: correlation between mammographic calcifications and tumor subtype, *AJR Am J Roentgenol* 159:483, 1992.

110. Kinkel K et al: Focal areas of increased opacity in ductal carcinoma in situ of the comedo type: mammographic-pathologic correlation, *Radiology* 192:443, 1994.

111. Boyages J et al: Factors associated with local recurrence as a first site of failure following the conservation treatment of early breast cancer, *Recent Results Cancer Res* 115:92, 1989.

112. Eberlein TJ et al: Predictors of local recurrence following conservative breast surgery and radiation therapy: the influence of tumor size, *Arch Surg* 125:771, 1990.

113. Osteen RT et al: Early breast cancer: predictors of breast recurrence for patients treated with conservative surgery and radiation therapy, *Radiother Oncol* 19:29, 1990.

114. Schnitt SJ et al: Pathologic findings on reexcision of the primary site in breast cancer patients considered for treatment by primary radiation therapy, *Cancer* 59:675, 1987.

115. Vicini FA et al: Recurrence in the breast following conservative surgery and radiation therapy for early-stage breast cancer, *J Natl Cancer Inst Monogr* 11:33, 1992.

116. Stomper PC, Margolin FR: Ductal carcinoma in situ: the mammographer's perspective, *AJR Am J Roentgenol* 162:585, 1994.

117. Graham RA et al: The efficacy of specimen radiography in evaluating the surgical margins of impalpable breast carcinoma, *AJR Am J Roentgenol* 162:33, 1994.

118. Lagios MD et al: Duct carcinoma in situ: relationship of extent of noninvasive disease to the frequency of occult invasion, multicentricity, lymph node metastases, and short term treatment failures, *Cancer* 50:1309, 1982.

119. Gluck BS et al: Microcalcifications on postoperative mammograms as an indicator of adequacy of tumor excision, *Radiology* 188:469, 1993.

120. Sickles EA: Mammographic features of 300 consecutive nonpalpable breast cancers, *AJR Am J Roentgenol* 146:661, 1986.

121. Wilhelm MC et al: The changing mammogram: a primary indication for needle localization biopsy, *Arch Surg* 121:1311, 1986.

122. Bassett LW, Shayestehfar B, Hirbawi I: Obtaining previous mammograms for comparison: usefulness and costs, *AJR Am J Roentgenol* 163:1083, 1994.

123. Bassett LW et al: Clinical Practice Guideline No 13. AHCPR Publication No. 95-0632. Rockville, MD, 1994, Agency for Health Care Policy and Research, Public Health Service, US Department of Health and Human Services.

124. Kopans DB et al: Asymmetric breast tissue, *Radiology* 171:639, 1989.

125. Adler DD, Rebner M, Pennes DR: Accessory breast tissue in the axilla, *Radiology* 163:709, 1987.

126. Kalisher L, Chu AM, Peyster RG: Clinicopathological correlation of xeroradiography in determining involvement of metastatic axillary nodes in female breast cancer, *Radiology* 121:333, 1976.

127. Gisvold JJ et al: Breast biopsy: a comparative study of stereotaxically guided core and excisional techniques, *AJR Am J Roentgenol* 162:815, 1994.

128. Meyer JE et al: Occult breast abnormalities: percutaneous preoperative needle localization, *Radiology* 50:335, 1984.

129. Rasmussen OS, Seerup A: Preoperative radiographically guided wire marking of nonpalpable breast lesions, *Acta Radiol Diagn (Stockh)* 25:13, 1984.

130. Moskowitz M: Impact of a priori medical decisions on screening for breast cancer *Radiology* 171:605 1989.

131. Howard J: Using mammography for cancer control: an unrealized potential, *CA Cancer J Clin* 33:33, 1987.

132. Cyrlak D: Induced costs of low-cost screening mammography, *Radiology* 68:661, 1988.

133. Linver MN et al: The mammography audit: a primer for the mammography quality standards act (MQSA), *AJR Am J Roentgenol* 165:19, 1995.

134. Murphy WA, Destouet JM, Monsees BS: Professional quality assurance for mammography screening programs, *Radiology* 175:319, 1990.

135. Sickles EA et al: Medical audit of a rapid-throughput mammography screening practice: methodology and results of 27,114 examinations, *Radiology* 175:323, 1990.

136. Bassett LW et al: Prevalence of carcinoma in palpable vs impalpable mammographically-detected lesions, *AJR Am J Roentgenol* 157:21, 1991.

137. Threatt B et al: Percutaneous needle localization of clustered microcalcifications prior to biopsy, *AJR Am J Roentgenol* 121:829, 1974.

138. Egan JF, Sayler CB, Goodman MJ: A technique for localizing occult breast lesions, *CA Cancer J Clin* 26:32, 1976.

139. Homer MJ: Nonpalpable breast lesion localization using a curved-end retractable wire, *Radiology* 157:259, 1985.

140. Kopans DB, Meyer JE: Versatile spring hookwire breast lesion localizer, *AJR Am J Roentgenol* 138:586, 1982.

141. Kwasnik EM, Sadowsky NL, Vollman RW: An improved system for surgical excision of needle-localized nonpalpable breast lesions, *Am J Surg* 154:476, 1987.

142. Bauermeister DE, Hall MH: Specimen radiography: a mandatory adjunct to mammography, *Am J Clin Pathol* 59:782, 1973.

143. Gallager HS: Breast specimen radiography: obligatory, adjuvant and investigative, *Am J Clin Pathol* 64:759, 1975.

144. Stomper PC et al: Efficacy of specimen radiography of clinically occult noncalcified breast lesions, *AJR Am J Roentgenol* 151:43, 1988.

145. D'Orsi CJ: Management of the breast specimen, *Radiology* 194:297, 1995.

146. Surratt JT, Monsees BS, Mazoujian G: Calcium oxalate microcalcifications in the breast, *Radiology* 181:141, 1991.

147. Rebner M et al: Paraffin tissue block radiography: adjunct to breast specimen radiography, *Radiology* 173:695, 1989.

148. D'Orsi CJ et al: Breast specimen microcalcification: radiographic validation and pathologic-radiologic correlation, *Radiology* 280:396, 1991.

149. Azevado E, Svane G, Aver G: Stereotactic fine needle biopsy in 2594 mammographically-detected nonpalpable lesions, *Lancet* 1:1033, 1989.

150. Hendrick RE, Parker SH: *Stereotaxic imaging in syllabus: RSNA categorical course in physics,* Chicago, 1993, Radiological Society of North America.

151. Gordon PB, Goldenberg SL, Chan NH: Solid breast lesions: diagnosis with US-guided fine-needle aspiration biopsy, *Radiology* 189:573, 1993.

152. Mitnick J et al: Stereotaxic localization for fine-needle aspiration breast biopsy, *Arch Surg* 126:1137, 1991.

153. Hayes MK et al: Mammographically-guided fine-needle aspiration cytology of the breast: reducing the rate of insufficient specimens, *AJR Am J Roentgenol* 167:381, 1996.

154. Masood S: Occult breast lesions and aspiration biopsy: a new challenge, *Diagn Cytopathol* 9:613, 1993.

155. Helvie MA et al: Radiographically guided fine-needle aspiration of nonpalpable breast lesions, *Radiology* 174:657, 1990.

156. Jackson VP: The status of mammographically-guided fine needle aspiration biopsy of nonpalpable breast lesions, *Radiol Clin North Am* 30:139, 1992.

157. Layfield L et al: Mammographically guided fine-needle aspiration biopsy of nonpalpable breast lesions, *Cancer* 68:2007, 1991.

158. Löfgren M, Andersson I, Lindholm K: Stereotactic fine-needle aspiration for cytologic diagnosis of nonpalpable breast lesions, *AJR Am J Roentgenol* 154:1191, 1990.

159. Elvecrog EL, Lechner MC, Nelson MJ: Nonpalpable breast lesions: correlation of stereotaxic large-core needle biopsy and surgical biopsy results, *Radiology* 188:453, 1993.

160. Bassett LW et al: Stereotactic breast CNB: report of the Joint Task Force of ACT, ACS, COAP, *CA Cancer J Clin* 166:341, 1997.

161. Brenner RJ et al: Percutaneous CNB: effect of operator experience and number of samples on accuracy, *AJR Am J Roentgenol* 166:341, 1996.

162. Dershaw DD et al: Nondiagnostic stereo CNB: results of rebiopsy, *Radiology* 204:485, 1996.

163. Jackman RJ et al: Atypical ductal hyperplasia diagnosed at stereotactic breast biopsy: improved reliability with 14-guage, directional, vacuum-assisted biopsy, *Radiology* 204:485, 1997.

164. Parker SH, Klaus AJ: Performing CNB with a directional, vacuum-assisted biopsy instrument, *Radiographics* 17:1233, 1997.

165. Philpotts LE et al: Comparison of rebiopsy rates after stereotactic core needle biopsy of the breast with 11-G vacuum suction probe vs. 14-G automatic gun, *AJR Am J Roentgenol* 172:683, 1999.

166. Parker SH: When is core biopsy really core? *Radiology* 185:641, 1991.

167. Lindfors KK, Rosenquist CJ: Needle core biopsy guided with mammography: a study of cost-effectiveness, *Radiology* 190:217, 1994.

168. Scanlon EF: The case for and against two-step procedures for the surgical treatment of breast cancer, *Cancer* 53:677, 1984.

169. Reynolds HE: Core needle biopsy of challenging benign breast conditions: a comprehensive literature review, *AJR Am J Roentgenol* 174:1245, 2000.

170. Jackman RJ et al: Stereotaxic large-core needle biopsy of 450 nonpalpable breast lesions with surgical correlation in lesions with cancer or atypical hyperplasia, *Radiology* 193:91, 1994.

171. Liberman L et al: Atypical ductal hyperplasia diagnosed at stereotaxic core biopsy of breast lesions: an indication for surgical biopsy, *AJR Am J Roentgenol* 164:1111, 1995.

172. Tabár L, Dean PB, Péntek Z: Galactography: The diagnostic procedure of choice for nipple discharge, *Radiology* 149:31, 1983.

173. Threatt B, Appleman HD: Mammary duct injection, *Radiology* 108:71, 1973.

174. Cardenosa H, Doudna C, Eklund GW: Ductography of the breast: technique and findings, *AJR Am J Roentgenol* 162:1081, 1994.

175. Wild JJ, Neal D: The use of high-frequency ultrasonic waves for detecting changes of texture in the living tissue, *Lancet* 1:655, 1951.

176. Jellins J et al: Ultrasonic gray scale visualization of breast disease, *Ultrasound Med Biol* 1:393, 1975.

177. Kobayashi T: Diagnostic ultrasound in breast cancer: analysis of retrotumorous echo patterns correlated with sonic attenuation by cancerous connective tissue, *J Clin Ultrasound* 7:471, 1979.

178. Cole-Beuglet C et al: Ultrasound mammography: a comparison with radiographic mammography, *Radiology* 139:693, 1981.

179. Cole-Beuglet C et al: Ultrasound analysis of 104 primary breast carcinomas classified according to histopathologic type, *Radiology* 147:191, 1983.

180. Kopans DB, Meyer JE, Lindfors KK: Whole-breast ultrasound imaging: four-year follow-up, *Radiology* 157:505, 1985.

181. Sickles EA, Filly RA, Callen PW: Breast cancer detection with sonography and mammography: comparison using state of the art equipment, *AJR Am J Roentgenol* 140:843, 1983.

182. Feig SA: The role of ultrasound in a breast imaging center, *Semin Ultrasound CT MR* 10:90, 1989.

183. Sickles EA, Filly RA, Callen PW: Benign breast lesions: ultrasound detection and diagnosis, *Radiology* 151:467, 1984.

184. Evans WP: Fine-needle aspiration cytology and core biopsy of nonpalpable breast lesions, *Curr Opin Radiol* 4:130, 1992.

185. Gordon PB, Goldenberg LS: Malignant breast masses detected only by ultrasound: a retrospective review, *Cancer* 76:626, 1995.

186. Jackson VP: Management of solid breast nodules: what is the role of sonography? *Radiology* 196:14, 1995.

187. DeBruhl ND et al: Silicone breast implants: US evaluation, *Radiology* 189:95, 1993.

188. Gorczyca DP et al: Silicone breast implant ruptures in an animal model: comparison of mammography, MR imaging, US and CT, *Radiology* 190:227, 1994.

189. Fajardo LL et al: Detection of breast abnormalities on teleradiology transmitted mammograms, *Invest Radiol* 25:1111, 1990.

190. Thurfjell EL, Lernevall KA, Taube AAS: Benefit of independent double reading in a population-based mammography screening program, *Radiology* 191:241, 1994.

191. Vyborny CJ: Can computers help radiologists read mammograms? *Radiology* 191:315, 1994.

192. Vyborny CJ, Giger ML: Computer vision and artificial intelligence in mammography, *AJR Am J Roentgenol* 162:699, 1994.

193. Shtern F: Digital mammography and related technologies: A perspective from the National Cancer Institute, *Radiology* 183:629, 1992.

194. Turner DA, Alcorn FS, Adler YT: Nuclear magnetic resonance in the diagnosis of breast cancer, *Radiol Clin North Am* 26:673, 1988.

195. Heywang SH et al: MR imaging of the breast using gadolinium-DTPA, *J Comput Assist Tomogr* 10:199, 1986.

196. Heywang-Kobrunner SH: Contrast-enhanced MRI of the breast-overview after 1250 patient examinations, *Electromedica* 2:43, 1993.

197. Harms SE et al: Fat-suppressed three-dimensional MR imaging of the breast, *Radiographics* 13:247, 1993.

198. Kaiser WA, Zeitler E: MR imaging of the breast: fast imaging sequences with and without Gd-DTPA, *Radiology* 170:681, 1989.

199. Lewis-Jones HG, Whitehouse GH, Leinster SJ: The role of MRI in the assessment of local recurrent breast carcinoma, *Clin Radiol* 43:197, 1991.

200. Orel SG et al: Suspicious breast lesions: MR imaging with radiologic-pathologic correlation *Radiology* 190:485, 1994.

201. Harms SE et al: MR imaging of the breast with rotating delivery of excitation off resonance: clinical experience with pathologic correlation, *Radiology* 186:493, 1993.

202. Adler LP et al: Evaluation of breast masses and axillary lymph nodes with (F-18) 2-Deoxy-2-fluoro-D-glucose PET, *Radiology* 187:743 1993.

203. Khalkhali I et al: Scintimammography: the complementary role of Tc-99m sestamibi prone breast imaging for the diagnosis of breast carcinoma, *Radiology* 196:421, 1995.

204. Khalkhali I et al: Prone scintimammography in patients with suspicion of carcinoma of the breast, *J Am Coll Surg* 178:491, 1994.

205. Love SM, McGuigan KA, Chap L: The Revlon/UCLA Breast Center Practice Guidelines for the Treatment of Breast Disease, *Cancer J* 2:2, 1996.

206. Winchester DP, Cox JD: Standards for breast-conservation treatment, *CA Cancer J Clin* 42:134, 1992.

207. Orel SG et al: Breast cancer recurrence after lumpectomy and irradiation: role of mammography in detection, *Radiology* 183:201, 1992.

208. Fajardo LL, Roberts CC, Hunt KR: Mammographic surveillance of breast cancer patients: should the mastectomy site be imaged? *AJR Am J Roengentol* 161:953, 1993.

209. Jain S et al: Patterns of metastatic breast cancer in relation to histologic type, *Eur J Cancer* 29:2155, 1993.

210. Patanaphan V, Salazar OM, Risco R: Breast cancer: metastatic patterns and their prognosis, *South Med J* 81:1109, 1988.

211. Muss HB et al: Perceptions of follow-up care in women with breast cancer, *Am J Clin Oncol* 14:55, 1991.

212. Loomer L et al: Postoperative follow-up of patients with early breast cancer, *Cancer* 67:55, 1991.

213. American Joint Committee on Cancer: *Manual for staging cancer,* Philadelphia, 1992, JB Lippincott.

214. Del Turco MR et al: Intensive diagnostic follow-up after treatment of primary breast cancer, *JAMA* 271:1593, 1994.

215. Impact of follow-up testing on survival and health-related quality of life in breast cancer patients: a multicenter randomized controlled trial—The GIVIO investigators, *JAMA* 271:1587, 1994.

216. O'Mara RE: Bone scanning in osseous metastatic disease, *JAMA* 229:1915, 1974.

217. Khansur T et al: Evaluation of bone scan as a screening work-up in primary and local-regional recurrence of breast cancer, *Am J Clin Oncol* 10:167, 1987.

218. Ciatto S et al: Preoperative staging of primary breast cancer: a multicenter study, *Cancer* 61:1038, 1988.

219. Coleman RE, Rubens RD, Fogelman I: Reappraisal of the baseline bone scan in breast cancer, *J Nucl Med* 29:1045, 1988.

220. Kunkler IH, Merick MV, Rodger A: Bone scintigraphy in breast cancer: a nine-year follow-up, *Clin Radiol* 36:279, 1985.

221. McNeill BJ et al: Preoperative and follow-up bone scans in patients with primary carcinoma of the breast, *Surg Gynecol Obstet* 147:745, 1978.

222. Bassett LW, Giuliano AE, Gold RH: Staging for breast carcinoma, *Am J Surg* 157:250, 1989.

223. Loprinzi CL: It is now the age to define the appropriate follow-up of primary breast cancer patients, *J Clin Oncol* 12:881, 1994.

224. Schaner EG et al: Comparison of computed tomography and conventional whole lung tomography in detecting pulmonary nodules: a prospective radiologic-pathologic study, *AJR Am J Roentgenol* 131:51, 1978.

225. Didolkar MS et al: Accuracy of roentgenograms of the chest in metastases to the lungs, *Surg Gynecol Obstet* 144:903, 1977.

226. Vestergaard A et al: The value of yearly chest x-ray in patients with stage I breast cancer, *Eur J Cancer Clin Oncol* 25:687, 1989.

227. Bernardino ME et al: Diagnostic approaches to liver and spleen metastases, *Radiol Clin North Am* 20:469, 1982.

228. Friedman ML, Esposito FS: Comparison of CT scanning and radionuclide imaging in liver disease, *CRC Crit Rev Diagn Imaging* 14:143, 1980.

229. Yeh H, Rabinowitz JG: Ultrasonography and computed tomography of the liver, *Radiol Clin North Am* 18:321, 1980.

230. Weiner SN, Sachs SH: An assessment of positive liver scanning in patients with breast cancer, *Arch Surg* 113:126, 1978.

231. Ferrucci JT: Leo G. Rigler lecture: MR imaging of the liver, *AJR Am J Roentgenol* 147:1103, 1986.

232. Russell EJ et al: Multiple cerebral metastases: detectability with Gd-DTPA-enhanced MR imaging, *Radiology* 165:609, 1987.

233. Weisberg LA: The computed tomographic findings in intracranial metastases due to breast carcinoma, *Comput Radiol* 10:297, 1986.

234. Bentson JR, Steckel RJ, Kagan AR: Diagnostic imaging in clinical cancer management: brain metastases, *Invest Radiol* 23:335, 1988.

235. Khansur T et al: Preoperative evaluation with radionuclide brain scanning and computerized axial tomography of the brain in patients with breast cancer, *Am J Surg* 155:232, 1988.

236. Brant-Zawadzski M: MR imaging of the brain, *Radiology* 166:1, 1988.

237. Davis PC et al: Diagnosis of cerebral metastases, *AJNR Am J Neuroradiol* 12:293, 1991.

32

The Kinetics of Neoplastic Growth and Interval Breast Cancer

JOHN C. MANSOUR

JOHN E. NIEDERHUBER

Chapter Outline

The Cell Cycle

The rate of growth of the primary breast cancer and its metastases is a major determinant of survival. Breast cancer cells, like other tumor cells, undergo binary division, grow to a certain point, and then repeat the division—a process known as the *cell cycle*. This cycle of cell division is divided into four stages: G_1, S (DNA synthesis), G_2, and M (mitosis/meiosis) (Figure 32-1). G_1 is the gap between completion of cell division and the beginning of the next round of DNA synthesis in the S phase. The two daughter cells generated by mitosis reside in either G_1 or G_0 (the resting state) and retain a diploid set of chromosomes.

Cells in culture usually spend several hours in G_1. For example, NIH-3T3 cells generally have a G_1 of 6 hours. However, the G_1 transit time is highly variable, even from one cell to another in the same culture. During G_1 the cell is most affected by external conditions. Studies of cell cycle kinetics suggest that a specific control event, called a *restriction point* (R), exists within the G_1 stage, and this control point determines whether the cell can progress to DNA synthesis (S phase).[1]

The R divides G_1 into two parts, termed the *prerestriction point phase* and the *postrestriction point phase*. The prerestriction phase of G_1 depends on the presence of growth factors, whereas the postrestriction phase is growth factor independent.[2,3] The growth factors required for prerestriction phase progression are all cell type–specific.[3] Once the restriction point is triggered, the remaining phases of the cycle are independent of extracellular factors. As noted, the most variable period of the cell cycle is the first gap, G_1. The cell responds to intrinsic and extrinsic signals that trigger entry into the S phase.[1,4] If the cell is not triggered to DNA synthesis, it may be shunted into a resting state termed G_0, from which the cell can reenter G_1 when conditions are appropriate. It appears to be rare for tumor cells to enter G_0. During the S phase, cells synthesize DNA and chromosome replication begins. The average duration of the S phase of NIH-3T3 cells in culture is 8 hours, and at the completion of DNA synthesis, the cell has replicated its entire complement of genetic material and has two diploid sets of chromosomes.

The S phase is followed by a second gap (G_2) that averages approximately 3 hours for NIH-3T3 cells in culture. The daughter chromosomes generated during the S phase remain intimately associated with their partners until mitosis. During G_1, S, and G_2 (the interphase of the cell cycle), RNA and protein synthesis are steadily increasing, with duplication of all organelles, including ribosomes and mitochondria. Mitosis, the shortest segment of the cycle, is the process by which the cell distributes two sets of identical chromosomes to the two daughter cells. Recent investigations of cell cycle regulation have established that similar mechanisms are responsible for taking the cell from G_1 to S and from G_2 to M. These systems have been termed *checkpoint control genes*.[5] The checkpoint control systems are responsible for ensuring the integrity of DNA replication (G_1 to S) and the accuracy of chromosomal segregation (G_2 to M; see Figure 32-1).[5]

The checkpoint controls of the cell cycle operate as positive-negative switches. The protein products of the checkpoint control genes determine whether the cell is ready to progress to the next phase. In addition, they are capable of editing and repairing defective genetic information to make the cell ready for transition. Thus loss of the G_1/S checkpoint can lead to genomic instability and the transition of the cells toward a malignant phenotype.[5,6]

An example of how the G_1/S checkpoint functions can be seen in studies of the role of the *p53* gene, a transcriptional activator, in mammalian cell G_1/S arrest.[7,8] In these experiments, mammalian cells treated with gamma irradiation to cause DNA damage show increased levels of p53 protein and G_1/S arrest. Mammalian cells with mutant p53 alleles fail to undergo G_1/S arrest when irradiated.[9]

In addition to the DNA repair enzymes operating at the checkpoints described, the *cyclin-dependent kinases* (cdks) also control cell cycle progression. *Cdks* bind cyclin, cause phosphorylation, and are inhibited by cyclin-dependent kinase inhibitors. The *cdks* have been grouped into six families according to the point in the cell cycle where they function.[10,11] Cyclin families C, D, and E act at the G_1/S transition, whereas B1 and B2 act at the G_2/M interphase. The cyclin A group, unlike the other families, is present throughout the S and M phases.

The best estimates for cell cycle time of human solid tumors (including breast cancer) were obtained using the percentage-labeled mitosis method. These estimates indicate that 90% of tumors' cell cycle times fall within 15 and 120 hours (median, 48 hours).[12] The duration of the S phase is less variable, with 90% between 9.5 and 24 hours (median, 16 hours). Although the duration of the cell cycle may vary significantly from one cell to another within a tumor, there appears to be less variation based on tumor histology. In fact, differences in cell cycle time cannot explain the much greater variation observed for actual tumor doubling time (DT).

Breast Cancer and the Cell Cycle

Disruptions of the tightly regulated mechanisms of cell cycle control are common in many tumors, including breast cancers. Some of these mechanisms central to

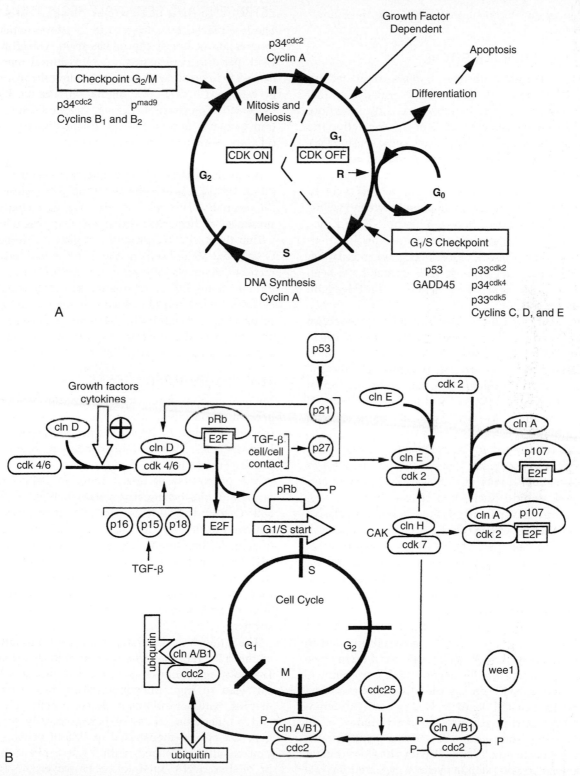

FIG. 32-1 **A,** This model of cell cycle control attempts to illustrate how different components ready the cell for division and control for accurate duplication of DNA; cdks are phosphorylated to become active and dephosphorylated to become inactive. Specific proteolysis of key proteins also serves to inactivate specific proteins at appropriate steps in the cycle. **B,** A schematic of the relationships of the many proteins involved in the cell cycle is shown to provide some insight into the degree of complexity associated with the process. Understanding these complex pathways and internal cycles governing progression through the process of cell division is the subject of intense investigation, which continues to evolve. This illustration also serves to indicate the vast array of opportunities for abnormal function that may lead to patterns of cancerous growth. *(**B,** from Stein GS et al:* Exp Hematol *23:1053, 1995.)*

breast cancer development are described in the following sections.

CYCLINS AND CDK INHIBITORS

Cells proceed from G_1 through S phase regulated by cyclins, cdks, and cdk inhibitors. Normally, cyclins complex with cdks to initiate S phase. Cdk inhibitors typically arrest the cell cycle at G_1 or G_0, preventing the cells from entering S phase when cells sense DNA damage. Cyclin levels are tightly regulated and vary widely throughout the cell cycle. In contrast, cdk levels remain relatively constant throughout the cell cycle. In tumor cells the controlled interaction between cyclins, cdks, and cdk inhibitors becomes disrupted. This dysregulation can be caused by cyclin overexpression, malfunction of cdk inhibitors, or loss of negative regulation. In breast cancer cells, at least three cyclins have been implicated in cell cycle dysregulation: cyclin D1, cyclin E, and cyclin D2.

Cyclin D1 in normal cells complexes with cdk4/cdk6 and phosphorylates the retinoblastoma protein (pRB) gene product.[13,14] The phosphorylated and inactivated pRB releases the transactivation factor E2F, thereby triggering entry into S phase. The cdk inhibitor, *p16*, can inactivate the cyclin-cdk4/cdk6 complexes and halt cell cycle progression.[15] Similarly, cyclin E complexes with cdk2 to initiate S phase.[16]

In a study measuring cyclin D1 expression in variously differentiated breast cancer cells, cyclin D1 was normally expressed in normal breast cells, ductal hyperplasia, and atypical ductal hyperplasia. In intraductal carcinoma, ductal carcinoma in situ (DCIS), and invasive ductal carcinoma cells, cyclin D1 was overexpressed in 44% to 72% of the cells.[17] Cyclin D1 is overexpressed in estrogen receptor (ER)-positive cells when undergoing estrogen-induced mitogenic activity.[17-19] In contrast, in ER-negative cells, cyclin E is overexpressed and cyclin D1 is normally expressed.[18,20,21]

Cyclin E is overexpressed in up to 25% of breast cancer samples analyzed with Western blotting and in 10 out of 10 breast cancer cell lines. Most of these overexpressing tumors were ER negative.[21] The overexpression of cyclin E has been associated with an increased risk of recurrence and death, as well as poorly differentiated tumors and increased proliferative index.[19,21] In an interesting series of cell culture experiments, researchers inactivated cyclin D1 with *p16*. Concomitant exogenous overexpression of cyclin E bypassed the role of cyclin D1 and led to pRB phosphorylation and cell cycle progression.[16,20]

In contrast to the role played by these positive regulators of the cell cycle, cyclin D2 mRNA and protein levels are normally increased during periods of growth arrest.[22] However, cyclin D2 levels are undetectable in almost all examined breast cancer cell lines.[23]

ESTROGENS AND CELL CYCLE REGULATION

The role played by estrogens in the development and progression of breast cancer has been widely studied. Work performed primarily in cell culture experiments has led to interesting findings regarding the role played by estrogens in cell cycle regulation. The mechanisms by which 17β-estradiol (E_2) can induce G_1 to S phase transition and increase S phase fraction in breast cancer cells are related to the cyclin dysregulation described earlier.

As mentioned previously, overexpression of cyclin D1 in breast cancer cells is strongly associated with ER positivity. This relationship may be related to the presence of imperfect estrogen response elements within the cyclin D1 promoter region.[24] Adding E_2 to G_1-arrested MCF-7 cells results in a twofold to fivefold increase in levels of cyclin D1 mRNA and protein within 6 hours.[25-28] E_2 treatment also led to activation of cyclin D1-cdk4 complexes and decreased the activity of p27[KIP1], a cdk inhibitor.[29] MCF-7 cells treated with antiestrogens demonstrate G_1 arrest and decreased expression of cyclin D1.[30,31]

TUMOR-SUPPRESSOR GENES

Many alterations in the expression of tumor-suppressor genes and cdk-inhibitor genes have been implicated in the development of breast cancer. *p53*, pRB, and *p16* have the most clearly defined roles in breast cancer tumorigenesis.

The proportion of breast cancers positive for *p53* on immunohistochemistry varies between 14% and 58%. One study has demonstrated that whereas 23% of noncomedo (low-grade) DCIS were *p53* positive, 42% of comedo (high-grade) DCIS were p53 positive.[32] The high levels of p53 protein are correlated with increased proliferation rate.[33] Some authors have even suggested that specific breast cancer *p53* mutations are associated with doxorubicin chemoresistance and diminished survival.[34,35]

The retinoblastoma (RB) gene is a central participant in the cell cycle dysregulation seen in breast cancers. Disrupted regulation of cyclins, cdks, and cdk inhibitors can lead to hyperphosphorylation and inactivation of pRB, with a resultant increase in cell cycle transit and proliferation.[33] Loss of heterozygosity in the RB gene has been demonstrated in 25% of primary breast cancers and correlated with high S-phase fraction, as well as DNA aneuploidy. However, no relationship between RB alterations and survival has been proved.[36]

The cdk inhibitor, *p16*, primarily acts at cdk4/cdk6 complexes to interrupt cell cycle progression.[37] Homozygous deletions of the 9p21-22 chromosomal subregion normally coding for *p16* have been found in immortalized MCF-10F cells.[38] Approximately half of all primary breast tumors in one study were focally or totally negative for p16 expression.[37] These results may be explained by the finding of hypermethylation in the p16 coding sequence of 30% of breast cancers.[39]

TELOMERASE

Telomerase is a holoenzyme that maintains telomere length by means of a reverse transcriptase and an RNA sequence complementary to telomeric repeats. This mechanism inhibits degradation of the 3' end of DNA and subsequent cellular senescence. Telomerase is present in up to 90% of breast cancers and has been associated with cyclin D1 and cyclin E overexpression.[40] The association between telomerase and more aggressive tumor phenotypes has been demonstrated in numerous studies; however, controversy persists as to whether this is translated into worse prognosis. The activation of telomerase, dysregulation of cyclins D1 and E, and increased frequency of p53 mutations are seen most commonly in the early stages of tumorigenesis, up to and including low-grade DCIS.[41]

Breast Cancer Growth Kinetics

In 1963 Gershon-Cohen, Berger, and Klickstein[42] reported 18 patients who had not undergone immediate biopsy until two or more mammograms had been obtained. An additional case from the Ellis Fischel Cancer Hospital was added and used to calculate a median observed DT of 120 days (range, 23 to 209 days).[43] One study reported 147 breast cancers that had been imaged with 388 serial mammograms before definitive treatment was undertaken.[44] The observation time in this study ranged from 2 months to 11 years (average, 27 months). Measured tumor volume DTs were 44 to 1869 days (average, 212 days). From these observations, the authors concluded that the smallest lesion detectable with mammography would be 1 to 2 mm in diameter, or about 20 doublings. Growth from this size to 10 mm required, on average, 4 additional years and a total of 20 years from initial transformed cell to a 2-cm tumor.

The growth rate of the primary breast cancer and its metastases is determined by a complex set of interrelated events that are a balance between cell gain and cell loss. Cell gain is determined by the fraction of tumor cell mass that is actively dividing and by the time each dividing cell spends completing the cell cycle. Using techniques described later in this chapter, investigators can estimate the fraction of breast tumor cells that are actively dividing. In an analysis of 1000 breast tumors by Dressler and colleagues,[45] investigators found that the median proportion of cells in S phase was 2.6% if the tumors were diploid and 10.4% if they were aneuploid.

While growing, the tumor is also losing cells through cell death and via shedding into the vascular or lymphatic circulation or into an adjacent body cavity. Thus the actual measured tumor DT represents a net effect of all these concurrent processes. For various tumors, including breast tumors, it has been possible to measure cell cycle time, and serial measurements of imaged tumor masses have provided direct information about actual tumor DT.

Spratt and colleagues combined mammographic measurements, thymidine-labeling techniques, and mathematical modeling to estimate growth patterns of primary human breast cancers. Using the Louisville data from the Breast Cancer Detection and Demonstration Project (BCDDP), these authors described growth patterns of breast tumors during different stages of tumor development.[46]

Direct observations of cancers detected on two different mammograms provided estimates of growth rates for tumors large enough to be visible mammographically. Interestingly, the authors were also able to estimate the growth rates of predetectable tumors. Duration before detection was estimated by dividing the prevalence at the first screening by the annual incidence rate in subsequent years. With this information, the authors calculated tumor DT in the predetectable phase. The DTs for predetectable tumors were much shorter than those for tumors large enough to be seen on mammography. By the time tumors are seen on mammography, their growth rate is already slowing.

These findings support the conclusion that breast cancer growth is best described as a gompertzian function. A cancer that demonstrates gompertzian growth initially grows rapidly, but as its size increases, its growth curve is downwardly concave and approaches a horizontal asymptote. This growth pattern can be explained by a number of factors that alter the growth rate of human tumors. As the tumor grows, portions may outgrow the blood supply and develop areas of necrosis or ischemia. Thus the rate of cell proliferation may vary even within the tumor. In the case of breast cancer, growth is also influenced by hormonal mechanisms—namely estrogens and other growth factors—both stimulatory and inhibitory.

This model was specifically proposed for breast cancer and predicts distinctly unique periods of gompertzian growth separated by plateaus of no growth. Most of the plateaus occur in either the preclinical phase or after the tumor size has reached a point where the tumor would be detected and removed. On the basis of observations, these growth plateaus may last from a few months to as long as 8 years.[47,48]

The conclusion that tumors do not always grow at a constant rate seems quite plausible to the clinician treating breast cancer. In clinical practice, deviations from constant growth are regularly observed. Irregular growth seems an appropriate explanation when considering that growth of a spontaneous human breast cancer is a balance of progressive genetic alterations within the cancer, hormonal changes in the patient, tumor cell necrosis, tumor cell apoptosis, immune modulation, and host defenses from surrounding healthy tissues.

The potential slowing of growth as size increases makes it difficult to determine the date of tumor origin by simply extrapolating from observed DT. It is also important to note that although a given tumor type may have different DTs in different patients, the various metastatic lesions in an individual patient tend to show a very uniform rate of growth, a rate that is generally more rapid than that of the original primary lesion.[12]

In the early 1970s, investigators introduced the technique of tritiated thymidine labeling of tumor cell DNA during the S phase. This technique for identifying specific cells in the process of dividing is based on the fact that cells synthesize DNA only during active division and take up thymidine. Providing the dividing cells with a source of radiolabeled thymidine makes it possible to identify these cells. Labeled cells are exposed to a plate coated with a photographic emulsion, and the radioactive cell nuclei are counted. This ratio of labeled to unlabeled cells is termed the *labeling index* (LI) and provides an estimate, in vitro, of the potential tumor DT.[49-53] Of course, cell loss in growing tumors may be relatively low or may be in excess of 90% of the rate of cell production, thus making the actual DT longer than predicted by the measured LI.[52] Nevertheless, in clinical observations, LI correlates well with actual DT.

The Institut Gustave-Roussy has reported the measurement of the LI in 128 consecutive breast cancers. Their results, initially reported in 1975 and updated several times, have shown a higher LI in patients with relapse.[50,52,53] Other studies examining large numbers of patients have reached a similar conclusion.[54-56] Subjecting LI to multivariate analysis has shown that its prognostic impact on relapse and death is independent of stage, tumor size, and nodal involvement. The LI does show a strong correlation with nuclear and histologic grades.[50,51,56]

Silvestrini and colleagues[56] determined the LI on fresh tumors of 258 node-negative patients (stages T_1, T_2, and T_{3a}) treated with radical mastectomy. In their study, the probability of a 6-year, relapse-free survival was 80.5% for patients with a low LI and 59.6% for those with a high LI ($p = .00004$).[56] Tubiana and Koscielyn[52] point out that the low incidence of relapse in the low-LI patients cannot be solely the result of differences in growth rates but must partly reflect differences in metastasizing potential.

The application of DNA flow cytometry and image cytometry has provided a more accurate assessment of the number of tumor cells in S phase.[57] Furthermore, by substituting bromodeoxyuridine (BrdU) for tritiated thymidine, the labeled cells can be detected by an anti-BrdU antibody. Thus it is possible to determine the proportion of cells engaged in a cell cycle, the duration of the cycle, and the DNA ploidy of the breast tumor.[58]

Data indicate that breast cancers with diploid DNA content tend to be of low histologic grade and high ER content, whereas tumors with higher DNA ploidy are more anaplastic and low in receptor content.[58-60] As a result, simultaneous measurement of these prognostic indicators provides a useful method of identifying the subsets of patients at increased risk.

Natural History of Breast Cancer

It has been possible to use the large, population-based, randomized breast cancer screening trials to study a broader range of questions about the biology of breast cancer. The analysis of the observed prevalence of cancer detected at the time of a given screen and the incidence of cancers discovered during the intervals between screens has provided insight into the kinetics of breast cancer cell growth and the biologic activity (metastatic potential) of the disease. During the asymptomatic preclinical phase of breast cancer growth, there is a time when the *prevalent cancer* has reached a size that is detectable with screening mammography. The time point is determined by a number of variables, including the rate of tumor cell growth, the suitability of the breast for optimal imaging, the sensitivity of equipment used, and the skill of the physician interpreting the results.

The interval between the time of detection by screening and the time when the cancer becomes clinically incident (*incident cancer*) is defined as the *lead-time* (Figure 32-2). Thus the longer the lead-time is, the better the prognosis is. Lead-time, of course, depends on how long a breast cancer is in the preclinical or asymptomatic phase but is detectable with screening. The longer this preclinical phase of detectable cancer is, the longer is the lead-time.

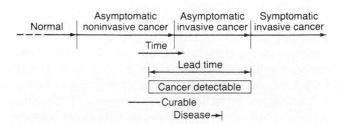

FIG. **32-2** A model of breast cancer progression. Estimates suggest that mammography is capable of detecting tumors once they have reached 1 to 2 mm in diameter.

If the breast cancer has developed to the point where it is incurable at the time of the screening, the time between diagnosis and death is prolonged only by the lead-time. In this case, earlier detection does not affect time of death. It is also possible that screening may detect breast cancers that have a long asymptomatic, noninvasive phase; some of these might never have become clinically detectable *(length bias sampling)*; thus their detection with screening would have little impact on breast cancer mortality.

Using the Health Insurance Plan (HIP) study, Walter and Day estimated lead-time at 1.387 years for breast cancer detected in the first year of screening.[61,62] In subsequent years, the number of cases found at screening diminished, presumably as the number of prevalent cases in the screened population gradually decreased. Table 32-1 summarizes the findings of a number of investigators who have determined the preclinical phase and the lead-time. As can be seen, there is a large variation in estimates of lead-time, ranging from 0.4 to 3.0 years. This large variation is undoubtedly the result of using numerous unverified assumptions in the calculations and a great diversity of mathematical approaches. In addition, some authors used data from the BCDDP, a nonrandomized screening study, for their calculations of lead-time. The best estimate of lead-time for cancers detected with mammography appears to be the one calculated by Walter and Day: 1.7 years for each screened period.[62,71]

Studies of a large group of breast cancer patients at the Institut Gustave-Roussy divided cancers according to their volume at surgical excision and plotted for each subset of volumes the actuarial cumulated proportion of patients with metastases as a function of time from treatment up to 25 years. From their extensive analysis of these data, the investigators concluded that the capacity for lymphatic spread is acquired much earlier than the capacity for hematogenous spread. In rapidly growing tumors, initial axillary node invasion was estimated in their model to have occurred when the primary tumor was 2 to 3 mm in diameter, and distant metastasis was estimated to have occurred with tumor diameter smaller than 1.5 cm.[72,73] This differed markedly from what was observed for tumors with a slow growth rate, where the predictions for axillary node invasion and distant metastasis were for tumors with diameters of 4 and 6 cm, respectively.

The ability to use screening mammography to diagnose breast cancer early during the lead-time, when it is either noninvasive or early in its invasive growth, emphasizes the importance of assessing the biologic parameters for each tumor. It is now possible to determine the patient's risk for occult metastases by assessing tumor growth rate, histologic grade, receptor content, the presence or absence of specific gene markers, and DNA ploidy. From such a profile it will be possible to predict the patient's position on the risk curve and thus select the appropriate surgical and adjuvant therapy. Certain genetic markers may even provide guidelines that will further increase the benefit of specific screening.

Interval Breast Cancers

In the large, population-based, randomized screening trials designed to evaluate the efficacy of mammography in detecting early occult breast cancer, a subset of women had their cancers diagnosed after a negative mammogram but before the next scheduled screening examination.[74-81] Fortunately, the incidence of

---

TABLE 32-1 Analysis of Preclinical Phase of Breast Cancer

REPORT	DATABASE	ESTIMATED MEAN PRECLINICAL DURATION (yr)	ESTIMATED MEAN LEAD-TIME (yr)
Hutchison and Shapiro[62a]	HIP	1.7	0.85
Zelen and Feinleib[63]	HIP	2.4	2.4
Shapiro et al[64]	HIP	1.3	0.65
Tallis and Sarfaty[65]	Melbourne Cancer Registry	1.8	—
Seidman[66]	BCDDP	—	1.4
Fox et al[67]	BCDDP	—	3.0
Albert et al[68]	HIP	1.8	—
Shwartz[69]	HIP, BCDDP	—	1.9
Dubin[70]	HIP	—	0.4
Walter and Day[61,62]	HIP	1.7	1.7

From Walter SD, Day NE: *Am J Epidemiol* 118:865, 1983.
BCDDP, Breast Cancer Detection Demonstration Project study; *HIP*, Health Insurance Plan study.

these *interval* cancers in the screened population is low (approximately 12%), which in itself is a measure of the effectiveness of mammography as a screening tool.[71,76,82,83] Concern has always existed that these interval breast cancers represent tumors with a shorter DT and therefore a more aggressive metastatic potential.[78,82,84-89] The question of a biologic difference between interval cancers and cancers detected on screening has been further confused by the possibility that there exists among screen-detected cancers an excess of slow-growing tumors.[90-93] These observations have led some to suggest that interval cancers should be treated more aggressively.[86]

Recent reports indicate that interval cancers have a similar prognosis to that of identically staged cancers diagnosed in an unscreened population.[44,79,94-98] These observations are at odds with the frequently stated hypothesis that the more rapid growth rate of the interval cancer gives them greater metastatic potential than cancers in the unscreened population. As might be expected, survival for those whose breast cancers are detected on screening is significantly better than for those with interval cancers. Although it is tempting to compare the survival of patients with interval cancers with those whose cancers are detected at regularly scheduled screening examinations, this comparison would introduce significant length bias sampling error.

These observations suggest that a faster growth rate for interval breast cancers is not associated with a greater risk for metastases and a worse prognosis and that the growth rate of interval cancers is not significantly different from that of cancers detected in the unscreened control population. Obviously, the significance of interval cancers and the relationship of growth rate to prognosis relate directly to decisions about appropriate therapy.

Although a number of screening trials have provided data on the incidence of interval breast cancers, much of our initial information concerning interval cancers and their relative risks came from two large, randomized trials: the HIP study of New York and the Swedish two-county study.[79,80] The Swedish trial contributed significantly to this subject because it was designed with longer screening intervals. The longer time between screens made it possible to study the effect of interval length on the incidence of interval cancers and their clinical stage. The authors recognized that the proportion of cancers detected as interval cancers, and the prognosis (i.e., stage) of those with cancers diagnosed at the next screening are what determine an acceptable interval between screens. Thus the design of the Swedish study, with longer screening intervals, provided the first opportunity to look at these important factors in greater detail.

The first breast cancer screening trial to use randomization in its design was the HIP study, initiated in 1963.[79,91] Two systematic random samples of 31,000 women aged 40 to 64 years were selected from HIP, a comprehensive prepaid group practice in New York. Following an initial screening examination, the study group women were offered three additional examinations, one per year. The control group was not screened, and its members continued to receive their usual medical care. By the end of 10 years, the screened group's mortality from breast cancer was approximately 30% lower than that of the control group.[79] Interestingly, the small number of interval cancers diagnosed in the HIP study group had the same case-fatality rate as that of the control group.[79]

The Swedish two-county study is even more enlightening because of its design and because it used the many technical advances in mammography that occurred since the 1960s. The Swedish trial began in 1977 and involved 162,981 women aged 40 or older who were randomly assigned to study or control groups on a population-block basis drawn from local parishes in two Swedish counties.[80] Between the first and second screenings, the average interval was 33 months for women 50 years and older and 24 months for women younger than 50 years. The average interval between the second and third examinations was 24 months for all age groups. Compliance for three screening examinations was quite good: 89.2%, 83.3%, and 84.0%, respectively. The study has another interesting design feature that incorporated screening of the control population after completion of the third round of screening for those aged 50 or older and after the fourth screen for those younger than 50 years.

In 1986 the Swedish group reported that during the first 7 years of screening 104 of 465 breast cancers presented as interval cancers.[96] Of the 104, 10 were in situ and were excluded from analysis. In addition, a blinded radiologic review of the cases revealed only six cancers that were missed on prior screening. These 88 true interval cancers were compared with 178 breast cancers in the control group.

Overall, the survival rate was higher in the interval cancer group than in the control cancers, but this difference was not significant.[96] A similar trend of greater difference was observed when comparing the disease-free intervals. These observations remained true even with a proportional hazards analysis, which introduced age, tumor size, axillary node involvement, and TNM (tumor, node, metastasis) stage into the analysis. Furthermore, when the authors analyzed the time between last screening and diagnosis of the interval cancer by the proportional hazards model, they could not demonstrate that the length of this interval was related to prognosis.[97] Thus these findings confirmed the observations in the earlier HIP study. The Swedish trial also observed that the proportion of deaths among women who refused screening increased rapidly with age, reaching 50% in the 70- to 74-year-old group, whereas the proportion of deaths in the interval cancer group decreased rapidly with age.[80] In their analysis of the screened population, the authors observed just the opposite. In this population, more than 50% of deaths from breast cancer in the 40- to 49-year-old group were from interval cancers.

It is important to examine the incidence of interval cancers based on the length of time between screenings and the age of the screened population. To do this, the Swedish group determined the incidence of breast cancers each year in the randomly selected control population. This provided the basis for estimating the number of cases that should be detected by screening each year. The ratio of the number of cases observed and the number expected (i.e., the number predicted from the control population) gives the *proportional incidence* of interval cancers.

The difference between the proportional incidence of interval cancers in the 40- to 49-year-old and the 50- to 69-year-old age groups was significant. In the younger women, screening detected 62% of the cancers that would have surfaced in the first 12 months and only 32% of the cancers predicted for the second 12 months. In contrast, the screening examination detected 87% for the first and 71% for the second 12 months in the 50- to 69-year-old group.[80,99] The Swedish trial also found that the proportion of stage II cancers in the interval cases, 57.5%, was essentially the same as it was for the cancers diagnosed in the control group of 59.2%. In this study, age had no effect on the percentage of stage II cases in either group.[99]

The results of the HIP and Swedish randomized trials support the conclusion that the prognosis of interval cancers is the same as that of similarly staged cancers diagnosed in an unscreened population. Although interval cancers may be faster-growing tumors, no evidence can be found that patients with interval cancers, when compared with unscreened women, are at greater risk for a more rapid course of systemic dissemination and death. Clearly, the value of screening is in the earlier stage of cancers detected at repeat screening, especially with increasing age (38% stage II, age 40 to 49 years; 25% stage II, age 50 to 59 years; and 17% stage II, age 60 to 69 years). It should be noted that the Swedish study consisted of only a single film of the breast instead of the standard two views. Therefore the incidence of interval cancer can be expected to be even lower when annual two-view screening mammography combined with physical examination of the breast is done. In addition, shorter-interval follow-up is often indicated when uncertainties arise. Overall, with an optimal screening program, the incidence of interval cancers can still be expected to be about 12%.[83,100]

Survival of Patients with Interval Breast Cancers

With more than 25 years of experience conducting mammographic screening trials, a number of investigators have reviewed these databases to determine whether true interval cancers represent a more aggressive subgroup of breast cancer with a poor prognosis.* Worse survival might be expected for those with interval cancers because there is evidence that screen-detected cases contain an excessive proportion of slow-growing tumors and that interval cancers have a faster growth rate and carry markers of unfavorable prognosis.[6,62,84,104,105]

In contrast to what might be expected, multiple reports have demonstrated that survival for patients with interval breast cancer is no worse than that for unscreened control patients.[42,75,94,106] As might be anticipated, because of the significant differences in trial design, it is difficult to interpret these results and to make comparisons between studies. For example, there has been a notable variation in length of screening interval (from 12 months to 4 years) as well as differences in criteria for selecting controls. More recent studies have carefully reviewed each case of interval breast cancer in an attempt to subgroup interval cancers and to identify those that are true interval cancers and not screening errors.†

The screening program of Stockholm identified 130 cases that were determined to be true interval cancers.[95] These patients were compared with 142 patients with cancers diagnosed clinically in the control population during the same study period. Multiple regression analyses found no differences between the two study groups when comparing tumor size, stage distribution, and mean age. The interval cancer group, however, contained more women in the younger age group. With up to 8 years of follow-up, the stage-by-stage survival was consistently higher for patients with interval cancers. These results are similar to those reported in the Swedish trial and the HIP study, where no statistical difference in survival was found between patients with interval cancers or control cancers.[79,96] These studies, however, did not compare survival rate stage by stage and did not classify the interval cancers into subgroups. When these various studies looked at the length of the interval between the negative screen and the clinical diagnosis of an interval cancer, no significant survival difference was found.[95,96]

The Diagnostisch Onderzoek Mammacarcinoam (DOM) program, a population-based, nonrandomized screening trial located in Utrecht, Netherlands, reported survival results for 75 interval breast cancers occurring

---

*References 64, 82, 86, 89, 95, 99-103.
†References 76, 82, 83, 95, 102, 107, 108.

within 2 years of a negative screen.[102] Review of each case determined that 58 of the 75 interval breast cancers could be considered true interval cancers. The 10-year survival for patients with these 58 true interval cancers was 58%, just slightly worse than for the 17 patients in the missed (false-negative) interval cancer subgroup, whose 10-year survival was 67% (*p* = .38). The authors concluded that there was no difference in survival between patients with true interval cancers or cancers in an unscreened population (Figure 32-3).[102]

As a result of these analyses of the prognosis for interval cancers, other investigators began looking for differences in the presentation of these cancers and for differences in their biology. For example, in a review of 64 interval cancers from the New Mexico Mammography Project published in 2000, the authors compared tumor proliferation and *p53* expression to an age- and ethnicity-matched group of patients with cancers detected on screening.[109] The authors found that interval cancers were more likely to have a high proportion of Ki-67–positive proliferating cells and *p53* expression. Consistent with these data, the interval cancers also had a higher histologic grade than cancers detected on screening. In the Swedish two-county study, as well as the DOM screening program, interval cancers exhibited increased S-phase levels and aneuploidy compared with screen-detected tumors.[110,111]

Because interval cancers are cancers that are diagnosed after a normal screening examination, it is reasonable to question whether these patients have more dysplastic mammographic patterns and tumor histologic patterns known to be difficult to image. Ikeda and colleagues, in analyzing the Malmö mammographic screening trial, found that 36.5% of their interval cancers occurred in patients with a P2 Wolf pattern and 23% in those with a dysplastic (DY) pattern.[112,113] They also found that 15% were lobular cancers and 38% were invasive comedo carcinoma, medullary, or mucinous cancers. These are breast cancer histologic types known to be difficult to image at an early stage.

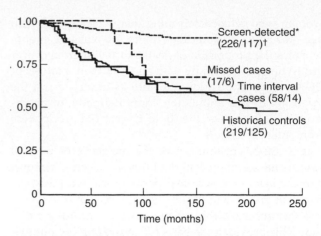

FIG. **32-3** Kaplan-Meier survival of breast cancer by mode of detection. *Corrected for lead-time. †Number of breast cancer cases at start after 10 years of follow-up. *(From Brekelmans CT et al: Eur J Cancer 31:1830, 1995. Copyright 1995, Elsevier Science Ltd, The Boulevard Langford Lane, Kidlington OX5 #26B, UK.)*

Koivunen and colleagues[100] found 74% of the mammograms of interval breast cancers in the BCDDP screening project at the Ellis Fischel Cancer Hospital to be of the P2 and DY patterns. The incidence of DY patterns in these two reports on interval breast cancers were 23% and 30%, respectively, only slightly higher than that reported for screen-detected cancers (Table 32-2).[113,114,116] From these reports on interval breast cancer, it appears safe to conclude that they are no more lethal cancers but are somewhat more difficult to image.

Several reports have analyzed the interval cancers in their screening programs in an effort to identify specific risk factors.[60,117,118] From these reports the following characteristics are identified:

- Younger women have a higher incidence than older women.
- Leaner and taller women have a higher incidence.
- Interval cancer occurs more frequently in women who have artificial menopause.

TABLE **32-2**	Wolfe's Mammographic Classification of Several Published Breast Cancer Series					
PUBLISHED SERIES	NO. OF PATIENTS	N (%)	P1 (%)	P2 (%)	DY (%)
Wolfe, 1976 (screened population)[113]	5284	41	26	26	7
Wolfe, 1976 (cancer patients)[113]	40	7.5	15	57.5	20
Verbeek et al, 1984[116]	20	30	30	40	0
Gravelle et al, 1986[114]	31	3	10	65	23
Compilation of above three series[113-115]	91	11	16.5	56	16.5
Ikeda et al, 1992 (interval cancers)[112]	96	4	36.5	36.5	23
Koivunen et al, 1994 (interval cancers)[100]	23	9	17	44	30

From Koivunen D et al: *Am J Surg* 168:538, 1994. Copyright 1994 by Excerpta Medica Inc.
N, No ductal prominence; *P1*, prominent ducts were confined to the anterior quarter of the breast; *P2*, extensive ductal prominence; *DY*, confluent density sufficient to obscure detail of underlying parenchyma.

- Interval tumors are more likely to be ER negative.
- Patients in whom interval cancers develop more often have a history of benign breast disease.
- Patients with interval cancers are more likely to have a P2 or DY mammographic pattern.
- Patients with interval cancers more frequently have tumors that are difficult to image.

Table 32-3 is a summary of the epidemiologic, radiologic, and histologic characteristics of true interval breast cancers compared with screen-detected cancers found on first round in the DOM program.[117]

Thus, although true interval cancers do not have a worse prognosis than cancers in an unscreened population, women who develop interval cancers clearly have

a different profile of risk factors. Interval cancers seem to include a subgroup of rapidly proliferating cancers when compared with those detected with screening mammography. How this difference could relate to earlier diagnosis and prevention remains to be determined by further study.

Interval Breast Cancer as an Indicator of Screening Sensitivity

It is important to recognize that the standards for optimal breast cancer screening continue to evolve (Figure 32-4). This evolution is significantly influenced by the ongoing improvements in the technical quality

TABLE 32-3 Epidemiologic, Radiologic, and Histologic Characteristics of Cancers Detected at First Screening (Reference Group) and "True" Interval Breast Cancers (Detected after One or More Screening Rounds)

VARIABLE	SCREEN-DETECTED CANCERS FIRST ROUND (n = 258)	"TRUE" INTERVAL CANCER (n = 105)	"TRUE" INTERVAL CANCER DETECTED AFTER FIRST SCREENING (n = 57)
Anthropometric variables: mean (in parantheses: SEM)			
Weight (kg)	70.5 (0.78)	68.6 (1.02)	67 (1.29)
Height (cm)	163.4 (0.41)	165.3 (0.67)*	166.1 (0.90)*
Quetelet's index (kg/m²)	26.4 (0.29)	25.3 (0.43)*	24.7 (0.49)*
Other epidemiologic and histologic characteristics: percentage (in parentheses: count)			
<50 yr at last screening	10.1 (258)	26.7 (105)*	45.6 (57)*
Premenopausal	27.5 (255)	35.0 (100)†	56.6 (53)*
Artificial menopause	7.6 (185)	24.6 (65)*	30.4 (23)*
Ever used oral contraceptives	16.7 (258)	28.6 (105)*	42.1 (57)*
Ever used estrogen replacement therapy	5.1 (254)	10.1 (99)†	5.9 (51)
History of benign breast disease	5.0 (258)	17.1 (105)*	19.3 (57)*
First-degree family member with breast cancer	17.4 (258)	12.4 (105)	12.3 (57)
Childless	19.5 (256)	21.9 (105)	24.6 (57)
Ever smoked	36.3 (152)	37.7 (77)	53.3 (30)†
Dense breast tissue	40.6 (256)	40.2 (105)	33.3 (57)
Estrogen receptor negative	26.3 (95)	34.3 (35)	66.7 (9)*
Axillary node involvement	26.9 (245)	52.9 (102)*	55.4 (56)*
Tumor stage‡ A	60.8 (245)	36.3 (102)*	37.5 (56)*
B	12.2	10.8	7.1
C	20.8	29.4	25.0
D	6.1	23.5	30.4
Histology:			
DCIS	12.8 (258)	3.7 (105)*	3.5 (57)*
Invasive	87.2	96.3	96.5

As a comparison, values for "true" interval cancers detected after first screening are listed in the last column.
From Brekelmans CT et al: *Breast Cancer Rev Treat* 30:223, 1994.
DCIS, Ductal carcinoma in situ.
*Denotes groups significantly different from screen detected cancers at the 0.05 level.
†Denotes groups significantly different from screen detected cancers at the 0.10 level.
‡*A,* tumor size <21 mm, node negative; *B,* tumor size >20 mm, node negative; *C,* tumor size <21 mm, node positive; *D,* tumor size >20 mm, node positive.

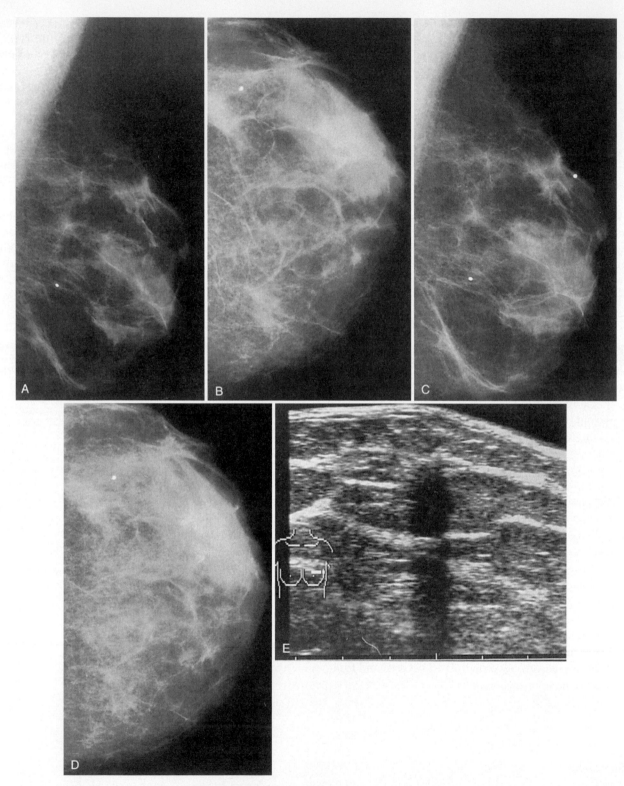

FIG. **32-4** These mammograms provide an excellent example of the subgroup of interval breast cancers that fail to image on conventional film/screen mammography. The patient is 52 years old and undergoing regularly scheduled yearly breast mammography and examination. Her yearly mammographic examination in June 1994 was negative (**A** and **B**), as was her physical examination. A stable mammographic pattern was unchanged from previous years, and there were no suspicious or questionable findings. The patient returned 3 months later concerned about a change in her self-examination. She directed the surgeon and the radiologist to a specific area in the upper outer quadrant of the left breast. Repeat mammography with a BB skin marker on September 14, 1994, was unchanged and again negative (**C** and **D**). However, ultrasound demonstrated a solid lesion measuring 8.6 mm (**E**). A biopsy documented the presence of grade II infiltrating ductal carcinoma measuring 1.5 cm in diameter with associated cribriform ductal carcinoma in situ. The patient was treated with breast conservation.

of film/screen mammography and the experience of radiologists dedicated to breast cancer screening.[119] These advances, plus ultrasound and stereotactic fine-needle aspiration of uncertain x-ray abnormalities, are expected to have a positive effect on further decreasing false-negative screening results and breast cancer mortality. Unfortunately, this positive impact on mortality cannot be measured for at least 7 years from the time a technical change or improvement in screening is introduced.[44,75,80,81] This long lag time before a benefit can be measured has necessitated the use of other methods of determining benefit. One method is calculating the incidence of interval cancers.[71,120] This incidence serves as an indicator of screening sensitivity.

Unfortunately, the group of interval cancers in any screening center is not always a true number but rather consists of cancers that were present at the time of screening that were missed for some reason and also includes newly developed true interval cancers. Several authors have reviewed mammograms of patients with interval cancer and classified the interval cancers into (1) screening error (18% to 29%), (2) minimal sign present (30% to 40%), (3) radiographically occult (33% to 58%), and (4) radiographically occult even at diagnosis (7% to 16%).[82,98,112,121] Ikeda and colleagues[112] suggested dividing interval cancers into three groups: true, unrecognized, and observable error.

The incidence of screening error is an important factor because it delays treatment by the length of the screening interval for this group of patients. Van Dijck and colleagues[83] looked at data from their population-based screening project in the Netherlands, which began in 1975 with a biennial mammogram (Table 32-4). They studied two groups of patients. The first group consisted of 41 patients with interval cancer diagnosed after a negative screen on the seventh round (1987 to 1988) but before their eighth screen. The second group consisted of 57 patients with breast cancers detected during the eighth round of screening (1989 to 1990).[83] Of the screen-detected cancers, a careful review determined that 9% were missed on the prior screen and thus were true false-negative or screening errors. In fact, in

nearly half of the eighth-round screen-detected cancers, minimal signs of cancer were thought to be present at round seven. Of the interval cancers, 18% were determined on review to be screening errors, 28% had minimal signs of cancer, 42% were radiographically occult, and 12% of the interval cancers still had no evidence of x-ray changes at diagnosis.[83]

Taplin and associates[122] examined the incidence of interval breast cancers among women enrolled in a regional breast cancer screening program. These authors discovered that interval cancers were more likely following images with poor positioning (odds ratio, 2.57; 95% confidence interval 1.28 to 5.52) or poor overall image quality ($p = .037$).[122]

The question that arises from these studies is, What constitutes adequate review to minimize false-negative findings? Compiling the information available suggests that optimal review occurs when a majority opinion is based on the interpretations of six reviewers (minimum of three) and when reviewers are looking at a mix of normal films and films with signs of cancer.[78]

It is important that screening programs establish a standard for mammographic technique, film review, and patient follow-up.[123,124] Annual screening minimizes the negative impact of screening errors. In addition, having films reviewed by at least three radiologists and developing a standard procedure for rigorous radiographic review of cases in which minimal radiographic signs of possible cancer are found will minimize screening errors and false-negative results.[76] At the very least, cases with minimal radiographic signs should have an even shorter interval of follow-up, such as 4 to 6 months (Box 32-1).

Perhaps the best way to compare the various reports on interval breast cancer is to express interval cancer rates in terms of the number of women examined and the number of mammographic screenings performed. For example, the HIP study had an interval cancer rate of 1.45 per 1000 women screened; the BCDDP in the United States had a rate of 1.93 per 1000 women; the Canadian National Breast Screening Study rate was 2.4 per 1000 women; the Nijmegen (Netherlands) study

TABLE 32-4 Interval Breast Cancer: Classification of Previous Screening Mammograms

		CLASSIFICATION OF PREVIOUS SCREENING MAMMOGRAMS			
INVESTIGATORS	CASES (N)	SCREENING ERROR (%)	MINIMAL SIGN (%)	RADIOGRAPH OCCULT (%)	RADIOGRAPH OCCULT AT DIAGNOSIS (%)
Martin et al.[108]	48	29	38	33	—
Von Rosen et al.[89]	42	24	33	36	7
Frisell et al.[77]	60	20	28	52	—
Peeters et al.[98]	153	26	—	58	16

Modified from van Dijck JA et al.: *Cancer* 72:1933, 1993. Copyright © 1993 American Cancer Society. Reprinted by permission of Wiley-Liss, Inc., a subsidiary of John Wiley & Sons, Inc.

BOX 32-1 Guidelines for Optimal Breast Cancer Screening

GOALS
- Minimize false-negative findings during screen
- Minimize incidence of true interval cancers

METHODS
- Two-view film/screen mammography
- Clinical breast examination
- Magnification views of questionable findings
- Screenings at 1-yr intervals
- Mammograms reviewed by three radiologists
- Short follow-up at 3 to 4 mo for patients with uncertain findings
- Identification of patients with greater risk for developing interval cancer

---

rate was 2.54 per 1000 women; and in the British Columbia screening program, the rate was 0.97 per 1000 women screened.[10,106,125-129] From these data the lowest incidence of true interval cancers occurs with 12-month screening intervals and a minimum of two views at mammography. The clinical trials clearly supported the importance of using the incidence of true interval cancers as a measure of screening excellence and patient benefit.

REFERENCES

1. Pardee AB: A restriction point for control of normal animal cell proliferation, *Proc Natl Acad Sci USA* 11:1286, 1974.
2. Reddy GP: Cell cycle: regulatory events in G_1-S transition of mammalian cells, *J Cell Biochem* 54:379, 1994.
3. Sherr CJ: G_1 phase progression: cycling on cue, *Cell* 79:551, 1994.
4. Brooks RF, Bennet DC, Smith JA: Mammalian cell cycles need two random transitions, *Cell* 19:493, 1980.
5. Murray A: Cell cycle checkpoints, *Curr Opin Cell Biol* 6:872, 1994.
6. Hoffman I, Karsenti E: The role of cdc25 in checkpoints and feedback controls in the eukaryocytic cell cycle, *J Cell Sci* 18:75, 1994.
7. Prive C: Doing the right thing: feedback control and p53, *Curr Opin Cell Biol* 5:214, 1993.
8. Zambetti GP et al: Wild type p53 mediates positive regulation of gene expression through a specific DNA sequence element, *Genes Dev* 6:1143, 1992.
9. Kastan MB et al: Participation of p53 protein in the cellular response to DNA damage, *Cancer Res* 51:6304, 1991.
10. Pines J: Cell proliferation and control, *Curr Opin Cell Biol* 4:144, 1992.
11. Sherr C: Mammalian G_1 cyclins, *Cell* 73:1059, 1993.
12. Tubiana M, Malaise EP: Growth rate and cell kinetics in human tumors: some prognostic and therapeutic implications. In Symington T, Carter RL (eds): *Scientific foundations of oncology*, London, 1976, Heinemann.
13. Hinds PW et al: Regulation of retinoblastoma protein functions by ectopic expression of human cyclins, *Cell* 70:993, 1992.
14. Kato JY et al: Direct binding of cyclin D to the retinoblastoma gene product and pRB phosphorylation by the cyclin D-dependent kinase: Cdk4, *Genes Dev* 7:331,1993.
15. Medema RH et al: Growth suppression by p16inkH requires functional retinoblastoma protein, *Proc Natl Acad Sci USA* 92:6289, 1995.
16. Harwell RM et al: Processing of cyclin E differs between normal and tumor breast cells, *Cancer Res* 60:481, 2001.
17. Umekita Y, Yoshida H: Cyclin D1 expression in ductal carcinoma in situ, atypical ductal hyperplasia and usual ductal hyperplasia: an immunohistochemical study, *Pathol Int* 50:527, 2000.
18. Foster JS et al: Multifaceted regulation of cell cycle progression by estrogen: regulation of cdk inhibitors and Cdc25A independent of cyclin D1-Cdk4 function, *Mol Cell Biol* 21:794, 2001.
19. Scott KA, Walker RA: Lack of cyclin E immunoreactivity in non-malignant breast and association with proliferation in breast cancer, *Br J Cancer* 76:1288, 1997.
20. Gray-Bablin J et al: Cyclin E, a redundant cyclin in breast cancer, *Proc Natl Acad Sci USA* 93:15215, 1996.
21. Nielsen NH et al: Cyclin E overexpression, a negative prognostic factor in breast cancer with strong correlation to oestrogen receptor status, *Br J Cancer* 74:874, 1996.
22. Evron E et al: Loss of cyclin D2 expression in the majority of breast cancers is associated with promoter hypermethylation, *Cancer Res* 61:2782, 2001.
23. Singletary E: A working model for the time sequence of genetic changes in breast tumorigenesis, *J Am Coll Surg* 194:202, 2002.
24. Altucci L et al: 17beta-estradiol induces cyclin D1 gene transcription, p36D1-p34cdk4 complex activation and p105Rb phosphorylation during mitogenic stimulation of G(1)-arrested human breast cancer cells, *Oncogene* 12:2315, 1996.
25. Ahamed S et al: Signal transduction through the Ras/Erk pathway is essential for the mycoestrogen zearalenone-induced cell-cycle progression in MCF-7 cells, *Mol Carcinog* 30:88, 2001.
26. Dees C et al: Dietary estrogens stimulate human breast cells to enter the cell cycle, *Environ Health Perspect* 105(suppl 3): 633, 1997.
27. Planas-Silva MD, Weinberg RA: Estrogen-dependent cyclin E-Cdk2 activation through p2 redistribution, *Mol Cell Biol* 17:4059, 1997.
28. Prall OWJ et al: Estrogen-induced activation of Cdk4 and Cdk2 during G1-S phase progression is accompanied by increased cyclin D1 expression and decreased cyclin-dependent kinase inhibitor association with cyclin E-Cdk2, *J Biol Chem* 272:10882, 1997.
29. Foster JS, Wimalesena J: Estrogen regulates activity of cyclin-dependent kinases and retinoblastoma protein phosphorylation in breast cancer cells, *Mol Endocrinol* 10:488, 1996.
30. Carroll JS et al: A pure estrogen antagonist inhibits cyclin E-Cdk2 activity in MCF-7 breast cancer cells and induces accumulation of p130-E2F4 complexes characteristic of quiescence, *J Biol Chem* 275:38221, 2000.
31. Reddel RR et al: Factors affecting the sensitivity of T-47D human breast cancer cells to tamoxifen, *Cancer Res* 44:2398, 1984.
32. Querzoli P et al: Modulation of biomarkers in minimal breast carcinoma, *Cancer* 83:89, 1998.

33. Landberg G, Roos G: The cell cycle in breast cancer, *APMIS* 105:575, 1997.
34. Aas T et al: Specific p53 mutations are associated with de novo resistance to doxorubicin in breast cancer patients, *Nature Med* 2:811, 1996.
35. Börresen AL et al: TP53 mutations and breast cancer prognosis: particularly poor survival rates for cases with mutations in the zinc-binding domains, *Genes Chromosomes Cancer* 14:71, 1995.
36. Borg A et al: The retinoblastoma gene in breast cancer: allele loss is not correlated with loss of gene protein expression, *Cancer Res* 52:2991, 1992.
37. Geradts J, Wilson PA: High frequency of aberrant p16 (INK4A) expression in human breast cancer, *Am J Pathol* 149:15, 1996.
38. Russo J et al: Biological and molecular basis of human breast cancer, *Front Biosci* 3:D944, 1998.
39. Herman JG et al: Inactivation of the CDKN2/p6/MTS1 gene is frequently associated with aberrant DNA methylation in all common human cancers, *Cancer Res* 55:4525, 1995.
40. Hiyama E et al: Telomerase activity in human breast tumors, *J Natl Cancer Inst* 88:116, 1996.
41. Landberg G et al: Telomerase activity is associated with cell cycle deregulation in human breast cancer, *Cancer Res* 57:549, 1997.
42. Gershon-Cohen J, Berger SM, Klickstein HS: Roentgenography of breast cancer moderating concept of "biologic predeterminism," *Cancer* 16:961, 1963.
43. Spratt JS, Spratt JA: Growth rates. In Donegan NL, Spratt JS (eds): *Cancer of the breast*, Philadelphia, 1979, WB Saunders.
44. Collette C et al: Evaluation of a breast cancer screening programme—the DOM project, *Eur J Cancer* 28A:1985,1992.
45. Dressler LG et al: Identifying breast cancer patients for adjuvant therapy by DNA flow cytometry and steroid receptors; a 1000 patient study. Proceedings of the twenty-second annual meeting of ASCO, Los Angeles, May 4-6, 1986.
46. Spratt JS, Meyer JS, Spratt JA: Rates of growth of human neoplasms: part II, *J Surg Oncol* 61:68, 1996.
47. Retsky MW et al: Is gompertzian or exponential kinetics a valid description of individual human cancer growth? *Med Hypothesis* 33:95, 1990.
48. Retsky MW et al: Prospective computerized simulation with nine sets of biological and clinical data, *Cancer Res* 47:4982, 1987.
49. Fournier D, Von Cubli F, Barth V: Growth rates of 147 mammary carcinomas, *Cancer* 45:2198, 1980.
50. McGurrin JF et al: Assessment of tumor cell kinetics by immunohistochemistry in carcinoma of the breast, *Cancer* 59:1744, 1987.
51. Meyer JS, Hizon B: Advanced stage and early relapse of breast carcinomas associated with high thymidine labeling indices, *Cancer Res* 39:4042, 1979.
52. Tubiana M, Koscielyn S: Cell kinetics, growth rate and the natural history of breast cancer: the Heuson Memorial Lecture, *Eur J Cancer Clin Oncol* 24:1879, 1983.
53. Tubiana M et al: The long-term prognostic significance of the thymidine labelling index in breast cancer, *Int J Cancer* 33:441, 1987.
54. Meyer JS et al: Prediction of early course of breast carcinoma by thymidine labeling, *Cancer* 51:1879, 1983.
55. Meyer JS et al: Breast carcinoma cell kinetics, morphology, stage and host characteristics: a thymidine labeling study, *Lab Invest* 54:41, 1986.
56. Silvestrini R et al: Cell kinetics as a prognostic marker in locally advanced breast cancer, *Cancer Treat Rep* 71:375, 1987.
57. McDivitt RW, Stone KR, Meyer JS: A method for dissociation of viable human breast cancer cells that produces flow cytometric kinetic information similar to that obtained by thymidine labeling, *Cancer Res* 44:2628, 1984.
58. Dean PN et al: Cell-cycle analysis using a monoclonal antibody to BrdUrd, *Cell Tissue Kinet* 17:427, 1984.
59. Coulson PB et al: Prognostic indicator including DNA histogram type, receptor content and staging related to human breast cancer survival, *Cancer Res* 44:4187, 1984.
60. Dieterich B et al: The prognostic value of DNA ploidy and S-phase estimate in primary breast cancer: a prospective study, *Int J Cancer* 63:49, 1995.
61. Day NE, Walter SD: Simplified models of screening for chronic disease: estimation procedures from mass screening programmes, *Biometrics* 40:1, 1984.
62. Walter SD, Day NE: Estimation of the duration of a preclinical disease state using screening data, *Am J Epidemiol* 118:865, 1983.
62a. Hutchison GB, Shapiro S: Lead time gained by diagnostic screening for breast cancer, *J Natl Cancer Inst* 41:665, 1968.
63. Zelen M, Feinlab M: On the theory of screening for chronic diseases, *Biometrika* 56:601, 1969.
64. Shapiro S, Strax P, Venet L: Periodic breast cancer screening in reducing mortality from breast cancer, *JAMA* 215:1777, 1971.
65. Tallis GM, Sarfaty G: On the distribution of the time to report cancers with application to breast cancer in women, *Math Biosci* 19:371, 1974.
66. Seidman H: Screening for breast cancer in younger women: life expectancy gains and losses, *CA Cancer J Clin* 27:66, 1977.
67. Fox SH et al: Benefit/risk analysis of aggressive mammographic screening, *Radiology* 128:359, 1978.
68. Albert A, Gertman PM, Louis TA: Screening for the early detection of cancer. 1. The temporal natural history of a progressive disease state, *Math Biosci* 40:1, 1978.
69. Shwartz M: An analysis of the benefits of serial screening for breast cancer based upon a mathematical model of the disease, *Cancer* 41:1550, 1978.
70. Dubin N: Benefits of screening for breast cancer: application of a probabilistic model to a breast cancer detection project, *J Chron Dis* 32:145, 1979.
71. Day NE, Williams DR, Khaw KT: Breast cancer screening programmes: the development of monitoring and evaluation system, *Br J Cancer* 59:954, 1989.
72. Koscielny S et al: Breast cancer, relationship between the size of the primary tumor and the probability of metastatic dissemination, *Br J Cancer* 49:709, 1984.
73. Koscielny S, Tubiana M, Valleron AJ: A simulation model of the natural history of human breast cancer, *Br J Cancer* 52:515, 1985.
74. Andersson I, Janzon L, Sigfirsson BF: Mammographic breast cancer screening: a randomized trial in Malmo, Sweden, *Maturitas* 7:21, 1985.
75. Collette HJ et al: Evaluation of screening for breast cancer in a non-randomized study (the DOM project) by means of a case-control study, *Lancet* i:1224, 1984.
76. Duncan AA, Wallis MG: Classifying interval cancers, *Clin Radiol* 50:774, 1995.
77. Frisell J et al: Randomized mammographic screening for breast cancer in Stockholm, *Breast Cancer Res Treat* 8:45, 1986.

78. Panoussopoulos D, Chang J, Humphrey LJ: Screening for breast cancer, *Ann Surg* 186:356, 1977.

79. Shapiro S et al: Ten to fourteen year effect of screening on breast cancer mortality, *J Natl Cancer Inst* 69:349, 1982.

80. Tabar L et al: Reduction in mortality from breast cancer after mass screening with mammography: randomized trial from the breast cancer screening working group of the Swedish National Board of Health and Welfare, *Lancet* i:829, 1985.

81. Verbeek AL et al: Reduction of breast cancer mortality through mass screening with modern mammography: first results of the Nijmegan project, 1975-1981, *Lancet* i:1222, 1984.

82. Frisell J et al: Analysis of interval carcinomas in a randomized screening trial in Stockholm, *Breast Cancer Rest Treat* 3:219, 1987.

83. van Dijck JA et al: The current detectability of breast cancer in a mammographic screening program: a review of the previous mammograms of interval and screen-detected cancers, *Cancer* 72:1933, 1993.

84. Andersson I et al: Mammographic screening and mortality from breast cancer: the Malmo mammographic screening trial, *BMJ* 297:943, 1988.

85. Andersson I: What can we learn from interval carcinomas? *Recent Results Cancer Res* 90:161, 1984.

86. DeGroote R et al: Interval breast cancer: a more aggressive subset of breast neoplasias, *Surgery* 94:543, 1983.

87. Heuser L, Spratt JS, Polk HC: Growth rates of primary breast cancer, *Cancer* 43:1888, 1979.

88. Heuser LS et al: The association of pathologic and mammographic characteristics of primary human breast cancers with "slow" and "fast" growth rates and with axillary lymph node metastases, *Cancer* 53:96, 1984.

89. von Rosen A et al: Assessment of malignancy potential in so-called internal mammary carcinomas, *Br Cancer Res Treat* 6:221, 1985.

90. Joensuu H, Toikkanen S, Klemi PJ: Histopathologic features, DNA content and prognosis of breast carcinomas found incidentally or in screening, *Br J Cancer* 64:588, 1991.

91. Kallioniemi OP et al: DNA flow cytometric analysis indicates that many breast cancers detected in the first round of mammographic screening have a low malignant potential, *Int J Cancer* 42:697, 1988.

92. Klemi PH et al: Aggressiveness of breast cancers found with and without screening, *BMJ* 304:467, 1992.

93. Love RR, Camilli AE: The value of screening, *Cancer* 48:489, 1981.

94. Brekelmans CT et al: Survival in interval breast cancer in the DOM screening programme, *Eur J Cancer* 31:1830, 1995.

95. Frisell J et al: Interval cancer and survival in a randomized breast cancer screening trial in Stockholm, *Breast Cancer Res Treat* 24:11, 1992.

96. Holmberg LH et al: Survival in breast cancer diagnosed between mammographic screening examinations, *Lancet* 2:27, 1986.

97. Moss SM et al: Survival of patients with breast cancer diagnosed in the United Kingdom trial of early detection of breast cancer, *J Med Screen* 1:193, 1994.

98. Peeters PH et al: The occurrence of interval cancers in the Nijmegen screening programme, *Br J Cancer* 59:929, 1989.

99. Tabar L et al: Update of the Swedish two-county program of mammographic screening for breast cancer, *Radiol Clin North Am* 30:187, 1992.

100. Koivunen D et al: Interval breast cancers are not biologically distinct—just more difficult to diagnose, *Am J Surg* 168:538, 1994.

101. Alexander FE et al: The Edinburgh randomized trial of breast cancer screening: results after 10 years of follow-up, *Br J Cancer* 70:542, 1994.

102. Bland KI et al: Analysis of breast cancer screening in women younger than fifty years, *JAMA* 10:1037, 1981.

103. Heuser L et al: Relations between mammary cancer growth kinetics and the intervals between screenings, *Cancer* 43:857, 1979.

104. DeWaard F et al: The DOM project for the early detection of breast cancer, Utrecht, Netherlands, *J Chron Dis* 37:1, 1984.

105. Kamb A et al: A cell cycle regulator potentially involved in genesis of many tumor types, *Science* 264:436, 1994.

106. Shapiro S: Evidence on screening for breast cancer from a randomized trial, *Cancer* 39:2772, 1977.

107. Bird RE, Wallace TW, Yankaskas BC: Analysis of cancers missed at screening mammography, *Radiology* 184:613, 1992.

108. Martin JE, Moskowtiz M, Milbrath JR: Breast cancer missed by mammography, *Am J Radiol* 132:737, 1979.

109. Gilliland F et al: Biologic characteristics of interval and screen-detected breast cancers, *J Natl Cancer Inst* 92:743, 2000.

110. Amerlov C et al: Breast carcinoma growth rate described by mammographic doubling time and S-phase fraction: correlations to clinical and histopathological factors in a screened population, *Cancer* 70:1928, 1992.

111. Hatschek T et al: Cytometric characterization and clinical course of breast cancer diagnosed in a population-based screening program, *Cancer* 64:1074, 1989.

112. Ikeda DM et al: Interval carcinomas in the Malmo mammographic screening trial: radiographic appearance and prognostic considerations, *AJR Am J Roentgenol* 159:287, 1992.

113. Wolfe JN: Risk for cancer development determined by mammographic parenchymal patterns, *Cancer* 37:2486, 1976.

114. Gravelle IH et al: A prospective study of mammographic parenchymal patterns and risk of breast cancer, *Br J Radiol* 59:487, 1986.

115. Tabar L et al: What is the optimum interval between mammographic screening examinations? An analysis based on the latest results of the Swedish two-county breast cancer screening trial, *Br J Cancer* 55:547, 1987.

116. Verbeek AL et al: Mammographic breast pattern and the risk of breast cancer, *Lancet* i:591, 1984.

117. Brekelmans CT et al: The epidemiological profile of women with an interval cancer in the DOM screening programme, *Breast Cancer Res Treat* 30:223, 1994.

118. Whitehead J, Cooper J: Risk factors for breast cancer by mode of diagnosis: some results from a breast cancer screening study, *J Epidemiol Comm Health* 43:115, 1989.

119. Bassett LW, Manjikian V, Gold RH: Mammography and breast cancer screening, *Surg Clin North Am* 70:775, 1990.

120. Kee F, Gorman D, Odling-Smee W: Confidence intervals and interval cancers…needles in haystacks? *Public Health* 106:29, 1992.

121. Buchanan JB, Spratt JS, Henser LS: Tumor growth, doubling times, and the inability of the radiologist to diagnose certain cancers, *Radiol Clin North Am* 21:115, 1983.

122. Taplin SH et al: Screening mammography: clinical image quality and the risk of interval breast cancer, *Am J Roentgenol* 178:797, 2002.

123. Muir Gray JA: *A draft set of criteria for evaluation and quality assurance*, 1990, Screening Publications.
124. Patnick J, Muir Grey JA: *Guidelines on the collection and use of breast cancer data*, London, 1993, NHSBSP Publications.
125. Burhenne HJ et al: Interval breast cancers in the screening mammography program of British Columbia: analysis and classification, *AJR Am J Roentgenol* 162:1067, 1994.
126. Holland R et al: So-called interval cancers of the breast, *Cancer* 49:2527, 1982.
127. Miller AB et al: Canadian National Breast Screening Study: 1. Breast cancer detection and death rates among women aged 40-49 years, *Can Med Assoc J* 147:1459, 1992.
128. Miller AB et al: Canadian National Breast Screening Study: 2. Breast cancer detection and death rates among women aged 50 to 59 years, *Can Med Assoc J* 147:1477, 1992.
129. Seidman H et al: Survival experience in the breast cancer detection demonstration project, *CA Cancer J Clin* 37:258, 1987.

CHAPTER

33

Stereotactic Imaging and Breast Biopsy

DAVID S. ROBINSON
MAGESH SUNDARAM

Chapter Outline

The stereotactic x-ray–guided technique, developed for mammography-directed fine-needle aspiration in 1977,[1] has evolved in the past quarter century to a rapid and accurate core biopsy.[2] A large, progressively growing volume of screening mammograms in North America and in Europe has resulted in the discovery of an increasing number of nonpalpable findings requiring a tissue diagnosis.[3] This in turn created a competitive market that has driven technologic advances both in imaging and in biopsy instrumentation. Of the estimated 1.3 million breast biopsies performed in the United States in 2003, between 25% and 33% were image-guided core biopsies and half of those used a stereotactic mammographic technique.[4]

Stereotactic Biopsy Procedure

Although the procedure may be performed with the patient either upright[5] or prone,[6] most stereotactic tables are set in the prone position for patient stability. It is estimated that there are 3000 prone tables in North America, 200 in Europe, and fewer in the rest of the world.[3] The number of upright units is unknown, but this technique is more widely accepted in Europe than in North America. Welle and colleagues[7] describe a variation of an upright unit with the patient positioned in the lateral decubitus position.

The prone tables are produced by Fischer Imaging, Inc. (Denver, CO) and Lorad (Danbury, CT). Upright units for stereotactic biopsies are produced by several companies as "add-on" accessories to existing mammography equipment.

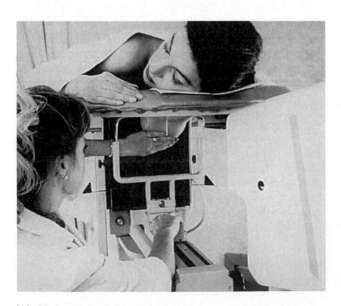

FIG. **33-1** Positioning the patient on the stereotactic table.

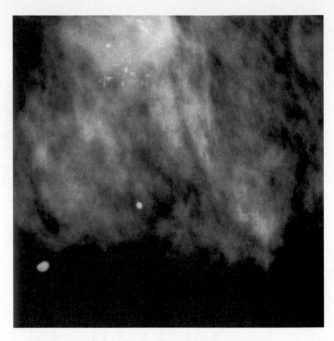

FIG. **33-2** Scout image with a microcalcification in the upper central area of the field.

On the prone table, the patient's breast, passing through a circular port (Figure 33-1), is held between the compression paddle and the charge-coupled device (CCD) plate. Digital imaging has replaced film, and this advancement from an analog to a digital image has reduced the acquisition time for each image from 7.5 minutes to 4 seconds. After a scout image confirms the mammographic lesion from which a biopsy specimen will be obtained within the 5 × 5 cm working window (Figure 33-2), offset views are taken 15 degrees to the right and to the left of the central axis for a 30-degree arc. The computer, using the two angled views in the same plane, then generates the three-dimensional coordinates of the target selected by the observer (Figure 33-3). This three-dimensional position is transferred to the stereotactic table, where small motors align the vertical and horizontal positions (X and Y coordinates) of the biopsy sled and inform the operator of the depth, or Z coordinate. The depth is then set by the operator, who has some discretion regarding placement. A local skin anesthetic is used, followed by a deeper series of injections parallel to the proposed path of the instrument (Figure 33-4); then a small incision allows insertion of the biopsy instrument. Its position within the lesion is confirmed with two more offset images at a 30-degree arc, with a subsequent electronic display of the target marker over the biopsy instrument's position. This allows highly accurate placement of the biopsy instrument to the target, to within a millimeter of where the instrument appears on the image.

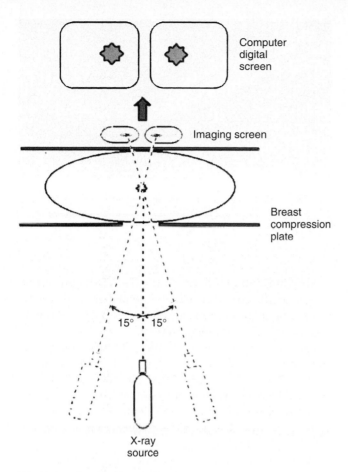

FIG. 33-3 Triangulation of depth of lesion using two views.

TABLE 33-1	Stereotactic Biopsy Instruments
TRADE NAME	**MANUFACTURER**
Vacuum-assisted core	
Mammotome	Ethicon Endo-Surgery, Cincinnati, OH
ATEC	Suros, Indianapolis, IN
Radiofrequency cutting, single excision	
en-bloc	Neothermia Corporation, Natick, MA
Large core	
SiteSelect	Imagyn Medical Technologies, Irvine, CA
Axial, side-biting biopsy instrument	
Magnum gun and needle	C.R. Bard, Inc., Murray Hill, NJ

The current choice of biopsy instruments holds an expanding array of options (Table 33-1). Fundamentally, these may be divided into three varieties: (1) side-biting, single-core, mechanical spring–release instruments, which are made by several manufacturers; (2) vacuum-assisted, side-suctioning core instruments; and (3) axial core instruments.

The side-biting (Magnum, C.R. Bard, Inc., Murray Hill, NJ) instrument (Figure 33-5) is doubly spring loaded. After its position has been confirmed, the instrument is fired first, sending the solid trocar with one side hollowed out into the tissue. That firing in turn releases a spring driving the overlying cutting sheath that passes over the hollowed out area, thus taking the core. Then the entire instrument is removed, the core is taken from it, and the process is repeated. A 14-guage size is considered optimal.

The vacuum-assisted, side-suctioning instrument (either Mammotome, Ethicon Endo-Surgery, Cincinnati, OH [Figure 33-6] or ATEC, or Automated Tissue Excision and Collection, Suros Surgical Systems, Indianapolis, IN [Figure 33-7]) is placed so that the vacuum port is adjacent to or within the tissue on which a biopsy is to be performed. After mammographic confirmation, suction is applied, bringing the tissue through the side window into the biopsy chamber. A central coring devise, then traveling more than

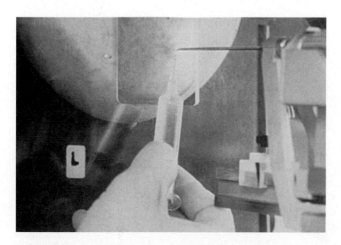

FIG. 33-4 Stereotactic needle placement is performed on the breast with the patient under local anesthesia.

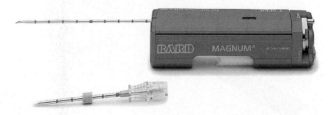

FIG. 33-5 Bard Magnum. *(Courtesy C.R. Bard, Inc., Murray Hill, NJ.)*

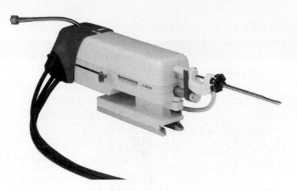

FIG. **33-6** Mammotome. *(Courtesy Ethicon Endo-Surgery, Inc., a Johnson & Johnson company, Cincinnati, OH.)*

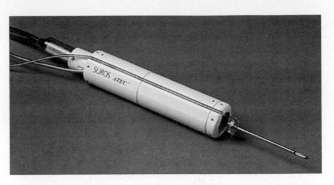

FIG. **33-7** ATEC (Automated Tissue Excision and Collection). *(Courtesy Suros Surgical Systems, Inc., Indianapolis, IN.)*

1200 RPM, is advanced in the chamber to take a specimen. Before the core is removed, the instrument, still at the same depth, is turned to take another specimen. Serially turning the port allows a biopsy cavity of up to 1.5 cm to be milled in this manner.

The axial coring devices, en-bloc (Neothermia Corporation, Natick, MA [Figure 33-8]) and SiteSelect (Imagyn Medical Technologies, Irvine, CA [Figure 33-9]), take their specimens through the end of the instrument. After the en-bloc device is passed through a skin incision, the end of the introducer easily transcends the breast tissue because of a radiofrequency cutting device at its tip. When the tissue for biopsy is reached, the operator activates a circular radiofrequency-charged metallic cutting wire, advanced forward by four metal bands that come together, centrally forming a "basket." The peanut-shaped sample, 20 mm across its axial diameter, is then removed and submitted as a single specimen.

The SiteSelect device (replacing the ABBI, which is no longer produced) takes a 22-mm diameter axial core by advancing a cutting tube around or through the lesion. Again, a single sample is removed.

For any of the instruments, after placement, its position is confirmed with paired stereo images (Figure 33-10). If a spring-fired mechanical system is used, after confirmation, each additional core is taken without additional imaging by removing the core and refiring the device again for each specimen. A vacuum-assisted device requires a single placement, after which cores are obtained by rotating the open tissue acquisition bay. On completion of the procedure and after partial withdrawal, either a single axial image or stereo views are taken for comparison with the initial images to confirm the adequacy of sampling (Figure 33-11). When microcalcifications are sampled for biopsy, the specimens are radiographed to confirm the removal of the calcifications

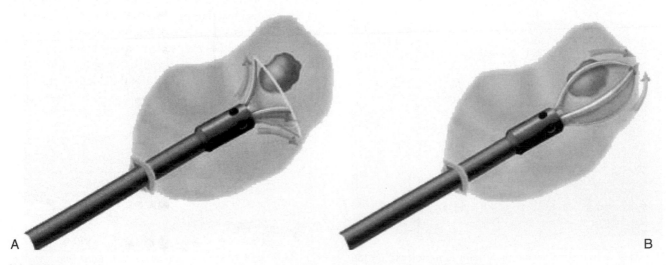

A   B

FIG. **33-8** **A** and **B,** Axial coring device, en-bloc. *(Courtesy Neothermia Corporation, Natick, MA.)*

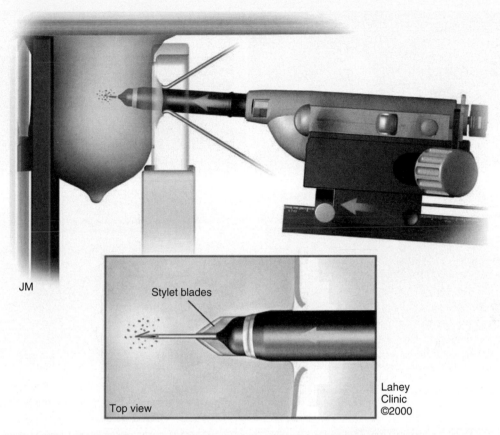

JM

Stylet blades

Top view

Lahey
Clinic
©2000

FIG. **33-9** SiteSelect. *(Courtesy Imagyn Medical Technologies, Irvine, CA.)*

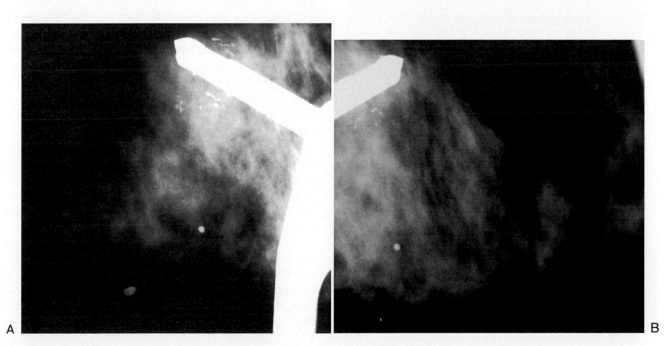

A

B

FIG. **33-10** **A** and **B**, Stereotactic needle in postfire position.

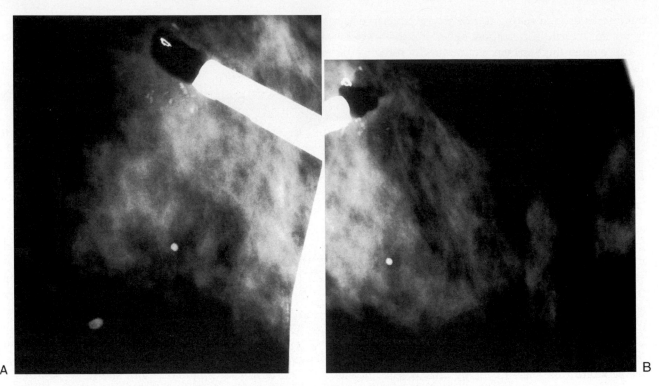

A   B

FIG. **33-11** **A** and **B,** Desired lesion has been accurately sampled with stereotactic biopsy.

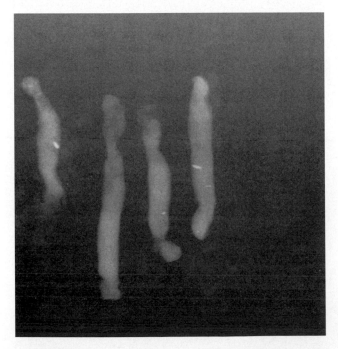

FIG. **33-12** Confirmation of removal of microcalcifications with tissue specimen x-ray study.

(Figure 33-12). This also allows those cores containing microcalcifications to be selected and submitted separately to ease the pathologist's search.

At the end of a procedure, when using an 11-gauge device or larger, many practitioners place a tissue marking clip (MicroMark, Ethicon Endo-Surgery, Cincinnati, OH)[8] (see Figure 3-11, *A*) or a radiopaque and ultrasound-visible gelatin marker (Gel Mark, SenoRx, Aliso Viejo, CA).[9] Although clips are easily seen, there have been reports of their movement.[10,11]

A specimen image should always be obtained to confirm that the area of concern was adequately sampled for biopsy, and if a clip or marker is used, it will demonstrate in the patient the position of the biopsy site on an image taken of the breast after the procedure. Postprocedural, full-field craniocaudal and mediolateral oblique mammograms will confirm that the site sampled for biopsy matches the location of the lesion recognized on the diagnostic mammogram.

Once identified with stereotactic biopsy, a cancer must be treated surgically. If the patient chooses a mastectomy, there is no issue; however, if a partial mastectomy (lumpectomy) is to be performed, relocation of the biopsy site following a stereotactic breast biopsy becomes important. In most circumstances, only a short time will have elapsed between the stereotactic biopsy and the lumpectomy. Recognition of the same landmarks used in setting up the biopsy can serve as a guide for needle localization and definitive excision because often there is mammographically recognizable tissue perturbation or a small fluid collection or hematoma at the site of the original biopsy. The presence of a titanium clip or Gel Mark pellet previously placed at the time of the biopsy is an excellent marker for a wire localization if a lumpectomy is performed.

Indications for Stereotactic Biopsy

The indications for stereotactic biopsy are the same as those for needle localization with mammographic guidance: either a nonpalpable suspicious focus of microcalcifications or a suspicious solid tissue density seen mammographically. Multiple areas to be sampled for biopsy in more than one quadrant are especially suitable to this technique because of the decreased morbidity compared with that of an open approach. Unique to the stereotactic technique, but rarely needed, is its ability to sample a lesion seen only on one view of the standard dual-view mammograms; that is, the site of concern may be seen on either the mediolateral or the craniocaudal view, but it cannot be found on both. Because the stereotactic approach makes two observations from different perspectives in the *same* plane, sampling of a lesion seen from one mammographic perspective is possible.

One special application of the stereotactic technology is its ability to safely sample a suspicious lesion adjacent to an augmentation prosthesis. The lesion and the breast implant can be quickly imaged after the device has been gently inserted and intermittently viewed during placement. Consequently, a core biopsy may reduce a patient's risk for implant perforation compared with a "blind," freehand needle placement.

Also because of its ease and lower morbidity, the risk/benefit ratio of a stereotactic biopsy may weigh in favor of sampling a lesion classified as breast imaging reporting and data system (BI-RADS) 3, "probably benign," with a recommended radiologic follow-up in 6 months but not one for which an open breast biopsy with needle localization is recommended. When the anxious patient is informed that the lesion reported is not suspicious enough for a biopsy to be done but that the radiologist is still concerned enough to ask her to return for repeat mammograms, she may insist on a tissue diagnosis to exclude malignancy. A stereotactic biopsy can establish that diagnosis and relieve the anxiety quickly, at lower cost[12,13] and with less morbidity than an open biopsy. Of note, BI-RADS 1 and 2 mammograms rarely require tissue diagnosis. A biopsy is almost always performed for BI-RADS 4 lesions, and a core biopsy is done for BI-RADS 5 lesions, except when excisional biopsy as a therapeutic lumpectomy is planned for a small lesion following needle localization.

Contraindications to Stereotactic Biopsy

Because the stereotactic procedure requires that the patient lie absolutely still in a prone position for 20 to 45 minutes, older patients with cervical or shoulder arthritis, the very anxious who may tend to move, and those with a cough are better treated in a supine position using either an ultrasound-guided core biopsy or an open biopsy in an operating room after needle localization. In theory, once the lesion is stereotactically targeted by the computer system, the patient actually could leave the table and let the machinery, unknowing, fire into space. More realistically, if the patient moves even a fraction of an inch, the machinery will obtain a sample from the wrong site, not sampling the imaged density. Occasionally, a patient may move just enough that the stereo pair images of the instrument's position will be out of alignment with the target selected for biopsy. If movement is even suspected at any time during the procedure, it should be confirmed with two new offset views. If the patient has moved, these images can be used as new target images or the process can be started again from the beginning.

Patients weighing more than 300 pounds are not stereotactic candidates because the tables are not built or licensed to hold more than that weight. Although it has been suggested that the operator could perform the procedure sitting on the floor with the table lowered to its base, prone table engineers have indicated that the horizontal positioning gears cannot tolerate this weight as well.

Lesions very close to the chest wall or in the mammary tail of Spence are also difficult to sample using a stereotactic technique, but by passing the patient's arm and shoulder through the port with the breast, more posterior tissues may often be brought into view. If the area of concern still cannot be seen after several attempts in different positions, again the patient will be better served through either an ultrasound-guided biopsy of a mass or mammographic placement of a guidewire to a cluster of suspicious microcalcifications and an open biopsy. Sampling of the wrong site because "it could be" the area of interest is of disservice both to the operator and the patient.

Accuracy of Core Biopsy

Parker and associates[14] reported the accuracy of stereotactic core biopsy in 4744 lesions that underwent stereotactic biopsy with 14-gauge core samples. Confirmation was obtained either through a subsequent excisional biopsy or through follow-up mammograms in 4 to 6 months: approximately 80% of the patients completed follow-up analysis. Twelve instances of false-negative findings were discovered initially (12 of 4744 = 0.25%), and four additional lesions were found on subsequent analysis (total false-negative findings of 0.39%).[2] Other reports of 14-gauge automated instruments range from 2.9% to 7.8%. Pfarl and co-workers[2] report a 3.3% false-negative rate for 11-guage vacuum-assisted core biopsy. In comparison, the rate of false-negative findings for excisional biopsy ranges from 0.5% to 20%, with an average of 1% to 3%.[15] Consequently, stereotactic core biopsy is as accurate as an open biopsy following needle localization.

Tissue Diagnosis: Core Diameter and Sample Size

The size of each core and the number of cores taken are important. The amount of tissue removed by stereotactic biopsy to establish an accurate diagnosis of malignancy has been well investigated. Fine-needle aspiration has given way to core sampling as a more accurate technique. Earlier publications evaluating mechanical core biopsies taken with 18-, 16-, and 14-gauge needles have found the 14-gauge core sample to be the most accurate size.[16] The Mammotome vacuum-assisted coring device removing 14-, 11-, or 8-gauge cores to a 15-mm diameter hole and the ATEC vacuum-assisted device removing 10- or 9-gauge cores, milling a cavity to a 20-mm diameter, are similar in their accuracy.[6] At present, most operators use an 11-gauge instrument that has a 3.3% false-negative rate, lower than that of 14-guage automated core devices.[2] For the spring-loaded Magnum system, Liberman and colleagues[17] have suggested that at least five 14-gauge cores need to be taken for accurate sampling; if microcalcifications are the target, more may be needed to remove the calcifications. Vacuum-assisted cores are larger and may assist in a more accurate diagnosis. The minimal number of cores should be similar.

Pathologic Diagnostic Difficulties

One of the most difficult histologic determinations of a core biopsy is distinguishing atypical ductal hyperplasia (ADH) from ductal carcinoma in situ (DCIS)[18,19] and further distinguishing DCIS from an invasive ductal carcinoma.[20] Between 16% and 44% of ADH diagnoses based on a 14-gauge mechanically automated core biopsy are later changed to a diagnosis of ductal

carcinoma after an open excisional biopsy[6]; although that can be decreased to a between 4% and 19% with an 11-gauge vacuum-assisted core biopsy,[6] still a significant number of patients with ADH would have had DCIS missed had they undergone a core biopsy alone. Infiltrating ductal carcinoma is also underdiagnosed as DCIS between 15% and 36% of the time based on a 14-gauge mechanical core biopsy,[20] and again, although this decreases to between 4%[21] and 18%[22] with an 11-gauge core biopsy, a group of patients with invasive cancer also would have been missed had they undergone core biopsy alone. Therefore all cases of ADH and DCIS should be followed by an open biopsy.

Other, less common lesions at risk are papillary lesions and radial scars. Philpotts and associates[23] report that papillary lesions diagnosed as "benign papilloma" based on core biopsy retained a benign designation on reexcision, whereas 3 of 4 "suspicious" papillary lesions proved to be papillary carcinomas. In their series of core biopsies of eight radial scars, none showed any evidence of cancer on reexcision. These authors recommend excision of all lesions that are "suspicious for malignancy," as well as those with "atypical" or unusual histologic findings; they further suggest that "benign papillary lesions" and radial scars need not be excised.

Complications of Stereotactic Biopsy

As with all technical advances, an understanding of the limitations, pitfalls, and potential problems comes to light with use. Several of these problems and, where possible, their remedies are addressed from this growing experience and from other authors. The classic, expected surgical complications of infection and bleeding occur rarely with the stereotactic technique.

INFECTIONS

In a comprehensive search for infections after stereotactic biopsy, no reference can be found in the scientific literature. One source suggests that the infection rate may be 0.1%, but no reference is cited. On gathering the collected experience of several practitioners who have performed more than 10,000 stereotactic biopsies cumulatively, poststereotactic infections are exceedingly rare.[24] Still, sterile technique should be maintained, with recognition of the close quarters in which the biopsies are taken from beneath the table.

BLEEDING AND HEMATOMA

Clinically problematic hematomas and bleeding are uncommon, but just as they can be expected from any invasive procedure, they may also occur during a stereotactic biopsy. To decrease this risk, patients should discontinue taking aspirin and other anticoagulants at least 4 days, or better yet 1 week, before the biopsy. To the contrary, Melotti and Berg[25] describe no greater incidence or increased size of hematoma in anticoagulated patients than they found in patients not taking anticoagulants who underwent breast core biopsies. That not withstanding, discontinuance when possible remains the most prudent course. Here one of the low-molecular-weight heparin fragments may be substituted several days ahead and discontinued 4 to 6 hours before the biopsy.

In considering another pitfall leading to bleeding or hematoma, if a blood vessel appears in the working field, the operator must determine whether that vessel is in the path of the biopsy instrument. By selecting the site to be sampled as the first target and the vessel as a second target, the operator, with a quick look at the numerical depth, or Z axis, of each, can determine whether the vessel is in front of or behind the lesion to be sampled. If it is far enough behind the lesion, there should be no problem. Another method of avoiding passage of the biopsy instrument through a vessel can be achieved by turning the breast until the vessel lies out of the path of the biopsy instrument.

In summary, although hematoma and bleeding do occur, large hematomas and uncontrolled bleeding are uncommon. Even with increased use of large-diameter, stereotactic biopsy devices, the incidence of hematoma and bleeding has not increased. Applying firm compression to the site after the procedure greatly reduces the incidence of hematoma and ecchymosis.

SEEDING THE TRACK

The question of seeding cancer cells in the instrument's track with any percutaneous biopsy of a malignancy raises concern. Smith[26] estimates the risk of cancer seeding to be approximately 1 in 20,000 (0.005%) for fine-needle aspiration with 20- to 23-gauge needles. With larger needles, one might expect a greater number of track seedings. In a histologic analysis of biopsy tracks of patients with newly diagnosed cancer who were undergoing lumpectomy or mastectomy after a core biopsy, Diaz, Wiley, and Venta[27] reported that about one third of 352 patients had tumor cell displacement in the track; this finding decreased over time. Davies, Honni, and D'Costa[28] described mammary epidermoid inclusion cysts after wide-core needle biopsies, and Liberman and co-workers[29] have reported epithelial displacement after stereotactic, 11-gauge vacuum-assisted core biopsy. Still, to date, there has not been one report of a clinical growth thought to be caused by a stereotactic core breast biopsy. In that regard, for several decades palpable breast cancers have been sampled for biopsy using Tru-Cut, and seeding in this circumstance has not been recognized as a significant clinical problem. Logically, this event should not occur with any greater frequency simply because the lesion is nonpalpable.

NO VACUUM

One relatively minor problem that can occur with a vacuum-assisted core biopsy of a lesion lying in the subcutaneous breast parenchyma is inadequate vacuum because of a leak. When the lesion is so superficial that the acquisition port lies with part of the bay outside the skin, a vacuum cannot be created to pull tissue into the chamber. This can be overcome in many cases by pulling the skin outward with a skin hook.

Pitfalls and Potential Problems

The sources of potential problems surrounding stereotactic breast biopsy fall into categories stemming from the patient, the disease, the technology, the operator, or a combination thereof.

LOST CALCIFICATIONS

Friedman and associates[30] have described retrieval of lost microcalcifications, not found in core specimen radiograms but clearly removed from the patient, by flushing and filtering debris from the tubing and vacuum reservoir after core biopsies. When any biopsy tissue contains microcalcifications, a confirmatory specimen radiogram should accompany that specimen to the pathologist, who should be so notified and asked to report the histologic presence or absence of microcalcifications. If microcalcifications cannot be found histologically, the paraffin blocks should be radiographed. If no microcalcifications are found either on specimen imaging, by microscopic analysis (including light polarization to look for unstained calcium oxalate crystals), or in the paraffin blocks, the patient should have another mammogram and additional biopsy done if necessary. After each core procedure, the patient should have craniocaudal and mediolateral oblique views to confirm both that the marker has been placed and that the proper site was sampled. A follow-up mammogram should be performed 3 to 6 months after the biopsy to evaluate the biopsy site. This confirms that the proper site was sampled, and it prevents later confusion when annual mammograms recognize the tissue perturbation caused by the biopsy itself.

IMAGING

Prone stereotactic imaging differs from standard mammographic imaging in the position of the breast. Whereas standard mammograms in craniocaudal and mediolateral-oblique projections are taken with the patient seated, prone stereotactic images are of a prone-dependent breast passed through the table. After one becomes familiar with stereotactic imaging, this issue is of little consequence, but when expected landmarks do not reveal the lesion's position or it has apparently been displaced, positioning may be the cause. One way to enhance proper orientation is to align the mammogram on a nearby viewbox to the position of the patient as she is on the stereotactic table.

TRANSPORTED MASS

A medial density on a mammogram may appear to be transported to the lateral aspect of the breast on stereotactic imaging. In this circumstance, a mass that is "clearly" the site to be sampled appears to have moved from an inner quadrant, as seen on the mammograms, to an outer quadrant on the stereotactic screen. The explanation for this optical illusion is unclear, but the most likely source of this problem is positioning of the patient. Any small amount of torque on the breast itself leading to shearing of one imaged plane over another may appear to transport a mass to the wrong quadrant. This problem may occur even in the hands of an experienced mammographic technologist.

VANISHING LESION

Occasionally, a lesion seen mammographically cannot be found at the time of proposed stereotactic biopsy. This is more likely to occur when attempting to sample very faint calcifications or a solid lesion in a very dense breast. It may also occur when trying to sample a finding that appears in one view but not in the other. The first course of action is a careful review of the mammograms to ensure that the site in the breast to be sampled is in the working field of view. This may require readjustment of the patient in the proper perspective (craniocaudal, mediolateral-oblique, or true mediolateral). If that offers little benefit and the lesion can be seen on both the standard craniocaudal and the mediolateral views, the unsuccessful perspective should be shifted to its orthogonal counterpart. If neither perspective identifies the lesion on a CCD screen, the field of view can be broadened by taking an analog film with the Bucky grid; such "a wide-angle, full-field view" may help the physician locate the lesion. Then once the target has been identified, a biopsy can be performed after returning to the narrower, digital field. If it cannot be located at all using a stereo approach, the site may be selected by a needle localization with a straight needle or placement of a skin marker, using an analog seated approach with an alpha-numeric grid and then targeting that needle or skin marker when the patient returns to the stereo table. If this does not work, consideration should be given to a needle localization and an open biopsy; alternatively, the patient should undergo repeat mammography again in 3 months.

UNCLEAR DENSITY

A density seen on an upright mammogram may not appear as clearly when the patient is on the stereotactic table. The decision to sample a radiographically observed image is based on its recognition as a possible cancer. At the time of stereotactic biopsy, if the lesion cannot be clearly identified as the same one seen on the mammogram, the biopsy should not be performed. Although it may be tempting to obtain a sample because the patient is willing and anxious and the operator's time is committed, those factors should not be seductive in performing a biopsy of a site that just "appears to be" the target. A pathology report of benign findings in this case may give the patient and the operator a false sense of security because the lesion with which the patient presented is not the site sampled. It would be better to bring the patient back for repeat mammograms; at that point, if a biopsy is still indicated and it is difficult to confirm stereotactically, a standard needle localization and open breast biopsy should be performed. In any event, the procedure at the time of stereotactic biopsy should be abandoned if the lesion cannot be conclusively identified as the target of concern.

ONE STEREO VIEW–ONLY LESION

After the offset views (15 degrees to the right and to the left) are obtained, the biopsy site is mathematically targeted from a 30-degree arc of difference. If the lesion can be seen on the scout image and on only one of the offset views but not the other, the scout image may replace one of the offset views. Now two views with a 15-degree arc of separation provide enough perspective to determine the depth of the lesion through a "target-on-scout" approach.

STRIKETHROUGH

Strikethrough is a product of the patient's anatomy and the technology. A patient with very thin or ptotic breasts may not have an adequate tissue depth after compression to permit the biopsy needle to move safely without passing entirely through the breast to strike the imaging plate behind. In addition, a patient whose lesion lies close to the skin surface against the imaging screen may also be subject to the same problem. Strikethrough can be prevented through several approaches.

When a vacuum-assisted device is being used, instead of firing it into place, it may be gently placed in a postfired position and the tissue acquisition bay may be set to sample most of the target just short of its usual depth. This allows the operator to sample part of the lesion, even if it is "short." With a Magnum needle, the "throw" is 23 mm. The needle is constructed so that the hollowed-out portion of the solid trocar begins 5 mm back from the tip, and the needle is usually withdrawn

5 mm before firing. Often, a greater withdrawal can still capture enough of the lesion for diagnosis. If that is inadequate, repositioning the patient at an orthogonal 90-degree position may resolve the problem. The Lorad engineers have solved this problem by revolving the biopsy entry site and the CCD plate 180 degrees, bringing the lesion to the surface opposite the imaging plate. For the very thin breast, the Fischer bioengineers have taken a different approach; a lateral "arm" is placed to perform a biopsy from the side, orthogonal to the axial view, and computation. If neither of those can be used, a second compression paddle may be placed between the undersurface of the breast and the imaging plate, with the biopsy window directly behind the lesion. Then, with the skin injected at both entry and possible exit sites, if the needle passes through, it will enter an air space in front of the imaging plate.

Summary

Stereotactic core biopsy is a safe, reliable approach for obtaining breast tissue for diagnosis. The indications are largely the same as those for needle localization. There are few limitations and complications. The technique, instruments, indications, contraindications, and possible complications have been discussed. It is certain that the venue of this approach will continue to expand.

REFERENCES

1. Bolmgren J, Jacobsen B, Nordenstrom B: Stereotactic instrument for needle biopsy of the mamma, *AJR Am J Roentgenol* 129:121, 1977.
2. Pfarl G et al: Stereotactic 11-gauge vacuum assisted breast biopsy: a validation study, *AJR Am J Roentgenol* 179:1503, 2002.
3. Cady B et al: The new era in breast cancer, *Arch Surg* 131:301, 1996.
4. Nields M: Personal communication, February 2003.
5. Caines JS et al: Stereotactic needle core biopsy of breast lesions using a regular mammographic table with an adaptable stereotaxic device, *AJR Am J Roentgenol* 163:317, 1994.
6. Liberman L: Percutaneous image-guided core breast biopsy, *Radiol Clin North Am* 40:483, 2002.
7. Welle GJ et al: Stereotactic breast biopsy: recumbent biopsy using add-on upright equipment, *AJR Am J Roentgenol* 175:59, 2000.
8. Burbank F, Forcier N: Tissue marking clip for stereotactic breast biopsy: initial placement accuracy, long-term stability, and usefulness as a guide for wire localization, *Radiology* 205:407, 1997.
9. Parker SH: Long term mammographic follow-up of the gelatin pledget/metallic marker combination. Presentation at the Radiological Society of North America (RSNA), 88th Scientific Assembly and Annual Meeting, Chicago, December 2002.
10. Philpotts LE, Lee CH: Clip migration after 11-gauge vacuum-assisted stereotactic biopsy: case report, *Radiology* 222:794, 2002.
11. Burnside ES, Sohlich RE, Sickles EA: Movement of a biopsy-site marker clip after completion of stereotactic directional vacuum-assisted breast biopsy: case report, *Radiology* 221:504, 2001.
12. Lee CH et al: Cost-effectiveness of stereotactic core needle biopsy: analysis by means of mammographic findings, *Radiology* 202:849, 1997.
13. Liberman L, Lsama MP: Cost-effectiveness of stereotactic 11-gauge directional vacuum-assisted breast biopsy, *AJR Am J Roentgenol* 175:53, 2000.
14. Parker SH et al: Percutaneous large-core breast biopsy: a multi-institutional study, *Radiology* 193:359, 1994.
15. Kopans DB: Unpublished presentation to a symposium on stereotactic breast biopsy at the Clinical Congress of the American College of Surgeons, October 1995.
16. Parker SH et al: Stereotactic breast biopsy with a biopsy gun, *Radiology* 176:741, 1990.
17. Liberman L et al: Stereotaxic 14-gauge breast biopsy: how many core biopsy specimens are needed? *Radiology* 192:793, 1994.
18. Rao A et al: Atypical ductal hyperplasia of the breast diagnosed by 11-gauge directional vacuum-assisted biopsy, *Am J Surg* 184:534, 2002.
19. Brem RF et al: Atypical ductal hyperplasia: histologic underestimation of carcinoma in tissue harvested from impalpable breast lesions using 11-gauge stereotactically guided directional vacuum-assisted biopsy, *AJR Am J Roentgenol* 172:1405, 1999.
20. Jackman RJ et al: Stereotactic breast biopsy of nonpalpable lesions: determinants of ductal carcinoma in situ underestimation rates, *Radiology* 218:497, 2001.
21. Meyer JE et al: Large-core needle biopsy of nonpalpable breast lesions, *JAMA* 281:1638, 1999.
22. Rubin E et al: Needle-localization biopsy of the breast: impact of a selective core needle biopsy program on yield, *Radiology* 195:627, 1995.
23. Philpotts LE et al: Uncommon high-risk lesions of the breast diagnosed at stereotactic core-needle biopsy: clinical importance, *Radiology* 216:831, 2000.
24. Parker SH, Israel P: Personal communication, February 1997.
25. Melotti MK, Berg WA: Core needle biopsy in patients undergoing anticoagulation therapy: preliminary results, *AJR Am J Roentgenol* 174:245, 2000.
26. Smith EII: The hazards of fine needle aspiration biopsy, *Ultrasound Med Biol* 10:629, 1984.
27. Diaz LK, Wiley EL, Venta LA: Are malignant cells displaced by large-gauge needle core biopsy of the breast? *AJR Am J Roentgenol* 173:1303, 1999.
28. Davies JD, Nonni A, D'Costa HF: Mammary epidermoid inclusion cysts after wide-core needle biopsies, *Histopathology* 31:549, 1997.
29. Liberman L et al: Epithelial displacement after stereotactic 11-gauge directional vacuum-assisted breast biopsy, *AJR AM J Roentgenol* 172:677, 1999.
30. Friedman PD et al: Retrieval of lost microcalcifications during stereotactic vacuum-assisted core biopsy, *AJR Am J Roentgenol* 180:275, 2003.

34

Cytologic Needle Samplings of the Breast: Techniques and End Results

HEATHER M. BROWN

EDWARD J. WILKINSON

SHAHLA MASOOD

Chapter Outline

History of Breast Fine-Needle Aspiration

The use of fine-needle aspiration (FNA) for the diagnosis of tumors is attributed to Martin and Ellis,[1] who in 1930 published their classic study on this procedure. The work on FNA was prompted by James Ewing, who objected to preliminary surgical excision of breast tumors because of concern regarding the dissemination of the tumor by biopsy.[2] The procedure, however, did not gain acceptance for a variety of reasons, one being concern about tumor spreading as a result of needle puncture. Tumor growing out of the needle tract had been reported to occur in only a few, but highly influential, cases.

It required the careful and comprehensive work on FNA by Franzen and Zajicek[3] to reintroduce the procedure. Their publications, from 1967 through 1974, were influential in renewing interest in FNA in the United States and elsewhere.[3-5] Subsequently, cost and reduced hospital utilization were major factors stimulating interest in breast FNA. Breast FNA is more rapid and cost effective than breast open surgical biopsy.[6] Improved understanding of the biology of malignant tumors has also provided a rationale for the reintroduction of FNA. Follow-up studies comparing women who underwent FNA of breast tumors with those who did not revealed no significant differences in recurrence or survival rates.[7-9]

Many different terms for FNA have appeared in the literature (Table 34-1). For the purpose of clarity, the acronym *FNA* and the term *fine-needle aspiration* are used throughout this text. This term has the advantage of including needle size ("fine needle") and technique ("aspiration") to clearly distinguish the procedure from needle biopsy, with which it might otherwise be confused. Indeed, *FNA* is the most commonly used term.

Comparison of Fine-Needle Aspiration to Core Needle Biopsy

The results of FNA have been compared with those of core needle biopsy, typically 14- to 18-gauge needle. The reported diagnostic accuracy for FNA of breast tumors has ranged from 77% to 99%.[10] In experienced hands, sensitivity can approach 96% and specificity 99%.[10] Some authors have found the sensitivity of FNA of detecting a malignant breast neoplasm to be higher than that for core needle biopsy.[11] Although sensitivity and specificity for core needle biopsy and FNA are fairly comparable, it has been reported that core needle biopsy results in fewer "suspicious for malignancy" diagnoses.[12]

Ultrasound-guided FNA of nonpalpable breast lesions is also thought to be a sensitive and specific means of diagnosis.[13] One study reviewed the literature and analyzed data on more than 3000 cases of FNA of nonpalpable breast lesions with histologic follow-up and showed comparable results of FNA of palpable and nonpalpable lesions.[14] One limitation of FNA of nonpalpable lesions is a somewhat higher rate of insufficient samples than with palpable breast lesions.[14-16] Use of more recent technologies such as ultrasound-guided mammotome vacuum biopsy of impalpable breast lesions has shown higher sensitivity and specificity than FNA cytology alone.[17]

The large needle biopsy is a more painful procedure than FNA and may leave a parenchymal scar. FNA is generally better tolerated by the patient than is core biopsy.[14] Breast FNA has proved useful in the follow-up of women who present with postoperative masses after lumpectomy[18] and in diagnosing axillary metastases and recurrent chest wall lesions.[19]

TABLE 34-1	Equivalent Terms Used to Describe FNA for Cytologic Study
Needle aspiration biopsy (NAB)	
Fine-needle aspiration (FNA)	
Fine-needle aspiration cytology	
Fine-needle aspiration biopsy	
Fine-needle biopsy	
Aspiration biopsy	
Aspiration cytology	
Aspiration biopsy cytology	
Thin-needle aspiration biopsy	

Evaluation of Breast Masses with Fine-Needle Aspiration

GENERAL PRINCIPLES

A basic principle of FNA is that it is usually not performed unless there is a palpable mass or a mass that has been identified with mammography or a similar screening procedure. There is no reason to attempt needle aspiration of nonspecific changes in the breast or to use FNA as a screening technique on a breast that is clinically and mammographically interpreted as negative. FNA of nonpalpable breast lesions may be best suited to cases that mammographically are of low suspicion, because of its strong negative predictive value.[20] In addition, multifocal disease in the breast may best be approached by FNA when nonpalpable lesions are involved.[20] A definite advantage of FNA over core biopsy is that it enables the pathologist to determine on site the adequacy of sampling, and in many cases, FNA and biopsy may be complementary. The combination of physical examination, mammography, and FNA (the so-called triple test) yields a diagnostic accuracy approaching 100%.[21-23] A negative FNA finding in the presence of a palpable mass, however, does not exclude tumor when the mass is clinically suspect.

LOCALIZATION OF THE BREAST MASS AND PALPABLE LYMPH NODES

Following identification of a palpable breast mass, FNA can be performed in an outpatient setting. The procedure usually does not require administration of an anesthetic (although some prefer a local anesthetic). If the mass is identified by mammography and is not palpable, a stereotactical method, with or without ultrasound, or some other guidance method is necessary to place the needle into the suspect lesion.

The evaluation of palpable masses and lymph nodes is approached in essentially the same manner. It is necessary to fix the mass or lymph node between the palpating fingers to hold it in place as the needle is inserted. Deep, freely moveable, barely palpable masses or lymph nodes are extremely difficult to aspirate, and generally it is best not to attempt FNA in such cases.

When lymph nodes are aspirated, we prefer to examine an air-dried Diff-Quik (American Scientific Products, McGaw Park, IL) smear at the bedside. If tumor is not identified or if lymphoma is considered a possibility, additional cellular material is collected in Eagle's medium for flow cytometry and assay for appropriate cell markers. In addition, cultures of the aspirate are performed if inflammation is suggested by clinical evidence or by evaluation of the aspirate.

COMPLICATIONS

The risk of tumor growing out of the needle tract has been described; this occurrence has been noted primarily in cases of bone tumor. This risk is markedly influenced by two factors. The first is needle size. The needles used in reported cases were usually large, ranging from 12 to 16 gauge. Needles of this size are commonly used for core needle biopsy, and a variety are available for this purpose; however, such large needles are unnecessary for FNA cytology. There is no

reason to use a needle any larger than 20 gauge, and often needles that are gauge 22 or smaller are satisfactory. These smaller needles are not associated with tumor spread into the needle tract. Moreover, the risk of needle-tract involvement by tumor following FNA is eliminated when the needle tract is excised when the tumor is surgically removed. The surgical approach to a breast mass, whether lumpectomy or mastectomy, can usually readily encompass the skin puncture site and needle tract resulting from the breast FNA.

Both acute mastitis and pneumothorax can occur as complications of breast FNA, but these complications are rare.[9,24] Hematomas may occur after FNA of the breast and can result in false-positive mammographic studies.

APPROACH TO THE PATIENT

The FNA procedure should be explained to the patient and informed consent obtained. For most women, breast FNA is less painful than venipuncture, a procedure with which women who have regular medical care are familiar. There is usually no need for anesthesia, although some physicians prefer to inject a small amount of local anesthetic (1 ml of 1% lidocaine or equivalent) into the skin at the site of the subsequent needle puncture. Usually a 27- or 29-gauge needle is used for the local anesthetic procedure. This anesthetic procedure may have more disadvantages than advantages. The major disadvantage is that if excessive amounts of anesthetic are injected or if hematoma results, the mass may be obscured to palpation and thus the probability of a successful FNA is reduced. Adverse effects, including anaphylaxis, may also occur from local anesthesia. Aspiration through the areolar region can be very painful, and if the placement of a needle in this area cannot be avoided, local anesthesia should be used.

The skin is usually prepared for FNA with 70% alcohol or an iodine solution. The proposed needle site is air-dried thoroughly before aspiration. Slides for the aspirate should be properly labeled with the patient's name, and an appropriate requisition form for the cytopathology laboratory should be completed. We prefer to have a cytotechnologist available at bedside to prepare the slides and to quick-stain representative air-dried and alcohol-fixed slides to evaluate the adequacy of the aspirate.

We prefer a 20-ml syringe within a syringe holder, which enables the physician performing the FNA to control the syringe and needle with one hand while positioning and holding the breast mass with the opposite hand. Smaller syringes, manipulated by hand without a syringe holder, can also be used.[8] A number

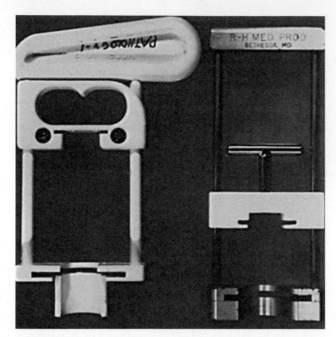

FIG. **34-1** Two commonly used syringe holders for fine-needle aspiration.

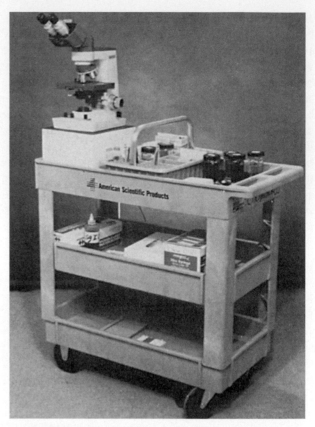

FIG. **34-2** Cytology cart prepared for fine-needle aspiration cytology.

of syringe holders are available (Figure 34-1). Some of these syringe holders can be sterilized if desired, and some can be heat-autoclaved. It is an uncommon practice to sterilize the syringe holder, except within an operating room setting. Usually only the syringe, needles, and local anesthetic are sterile. Disposable syringe holders significantly add to the cost of the procedure but may be a practical solution in some circumstances.

Once the patient is informed, the consent is signed, the needle site is prepared, the slides are appropriately labeled, the syringe is placed into the syringe holder, and the patient is positioned ideally for optimal access to the breast mass, the needle aspiration may be performed.

At the University of Florida, a prepared cart is taken to the patient's bedside or clinic station (Figure 34-2). The cart contains the following:

Microscope (to assess specimen adequacy at the time of the procedure)

Glass slides, pretreated (for improved cell-glass adherence)

Gloves

20- to 25-gauge needles (and 27- or 29-guage if local anesthesia is anticipated)

Alcohol or povidone-iodine (Betadine) swabs (to cleanse skin)

Band-Aids

Gauze pads

Several (at least 6) sterile syringes (10 or 20 ml)

Needle holder

Two tubes (10 ml each) of tissue culture medium (Eagle's, also known as Cellgro or RPMI)

One tube of CytoLyt solution (30 to 40 ml)

Requisition forms

Paper towels

Black pen to fill out the requisition and to label samples, and a pencil to write on slides

Two Coplin jars with 95% ethanol to fix smear (or spray fixative may be used)

Three Coplin jars with methanol and Diff-Quik solutions I and II

Hemostat (to remove needle from syringe, if necessary, or to hold glass slides while staining)

One Coplin jar of water (to rinse slides after staining)

FNA TECHNIQUE

In most women a 1.5-inch, 20- to 25-gauge needle will be adequate for FNA of a breast mass. Very small needles (27 gauge) may be useful for small targets. In addition, smaller needles (especially 25 gauge) may increase the cellular yield from lesions with dense or fibrotic stroma. Aspiration at the periphery of a fibrotic lesion may also increase the yield.[25] If fluid is obtained, a larger needle can be used to drain the cyst. We prefer to withdraw 5 cc of air into the 20-ml syringe before attaching the needle to the syringe. The advantage of this practice is that following the procedure the air can be used to express the needle contents onto the slides without the syringe being removed from the needle.

Aspiration is performed as follows:

1. With the needle in the syringe and the syringe in the holder, withdraw the plunger of the syringe to the 5-ml mark.

2. Holding the breast mass in a fixed position with one hand, advance the needle (usually by holding the syringe in the holder) into the mass.

3. Once the needle is in the mass, place full suction on the syringe (move the plunger to the 20-ml position) and move the needle slowly back and forth within the mass (Figure 34-3). Moving the needle along a single needle tract will give a satisfactory cellular yield in most cases.[26]

4. Keep the needle tip within the mass and full suction on the syringe until you can see material coming into the hub of the needle (Figure 34-4). The principle is to fill the needle, not the syringe, with cells. One needle can hold more than 100,000 cells, and this is usually adequate for cytologic diagnosis.[27]

5. Once material is seen at the hub of the needle, release the suction and return the plunger to the 5-ml mark.

6. Withdraw the needle (still attached to the syringe) and express the needle contents onto the glass slides. The needle should touch the surface of the slide so that air-drying of the sample is avoided. A small amount of material, usually a drop not exceeding 5 mm in diameter, should be expressed onto the slide (Figure 34-5).

It is usually preferable to place aliquots of the sample on several slides. The slides should lie flat on a paper towel placed on a firm surface such as a tabletop. Do not have a technologist or an assistant hold the slides because of the risk of a needlestick injury. If not all of the sample expresses from the needle, simply remove the needle from the syringe, withdraw the plunger to the 20-ml mark to fill the syringe with air, and reexpress the material by forcing air through the needle. Alternatively, one can flush the needle and syringe in tissue culture medium and load up a fresh syringe and needle.

We prefer using Eagle's tissue culture medium to rinse the needle and syringe and to ensure that all of the cellular material is harvested. In the cytopathology laboratory, cells are collected from the medium with Nuclepore filtration or cytocentrifugation, or they are prepared for a cell block for paraffin embedding. Centrifugation depends on the amount of cellular material within the washings.

It is important to realize that a cytologic sample placed in tissue culture medium can be used for ancillary tests in which fresh, unfixed cells are necessary (e.g., flow cytometry in a case of potential lymphoma). Medium such as CytoLyt contains a cell fixative, and therefore the cells are unrecoverable for techniques that require fresh cells after they've been placed in this solution.

For palpable lesions, the recommended number of needle passes for an adequate specimen is three to five. Lesions larger than 3 cm may require additional sampling of different areas of the tumor.[28] Pennes, Naylor, and Rebner[29] systematically examined the cellular yield for each FNA pass performed. They found that the first pass usually yielded sufficient material for a benign or malignant cytologic diagnosis, with small incremental yields on subsequent passes. After four passes, the gain for palpable lesions was very small, and

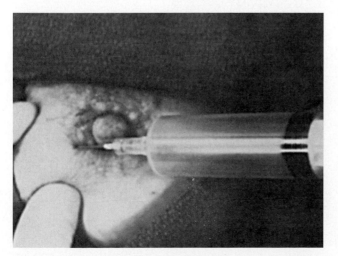

FIG. **34-3** Needle in mass, with full suction on the syringe.

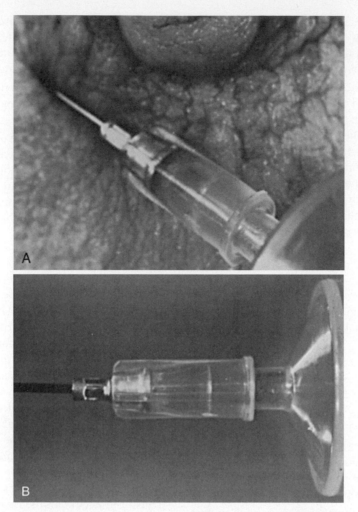

FIG. 34-4 A, Breast aspirate material within the hub of the needle. B, Close view demonstrating cellular material within the needle hub.

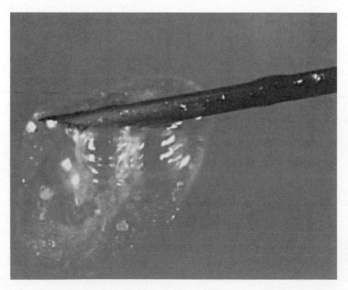

FIG. 34-5 Aspirate material placed on the slide.

for lesions smaller than 1 cm, there was no added gain after three passes.

Specimen adequacy for breast FNA remains a somewhat controversial issue. The most recent recommendations from a National Cancer Institute (NCI)-sponsored conference on breast FNA stated that there should be no specific requirements for a minimal number of ductal cells to determine specimen adequacy but that adequacy should be determined by the following[23]:

1. The opinion of the aspirator that the cytologic findings are consistent with the clinical findings and that the lesion was sampled adequately
2. The opinion of the pathologist that the smears do not have significant artifact or distortion and can be interpreted

It was also recommended that the microscopic description in the cytopathology report comment on the presence and amount of epithelial cells in addition to the nonepithelial components.[23]

For nonpalpable lesions, stereotactic guidance and sampling of the lesion by a radiologist consists of biopsy, FNA, or both. Generally, three to five separate guided aspirations or needle biopsies are performed for nonpalpable masses. One current recommendation is to obtain at least six samples from three sites within an area of microcalcifications when dealing with a nonpalpable lesion.[20] In a study in which needle biopsy results were compared with findings when cytologic samples were obtained by flushing the needle after removal of the biopsy core, there was no improvement in detection of carcinoma from the additional needle cytologic sample.[30]

PREPARATION OF SLIDES FROM FNA

Opinions vary on how to make preparations from needle aspirate material.[8,26,31,32] We prefer the "book opening" technique, which limits air drying and smear artifacts and produces "mirror-image" slides that are useful when both air-dried and alcohol-fixed materials are prepared. Once a drop of needle aspirate is placed on the slide, a second slide is laid on top and gentle pressure is exerted on the cover slide (Figure 34-6). When this is done, the cellular sample will be seen to spread out between the two glass slides (see Figure 34-6). The slides are then turned apart, as if opening a book (Figure 34-7). This technique preserves cell group orientation and avoids the smear artifact that can make interpretation difficult.

At the University of Florida, both air-dried and 95% ethanol–fixed slides are prepared. Opinions differ as to the advantages and disadvantages of air-dried versus alcohol-fixed material. Both air-dried slides and alcohol-fixed slides can be prepared and stained with Diff-Quik or a similar stain within a few minutes at the patient's bedside. We use such preparations to evaluate the adequacy of the smear. Air-dried slides give good cytoplasmic and cell orientation detail but lack the nuclear detail available with alcohol-fixing. Unlike air-dried slides, alcohol-fixed slides can be used for immunohistochemical stains.

Some data indicate that when the pathologist is given full responsibility to both perform and interpret the FNA, the frequency of false-negative results is at a minimum (0.7%), whereas when surgeons perform the FNA, the false-negative rate is 22.8%.[26] This higher rate

F I G. **34-6** Book-opening technique of cellular preparation of the fine-needle aspiration sample. First, a second slide is placed over the slide containing the sample. The cellular material can be seen spreading out between the two slides with slight pressure.

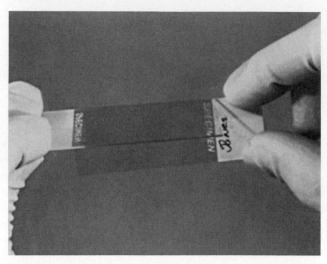

FIG. **34-7** Book-opening technique. The two slides are turned apart, as in opening a book.

of false-negative results occurs primarily because the needle aspiration technique and slide preparation pose various pitfalls for the surgeon. Although we offer to perform FNA as part of the pathology service, most breast FNAs are performed by the patients' surgeons. The cytotechnologist can be available to prepare the smears and evaluate for cellular adequacy at the time of the aspiration.

Fine-Needle Aspiration Diagnostic Terminology

The breast FNA diagnosis should fall into one of five categories[33,34]:

1. Benign (i.e., no evidence of malignancy)
2. Atypical/indeterminate (i.e., nondiagnostic cellular findings)
3. Suspicious for malignancy/probably malignant (i.e., cellular findings are suggestive of malignancy because of significant atypia or architectural distortion but quantitatively are insufficient for a definitive diagnosis of malignancy)
4. Malignant (i.e., cellular findings are diagnostic of malignancy, necessitating further classification of tumor by subtype and nuclear grade)
5. Unsatisfactory for evaluation (i.e., secondary to scant cellularity, air-drying artifact, obscuring blood or inflammation, or some other inadequacy)

The stratification of the malignant category into two, "probable cancer" (category 3) versus "definite cancer" (category 4), recognizes the heterogeneity of breast lesions. The major point is that there is clinical utility in separating those cases in which a definitive diagnosis can be made with FNA from those that cannot.[35,36] It is advocated that those cases that are definitively thought to represent cancer on FNA be placed in the "malignant" or "definite cancer" category with a statement that definitive intervention may be made without further diagnostic procedures (specifically tissue biopsy). A diagnosis of "suspicious" or "probable cancer" should include a statement prompting further investigation of the lesion before definitive therapy.[35] In doing so, the occurrence of false-positive diagnoses based on FNA results should be virtually eliminated. Most cases diagnosed as "probable cancer" based on FNA results are malignant on subsequent tissue biopsy, although they are often low-grade lesions that may be difficult to diagnose as malignant with FNA.

Interpretation of Cytopathologic Findings of Breast Fine-Needle Aspirates

GENERAL DIAGNOSTIC CYTOLOGIC CRITERIA

Benign Breast Disease. Normal structures of the breast include major lactiferous ducts, branched ducts, lobules, and connective tissue stroma. When normal breast tissue is aspirated, the cellular yield is quite low;

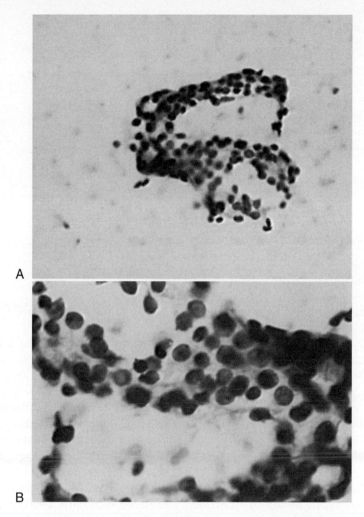

FIG. **34-8 A,** Benign group of ductal epithelial and myoepithelial cells. (×400.) **B,** Benign ductal epithelial cells and benign myoepithelial elements. (×1000.)

sometimes smears are hypocellular or acellular smears. More than one type of cell is evident in epithelial cell groups, representing a mix of ductal and myoepithelial cells.

The specific cellular characteristics found in benign breast disease (Figure 34-8) are summarized in Table 34-2. Although there are some rare exceptions, such as when nucleoli are found in the cells of lactating adenoma, if these features are identified in an adequate and well-prepared sample, they are characteristic of most benign processes within the breast.

Multiple needle aspiration passes may be necessary to increase the cellular yield in cases of benign breast disease, because benign diseases usually produce hypocellular samples. The cellularity of the aspirate also depends on the quantitative proportion of cells and fibrous stroma.

In addition to sheets of ductal cells, FNA specimens from patients with benign breast disease also show variable numbers of myoepithelial cells composed of single, bare nuclei (i.e., nuclei devoid of cytoplasm) (Figure 34-9). These nuclei have a bipolar shape, a smooth and distinctive nuclear profile, a compact chromatin pattern, and an indistinct nucleolus. The presence of naked, bipolar nuclei in a smear is a good indicator that the lesion is probably benign.[25]

TABLE 34-2	Common Cellular Features of Benign Breast Disease
Sheets or monolayers of cohesive, orderly ductal epithelial cells/few single cells (excluding myoepithelial cells)
Usually a hypocellular specimen
Variable cell types are present
Uniformity in nuclear size
Nuclear size about 1-1.5 times that of red blood cells
Smooth nuclear membranes, fine and evenly distributed chromatin
Absent or inconspicuous nucleoli
Absence of necrosis
Presence of myoepithelial cells mixed with epithelial cells

Malignant Breast Disease. Increased cellularity, loss of cellular cohesion, nuclear pleomorphism, anisonucleosis (Figure 34-10), and a coarse chromatin pattern are the predominant features of malignant lesions. Macronucleoli are associated with malignancy, but their absence does not indicate benignity. Micronucleoli are common in both benign and malignant lesions and cannot be used as a reliable indicator of malignancy. The presence of myoepithelial cells in the smears is significant because these cells are typically not found in cases of malignancy.

Some common cellular features are shared by breast adenocarcinomas of different types, as summarized in Table 34-3.

BENIGN LESIONS/CHANGES OF THE BREAST

Fibrocystic Changes. The histopathologic heterogeneity of this diverse group of benign changes results in variable appearances in FNA smears.[37] Lesions that are essentially fibrous or fatty produce hypocellular smears. Epithelial hyperplasias produce more cellular smears, with cellular groups bearing the benign characteristics and ductal cell populations described previously (Figure 34-11). Depending on the degree of hyperplasia, nuclear crowding and overlapping may occur, with irregular nuclear placement. The nuclei maintain relative uniformity. There is no tendency for the cells to disassociate, and isolated, intact, single abnormal

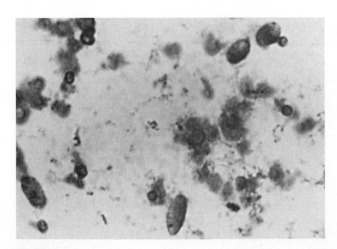

FIG. 34-9 Bare nuclei.

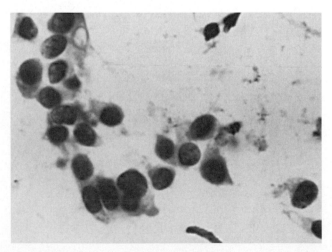

FIG. 34-10 Cell groups and single cells with characteristic cellular features of adenocarcinoma of the breast.

TABLE **34-3**   Common Cellular Features of Breast Carcinoma

Dyscohesive and disorderly cellular groups/presence of isolated, single cells

Usually a highly cellular specimen

Single cell population

Variation in nuclear size from cell to cell (anisonucleosis)

Enlarged nuclei (>2 times the size of a red blood cell)

Irregular nuclear membranes, coarse and clumped chromatin

Prominent nucleoli or macronucleoli

Necrosis often present

Absence of myoepithelial cells in the cell groupings

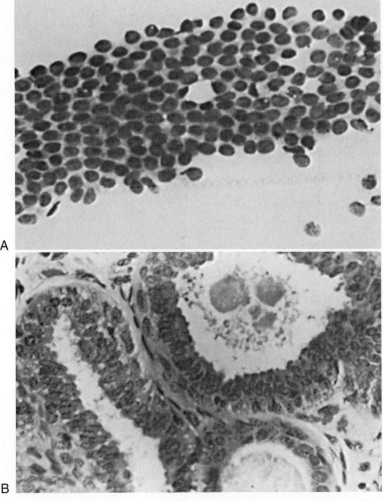

FIG. **34-11** **A,** Ductal epithelial hyperplasia, FNA. (×400.) **B,** Ductal epithelial hyperplasia, tissue biopsy corresponding to FNA in **A.** (×400.)

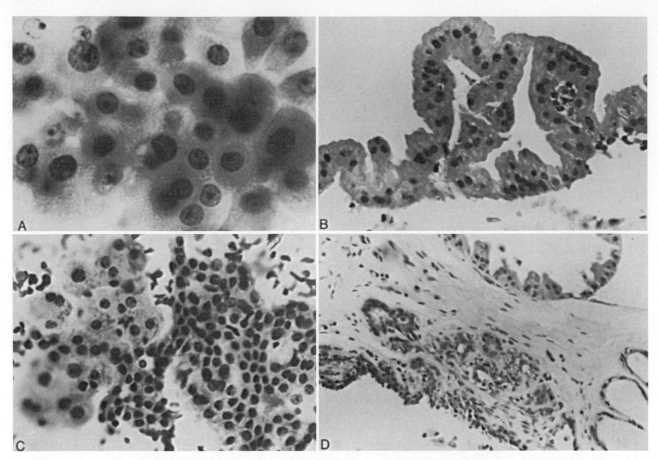

FIG. **34-12** **A,** Apocrine metaplasia. (×1000.) **B,** Apocrine cyst lining epithelium, tissue biopsy corresponding to FNA from **A.** (×400.) **C,** Apocrine metaplastic and ductal hyperplastic cellular groups. (×400.) **D,** Apocrine metaplasia with adjacent ductal epithelium, tissue biopsy corresponding to FNA from **C.** (×200.)

cells are generally absent. Bare nuclei vary from few to moderate in number.

Large cells of polygonal shape with a large nucleus and a single, prominent central nucleolus are characteristic of apocrine metaplasia. Cytoplasm is prominent and often amphoteric (Figure 34-12).

Apocrine cells in metaplasia and hyperplasia often occur singly and are an exception to the general cytologic criterion that a lack of cohesiveness in FNA smears is evidence of malignancy. These findings are distinguishable from those in apocrine cell carcinoma of the breast, which can also be recognized on FNA.

Cysts usually produce fluid on FNA, and the "mass" may no longer be palpable following the aspiration. The fluid may be seen as finely granular background material on both air-dried and alcohol-fixed slides. Cellular components include macrophages, hyperplastic ductal cells, and apocrine cells (Figure 34-13).[38] The epithelial

cells may show reactive or degenerative atypia.[25] In general, the fluid from benign cysts is clear to mildly cloudy and green to yellow. There is always the possibility of an associated carcinoma in a cyst wall. If a cyst is aspirated, a follow-up mammogram may be helpful to visualize the tissue surrounding the collapsed cyst, because cysts can obscure adjacent small neoplasms or calcifications on mammography.[39] Whenever a cystic lesion is aspirated, it is important to determine whether a residual mass remains; if a mass does remain, it is advisable to obtain a repeat FNA of the palpable mass or to perform a surgical biopsy. Fluid that is bloody, dark brown, opaque, or viscous may be present with a benign lesion; however, almost all cysts that form as a result of tumors are bloody. Cytologic examination of cyst fluids should be limited to those that are blood-stained, and it is recommended that, as a cost-effective method, routine cytologic examination not be performed on all breast fluids.[40]

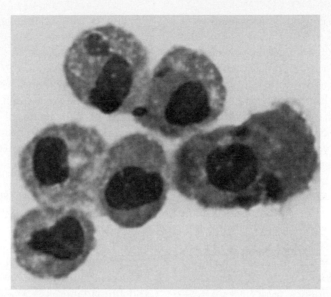

FIG. **34-13** Cyst cellular contents showing macrophages. (×1000.)

Fat Necrosis. In fat necrosis the aspirate usually consists of milky or oily fluid; fat is easily recognizable microscopically as macroglobules and microglobules, particularly on air-dried slides prepared with Wright's stain. Ductal cells are few and cohesive. Macrophages may appear atypical, with large nuclei, multinucleation, prominent nucleoli, and hyperchromasia; chronic inflammatory cells may also be present. Markedly reactive ductal epithelial cells may be seen in the sample, and because of the necrosis, the overall picture may resemble carcinoma. It is a common pitfall to misdiagnose carcinoma; adhering to strict cytologic criteria for carcinoma can usually help prevent this.

Mastitis

Acute. Acute mastitis usually occurs during breast-feeding and is caused by bacterial organisms, including staphylococci and streptococci. The fine-needle aspirate usually yields yellow, purulent-appearing material with acute inflammation, multinucleated giant cells, debris, and fat necrosis (Figure 34-14).[25] Epithelial elements may show inflammatory or reparative atypia[25] that should not be overinterpreted as atypia associated with malignancy. To aid in the differential diagnosis, breast carcinoma, even inflammatory carcinoma, is seldom associated with acute inflammation.[25]

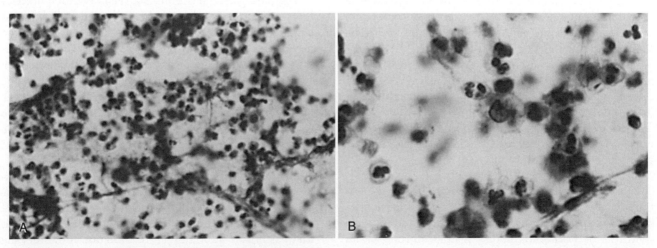

FIG. **34-14** **A,** Acute mastitis. (×200.) **B,** Acute mastitis. (×1000.)

Chronic. Chronic mastitis is usually associated with duct ectasia or plasma cell mastitis. The fine-needle aspirate usually obtains thick secretions that microscopically correspond to amorphous or granular material.[25] Epithelial proliferation is generally not a part of chronic mastitis.[25] The inflammatory infiltrate is generally plentiful and composed of plasma cells and macrophages, with or without multinucleated giant cells.

Granulomatous. Granulomatous mastitis may be caused by tuberculosis, fungus, cat-scratch disease, foreign bodies (e.g., sutures), silicone injections, or leaking breast implants, among other things.[25] The FNA usually shows granulomas and/or multinucleated giant cells, with or without the causative agent.[25]

Pregnancy and Lactation-Associated Changes. Aspirates from benign lesions of the breast under gestational or lactational influence may be hypercellular, and nuclear changes such anisonucleosis and prominent nucleoli can be seen.[41] Therefore, to avoid a false-positive diagnosis of malignancy, these changes must be considered with the knowledge that the aspirate is from a patient who is pregnant or lactating. Most aspirates from pregnant and/or lactating women are benign, with findings consistent with pregnancy or lactation. These changes include foamy cytoplasm as a result of milk fat vacuolization, the presence of fat droplets, and dispersed naked nuclei secondary to the fragile nature of the vacuolated cytoplasm.[25] Breast masses in pregnancy and lactation are most often benign lactating adenomas. These adenomas are characterized on FNA by hypercellular smears that may contain blood and amorphous debris that could be misinterpreted as necrotic material. Cell groupings lack cohesion, and individual intact cells may be present; because the cells are engaged in making milk, they have active, enlarged nuclei (usually up to two times the size of a red blood cell) and prominent nucleoli.[25] The differential diagnosis is based on the presence of abundant fatty material in the background, uniformity of nuclear shape, and nuclear enlargement to no more than two times the size of a red blood cell. Although breast cancer is relatively rare during pregnancy, it is the second most common malignancy diagnosed during pregnancy.[25] The FNA biopsy of breast cancer during pregnancy or lactation shows typical cytologic features of malignancy such as poorly cohesive, pleomorphic cells with enlarged nuclei, irregular nuclear membranes, and mitotic activity.[42]

Silicone Breast Implant Cytology. Needle aspiration of the fluid within the bursae-like space that surrounds silicone implant capsules, prepared by cytocentrifuge preparation, can demonstrate silicone within foreign body giant cells, especially if the capsule of the implant is leaking. Fourier transform infrared microscopy can be used for the positive identification of silicone in such cases.[43]

Subareolar Abscess. Subareolar abscess is a breast abscess that may be related to duct ectasia. The aspiration consists of thick material with numerous neutrophils, anucleate and nucleated squamous cells and multinucleated giant cells.[25] Very reactive ductal epithelial cells that may resemble significant cellular atypia may be present.

Sclerosing Lesions/Radial Scar. The cytologic characteristics of a radial scar or complex sclerosing lesion are relatively nonspecific and include benign epithelial cell clusters, apocrine and foam cells, and bipolar naked nuclei—all features that may be seen in other benign breast lesions, including fibrocystic change and fibroadenoma.[44] The radiologic appearance of the lesion is important in arriving at the proper diagnosis by cytology.[44]

Nodular Fasciitis and Inflammatory Pseudotumor within the Breast. Both nodular fasciitis and inflammatory pseudotumor may present clinically as a suspicious-looking breast mass. On FNA the nuclear features of malignancy are typically absent. Small groups of spindled cells may be seen; these cells usually have relatively uniform nuclei and lack significant nuclear pleomorphism. A storiform cell pattern and myxoid cellular features may be seen. Biopsy may be necessary to distinguish from spindle cell tumors.[45]

Benign Tumors

Fibroadenoma. Fibroadenoma is a benign proliferation of both epithelial and stromal elements, and typically the stromal elements predominate. Characteristically, the cellular yield from fibroadenomas on FNA is quite abundant, with numerous broad sheets of regularly arranged epithelial cells ("antler horns") (Figure 34-15). The nuclei of the epithelial cells are slightly larger than those of normal ductal cells; they are uniform in size and shape and have a finely granular chromatin pattern and one or two small nucleoli. Large numbers of bare, bipolar nuclei are also present[25] and are best appreciated at medium scanning power as abundant small dark dots. The third characteristic component to the fibroadenoma is the stroma, which is best seen with Wright's stain as metachromatic and fibrillar material.

Fibroadenomas share many similarities with fibrocystic change, and the two may occasionally be cytologically indistinguishable.[46] In general, fibroadenomas are more cellular than fibrocystic change, with more stromal tissue and more numerous bare nuclei. Fibrocystic change tends to show greater abundance of apocrine

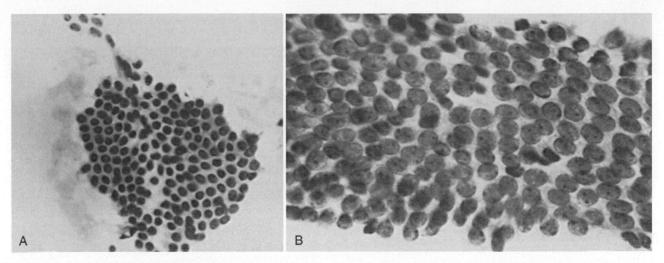

FIG. **34-15 A,** Fibroadenoma. (×400.) **B,** Fibroadenoma. (×1000.)

metaplasia and foam cells than the fibroadenoma. Epithelial atypia is common in fibroadenomas, and its recognition in a smear that otherwise looks like fibroadenoma is important to avoid a false-positive diagnosis of malignancy.[46] Carcinoma of the breast may rarely be found in a fibroadenoma.[47]

Tubular Adenoma. Aspirates from this relatively uncommon lesion, which may be clinically indistinguishable from a fibroadenoma, typically show sparse to moderate cellularity composed of three-dimensional balls of cells and/or cylindrical tubules.[48] The nuclei of these cells are uniform and bland, in contrast to those in tubular carcinoma.[48] The cytoplasm may contain intracytoplasmic granules in Giemsa-stained smears.[48]

Intraductal Papilloma. Aspirates from intraductal papillomas can be similar to fibroadenomas. Clinical information such as nipple discharge or a central/subareolar lesion should alert the pathologist to the possibility of a papilloma when the smears resemble a fibroadenoma (Figure 34-16).[31]

Characteristic but inconsistent findings of a papilloma include the following:

1. Complex cohesive papillary groups of hyperplastic ductal cells with fibrovascular cores

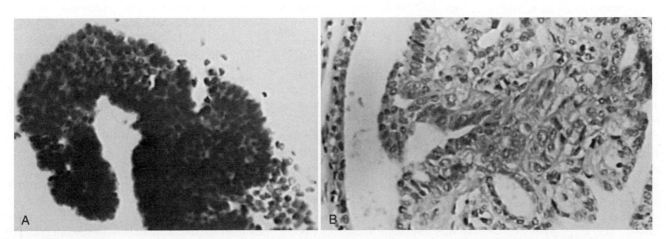

FIG. **34-16 A,** Intraductal papilloma. (×400.) **B,** Intraductal papilloma in biopsy corresponding to cytologic study **(A).** (×400.)

TABLE 34-4 Cytologic Criteria Grading System for Interpretation of Mammographically Guided
FNA Biopsies

CELLULAR ARRANGEMENT	CELLULAR PLEOMORPHISM	MYOEPITHELIAL CELLS	ANISONUCLEOSIS	NUCLEOLI	CHROMATIN CLUMPING	SCORE
Monolayer	Absent	Many	Absent	Absent	Absent	1
Nuclear overlapping	Mild	Moderate	Mild	Micronucleoli	Rare	2
Clustering	Moderate	Few	Moderate	Micronucleoli and/or rare macronucleoli	Occasional	3
Loss of cohesion	Conspicuous	Absent	Conspicuous	Predominantly micronucleoli	Frequent	4

From Masood S et al: *Cancer* 66:1480, 1990. Copyright © 1996 American Cancer Society. Reprinted by permission of Wiley-Liss, Inc., a subsidiary of John Wiley & Sons, Inc.

2. Large numbers of foamy macrophages, indicating a cystic area where the papilloma protrudes

Nipple Adenoma. On FNA, nipple adenoma appear similar to a fibroadenoma with a cellular yield composed of cohesive clusters of uniform cells and naked oval nuclei.[35] The cells may show some dissociation, but minimal nuclear pleomorphism.[25]

Granular Cell Tumor. Granular cell tumors can occur in and around the breast and may present as a lump that clinically and radiologically simulates malignancy. Aspirates show moderately cellular smears with clusters of cells and individual cells with abundant, granular cytoplasm; prominent cytoplasmic granularity; and small, round to oval central nuclei.

Cytologically, because of the abundant, granular cytoplasm, histiocytes and apocrine cells are within the differential diagnosis of an aspirate of the cells of a granular cell tumor. In these cases, knowledge of the clinical and radiologic findings is important. If cell block material is available, immunohistochemical staining for S-100 protein may be helpful.

CYTOPATHOLOGIC GRADING SYSTEM TO EVALUATE BREAST FNA SPECIMENS

The association between so-called fibrocystic disease and increased risk of breast cancer has been recognized for many years. However, morphologic classification of fibrocystic disease into reproducible and prognostically relevant categories was delayed until Dupont and Page reported the results of their study in 1985.[50] They evaluated the relative risk of subsequent development of breast cancer in patients with "fibrocystic disease" diagnosed on the basis of histologic features of biopsy specimens. The term *fibrocystic disease* was replaced with *fibrocystic change*, and the new terms *nonproliferative*

breast disease, proliferative breast disease without atypia, and *proliferative breast disease with atypia (atypical hyperplasia)* were introduced.

A grading system to define the cytologic features of proliferative and nonproliferative breast disease and to differentiate between atypical hyperplasia and carcinoma is presented in Table 34-4. This grading system is based on the cellular arrangement, the degree of cellular pleomorphism and anisonucleosis, the presence of myoepithelial cells and nucleoli, and the chromatin pattern. Values ranging from 1 to 4 are assigned to each criterion, and a score based on the sum of the individual values is calculated for each case. Cellular smears used to create this system were from a prospective study of mammographically guided FNAs of 100 nonpalpable breast lesions. The reliability of this grading system was assessed by comparing the cytologic interpretation with the histologic diagnosis from the corresponding needle-localization excisional biopsies. The results showed a high degree of concordance between the two approaches (Tables 34-5 and 34-6).[51,52]

The significance of benign breast disease depends on the presence of proliferation and atypia.[53] Although there are some distinguishing cytologic features, the categorization of benign breast disease ranging from nonproliferative to proliferative with atypia is not always reliable based on cytologic analysis.

Nonproliferative breast disease is characterized by relatively low cellularity, monolayered cell arrangements, and a lack of nuclear overlapping and atypia. Foam cells, apocrine cells, naked single cells, and fragments of stromal cell groups are frequently observed. The ductal cells have regular nuclei with a fine chromatin pattern without appreciable nuclear overlap. Nucleoli are uncommon. Myoepithelial cells are common and easily identified (Figures 34-17 and 34-18).

TABLE **34-5** Cytologic Findings Compared with Histologic Diagnosis in 100 Mammographically Suspect Cases

CYTOLOGY	NO. OF CASES	NONPROLIFERATIVE BREAST DISEASE	PROLIFERATIVE WITHOUT ATYPIA	PROLIFERATIVE WITH ATYPIA	CARCINOMA IN SITU LCIS	DCIS	INVASIVE CANCER
Insufficient	9	7	2	—	—	—	—
Nonproliferative breast disease	34	29	4	—	1*	—	—
Proliferative without atypia	17	—	15	2	—	—	—
Proliferative with atypia	23	—	—	21	1*	1*	—
Carcinoma	17	—	—	—	—	5	—
TOTAL	100	36	21	23	2	6	12

From Masood S et al: *Cancer* 66:1480, 1990. Copyright © 1990 American Cancer Society. Reprinted by permission of Wiley-Liss, Inc., a subsidiary of John Wiley &. Sons, Inc.
DCIS, Ductal carcinomma in situ; *LCIS*, lobular carcinoma in situ.
*False-negative cytologic interpretations.

TABLE **34-6** Concordance between Cytologic Evaluation versus Histologic Diagnosis in 100 Mammographically Guided Fine Needle Aspirates

DIAGNOSIS	NO. OF CASES	CONCORDANCE (%)
Nonproliferative breast disease	29/34	85
Proliferative breast disease without atypia	15/17	88
Proliferative breast disease with atypia	21/23	91
Cancer	17/20	85

Modified from Masood S et al: *Cancer* 66:1480, 1990. Copyright © 1990 American Cancer Society. Reprinted by permission of Wiley-Liss, Inc., a subsidiary of John Wiley & Sons, Inc.

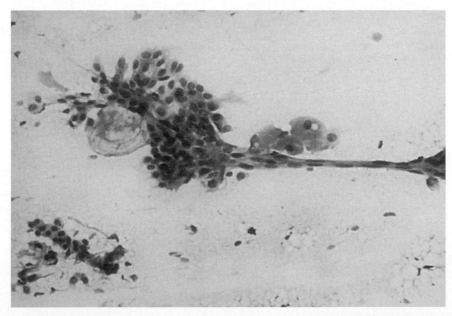

FIG. **34-17** Cytology of nonproliferative breast disease: cluster of ductal epithelial cells with apocrine cells and minute fragments of stroma. (Papanicolaou stain, ×200.) *(From Masood S et al: Diagn Cytopathol 7:581, 1991. Reprinted by permission of Wiley-Liss, Inc., a subsidiary of John Wiley & Sons, Inc.)*

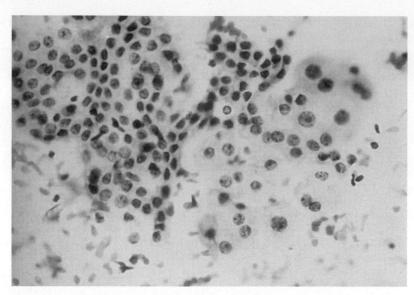

FIG. **34-18** Nonproliferative breast disease. Duct epithelial cells and apocrine metaplasia. (Papanicolaou stain, ×200.) *(From Masood S:* Breast J *1:210, 1996.)*

Nonproliferative breast disease is characterized by relatively low cellularity, monolayered cell arrangements, and a lack of nuclear overlapping and atypia. Foam cells, apocrine cells, naked single cells, and fragments of stromal cell groups are frequently observed. The ductal cells have regular nuclei with a fine chromatin pattern without appreciable nuclear overlap. Nucleoli are uncommon. Myoepithelial cells are common and easily identified (Figures 34-17 and 34-18).

Some cytologic overlap does exist between nonproliferative and proliferative disease because of the spectrum of changes that may be observed in the two conditions.[54]

Proliferative breast disease is a morphologic continuum that includes hyperplasia with and without atypia and carcinoma in situ.[55]

Proliferative breast disease without atypia differs from nonproliferative breast disease in that it has a higher

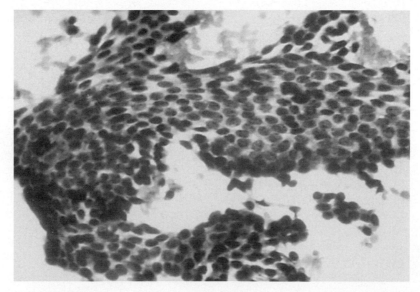

FIG. **34-19** Proliferative breast disease without atypia. Crowded cluster of ductal epithelial cells with overriding of the nuclei. (Papanicolaou stain, ×400.) *(From Masood S et al:* Diagn Cytopathol *7:581, 1991. Reprinted by permission of Wiley-Liss, Inc., a subsidiary of John Wiley & Sons, Inc.)*

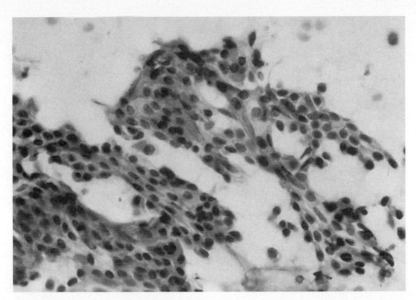

FIG. **34-20** Proliferative breast disease without atypia. Dual population of cells. Uniform hyperplastic ductal cells and smaller, darker myoepithelial cells. (Papanicolaou stain, ×400.) *(From Masood S et al: Diagn Cytopathol 7:581, 1991. Reprinted by permission of Wiley-Liss, Inc., a subsidiary of John Wiley & Sons, Inc.)*

cell yield and more cellular groups. Crowded clusters of epithelial cells with conspicuous overriding of the nuclei characterize this entity. Micronucleoli are occasionally seen (Figures 34-19 and 34-20).

Proliferative breast disease with atypia shows some but not all of the features of malignancy.[56] It is characterized cytologically by the rich cellularity and multiple clusters of atypical epithelial cells. There is loss of polarity with marked overriding of the nuclei. Nuclei display a coarse, irregular chromatin pattern, and nucleoli are conspicuous. These features are worrisome and may be difficult to distinguish from those of carcinoma. In atypical hyperplasia, intermingled with the crowded epithelial cells are spindle cells with morphologic

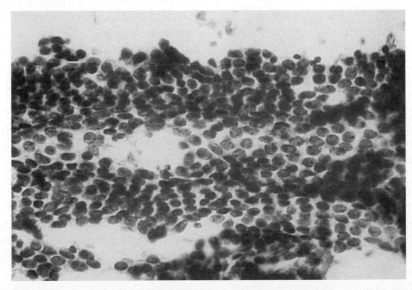

FIG. **34-21** Proliferative breast disease with atypia (atypical hyperplasia). Conspicuous overriding of the nuclei with cytologic atypicality. (Diff-Quik, ×200.) *(From Masood S: Breast J 1:210, 1996.)*

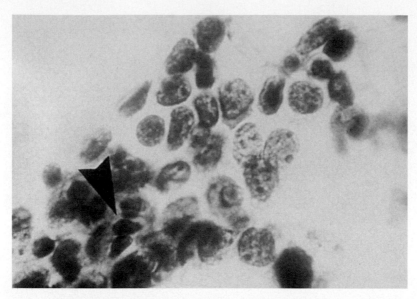

FIG. 34-22 Cluster of highly atypical cells with features simulating those of carcinoma. However, the presence of myoepithelial cells *(arrow)* excludes the possibility of a neoplasm. (Papanicolaou stain, ×1000.) *(From Masood S: Breast J 1:210, 1996.)*

Follow-up studies indicate that false-negative results of FNA of palpable breast lesions may occur in the cytomorphologic differentiation between atypical hyperplasia and low-grade breast carcinomas. However, these false-negatives may not pose a significant problem, because most investigators advocate excisional biopsy for any case that is diagnosed as atypical hyperplasia and is suspicious-looking or inconclusive for carcinoma.[52,56,64-68]

The potential value of cytologic recognition of atypical hyperplasia by FNA is in identifying women at high risk for breast cancer. This use of FNA has clinical implications in the design of chemoprevention trials.[69] The breast is uniquely suited to sampling by FNA. If adequately cellular, aspirates can be used to assess potential risk by means of additional tests such as those for DNA ploidy, proliferation rate (e.g., S-phase fraction, Ki-67), hormone receptors, oncogenes, and tumor-suppressor genes.[69-71]

Ductal Carcinoma In Situ. Aspirates of ductal carcinoma in situ (DCIS) have variable cytologic features, reflecting the tumor's morphologic diversity and whether the tumor is of a comedocarcinoma or non-comedo carcinoma type.

Comedocarcinoma. FNA samples of DCIS, comedo-type are usually cellular and display loosely cohesive clusters of malignant cells with individual cell necrosis. Nuclear membrane irregularities, nuclear pleomorphism, chromatin clumping, and large nucleoli are often present. Nuclear pleomorphism and irregularly shaped nucleoli are characteristic features of comedocarcinoma. No myoepithelial cells are present (Figure 34-23).

Noncomedocarcinoma. The cellularity of the aspirates from noncomedo-type DCIS varies. The aspirates show a monomorphic cell population of small to medium epithelial cells arranged singly or in loosely cohesive clusters. The cell clusters may have a solid, cribriform, or papillary pattern with no myoepithelial cell differentiation (Figure 34-24).

DUCTAL CARCINOMA IN SITU VERSUS INVASIVE CARCINOMA

Cytologic discrimination between DCIS and invasive carcinoma is very difficult, and although some features may suggest invasion,[72] it is not possible to reliably make this distinction. Invasive lesions are more cellular and more frequently display loss of cell cohesion. The clinical presentation and radiologic features can complement the findings of the breast aspiration and assist one in making a correct diagnosis. Recognition of the cytologic features of certain subtypes of invasive carcinoma, such as mucinous, medullary, or sarcomatoid, can generally be identified with FNA.[73]

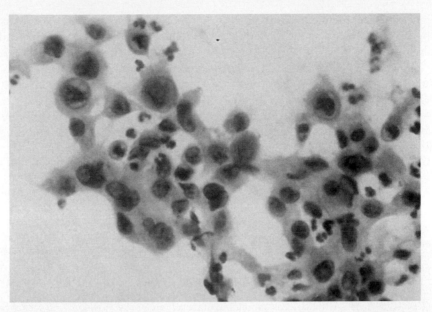

FIG. **34-23** Aspirate of comedocarcinoma shows pleomorphic population of neoplastic cells, with evidence of individual cell necrosis. (Hematoxylin and eosin, ×400.) *(From Masood S: Breast J 1:210, 1996.)*

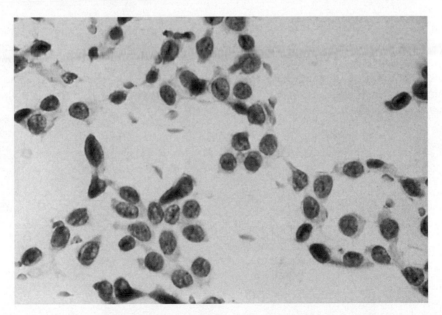

FIG. **34-24** Aspirate from noncomedo carcinoma shows loosely cohesive clusters of bland-appearing epithelial cells forming a cribriform pattern. (Papanicolaou stain, ×200.) *(From Masood S: Breast J 1:210, 1996.)*

In summary, generally, it is impossible to distinguish in situ and infiltrating ductal carcinomas by FNA with use of cellular morphology alone.[56]

Invasive Adenocarcinoma, Not Otherwise Specified. The usual invasive adenocarcinoma of the breast clinically presents as an ill-defined, hard nodule firmly attached to the adjacent breast tissue. Depending on the degree of fibrous response, aspirates can be hypocellular, and examiners must be sensitive to the adequacy of the specimen. The diagnosis depends on finding the usual malignant criteria, including hypercellularity, cellular lack of cohesion, single cells, characteristic cell groupings, monomorphism, anisonucleosis, nuclear hyperchromasia, and membrane changes. Prominent nucleoli are frequently observed. Nuclear molding, overriding, and crowding are also commonly observed (Figure 34-25).

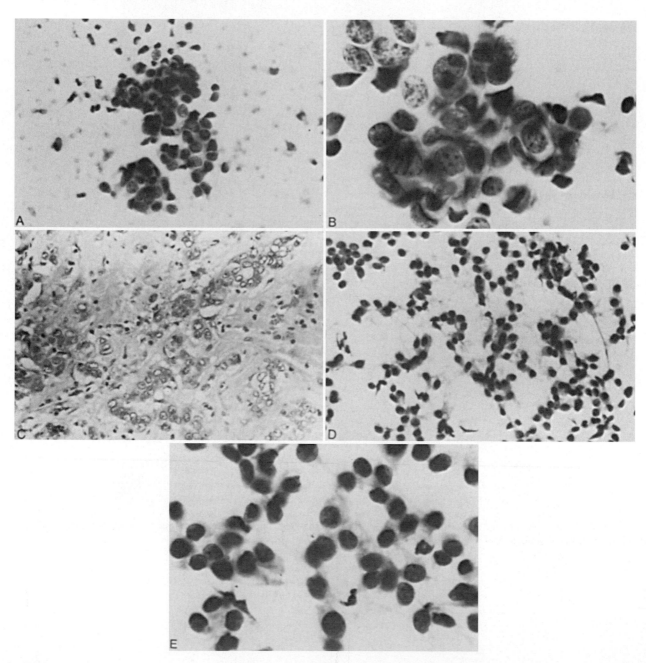

FIG. **34-25 A,** Invasive adenocarcinoma. (×400) **B,** Invasive adenocarcinoma (×1000.) **C,** Invasive adenocarcinoma in biopsy corresponding to **A** and **B**. (×400.) **D,** Invasive adenocarcinoma. (×250.) **E,** Invasive adenocarcinoma. (×400.)

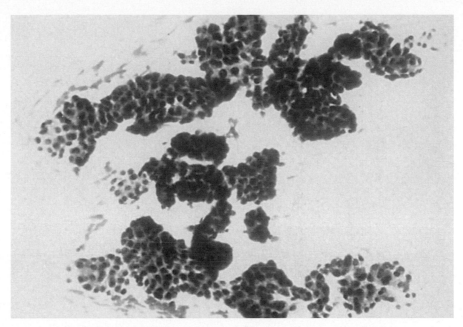

FIG. **34-26** Cytomorphology of atypical lobular hyperplasia (lobular hyperplasia): acinar proliferation consisting of small cells with a uniform appearance. (Papanicolaou stain, ×100.) *(From Johnston W [ed], Cytopathology of the breast, Chicago, 1995, ASCP Press).*

Lobular Neoplasia. The cytologic distinction between atypical lobular hyperplasia, lobular carcinoma in situ, and infiltrating lobular carcinoma is difficult. Aspirates of atypical lobular hyperplasia and lobular carcinoma in situ show loosely cohesive groups of small, uniform cells with eccentric regular nuclei, and occasional intracytoplasmic lumina. The nuclei are hyperchromatic, with a fine chromatin pattern and inconspicuous nucleoli. Occasionally, small groups of cells that form three dimensional cell groups may be seen (Figures 34-26 and 34-27). Aspirates from infiltrating lobular carcinoma have

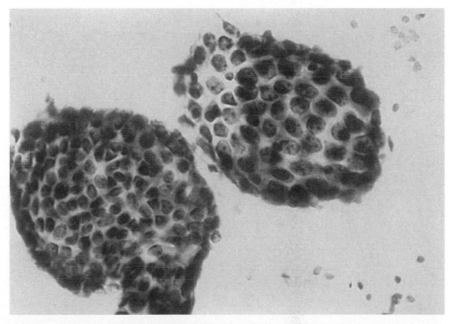

FIG. **34-27** Atypical lobular hyperplasia (lobular neoplasia). "Cell balls" simulating acini. (Papanicolaou stain, ×400.) *(From Masood S: Breast J 1:210, 1996.)*

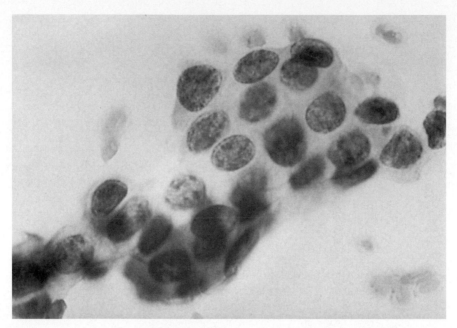

F I G. **34-28** Infiltrating lobular carcinoma. Loosely arranged, uniform-appearing epithelial cells. (Diff Quik, ×400.) *(From Masood S: Breast J 1:210, 1996.)*

similar cytomorphologic features but are more cellular.[56] The cells may also occur in small groups or "Indian file" cords, or they may occur as single cells.[56] Occasionally, signet ring cells may also be seen (Figures 34-28 and 34-29). Cellular aspirates that contain a significant number of small, uniform cells characteristic of infiltrating lobular carcinoma can be diagnosed accordingly. Patients whose aspirates show scant cellularity that is consistent with lobular neoplasia should undergo an excisional biopsy for definitive diagnosis.

Lobular Carcinoma. Invasive lobular carcinoma has recognized histologic subtypes: classic, alveolar,

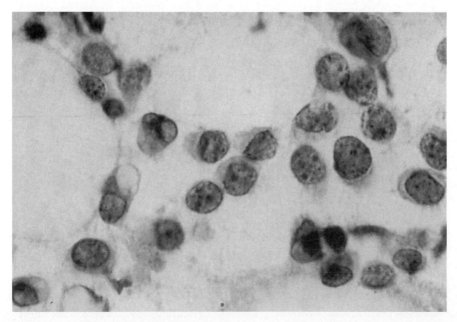

F I G. **34-29** Infiltrating lobular carcinoma. Discohesive population of small tumor cells with a few signet ring forms. (Papanicolaou stain, ×400.) *(From Masood S: Breast J 1:210, 1996.)*

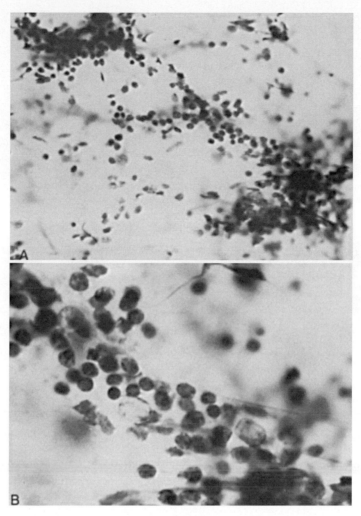

FIG. 34-30 **A,** Lobular carcinoma. (×250.) **B,** Lobular carcinoma. (×400.)

mixed, solid, and pleomorphic types.[73,74] The latter type may be confused cytologically with ductal carcinoma because of its pleomorphic cytologic features.[75] Characteristic cytologic features of nonpleomorphic lobular carcinoma include smears of low cellularity, small- to medium-sized isolated single cells (8 to 12 microns),[76] a small amount of ill-defined cytoplasm, minimal pleomorphism, uniform chromatin, and small nucleoli[76,77] (Figure 34-30). Indian filing of the cells, considered a characteristic finding in invasive lobular carcinoma, is observed in approximately one third of cases and, when present, tends to be focal.[76]

Pleomorphic lobular carcinoma has a high nuclear grade with nuclear pleomorphism. These are important tumors to identify in that they are associated with a shorter disease-free interval and lower survival rate than is lobular carcinoma of the usual type.[78] Because of the similar cytologic features with ductal carcinoma,

the FNA diagnosis of pleomorphic lobular carcinoma is usually presumptive and the final histopathologic tumor classification may require biopsy.

Medullary Carcinoma. Medullary carcinomas contain medium to large cells with little intracellular cohesion, abundant cytoplasm (sometimes resembling squamous carcinoma), and marked nuclear abnormalities, including nucleoli and nuclear membrane folding.[31] Necrotic material, lymphocytes, and plasma cells may be found within the background (Figure 34-31).

Mucinous (Colloid) Carcinoma. Mucinous carcinomas of the breast are a subtype of breast cancer with a particularly good prognosis. They are associated with mucous secretion, and aspirates are typically cellular. The tumor cells are frequently arranged in compact

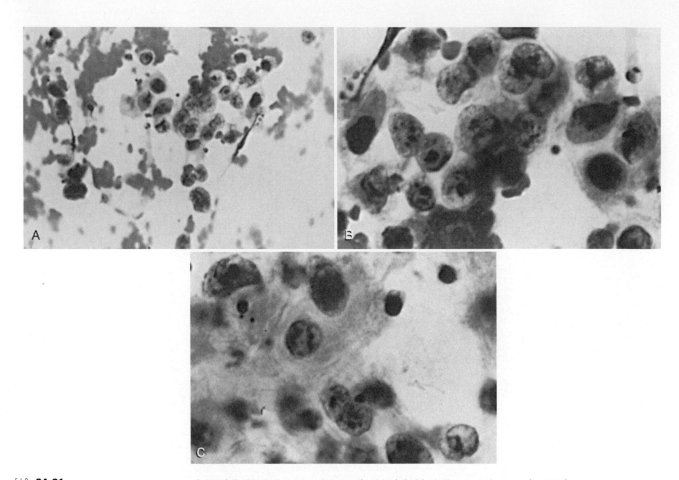

FIG. **34-31** **A,** Medullary carcinoma. (×250.) **B,** Medullary carcinoma. (×1000.) **C,** Medullary carcinoma. (×1000.)

three-dimensional groups ("balls") with numerous single cells and demonstrate a mild to moderate degree of nuclear pleomorphism (Figure 34-32). The characteristic mucinous background may be lost if only filter material is available for cytologic review.[79] The mucin is readily detected with Romanovsky-type stains on air-dried smears but is also fairly easily recognized with the Pap stain.[80] It may be difficult to distinguish a mucinous carcinoma from a benign mucocele if the smears are hypocellular and show cells with minimal cytologic atypia and mucin. These cases should likely be diagnosed as inconclusive on FNA with a recommendation for further investigation of the lesion (i.e., biopsy).[10] Mucinous carcinomas may be mixed with other adenocarcinoma cell types that may not be evident on FNA. Because this finding will influence prognosis and therapy, definitive diagnosis requires study of the excised tumor.[81]

Tubular Carcinoma. Tubular carcinomas are well-differentiated carcinomas that maintain cell cohesion and have minimal nuclear abnormalities.[82] Because malignancy in breast cytology is often diagnosed on the basis of high cellularity, dyscohesive tumor cells, and nuclear atypia, the diagnosis of tubular carcinoma on cytology can be difficult. Characteristic glandular structures are usually found within the FNA smear and appear in groupings.[83] Tubular structures are also characteristic with a central lumen.[25] Nuclear enlargement, evident on comparison with benign ductal cells, is a consistent finding.[8,31] Other features that may suggest the diagnosis of tubular carcinoma include irregular nuclear membranes and intracytoplasmic lumens.[25] Myoepithelial cells are often considered a sign of a benign lesion in the breast; however, they may be present in tubular carcinoma.[83] A firm diagnosis of cancer may require tissue biopsy.[25]

Inflammatory Carcinoma. Knowledge of the distinctive clinical presentation of inflammatory carcinoma is essential for appropriate diagnosis by FNA. Aspirates are usually cellular, with all the malignant cytologic criteria (Figure 34-33) usually found in breast adenocarcinoma.[31] Inflammatory carcinoma is not a specific

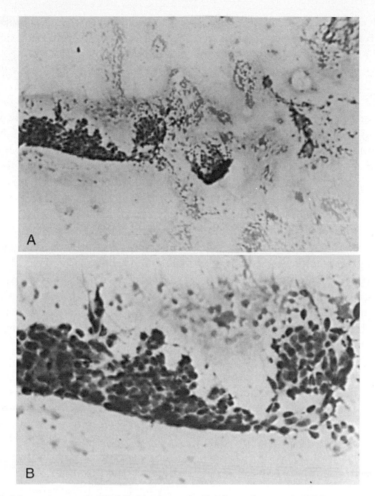

FIG. **34-32** **A**, Mucinous (colloid) carcinoma. (×250.) **B**, Mucinous (colloid) carcinoma. (×400.)

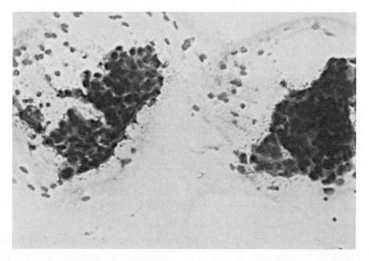

FIG. **34-33** Inflammatory carcinoma. Aspirate from reddened periareolar skin. Clusters of monomorphic cells are present with cellular features of adenocarcinoma.

tumor type but rather a distinctive clinical presentation. The tumor type is typically invasive adenocarcinoma, NOS.

Mammary Paget's Disease. Smears prepared from scrapings from the nipple in Paget's disease show a background of keratinous debris, inflammatory cells, and benign squamous cells of skin origin. The Paget cells are intraductal or invasive ductal adenocarcinoma in origin and show those cytologic characteristics.[25]

Other Breast Carcinoma Types. Papillary neoplasms include the benign papilloma (previously discussed) and noninvasive and invasive papillary carcinomas. These lesions are composed of papillary groups with fibrovascular cores. Papillary carcinomas tend to be less cohesive than benign papillomas with greater numbers of single cells and greater nuclear pleomorphism. However, it can be difficult to cytologically distinguish benign papilloma from papillary carcinoma, and when a papillary neoplasm is suspected based on FNA analysis, the recommendation should be for tissue biopsy or excision of the lesion for definitive diagnosis.[25]

Squamous carcinoma may arise as a primary tumor within the breast, and its diagnosis by FNA has been described.[84,85] Groups and sheets of atypical squamous cells are usually seen, with keratin or dyskeratosis being an important diagnostic feature.

Secretory carcinoma of the breast is rare; however, cytologic findings after FNA have been observed. Distinctive features include sheets and "grapelike" clusters of neoplastic cells, with granular cytoplasm, cytoplasmic vacuolization,[86,87] and signet ring cell formation.[88]

Carcinoma of the breast with osteoclast-like stromal giant cells has been identified on breast FNA.[90] Characteristically, multinucleated giant cells are mixed with an invasive breast carcinoma. The giant cells have been identified as being of histiocytic origin.

Metaplastic carcinomas are a heterogeneous group of breast neoplasms that have adenocarcinoma admixed with areas of spindle, squamous, osseous, or chondroid differentiation.[73] The spindle cells can be confirmed as epithelial in origin with the use of immunohistochemical stains for cytokeratins (versus a true carcinosarcoma, in which the spindle cells are considered mesenchymal in origin and would be immunoreactive for mesenchymal markers, not epithelial markers).[73]

Neuroendocrine differentiation may be seen in approximately 3% to 21% of mammary carcinomas as focal argyrophilic granules.[73] Argyrophilia, carcinoid pattern, and neuroendocrine differentiation have all been reported in human breast carcinoma.[73,90] Breast carcinoid typically is composed of monomorphic small cells with minimal nuclear pleomorphism and minimal nuclear membrane irregularities,[25] which must be distinguished from the bland cells of lobular carcinoma.

Apocrine carcinoma, an unusual variant of ductal carcinoma, is composed of large apocrine cells with abundant granular eosinophilic cytoplasm and central large nuclei with prominent nucleoli. On needle aspiration these tumors yield numerous cells with apocrine features, including large size (15 to 20 μm) and abundant granular cytoplasm (Figure 34-34). The cytoplasm is typically well delineated in isolated cells but rather indistinct in cell groupings. Nuclear anisocytosis and prominent nucleoli, often occupying half of the nuclear volume, are usually seen.[8] Apocrine carcinoma versus apocrine metaplasia with atypia can be difficult by cytology, and the two entities may coexist.[92] In general, apocrine carcinoma has larger nuclei (>12 microns) and more marked nuclear abnormalities than atypical apocrine metaplasia.[91]

Phyllodes. Phyllodes tumor is a biphasic tumor characterized by proliferation of both epithelial and stromal elements that encompasses a spectrum of benign to malignant tumors. Malignant criteria are based on the stromal characteristics and include stromal cellularity, cellular atypia, mitotic activity, and tumor margins. The aspirate is usually cell rich, with stromal elements predominating, including cohesive clusters; bare nuclei are also evident. Fibroadenomas and low-grade phyllodes tumors share similar characteristics on FNA.[92] Stromal hypercellularity is often used to distinguish fibroadenoma from phyllodes tumor; however, hypercellular areas can occur in fibroadenomas and therefore should not be used as the sole criterion.[92] One study of fibroadenomas and phyllodes tumors on FNA reports using the proportion of background individual long spindle nuclei amid the dispersed (oval) stromal cells as a more reliable discriminator between the two lesions.[92] Typically, the distinction between a fibroadenoma and a malignant phyllodes is straightforward on FNA[92] because of the nuclear atypia and mitotic activity seen in the latter.

CYTOPATHOLOGIC EVIDENCE OF SOFT TISSUE TUMORS AND SARCOMAS OF THE BREAST

Primary schwannoma (benign neurilemmoma) of the breast has been reported in which the needle aspirate contained clusters of spindle-shaped cells and Verocay bodies. The tumor cells were immunoreactive for S-100 antigen.[93] Sarcomas of the breast arise from the mesenchymal component and are relatively rare.

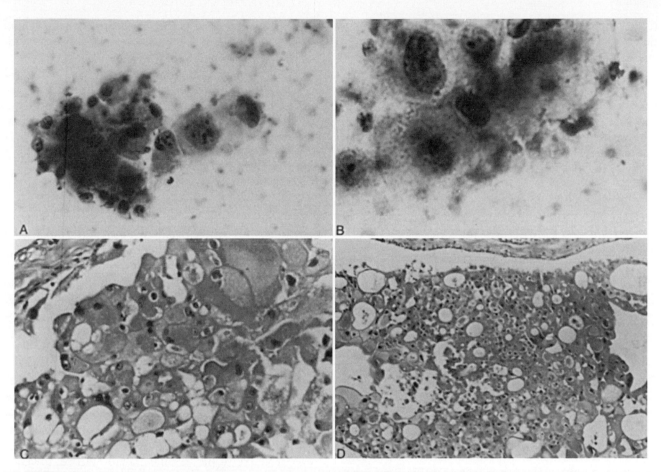

FIG. **34-34** **A,** Apocrine carcinoma. (×400.) **B,** Apocrine carcinoma. (×1000.) **C,** Apocrine carcinoma, tissue biopsy corresponding to FNA from **A** and **B.** (×400.) **D,** Apocrine carcinoma, tissue biopsy corresponding to FNA from **A** and **B.** (×250.)

Numerous primary sarcomas of the breast have been described on FNA, including liposarcoma,[94] malignant myoepithelioma,[95] leiomyosarcoma,[96] and angiosarcoma.[97] These tumors are characterized on FNA by clusters of spindle cells, usually with malignant nuclear features. Immunohistochemical studies are of great value, and a cell block for paraffin sections from one or more aspirates is of special value in performing the immunohistochemical studies. The differential diagnosis includes fibroma and other benign spindle cell tumors, as well as nonneoplastic conditions that may produce palpable masses, including nodular fasciitis, inflammatory pseudotumor, and granulation tissue.[45]

FNA samples from angiosarcomas of the breast usually have a bloody background; tumor cells are sparse and difficult to identify. This is particularly true in low-grade angiosarcomas, in which the malignant endothelial cells have little tendency to proliferate in solid clusters.[97] These tumors are rich in factor VIII, which can be identified within the malignant endothelial cells by using immunohistochemical techniques. The spindled cells of angiosarcoma must be distinguished from granulomatous tissue or fibroblasts, which do not contain factor VIII or ulex europaeus antigen, both of which are present in the spindle cells of angiosarcoma.

Primary rhabdomyosarcoma of the breast has been identified with FNA.[98] Large, striated cells and rhabdomyoblasts may be seen. Immunohistochemical detection of desmin, actin, myosin, and myoglobulin may assist in the identification of these tumors.

The Male Breast

GYNECOMASTIA

FNA of the male breast may be useful to rule out malignancy, especially if the patient presents with a unilateral or progressively enlarging discrete lesion.[99] The cellularity of an aspirate from a male patient with gynecomastia is often scant but may be abundant. Aspiration usually shows cohesive groups of bland or mildly atypical ductal cells, occasional single epithelial cells, bipolar naked nuclei, fibromyxoid stromal fragments, foamy histiocytes, and apocrine metaplasia.[99,100] Features that may cause diagnostic difficulty include increased cellularity and cell atypia as seen during the proliferative phase of gynecomastia.[99] However, these features are distinguishable from primary breast carcinoma of the male breast.[101]

CANCER

Primary breast cancer in men is usually of ductal type and cytologically is identical to ductal carcinoma of the female breast.[101]

Extramammary Tumors Metastatic to the Breast

Metastases to the breast are rarely the presenting symptom of an extramammary malignancy. However, clinically and radiographically they can simulate primary breast malignancy.[102] Most commonly, tumors that metastasize to the breast include lymphoma, carcinoma (e.g., lung, ovary, cervix, endometrium, stomach), and melanoma.[102] Tumors metastatic to the breast can cytologically range from a pattern not seen in primary breast cancers to indistinguishable from a primary breast carcinoma.[102] Therefore clinical history and review of previous pathologic material is essential in establishing the proper diagnosis.

Immunohistochemical and Immunofluorescence Procedures in Fine-Needle Aspiration

IMMUNOHISTOCHEMICAL TECHNIQUES IN THE STUDY OF BREAST CARCINOMA

Immunohistochemical techniques have become a powerful adjunctive diagnostic tool in surgical pathology and are now widely used. These techniques can provide information about the histogenesis of a variety of neoplasms with use of various tissue-specific markers, for example, distinguishing a poorly differentiated neoplasm as carcinoma, sarcoma, or lymphoma.

Demonstration of a myoepithelial layer with immunohistochemical markers to actin may be helpful in discriminating benign from malignant breast lesions.

Actin is a contractile protein present in muscular and normovascular cells. Malignant breast neoplasms typically lack a myoepithelial (actin positive) layer.

Immunohistochemical studies are often performed on the surgically removed breast specimen. However, a recent study showed good correlation between immunostaining of cell block material from FNA and on the corresponding surgically resected tumor tissue. Immunohistochemical markers studied on the cell block material included ER/PR, the cell proliferation marker Ki-67 (MIB-1), p53, and c-erb-B-2 (HER2/neu). The conclusion of this study was that cell block material prepared from an FNA of primary or metastatic breast cancer can be useful when planning neoadjuvant treatment (i.e., surgical excision of the lesion is not indicated).[103]

Fluorescence in situ hybridization (FISH), which is a validated method for detecting amplification of the HER2/neu gene, has recently been used on cytologic touch imprint preparations and has been found to be reliable.[104]

FALSE-NEGATIVE FNA RESULTS

A false-negative result is a negative result in the presence of tumor. In the literature, the false-negative rate of FNA of the breast ranges from 0.7% to 22%.[79,105] This figure is variable and depends on whether only satisfactory cellular smears were considered for a false-negative diagnosis (i.e., the lesion in question was sampled). Geographic miss of the lesion is one of the most common reasons for a false-negative diagnosis. A false-negative diagnosis can depend on several different factors, including experience of the aspirator; experience of the pathologist interpreting the cytologic sample; and tumor characteristics, such as size (especially lesions <2 cm),[105] amount of desmoplasia or fibrosis associated with the tumor (more fibrotic tumors are less likely to yield cells), and degree of tumor differentiation. The tumor type may be a factor. For example, failure to recognize a well-differentiated tumor as malignant may be the source of a false-negative diagnosis. For example, because of its bland cytologic features and diffuse growth pattern, lobular carcinoma is associated with a generally higher false-negative rate than other breast tumor types.[19] In addition, lobular carcinomas often yield hypocellular or inadequate samples,[106] with a reported higher false-negative rate when compared with FNA of ductal carcinoma. Similar difficulty may be encountered in recognizing tubular carcinoma as malignant on FNA because of its bland cytologic features.[48,107]

Steps that can be taken to reduce false-negative results include having pathology assistance in performing the aspirate so that the sample can be assessed for adequacy and the appropriate smears can be made for optimum cytologic evaluation. In the experience of Oertel,[26] the lowest false-negative rate (0.7%)

was observed when the pathologist performed the aspirate.

When multiple slides are made, unless the findings obviously indicate a tumor, a final diagnosis of negative requires careful screening of all cytologic material available for study. Any preliminary (bedside) negative diagnostic statement should imply that the final diagnosis is pending review of all cytologic material obtained. When there are suspicious clinical or radiologic findings despite a negative FNA result, further diagnostic procedures may be in order.

FALSE-POSITIVE FNA RESULTS

A false-positive result is a positive diagnosis for tumor when no tumor is present. False-positive findings have ranged from 0% to 11%.[10] However, with experienced cytopathologists, the reported false-positive rate is similar to that of frozen section (approximately 0.1% to 0.2%).[10]

False-positive results can sometimes be avoided by being aware of the clinical history and physical findings. FNA interpretative difficulties may occur when benign samples show features that typically characterize malignant tumors, such as high cellularity, cellular atypia, and loss of cell cohesion.[10] Apocrine cysts may show significant cytologic atypia in the apocrine cells, and the approach to apocrine lesions should be made with caution.[10] Other sources of false-positive diagnoses may be hematomas, subareolar abscesses, fat necrosis, irradiation, fibroadenomas, gynecomastia, papillomas, pregnancy-associated hyperplasia, and granulation tissue. All of these have been misinterpreted as malignancy on FNA by experienced pathologists.[26,31,108,109] Fulfillment of diagnostic cytologic criteria for malignancy is necessary to avoid false-positive results. If the FNA lacks adequate evidence for malignancy but reveals cellular findings such as single isolated cells and significant atypia suggestive of carcinoma, it is best to report the results as "suspicious" but not diagnostic, with a comment regarding the problem and a discussion of these findings with the surgeon.

Because of the small possibility of false-positive diagnosis, mastectomy should never be performed based on cytologic material alone but rather on the combination of clinical, radiologic, and pathologic evidence.[25]

REFERENCES

1. Martin HE, Ellis EB: Biopsy by needle procedure and aspiration, *Ann Surg* 92:169, 1930.
2. Silver CE et al: Needle aspiration cytology of tumors at various body sites, *Curr Probl Surg* 22:1, 1985.
3. Franzen S, Zajicek J: Aspiration biopsy in diagnosis of palpable lesions of the breast: critical review of 3479 consecutive biopsies, *Acta Radiol Ther Phys Biol* 7:241, 1968.
4. Zajicek J: Introduction to aspiration biopsy, *Monogr Clin Cytol* 4:1, 1974.
5. Zajicek J et al: Aspiration of mammary tumors in diagnosis and research: a critical review of 2,200 cases, *Acta Cytol* 11:169, 1967.
6. Rimm DL et al: Comparison of the costs of fine needle aspiration and open surgical biopsy as methods for obtaining a pathologic diagnosis, *Cancer* 81:51, 1997.
7. Berg JW, Robbins GF: A late look at the safety of aspiration biopsy, *Cancer* 15:826, 1962.
8. Kline TS: *Handbook of fine needle aspiration biopsy cytology,* ed 2, New York, 1988, Churchill Livingstone.
9. Rosemond GP, Maier WP, Brobyn TJ: Needle aspiration of breast cysts, *Surg Gynecol Obstet* 128:351, 1967.
10. Sneige N: Fine needle aspiration of the breast: a review of 1,995 cases with emphasis on diagnostic pitfalls, *Diagn Cytopathol* 9:106, 1993.
11. Ballo MS, Sneige N: Can core biopsy replace fine needle aspiration cytology in the diagnosis of palpable breast carcinoma: a comparative study of 124 women, *Cancer* 78:773, 1996.
12. Westenend PJ et al: A comparison of aspiration cytology and core needle biopsy in the evaluation of breast lesions, *Cancer* 93:146, 2001.
13. Boerner S et al: Ultrasound-guided fine-needle aspiration (FNA) of nonpalpable breast lesions: a review of 1885 FNA cases using the National Cancer Institute-supported recommendations on the uniform approach to breast FNA, *Cancer* 87:19, 1999.
14. Masood S: Occult breast lesions and aspiration biopsy: a new challenge, *Diagn Cytopathol* 9:613, 1993.
15. Pisano ED et al: Rate of insufficient samples for fine needle aspiration for nonpalpable breast lesions in a multicenter clinical trial: the Radiologic Diagnostic Oncology Group 5 study, *Cancer* 82:679, 1998.
16. Pisano ED et al: Fine needle aspiration biopsy of nonpalpable breast lesions in a multicenter clinical trial: results from the radiologic diagnostic oncology group V, *Radiology* 219:785, 2001.
17. Meloni GB et al: Ultrasound-guided mammotome vacuum biopsy for the diagnosis of impalpable breast lesions, *Ultrasound Obstet Gynecol* 18:520, 2001.
18. Ku NN et al: Role of fine needle aspiration cytology after lumpectomy, *Acta Cytol* 38:927, 1994.
19. Kim A et al: Fine needle aspiration cytology of the breast: experience at an outpatient breast clinic, *Acta Cytol* 44:361, 2000.
20. Symmans WF et al: What is the role of cytopathologists in stereotaxic needle biopsy diagnosis of nonpalpable mammographic abnormalities, *Diagn Cytopathol* 24:260, 2001.
21. Salami N et al: Triple test approach to inadequate fine needle aspiration biopsies of palpable breast lesions, *Acta Cytol* 43:339, 1999.
22. Steinberg JL et al: Combined fine needle aspiration, physical examination and mammography in the diagnosis of palpable breast masses: their relation to outcome for women with primary breast cancer, *Can J Surg* 39:302, 1996.
23. Tabbara SO et al: Changing trends in breast fine-needle aspiration: results of the Papinicolaou Society of Cytopathology survey, *Diagn Cytopathol* 22:126, 2000.
24. Kaufman Z et al: Pneumothorax: a complication of fine needle aspiration of breast tumors, *Acta Cytol* 38:737, 1994.
25. DeMay RM: *The art and science of cytopathology,* Chicago, 1996, ASCP Press.

26. Oertel YC: *Fine needle aspiration of the breast,* Boston, 1987, Butterworths USA.

27. Wilkinson EJ et al: Potential value of fine needle aspiration in the cytologic and cytometric analysis of bone and soft tissue tumors, *Lab Invest* 48:93A, 1983.

28. Sneige N et al: A plea for uniform terminology and reporting of breast fine needle aspirates: M.D. Anderson Cancer Center proposal, *Acta Cytol* 38:971, 1994.

29. Pennes DR, Naylor B, Rebner M: Fine needle aspiration of the breast, *Acta Cytol* 34:673, 1989.

30. Grant LD, Wilkinson EJ, Steinbach B: Combined cytologic and biopsy results with the biopty gun: stereotactic biopsies of nonpalpable lesions. Presented at the ASCP/CAP Spring Meeting, Orlando, FL, April 1995.

31. Frable WJ: *Thin needle aspiration biopsy,* Philadelphia, 1983, WB Saunders.

32. Howat AJ et al: Fine needle aspiration cytology of the breast: a review of 1,868 cases using the Cytospin method, *Acta Cytol* 38:939, 1994.

33. The uniform approach to breast fine needle aspiration biopsy: National Cancer Institute Fine-Needle Aspiration of Breast Workshop Subcommittees, *Diagn Cytopathol* 16:295, 1997.

34. The uniform approach to breast fine needle aspiration biopsy: a synopsis, *Acta Cytol* 40:1120, 1996.

35. Casey TT et al: Stratified diagnostic approach to fine needle aspiration of the breast, *Am J Surg* 163:305, 1992.

36. Page DL, Johnson JE, Dupont WD: Probabilistic approach to the reporting of fine-needle aspiration cytology of the breast, *Cancer* 81:6, 1997.

37. Maygarden SJ et al: Subclassification of benign breast disease by fine needle aspiration cytology: comparison of cytologic and histologic findings in 265 palpable breast masses, *Acta Cytol* 38:115, 1994.

38. Takeda T et al: Aspiration cytology of breast cysts, *Acta Cytol* 26:37, 1982.

39. Squires JE, Betsill WL: Intracystic carcinomas of the breast, *Acta Cytol* 25:267, 1981.

40. Ciatto S, Cariaggi P, Bulgaresi P: The value of routine cytologic examination of breast cyst fluids, *Acta Cytol* 31:301, 1987.

41. Gupta RK et al: Fine-needle aspiration cytodiagnosis of breast masses in pregnant and lactating women and its impact on management, *Diagn Cytopathol* 9:156, 1993.

42. Mitre BK, Kanbour AI, Mauser N: Fine needle aspiration biopsy of breast carcinoma in pregnancy and lactation, *Acta Cytol* 41:1121, 1997.

43. Caffee HH, Hardt NS, LaTorre G: Detection of breast implant rupture with aspiration cytology, *Plastic Reconst Surgery* 95:1145, 1995.

44. Bonzanini M et al: Cytologic features of 22 radial scar/complex sclerosing lesions of the breast, three of which are associated with carcinoma: clinical, mammographic, and histologic correlation, *Diagn Cytopathol* 17:353, 1997.

45. Powers CN, Berardo MD, Frable WJ: Fine-needle aspiration biopsy: pitfalls in the diagnosis of spindle-cell lesions, *Diagn Cytopathol* 10:232, 1994.

46. Lopez-Ferrer P et al: Fine needle aspiration cytology of breast fibroadenoma: a cytohistologic correlation of 405 cases, *Acta Cytol* 43:579, 1999.

47. Simpson RH et al: Carcinoma in a breast fibroadenoma, *Acta Cytol* 31:313, 1987.

48. Shet TM, Rege JD: Aspiration cytology of tubular adenomas of the breast: an analysis of eight cases, *Acta Cytol* 42:657, 1998.

49. McCluggage WG et al: Fine needle aspiration cytology (FNAC) of mammary granular cell tumour: a report of three cases, *Cytopathology* 10:383, 1999.

50. Dupont WD, Page DL: Risk factors for breast cancer in women with proliferative breast disease, *N Engl J Med* 312:146, 1985.

51. Masood S et al: Prospective evaluation of radiologically directed fine-needle aspiration biopsy of nonpalpable breast lesions, *Cancer* 66:1480, 1990.

52. Masood S et al: Cytologic differentiation between proliferative and nonproliferative breast disease in mammographically guided fine needle aspirates, *Diagn Cytopathol* 7:581, 1991.

53. Lee WY, Wang HH: Fine needle aspiration is limited in the classification of benign breast diseases, *Diagn Cytopathol* 18:56, 1998.

54. Sidawy MK et al: The spectrum of cytologic features in nonproliferative breast lesions, *Cancer* 93:140, 2001.

55. Sidawy MK et al: Interobserver variability in the classification of proliferative breast lesions by fine-needle aspiration: results of the Papanicolaou Society of Cytopathology study, *Diagn Cytopathol* 18:150, 1998.

56. Silverman JF et al: Can FNA biopsy separate atypical hyperplasia, carcinoma in situ, and invasive carcinoma of the breast? Cytomorphologic criteria and limitations in diagnosis, *Diagn Cytopathol* 9:713, 1993.

57. Masood S, Lu L, Assaf-Munasifi N: Application of immunostaining for muscle specific actin in detection of myoepithelial cells in breast fine needle aspirates, *Diagn Cytopathol* 13:71, 1995.

58. Crissman JD, Visscher DW, Kubus J: Image cytophotometric DNA analysis of atypical hyperplasias and intraductal carcinomas of the breast, *Arch Pathol Lab Med* 114:1249, 1990.

59. Teplitz RL et al: Quantitative DNA patterns in human preneoplastic breast lesions, *Anal Quant Cytol Histol* 12:98, 1990.

60. Norris HJ, Bahr GF, Mikel UV: Quantitative DNA patterns in human preneoplastic breast lesions, *Anal Quant Cytol Histol* 12:98, 1990.

61. King ER, Chen KL, Duarte L: Image cytometric classification of premalignant breast disease in fine-needle aspirates, *Cancer* 62:114, 1988.

62. King EB et al: Characterization by image cytometry of duct epithelial proliferative disease of the breast, *Mod Pathol* 4:291, 1991.

63. Masood S: HER-2/neu oncogene expression in atypical ductal hyperplasia, carcinoma in situ and invasive breast cancer, *Mod Pathol* 4:12A, 1991.

64. Masood S, Hardy NM, Assaf-Munasifi N: Cytologic grading system in diagnosis of high-risk and malignant breast lesions: merits and pitfalls, *Acta Cytol* 38:797, 1994 (abstract).

65. Sneige N, Staerkel GA: Fine-needle aspiration cytology of ductal hyperplasia with and without atypia and ductal carcinoma in situ, *Hum Pathol* 25:485, 1994.

66. Abendroth CS, Wang HH, Ducatman BS: Comparative features of carcinoma in situ and atypical ductal hyperplasia of the breast on fine-needle aspiration biopsy specimens, *Am J Clin Pathol* 96:654, 1991.

67. Stanley MW, Henry-Stanley MJ, Zera R: Atypia in breast fine needle aspiration smears correlates poorly with the presence

of a prognostically significant proliferative lesion of ductal epithelium, *Hum Pathol* 24:630, 1993.

68. Masood S: Cytomorphology of fibrocystic change, high-risk, and premalignant breast lesions, *Breast J* 1:210, 1995.
69. Boone CW, Kelloff G: Biomarkers of premalignant breast disease and their use as surrogate endpoints in clinical trials of chemopreventive agents, *Breast J* 1:228, 1995.
70. Visscher D: Biomarkers of proliferative breast disease, *Breast J* 1:222, 1995.
71. Fabian CJ, Kamel S, Kimler BF: Potential use of biomarkers in breast cancer risk assessment and chemoprevention trials, *Breast J* 1:236, 1995.
72. McKee GT, Tambouret RH, Finkelstein D: Fine needle aspiration cytology of the breast: invasive vs. in situ carcinoma, *Diagn Cytopathol* 25:73, 2001.
73. Tavassoli FA: *Pathology of the breast,* ed 2, New York, 1999, McGraw-Hill.
74. Fleming H, Tang SK: An unusual variant of lobular breast carcinoma: a case report, *Acta Cytol* 38:767, 1994.
75. Katz RL: A turning point in breast cancer cytology reporting: moving from callowness to maturity, *Acta Cytol* 38:881, 1994.
76. Jayaram G et al: Cytologic appearances in invasive lobular carcinoma of the breast: a study of 21 cases, *Acta Cytol* 44:169, 2000.
77. Greeley CF, Frost AR: Cytologic features of ductal and lobular carcinoma in fine needle aspirates of the breast, *Acta Cytol* 41:333, 1997.
78. Dabbs DJ, Grenko RT, Silverman JF: Fine needle aspiration cytology of pleomorphic lobular carcinoma of the breast: duct carcinoma as a diagnostic pitfall, *Acta Cytol* 38:923, 1994.
79. Wilkinson EJ et al: Fine needle aspiration of breast masses; analysis of 276 aspirates, *Acta Cytol* 33:613, 1989.
80. Dawson AE, Mulford DK: Fine needle aspiration of mucinous (colloid) breast carcinoma: nuclear grading and mammographic and cytologic findings, *Acta Cytol* 42:668, 1998.
81. Palombini L et al: Mucoid carcinoma of the breast on fine-needle aspiration biopsy sample: cytology and ultrastructure, *Appl Pathol* 2:70, 1984.
82. Torre M, Lindholm K, Lindgren A: Fine needle aspiration cytology of tubular breast carcinoma and radial scar, *Acta Cytol* 38:884, 1994.
83. Gupta RK, Dowle CS: Fine needle aspiration cytology of tubular carcinoma of the breast, *Acta Cytol* 41:1139, 1997.
84. Hsiu JG et al: A case of pure primary squamous cell carcinoma of the breast diagnosed by fine needle aspiration biopsy, *Acta Cytol* 29:650, 1985.
85. Lazarevic B, Katatikarn V, Marks RA: Primary squamous cell carcinoma of the breast: diagnosis by fine needle aspiration cytology, *Acta Cytol* 28:321, 1984.
86. Shinagawa T et al: Secretory carcinoma of the breast: correlation of aspiration cytology and histology, *Acta Cytol* 38:909, 1994.
87. Pohar-Marinsek Z, Golouh R: Secretory breast carcinoma in a man diagnosed by fine needle aspiration biopsy: a case report, *Acta Cytol* 38:446, 1994.
88. d'Amore ES et al: Secretory carcinoma of the breast: report of a case with fine needle aspiration biopsy, *Acta Cytol* 30:309, 1986.
89. Pettinato G et al: Carcinoma of the breast with osteoclast-like giant cells: fine-needle aspiration cytology, histology and electron microscopy of 5 cases, *Appl Pathol* 2:168, 1984.
90. Ni K, Bibbo M: Fine needle aspiration of mammary carcinoma with features of a carcinoid tumor: a case report with immunohistochemical and ultrastructural studies, *Acta Cytol* 38:73, 1994.
91. Yoshida K et al: Apocrine carcinoma vs. apocrine metaplasia with atypia of the breast: use of aspiration biopsy cytology, *Acta Cytol* 40:247, 1996.
92. Krishnamurthy S et al: Distinction of phyllodes tumor from fibroadenoma: a reappraisal of an old problem, *Cancer* 90:342, 2000.
93. Bernardello F et al: Breast solitary schwannoma: fine-needle aspiration biopsy and immunocytochemical analysis, *Diagn Cytopathol* 10:221, 1994.
94. Foust RL, Berry III AD, Moinuddin SM: Fine needle aspiration cytology of liposarcoma of the breast: a case report, *Acta Cytol* 38:957, 1994.
95. Tamai M, Nomura K, Hiyama H: Aspiration cytology of malignant intraductal myoepithelioma of the breast: a case report, *Acta Cytol* 38:435, 1994.
96. Szekely E et al: Leiomyosarcoma of the female breast, *Pathol Oncol Res* 7:151, 2001.
97. Carson KF et al: Pitfalls in the cytologic diagnosis of angiosarcoma of the breast by fine-needle aspiration: a case report, *Diagn Cytopathol* 11:297, 1994.
98. Torres V, Ferrer R: Cytology of fine needle aspiration biopsy of primary breast rhabdomyosarcoma in an adolescent girl, *Acta Cytol* 29:430, 1985.
99. Amrikachi M et al: Gynecomastia: cytologic features and diagnostic pitfalls in fine needle aspirates, *Acta Cytol* 45:948, 2001.
100. Gupta RK et al: Incidence of apocrine cells in fine needle aspirates: a study of 100 cases, *Diagn Cytopathol* 22:286, 2000.
101. Sneige N et al: Fine needle aspiration cytology of the male breast in a cancer center, *Diagn Cytopathol* 9:691, 1993.
102. Deshpande AH et al: Aspiration cytology of extramammary tumors metastatic to the breast, *Diagn Cytopathol* 21:319, 1999.
103. Briffod M, Hacene K, Doussal VL: Immunohistochemistry on cell blocks from fine needle cytopunctures of primary breast carcinomas and lymph node metastases, *Mod Pathol* 13:841, 2000.
104. Moore JG et al: HER-2/neu gene amplification in breast imprint cytology analyzed by fluorescence in situ hybridization: direct comparison with companion tissue sections, *Diagn Cytopathol* 23:299, 2000.
105. O'Malley F et al: Clinical correlates of false negative fine needle aspirations of the breast in a consecutive series of 1,005 patients, *Surg Gynecol Obstet* 176:360, 1993.
106. Abdulla M et al: Cellularity of lobular carcinoma and its relationship to false negative fine needle aspiration results, *Acta Cytol* 44:625, 2000.
107. Arisio R et al: Role of fine needle aspiration biopsy in breast lesions: analysis of a series of 4,110 cases, *Diagn Cytopathol* 18:462, 1998.
108. Silverman JF et al: Fine needle aspiration cytology of subareolar abscess of the breast: spectrum of cytomorphologic findings and potential diagnostic pitfalls, *Acta Cytol* 30:413, 1986.
109. Greenberg ML, Middleton PD, Bilous AM: Infarcted intraductal papilloma diagnosed by fine-needle biopsy: a cytologic, clinical, and mammographic pitfall, *Diagn Cytopathol* 11:188, 1994.

35

Breast Ductoscopy

WILLIAM C. DOOLEY

Current screening methods for breast cancer involve clinical breast examination and mammography. Using these methods has resulted in a recent decrease in the age-adjusted death rate from breast cancer as the percentage of patients diagnosed with in situ and small early-stage breast cancers has increased.[1] Clinical examination usually finds only scirrhous masses within the breast, which are a result of the body's scar reaction to an invasive cancer. Furthermore, clinical examination detects few masses smaller than 1 cm, which have the highest survival rates for invasive breast cancers. Mammography detects breast cancers by revealing either density/architectural distortions of breast tissue or suspicious microcalcifications. In the dense architectural distortion, tumors are identified primarily by the schirrous immune response to an invasive cancer. Ductal cancers, which are more likely to possess such a schirrous response, are most commonly seen, and lobular cancers, which occasionally lack this scarring response, are poorly seen or missed more often. Microcalcifications form in response to ducts filled with proliferative cells. Often these cells have so distended the ducts that oxygen delivery to the center of the duct is compromised and central necrosis is the process present in the vicinity of the calcifications. To get to this stage the duct is massively distended from its baseline diameter (200 to 600×). Clearly ductal carcinoma in situ (DCIS) can often be identified in patches of suspicious microcalcification, but even then we are detecting a process that has been present for many generations.[2] Our current methods allow breast cancers to be detected late in the clinical evolution of the neoplastic process and all too often when cancers have already begun to metastasize. Estimates from the American Cancer Society suggest that if all women older than age 50 were to adhere to screening recommendations for annual mammography and clinical breast examination, the deaths from breast cancer in the United States would fall by only about 25%.[3] New strategies are needed to make a bigger dent in this death rate.[4]

In Japan, fewer women present with mammographic abnormalities and greater numbers present with breast cancers either causing a clinical mass or bloody nipple discharge. In fact, the incidence of nipple discharge as the presenting symptom of breast cancer is much higher in all Oriental populations. Okazaki and colleagues[5] used a single optical fiber microendoscope to demonstrate the ability to examine the central breast and often isolate the cause for symptomatic nipple discharge. The Japanese experience was limited, however, because of scope size, limitations of air insufflation to distend the ducts, and fragility of the single fiber scopes. Despite these limitations, breast ductoscopy increased in popularity in Japan, Korea, and China over the following decade.[6-10] Few Western investigators were successful at navigating beyond the first 2 to 3 cm, and image quality

was so poor that the technique failed to gain acceptance.[11] However, American manufacturers began to develop multifiber submillimeter endoscopes during the 1990s; the images from these endoscopes optically surpassed those from the single-fiber microscopes used in the earliest mammary ductoscopies.[12,13]

By the late 1990s, chemoprevention studies showed the first real success with the National Surgical Adjuvant Breast and Bowel Project (NSABP) P-01 study.[14] These studies defined high risk through the Gail model—depending greatly on close family history, menstrual history, and breast biopsy history. Still, many patients in whom breast cancer ultimately develops have a low Gail model risk. Even with this limitation in selecting patients who are at risk for breast cancer for enrollment in the chemoprevention trial, tamoxifen was shown to substantially decrease the incidence of new cancers. When subsets were analyzed, the group of women with atypical hyperplasia as their primary risk factor had the greatest reduction in new cancer incidence. Although the caveats of subset analysis apply, this does strongly suggest that the best target for chemoprevention might be the stages of hyperplasia and/or atypical hyperplasia. Unfortunately, none of our standard methods of breast cancer screening are optimized to detect hyperplastic noncancerous lesions. These women have been identified as being high risk based on previous unrelated biopsies in which the hyperplasia presence in the specimen was unexpected.

Finally, chemoprevention studies have been hampered by having to wait for the development of a mammographic or clinical breast cancer to prove usefulness. There have been no standard agreed-on biologic intermediates that predict chemoprevention success.[15-17] If we could screen for hyperplastic changes likely to progress, this same technology could be used to monitor women in prevention studies and could potentially be used as that biologic intermediary. To get us out of our current stalemate with diagnosis 66% of breast cancer as invasive, we need to look to the promise of prevention of breast cancer—the 85% reduction with tamoxifen in new events in those with atypical hyperplasia as their increased risk factor for breast cancer.[14] To achieve this, we need to screen for the lesions most sensitive to prevention and prove that we can reverse them or at least stop them from further progression toward breast cancer.

In an effort to develop and define a new method for detection of atypical hyperplasia in the breast, a multicenter clinical trial of a new procedure—ductal lavage—for collecting ductal epithelial cells was designed.[18] In this study, ductal lavage was compared with nipple aspiration with regard to safety, tolerability, and ability to detect abnormal breast epithelial cells in women at high risk for breast cancer who have nonsuspicious mammogram and clinical breast examination results. Women enrolled were at high risk for breast cancer as defined by Gail model risk or a history of contralateral breast cancer and underwent nipple aspiration followed by lavage of fluid-yielding ducts. All statistical tests were two-sided. We enrolled 507 women, including 291 (57%) with a history of breast cancer and 199 (39%) with a 5-year Gail model risk for breast cancer of 1.7% or greater. Nipple aspirate fluid (NAF) samples were evaluated cytologically for 417 women, and ductal lavage samples were evaluated for 383 women. Only 27% of subjects had NAF samples adequate for diagnosis, whereas 78% of subjects had adequate ductal lavage samples. A median of 13,500 epithelial cells per duct (range, 43 to 492,200 cells) was collected with ductal lavage, compared with a median of 120 epithelial cells per breast (range, 10 to 74,300) collected with nipple aspiration. Of women in whom a ductal lavage specimen was obtained, 24% (92 of 383) had abnormal cells that were mildly (17%) or markedly (7%) atypical. Two subjects had ductal lavage samples with malignant cells. Ductal lavage detected abnormal intraductal breast cells 3.2 times more often than nipple aspiration (79 versus 25 breasts; McNemar's test, $p < .001$). No serious procedure-related adverse events were reported. Using a visual pain scale, subjects reported tolerating NAF well. In conclusion, large numbers of ductal cells can be collected with ductal lavage and can then be used to detect atypical cellular changes within the breast. Ductal lavage is a safe and well-tolerated procedure and is a much more sensitive method of detecting cellular atypia than nipple aspiration.[18,19]

This study raised then an important new clinical problem. Repeated lavage of the same duct can be performed and show persistent severe/malignant atypia in 7% of cases of women with normal mammogram and physical examination results. Even when adding ultrasound, Miraluma, and magnetic resonance imaging, other abnormalities were rarely found. Remembering an earlier Japanese experience with ductoscopy[5-10] and combining those techniques with newer American submillimeter scopes and the techniques of ductal distention developed during the lavage trial, researchers undertook a systematic investigation of the potential of ductoscopy to find these lesions.[12] In each of the initial 12 patients with severe atypia, an intraluminal lesion was found; when biopsy was performed, the lesion had the same cytologic cell appearance as the lavaged atypical cells. The cancers found were all in situ, and the noncancerous lesions usually showed severe atypical hyperplasia.

In the course of the lavage research, it was recognized that fluid could often be produced from ducts in the same quadrant of the breast as a newly diagnosed breast cancer. Cytologic analysis could occasionally confirm the presence of tumor cells. Current surgical methods are limited in intraoperative imaging (ultrasound and palpation) during breast conservation procedures. Unsuspected extensive intraductal component (EIC) and more extensive disease are often found in the final pathology of the intended wide excision. It was hypothesized that such fluid-producing ducts would likely connect to the site of the known cancerous/precancerous lesion and that endoscopic evaluation of such ducts might reveal unsuspected additional disease. To test this, women from a single surgeon's practice undergoing lumpectomy for breast conservation from January 2000 to August 2001 were evaluated for fluid production from the nipple at the time of lumpectomy. If a fluid-producing duct was identified in the same quadrant as the lesion, it was cannulated and dilated using local anesthetic; endoscopy was then performed using a 0.9-mm Acueity microendoscope. Of the 201 patients (16 atypical ductal hyperplasia, 52 DCIS, and 133 stage I or II breast cancers) from which fluid could be obtained, 150 (74.6%) could be successfully dilated and their breast ducts navigated beyond multiple divisions. Additional lesions outside the anticipated lumpectomy were identified in 41% (83) of cases. If endoscopy was successful, the chances for a positive margin in DCIS or invasive cancer fell from 23.5% to only 5.0%. Margins were positive in the nipple direction in only 1 of the 150 cases of successful endoscopy. Endoscopy proved to be a useful adjunct in this series of patients because it identified all cases of EIC in early-stage breast cancer and identified additional noncontiguous DCIS in more than half of the patients with stage 0 lumpectomy who underwent endoscopy (Figures 35 1 to 35 4). Routine operative breast endoscopy has a great potential to reduce the need for reexcision lumpectomy for initial positive margins. It also finds substantially more cancerous and precancerous disease than anticipated by routine preoperative mammography and ultrasound.[20]

The intraductal approaches to screening with lavage and endoscopy allow collection of both fluid and cells from proliferative epithelial surfaces in the breast. Prior studies suggest that early, relatively large karyotypic events occur in the evolution of a breast cancer.[21] These are often associated with hypermethylation of numerous genes. Cells collected from lavage and endoscopy specimens of the breast ducts were tested with methylation-specific polymerase chain reaction (PCR) (MSP). Methylated alleles of cyclin D2, *RAR-β*, and *Twist* genes were often detected in fluid from mammary ducts containing endoscopically visualized carcinomas (17 of 20 cases) and DCIS (2 of 7 cases) but rarely in ductal lavage fluid from healthy ducts (5 of 45 cases). Two of the women with healthy mammograms whose ductal lavage fluid contained methylated markers and cytologically abnormal cells were subsequently diagnosed as having breast cancer. Furthermore, this study demonstrated that carrying out methylation-specific PCR in these fluid samples from lavage or endoscopy may provide a sensitive and powerful addition to mammographic or cytologic screening for early detection of breast cancer.[22]

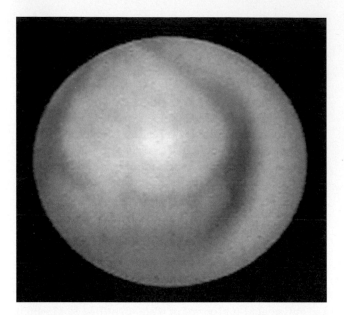

FIG. **35-1** Papilloma.

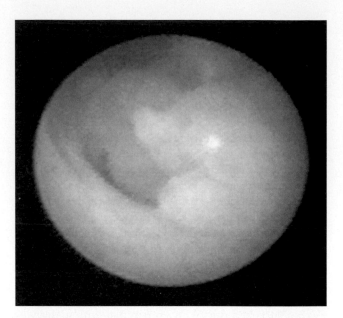

FIG. **35-2** Papillomas.

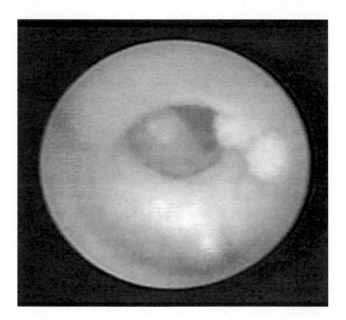

FIG. **35-3** Low-grade ductal carcinoma in situ.

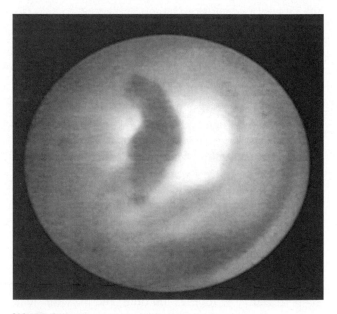

FIG. **35-4** High-grade ductal carcinoma in situ.

The two new resources of ductal lavage and endoscopy now need to be refined and developed into the tools that will allow clinicians to screen for, diagnose, and monitor premalignant disease in the breast. Both lavage and endoscopy are time consuming and dependent on a relatively high skill level of the operator, much like gastrointestinal endoscopy. Both may currently be appropriate for patients at highest risk for breast cancer, but they are not the answer for mass screening. Through examination of the cells and protein obtained from ducts with premalignant and malignant disease, molecular markers of increased risk for atypia may be identified, which are more feasible to test on the few microliters of NAF. By identifying women with suspicious or increased risk by nipple aspirate, the workup can continue with lavage to identify the ductal system producing these changes and then with endoscopy to find the lesions and perform a biopsy.

The burning clinical questions of both lavage and endoscopy is how to best incorporate them into clinical practice. Ductoscopy has a direct and obvious application to investigations of symptomatic nipple discharge. It provides immediate visual intraductal information and direct localization, through transillumination, of the suspect lesion. Beyond this situation, the future of these technologies is less clear. Research that examines the strengths and weaknesses of each technique by collecting data from multiple surgeons performing these techniques at multiple centers is required. The initial lavage study enrolled only patients with breasts considered high risk and that were normal as determined with mammography and clinical examination. It detected significant amounts of atypia cytologically and a few breast cancers. However, this study does not have any comparative data with our traditional screening methods to determine direct comparison to standard screening of physical examination and mammography. Ductoscopy has potential to allow surgeons to visually direct lumpectomy procedures or even nonsurgical ablation by determining margin. It is limited because most of our currently identified breast cancers already obstruct the ducts and limit the ability to navigate the scope toward the nipple side only. The increased incidence of intraluminal disease seen endoscopically that was expected with traditional pathologic analysis may account for the regional recurrences following breast conservation. These same endoscopically abnormal lesions may be subclinical and may never progress rapidly enough to limit the patient's life. The hope of the intraductal approach to increase both our understandings of breast cancer initiation and progression and design better treatments is great but will be reached only through careful multiinstitutional research.

REFERENCES

1. Ries LAG et al (eds): SEER cancer statistics review, Bethesda, MD, 1973-1999, National Cancer Institute. Available at http://seer.cancer.gov/csr/1973_1999/. Accessed November 2002.
2. Tabar L et al: The natural history of breast carcinoma: what have we learned from screening? Cancer 86:449, 1999.
3. Thomas AG, Jemal A, Thun MJ: Breast cancer facts and figures, Atlanta, 2001, American Cancer Society.
4. Charting the course: priorities for breast cancer research—the report of the Breast Cancer Progress Review Group National Cancer Institute. Available at http://prg.nci.nih.gov/breast/default.html. Accessed November 2002.
5. Okazaki A et al: Fiberoptic ductoscopy of the breast: a new diagnostic procedure for nipple discharge, Jpn J Clin Oncol 21:188, 1991.
6. Yamamoto D et al: New diagnostic approach to intracystic lesions of the breast by fiberoptic ductoscopy, Anticancer Res 21:4113, 2001.
7. Yamamoto D et al: A utility of ductography and fiberoptic ductoscopy for patients with nipple discharge, Breast Cancer Res Treat 70:103, 2001.
8. Shen KW et al: Fiberoptic ductoscopy for breast cancer patients with nipple discharge, Surg Endosc 15:1340, 2001.
9. Matsunaga T et al: Mammary ductoscopy for diagnosis and treatment of intraductal lesions of the breast, Breast Cancer 8:213, 2001.
10. Okazaki A et al: Nipple discharge disorders: current diagnostic management and the role of fiber-ductoscopy, Eur Radiol 9:583, 1999.
11. Love SM, Barsky SH: Breast-duct endoscopy to study stages of cancerous breast disease, Lancet 348:997, 1996.
12. Dooley WC: Endoscopic visualization of breast tumors, JAMA 284:1518, 2000.
13. Dietz JR et al: Feasibility and technical considerations of mammary ductoscopy in human mastectomy specimens, Breast J 6:161, 2000.
14. Fisher B et al: Tamoxifen for prevention of breast cancer: report of the National Surgical Adjuvant Breast and Bowel Project P-1 Study, J Natl Cancer Inst 90:1371, 1998.
15. Wrensch MR et al: Breast cancer incidence in women with abnormal cytology nipple aspirates of breast fluid, Am J Epidemiol 135:130, 1992.
16. Fabian C et al: Short-term breast cancer prediction by random periareolar fine-needle aspiration cytology and the Gail risk model, J Natl Cancer Inst 92:1217, 2000.
17. Dupont WD, Page DL: Risk factors for breast cancer in women with proliferative breast disease, N Engl J Med 312:146, 1985.
18. Dooley WC et al: Ductal lavage for detection of cellular atypia in women at high risk for breast cancer, J Natl Cancer Inst 93:1624, 2001.
19. O'Shaughnessy JA et al: Ductal lavage and the clinical management of women at high risk for breast carcinoma: a commentary, Cancer 94:292, 2002.
20. Dooley WC: Routine operative breast endoscopy during lumpectomy, Ann Surg Oncol 10:38, 2003.
21. Gusev Y, Kagansky V, Dooley WC: Long-term dynamics of chromosomal instability in cancer: a transitional probability model, J Math Comput Model 33:1253, 2001.
22. Evron E et al: Detection of breast cancer cells in ductal lavage fluid by methylation-specific PCR, Lancet 357:1335, 2001.

XII

CLINICAL TRIALS: BIOSTATISTICAL APPLICATIONS

36

Design and Conduct
of Clinical Trials
for Breast Cancer

ALFRED A. BARTOLUCCI

KARAN P. SINGH

Chapter Outline

This chapter is intended to outline the important principles for the design and conduct of therapeutic clinical trials in breast cancer. Such trials have become extremely sophisticated and complicated. We do not cover every single aspect of these types of trials but highlight the major points.

This chapter concentrates on prospective clinical trials and does not focus on retrospective trials (the after-the-fact abstracting of data and data interpretation by investigators), except to say that retrospective trials are often tainted by biases inherent in the data and biases inherent in the investigators. Well-planned prospective trials ensure objectivity.

Spilker[1] indicates that biases, in general, occur as a consequence of the study design used, the tests used, the people involved in the study, the patients, and the analyses or perspectives used in interpreting the data. Sackett[2] attributes most biases to the investigator who designs, conducts, and analyzes the study. In this chapter we outline, in as much detail as possible, the various salient points of well-conducted breast cancer trials that avoid the problems of biases or other underlying shortcomings for which the trial can be criticized.

Three types of clinical trials are usually applied: phase I, phase II, and phase III clinical trials. Each of these types of trials is geared to a specific patient population, and the objectives may vary according to the type of sample under study. If these trials are conducted according to good scientific practice, they are said to be generalizable to the particular population for which they were designed. Phase IV studies, discussed later, are also sometimes used.

Phase I Studies

Phase I studies usually involve the determination of a generally safe or well-tolerated dose of a new drug by the patient. This is often referred to as a *maximally tolerated dose* in patients. The objective is to seek dose-limiting toxicity. The end points usually involved are commonly noted adverse reactions, characteristics of the drug, and perhaps characteristics of the drug at different dose levels. This involves identifying laboratory parameters affected by the drug. Spilker[1] refers to this as seeking an initial pharmacokinetic profile. A second objective, which is often serendipitous, is usually a determination of efficacy of the drug in some situations. Again, this depends on the therapy under study and the parameters of efficacy that are being considered in the particular population under study.

Phase II Studies

Phase II studies in breast cancer usually involve identifying tumor types for which the treatment appears promising. The major end point is generally the magnitude of efficacy (the level of response), which is discussed later. Other end points may include the duration of the effects produced (often referred to as *duration of response or survival*), the doses of the drug that are effective, and additional information on suitable dose regimens or schedules of the drug. Toxicities are also measured.

Phase III Studies

The purpose of phase III studies is to determine the effect of a new treatment relative to a standard therapy. These are often referred to as *comparative trials.* Another benefit of a phase III study is to determine the effect of a treatment relative to the natural history of the disease or to determine whether a new treatment is relatively as effective as a standard therapy but is associated with less morbidity or toxicity. Many special studies are commonly associated with phase III trials; these may include studies of demographic or environmental characteristics, particular patient clinical values (laboratory values), or other characteristics that may be influential in terms of prognostic significance of a particular therapy or group of therapies.

End points of phase III studies may include the evaluation of chemotherapeutic, radiotherapeutic, or surgical procedures. Other considerations may involve the activity of immunostimulants, biotherapeutic agents, antiemetics, and pain control agents and measurement of the quality of life during the conduct of the trial. It must also be remembered that the trials conducted are usually specific to a particular patient population. For example, phase I and II studies are sometimes conducted in refractory or relapsed types of patient populations. Phase III studies usually involve early-stage disease or metastatic disease, depending on the end points of interest.

Phase IV Studies

The phase IV study is less scientific than the phase III study and usually involves the safety, tolerance, and efficacy of the drug in the general population of patients for whom the drug or therapy is intended. Once the therapy has become "standard" practice, early indications of unexpected or expected beneficial activities can be studied further in the general population. Phase IV studies usually involve postmarketing surveillance, epidemiology, and the marketing of therapeutic agents. Thus in these studies, the science is now extended to the general population for treatment of a specific disease, which in our case is breast cancer.

Protocol Design from the Statistical Perspective

CONTENT OF EXPERIMENTAL DESIGN

All well-planned strategies involve a protocol. In a breast cancer clinical trial, this is a written document detailing the scientific questions to be reviewed, giving a justification for the type and number of patients to be studied and a scientific basis for the study. The elements of a protocol typically include objectives, background and rationale, therapeutic agents, patient selection criteria, studies to be done, stratification and randomization procedures, treatment regimens, toxicity and dosage estimates, evaluation of response, reporting procedures, and statistical considerations.

Objectives. Objectives are well-stated hypotheses addressing the types of questions the protocol is designed to address. Usually just before the objectives or following the objectives or sometimes in the appendices of a protocol, a schema, which is a schematic diagram showing an overview of the study design, may be included. It is important to list these study objectives specifically in the protocol. This enables all concerned to clearly understand the research plan. As discussed later, the objectives also help determine the size of the study (the numbers of patients and controls), depending on the type of study that is being conducted. Unfortunately, for a number of trials that are published, the stated sample size is never fully met, often because of extenuating circumstances. However, studies are often ended too early with inadequate numbers, and as a result, the conclusions can be questionable. The objectives of the study usually include the elements outlined in the phase I, II, and III trial descriptions. Thus in a phase I trial, the question is one of dose-limiting toxicity (the maximal dose to obtain a toxic effect). The objective then is to move on to a phase II study and to conduct a response or efficacy trial, in which the maximal tolerable dose is often indicated and the objective changes from determination of toxicity to evaluation of treatment efficacy. Once the phase II objective is met and it is found that the treatment in question does have satisfactory efficacy, the study will move on to a phase III trial, which involves a comparative study. Two or more treatments or therapeutic modalities are then tested against one another to determine which is the most efficacious in the patient population under study.

Background and Rationale. The background and rationale of a proposed protocol include previous studies that have attested to the therapeutic efficacy of a particular treatment or combination of treatments; as a result, these treatments or combinations have been given a "green light" to be studied further in a particular patient sample of interest. The background and rationale section of a protocol is often filled with many references, much past data, and good scientific indications for the proposed study. The background and rationale of a phase III study could include data from phase I and phase II studies as a prelude to the present design.

Therapeutic Agents. Therapeutic agents are usually the agents or modalities (e.g., surgery, radiation, immunotherapy, chemotherapy) that will be used in the protocol. In chemotherapy the section on therapeutic agents usually includes a description of the chemical aspects of the drugs under consideration, the routes of administration, and known side effects. The surgery section may include a detailed description of the type of surgery required. In the case of breast cancer this may include a description of a segmental, total, modified, or radical mastectomy, for example. The radiation therapy section usually includes the procedure for the type of radiation to be delivered and the sites, dosage, timing, and the toxicity that is expected to be encountered.

CRITERIA FOR PATIENT SELECTION

The patient eligibility criteria section is an extremely important section of the protocol because it usually describes the types of patients who may benefit from the types of therapies under study. As a result, the protocol treatments, if successful, can then be extended to the general patient population with the characteristics of the patients in the particular sample under study in the protocol.

The patients identified for a particular protocol should be those who would most likely benefit from the new therapy or therapies under study. The eligibility limitations can be altered as a result of phase I and phase II trials, in which the objectives may extend beyond a particular patient sample. For example, eligibility criteria may include the tumor type that is under study—in our case, breast cancers. Therefore the protocols would be targeted toward women with breast cancer. The eligibility criteria may further be refined to include a certain stage of breast cancer. The criteria may also restrict the type of past therapy that patients under study would be allowed to have had before coming into a particular protocol. There may be specifications as to the time limit in which a patient can be entered on protocol following certain procedures. For example, in adjuvant breast studies there may be limitations on the number of days a patient may enter a protocol for chemotherapy following surgery or radiation therapy. The eligibility criteria may extend to a patient's physiologic function. This would include, for example, adequate absolute granulocyte count, adequate bilirubin and blood urea nitrogen (BUN), and absence of infection or septicemia.

The criteria for patient selection of the protocol or document may also list a number of reasons why patients would be ineligible for a study. For example, if a woman is coming into a breast cancer protocol, she may be ineligible if she has had a previous history of cancer other than breast cancer. Especially in the adjuvant setting, the objective of a protocol may be to determine the effect on prolongation of life with chemotherapy following surgery, and a woman may be ineligible if she has had any previous chemotherapy. The same may apply to those who have received previous radiation, especially if there is a radiotherapy (RT) question in the protocol. In the case of metastatic disease, sometimes the protocol is restricted to the sites of disease and to types of previous therapies that the patient has received. Sometimes preexisting conditions also disqualify a patient from a study.

It was previously stated that the eligibility criteria are set so that the results of the study under question may be generalized to a broader population of individuals. There are often problems with eligibility criteria. If the criteria are too narrow, the study may yield results that are not generalizable beyond the patients of the restricted types that have been included. A balance must be struck between attaining a homogeneous group to answer the protocol question and having a general group so that the results of the study can be applied to a broad population base. This has political, ethical, and scientific implications. Simon[3] gives a good discussion of this type of controversy.

STUDIES TO BE DONE

The section on the studies to be done usually includes the clinical workup and follow-up of patients during the course of the protocol. This may involve, for example, physical examinations, laboratory readings, or computed tomography (CT) scans. Typically, the timing and requirements of these are described. The statistical issues involved here are to ensure that all patients are supported and evaluated the same way on protocol, thus protecting the reliability of study results.

STRATIFICATION AND RANDOMIZATION PROCEDURES

For phase I and phase II studies, stratification and randomization procedures are not usually important. The only criterion for stratification in a phase II study is usually the inclusion of several types of populations of patients to determine whether a treatment is efficacious within these particular populations. For example, stratification might be done according to stage of disease to test a treatment within those subgroups for efficacy.

Randomization and stratification are most important in phase III randomized trials. Randomization is the "random" allocation of patients to the various treatments under study. The technique used in randomization may be simple or complex, depending on the protocol. The purpose is to ensure that all patients in a study have an equally likely chance to be allocated to the treatments under consideration. Patients are usually stratified according to specific criteria based on patient characteristics believed to be related to response to therapy. For example, in an adjuvant breast cancer study, patients may be stratified by the number of positive axillary lymph nodes. Some patients may present at surgery with limited metastatic disease in the axilla (one to three positive nodes). Others may present with more extensive axillary disease (four or more positive nodes). To ensure that patients allocated to the treatments under consideration are not allocated disproportionately, randomization within the nodal status is often done.

Suppose treatments A and B were to be tested to determine which was more efficacious in prolonging disease-free survival (DFS) or overall survival. Patients with one to three positive nodes would be randomized to A or B, and those presenting with four or more positive nodes would also be randomized to either A or B. The strategy is to ensure that approximately 50% of the patients with one to three positive nodes are allocated to A and 50% are allocated to B and likewise for patients with four or more positive nodes. This approach guards against the possibility of one of the treatments being applied to most patients within either nodal status and thus possibly biasing the results of the study in favor of A or B.

Randomization and stratification are usually described in a bit of detail in the written protocol. Researchers may stratify by a number of factors, but it must be remembered that the subgroups created are the number of randomization arms multiplied by the number of possible combinations of stratification grouping. It is easily possible for this to become very complex. Randomization, stratifications, and justifications for stratifications are usually written into a treatment protocol.

TREATMENT REGIMENS

The treatment regimen section of the protocol includes the timing and dosage of therapy to be given in a particular study. This includes the timing and dosage of chemotherapy and timing and dosage of radiation therapy. If surgery is involved, the surgical procedures are often outlined or at least referenced for the respective surgeons who will participate in the study.

TOXICITY AND DOSAGE ESTIMATES

The toxicity and dosage estimates part of the protocol involves the expected toxicities and the types of treatments, adjustments, delays, and modifications required to accommodate these toxicities. This section of the protocol may also involve statements regarding the notification of appropriate personnel should unexpected or life-threatening toxicities be encountered. This administrative procedure is necessary so that others who are writing similar protocols or wish to pursue similar studies will be aware of the types of problems that they may encounter during the course of their particular study. Toxicities are usually graded as to severity according to specific criteria included either in this section of the protocol or in the appendices.

EVALUATION OF RESPONSE

The type of response that an investigator wishes to evaluate depends on the type of trial being conducted and the type of question under study. For example, as discussed previously, a phase I trial measures responses to determine the correct dosage to limit toxicity. A phase II trial usually measures tumor shrinkage, and appropriate types of procedures for measuring tumor response are often indicated in the protocol. In some circumstances, phase II studies have measured disease-free intervals (DFIs) or prolonged survival. This is not really the purpose of a phase II study, but some trials have added these as secondary end points to determination of tumor response to treatment.

A phase III trial may study tumor shrinkage or DFI. Metastatic disease protocols often measure tumor response to treatment. Basically, a tumor or group of tumors within an individual is sited for observation, and during the course of the therapy, whether the tumor has responded to therapy and the degree of response (the amount of shrinkage in the tumor) is determined.

Phase III adjuvant studies, which, for example, determine the effect of chemotherapy on prolongation of DFS after surgical removal of a tumor, often have the end point of DFI or overall survival. The analysis section considers both metastatic and adjuvant phase III studies. The DFI in the adjuvant protocol is usually defined as beginning when the patient has either received surgery or has started on protocol and ending when the disease or tumor recurs, either during the progress of the adjuvant therapy or after therapy is completed. Evaluation of the response often coincides with the "Studies to Be Done" section. For example, a chest x-ray film, bone scan, or liver scan may be used to determine whether disease has recurred. In addition, these are used throughout the protocol to evaluate the progress of the patient. It is most important that the dates of evaluations and their results be recorded during the course of a study so that an accurate assessment can be made of the relative efficacy of various treatments and their effect on the end points or the responses to be evaluated.

REPORTING PROCEDURES

The reporting procedures involve the timely notification of a central office or reviewing organization about the progress of the patients on study. Summary results of a patient's progress are usually required within certain specified periods as the study progresses. Indications or provisions in the reporting procedures are usually made if a recurrence occurs before a scheduled reporting time. It is just as important for reporting procedures to be followed as it is for response criteria and timing to be followed so that fair comparisons can be made among therapeutic strategies in the evaluation of certain tumor types. It has become an extremely important and sensitive quality control issue to accurately maintain the files of patients both at the site of treatment and at some central location so that the integrity of all data received, reported, and analyzed can be ensured.

In both metastatic breast cancer studies and adjuvant breast cancer studies, all patients are usually followed at regular intervals until death, and all reporting procedures with all relevant details are expected to be carried out until that time or until the question in the protocol has been satisfactorily answered. In adjuvant trials, a median DFI (the time at which approximately half the patients are still disease free) may be as long as 5 or 10 years, and the follow-up status and reporting procedures can go on for a very long time. The reporting of a study not only in publication form but also in case record form can involve much time and expense. The questions studied and the patient population considered must be of sufficient scientific and practical interest to justify undertaking such a commitment.

Statistical Considerations. Previous sections have dealt with specific statistical objectives and their impact on the other sections of the protocol. The statistical considerations section of the protocol basically outlines the experimental design in terms of the stratification and randomization of the patients. This section restates the objectives and the hypotheses of the protocol associated with the objectives.

Based on the objectives, the sample size requirements (number of patients needed for the study) are then derived and reviewed. Other topics in the statistical considerations include the expected time frames and the proposed analyses of the particular study.

The statistical considerations follow from the protocol document and should be consistent with the entire document. For example, if the objective is a phase III question, the sample size as stated in the statistical section should not be that for a phase II study. The sample size usually follows closely from the objectives of the study. In a phase III trial the objective may be to study the DFI and survival of patients who have undergone radical mastectomy for carcinoma of the breast with positive axillary nodes; patients are randomized to one of three adjuvant therapies. The statistical consideration then assumes the null hypothesis that the three therapies (A, B, and C) are equally effective with respect to the length of DFI and overall survival. The null hypothesis is often stated as follows:

H: The three therapies are equally efficacious.

The alternative is often stated as follows:

H: At least one therapy is different.

The alternative hypothesis can also be stated as A being better than B or C, B being better than C or A, or C being better than A or B. A particular alternative or combination of alternatives may be appropriate for the therapeutic agents under the study.

The statistical literature contains several methods for determining the appropriate numbers of patients for each treatment group to have a valid clinical trial.[3-11] Sample size considerations often take into account the duration or the expected duration of a study[7] and also depend on the type of analysis that will be conducted in a particular study. For example, in a metastatic disease protocol with a response objective, the response can be defined in several ways. In measuring tumor response or tumor shrinkage, a complete response (CR) is considered complete disappearance of the tumor. A partial response (PR) is considered a shrinkage totaling at least 50% of the tumor diameter. Tumor shrinkage can be controversial because it depends on the actual types of measurement and measurement instrumentations that are used in the study. A stable response (S) is usually considered to be either no change in the tumor or a tumor shrinkage of less than 50%. Tumor progression indicates that the tumor has not responded to therapy or has increased in size or new tumors have been found. Sample size considerations become important when comparing the ability of two regimens to shrink a tumor in size. The null hypothesis for comparing two treatments with respect to their degree of efficacy is often stated as follows:

$$H : P_A = P_B$$

This is often used in a null hypothesis to state that the two treatments are equal with respect to the proportion of individuals in which a response will be achieved. The variable denotes the proportion of response and is often considered the combination of both the CRs and PRs. There are many techniques for comparing these proportions and for reaching conclusions about the superiority of one treatment to another in its ability to shrink the tumor. A comprehensive outline of these techniques can be found in Bartolucci.[12]

The sample size in a clinical trial, depending on the end point or objective, is determined by the magnitude of the expected differences between A and B at the initiation of the clinical trial. Usually, the greater the magnitude is, the fewer patients required in each of the two treatment arms. The sample size required in each treatment arm also depends on statistical issues such as the size and power of the statistical procedure used to test the null hypothesis. The size of the test or alpha level is usually set at .05. This is the probability of rejecting the null hypothesis when, in fact, it is true. This is also commonly called the *type I error*. The *p* value often quoted in the literature is compared with this alpha level, which statisticians use to determine the sample size of the test.

The other statistical consideration in determining sample size, the power of the test, is the probability of rejecting the null hypothesis when, in fact, it is false. This is analogous to the probability of declaring the two treatments to be different at a given magnitude when in reality they are different. The complement of the power is called the *type II error*. This is the probability of not rejecting the null hypothesis when, in fact, it is false. When the sample size is computed, both type I and type II errors should be minimized; through minimization of the type II error, the power of the test is maximized. The power is usually set to be at least 80% to 95% in most trials. The literature often indicates a *p* value or significance level associated with the results of a clinical trial, but the power of the test is also important. It is possible with inadequate sample size to get a significant *p* value yet achieve inadequate power.

End points such as survival and DFS can also be considered in the conduct of statistical tests. The statistical procedures are different than those just considered with respect to their methodology of computation, but the underlying theory of limiting type I and type II errors holds throughout. Also it should be noted that a conventional type I error of .05 is not always appropriate. A statistician should be consulted to determine whether the alpha level should be increased or decreased for the questions being asked.

The statistical considerations section should also contain a paragraph or two stating the types and timing of analyses according to the stated objectives of the protocol. Later sections in this chapter discuss various types of analyses that are appropriate for either metastatic or adjuvant breast cancer protocols.

Other Protocol Sections. Other sections of a treatment protocol usually include a bibliography or references for the background of the protocol design, a list of investigators who are authoring the study, and an example of a consent form. The consent form usually seeks the patient's permission to participate in the study, summarizes the study's purpose, and outlines the risks and benefits of the therapeutic alternatives.

Tools for Conducting Breast Cancer Trials

The essence of a good clinical trial is a strong and knowledgeable team of individuals experienced in the procedures that have been discussed. These individuals also contribute to the development and implementation of the tools necessary to conduct a well-designed breast cancer clinical trial. This section discusses the specific tools necessary for designing and implementing a clinical trial and the organization needed to put such a trial in place. One such tool is the data collection form on which information relevant to the clinical trial is transcribed. These data collection instruments must be designed once the study objectives have been defined. Again, we see the pivotal value of the study objectives. The types of forms follow the same sequence or order as that used for the collection of information as the patient progresses through the trial. The data collection and reporting schedules are summarized in the sections of the protocol entitled "Studies to Be Done" and "Reporting Procedures." Everything done in a clinical trial, from data collection to analysis, depends on the written protocol.

DATA COLLECTION FORMS

On-Study Form. Once a patient is randomized and registered in the trial, the on-study form is completed. It contains patient information such as basic demographics, past treatment history, initial laboratory workup, tumor measurements, sites of disease, and clinical stage of disease. Sometimes, depending on the study, information particular to the eligibility or stratification criteria may be requested on this form. For example, for adjuvant breast studies, information about axillary staging is requested on the form and the date of primary surgery and type of surgery (radical mastectomy, modified radical mastectomy, or segmental mastectomy).

Flow Sheet. The information to be entered on the flow sheet depends on the study and usually includes dates and dosages of therapies given, basic patient clinical data, laboratory data, the tests or procedures to be done, and the results of those procedures. These tests and procedures are usually recorded on a periodic basis (i.e., weekly, biweekly, or monthly), depending on the instructions given in the protocol and the timing of the treatment and suggested delays according to the toxicity

criteria in the protocol. This is usually very detailed information during the course of the patient's treatment on study.

Response or Summary Form. The response form contains information summarizing the patient's progress on study with respect to the end points discussed in the protocol. Such information includes the DFS (usually disease free or not disease free), survival information (either dead or last known date alive), and response criteria if a tumor measurement is required (i.e., CR, PR, S, or progression). For breast cancer clinical trials, specific information such as the sites of relapse may also be included on this form. As time progresses, the protocol may require that this form be updated occasionally should a patient's status change, usually to coincide with the completion of specific cycles of therapy. The reporting procedures of the protocol dictate when and how often this particular form is to be completed and submitted for central review.

Follow-Up Form. The follow-up form is normally completed and submitted every 6 months or yearly, depending on the protocol, and contains information concerning the patient's end point status (i.e., recurrence date, death date, or last known date alive), and possible subsequent therapy. In some respects this form may overlap with the response form, and in some circumstances it may not be very detailed. Again, an example is given in the appendix.

Other Forms. This has been a brief overview of the major types of forms that may be required by the protocol document. There are, however, other specialized forms. For example, in an adjuvant breast study, a surgical report detailing the type of surgery and other relevant information may be required. A radiation summary form may also be required if radiation was part of the treatment plan. A pathology form may be necessary for documentation of the diagnosis. A pathology form and radiation summary may also be required for a metastatic breast disease protocol in certain circumstances.

Computerized Database. Patients are usually entered on study via a remote site (e.g., hospital, private practice, university medical center). Eligibility or patient selection criteria are checked at these remote sites but are also checked at a central administrative and statistical organization experienced in study design, data collection, quality control, and data computerization. All the data relevant to a particular protocol are reported to this central organization for appropriate synthesis, checking, analysis, and reporting. All forms are entered centrally on a computer database for report generation; the ultimate goal is publication of the trial.

The central collection of forms can become cumbersome and time consuming. Several investigators have been working on systems commonly called *distributed database systems*. This involves not only collection at a remote site but also data entry directly into a personal computer or computer terminal with communication (e.g., diskette, phone line) to the host computer (personal computer, minicomputer, or main frame) at the central location. With current software and technology, much of this is feasible and can be implemented. This type of a system allows for instant data checking, processing, and feedback queries regarding missing, inconsistent, or out-of-range data. Thus data are always available and can be checked much more rapidly than if handled through the postal service. Techniques have been developed to assist investigators with this type of data transmission and checking procedures. Bartolucci[13] described the application of these techniques to oncologic clinical trials. The technology is not only available but is also constantly being updated.

Computerization of any database is a costly and time-consuming undertaking. Therefore these trials must always be approached with much caution and great organization. The protocol's importance to a well-organized clinical trial cannot be overemphasized. It affects every aspect of the trial (e.g., the general conduct and organization of the trial from start to finish, the results and reporting of the trial, and finally, the publication of the trial for public scrutiny and evaluation).

Quality Control Procedures. We have already established that patients entered on breast cancer clinical trials (and other types of trials) can be from multiple sites (e.g., hospitals, private practices, university medical centers) and that the trial is centrally administered. Multiple-site participation is usually necessary because a clinical trial requires many more patients than can normally be obtained at a single site in a reasonable amount of time. A phase III trial should not take longer than 3 to 5 years for patient entry (with less time for phase I or II trials—usually 2 years or less).

The central organization that is responsible for the conduct of the trial (design, data collection, database management, and analysis) is usually staffed by individuals who are an educational resource for quality control. Quality control is defined here as monitoring of the study to guarantee a number of assurances (e.g., that only eligible patients are entered, that forms are completed properly by the contributing investigator or by data personnel, that data are submitted in a timely manner, that all data are accurate and complete). To achieve this high quality of data accuracy, the central staff publishes general data collection guidelines that may be amended to accommodate protocols asking for specialized data or end points. This is usually called a

procedures document or *manual* and is made available to all study participants. Contents of the document usually include methods for manual data entry and checks. Usually, additional computerized checks of the data are made centrally and are often referred to as *edit, consistency,* or *range* checks. Quality control in breast cancer trials also includes confirmation of correct treatment being delivered. Often, the patient's case record and forms are further checked by a surgeon, chemotherapist, radiologist, and pathologist not treating the patient to ensure that the patient was followed with respect to the procedures of treatment delivery detailed for each modality in the protocol. Again, failure to comply with protocol guidelines with respect to these quality control procedures has serious implications for the interpretation of the outcome of any study.

Analyses of Clinical Breast Studies

Analyses examples are confined to oncologic trials, although the techniques apply broadly. Two well-designed clinical trials, one a study of metastatic breast cancer and the other a study of adjuvant breast disease, are examined.

METASTATIC BREAST CANCER STUDY

The Southeastern Cancer Study Group Protocol of metastatic breast cancer (a phase III trial) involved a randomized comparison between two chemotherapeutic combinations in women with metastatic breast cancer. The objective of the study was to determine the complete and partial response rates of metastatic breast carcinoma to the regimens listed in Table 36-1. The treatment plan is also given in Table 36-1. Treatment duration was approximately 25 weeks.

This was a multiinstitutional study with 16 institutions participating. Patients were assigned to either regimen A or B (see Table 36-1) after eligibility was confirmed and the patient had signed an informed consent. Eligibility criteria included the following:

1. All patients with metastatic breast adenocarcinoma with at least one measurable tumor mass (excluding radiographic bone lesions, previously irradiated lesions, liver scan abnormalities, and pleural effusion) who had not received any of the six drugs (or other alkylating agents) in the trial were eligible provided symptoms were present or there had been a recent enlargement of a metastatic lesion. Patients with elevated bilirubin levels before the study were not eligible.

   Patients with radiographic bone lesions as their only manifestation were eligible for entry on regimen A. They were not randomized.

TABLE **36-1**	Combination Chemotherapy Regimen

REGIMEN	DOSAGE	
A (CAF)		
Cyclophosphamide	500 mg/m² IV (day 1)	
Adriamycin	50 mg/m² IV (day 1)	q3wk
Fluorouracil	500 mg/m² IV (day 1)	
B (CMFVP)		
Cyclophosphamide	400 mg/m² IV (day 1)	
Methotrexate	30 mg/m² IV (days 1, 8)	
Fluorouracil	400 mg/m² IV (days 1, 8)	q28days
Vincristine	1 mg IV (days 1, 8)	
Prednisone	20 mg qid PO (days 1-7)	

Their survival was compared with that of the other patients entered on regimen A. They were evaluated for response at 6 weeks.

Patients with local recurrence at the mastetomy site, with or without ipsilateral supraclavicular or axillary nodes, with or without bone metastasis by bone scan or by x-ray film and liver scan were eligible for entry on regimen A. They were not randomized. They were evaluated for response at 6 weeks.

2. Premenopausal patients, defined as women who were still menstruating, had been amenorrheic less than 1 year, or had had a hysterectomy but were still younger than 50 years, were not eligible unless there had been previous ovarian ablation by surgery or radiation.

3. Following oophorectomy, patients were eligible no sooner than 3 weeks after surgery with progressive disease and 10 weeks after surgery with unresponsive (i.e., stable) disease.

4. At least 3 weeks must have lapsed following discontinuation of any hormone therapy, and there had to be evidence of stable or progressive disease

(e.g., patients with regressing disease following discontinuation were ineligible).

5. Patients with a bilirubin level greater than 1.2 mg/dl, and absolute granulocyte count of less than 1500 mm³, or platelet count less than 100,000/mm³ were not eligible.

6. Patients with skeletal metastases must have undergone a bone marrow biopsy. If there was tumor involvement, the patient was treated with a 50% dose of all drugs except vincristine and prednisone. They were analyzed separately, along with patients who had only bone disease and no other measurable lesions. The dosage was escalated 25% with each subsequent course if grade I toxicity had not occurred.

The analysis of this study involves only the randomized patients and not the nonrandomized bone lesion cases.

Table 36-2 lists the response status of the 306 eligible patients entered on study. The statistical considerations of the study as originally designed required approximately a 20% difference in complete plus partial response rates between the two combinations, with an alpha level of 0.05 and power of 80%. This required approximately 110 to 120 patients on each treatment arm. The study clearly met its objective.

There were 160 patients assigned to each arm, but response data were not available on 4 subjects on arm A and 10 subjects on arm B. The response rate of A was 74 per 156 (47.4%) and on B was 52 per 150 (34.7%), or approximately a 13% difference. This had a significance level of .025, denoted as $p = .025$, which meant that if the two regimens were equal in their ability to induce a response, the chance of observing a difference was 2.5%. Thus they were not equivalent in their ability to induce a response. The power appears to be adequate (approximately 90%). Thus statistically we can say that A was superior to B. However, an important consideration is clinical significance. There was significantly more morbidity associated with regimen A than with regimen B. Future studies will have to consider the risk/benefit ratios of such therapies (see Spilker[1]).

End points such as survival time (time from entry in study to death) and duration of disease control (time from entry in study to observed progression) are given in Figures 36-1 and 36-2. There was no advantage with either regimen. The median survival (the point in time at which

TABLE **36-2**	Response Status of 306 Patients in Metastatic Breast Cancer Study

REGIMEN	ELIGIBLE	COMPLETE RESPONSE	PARTIAL RESPONSE	STABLE	PROGRESSION
A (CAF)	156	23	51	37	45
B (CMFVP)	150	7	45	40	58

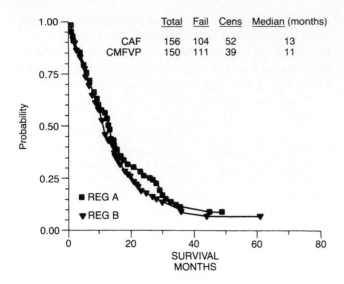

	Total	Fail	Cens	Median (months)
CAF	156	104	52	13
CMFVP	150	111	39	11

■ REG A
▼ REG B

FIG. **36-1** Time from date on study: all induction entries.

approximately 50% of the sample were still alive or free of progression) is equivalent on both regimens.

This is a general overview of a study from its stated objectives to the primary analysis. Often, large phase III studies such as this one would probe the data further to impose a regression structure to determine, for example, which underlying variables (e.g., site of metastasis, patient demographics, initial laboratory workup) most influenced the response or survival outcome. Such was done with this study. Smalley and colleagues[14,15] discuss in detail the clinical patterns of metastases found in this study; further detail can be found in Smalley and Bartolucci.[16]

The techniques used to analyze regression relationships are well established.[17-21] However, results should be

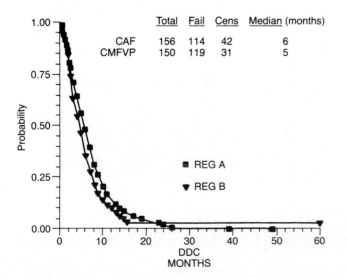

	Total	Fail	Cens	Median (months)
CAF	156	114	42	6
CMFVP	150	119	31	5

■ REG A
▼ REG B

FIG. **36-2** Duration of disease: all induction entries.

interpreted with caution. One shortcoming in these types of analyses is that there may be insufficient numbers of observations compared with the variables considered in the regression equation.[22] One guideline is to have at least 10 to 15 times as many observations as variables. A thorough statistical evaluation of all planned methodology is advised before any attempt to analyze the database. The safest and most reliable analyses usually are those for which the study was originally designed.

ADJUVANT BREAST DISEASE STUDY

In 1976 the Southeastern Cancer Study Group initiated a trial to compare the DFI and survival of patients who had undergone radical or modified radical mastectomy for breast carcinoma with positive axillary nodes; patients were randomized to one of three adjuvant therapies:

1. Short-term chemotherapy: six cycles of cyclophosphamide, methotrexate, and 5-fluorouracil (CMF)
2. Long-term chemotherapy: 12 cycles of CMF
3. Radiation therapy plus short-term chemotherapy: six cycles of CMF

A secondary objective was to compare the tolerance of patients in each of the regimens. The objectives here were different than in the previous example because a different population of women was involved. The eligibility criteria for patient selection for this study included the following:

1. Women of all ages with proven stage II carcinoma of the breast who had undergone radical or modified radical mastectomy and whose pathologic specimens had shown one or more positive axillary nodes, regardless of level, were eligible. Stage II was defined as any combination of T_{1a}, T_{1b}, T_{2a}, T_{2b}, T_{3a}, N, N_{1a}, or N_{1b}, according to the International Staging System. The staging was defined in the appendix of the protocol.
2. Patients were entered on study within 56 days of standard or modified radical mastectomy and after complete healing of the surgical wound.
3. Patients were eligible if they had adequate physiologic function, defined as absolute granulocyte count of greater than $1500/mm^3$ or platelets greater than $100,000/mm^3$, bilirubin levels less than 1.2 mg/dl, BUN less than 25% or creatinine less than 1.2 mg/dl, and absence of infection or septicemia.

The following were ineligible for study:

1. Patients with a history of cancer in the other breast
2. Patients who had received prior chemotherapy or hormone therapy for breast cancer

3. Patients who had received prior radiation therapy
4. Patients with inflammatory carcinoma of the breast
5. Patients with residual foci of metastatic disease as judged by careful physical examination and by appropriate studies (chest x-ray film, liver scan, and bone scan)
6. Patients who did not meet listed criteria for adequate physiologic function
7. Patients whose personal circumstances did not permit adequate treatment and follow-up as outlined
8. Patients with preexisting medical conditions that would make them poor candidates for adjuvant therapy

The details of the treatment plan are not discussed here, except to say that the timing of a cycle was approximately 1 month. The study was stratified by nodal status (one to three positive axillary nodes versus four or more), premenopausal versus postmenopausal status, interval after surgery (<28 days versus 28 to 56 days), and type of mastectomy (radical versus modified radical). For a complete discussion of this study, see Velez-Garcia and associates.[23]

The study initially included regimens A (short-term chemotherapy) and B (long-term chemotherapy) within the women with one to three positive nodes and regimens A, B, and C (radiation plus short-term chemotherapy) within the women with four or more positive nodes. Later, the study was revised to include only regimens A and C in the women with four or more positive nodes. Twenty-four institutions participated in this study.

The objectives of this study dictated that the sample size in each nodal stratum be between 200 and 240 patients. With an alpha level of .05 and power of 80%, the alternative hypothesis stated that the 12-month CMF regimen would reduce the relapse rate at 2 years from 30% to 10% in the group with one to three positive nodes. For the group with four or more positive nodes, the addition of radiotherapy was hypothesized to reduce the 2-year relapse rate by the same magnitude (30% to 10%).

Table 36-3 lists the patient characteristics by the strata set out in the protocol; clearly the accrual objectives were met. There were 301 eligible entries in the group with one to three positive nodes and 241 eligible entries in the group with four or more positive nodes. These numbers do not include the 55 patients on the long-term chemotherapy arm in the group with four or more positive nodes.

Figures 36-3 to 36-6 show no statistical advantage of any of the regimens with respect to DFI or survival. This was a case in which the null hypothesis was not rejected. Some may argue that further subsetting of the

data is required to ferret out statistical differences among the strata of interest. This is precisely the situation to avoid because the study was not designed to accommodate and the objectives did not hypothesize a subgrouping effect. At best, trends in the data can be investigated, as shown in Figure 36-7. Even if a statistical difference is seen in regimen A versus regimen C in the DFI of premenopausal woman with four or more positive nodes, there are only two avenues to take. One is to conclude that statistical significance has been reached by pure chance. This is the multiplicity issue in statistics, which says that if subsets of data continue to be analyzed, a significant result may be found by chance and the conclusions are more superficial than real. In this study the 95% confidence intervals around these curves overlapped; thus the difference was not as real as it appeared. This can be avoided by using the regression techniques discussed previously with the appropriate cautions outlined. This way we can determine whether treatment adjusted for menopausal status and nodal status was a determinant in the DFI. The problem of multiplicity in analyses has been discussed by Bartolucci.[12]

The other avenue to pursue given such a finding is to investigate this phenomenon further in a clinical trial of premenopausal women with four or more positive nodes. If this result were real, it might be used to set up an entirely new clinical trial with precisely stated objectives, thus leading to adequate sample size. However, the narrowness of the eligibility criteria might preclude the feasibility of conducting such a trial.

As previously stated, a secondary objective of the study was to compare the tolerance of patients for each of the regimens. Table 36-4 summarizes these results. The following is an example of the type of toxicity report found in most such studies.

Of the 597 eligible cases, 548 have toxicity evaluations on file. Toxicities are reported as mild, severe, and life threatening. No lethal toxicity has been reported during protocol therapy, and no deaths secondary to therapy are known to have occurred in patients off study. Toxicities reported appear in Table 36-4. Other reported adverse events are at 6 months: chemoweight, tearing of eyes, fatigue, hot flashes, conjunctivitis, anorexia, vaginal yeast infection, and tinnitus; 12 months: chemoweight, folliculitis, conjunctivitis, fatigue, nasal mucositis, corneal ulcerations, and mucositis; RT and 6 months: chemoanxiety, tearing of eyes, and fatigue.

In summary, studies must be designed and reported in such a way as to prevent reporting and publishing misleading anecdotes. This section has discussed two examples of studies generated from well-designed protocols, with significant results confirmed by a check on the power of the statistical procedures and with results reported as stated in the objectives.

TABLE 36-3 | Characteristics of Patients in Adjuvant Breast Disease Study

	1 TO 3 NODES				4 + NODES					
	6 mo		12 mo		6 mo		12 mo		RT + 6 mo	
	NO.	%	NO.	%	NO.	%	NO.	%	NO.	%
PREMENOPAUSAL										
Number of cases	70	100	70	100	49	100	22	100	48	100
Type of surgery										
Radical	18	26	12	17	9	18	6	27	9	19
Modified radical	52	74	58	83	40	82	16	73	39	81
Time from surgery										
<28 days	19	27	19	27	14	29	11	50	13	27
≥28 days	51	73	51	73	35	71	11	50	35	73
Age										
<40	31	44	24	34	24	49	9	41	21	44
≥40	39	56	46	66	25	51	13	59	27	56
TNM stage										
$T_1 + T_2$	58	82	53	76	40	82	15	68	31	65
T_3	6	9	12	17	8	16	5	23	12	25
Unknown	6	9	5	7	1	2	2	9	5	10
Performance status										
<70%	1	1	0	0	0	0	2	9	1	2
≥70%	69	99	67	96	48	98	19	86	46	96
Unknown	0	0	3	4	1	2	1	5	1	2
Estrogen receptor status										
Yes	24	34	27	39	20	47	4	18	13	27
No	15	21	10	14	8	19	2	9	8	17
Unknown	31	44	33	47	21	34	16	73	27	56
Number of nodes +										
4-6					16	33	7	32	16	33
7-12					22	45	7	32	15	31
≥12					11	22	8	36	17	36
POSTMENOPAUSAL										
Number of cases	85	100	76	100	73	100	33	100	71	100
Type of surgery										
Radical	11	13	12	16	15	21	11	33	11	15
Modified radical	74	87	64	84	58	79	22	67	60	85
Time from surgery										
<28 days	27	32	21	28	25	34	13	39	20	28
≥28 days	58	68	55	72	48	66	20	61	51	72
Age										
<40	1	1	2	3	0	0	1	3	0	0
≥40	83	98	74	97	73	100	32	97	70	99
Unknown	1	1	0	0	0	0	0	0	1	1
TNM stage										
$T_1 + T_2$	72	85	66	87	50	69	24	73	47	66
T_3	5	6	4	5	16	22	5	15	14	20
Unknown	8	9	6	8	7	9	4	12	10	14
Performance status										
<70%	1	1	0	0	0	0	0	0	1	1
≥70%	79	93	74	97	71	97	31	94	66	93
Unknown	5	6	2	3	2	3	2	6	4	6

TABLE **36-3** Characteristics of Patients in Adjuvant Breast Disease Study—cont'd

| | 1 TO 3 NODES | | | | 4 + NODES | | | | | |
| | 6 mo | | 12 mo | | 6 mo | | 12 mo | | RT + 6 mo | |
	NO.	%	NO.	%	NO.	%	NO.	%	NO.	%
Estrogen receptor status										
Yes	34	40	27	36	24	33	11	33	34	34
No	7	8	14	18	7	10	2	6	13	18
Unknown	44	52	35	46	42	57	20	61	34	48
Number of nodes +										
4-6					34	47	13	39	30	42
7-12					15	21	9	27	22	31
≥12					24	32	11	34	19	27

Overview of Several Controversies

RANDOMIZATION

The controversy over randomization concerns two types of randomization: conventional randomization and prerandomization. Conventional randomization occurs when the patient has been demonstrated to be eligible, has had the details and purposes of the study explained, and has signed an informed consent document. Included in the explanation of the details of the study are the possible risks and benefits of the therapeutic alternatives. The patient can refuse to participate in the study at any time—even before signing the informed consent. Thus there may not be any record of the patient even being approached for the study, and most written protocols do not require investigators to keep an accounting of all eligible patients who were approached and subsequently refused to participate.

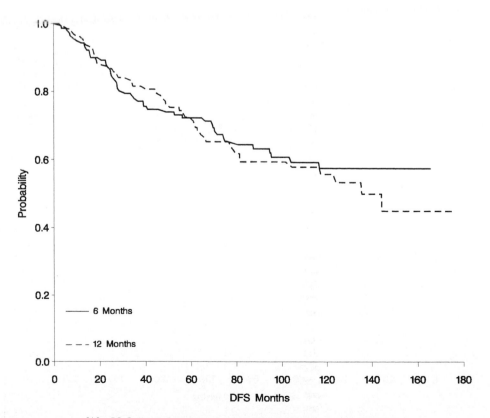

FIG. **36-3** Disease-free survival *(DFS)* time: one to three nodes.

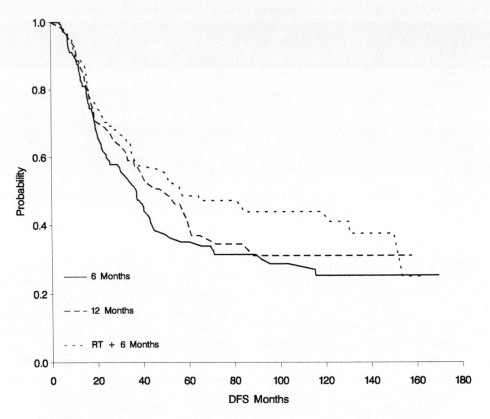

FIG. **36-4** Disease-free survival *(DFS)* time: four or more nodes. *RT,* Radiotherapy.

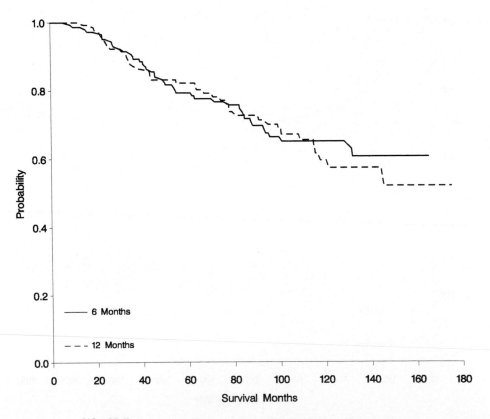

FIG. **36-5** Survival time from date on study: one to three nodes.

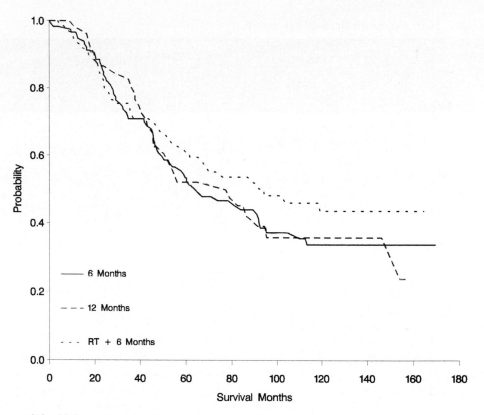

FIG. **36-6** Survival time from date on study: four or more nodes. *RT,* Radiotherapy.

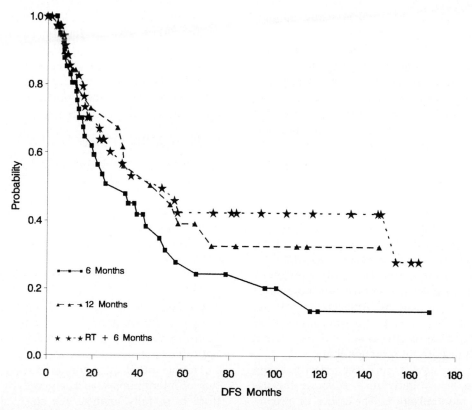

FIG. **36-7** Disease-free survival *(DFS)* time: four or more nodes, premenopausal patients. *RT,* Radiotherapy.

TABLE 36-4 | Toxicities in Adjuvant Breast Disease Study

	NUMBER OF PATIENTS								
	258			187			103		
	6 mo (%)			12 mo (%)			RT + mo (%)		
TOXICITY	MILD	SEVERE	LOW TOLERANCE	MILD	SEVERE	LOW TOLERANCE	MILD	SEVERE	LOW TOLERANCE
Hemoglobin	12	1	—	16	2	—	8	1	—
Granulocytes	39	21	2	43	19	2	34	11	—
Platelets	11	3	—	18	4	2	12	2	—
Cardiovascular	<1	—	—	1	—	—	—	—	—
Oral	9	4	1	3	6	1	4	2	2
Gastrointestinal	28	11	1	28	13	5	32	9	1
Liver		2	—	2	4	—	2	1	—
Central nervous system	<1	<1	<1	1	—	—	2	1	—
Skin and hair	28	3	—	25	3	—	22	4	—

RT, Radiotherapy.

Prerandomization occurs when the physician randomly assigns the patient to treatment after determining eligibility but before discussing the study and its implications with the patient and obtaining informed consent. This approach eliminates the uneasiness experienced by most physicians when they have to obtain the patient's consent to participate in the trial but are not able to tell the patient what treatment will be administered, something that makes many patients unwilling to participate. Many physicians argue that some clinical trials cannot be accomplished without the accrual enhancement technique of prerandomization. A variation of this technique, called the *randomized-consent design*, has been discussed by Zelen.[24] Both Zelen[24] and Ellenberg[25] have reported the negative implications of this procedure. A particular statistical concern is the refusal rate of patients with this type of design and the adverse impact it has on the overall efficiency of the study. To achieve a valid study, the accrual has to be inflated to accommodate the study efficiency lost by refusal to receive the assigned treatment. For example, if the refusal rate on a prerandomized study is 10%, the overall accrual has to be increased by almost 60%. This assumes an overall selection bias when, for example, patients on a two-arm study have a prognosis that prompts them to choose one treatment in favor of another.[25] The National Surgical Adjuvant Breast and Bowel Project (NSABP) used prerandomization in its study comparing total mastectomy with segmental mastectomy with or without radiation therapy.

Because of the statistical controversy associated with prerandomization, many individuals advocate the use of conventional randomization. The critics of prerandomization are often accused of not having had adequate experience with large-scale cooperative group trials and the problems associated with obtaining adequate accrual. Also, prerandomization is a victim of its own technique. With prerandomization, the rate of refusal for a study is known because a random assignment is recorded and registered. However, with conventional randomization, the patient's refusal may not be recorded. Therefore the refusal rate can be just as frequent and biased in a conventionally randomized study as in a prerandomized study, and it may go undetected. Regardless of the randomization technique used, the patient is of primary concern. Honest and open discussions of all options, risks, and benefits are necessary. If a patient's physician believes that a particular treatment option is best for a patient, a randomized trial may not be appropriate.

SUBSET AND INTERIM ANALYSES

A previous section discussed the problem of multiple testing (i.e., looking for significant comparisons in subsets of the data). The danger is that of achieving statistical significance purely by chance. For example, the chance of committing at least one type I error at alpha level ($\alpha = .05$) when c + 10 tests are conducted is as follows:

$$1 - (1 - \alpha)^c = 1 - (1 - .05)^{10} = .40$$

The accommodation of the many factors in a patient sample and their associated influence on the major end points of the study can be best dealt with by using the appropriate analytic tools.[18,19]

Another problem in the analysis of clinical trials is that of interim analysis. The generally accepted procedure is to fully analyze the study at its conclusion because type I error can be increased by repeated testing (interim analyses) throughout the course of the trial.[26,27] Interim analyses can be misleading because differences in treatment response could be noted for patients entered early on the trial who may be of a different prognostic characterization than those entered later on the trial. Interim analyses can cause unjustified early termination of a trial for the reasons stated. Also these misleading results can influence the rate of accrual to a study, cause individual physicians to adopt a particular treatment strategy prematurely, and influence the way particular study end points are evaluated. Peto[28] has suggested techniques for terminating clinical studies early on the basis of highly statistically significant *p* values. Also see Lan and DeMets.[29]

NONRANDOMIZED CONTROLS

The use of nonrandomized (historical) controls in clinical trials is primarily an economic move to expedite the initiation and completion of those trials. Gehan and Freireich[30] have discussed the rationale and conditions for the use of nonrandomized controls. The success of the technique depends on the success of matching concurrent and historical groups based on relevant prognostic variables. This can be tenuous because archived prognostic data may not be available and certain underlying prognostic data influencing the results may be unknown to those analyzing the data. However, Makuch and Simon[8,31] have discussed the sample size requirements for using this technique if the use of historical data is relevant.

META-ANALYSIS

Meta-analysis, although not new, has recently been advocated by Peto[28] as a possible technique in analyzing results from many studies. One of the purposes of this technique is to decide the future direction in the study of a disease. See Fossatti and colleagues.[32] The technique involves the continued analysis of past studies in the literature for a particular type and stage of cancer. Combining the results of many small trials using similar therapies for a particular disease allows the past sample size and power of the studies to be increased. This may allow more definitive conclusions concerning the relative efficacy of past treatments. This technique suffers from many of the same pitfalls found in the technique using historical controls (possible prognostic incomparability of the samples and possible lack of relevant demographic or clinical information).

QUALITY OF LIFE

Another issue not yet discussed is that of the quality of life. Many clinical groups include this assessment as part of the clinical protocols. End points such as response and survival may be of primary clinical interest. However, other health-related professionals, such as psychologists and nutritionists, are now becoming important partners in the conduct of clinical trials. Methodologic tools are constantly being developed and tested to assess the psychologic well-being of patients on study. This is especially important in trials in which the overall mortality over time may be decreased, but the morbidity becomes a real detriment to the patient. Future reports of clinical studies are likely to incorporate an ever-increasing analysis of the quality of life.

REFERENCES

1. Spilker B: *Guide to clinical interpretation of data*, New York, 1986, Raven.
2. Sackett DL: Biases in analytic research, *J Chronic Dis* 32:51, 1979.
3. Simon R: Design and conduct of clinical trials. In DeVita VT Jr, Hellman S, Rosenberg SA (eds): *Cancer: principles and practice of oncology*, Philadelphia, 1982, Lippincott.
4. Cassagrande JT, Pike MC, Smith PG: An improved formula for calculating sample sizes for comparing two binomial distributions, *Biometrics* 34:483, 1978.
5. Fleiss JL: *Statistical methods for rates and proportions*, New York, 1973, Wiley.
6. Gehan EA: The determination of the number of patients required in a preliminary and followup trial of a new chemotherapeutic agent, *J Chronic Dis* 13:346, 1961.
7. George SL, Desu MM: Planning the size and duration of a clinical trial studying the time to some critical event, *J Chronic Dis* 27:15, 1974.
8. Makuch R, Simon R: Sample size requirements for evaluating a conservative therapy, *Cancer Treat Rep* 62:1037, 1978.
9. Pocock SJ: *Size of cancer clinical trials and stopping rules*, *Br J Cancer* 38:757, 1978.
10. Schoenfeld DA, Gelber RD: Designing and analyzing clinical trials which allow institutions to randomize patients to a subset of the treatments under study, *Biometrics* 35:825, 1979.
11. Zelen M: *Aspects of the planning and analysis of clinical trials in cancer: a survey of statistical design and linear models*, New York, 1975, North Holland.
12. Bartolucci AA: Estimation and comparison of proportions. In Buyse M, Sylvester R, Staquet M (eds): *Cancer clinical trials. Methods and practice*, Oxford, 1984, Oxford University Press.
13. Bartolucci AA: *The role of microcomputers in clinical trials*. The Southeastern Cancer Study Group experience, Community Clinical Oncology Program Workshop, Bethesda, MD, 1983, National Cancer Institute.
14. Smalley RV et al: A comparison of cyclophosphamide, adriamycin and 5-fluorouracil (CAF) and cyclophosphamide, methotrexate, 5-fluorouracil, vincristine, prednisone (CMFVP) in patients with advanced breast cancer. A Southeastern Cancer Study Group project, *Breast Cancer Res Treat* 3:209, 1983.
15. Smalley RV et al: Southeastern Cancer Study Group: breast cancer studies 1972-1982, *Int J Radiat Oncol* 9:1867, 1983.
16. Smalley RV, Bartolucci AA: Variations in responsiveness and survival of clinical subsets of patients with metastatic breast cancer to two chemotherapy combinations, *Eur J Cancer* 16(suppl 1):141, 1980.
17. Bartolucci AA, Fraser MD: Comparative step up composite tests for selecting prognostic indicators associated with survival, *Biomet J* 19:437, 1977.

18. Cox DR: *Analysis of binary data,* Methuen Monograph Series, London, 1970, Methuen.

19. Cox DR: Regression models and life tables (with discussion), *J R Statist Soc B* 34:187, 1972.

20. Fraser MD, Bartolucci AA, Smith WA: A Bayesian decision procedure for selecting prognostic variables associated with survival, *Biomet J* 37:463, 1995.

21. Lee ET: A computer program for linear logistic regression analysis, *Comput Prog Biomed* 4:80, 1974.

22. Marascuilo LA, Levin JR: *Multivariate statistics in the social sciences: a researcher's guide,* Pacific Grove, CA, 1983, Brooks/Cole.

23. Velez-Garcia E et al: Postsurgical adjuvant chemotherapy with or without radiotherapy in women with breast cancer and positive axillary nodes. A Southeastern Cancer Study Group Trial, *Eur J Cancer* 28A:1833, 1992.

24. Zelen M: A new design for randomized clinical trials, *N Engl J Med* 300:1242, 1979.

25. Ellenberg SS: Randomization designs in comparative clinical trials, *N Engl J Med* 310:1404, 1984.

26. Peto R et al: Design and analysis of randomized clinical trials requiring prolonged observation of each patient. 1. Introduction and design, *Br J Cancer* 34:585, 1976.

27. Peto R et al: Design and analysis of randomized clinical trials requiring prolonged observation of each patient. 2. Analysis and examples, *Br J Cancer* 35:1, 1977.

28. Peto R: Clinical trial methodology, *Biomedicine* 28:24, 1978.

29. Lan GNK, DeMets DL: Discrete sequential boundaries for clinical trials, *Biometrika* 70:659, 1983.

30. Gehan EA, Freireich EJ: Non-randomized controls in cancer clinical trials, *N Engl J Med* 290:198, 1974.

31. Makuch RW, Simon R: A note on the design of multi-institution three treatment studies, *Cancer Clin Trials* 1:1301, 1978.

32. Fossatti, R et al: Cytotoxic and hormonal treatment for metastatic breast cancer: a systematic review of published randomized trials involving 31,510 women, *J Clin Oncol* 5:728, 2001.

XIII

SURGERY FOR BENIGN AND MALIGNANT DISEASES OF THE BREAST

37

Evolution of Surgical Principles and Techniques for the Management of Breast Cancer

ERIC R. FRYKBERG

KIRBY I. BLAND

Chapter Outline

To understand a science it is necessary to know its history.   Auguste Comte (1798-1857)

Let us not lightly cast aside things that belong to the past, for only with the past can we weave the fabric of the future.   Anatole France (1844-1924)

Those who cannot remember the past are condemned to repeat it.   George Santayana (1863-1952)

We see so far, because we stand on the shoulders of giants.   Sir Isaac Newton (1643-1727)

Ancient Records

The ancient recordings of historical aspects of carcinoma of the breast document the development of thought regarding its biology and pathophysiology and the application of these concepts to rational treatment. Its description in the earliest medical literature indicates that this disease has always been the relatively common and virulent entity that we know today.

The Edwin Smith Papyrus is thought to date from between 3000 BC and 2500 BC. Believed to have been written by the first known physician, Imhotep, it contains the oldest known reference to tumors or ulcers of the breast.[1-4] Herodotus (ca. 484-425 BC) credited the Persian physician Democedes (ca. 525 BC) with the successful treatment of a breast tumor that had already ulcerated and spread in Atossa, daughter of Cyrus and wife of Darius.[2,3,5] This may be the first description of local and metastatic spread of cancer, although the fact that it was apparently cured raises doubt that it was a malignancy.[2,6] The hindrance of early diagnosis by a woman's fear and cosmetic considerations, a problem that persists to the present day, is also demonstrated by this anecdote.[3]

Hippocrates, the Father of Medicine (ca. 460-370 BC), made two references to apparently advanced cases of breast malignancy[2,3,7]:

> The whole body becomes emaciated....When they have gone as far as this, they do not recover, but die of this disease.

This probably also represents an early reference to metastatic breast carcinoma. Hippocrates was the first to distinguish benign from malignant breast neoplasms, applying the latter term to any growth that spread and caused death.[6] He advocated withholding any treatment for "hidden" or deep-seated breast tumors (presumably referring to those that did not yet involve the overlying skin) in view of his observations that medical therapy caused a "speedy death, but to omit

treatment is to prolong life." Some have interpreted these hidden cancers to mean those occurring within the body (i.e., metastatic lesions), for which this caution is logical.[7] There is no evidence that surgery was then applied to this disease.

Aulus Cornelius Celsus (ca. 30 BC-38 AD), in his work *De Medicina*, demonstrated remarkable insight into the natural history of cancer, particularly as it applied to the breast.[3,8] He provided one of the first descriptions of the "dilated tortuous veins" that typically surround a tumor,[2] which later led Galen to liken the lesion to a crab and to apply the label of *cancer*. Celsus described four stages in the clinical evolution of breast cancer, the first of which (*cacoethes*) represented either early malignancy or a benign premalignant lesion. He advised treatment only at this stage, first with caustics, followed by surgical excision and cauterization if symptoms improved. Like his Egyptian and Greek predecessors, he advised against any treatment for the three more advanced stages of malignancy, because any surgery seemed to "irritate" the process and hasten the patient's demise. It is evident that extensive surgery was commonly carried out for breast carcinoma in this ancient Roman period. Celsus advised against removal of the pectoral muscles if breast amputation was done. He thus indicated the benefits of early detection and treatment and the dangers of surgery for locally advanced disease that were ultimately confirmed some 2000 years later.[2,3,6,7]

Galen (ca. 131-203 AD) was a Greek physician whose abundant works on medicine centered around the humoral principle of disease first elaborated by Hippocrates. He asserted that cancer was a local manifestation of "melancholia" caused by an excess of black bile in the body. He noted that most cases of breast carcinoma occurred in postmenopausal females. Such a concept represents perhaps one of the earliest views of breast malignancy as a systemic disease that required systemic treatment and served to explain its poor prognosis at that time.[9] Galen recommended surgical excision of the diseased breast if it was amenable to removal. In what may be the first description of an operation for cancer of any kind, he advised incising the breast through healthy, uninvolved tissue to widely encompass the whole tumor without leaving behind "a single root" that would allow recurrence. He also advised against the use of either ligatures or cautery, because free flow of blood was thought to maximize the drainage of black bile and thus minimize the chance of local recurrence and spread.[2,3,7]

The Greek physician and surgeon Leonides, who worked in the great school of Alexandria around 180 AD, provided the first detailed factual description of a mastectomy as it was widely practiced at that time. He, like Galen, advocated wide excision of the tumor through normal tissues, but he used cautery to both stem the bleeding and eradicate the disease. The common association of enlarged axillary nodules with breast cancer was noted in his writings.[2,4] He was the first to describe nipple retraction as a clinical sign of breast cancer. He advised against surgical intervention in cases of locally advanced disease and also advocated systemic "detoxification of the body" in both the preoperative and postoperative phases of treatment.[3,7,10] His practice of performing mastectomy by alternate incision and cautery persisted largely unchanged for at least the next 1500 years.

Progress was made in these ancient times toward understanding the pathophysiology of breast carcinoma and developing some of the basic surgical treatment principles that we still follow today. In the next several centuries further progress was scant, and some concepts were even forgotten.

Medieval and Renaissance Periods

The humoral theory of disease prevailed throughout the Dark Ages, and rigid adherence to Galen as the ultimate authority in medical matters prevented any further innovations in the treatment of breast carcinoma. A conservative and nihilistic view of this disease process was held by virtually all medical practitioners. The influence of the Church on all scholarly matters in this era is suggested by the fact that the Council of Tours in 1162 banned the "barbarous practice" of surgery for breast tumors.[2] The treatises of the Spanish-Arabian surgeon Albucaisis (ca. 1013-1106) and the French surgeons Henri de Mondeville (ca. 1260-1320) and his pupil Guy de Chauliac (ca. 1300-1367) reflected Galen's approach to breast cancer in advocating only a limited role for surgery for tumors that could be completely removed.[11] Lanfranc (ca. 1296), the Father of French Surgery, practiced the same technique for mastectomy that Leonides had described 1100 years before and was largely responsible for this operation's becoming the standard treatment for breast cancer in the larger schools of medicine in Europe.[2-4]

As the Renaissance philosophy of enlightenment and learning spread throughout Europe in the fifteenth and sixteenth centuries, many of the principles that eventually led to the modern era of breast cancer treatment were developed or rediscovered. At the same time, however, several extreme and irrational modes of treatment persisted. Incising into a diseased breast and through tumor in a piecemeal approach to removing the malignancy appears to have been commonly practiced during this period. The poor results of this practice, in terms of the rapid recurrence of ulcerating tumors, led Fabricius ab Aquapendente (1537-1619), the

famed Italian surgeon and anatomist who was William Harvey's teacher, to condemn partial excision as worthless. He performed radical excisions of the entire breast, but only when the patient requested it.[2,3,12] This idea recalled the advice of Galen and Leonides that breast tumors be widely excised through normal tissue and represented an important conceptual basis for the ultimate evolution of the modern mastectomy.

Ambrose Pare (1510-1590), the French military surgeon and Father of Modern Surgery, widely excised smaller tumors, using sulfuric acid instead of hot cautery to control bleeding. The observation of the probable relationship between breast carcinoma and swelling of the axillary glands was an important advance credited to Pare.[4] His pupil, Bartholemy Cabrol, took a more radical approach to breast cancer by advocating mastectomy and removal of the underlying pectoral muscles, as did Jacques Guillemeau (1550-1601) and Michael Servetus (1509-1553). Servetus, a Spanish surgeon who was burned at the stake by Calvinists, was also perhaps the first to recommend that axillary lymph nodes be removed along with the radical excision of the breast in the treatment of breast carcinoma.[4,12] This idea was also advanced by the Italian surgeon Marcus Aurelius Severinus (1580-1659), who was perhaps the first author since Hippocrates to emphasize the distinction between benign and malignant breast tumors. He also recommended excision of benign lesions to prevent their developing into cancers.[3]

The sixteenth and seventeenth centuries were marked by a variety of innovations in the technique of mastectomy for breast cancer that led to a more efficient, thorough, and swift operation in this preanesthetic era. Wilhelm Fabry von Hilden, also known as Fabricius Hildanus (1560-1624), a German surgeon taught by Vesalius, emphasized the need for tumors to be mobile if the patient were to be a candidate for surgery and to avoid leaving behind "sprouts," asserting[13]:

But before everything we must carefully make out whether the tumour can be shifted and moved from one point to another, and whether it can be radically excised. For the operation will be fruitless if any part of the tumour, however minute—nay, even the membranes in which tumours of this sort are usually enveloped—be left behind. For the disease sprouts up again, and becomes more malignant than ever, while there is no hope that we can remove what remains behind by cauterising.

Fabry also removed axillary lymph nodes as a part of his procedure.[2,4,14,15]

One of the first surgical attempts to allow healing by direct union of the incised skin edges following mastectomy was recorded by Van der Mullen in 1698. The fact that this patient died contributed to the controversy over the safety of primary wound closure.[7]

Threshold of the Modern Period

One of the greatest impediments to the advancement of knowledge of the treatment of breast carcinoma through these years was in the failure of physicians to keep comprehensive records of their results, the absence of scientific analysis of such results, and the poor communication among physicians. With the advent of the Age of Enlightenment in the eighteenth century, this situation began to change. The great hospitals of Paris and London became centers of scholarly study in both theoretical and practical aspects of medicine. Formal lectures in anatomy and surgery were instituted, prizes were awarded for scientific research, and in 1731 one of the first surgical societies was founded in France, the Academie de Chirurgie.[7] Its publication, *The Memoires*, was the first journal devoted entirely to surgery, and it pioneered the spread of surgical knowledge throughout Europe.

The systemic theory of origin of breast carcinoma persisted during this period, although derangements of the newly discovered and described lymphatic system replaced Galen's black bile as the stimulating agent.[3,6] John Hunter (1728-1793), a proponent of this idea, believed that cancer made its appearance wherever lymph coagulated. He also believed, however, that a local component of disease origin was important in the treatment of breast carcinoma, which required wide excision beyond the grossly visible disease if recurrences were to be avoided.[16] This marked the beginning of a trend toward more aggressive and thorough local treatments that ultimately led to greatly improved results for women afflicted with breast cancer. The report of Guillaume de Houpeville in 1693, describing his removal of a breast with surrounding healthy tissue and the underlying pectoral muscle, indicated a revival of the radical operation first advocated 150 years before by Cabrol, Guillemeau, and Servetus.[4]

One of the greatest contributions to this changing attitude was made by the French surgeon Henri Francois LeDran (1685-1770), who practiced at the Hôpital St. Come. He courageously repudiated the classic humoral theory of Galen, which was still firmly entrenched in the contemporary teachings of medical schools, by asserting in 1757 that breast cancer began in its earliest stages as a local process within the breast proper. As it grew, he believed it spread initially to the regional axillary lymphatics and then to distant sites through the general circulation.[17] He thus claimed, "we may hope for a perfect cure" by aggressive surgical ablation in its earliest stages. This presaged the benefits of early detection of this disease that were to be well demonstrated more than 200 years later,[18,19] as well as the benefits of a wide surgical resection of disease that

were to be so famously demonstrated by Halsted 150 years later.[20] LeDran's operation included the dissection of enlarged axillary lymph nodes, as previously advocated by Servetus, Severinus, and Fabry. He also recognized the dismal prognostic implications of axillary lymph node involvement with the malignant process.[3,4,6,7] The results of these efforts can only be surmised by LeDran's vague statement, characteristic of this period, that he carried out "a great number" of such operations, "many" with success.

Jean Louis Petit (1674-1750), LeDran's contemporary, was a prominent French surgeon and the first director of the Academie Francaise de Chirurgie (Figure 37-1). He is credited as the first to introduce an improved operation for breast carcinoma with the goal of curing rather than simply removing an inevitably fatal tumor.[2-4,10,21] His book, *Traites des Operations*, was not published until 24 years after his death. In it, he recommended total removal of the breast and of any enlarged axillary lymph nodes, as well as the pectoralis major muscle if it was involved by tumor. It is unclear whether the lymph nodes were removed in continuity, but he did begin the operation by removing them.[7] He discouraged the practice of partial or piecemeal removal of tumor and breast tissue that was so prevalent at the time and asserted, "the roots of a cancer (of the breast) were the enlarged lymphatic glands." This principle of wide

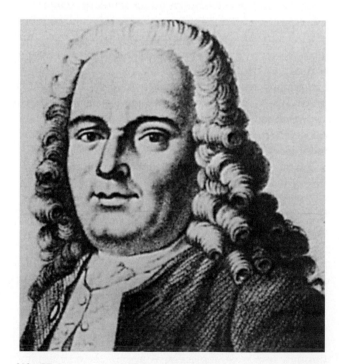

FIG. 37-1 Jean Louis Petit (1674-1750), the French surgeon who was the first to apply surgical intervention as a curative modality for breast carcinoma. *(From Robinson JO: Am J Surg 151:317, 1986. Adapted with permission from Excerpta Medica, Inc.)*

excision without incising, or even viewing, the tumor itself recalls the original philosophy set forth by Galen.

Although Petit's operation may be considered the direct forerunner of the modern radical mastectomy in both principle and technique, it did differ principally in the amount of skin removed. He advised leaving the greater portion of overlying skin, and even the nipple, and dissecting breast tissue out from beneath it. His pupil and colleague, Rene Garangeot (1688-1760), was largely responsible for preserving and spreading the teachings of this eminent surgeon who was so far ahead of his time. Garangeot explained the rationale for skin preservation in mastectomy in his own book, *Traites des Operations de Chirurgie* (1720):

Sewing up the lips of the wound immediately after operation, as was practiced by J. L. Petit, is not only the safest method of arresting hemorrhage but is also the quickest way of healing the wound and preventing the return of the cancer.

It probably also served to reduce the considerable number of infectious complications associated with the typically large and open wounds that most surgeons of that era left, although no definitive results were ever published.[10] Petit did recognize the necessity of removing any skin directly involved by the cancer.[21]

This further reinforced the principle of wide excision of all clinically evident malignancy. He also recognized the poor prognosis of cervical and supraclavicular lymph node involvement.[3,4]

These principles of breast carcinoma beginning as a localized disease process and necessitating wide excision of the entire breast and surrounding tissues if cure was to be achieved gained momentum during this period. Lorenz Heister (1683-1758), a famous German surgeon, used a guillotine device to amputate the entire breast. He was also aware of the morbid implications of axillary lymph node involvement. Removal of axillary contents, the pectoralis major muscle, and even portions of the chest wall if necessary, for excision of the gross tumor were recommended by him in conjunction with mastectomy.[4,22] Bernard Peyrilhe (1735-1804) also embraced the concept that breast cancer began as a local disease in the breast and later spread by way of the lymphatics.[23] Like Heister and Petit, he advocated the total removal of a cancerous breast along with the axillary contents and pectoralis major muscle.[6,7]

Samuel Sharpe, an English surgeon, advocated a similarly aggressive approach in his *Treatise on the Operations of Surgery*, published in 1735. He recommended removing the entire breast through a longitudinal incision for small tumors, although an oval segment of skin was taken for larger tumors, to facilitate the dissection. He claimed that the breast should be cleaned away from the pectoral fascia and that this operation was impractical if the tumor involved the pectoral muscles. The necessity of removing any "knobs" in the armpit was also asserted by Sharpe.[4,13,15]

Benjamin Bell (1749-1806), surgeon to the Edinburgh Royal Infirmary, not only advocated a radical operation for all breast tumors but also emphasized the importance of early diagnosis.[3,4,10,24] He echoed Petit's views in his book, *A System of Surgery* (1784), in which he wrote[25]:

When practitioners have an opportunity of removing a cancerous breast early, they should always embrace it, that as little skin as possible should be removed, and that the breast should be dissected off the pectoral muscle, which ought to be preserved. If any indurated glands be observed, they should be removed and particular care should be given to this part of the operation. For unless all the diseased glands be taken away, no advantage whatever will be derived from it.

These principles of treatment of breast carcinoma remained the standard in Scotland for the next century.

Henry Fearon (1750-1825), a British surgeon of this period, also recognized the importance of early treatment of breast carcinoma and the unlikely probability of achieving this goal. In 1784 he asserted[16]:

The early period of the complaint is beyond all doubt the most favorable period for extirpating it, however patients can seldom be convinced that there is any necessity for an operation while the disease continues in a mild state.

In the latter years of the eighteenth century and the first half of the nineteenth century, a greater degree of conservatism and pessimism toward breast carcinoma pervaded the medical literature and the practice of many surgeons. This arose primarily from the poor results of the bold operations already described. Petrus Camper commented on the reluctance of most surgeons at that time to perform mastectomy for breast carcinoma; he reported in 1757, "not six times a year a breast was amputated with reasonable chance of cure" in Amsterdam, which had a population of 200,000.[4,7,26]

The first efforts to record and analyze the results of treatment of breast carcinoma occurred during this period and reinforced these pessimistic attitudes. Most of the literature consisted of case reports of mastectomy. Alexander Monro Senior (1697-1767) reviewed the cases of 60 patients with this disease who had been treated by contemporary methods and found only 4 patients free of disease after 2 years. Operative mortality alone was reported to be as high as 20%, predominantly from sepsis.[27]

The Scottish surgeon James Syme (1799-1870) wrote in 1842 in his *Principles of Surgery* that palliative procedures for breast carcinoma should be abandoned when axillary glands are involved or the tumor is too extensive or fixed to allow complete removal.[3,4,28] He found that surgery is more likely to "excite greater activity" of the tumor left behind, echoing the observations of Celsus nearly 1900 years earlier.

Sir James Paget (1814-1899) wrote in 1856 that breast carcinoma was such a hopeless disease that he doubted the substantial mortality and morbidity of its treatment could be justified.[29] He found that women with "scirrhous" breast carcinoma actually lived longer without surgical intervention than those who underwent attempts at surgical excision.[7] In 235 cases he had an operative mortality of 10% and had never seen a cure or a case in which recurrence was delayed beyond 8 years.[3,4]

The first hospital ward for indigent cancer patients opened in Middlesex Hospital in London in 1792.[7] The surgeon John Howard provided the major initiative in this effort by arguing that such a ward would not only benefit the patients themselves but also provide an opportunity to study the natural history of this disease, which could lead to improvements in treatment. Private endowments eventually allowed this goal to be realized by contributing to its development into perhaps the first modern cancer institute. From this establishment came some of the most important advances in our knowledge and experience with breast carcinoma in the ensuing years.

By the middle of the nineteenth century, the basic principles of surgical treatment of breast carcinoma had been laid down. Several surgeons had already performed what would later be called the *standard radical mastectomy;* however, there was no consistency among various surgeons or between different geographic regions in the overall management of this disease or in the specific operations performed. This can be attributed to a less than optimal mechanism for widespread communication and dissemination of ideas, ignorance of the basic pathology and pathophysiology of the malignant process, and the poor results of treatment, evident in the few scientific analyses available. Advances in these areas were necessary for the evolution of a truly effective and widely accepted treatment for breast carcinoma.

The Modern Era

Two major advances that paved the way for an effective operation for breast carcinoma were the discovery and development of general anesthesia and the dissemination of the germ theory of disease and principles of antisepsis.[7] These both occurred in the middle to late 1800s. One other series of scientific advances occurred during this same period that contributed to a basic understanding of tumor biology that many consider the

most important contribution to the ultimate development of a rational treatment for breast carcinoma. The widespread use of the microscope led to the birth of cell pathology, and such scientists as Raspail (1826), Schleiden (1838), Schwann (1838), Muller (1838), and Remak (1852) established the cell as the basic structural and functional unit of normal tissue, as well as of neoplasms.[3] The growth and behavior of malignancies were found by (among others) Virchow and Leydig to be caused primarily by cell division, thus removing cancer from the realm of body humors. Recamier first used the term *metastasis* in 1829 and described local tumor infiltration and venous invasion.[6] Rene Laennec (1781-1826) was the first to devise a classification of tumors based on scientific principles. Hannover (1843) and Lebert (1845) first described a *cancer cell*, which identified a malignancy and distinguished it from benign growths. Hannover also asserted that these cells could be found circulating in the blood and were responsible for distant metastases.[6,7] Thiersch (1822-1895) and Waldeyer (1872) established the epithelial origin of all carcinomas. These investigators also supported the mechanical theory of metastasis, asserting that emboli of cancer cells through the lymphatics and bloodstream are responsible for the spread of disease.[6]

These scientific advances fostered an enlightened atmosphere in the second half of the nineteenth century, which led to the reemergence of radical surgery for breast carcinoma. The increasing acceptance of the local theory of origin of this disease and the desire to eliminate its local recurrence further contributed to a decline in pessimistic and fatalistic attitudes and to the establishment of a more rational approach to management. Joseph Pancoast (1805-1882) was a professor of surgical anatomy at Jefferson Medical College in Philadelphia (Figure 37-2). He revived the teachings of Petit and Bell, advocating routine removal of the entire breast for tumors of any size and removal of axillary lymph nodes if they were clinically involved. His assertion that the axillary contents should be removed in continuity with the breast represented the first description of an en bloc resection.[7,10,24,30] This was not a widely held view at the time, as suggested by the fact that Pancoast's successor, Samuel D. Gross (1805-1884), believed, "the proper operation is amputation, not excision."[10] Gross taught that as much skin as possible should be preserved and that axillary lymph nodes should not be removed, in view of the hopelessness of a cure if they were involved.

A landmark paper by Charles Hewitt Moore (1821-1870) was presented before the Royal Medical and Surgical Society in London in 1867.[31] Moore was a surgeon to the Middlesex Hospital, where he observed several breast cancer patients who had been subjected to the various operations then being practiced for this disease and who had subsequently developed local

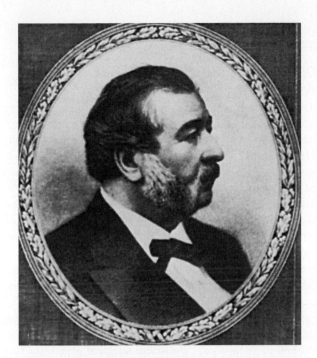

FIG. **37-2** Joseph Pancoast (1805-1882), the American surgeon who supported wide breast excision and first described en bloc axillary lymph node dissection. *(From Robinson JO: Am J Surg 151:317, 1986. Adapted with permission from Excerpta Medica, Inc.)*

recurrences. He postulated that these recurrences probably represented direct extension of the primary disease rather than new foci of malignancy. Thus they appeared to result from incomplete removal of the disease at the original operation rather than from a systemic predisposition. He advocated removal of the entire breast for any breast carcinoma, along with a wide margin of overlying skin, especially if there was any doubt about skin involvement by the tumor. Another principle set forth in this paper was to avoid cutting into the tumor or even seeing it in the course of resection—so as to prevent any of its cells from lodging in the wound. He also recommended removing diseased axillary glands en bloc with the breast, although he later stated that even normal-looking axillary lymph nodes can never be assumed to be healthy, suggesting that axillary dissection should be a routine part of the operation.[2,4,7,10] He did not recommend removing the pectoral muscles. He reported the placement of a drainage tube through the armpit as early as 1858.[10] Moore gave new impetus to the theory of local origin of breast carcinoma with this report, and his remarkable clinical insight into the underlying pathophysiology of this disease served as the foundation on which a standard and widely accepted operation would later be based.

Richard Sweeting, a British surgeon from Stratford, advocated the same principles of wide excision[32]:

For if a purely localized cancer is to be cured by incisions, and is sure to return if not completely removed, then we are more likely to succeed in proportion as our incisions are as deep and as extensive as is consistent with the patient's safety.

He reported three patients who were "cured" by this operation on follow-up of 7 months, 25 months, and 31 months, respectively.

Joseph Lister (1827-1912) of Edinburgh, Scotland, revolutionized the surgical approach toward breast carcinoma with his introduction of antiseptic techniques; he also supported the principles laid down by Moore. In 1870 he reported removing the entire breast in continuity with the axillary glands and was the first to describe division of the origins of both pectoral muscles to facilitate the axillary dissection.[33]

In 1877 William Mitchell Banks, surgeon to the Liverpool Royal Infirmary, emphasized the need to avoid the axillary recurrence that was often noted when the axillary nodes were left in situ. He reiterated Moore's observation that it was impossible clinically to judge axillary node involvement. Also described in his paper was the technique of first removing the breast until it was attached only to the axillary pedicle, which could then be meticulously dissected free of the axillary vein as far as the clavicle (thus recalling the advice of Sharpe more than a century before). He employed "undercutting" of the remaining skin to facilitate primary closure of the wound. He did not find it necessary to divide the pectoral muscles as Lister had but did subscribe to Lister's antiseptic techniques.[10,34] By 1902 he had performed this operation 300 times and documented the course of 175 patients. In his last 80 consecutive cases he reported only 1 operative mortality and several anecdotal reports of cure. He also expressed an opinion, which was to be shared increasingly by others in subsequent years, concerning the desirability of achieving earlier detection of breast carcinoma to improve the chances for cure[13]:

Have you ever imagined what the results would be if all cancers were thoroughly excised when they were no bigger than peas? But if this happy consummation is to be reached, it will not be by performing tremendous operations upon practically hopeless cases.

A German surgeon from Berlin, Ernst Küster (1839-1922), had practiced routine clearance of the axilla in conjunction with mastectomy since 1871.[35] A review of 95 recurrences in his series demonstrated only one in the axilla.[36] Halsted later credited Küster with being the first to advocate routine systematic axillary dissection.

Theodor Billroth (1824-1887), the famous professor of surgery in Vienna, elevated the practice of surgery to a scientific discipline. The overall mortality of his mastectomy operation was 15.7%, and it was 21.3% for cases with axillary dissection. With the introduction of antiseptic wound techniques, these rates were reduced to 5.8% and 10.5%, respectively. As was characteristic of most mastectomies of this period, 82% of Billroth's patients developed local recurrence, and only 4.7% had survived by the end of 3 years.[37,38]

Richard von Volkmann (1830-1889), a German professor of surgery from Halle, was among the first to apply histologic observations to the treatment of breast carcinoma. He advocated removal of a wide margin of skin, as well as a generous portion of underlying muscle if the tumor were fixed to it, and routinely removed the pectoral fascia.[39] In 38 cases of far-advanced disease, he reported a 14% 3-year survival rate and no local recurrence.[3]

Lothar Heidenhain (1860-1940), an assistant to Küster, reported the histologic observation of metastases in lymphatic channels running between the breast and pectoral muscle in two thirds of the cases of breast carcinoma.[40] Based on these observations, he routinely extended the surgical treatment of this disease to include the muscle.

Samuel Weissel Gross (1837-1889) endorsed the tenets of Pancoast and Moore advocating total mastectomy, including all skin covering the breast, routine axillary dissection, and excision of the pectoral fascia. This became known as the *dinner plate operation* because of the shape of the wound it left.[3,4,10] In his report of 207 patients, he demonstrated a 19.4% 3-year survival rate and a 53% rate of local recurrence, with only a 4.6% operative mortality.[41] He also showed that 87.5% of all nonpalpable axillary lymph nodes were actually involved with tumor, reinforcing his belief in the necessity for routine axillary dissection.

Sir Henry Butlin[4,15] recommended axillary dissection only when enlarged axillary glands could be palpated. His operative mortality rate (20%) and 3-year survival rate (5%) among 209 women whose axillas were opened were substantially worse than those rates (10% and 18%, respectively) among 101 women who did not undergo axillary dissection as part of their operation.

Johannes Adrianus Korteweg (1851-1930) was a Dutch professor of surgery who reviewed the operative mortality and cure rates of surgery for breast carcinoma from several European clinics.[42,43] The widely differing operative procedures and degrees of adherence to antiseptic techniques between various surgeons made comparison difficult and largely explained the range of differences in their respective results.[2] He postulated that some forms of breast carcinoma are more malignant than others, thus foreshadowing current knowledge of the individual differences in tumor biology and growth characteristics among patients with the disease. He noted the substantially higher 3-year survival rates in patients without axillary nodal involvement than in those *with* axillary involvement.

DEVELOPMENT OF THE STANDARD RADICAL MASTECTOMY

The evolution of a standardized, effective, and widely accepted operation for the treatment of breast carcinoma culminated with the efforts of William Stewart Halsted (1852-1922). Having completed his undergraduate education at Yale in 1874 and his medical education at Columbia in 1877, Halsted then spent 2 years (1878-1880) in Europe observing the practice of the noted surgeons of that era (Figure 37-3). For much of this period he worked in Vienna under Billroth, whose experience he later reviewed along with that of many other European surgeons. He developed a working knowledge of state-of-the-art surgical treatment of breast carcinoma, which predominantly involved Volkmann's operation. He returned to New York with a firm idea, based on his observations and analyses of the results of others, of what the appropriate surgical attack on this disease should encompass.[38] The high rates of local recurrence and low rates of survival of the operations performed by the prominent European surgeons led him to extend the concept of wide excision, based on the theory of local origin of breast carcinoma. Halsted

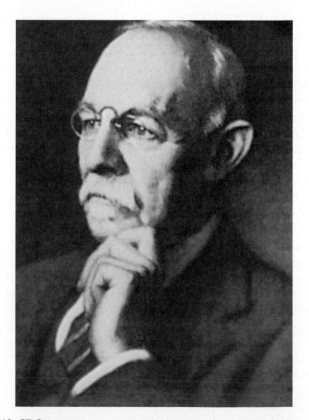

FIG. **37-3** William Stewart Halsted shortly before his death at age 70. *(Courtesy Johns Hopkins Hospital.)*

believed these poor results must be caused by an inadequate and inconsistent removal of tissue surrounding the tumor, thus failing to give the malignancy a wide enough berth to avoid leaving any cancer cells behind. He pronounced Volkmann's operation "a manifestly imperfect one."[44] Although Halsted's philosophy toward breast carcinoma was very much like that of Moore and Banks, he never referred to the work of these surgeons in his early reports. This was probably a result of the small circulation of the British journals in which they published.[10]

The major contribution that Halsted made in this area was his advocacy of the routine removal of the pectoralis major muscle (in addition to the entire breast) and meticulous clearing of the axillary tissue. He performed all of these maneuvers as an en bloc resection to avoid cutting across any cancer-involved tissues. He firmly believed that cancer spread entirely through the lymphatics and not through the bloodstream, having been influenced by Heidenhain's studies that showed a high incidence of microscopic involvement of the pectoral muscles with tumor cells.[45]

Halsted first performed his "complete operation" at Roosevelt Hospital in New York City in 1882. In 1883 he used it in "almost every case" of breast carcinoma, and it ultimately became known as the *radical mastectomy*.[38] His first 13 cases were summarized in an article he published on wound healing in 1891.[45] In 1894 he published his landmark study that described in detail both the operation he developed and the follow-up results from his first 50 patients.[44] There were no operative deaths in this series. The local recurrence rate of 6% (3 of 50 patients) and the 3-year survival (cure) rate of 45% stood in stark contrast to all of Halsted's contemporaries', which he meticulously analyzed in this same report (Table 37-1). He achieved his results in spite of his finding that 27 of

the 50 patients had been labeled *hopeless* or *unfavorable* on presentation, that all had axillary node metastases, and that 10% had supraclavicular node metastases. By modern standards, his actual local recurrence rate was 18%. A follow-up study of this population by Lewis and Rienhoff in 1932[46] reported this local recurrence rate to have increased to 31.5%, which still represented a substantial improvement at that time. Another perspective was provided in 1980 by Henderson and Canellos,[47] whose analysis of Halsted's data showed only 8% disease-free survival (DFS) at 4 years and no more than a 12% overall improvement in survival. Halsted himself continued to update his results, which he perceived as vindication of his original premise and reinforcement of the prevalent concept of breast carcinoma as a disease that arises locally and spreads exclusively via the lymphatics.[20,48]

Halsted's radical mastectomy involved wide excision of skin through a teardrop incision extending across the deltopectoral groove onto the arm, excision of the entire pectoralis major muscle, and simple division of the pectoralis minor muscle to expose the axillary contents for dissection (Figure 37-4). By the time of his follow-up report in 1898, he had extended the operation routinely to include excision of the supraclavicular lymph nodes and pectoralis minor muscle and immediate skin graft of all wounds.[48] He learned this latter technique from Thiersch, in Germany, and was one of the few in the United States at that time to have mastered it. Halsted also described the dissection of mediastinal nodes by his house surgeon, Harvey Cushing, in three cases of recurrent breast carcinoma, prompting his prediction that this would probably be a routine part of the primary operation in the future.

In 1907 Halsted reported before the American Surgical Association an update of his results on 232 patients who

TABLE 37-1 | Results of Surgical Treatment of Breast Carcinoma up to 1894

SURGEON	TIME	CASES (n)	LOCAL RECURRENCE (%)	3-YEAR CURE (%)
Banks	1877	46	—	20
Bergmann	1882-1887	114	51-60	20
Billroth	1867-1876	170	82	4.7
Czerny	1877-1886	102	62	18.8
Fischer	1871-1878	147	75	—
Gussenbauer	1878-1886	151	64	—
Konig	1875-1885	152	58-62	—
Küster	1871-1885	228	59.6	21.5
Lucke	1881-1890	110	66	16.2
Volkmann	1874-1878	131	60	11
Halsted	1889-1894	50	6	45

Compiled from Halsted WS: *Johns Hopkins Hosp Rep* 4:297, 1894-1895; and Cooper WA: *Ann Med His* 3:36, 1941.

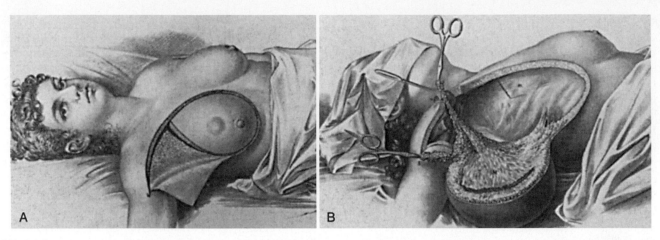

FIG. **37-4** **A** and **B**, Plates X and XI from Halsted's landmark 1894 paper (from Johns Hopkins Hospital Reports, 4:297, 1894-1895) showing his incision and dissection for the radical mastectomy. *(Courtesy Johns Hopkins Hospital.)*

underwent his complete operation at Johns Hopkins,[20] where he had served as professor of surgery since 1891. All patients in this series had been subjected to at least 3 years of follow-up. His operative mortality was 1.7% (4 patients), and only 18 patients had been lost to follow-up. The 27.6% of patients without axillary lymph node metastasis had substantially better outcomes than did those with nodal metastasis. Halsted was pessimistic in this paper about the efficacy of routine supraclavicular node dissection and had abandoned this practice for cases with no clinical evidence of axillary or neck disease.

This paper contained many of the fundamental precepts that are currently taken for granted. The number of recurrences found more than 3 years after primary treatment led Halsted to first advance the idea that perhaps at least 5 years of survival was a more appropriate measure of "cure." His data also clearly demonstrated the importance of axillary lymph node involvement as a prognostic factor and that the prognosis for breast carcinoma is related to its stage or level of advancement at the time of diagnosis and treatment. The poor outcome of patients with supraclavicular node involvement, regardless of the extent of surgery, suggested systemic dissemination.

All of these observations emphasized the advantages of early detection of breast carcinoma, a principle strongly advocated by Halsted and one of the most vigorous thrusts of current research[20]:

But women are now presenting themselves more promptly for examination, realizing that a cure of breast cancer is not only possible, but, if operated upon early, quite probable. Hence the surgeon is seeing smaller and still smaller tumors, cancers which give not one of the cardinal signs ... It would undoubtedly be possible for the expert to discover of the scirrhous growth earlier stages than he encounters, but unfortunately the tumor must first be recognized by the patient, and a scirrhous cancer large enough to attract her attention has quite surely already gone afield. Our problem, therefore, is to discover these tumors before the afflicted one can do so.

Halsted's operation resulted in the most significant improvement in survival and overall control of breast carcinoma that had occurred up to that time, which was reflected in its rapid and widespread adoption, by the turn of the century, as the standard treatment for this disease.[4] This was the first time in the long history of treatment of breast carcinoma that any single procedure was uniformly embraced. Halsted's 1907 paper, however, also contained the seeds of the eventual demise of the radical mastectomy some 70 years later. The fact that 23.4% of node-negative patients died of disseminated disease, despite having undergone the complete operation, provided the first indication that the theory of local origin does not adequately explain the underlying biology of this disease. Halsted was troubled by this observation. Further studies in subsequent years confirmed that more extensive local excision does not, in fact, improve the approximately 20% rate of relapse in patients with stage I disease.[49]

In 1894 a professor of surgery at the New York Postgraduate Medical School, Willy Meyer (1858-1932), reported the details of an operation very similar to Halsted's radical mastectomy before the Section on Surgery of the New York Academy of Medicine.[50] Meyer (Figure 37-5), born and educated in Germany, had independently conceived this operation based on the observations of Heidenhain and many of the other European surgeons who had also influenced Halsted. Meyer's report was given only 10 days after the publication of Halsted's landmark paper on the "complete operation," although Meyer had performed his first

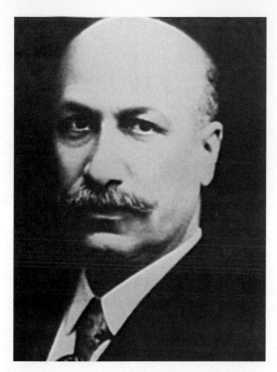

FIG. **37-5** Willy Meyer (1858-1932), German-born New York surgeon who conceived of and performed radical mastectomy independently of Halsted in 1894. *(From Ravitch MM: A century of surgery, vol 1, Philadelphia, 1980, JB Lippincott.)*

venture to hope that, by absolutely and continuously working everywhere around the seat of disease, by never trespassing on the belly of the muscles, and always removing the latter completely, this extremely gratifying result might also be secured by others.

Meyer published an update of the results of his operation after 10 years' experience with 72 procedures in 70 patients.[51] He reported 1.4% operative mortality. Of the 30 study patients with a 5- to 10-year follow-up, 8 (26.7%) were still alive, of whom 7 (23.3%) were disease free, and 1 had developed a regional recurrence 8 years after surgery. Thirty-five patients (52.3%) had died of their disease. Of those who died, 27 had distant metastases, accounting for 40.3% of all 67 traceable patients. Meyer concluded this paper, as he did in his original report, with an observation on the value of early detection[51]:

I am convinced that final results could be further improved only if we could get patients to come earlier for operation. The important task before us, therefore, is that of educating the public.... In view of the excellent results that can be obtained by radical operation ... physicians, too, should advise early operation, not only in the plainly recognizable cases, but also in the doubtful ones, rather than keep such patients under observation until the disease has become manifest beyond question, and, perhaps, developed to a stage where it is beyond surgical reach.

fully developed operation only 2 months before and had performed only six other similar operations since 1891. The basis of Meyer's operation, like Halsted's, was removal en bloc of the entire breast, pectoralis muscles, and axillary contents. He concluded[50]:

That this kind of radical operation will be "the" operation for the extirpation of carcinoma of the breast, there can be no doubt.... I

In the first decade of the twentieth century, several surgeons published their experiences with the radical mastectomy, indicating again how rapidly and widely it was accepted (Table 37-2). One of the most comprehensive such reports was published by J. Collins Warren of Boston in 1904,[52] describing the results of 100 consecutive cases of breast carcinoma accumulated during a 20-year period for which at least 3 years' follow-up was

| TABLE **37-2** | Results of Radical Operation for the Treatment of Breast Carcinoma Since 1904 |

AUTHOR	DATE	NO. OF CASES	OPERATIVE MORTALITY (%)	LOCOREGIONAL RECURRENCE (%)	5-YEAR SURVIVAL (%)
Warren[52]*	1904	100	2	6	12
Meyer[50]	1905	72	1.4	9	26.7
Greenough[54]*	1907	376	3.6	47.7	11.2
Halsted[20]	1907	232	1.7	19.5	30.9
Ochsner[53]*	1907	98	3	—	18.4
Lee et al[66]	1924	75	—	—	15
Harrington[68]	1929	2083	0.76	—	34
Jessop[105]	1936	217	3.2	—	48
Taylor and Wallace[57]	1950	2000	0.65	—	51

*Includes a mixture of cases, some of which were subjected to "complete" operations, others to lesser procedures.

available. There was only a 2% operative mortality among these patients. In following patients beyond 3 years, Warren found only a 12% cure rate at 5 years and 5% at 10 years, leading him to assert, "the 3-year limit does not by any means constitute an infallible test of cure." He found that 56% of all locoregional recurrences that occurred did so within 5 years of surgery, and 37% occurred within 2 years. This was perhaps the first indication that local recurrence is not necessarily the inevitable death sentence that past authors had suggested. A unique addition introduced by Warren was his insistence that a pathologist be present in the operating room throughout the procedure to confirm that all margins were free of tumor before the dissection was completed.

In 1907 Albert J. Ochsner of Chicago published the results of his surgical treatment of breast carcinoma in 98 patients who could be followed out of a total of 164 patients treated.[53] He reported 54 patients (55%) still alive at intervals of 1 to 13 years after surgery, 36 of these 54 patients having only a 5-year follow-up. Only 5 patients were alive 10 years or more after surgery. There was only 3% (5 of 164) operative mortality in this population (see Table 37-2). This paper typified the problems with many reports of this period in that it included patients with different stages of disease treated by different operative procedures.

Robert B. Greenough, a Boston surgeon on the faculty of Harvard Medical School, reported 416 primary operations for breast cancer, of which 376 patients (90%) could be traced for long-term follow-up.[54] The overall operative mortality was 3.6%, dropping from 5.1% in the first 5 years to only 2% in the last 5 years. The overall DFS rate at 3 years, excluding the palliative group, was 21%. In the last 5 years of the study, the DFS rate was 26%. The author noted that local recurrence was least likely to occur in those who had the widest and most complete primary resections. This paper documented several clinical features associated with a poor prognosis, all of which were later recognized to be ominous signs.[55,56] These included skin involvement, ulceration, axillary gland involvement, supraclavicular gland involvement (in which group there was not a single cure), bilateral cancer, and chest wall or axillary vein attachment.

In 1950 Taylor and Wallace updated this experience at Massachusetts General Hospital.[57] They analyzed 2500 cases of primary breast carcinoma, 2000 of whom had been treated by radical mastectomy. A greater degree of uniformity was apparent in this study population, because patients with Greenough's unfavorable factors were eliminated from study. The operative mortality decreased to 0.65%. They reported a 51% overall 5-year "cure" rate. Those without axillary node involvement

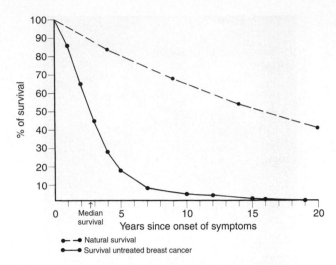

FIG. **37-6** Survival of women with untreated breast carcinoma. (*Modified from Bloom HJG et al:* BMJ *2:213, 1962.*)

had a 77% cure rate, whereas axillary involvement resulted in a 33% cure rate. Again, axillary node status was shown to be a significant prognostic factor. There was still a 76% cure rate when only one or two axillary nodes were involved.

These survival figures for breast cancer must be viewed in the context of what is known of the natural history of this disease. Bloom and associates in 1962 reviewed the clinical courses of 250 women with a confirmed diagnosis of breast carcinoma who had been admitted to the Middlesex Hospital Cancer Ward between 1805 and 1933 and were not treated.[58] He found a median survival of 2.7 years from onset of symptoms; 20% were alive at 5 years, 5% at 10 years, and approximately 1% were still alive at the end of 15 years (Figure 37-6). Thus in some series at the turn of this century radical mastectomy did not appear to affect survival at all.

THEORIES OF METASTATIC DISSEMINATION

The perceived means by which breast carcinoma spreads throughout the body has, appropriately, always influenced its primary surgical treatment. In the late nineteenth century, Thiersch and Waldeyer demonstrated that metastasis occurred through seeding of distant organs with cells of the primary tumor, by way of embolization through the lymphatics and bloodstream.[6] This formed the basis of the *mechanical theory* of tumor dissemination that was widely accepted at the beginning of the twentieth century.

William Sampson Handley (1872-1962), a British surgeon at London's Middlesex Hospital, made a meticulous study of the pathologic anatomy of the lymphatic circulation and cancer dissemination and applied his

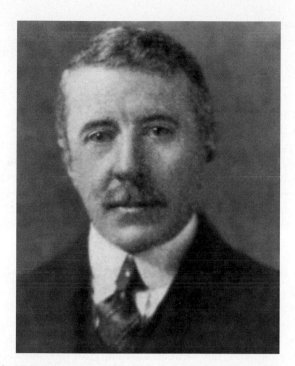

FIG. **37-7** William Sampson Handley (1872-1962), surgeon to Middlesex Hospital, whose permeation theory of breast cancer dissemination was embraced by Halsted. *(Courtesy Professor Irving Taylor, Department of Surgery, Middlesex Hospital, London, England.)*

observations to the clinical management of breast carcinoma (Figure 37-7). He believed that the lymphatics were the sole route by which this dissemination occurred, referring to earlier studies that indicated that bloodborne tumor cells are routinely destroyed because they stimulate a thrombotic process.[6,15] According to Handley's theory, regional lymph nodes act as filters for these permeating cancer cells, and only after the cells are able to grow beyond them are they capable of reaching the bloodstream for embolic spread. These principles contributed to the idea that breast cancer begins as a local process in the breast proper and then spreads in an orderly, incremental fashion first to the regional lymphatics and then to distant sites. This formed the conceptual basis for radical mastectomy because, according to this theory, complete ablation of all tissues through which the lymphatics travel provided the only chance of curing the disease as long as it had not already reached distant sites through the bloodstream. It also supported the practice of excising all tissues in continuity, so as not to cut across and disperse the tumor-filled regional lymphatics. Halsted embraced and endorsed Handley's theory, and its publication in Handley's first book on breast cancer in 1906 was a significant contribution to the management of this disease that affected surgical practice throughout the world.[4,20,59] Handley

recommended the modification of Halsted's operation to include smaller areas of skin and greater portions of the deep fascia, to more fully encompass the offending lymphatics.[2]

One of Halsted's major concerns, derived from the mechanical theory of tumor dissemination, was the danger of manipulating a breast tumor, especially for diagnostic purposes. Moore had voiced these same concerns some 30 years earlier. Halsted asserted[48]:

Tumors should never be harpooned, nor should pieces even be excised from malignant tumors for diagnostic purposes. Think of the danger of rapid dissemination of the growth from ... snipping off a piece of the tumor with scissors.

These concerns were supported by experimental evidence published in 1913 of tumor dissemination after manipulation of breast tumors in the Japanese waltzing mouse, although this was never corroborated in humans.[60]

The perceived necessity for a one-stage operation that encompassed both the diagnostic biopsy and a definitive procedure led to the development at Johns Hopkins of the frozen section examination. William H. Welch is credited with first using this technique in 1891 on a patient Halsted operated on for a benign breast tumor.[4]

Handley's permeation theory eventually was discredited in favor of the original theory of tumor cell embolization.[15] J. H. Gray showed in an extensive series of observations that cancer cells can be found only rarely along the entire course of a lymph channel, a well-known observation that Handley explained by postulating that an obliterative lymphangitis obscured cancer cells.[61,62] He also found that the deep fascia was virtually devoid of lymphatics, contrary to Handley's assertion. Abundant evidence also accumulated of the existence of cancer cells in the circulating blood, which is now believed to be the primary route of metastatic dissemination.[63] These changing attitudes toward the underlying biology of breast carcinoma were among many that in ensuing years led to a new appreciation of the extent of surgery necessary to control the disease.

RESULTS AND MODIFICATIONS OF RADICAL MASTECTOMY

Halsted made very little modification to his procedure during the 40 years that he performed it. Supraclavicular dissection, mediastinal dissection, and stripping of the fascia of the rectus and serratus muscles were all temporary additions that he eventually abandoned. In 1913 he published a fourth paper on breast cancer that summarized the technique and advantages of skin grafting in radical mastectomy, a part of the procedure to which he remained firmly committed.[38,64] His last paper, published in 1921, dealt with lymphedema of the arm after radical mastectomy.[65]

In 1924 Burton J. Lee, a surgeon at the Cornell Medical School in New York, published the first survival curve for treated breast carcinoma.[66] Of 87 cases, 75 were available for long-term follow-up, which showed a 15% 5-year recurrence-free survival. He advocated abandoning the 3-year standard for defining cure.

In 1929 Stuart W. Harrington of the Mayo Clinic updated the results of operation for primary breast carcinoma that had originally been reported by Judd and Sistrunk in 1914.[67,68] From 2083 operations, he reported an operative mortality of only 0.76%. Axillary lymph node involvement was confirmed to be "the most important factor in the prognosis" of breast carcinoma, a principle that has remained valid up to the present.[69-71] Harrington observed gradual improvement in survival from this operation up to 1915, which he attributed to "improvement and standardization of technic and the gradual increase of the operative procedure." After 1915 these results reached a plateau, indicating the limits of surgery for the disease. There was an 80% 3-year survival rate and a 53% 10-year survival rate among those treated with primary radical operation who had no axillary node involvement. These were the best results obtained up to that time.

Harrington made several observations in this paper that were to become important issues in the future. A group of 112 patients who had undergone inadequate forms of treatment before having a radical operation at the Mayo Clinic had substantially lower survival rates than those who underwent radical operation initially, demonstrating the validity of Moore's original thesis published more than 60 years earlier. For 51 patients with bilateral malignancy, the second malignancy did not have any additional adverse effect on survival. In 1092 cases, adding "roentgen ray" treatment to radical operation produced no demonstrable survival benefit, which was to be expected with the state of knowledge at that time.

Harrington understood that radiation therapy was strictly a modality for local control of disease and not a substitute for an incomplete or poorly executed operation. Because breast cancer is a systemic illness that ultimately kills, radiation treatment should have no effect on survival.

Harrington[68] also emphasized the benefits of early detection of disease, which were evident in his statistics relating survival to lymph node involvement. He stated:

The results in these cases can be greatly improved if operation is performed early in the course of the disease. If operation is delayed until the signs of malignancy are obvious, it is too late to expect much more than a palliative result. There are few, if any, single tumors of the breast in which delay in the institution of treatment is safe for the patient, and few physicians care to assume the responsibility of determining the presence or absence of malignancy by the physical characteristics of the tumor.

In 1927 William Sampson Handley (see Figure 37-7), still devoting his career at London's Middlesex Hospital to the investigation of breast carcinoma, published a report that revived an awareness of the internal mammary and mediastinal lymph node chains as a route of metastatic dissemination.[72] He observed that despite the lower incidence of local recurrence (especially in the axilla) following radical mastectomy, involvement of axillary lymph nodes with tumor was still predictive of death from disseminated disease. Most of the recurrences in his patients occurred along the sternal border of the excised breast. He concluded that these lymph nodes must be seeded with microscopic deposits of tumor quite early in the course of the disease. The extent of surgical treatment would have no effect on outcome for these patients unless the nodes were also treated. Handley did not believe that surgical excision was appropriate, in view of the time and morbidity it added to the radical mastectomy, but he did advocate routine placement of radium tubes along the sternal border as an adjunct to mastectomy. This practice resulted in improved DFS at 3 years. He also noted that local recurrences only rarely occurred in the sites where radium had been inserted.

After World War II, Handley's son, Richard S. Handley (1909-1984), published the results of his practice of routine biopsy of the internal mammary lymph nodes in all cases of breast carcinoma.[73] Among 119 patients, these nodes were involved with metastases in 34% of patients overall and in 48% of those with axillary lymph node metastasis. He believed this explained both the recurrence of disease when radical mastectomy is performed for early lesions and the fact that the lungs and pleura are the most common sites of distant metastasis.

The implications of Handley's observations that one third of all mastectomies are doomed to failure from the start led some surgeons to recommend treating breast carcinoma with an "extended" radical mastectomy, which included en bloc resection of the internal mammary lymph nodes. The first to do this routinely was the Italian surgeon Margottini in 1948, although Halsted had described this being done in three cases by his house surgeon, Harvey Cushing, in 1898.[48,74]

In 1952 Jerome Urban published his initial experience with radical mastectomy in continuity with en bloc internal mammary dissection at Memorial Hospital in New York.[75] He developed this procedure after observing that more than 70% of chest wall recurrences after radical mastectomy occurred in the medial parasternal area.[76] Although the short follow-up period did not allow any assessment of survival, Urban postulated significant improvement and even considered extending the procedure to supraclavicular dissection.

Wangensteen, Lewis, and Arhelger[77] had already been performing a "superradical" mastectomy, including supraclavicular, internal mammary, and mediastinal lymph node dissection. They found that 58% of their cases of operable breast carcinoma had internal mammary node involvement, but they were unable to demonstrate any significant improvement in survival with this procedure. Because of a 12.5% operative mortality, they abandoned the procedure for treating breast carcinoma.

Other series also demonstrated either no difference in overall results between simple mastectomy plus postoperative irradiation and extended radical mastectomy, or simply failure of internal mammary node dissection to improve survival.[78] These extended procedures never became widely accepted because of the absence of any clear benefit despite the substantial added risk; however, they are still used selectively in some centers.

During these same years the bilaterality of breast carcinoma became evident in a small percentage of cases, and victims of such disease were at greater risk of a second malignancy developing metachronously in the contralateral breast. In 1951 Pack advocated bilateral mastectomy for any unilateral breast malignancy, an idea that has continued to be sporadically advocated.[79] Robbins and Berg demonstrated that the cumulative risk of developing clinically evident contralateral breast carcinoma following ipsilateral disease was less than 1% per year, which is less than the incidence of clinically occult carcinoma in the opposite breast detected by routine blind biopsy.[80] Metachronous contralateral breast carcinomas have been shown to have no adverse impact on ultimate survival over that of the original primary breast carcinoma, perhaps owing to the more aggressive mammographic surveillance of these women, which results in earlier detection of these second lesions.[81]

BIOLOGY AND DETECTION OF EARLY BREAST CANCER

The potential improvement in survival through the detection of breast cancer in its earliest stages of development had been suggested by several investigators through the centuries, including Celsus, Severinus, LeDran, Fearon, Banks, Halsted, Meyer, and Harrington.* Since Astley Cooper first reported an association between benign breast changes and carcinoma in 1845, numerous clinical investigators have provided evidence that certain benign breast lesions progress to malignancy.[82] These observations led to the "transition

theory" of breast cancer development.[82,83] It has since been firmly established that epithelial hyperplasia, especially atypical hyperplasia, is the benign change that leads to breast cancer, although this progression is nonobligate.[82,84-89]

According to the transition theory, all cases of invasive breast carcinoma traverse a stage in which previously normal epithelial cells of the breast become malignant but have not yet invaded beyond their confining basement membranes.[89a] Several authors of the late nineteenth and early twentieth centuries published illustrations of the histology of this "noninvasive" stage of breast malignancy. Cheatle and Cutler asserted, "in these instances there is no doubt that these epithelial cells inside the normal boundaries are as histologically malignant as those that have transgressed them and are trespassing in the surrounding tissues."[90] In 1932 Broders first applied the term *in situ carcinoma* to this intermediate, noninvasive stage of cancer development, recognizing it as an independent entity, distinct from its benign precursors and invasive counterparts.[91] Broders also recognized the important opportunity for improved survival offered through detection of malignancy at this still-localized stage. This opportunity would not be exploited to any significant extent for breast cancers for another 50 years.

Joseph Colt Bloodgood (Figure 37-8), a surgeon at Johns Hopkins Hospital in the early twentieth century,

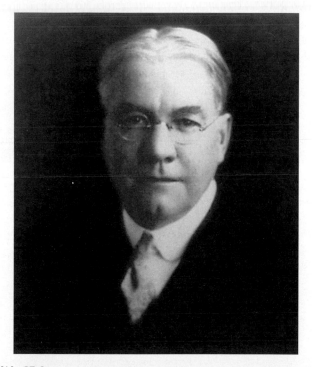

FIG. **37-8** Dr. Joseph Colt Bloodgood, who made important observations on the biology of early breast malignancies. *(Courtesy Johns Hopkins Hospital.)*

---

*References 2, 3, 6-8, 13, 16, 17, 20, 51, 68.

published several investigations of the biology and clinical behavior of the earliest forms of ductal carcinoma of the breast, which he termed "borderline breast tumors."[92] His histologic illustrations are now recognized as typical examples of ductal carcinoma in situ of the breast. Bloodgood was the first to describe both the excellent prognosis for this lesion and the importance of public education for improving survival from breast cancer by detecting it in this earliest noninvasive stage.[93]

The most effective modality for detecting breast carcinoma in its earliest forms, when treatment promises to be most successful, had its beginnings as early as 1913. Salomon then first applied radiography to the study of breasts.[94] By 1960 Egan demonstrated this new technique of mammography to be sufficiently effective and standardized to be clinically applicable to a large population.[95] Several prospective randomized trials over the next 30 years consistently demonstrated that routine mammographic screening detects breast carcinoma at an earlier stage and, consequently, leads to as much as a 46% reduction in mortality, compared with standard physical examination.[18,19]

The increasing use of mammography in the United States during the 1980s resulted in substantial changes in the techniques used by surgeons to diagnose breast carcinoma. Standard open surgical biopsies could no longer be performed on the progressively smaller and nonpalpable lesions detected by mammography. Needle localization biopsy with specimen radiography evolved as the most common method to accurately localize and sample nonpalpable mammographically detected breast lesions (see Chapters 31 and 38).[96] The effectiveness of this technique at early diagnosis of breast cancer has been demonstrated in several published series that report an average yield of carcinoma in situ among all malignancies of more than 43% and fewer than 15% of invasive lesions that have axillary metastases (Table 37-3). These results are clearly superior to those of physical examination alone.[97]

Thanks largely to mammography, more than 80% of all breast carcinoma lesions in the United States are now smaller than 2 cm at the time of diagnosis. Early detection is therefore one of the most important factors that made possible the treatment of breast carcinoma with less extensive surgical procedures than were used in the first half of the twentieth century.

EMERGENCE OF LESS EXTENSIVE OPERATIVE PROCEDURES

The basic flaw in the theory of local disease origin was quickly manifested by the fact that surgery alone did not consistently yield high rates of cure, regardless of how extensive the procedure or early the diagnosis. Although survival at 3 years appeared to show an improvement over that with earlier procedures, longer follow-up revealed steadily diminishing rates. The efforts of many surgeons to extend the scope of the radical mastectomy indicated their recognition of its inadequacy as the sole treatment for breast carcinoma.

Lane-Claypon published the first epidemiologic analysis of the results of surgical treatment of breast carcinoma in 1928 and concluded that whatever improvement in survival may exist was primarily attributable to earlier diagnosis rather than to the radical mastectomy itself.[98] In a retrospective review of 20,000 operations for breast carcinoma in the medical literature, she showed

| TABLE 37-3 | Results of Biopsy of Nonpalpable Mammographically Detected Breast Lesions—1986-1992 |

INVESTIGATOR	NO. OF BIOPSIES (n)	MALIGNANCIES (n)	MALIGNANCIES (%)	IN SITU (n)	IN SITU (%)*	AXILLARY METASTASIS (n)	AXILLARY METASTASIS (%)†
Bauer et al[183]	2077	286	14	82	29	29/251	12
Franceschi et al[184]	1144	269	24	98	36.5	31/171	18
Landercasper et al[185]	203	44	22	29	66	5/24	21
Marrujo et al[186]	237	64	27	23	36	7/54	13
Perdue et al[187]	536	96	18	48	50	4/41	10
Poole et al[188]	148	21	14	5	24	3/19	16
Shroff et al[189]	246	43	17.5	13	30	5/31	16
Silverstein et al[190]	653	147	22.5	88	60	6/127	5
Skinner et al[191]	179	41	23	9	22	7/30	23
Symmonds et al[193]	499	72	14	13	18	7/62	11
Wilhelm et al[192]	1464	264	18	178	67	18/78	23
TOTALS	7386	1347	18	586	43.5	122/888	13.7

*Percentage of all malignancies.
†Ratio (percentage) of cases of axillary metastasis to number of cases treated with axillary dissection.

43% 3-year survival and 33% 5-year survival for those subjected to radical mastectomy. Those treated with less extensive operations had 3-year survival of only 29%. Also shown was a twofold increase in survival in the absence of lymph node involvement.[7]

The noted New York pathologist James Ewing was also pessimistic about the true value of radical mastectomy during this period, agreeing that the relatively good survival in most reports was more likely attributable to early detection than to the surgery. He was concerned that this operation was being performed too often for relatively harmless and sometimes benign lesions, whereas ultimately it seemed to make little difference to mortality for those with very aggressive and advanced lesions.[4,99]

The pessimistic extreme was represented by Park and Lees, who in 1950 published an extensive and elegant analysis of treatment results for breast carcinoma.[100] They cautioned that the variability of individual tumor growth rates may render survival rates meaningless and that the available forms of treatment were unlikely to alter mortality rates, because the rates were largely related to distant metastases. They concluded that there was no firm evidence that treatment had any effect whatsoever on survival.

The evident shortcomings of surgical treatment of breast carcinoma led some to consider using less extensive procedures in conjunction with other modalities to spare patients unnecessary tissue loss. Radiation therapy was one of the first adjunctive modalities applied to breast carcinoma for this purpose, having first been used in this way by Emile Grubbe in Chicago within 2 months of the discovery of x-rays by Wilhelm Roentgen in 1895.[101] In 1917 Janeway described the use of interstitial irradiation instead of mastectomy for operable breast carcinoma, finding it an acceptable alternative for patients who refused surgery or for those tumors that were not amenable to surgical ablation.[102]

Geoffrey Keynes, a surgeon at St. Bartholomew's Hospital in London, began applying radium needles to the treatment of breast carcinoma in 1922.[4,15] He treated only advanced, inoperable cases at first but extended the use of the procedure as success became evident. In 1932 Keynes reported 171 cases treated during a 7-year period, pointing out some of the harmful effects of this method on both patient and physician.[103] In this report he also first speculated that radium might be more efficacious if the bulk of the tumor were first surgically removed. Several patients had been subjected to this combination of surgery and radiotherapy by 1937, when Keynes published his results from 250 patients for whom at least a 3-year follow-up was available.[104] Pathologic staging was not possible, because axillary dissections were not performed. There was a 71.4% 5-year survival rate for these patients and a 29% 5-year

TABLE 37-4	Grave Signs of Inoperability in Patients with Breast Carcinoma
Matted, enlarged, or fixed axillary nodes	
Skin edema	
Skin ulceration	
Chest wall fixation	
Matted, enlarged, or fixed axillary nodes	
Satellite skin nodules	
Supraclavicular node enlargement	
Arm edema	
Inflammatory carcinoma	

Data from Greenough et al: *Surg Gynecol Obstet* 3:39, 1907; and Haagensen CD, Stout AP: *Ann Surg* 118:859, 1032, 1943.

survival for those judged clinically to be stage II at presentation. This compared with 69% stage I and 30.5% stage II 5-year survivals among patients subjected to surgery alone, as reported in a contemporary series by Jessop.[105] This demonstrated for the first time the possibility that less extensive surgical ablation of breast carcinoma may provide acceptable results.[106]

Haagensen and Stout in 1943 defined the clinical features of breast carcinoma that predicted a poor outcome after radical mastectomy in terms of a prohibitively high rate of local recurrence and poor overall survival (Table 37-4).[55,56] Such cases were considered inoperable. This report recognizes the same limitations of surgery (especially for locally advanced disease) that such authorities as Banks, Moore, Petit, LeDran, and Hippocrates had espoused in centuries past.

After World War II, efforts to investigate the feasibility of less extensive operative procedures for breast carcinoma continued. High-voltage external-beam radiation was developed, allowing more effective and safer delivery of radiation to the breast with better cosmetic results. In 1948 Robert McWhirter, a surgeon at the Royal Infirmary in Edinburgh, Scotland, published the results of treatment of 1345 patients who presented with breast carcinoma between 1941 and 1945.[107] Simple mastectomy and radiotherapy were carried out in 757 patients whose disease appeared clinically to be localized to the breast. The surgery involved only limited skin excision and limited undermining of flaps, with no axillary dissection in the absence of clinically palpable nodes. Radiation was applied to the chest wall, axilla, and supraclavicular fields in a minimum dose of 3750 rad over 3 weeks. The 5-year survival rate for these patients was 62.1%, which was substantially better than that for women treated with radical mastectomy alone in most series.

McWhirter emphasized the validity of study techniques that are necessary to identify optimal treatment

die of the disease whatever combination of local treatment by surgery and irradiation is used, because in such a high proportion of cases the disease has passed outside the field of local attack when the patient first comes for treatment.

The abundant experimental and clinical evidence that has emerged in support of this hypothesis has led to the current acceptance of a diminished emphasis on locoregional treatment of this disease, as discussed previously, whereas systemically oriented modalities have been increasingly emphasized. Hormone manipulation was the first systemic therapy applied to breast carcinoma when Sir George Beatson of Glasgow performed oophorectomy for an advanced case in 1896.[153] Since then, hormone therapies of various types have continued to be used, showing promising, although less than optimal, results.[154] Cytotoxic chemotherapy became popular in the late 1950s and has since become a mainstay of adjuvant systemic therapy following surgical treatment and, as such, has demonstrated better survival than surgery alone.[49,155] Advances in molecular biology have led to the discovery of oncogenes, which offer the opportunity of perhaps manipulating the process of malignancy to prevent it altogether.[156] Adoptive immunotherapy is another form of systemic treatment involving the application of the lymphokine interleukin-2 to activate "killer" lymphocytes with antitumor activity; this is currently being investigated for clinical use and may represent the next generation of treatment for breast carcinoma.[157]

The surgeon has become an integral part of a multidisciplinary team who manages patients with breast carcinoma. This team includes the diagnostic radiologist, radiation oncologist, medical oncologist, and pathologist. The surgeon's role has evolved to diagnosing and ensuring the removal of all clinically evident disease so as to maximize the efficacy of radiation and systemic therapy. All members of this team must be committed to the total patient and to a thorough understanding of the disease process and of management options. Mastectomy is still a valid, and sometimes preferable, option for operable (stage I and II) breast carcinoma, as well as most cases of locally advanced disease judged to be amenable to operation.

In the future, axillary dissection may assume diminished importance for treatment of breast carcinoma. Recent studies have demonstrated that there is no survival advantage to the routine removal of axillary lymph nodes and that the only therapeutic advantage of this practice is a substantial reduction in the rate of regional axillary recurrence.[158,159] The clinical significance of axillary lymph node involvement, beyond its prognostic implications, has also been questioned.[159] It would therefore seem reasonable, because of the absence of data to suggest any detriment to survival, to perform axillary dissection only in patients who have palpable adenopathy or who develop such adenopathy after primary treatment.[160-162] However, most investigators still advocate routine axillary dissection in the treatment of primary breast carcinoma, in view of some persistent uncertainty as to benefit.[163-165] Sentinel lymph node biopsy has evolved as a reasonable compromise and is being used increasingly by surgeons (see Chapter 51).

The therapeutic challenge posed by noninvasive breast carcinoma will be faced increasingly in the future because of more frequent detection of these lesions, owing to the current emphasis on early detection of breast carcinoma and the use of mammography. In situ breast malignancies may be the one form of this disease that may still be governed by the precepts of the local origin theory, because by definition systemic dissemination should not yet have occurred at this stage (see Chapters 11, 48, and 49). Aggressive local treatment alone may thus be curative, as has been demonstrated in a number of studies.[19] The evidence of the natural history of lobular carcinoma in situ currently available suggests that it may best be managed expectantly and may be more of a marker of increased risk for future development of invasive carcinoma than an actual precursor of stage I.[166] Ductal carcinoma in situ appears to be a more ominous lesion that requires definitive surgery, although breast-sparing procedures with postoperative irradiation result in survival rates comparable with those of total mastectomy, which, as would be predicted at this stage of disease, approach 100%.[19,167]

Although mammography has resulted in the detection of early malignancies that appear to be highly curable, 80% of biopsies of nonpalpable breast lesions are currently benign (see Table 37-3). This has led to an emphasis on a more selective approach to biopsy of mammographic lesions to improve the yield of malignancies without missing any.[168] Nonoperative observation of certain mammographic lesions has been shown to be safe when followed reliably for interval change.[169] This finding promises to reduce substantially the number of unnecessary surgical biopsies and improve the cost-effectiveness of diagnosis of breast carcinoma (see Chapter 33).

Fine-needle aspiration (FNA) biopsy, introduced in 1930 for cytologic tissue diagnosis, assumed an increasingly prominent role in the diagnosis of breast masses during the 1980s.[170] It is now the recommended diagnostic modality of choice for palpable breast masses and has been applied successfully to the diagnosis of nonpalpable breast masses.[171] Stereotactic devices have also been successfully applied to the diagnosis of nonpalpable breast lesions, using either FNA biopsy or core biopsy techniques.[172,173] The accuracy of these methods is entirely comparable to that of open surgical biopsy, and they also promise to reduce the need for diagnostic surgery of breast lesions that carry an intermediate risk for malignancy.[173]

Locally advanced carcinoma of the breast is no longer considered inoperable, as originally asserted by Haagensen and Stout.[55,56] The introduction of multi-modality treatment, including preoperative induction, or neoadjuvant, chemotherapy followed by mastectomy and postoperative chemotherapy and radiation therapy, has greatly improved the resectability of these complex breast tumors, their local control, and these patients' survival.[174,175] Compelling evidence has also been reported that the substantial shrinking of these cancers afforded by neoadjuvant chemotherapy allows even breast conservation to be applied safely and successfully to them.[176-180]

Despite the abundance of compelling data from numerous prospective randomized trials on the validity and safety of breast conservation treatment of breast carcinoma,[141,143-146] only about 12% of all patients, and fewer than 30% of women with the most favorable T_1 tumors, receive this treatment in the United States.[181,182] This is largely a result of the reluctance of surgeons to abandon mastectomy, as well as to unfounded fears of radiation therapy on the part of patients. Widespread education of both surgeons and patients is needed if breast conservation is to achieve its full potential.[182]

As we come to the end of the twentieth century, breast carcinoma is increasingly regarded as a systemic disease. This same concept was shared by Imhotep, Hippocrates, Galen, and Hunter at the crest of many other cycles of belief and practice. Although these swings in philosophy during the past several centuries may appear arbitrary, they have actually occurred in response to advances in clinical experience and scientific knowledge. It is likely that the remarkable rate of scientific advances currently being made in this field will result in further shifts in conceptual and practical approaches to breast carcinoma in the future. We can hope that this cycle will culminate in an ideal management regimen for this complex disease process. This sentiment was expressed by Lewison in 1953[3]:

> The soundest predication of future progress must come from a realistic view of the past. Only by carefully examining our present precepts and practice can we intelligently plan for the future. Our resolute purpose must always be to promote the best interest of each individual patient, and not those of surgery, radiotherapy or chemotherapy.

Bernard Fisher, among others, has much contributed to achieving this purpose by developing and establishing the clinical trial, as McWhirter[108] had recommended. Such trials become the primary tool for testing hypotheses and determining optimal treatment for breast carcinoma. Fisher has asserted thus[49]:

Therapeutic strategies for breast cancer have evolved over time in step-wise fashion and are the result of biological information, which has led to a better understanding of this disease. It is logical to anticipate that this course will continue and that future gains will occur as a result of the testing of new biological hypotheses. Breast cancer management has been, is, and will be related to science and not to populism!

Interestingly enough, Fisher's sentiment on this issue closely echoes one of Virchow's many dictums, stated in 1896, as cited by DeMoulin[7]:

> Indeed, a great deal of industrious work is being done and the microscope is extensively used, but someone should have another bright idea!

This impatience with the status quo and commitment to shed light on the unknown will continue to advance the frontiers of our knowledge of breast carcinoma.

REFERENCES

1. Breasted JH: *The Edwin Smith surgical papyrus,* vol 1, Chicago, 1930, University of Chicago Press.
2. Cooper WA: The history of the radical mastectomy, *Ann Med Hist* 3:36, 1941.
3. Lewison EF: The surgical treatment of breast cancer: an historical and collective review, *Surgery* 34:904, 1953.
4. Robinson JO: Treatment of breast cancer through the ages, *Am J Surg* 151:317, 1986.
5. Herodotus: *The histories,* New York, 1967, Penguin.
6. Wilder RJ: The historical development of the concept of metastasis, *J Mt Sinai Hosp* 23:728, 1954.
7. De Moulin D: *A short history of breast cancer,* Boston, 1983, Martinus Nijhoff.
8. Celsus AM: *De medicina,* vol 2, Cambridge, 1953, Harvard University Press (Translated by WG Spencer).
9. Galen: De tumoribus praeter naturam. In Kuhn CG (ed): *Opera omnia,* vol 7, Lipsiae, 1821, C Knobloch.
10. Power D: The history of the amputation of the breast to 1904, *Liverpool Med Chir J* 42:29, 1934.
11. deMondeville H: *Die chirurgie des heinrich demondeville,* Berlin, 1892, A Hirschwald.
12. Wolff J: *Die lehre von der krebskrankenheit,* vol 1, Jena, 1907, G Fischer.
13. Banks WM: A brief history of the operations practised for cancer of the breast, *BMJ* 1:5, 1902.
14. Fabry W: *Observationum et curationum chirurgicarum centuriae,* cent II, Lugduni, 1641, IA Huguetan.
15. Keynes G: Carcinoma of the breast: a brief historical survey of the treatment, *St Bartholomew's Hosp J* 56:462, 1952.
16. Dobson J: John Hunter's views on cancer, *Ann R Coll Surg Engl* 1:176, 1959.
17. LeDran F: Memoire avec une precis de plusiers observations sur le cancer, *Mem Acad R Chir Paris* 3:1, 1757.
18. Shapiro S et al: Ten-to-fourteen year effect of screening on breast cancer mortality, *J Natl Cancer Inst* 69:349, 1982.
19. Seidman H et al: Survival experience in the Breast Cancer Detection Demonstration Project, *CA Cancer J Clin* 37:258, 1987.
20. Halsted WS: The results of radical operations for the cure of carcinoma of the breast, *Ann Surg* 46:1, 1907.

21. Petit JL: *Oeuvres completes,* section VII, Limoges, 1837, R Chapoulard.
22. Heister L: *General system of surgery,* part II, section 4, London, 1745, Innys.
23. Peyrilhe B: *Dissertatio academia de cancro,* Paris, 1774, De Hansy Jeune.
24. Degenshein GA, Ceccarelli F: The history of breast cancer surgery, part 1: early beginnings to Halsted, *Breast* 3:28, 1977.
25. Bell B: *A system of surgery,* vol 5, Edinburgh, 1791, Bell & Bradfute.
26. Doets CJ: De heelkunde van petrus camper 1722-1789, thesis, Leiden, 1948.
27. Monro A: Collections of blood in cancerous breasts. In *The works of Alexander Monro: published by his son Alexander Monro,* Edinburgh, 1781, Ch. Elliot.
28. Syme J: *Principles of surgery,* London, 1842, H Balliere.
29. Paget J: On the average duration of life in patients with scirrhous cancer of the breast, *Lancet* 1:62, 1856.
30. Pancoast J: *A treatise on operative surgery,* Philadelphia, 1852, R Hart.
31. Moore CH: On the influence of inadequate operations on the theory of cancer, *R Med Chir Soc London* 1:244, 1867.
32. Sweeting R: A new operation for cancer of the breast, *Lancet* 1:323, 1869.
33. Lister J: *Collected papers,* vol 2, Oxford, 1909, Clarendon Press.
34. Banks WM: A plea for the more free removal of cancerous growths, *Liverpool Manchester Surg Rep* 192, 1878.
35. Küster E: Zur behandlung des brustkrebses, *Arch Klin Chir* 29:723, 1883.
36. Schmid H: Zur statisk der mammacarcinome und der heitung, *Dtsch Z Chir* 26:139, 1887.
37. Billroth T: *Die krankheiten der brust drusen,* Stuttgart, 1880, F Enke.
38. Haagensen CD: The history of the surgical treatment of breast carcinoma from 1863-1921. In Haagensen CD (ed): *Diseases of the breast,* ed 3, Philadelphia, 1986, WB Saunders.
39. Volkmann R: *Beitrage zur chirurgie,* Leipzig, 1875, Breitkoff und Hartel.
40. Heidenhain L: Ueber die ursachen der localen krebsrecidive nach amputation mammae, *Arch Klin Chir* 39:97, 1889.
41. Gross SW: An analysis of two hundred and seven cases of carcinoma of the breast, *Med News* 51:613, 1887.
42. Korteweg JA: Die statistischen resultate der amputation des brustkrebses, *Arch Klin Chir* 38:679, 1889.
43. Korteweg JA: Carcinoom en statistiek, *Ned Tijdschr Geneeskd* 39:1054, 1903.
44. Halsted WS: The results of operations for the cure of cancer of the breast performed at the Johns Hopkins Hospital from June 1889 to January 1894, *Johns Hopkins Hosp Rep* 4:297, 1894-1895.
45. Halsted WS: The treatment of wounds with especial reference to the value of the blood clot in the management of dead spaces, *Johns Hopkins Hosp Rep* 2:255, 1890-1891.
46. Lewis D, Rienhoff WF: A study of the results of operations for cure of cancer of the breast performed at the Johns Hopkins Hospital from 1889-1931, *Ann Surg* 95:336, 1932.
47. Henderson IC, Canellos GP: Cancer of the breast: the past decade, *N Engl J Med* 302:17, 1980.
48. Halsted WS: A clinical and histological study of certain adenocarcinomata of the breast: and a brief consideration of the supraclavicular operation and of the results of operations for cancer of the breast from 1889 to 1898 at the Johns Hopkins Hospital, *Ann Surg* 28:557, 1898.
49. Fisher B et al: The contribution of recent NSABP clinical trials of primary breast cancer therapy to an understanding of tumor biology: an overview of findings, *Cancer* 46:1009, 1980.
50. Meyer W: An improved method of the radical operation for carcinoma of the breast, *Med Rec* 46:746, 1894.
51. Meyer W: Carcinoma of the breast: ten years' experience with my method of radical operation, *JAMA* 45:297, 1905.
52. Warren JC: The operative treatment of cancer of the breast: with an analysis of a series of one hundred consecutive cases, *Ann Surg* 40:805, 1904.
53. Ochsner AJ: Final results in 164 cases of carcinoma of the breast operated upon during the past fourteen years at the Augustana Hospital, *Ann Surg* 46:28, 1907.
54. Greenough RB, Simmons CC, Barney JD: The results of operations for cancer of the breast at the Massachusetts General Hospital from 1894-1904, *Surg Gynecol Obstet* 3:39, 1907.
55. Haagensen CD, Stout AP: Carcinoma of the breast. I. Criteria of operability, *Ann Surg* 118:859, 1943.
56. Haagensen CD, Stout AP: Carcinoma of the breast. II. Criteria of operability, *Ann Surg* 118:1032, 1943.
57. Taylor GW, Wallace RH: Carcinoma of the breast: fifty years experience at the Massachusetts General Hospital, *Ann Surg* 132:833, 1950.
58. Bloom HJG, Richardson WW, Harries EJ: Natural history of untreated breast cancer (1805-1933), *BMJ* 2:213, 1962.
59. Handley WS: *Cancer of the breast,* ed 2, New York, 1906, Paul B Hoeber.
60. Tyzzer EE: Factors in the production and growth of tumor metastases, *J Med Res* 28:309, 1913.
61. Handley WS: *Cancer of the breast and its operative treatment,* London, 1922, John Murray.
62. Gray JH: The relation of lymphatic vessels to the spread of cancer, *Br J Surg* 26:462, 1938.
63. Engell HC: Cancer cells in the circulating blood, *Acta Chir Scand* 201(suppl):1, 1955.
64. Halsted WS: Developments in the skin grafting operation for cancer of the breast, *JAMA* 60:416, 1913.
65. Halsted WS: The swelling of the arm after operations for cancer of the breast—elephantiasis chirurgica—its cause and prevention, *Bull Johns Hopkins Hosp* 32:309, 1921.
66. Ravitch MM: *A century of surgery,* vol I, Philadelphia, 1980, JB Lippincott.
67. Judd ES, Sistrunk WE: End-results in operation for cancer of the breast, *Surg Gynecol Obstet* 28:289, 1914.
68. Harrington SW: Carcinoma of the breast: surgical treatment and results, *JAMA* 92:208, 1929.
69. Valagussa P, Bonadonna G, Veronesi U: Patterns of relapse and survival following radical mastectomy, *Cancer* 41:1170, 1978.
70. Fisher B et al: Relationship of number of positive axillary nodes to the prognosis of patients with primary breast cancer: an NSABP update, *Cancer* 52:1551, 1983.
71. Sutherland CM, Mather FJ: Long-term survival and prognostic factors in breast cancer patients with localized (no skin, muscle, or chest wall attachment) disease with and without positive lymph nodes, *Cancer* 57:622, 1986.
72. Handley WS: *Cancer of the breast and its operative treatment,* London, 1922, John Murray.
73. Handley RS, Thackray AC: Internal mammary lymph chain in carcinoma of the breast: study of 50 cases, *Lancet* 2:276, 1949.
74. Margottini M: Recent developments in the surgical treatment of breast cancer, *Acta Unio Int Contra Cancrum* 8:176, 1952.

75. Urban JA: Radical excision of the chest wall for mammary cancer, *Cancer* 4:1263, 1951.

76. Urban JA, Baker HW: Radical mastectomy in continuity with en bloc resection of the internal mammary lymph-node chain: a new procedure for primary operable cancer of the breast, *Cancer* 5:992, 1952.

77. Wangensteen OH, Lewis FJ, Arhelger SW: The extended or super-radical mastectomy for carcinoma of the breast, *Surg Clin North Am* 36:1051, 1956.

78. Veronesi U, Valagussa P: Inefficacy of internal mammary node dissection in breast cancer surgery, *Cancer* 47:170, 1981.

79. Pack GT: Argument for bilateral mastectomy, *Surgery* 29:929, 1951.

80. Robbins GF, Berg JW: Bilateral primary breast cancers: a prospective clinicopathological study, *Cancer* 17:1501, 1964.

81. Singletary SE et al: Occurrence and prognosis of contralateral carcinoma of the breast, *J Am Coll Surg* 178:390, 1994.

82. Gallager HS, Martin JE: Early phases in the development of breast cancer, *Cancer* 24:1170, 1969.

83. Gallager HS, Martin JE: An orientation to the concept of minimal breast cancer, *Cancer* 28:1505, 1971.

84. Fisher ER, Shoemaker RH, Palekar AS: Identification of premalignant hyperplasia in methyl-cholanthrene–induced mammary tumorigenesis, *Lab Invest* 33:446, 1975.

85. Gullino PM: Natural history of breast cancer: progression from hyperplasia to neoplasia as predicted by angiogenesis, *Cancer* 39:2697, 1977.

86. Fisher ER: The impact of pathology on the biologic, diagnostic, prognostic, and therapeutic considerations in breast cancer, *Surg Clin North Am* 64:1073, 1984.

87. Gump FE: Premalignant diseases of the breast, *Surg Clin North Am* 64:1051, 1984.

88. Dupont WD, Page DL: Risk factors in women with proliferative breast disease, *N Engl J Med* 312:146, 1985.

89. Page DL et al: Atypical hyperplastic lesions of the female breast: a long-term follow-up study, *Cancer* 55:2698, 1985.

89a. Rosen PP: Lobular carcinoma in situ and intraductal carcinoma of the breast, *Monogr Pathol* 25:59, 1984.

90. Cheatle GL, Cutler M: *Tumors of the breast,* Philadelphia, 1931, JB Lippincott.

91. Broders AC: Carcinoma in situ contrasted with benign penetrating epithelium, *JAMA* 99:1670, 1932.

92. Bloodgood JC: Borderline breast tumors, *Ann Surg* 93:235, 1931.

93. Bloodgood JC: Cancer of the breast: figures which show that education can increase the number of cures, *JAMA* 66:552, 1916.

94. Salomon A: Beitrage zur pathologie und klinik der mammacarcinome, *Arch Klin Chir* 101:573, 1913.

95. Egan RL: Experience with mammography in a tumor institution: evaluation of 1000 studies, *Radiology* 75:894, 1960.

96. Kopans DB, Meyer JE: Versatile spring hookwire breast lesion localizer, *AJR Am J Roentgenol* 138:586, 1982.

97. Rosner D et al: Noninvasive breast carcinoma: results of a national survey by the American College of Surgeons, *Ann Surg* 192:139, 1980.

98. Lane-Claypon JE: *Report on the late results of operation for cancer of the breast: reports on public health and medical subjects No. 51,* London, 1928, Ministry of Health.

99. Ewing J: *Neoplastic diseases,* ed 3, Philadelphia, 1928, WB Saunders.

100. Park WW, Lees JC: The absolute curability of cancer of the breast, *Surg Gynecol Obstet* 93:129, 1951.

101. Grubbe EH: *X-ray treatment: its origin, birth, and early history,* St Paul, 1949, Bruce Publishing.

102. Janeway HH: *Radium therapy in cancer at memorial hospital,* New York, 1917, Hober.

103. Keynes G: The radium treatment of carcinoma of the breast, *Br J Surg* 19:415, 1932.

104. Keynes G: Conservative treatment of cancer of the breast, *BMJ* 2:643, 1937.

105. Jessop WH: Results of operative treatment in carcinoma of the breast, *Lancet* 2:424, 1936.

106. Porritt A: Early carcinoma of the breast, *Br J Surg* 51:214, 1964.

107. McWhirter R: The value of simple mastectomy and radiotherapy in the treatment of cancer of the breast, *Br J Radiol* 21:599, 1948.

108. McWhirter R: Should more radical treatment be attempted in breast cancer? *AJR Am J Roentgenol* 92:3, 1964.

109. Patey DH, Dyson WH: The prognosis of carcinoma of the breast in relation to the type of operation performed, *Br J Cancer* 2:7, 1948.

110. Patey DH: A review of 146 cases of carcinoma of the breast operated on between 1930 and 1943, *Br J Cancer* 21:260, 1967.

111. Handley RS, Thackray AC: Conservative radical mastectomy (Patey's operation), *Ann Surg* 170:880, 1969.

112. Williams IG, Murley RS, Curwen MP: Carcinoma of the female breast: conservative and radical surgery, *BMJ* 2:787, 1953.

113. Anonymous: *Report by the American College of Surgeons Commission on Cancer,* Chicago, 1982, ACS.

114. Moxley JH et al: Treatment of primary breast cancer: summary of the National Institutes of Health Consensus Development Conference, *JAMA* 244:797, 1980.

115. Maddox WA et al: A randomized prospective trial of radical (Halsted) mastectomy versus modified radical mastectomy in 311 breast cancer patients, *Ann Surg* 198:207, 1983.

116. Adair FE: Role of surgery and irradiation in cancer of the breast, *JAMA* 121:553, 1943

117. Crile G: Treatment of breast cancer by local excision, *Am J Surg* 109:400, 1965.

118. Crile G, Hoerr SO: Results of treatment of carcinoma of the breast by local excision, *Surg Gynecol Obstet* 132:780, 1971.

119. Hermann RE et al: Results of conservative operations for breast cancer, *Arch Surg* 120:746, 1985.

120. Tagart RE: Partial mastectomy for breast cancer, *BMJ* 2:1268, 1978.

121. Montgomery AC, Greening WP, Levene AL: Clinical study of recurrence rate and survival time of patients with carcinoma of the breast treated by biopsy excision without any other therapy, *J R Soc Med* 71:339, 1978.

122. Lagios MD et al: Segmental mastectomy without radiotherapy: short-term follow-up, *Cancer* 52:2173, 1983.

123. Anscher MS et al: Local failure and margin status in early-stage breast carcinoma treated with conservation surgery and radiation therapy, *Ann Surg* 218:22, 1993.

124. Schnitt SJ et al: The relationship between microscopic margins of resection and the risk of local recurrence in patients with breast cancer treated with breast-conserving surgery and radiation therapy, *Cancer* 74:1746, 1994.

125. Prosnitz LR et al: Radiation therapy as initial treatment for early stage cancer of the breast without mastectomy, *Cancer* 39:917, 1977.

126. Mustakallio S: Treatment of breast cancer by tumor extirpation and roentgen therapy instead of radical operation, *J Fac Radiol* 6:23, 1954.

127. Peters MV: Wedge resection and irradiation: an effective treatment in early breast cancer, *JAMA* 200:144, 1967.

128. Wise L, Mason AY, Ackerman LV: Local excision and irradiation: an alternative method for the treatment of early mammary cancer, *Ann Surg* 174:392, 1971.

129. Freeman CR et al: Limited surgery with or without radiotherapy for early breast carcinoma, *J Can Assoc Radiol* 32:125, 1981.

130. Vilcoq JR et al: The outcome of treatment by tumorectomy and radiotherapy of patients with operable breast cancer, *Int J Radiat Oncol Biol Phys* 7:1327, 1981.

131. Romsdahl MM et al: Conservation surgery and irradiation as treatment for early breast cancer, *Arch Surg* 118:521, 1983.

132. DuBois JB et al: Tumorectomy and radiotherapy in early breast cancer: a report on 392 patients, *Int J Radiat Oncol Biol Phys* 15:1275, 1988.

133. Harris JR et al: The use of pathologic features in selecting the extent of surgical resection necessary for breast cancer patients treated by primary radiation therapy, *Ann Surg* 201:164, 1985.

134. Leung S et al: Locoregional recurrences following radical external beam irradiation and interstitial implantation for operable breast cancer: a twenty-three-year experience, *Radiother Oncol* 5:1, 1986.

135. Delouche G et al: Conservation treatment of early breast cancer: long-term results and complications, *Int J Radiat Oncol Biol Phys* 13:29, 1987.

136. Stehlin JS et al: A ten year study of partial mastectomy for carcinoma of the breast, *Surg Gynecol Obstet* 165:191, 1987.

137. Haffty BG et al: Conservative surgery with radiation therapy in clinical stage I and II breast cancer: results of a 20-year experience, *Arch Surg* 124:1266, 1989.

138. Veronesi U et al: Conservative treatment of early breast cancer: long-term results of 1232 cases treated with quadrantectomy, axillary dissection, and radiotherapy, *Ann Surg* 211:250, 1990.

139. Fowble BL et al: Ten-year results of conservative surgery and irradiation for stage I and II breast cancer, *Int J Radiat Oncol Biol Phys* 21:269, 1991.

140. Hochman A, Robinson E: Eighty-two cases of mammary cancer treated exclusively with roentgen therapy, *Cancer* 15:670, 1960.

141. Fisher B et al: Eight-year results of a randomized clinical trial comparing total mastectomy and lumpectomy with or without irradiation in the treatment of breast cancer, *N Engl J Med* 320:822, 1989.

142. Fisher B, Redmond C: Lumpectomy for breast cancer: an update of the NSABP experience, *J Natl Cancer Inst Monogr* 11:7, 1992.

143. Veronesi U et al: Comparison of Halsted mastectomy with quadrantectomy, axillary dissection, and radiotherapy in early breast cancer: long-term results, *Eur J Cancer Clin Oncol* 22:1085, 1986.

144. Blichert-Toft M et al: A Danish randomized trial comparing breast-preserving therapy with mastectomy in mammary carcinoma: preliminary results, *Acta Oncol* 27:671, 1988.

145. Sarrazin D et al: Ten-year results of a randomized trial comparing a conservative treatment to mastectomy in early breast cancer, *Radiother Oncol* 14:177, 1989.

146. Van Dongen JA et al: Randomized clinical trial to assess the value of breast-conserving therapy in stage I and II breast cancer, EORTC 10801 trial, *J Natl Cancer Inst Monogr* 11:15, 1992.

147. Hellman S, Harris JR: The appropriate breast cancer paradigm, *Cancer Res* 47:339, 1987.

148. Clark RM et al: Breast cancer: a 21-year experience with conservative surgery and radiation, *Int J Radiol Oncol Biol Phys* 8:967, 1982.

149. Schnitt SJ et al: Pathologic findings on re-excision of the primary site in breast cancer patients considered for treatment by primary radiation therapy, *Cancer* 59:675, 1987.

150. Kurtz JM et al: Results of salvage surgery for mammary recurrence following breast-conserving therapy, *Ann Surg* 207:347, 1988.

151. Fisher B, Fisher ER: Transmigration of lymph nodes by tumor cells, *Science* 152:1397, 1966.

152. Fisher B, Fisher ER: The interrelationship of hematogenous and lymphatic tumor cell dissemination, *Surg Gynecol Obstet* 122:791, 1966.

153. Beatson GT: On the treatment of inoperable cases of carcinoma of the mamma: suggestions for a new method of treatment, with illustrative cases, *Lancet* 2:104, 1896.

154. MacMahon CE, Cahill JL: The evolution of the concept of the use of surgical castration in the palliation of breast cancer in premenopausal females, *Ann Surg* 184:713, 1976.

155. Bonadonna G, Valagussa P: Dose-response effect of adjuvant chemotherapy in breast cancer, *N Engl J Med* 304:10, 1981.

156. Nowell PC: Molecular events in tumor development, *N Engl J Med* 319:575, 1988.

157. Rosenberg SA et al: Observations on the systemic administration of autologous lymphokine-activated killer cells and recombinant interleukin-2 to patients with metastatic cancer, *N Engl J Med* 313:1485, 1985.

158. Fisher B et al: The accuracy of clinical nodal staging and of limited axillary dissection as a determinant of histological nodal status in carcinoma of the breast, *Surg Gynecol Obstet* 152:765, 1981.

159. Fisher ER, Sass R, Fisher B: Biologic considerations regarding the one- and two-step procedures in the management of patients with invasive carcinoma of the breast, *Surg Gynecol Obstet* 161:245, 1985.

160. Cady B, Stone MD, Wayne J: New therapeutic possibilities in primary invasive breast cancer, *Ann Surg* 218:338, 1993.

161. Haffty BG et al: Breast conservation therapy without axillary dissection: a rational treatment strategy in selected patients, *Arch Surg* 128:1315, 1993.

162. Silverstein MJ et al: Axillary lymph node dissection for T_{1a} breast carcinoma: is it indicated? *Cancer* 73:664, 1994.

163. Danforth DN: The role of axillary lymph node dissection in the management of breast cancer, *PPO Updates* 6:1, 1992.

164. Margolis DS et al: Aggressive axillary evaluation and adjuvant therapy for nonpalpable carcinoma of the breast, *Surg Gynecol Obstet* 174:109, 1992.

165. Recht A, Houlihan MJ: Axillary lymph nodes and breast cancer: a review, *Cancer* 76:1491, 1995.

166. Frykberg ER: Lobular carcinoma in situ of the breast, *Surg Gynecol Obstet* 164:285, 1987.

167. Recht A et al: Intraductal carcinoma of the breast: results of treatment with excisional biopsy and radiation, *J Clin Oncol* 3:1339, 1985.

168. Baute PB, Thibodeau M, Newstead G: Improving the yield of biopsy for nonpalpable lesions of the breast, *Surg Gynecol Obstet* 174:93, 1992.

169. Sickles EA: Periodic mammographic follow-up of probably benign lesions: results in 3,184 consecutive cases, *Radiology* 179:463, 1991.

170. Martin H, Ellis E: Biopsy by needle puncture and aspiration, *Ann Surg* 92:169, 1930.

171. Masood S et al: Prospective evaluation of radiologically directed fine-needle aspiration biopsy of nonpalpable breast lesions, *Cancer* 66:1480, 1990.

172. Dowlatshahi K et al: Nonpalpable breast lesions: findings of stereotaxic needle-core biopsy and fine-needle aspiration cytology, *Radiology* 181:745, 1991.

173. Morrow M et al: Preoperative evaluation of abnormal mammographic findings to avoid unnecessary breast biopsies, *Arch Surg* 129:1091, 1994.

174. Swain SM et al: Neoadjuvant chemotherapy in the combined modality approach of locally advanced nonmetastatic breast cancer, *Cancer Res* 47:3889, 1987.

175. Hortobagyi GN et al: Management of stage III primary breast cancer with primary chemotherapy, surgery, and radiation therapy, *Cancer* 62:2507, 1988.

176. Bonadonna G et al: Primary chemotherapy to avoid mastectomy in tumors with diameters of three centimeters or more, *J Natl Cancer Inst* 82:1539, 1990.

177. Khanna MM et al: Breast conservation management of breast tumors 4 cm or larger, *Arch Surg* 127:1038, 1992.

178. Singletary SE, McNeese MD, Hortobagyi GN: Feasibility of breast conservation surgery after induction chemotherapy for locally advanced breast carcinoma, *Cancer* 69:2849, 1992.

179. Schwartz GF et al: Induction chemotherapy followed by breast conservation for locally advanced carcinoma of the breast, *Cancer* 73:362, 1994.

180. Veronesi U et al: Conservation surgery after primary chemotherapy in large carcinomas of the breast, *Ann Surg* 222:612, 1995.

181. Nattinger AB et al: Geographic variation in the use of breast-conserving treatment for breast cancer, *N Engl J Med* 326:1102, 1992.

182. Tarbox BB, Rockwood JK, Abernathy CM: Are modified radical mastectomies done for T_1 breast cancers because of surgeon's advice or patient's choice? *Am J Surg* 164:417, 1992.

183. Bauer TL et al: Mammographically detected carcinoma of the breast, *Surg Gynecol Obstet* 173:482, 1991.

184. Franceschi D et al: Not all nonpalpable breast cancers are alike, *Arch Surg* 126:967, 1991.

185. Landercasper J et al: Needle localization and biopsy of nonpalpable lesions of the breast, *Surg Gynecol Obstet* 164:399, 1987.

186. Marrujo G, Jolly PC, Hall MH: Nonpalpable breast cancer: needle-localized biopsy for diagnosis, *Am J Surg* 151:599, 1986.

187. Perdue P et al: Early detection of breast carcinoma: a comparison of palpable and nonpalpable lesions, *Surgery* 111:656, 1992.

188. Poole GV et al: Occult lesions of the breast, *Surg Gynecol Obstet* 163:107, 1986.

189. Shroff JH, Lloyd LR, Schroder DM: Open breast biopsy: a critical analysis, *Am Surg* 57:481, 1991.

190. Silverstein MJ et al: Hooked-wire–directed breast biopsy and over penetrated mammography, *Cancer* 59:715, 1987.

191. Skinner MA et al: Nonpalpable breast lesions at biopsy: a detailed analysis of radiographic features, *Ann Surg* 208:203, 1988.

192. Wilhelm MC et al: Nonpalpable invasive breast cancer, *Ann Surg* 213:600, 1991.

193. Symmonds RE, Roberts JW: Management of nonpalpable breast abnormalities, *Ann Surg* 205:520, 1987.

38

Indications and
Techniques for Biopsy

MARSHALL M. URIST

KIRBY I. BLAND

Chapter Outline

Breast biopsy is one of the most common surgical procedures performed today. Advances in technology have changed this operation from primarily diagnostic to one that is more often therapeutic because larger tissue samples can now be obtained for diagnosis through large core needle biopsies.

Even though a presumptive diagnosis of breast cancer can be made from a patient's history and physical examination or from radiologic studies, the actual removal of tissue from the breast or from a metastatic site, followed by microscopic examination, is essential to confirm the diagnosis. Breast masses that appear benign have a real, although relatively small, probability of malignancy that cannot be ruled out until a biopsy is performed.[1,2] Open biopsy of a breast mass under general or local anesthesia is associated with relatively low morbidity and essentially no mortality. A 1980 study on the cost-effectiveness of breast cancer management demonstrated that screening costs are very high and that the most effective means of containing the economic cost of this illness is through targeted selection of high-risk patients for breast biopsy with local anesthesia.[3] Although many biopsies of "suspicious" breast lesions prove to be benign, certain clinical and mammographic features are associated with a high probability of malignancy.[4-10]

The history, physical examination, radiologic findings, and preoperative evaluation each influence the timing and the type of breast biopsy performed. Should the patient have cancer confirmed with biopsy, the information gained from the specimen is crucial to staging, assessment of prognosis, and selection of the appropriate therapy. Inconclusive or inaccurate data derived from insufficient tissue or a malpositioned biopsy incision can delay diagnosis, limit therapeutic options, and complicate definitive treatment.

Breast masses in adolescent and young adult women are often benign lesions that can be followed at specific intervals when the physical examination and ultrasound findings are concordant. Kopans and associates[11] evaluated the positive predictive value (PPV) and its variation with age for 4778 women who underwent biopsy for an occult mammographic abnormality. These authors did not detect abrupt changes in the PPV at any age for women aged 40 to 79 years, but diagnostic results increased steadily. This study affirms the existing evidence for the probability of disease at any age. The modeled PPV for cancer in these 4778 patients increased with age from approximately 12% at 40 years to 46% by 79 years.

For women older than 35 years, there are several clinical situations in which a biopsy is generally indicated. The first is the presence of a previously unrecognized three-dimensional mass that is anatomically distinct from the remainder of the breast tissue. Even though the mammogram and ultrasound show no evidence of an abnormality, the presence of a new mass is commonly an indication for biopsy. Criteria that should influence the surgeon's decision to perform the biopsy include mammographic findings that are suspicious for carcinoma,[12] a positive family history for breast cancer or previous personal history of breast cancer,[13] and physical findings (e.g., skin dimpling, peau d'orange, or clinically positive axillary nodes) indicative of neoplastic disease.[1] The second indication for breast biopsy is the presence of mammographic findings that are suggestive of, or compatible with, carcinoma.[8,12,14-19] These radiographic features include a mass, architectural distortion of the surrounding breast tissue that may suggest carcinoma, or clustered microcalcifications (see Chapter 31). In the absence of any physical abnormality, these findings are generally an indication for excisional biopsy of the nonpalpable lesion.

Nonpalpable Lesions

A "normal" breast may not present any physical signs of an underlying breast cancer but may harbor a neoplasm in the noninfiltrating (in situ) stage or, less often, as an occult infiltrating breast carcinoma.[7] Nonpalpable breast lesions are generally discovered on routine screening mammography, although incidental breast masses have been found on computed tomography (CT) and magnetic resonance imaging (MRI) scans of the chest.[20] In the past two decades, the widespread application of high-quality film/screen mammography has resulted in the detection of increasing numbers of nonpalpable breast lesions.[8] The radiographic criteria on which the decision to perform biopsy is based include (1) a localized soft tissue mass within the breast parenchyma; (2) architectural distortion, including contracture of trabeculae producing stellate alterations, with severe asymmetric periductal and lobular thickening; and (3) clustered microcalcifications, with or without the aforementioned features.[1,5,12] However, the diagnosis of breast cancer in younger women (aged 30 to 40 years) with mammography is limited, with a sensitivity of approximately 75%.[21] Younger women should be informed that mammography and physical examination have limitations in diagnosis and that presentation and detection of their cancers is often delayed.

PREOPERATIVE LOCALIZATION OF NONPALPABLE BREAST LESIONS

The widespread use of mammography has resulted in the detection of increasing numbers of suspicious but clinically occult lesions of the breast.[12] Such lesions represent more than half of the detected cancers in screening clinics and account for a substantial proportion of breast tumors investigated with biopsy. Despite the frequency and simplicity of mammographic identification of suspicious lesions, intraoperative localization with subsequent adequate excision presents challenging technical problems because the shape and position of the breast during compression mammography may be quite different from those seen by the surgeon in the operating room. This has led to the development of several methods for preoperative localization of nonpalpable lesions.[18,22-33] The aim of these methods is to facilitate complete removal of the tumor at the first attempt at excision while simultaneously minimizing the size of the resected specimen and shortening the duration of anesthesia. Radiologically guided, invasive, preoperative localization of nonpalpable breast lesions is a safe, simple, and established procedure that allows for accurate and expeditious biopsy that can often be performed with the patient under local anesthesia. Because nonpalpable breast masses are often discovered as clustered microcalcifications or architectural distortions, they may remain nonpalpable, even on examination of the resected specimen. Thus specimen radiographs are mandatory to document the removal of the suspect area and to facilitate histologic examination.[31,34-40]

Noninvasive Techniques. Noninvasive techniques for localization of mammographically suspicious breast lesions include visual estimation, external breast markers, coordinates plotted on a diagram of the breast,[33] stereomammograms,[22] grid compression devices, ultrasound, and CT-directed biopsy. The latter technique may be of value for the 5% of mammographically suspicious lesions detectable in only one mammographic view (craniocaudal or mediolateral). More recently, MRI-guided techniques have been used.[41] MRI has also been used successfully in patients with axillary nodal metastases and a normal mammogram. Although superficial lesions of the breast or lesions adjacent to the nipple may be localized adequately preoperatively with visual estimation, deeper suspect areas may require localization with invasive techniques. Stevens and Jamplis[33] were among the first investigators to describe preoperative localization of nonpalpable breast lesions with use of a "mammographic map" that established the relative position for the suspect area within the breast using coordinates. With this localization technique, a wedge biopsy with adequate margins could be obtained. These authors emphasized the need for radiologic confirmation of removal of the suspect lesion. Following "bread loafing" of the specimen and repeat roentgenography, the exact site of the suspect lesion may be localized and submitted for pathologic evaluation (Figure 38-1). Although this technique for localization of nonpalpable lesions was an

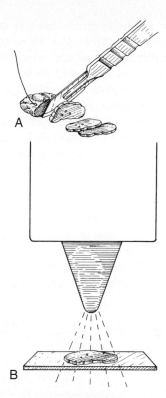

FIG. **38-1** **A,** "Bread loafing" of the biopsy specimen allows the exact site of the lesion to be determined and submitted for pathologic evaluation. **B,** After excision of the suspicious lesion, specimen radiography is completed to confirm the presence of the suspect lesion in the excised tissue.

improvement over blind biopsy methods, it was fraught with error and sampling of the suspect breast lesion was inaccurate.

Invasive Techniques. Localization of occult breast masses has markedly improved with the use of radiopaque needles and wires that can be radiographically guided into the breast.[27-29,42,43] Once inserted, the relative position of the device and the lesion is defined mammographically. The success of breast localization procedures requires close communication among the radiologist, surgeon, and pathologist to ensure that the suspicious site has been removed and that the pathologist has analyzed the correct area of the specimen.

RIGID NEEDLE LOCALIZATION

Needle localization methods that used needles placed percutaneously in the vicinity of the suspect mass as a biopsy guide were first described by Dodd.[44] However, this technique did not gain widespread acceptance until screening mammography achieved universal application. Variations of this technique have been reported by many radiologists[27,28] and became popular and routinely accepted in the late 1970s. Thereafter, Libshitz, Feig, and Fetouh[29] reported complete success in the removal of 83 suspicious breast lesions.

Technical problems with this method of localization include (1) movement of the inflexible needle during the time between placement and operation, even when the needle hub is taped or secured in place; (2) compression of the breast during mammography and localization, creating tissue stress that may alter the position of the needle, even when it is sutured in place; and (3) inadvertent dislodgement of the needle during the procedure leading to inadequate tissue sampling (false-negative results) or inadvertent transection of the tumor with incomplete removal of the suspect mass. Interest in this technique has declined because many of these problems were eliminated by the use of self-retaining flexible wires.

Hasselgren and associates determined that the frequency of a malignancy in nonpalpable breast lesions is affected by various factors, including patient age and mammographic features.[45,46] Using these discriminants allows selective biopsy to enhance diagnostic accuracy and cost-effectiveness.

NEEDLE-LOCALIZATION BIOPSY (SELF-RETAINING WIRE LOCALIZATION)

The two principal problems with rigid needle localization (the inflexibility of the stainless steel needle and the unreliability of the position of the needle following breast compression)[24] have been overcome by placing a flexible, hooked wire within the localizing needle, a technique first described by Frank, Hall, and Steer.[47] This procedure is commonly termed *needle localization biopsy*, even though the needle is usually removed once the wire is in place. Ideally, the hook lodges within or adjacent to the suspicious breast lesion and prevents dislodgement from the specimen (Figures 38-2 and 38-3). With the patient under local anesthesia, the rigid introducer

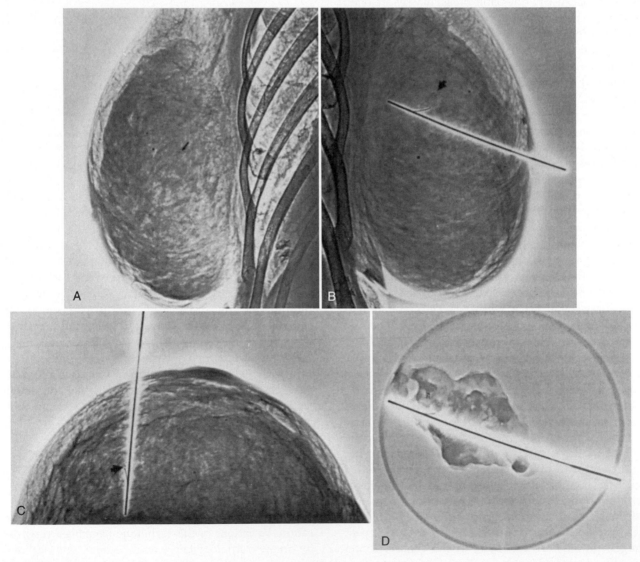

FIG. **38-2** Preoperative needle localization of a nonpalpable breast lesion **(A)** requires mediolateral **(B)** and craniocaudal **(C)** views of the breast. It is mandatory to obtain specimen mammography of the excised tissue **(D)**, preferably with the localization wire in place to confirm extirpation of the suspect lesion.

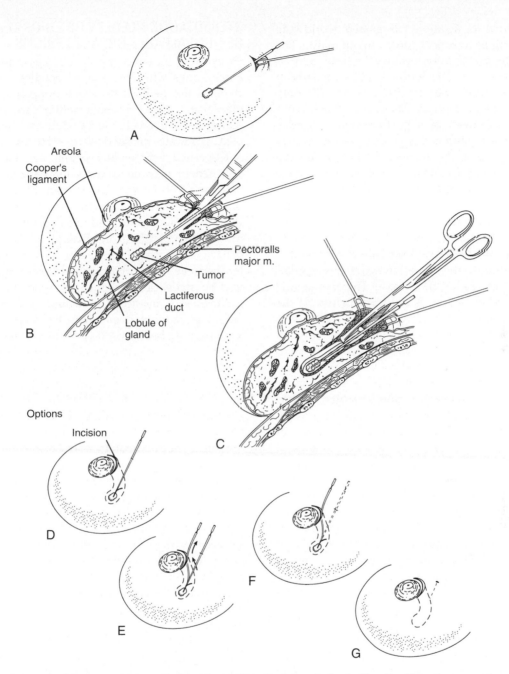

FIG. **38-3** Operative technique for needle localization biopsy: The suspicious lesion is "localized" on the mammogram immediately before surgery. **A,** During the operation the needle serves as a guide for the surgeon to perform the biopsy. **B,** Development of tissue planes circumferential and parallel to the localization wire. **C,** Controlled dissection of the wire, which is purchased with tissues using an Allis clamp. The suspicious lesion is incorporated in the dissection, which includes tissue beyond the tip of the hooked wire. Specimen radiography confirms excision of the suspicious, nonpalpable mammographically identified lesion. **Options. D,** Deeply localized, suspicious lesion approached via circumareolar incision. **E,** Wire is repositioned from percutaneous localized position to exit via incision. **F,** Dissection completed circumferentially and parallel to wire via circumareolar incision. **G,** Completed dissection with breast defect.

needle with the hooked wire within it is directed into the breast using biplanar mammographic or ultrasound guidance. The rigid needle is then removed, leaving the hooked wire in place. Because of its self-retaining feature, the wire is not easily withdrawn, advanced, or redirected. The incision should be placed directly over the mammographic abnormality, regardless of where the entry site of the wire is positioned. The direction of the dissection and

dimensions of the specimen are determined by the lesion size and the relative proximity of the wire to the lesion. If the incision does not pass through the entry site of the wire, it is necessary to identify the shaft of the wire proximal to the lesion and retract it into the wound. Resection then proceeds to encompass a volume of tissue with at least 1 cm of normal-appearing tissue outside of the mammographic abnormality.

Although wire localization has gained worldwide acceptance, some technical problems remain. The surgeon may have difficulty locating the flexible localization wire, especially if the lesion is approached via an incision remote from the suspicious mass. To help reduce this problem, Homer, Fisher, and Sugarman[42] advocate the placement of a postlocalization needle. This needle, or wire stiffener, is guided percutaneously by the surgeon over the flexible hooked wire. The rigidity of the needle facilitates palpation of its course during the operative procedure. Other modifications have added distance markers along the wire and a rigid segment that makes the tip easier to palpate intraoperatively.

Methods for preoperative localization represent a major contribution to the operative treatment of occult (nonpalpable) lesions of the breast. The therapeutic adequacy of this procedure is enhanced when (1) the diagnosis is made preoperatively with fine-needle aspiration (FNA) or core biopsy and (2) the surgeon plans to resect the lesion with a border of normal-appearing breast tissue. Cox and co-workers[48] estimate that more than 75% of patients who have diagnostic biopsy lesions (palpable or nonpalpable) harbor residual breast cancer. The success and effectiveness of any invasive breast localization procedure, decrease in operating time and expense, and reduced biopsy size are enhanced by an experienced surgeon working in close cooperation with the radiologist. Obtaining an intraoperative specimen radiograph after wire localization is strongly recommended to corroborate complete excision. However, Hasselgren, Hummel, and Fieler[45] observed a false-positive specimen x-ray film rate of 7.8% and a false-negative rate of 55%. Thus a postoperative mammogram is also important in most cases, especially when there is discordance between the mammogram, specimen radiograph, and pathology report.

STEREOTACTIC NEEDLE CORE BIOPSY OF NONPALPABLE BREAST LESIONS

Stereotactic mammographic devices and automated biopsy guns with core biopsy needles have radically changed the methods by which nonpalpable, mammographically detected abnormalities are managed. In many cases, stereotactic needle core breast biopsy (SNCB) obviates the need for open biopsy, costs less, and is associated with greater patient satisfaction.[49-55] The cost benefit may be greatest for patients with breast imaging reporting and data system (BI-RADS) 4 lesions rather than BI-RADS 5 tumors.[56] The analysis by Wallace's group[57] reiterated this view and further determined that SNCB is equivalent to needle-localized biopsy in the frequency of diagnosis of breast cancer. Furthermore, these investigators determined that there was no statistical difference between the two biopsy techniques in diagnosis for women younger than and older than 50 years. Even when all radiographic changes have been excised with the core biopsy technique, 10% or more patients may have additional neoplasia.[58]

Stereotactic mammographic devices use the principle of triangulation, which allows precise location of the breast lesion to be determined in three dimensions.[52] A 14-gauge cutting needle that fits into an automated, spring-loaded biopsy gun is used. A core of tissue, measuring approximately 2 to 2.5 mm in diameter, is obtained during the procedure.

The procedure consists of placing the patient prone on the stereotactic biopsy table with the breast dependent. The breast is compressed within the unit, and a scout film is obtained and evaluated. The skin of the breast is sterilized with povidone-iodine, and the region of the skin through which the biopsy needle will pass is anesthetized with lidocaine. Using computed calculations, the center of the lesion is determined and the needle is advanced into the breast after passing through the skin puncture site (Figure 38-4). The core biopsy needle is

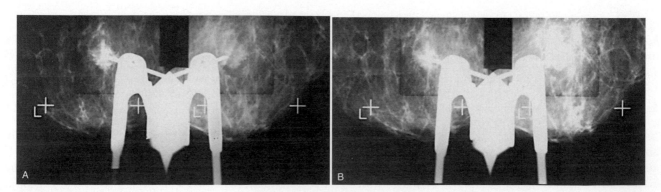

FIG. **38-4** Stereotactic image pair showing placement of the 14-gauge guide needle for stereotactic core biopsy. **A,** Prefire views with core needle in place in the center of the target lesion. **B,** Postfire views with the needle passing through the target, having sampled a core of the lesion.

advanced to the leading edge of the lesion, its position is verified, and the biopsy gun is fired. Vacuum-assisted core needle biopsy techniques allow fixation of the target area to the cutting surface of the needle resulting in even greater accuracy (Mammotome, Ethicon). After the tissue is retrieved, repeat views are obtained to document that the needle traversed or removed part or all of the lesion. The needle containing the tissue sample is then withdrawn. Additional cores can be obtained by targeting different areas within the index or other mammographic abnormalities. The cores are submitted for pathologic evaluation. After completion of the biopsy, pressure is held over the biopsy site to minimize bleeding and ecchymosis.

Core biopsy has also been found to be useful in the diagnosis of multiple synchronous neoplastic ipsilateral lesions in more than one site in the breast.[59] Repeat biopsy of patients undergoing SNCB, with results that are not concordant with initial imaging and histopathology of the suspicious lesion, is emphasized by Dershaw's group.[60] This practice to ensure corroboration of SNCB results is necessary for the technique to be optimally effective. Furthermore, pathologic incidence of atypical ductal hyperplasia diagnosed at SNCB requires open (needle-directed) biopsy to rule out associated ductal carcinoma in situ or invasive disease.[61]

SNCB can also be done to evaluate suspicious microcalcifications. The extracted core of tissue should be examined with specimen mammography to confirm the presence of microcalcifications within the biopsy. For patients whose core biopsy documents the presence of carcinoma, a definitive surgical procedure should be planned. As noted previously, when the core biopsy is equivocal or shows atypia, needle-localized breast biopsy should be performed. Liberman and colleagues[62] determined that 14-gauge SNCB achieved 99% diagnostic yield with five specimens obtained from masses. The same authors have shown that SCNB reduces the number of operations in patients with highly suspicious calcifications. Additional specimens may be essential to avoid false-negative results with the diagnosis of some calcified lesions.[61,63,64] Discordance is minimized by removing the entire mammographic abnormality, as opposed to obtaining a portion for diagnosis.[65] Larger areas of microcalcifications can be accurately resected by using bracketing wires to define the extent of changes.[66]

Patients who cannot lie prone or who cannot tolerate breast compression are not candidates for SCNB. In addition, if the breast compresses to less than 2 cm from the chest wall, biopsy may be inadvisable because the needle excursion is often slightly greater than 2 cm and injury to the chest wall and the pleura may occur. Complications of SCNB include hematomas, infections, possible tumor seeding of the biopsy track, and some discomfort during the procedure itself. The complication rate is acceptably low.

In good hands, the procedure can be done in 30 minutes, with a false-negative rate of less than 2%. SCNBs are associated with significant savings (possibly as much as $1000 per biopsy) compared with needle-localized biopsy.[67] A comprehensive review of stereotactic biopsy technique is included in Chapter 33.

ULTRASOUND-DIRECTED PERCUTANEOUS BIOPSY OF MAMMOGRAPHIC ABNORMALITIES

Ultrasound guidance is now used to facilitate breast biopsies using FNA, core needle biopsy, and open surgical excision. Ultrasound-guided FNA biopsy offers certain advantages over SCNB.[17,68] In the hands of an experienced operator, the procedure is tolerated extremely well by patients, fluid (e.g., from a small cyst) can be aspirated, and noncystic lesions can be sampled with great accuracy.[17,64] Samples obtained from FNA biopsy require evaluation by an expert cytopathologist and can be complicated by an inadequate specimen or by the inability to determine whether invasive carcinoma is present. Ultrasonography may not detect microcalcifications and is less accurate for solid masses smaller than 5 to 6 mm. The operator who performs the technique can select any site of entry on the skin. As the needle is advanced or moved, it is monitored in real time on the ultrasound monitor.

Complications of ultrasound-guided FNA include hematoma, infection, and failure to adequately sample the abnormality in question. Inadequate cytologic specimen requires additional attempts that, if unsuccessful, should be followed by core biopsy or needle-localized breast biopsy. False-negative and false-positive rates are acceptably low.

Ultrasound-guided large core needle biopsy can also be performed safely. New devices that include suction assistance and an automated firing mechanism provide a high-quality specimen using needles up to 11 gauge. Under ultrasonographic guidance, the tip of the needle is directed toward the abnormality. When the biopsy needle is appropriately positioned, the mechanism is fired, the needle is withdrawn, and the core is placed in formalin. The procedure can be repeated several times through an introducer that is first inserted to the proximal surface of the lesion, permitting rapid reinsertion and avoiding reintroduction through breast tissue. Ultrasound-guided biopsy is particularly useful in pregnant patients and in patients with lesions that cannot be visualized mammographically. In general, a negative result of needle biopsy or of core biopsy in the face of a worrisome physical finding or a suspicious mammographic abnormality should not delay definitive surgical removal.

Palpable Lesions

Although nonpalpable breast lesions require needle localization before definitive biopsy, palpable lesions may be "biopsied" by one of several techniques such as FNA, core needle biopsy, incisional biopsy, or excisional biopsy. The choice of the biopsy technique is influenced by the physical characteristics and size of the breast mass, the site of the suspicious lesion in the breast, the use of local or general anesthesia, and the method of treatment that would be chosen should a malignancy be confirmed. For example, a core needle biopsy of a large breast tumor performed with the patient under local anesthesia in a woman who presents with bony metastases provides histologic confirmation of the malignancy and adequate tissue for hormone receptor analysis before the initiation of chemotherapy. On the other hand, FNA biopsy of a suspicious mass done in an outpatient setting for a woman with clinical stage I breast cancer provides a diagnosis and allows the surgeon and the patient to discuss treatment strategies and options before the definitive surgical procedure.

COLLECTION OF SPECIMENS FOR CYTOLOGIC AND HISTOLOGIC EXAMINATION

Direct Smear. Specimens for exfoliative cytologic analysis in the patient with suspected Paget's disease of the breast may be obtained with direct smear of the weeping eczematoid lesion of the nipple. If the areola and surrounding skin is scaly and encrusted, a sterile glass slide can be used to scrape this area gently. The direct smear technique is simple and can be performed as an office procedure. Comprehensive management of nipple cytology and secretions is reviewed in Chapter 4.

Fluid Aspiration. Fluid from palpable breast cysts is simple to aspirate with a needle and syringe (Figure 38-5). If the cyst is not palpable, ultrasound may confirm its presence and can be used as a guide to direct the depth and location of the biopsy needle. The return of greenish brown fluid confirms the diagnosis of benign (nonproliferative) cystic disease and, unless otherwise indicated, should not be submitted for cytologic examination. Bloody cystic fluid, on the other hand, is more likely to indicate malignancy and therefore should always be examined cytologically, either by direct smear or after centrifugation of the aspirated contents. Palpable breast cysts should no longer be detectable after aspiration of their contents because the walls of the cyst collapse and conform to the configuration of contiguous breast tissues. If fluid is not obtained or the mass persists, further workup is required. If the mass resolves and later recurs, clinical and mammographic evaluations are also indicated.

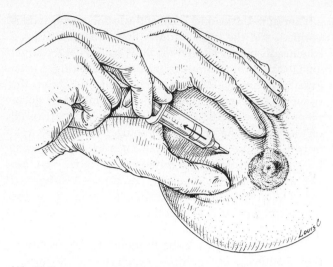

FIG. **38-5** Technique for aspiration of fluid from a breast cyst.

Fine-Needle Aspiration Biopsy. FNA biopsy of breast masses is a safe and reliable diagnostic technique that can be performed in the office using local anesthesia for palpable masses.[69,70] The skin overlying the palpable lesion is infiltrated with a local anesthetic. The breast lump is held relatively immobile, using one hand to gently but firmly stabilize the quadrant containing the mass. If the mass is not well defined, the procedure should be performed under ultrasound or mammographic guidance. FNA is facilitated using an "aspiration gun" to allow the operator to apply suction while maintaining the position of the needle tip in the mass. The procedure uses a 10- to 20-ml syringe and 22- or 25-gauge needle. The needle is inserted into the mass through the anesthetized skin, and suction is applied to the syringe. Moving the needle into the suspect lesion at various angles over an area of no more than 1 cm allows clumps of cells to be dislodged from the tumor, aspirated into the syringe, and submitted for cytologic examination (Figure 38-6). FNA is quite safe, although the operator performing the procedure must be cognizant of the relationship of the aspiration needle to the chest wall, because entry into the parietal pleura and iatrogenic pneumothorax is a potentially dangerous, although rare, complication. Following FNA biopsy, local pressure should be applied to the skin puncture site to prevent bleeding.

The diagnostic accuracy of FNA biopsy of breast masses approximates 80%.[70,71] False-positive results are unusual when the aspirated specimen is properly prepared and reviewed by a qualified cytopathologist. False-negative results are much more common, and it must be emphasized that the absence of malignant cells in the aspirate does not rule out the diagnosis of cancer. Thus any clinically or mammographically suspicious breast mass investigated with FNA biopsy that does not yield a diagnosis of malignancy must be subjected

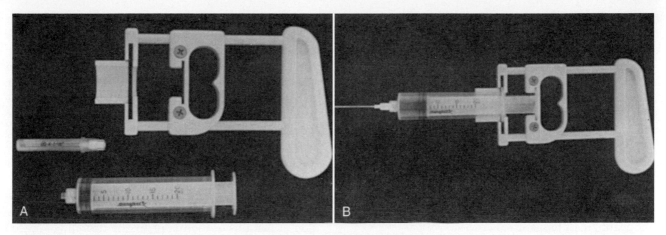

FIG. **38-6** **A** and **B**, Aspiration of a solid breast mass is best performed by using a cytology fine-needle "aspiration gun" (Cameco, Enebyberg, Sweden).

to further diagnosis by means of core needle biopsy or surgical excision. Although qualitative immunofluorescence monoclonal antibody techniques can be applied to the cytology specimen, hormone receptor and tissue marker studies are best performed on histologic specimens obtained by way of core needle biopsy. This technique can also be used to evaluate suspicious axillary lymph nodes.[72]

Cutting Needle Biopsy. The technique of biopsy with a needle that incises a core of tissue from the breast is termed *cutting needle biopsy* or *large-core needle biopsy.* Several types of automated biopsy needles are available (Figure 38-7). The false-positive diagnostic rate is lower with tissue procured with cutting needles than with FNA biopsy, because more tissue is retained and can be submitted for analysis. Doyle and associates[73] noted the specificity of large core needle biopsies to be 98%; sensitivity based on limited follow-up was 100%. A core biopsy that yields no malignant tissue cannot, however, be considered conclusively benign when only a portion of the mass has been sampled (sampling error). Thus, as with FNA biopsy, the cutting needle biopsy is most useful when the results are positive for malignancy. Cutting needles are 18 gauge or larger and thus require use of local anesthesia. Because the biopsy yields a core of solid tissue rather than clumps of cells, the potential

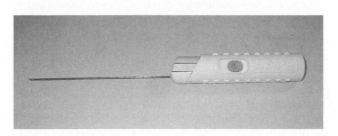

FIG. **38-7** Disposable 18-gauge core needle biopsy instrument (Bard).

risk for hemorrhage and tissue disturbance is greater than with needle aspiration methods. Care must be taken to avoid advancing the cutting needle beyond the suspect mass, lest the contiguous normal breast or chest wall be injured or implanted with malignant cells.

Incisional Biopsy. Incisional biopsy of a suspicious breast mass involves removal of a portion of the lesion, which is then submitted for pathologic examination. This type of biopsy has largely been replaced by core needle biopsy because adequate tissue can be obtained in all but the densest of tumors. The incisional biopsy should excise only the amount of tissue necessary for histologic confirmation of the diagnosis and for tissue receptor studies.

The biopsy site should be marked on the breast, typically in curvilinear fashion paralleling Langer's lines, to enable the surgeon to excise the entire scar and the primary neoplasm at the time of definitive surgical therapy (see Chapter 41). Meticulous attention to hemostasis is mandatory to avoid spreading potentially malignant cells. The technical aspects of incisional biopsy of breast masses are relatively simple and straightforward. Local anesthesia is infiltrated into the dermis of the planned skin incision, directly over the tumor. The actual biopsy of tumor is best performed with a scalpel because electrocautery may distort the histologic features of the specimen. Hemostasis with electrocautery is important because open tumor surfaces may bleed extensively.

Excisional Biopsy. As the terminology implies, excisional biopsy of a breast mass removes the entire lesion and generally includes a margin of normal breast tissue that surrounds it. Suspicious breast lesions that are apparent only on mammograms should be removed with excisional biopsy using preoperative needle localization.[74] Intraoperative localization with ultrasound can also be used if the mass is well seen with this technique. When possible, the diagnosis should be made preoperatively to facilitate a planned resection for cancer.

Diagnostic excisional biopsy should *not* be considered a substitute for planned removal of malignant lesions. Tafra, Guenther, and Giuliano[75] determined that biopsy specimens with residual tumor had larger median tumor diameters than those that had no residual disease (2 cm versus 1 cm, $p < .01$), were more likely to be associated with positive axillary nodes ($p < .001$), and were more likely to develop recurrence ($p < .025$). The authors suggest that any procedure less extensive than the planned surgical operation is liable to leave behind malignant breast tissue.

Lumpectomy (Segmental Mastectomy). When the National Surgical Adjuvant Breast and Bowel Project (NSABP) was implemented in the 1950s, the standard surgical treatment for carcinoma of the breast was modified radical or radical mastectomy. Surgeons had essentially no familiarity with "breast conservation surgery" or terms such as *tylectomy, lumpectomy, segmental mastectomy,* and *quadrantectomy.* Through a series of workshops and other educational tools, the participating NSABP surgeons were instructed in the methods mandated by the protocol. Lumpectomy with axillary dissection (levels I and II) followed by radiation therapy to the breast became the preferred surgical treatment for many carcinomas of the breast. With the introduction of sentinel lymph node biopsy, the extent of lymph node dissection has diminished; however, the principles of lumpectomy remain the same.

Lumpectomy, as the initial technique for biopsy of a suspicious breast mass, is now uncommon. For most masses, FNA or core needle biopsy is used to diagnose or confirm the diagnosis and allow planning for sentinel lymph node biopsy. When the diagnosis of cancer is established preoperatively, there is a higher probability that the lumpectomy specimen margins will be clear. A detailed review of the indications and techniques for conservation surgery is provided in Chapter 43.

Curvilinear incisions are recommended for most lumpectomies, regardless of the site of the primary breast lesion. Although some surgeons prefer radial incisions for lesions in the lower half of the breast, we use nonradial incisions in most patients, because the cosmetic results are equivalent or superior with curvilinear incisions that follow the breast contour parallel to Langer's lines. The surgeon must always be cognizant of the occasional necessity to convert a planned segmental mastectomy into a total mastectomy. Thus placement of breast incisions that are readily incorporated into cosmetically acceptable incisions for total mastectomy is important in planning the operative procedure.

It is helpful if the preoperative diagnosis of cancer has been established by needle aspiration biopsy or core biopsy. For breast lesions that require needle localization, the incision for lumpectomy should be placed directly over the lesion. Extensive tunneling through and elevation of contiguous breast tissue makes the procedure more difficult and may compromise the margin status.[76] In patients who have undergone an incisional biopsy or a biopsy with grossly positive margins, reexcision of the old scar and entire biopsy site is recommended to reduce the risk of local recurrence.

It is imperative to excise a margin of healthy breast tissue contiguous with the suspect mass. Careful palpation of margins of the tumor by the operating surgeon during excision provides a three-dimensional perspective on the lesion that is essential to ensure that the tumor is not violated and is excised within the sphere of extirpated breast tissue. This technique does not necessitate removal of a predetermined volume of normal tissue; the goal of the operative procedure is to obtain margins that are grossly free of tumor. Skin edges need not be undermined, and the pectoralis major fascia is not included in the resected margin unless the lesion is contiguous with or is fixed to the fascia. The specimen should be oriented in all dimensions, using a standard-ized method such as suture tags, colored dyes, or separate samples of tissue taken from the specimen or the sides of the defect created in the breast. The designations *cranial-caudal, medial-lateral,* and *superficial-deep* allow the surgeon to identify clearly the margins of the excised specimen for the pathologist. On occasion, the pathologist may complete frozen section tissue or cytologic analysis of the margins of biopsy specimens to ensure histologically clear margins. The pathologist's role is essential: confirming histologic diagnosis, establishing the presence of tumor-free margins, and submitting tissue for estrogen and progesterone receptor (ER/PR) analyses and other prognostic determinants (e.g., oncogene biochemical markers, ploidy, S phase). The surgeon must be cognizant of tumor orientation with respect to the wound and the chest wall during resection of the breast mass. The presence of a positive margin requires reexcision of any area in which the frozen section was histologically positive. When lumpectomy cannot achieve tumor-free margins (e.g., multifocality, multicentricity, multiple histologic types, diffuse microcalcifications), total mastectomy is performed.

After confirmation of tumor-free margins by the pathologist, meticulous hemostasis is achieved and wound closure is begun. Special attention is paid to closure of the wound, because tissue defects created with lumpectomy may produce a cosmetically unacceptable appearance that may be further exaggerated after completion of breast irradiation. Larger defects are preferably closed without tension in multiple layers using interrupted absorbable sutures. Some surgeons make no attempt to obliterate dead space, and others make no effort to drain this space.

SURGICAL BIOPSY OF THE BREAST

Only by removing a sample of breast tissue sufficient for histologic preparation can a diagnosis be made with ultimate confidence. The accuracy of pathologic information obtained is limited only by the accuracy of sampling and the morphologic interpretation. Because a negative biopsy result can be caused by sampling error, cancer cannot be excluded unless representative pathologic tissue is removed and examined thoroughly. This principle is most important, because therapy for cancer can be predicated only on histologic verification of its presence. Depending on histologic and mammographic findings, bilateral biopsy may be indicated. Simkovich and colleagues[77] determined that random contralateral breast biopsy is indicated with histologic confirmation of infiltrating lobular carcinoma. This treatment is considered debatable by many[78] and is reviewed comprehensively in Chapters 13, 14, and 47.

Breast biopsy is best performed in a surgical suite, under sterile conditions, and with techniques of local or general anesthesia. This may be done on an outpatient basis, but the setting depends on patient and physician preference. It is essential that incisions be cosmetically designed, because approximately 70% of breast biopsies confirm benign (proliferative and nonproliferative) disease. Because the lines of tension in the skin of the breast (Langer's lines) are generally concentric with the nipple (Figure 38-8), incisions that parallel these lines generally result in thin and cosmetically acceptable scars.[79] It is best to keep these incisions within the boundaries of potential incisions for future mastectomy or wide local excision, should those therapies be required for definitive treatment (Figure 38-9).[80] Principles for planning breast biopsy are further reviewed in Chapters 40 and 58. The most cosmetically acceptable scars result from circumareolar (curvilinear) incisions. Most centrally located subareolar lesions can be approached in this manner.

Once the patient is positioned comfortably on the operating table, the thorax is slightly elevated ipsilaterally to the suspect lesion (using folded sheets) and the arm is placed in a relaxed position on an armboard. Incisions commonly used for all quadrants are depicted in Figure 38-9. In general, dermal tension is concentric

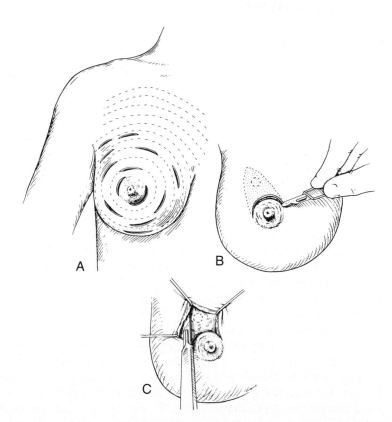

F I G. 38-8 Recommended locations of incisions for performing breast biopsy. **A,** The most cosmetically acceptable scars result from circumareolar incisions that follow the contour of Langer's lines. **B** and **C,** Technique for dissection of breast masses within 2 cm of the areolar margin. Thick skin flaps are advised to ensure cosmetically contoured and viable tissues about the areola.

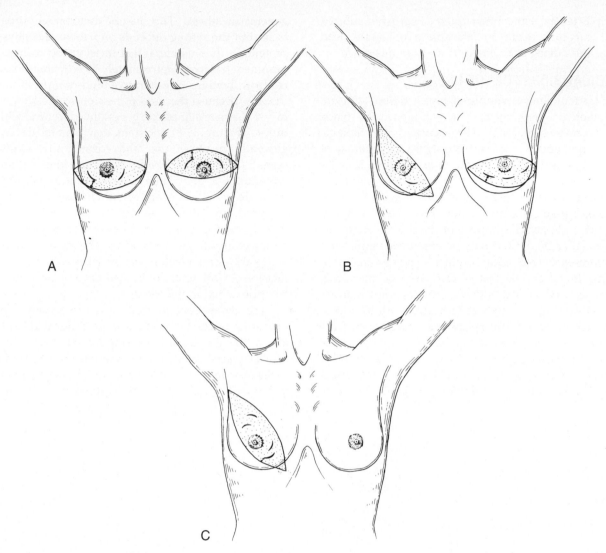

FIG. **38-9** Incisions for breast biopsy should be placed within the boundaries of skin flaps elevated for future mastectomy. **A,** Transverse Stewart mastectomy incision for total mastectomy. Margins of the mastectomy incision are developed at 1 to 2 cm from the margins of the curvilinear breast biopsy *(arrows).* **B** and **C,** Oblique and transverse mastectomy incisions are designed similarly for breast biopsy incisions in the lower one half of the breast. Circumareolar biopsy incisions are extirpated en bloc within the margins of the total mastectomy. Again, incisions are developed 1 to 2 cm from the margins of the breast biopsy *(arrows).*

with the nipple, becoming transverse over the sternum and diagonal toward the extreme upper lateral anterior chest. Periareolar and concentric lesions follow these lines of tension and therefore are optimally "aesthetic." The proposed incision is marked on the skin after the dimensions of the tumor are estimated, and local anesthesia is infiltrated into the dermis (cutis vera). Injection of anesthetic is made in the plane of the resection but not into the tumor itself, because this adds nothing to patient comfort.

After completion of the skin incision, dermal and subcutaneous bleeding is controlled and the incision is opened through the subcutaneous fat with sharp dissection to expose the tumor mass. Unless incisional biopsy is planned because of the size (>4 cm) of the neoplasm, every effort is made to avoid incision into

the tumor. Using sharp dissection guided by careful and gentle digital palpation, the operating surgeon excises the mass with a rim (1 to 2 cm) of normal breast parenchyma. If the diagnosis of cancer is not determined at histologic review of permanent sections, the entire mass should be removed.

After the specimen has been removed, attention to meticulous hemostasis with electrocautery or suture ligatures is mandatory. Catheter or Penrose drainage of the wound bed is unnecessary when adequate hemostasis is achieved. Drainage via suction methods had no impact on postoperative pain or long-term outcomes in the prospective analysis in the United Kingdom by Warren and co-workers.[81] Closure of the breast tissue defect is not mandatory, although we recommend closure when this can be performed without distortion of the shape of the breast. The subcutaneous tissues and skin are closed with absorbable sutures, and a light occlusive dressing is applied.

Goff and associates[82] observed the long-term impact of previous breast biopsy on breast cancer screening modalities in a prospective analysis. These investigators and others[83] concluded that excision at biopsy does not generally produce long-term changes that affect the interpretation of breast physical examination or mammography.

Choice of Anesthesia for One- and Two-Stage Procedures

The choice of anesthesia (local, local with sedation, or general) for breast biopsy depends on the following factors:

1. Presence of a lesion, palpable or nonpalpable
2. Age and general medical condition of the patient
3. Presumptive diagnosis
4. Necessity to procure adequate amounts of tissue for hormone receptor analysis before initiation of anticancer therapy
5. Type of biopsy (incisional, excisional, FNA) that the physician plans to perform
6. Location of the mass within the breast
7. Personal preference of the physician and the patient

In general, efforts should be made to avoid sequential general anesthesia when treating patients with a potentially malignant breast mass, although this is not always feasible or possible. For example, nonpalpable lesions that lie deep in the breast may be best excised with the patient under general anesthesia. In addition, an anxious patient who is apprehensive of undergoing the biopsy with local anesthesia may elect a general anesthetic if her medical condition is compatible with this technique.[84]

Biopsy as a separate procedure with the patient under general anesthesia should be avoided when needle biopsy, core needle biopsy, or open biopsy under local anesthesia, with or without sedation, can safely and comfortably be accomplished. The great majority of palpable and nonpalpable breast masses can be excised with local anesthesia and sedation, incurring minimal morbidity and no mortality, with substantial cost reduction.[85] Local agents such as lidocaine or bupivacaine are safe and effective and produce minimal discomfort after injection of the dermis and surrounding breast tissues. Contraindications to local anesthesia for breast biopsy generally include (1) a palpable or nonpalpable lesion deep within the breast parenchyma for which significant manipulation of tissue near the fascia is

anticipated; (2) an anxious, apprehensive patient or one who prefers to have the biopsy done while under general anesthesia; and (3) a patient with a breast mass suggestive of carcinoma who agrees to undergo biopsy, frozen section, and definite operative therapy, all during one procedure while under general anesthesia.

REFERENCES

1. Egan RL: Breast biopsy priority: cancer versus benign preoperative masses, *Cancer* 35:612, 1975.
2. Roses DF et al: Biopsy for microcalcification detected by mammography, *Surgery* 87:248, 1980.
3. Doberneck RC: Breast biopsy, a study of cost-effectiveness, *Ann Surg* 192:152, 1980.
4. Egan RL, McSweeney MB, Sewell CW: Intramammary calcifications without an associated mass in benign and malignant diseases, *Radiology* 137:1, 1980.
5. Egeli RA, Urban JA: Mammography in symptomatic women 50 years of age and under, and those over 50, *Cancer* 43:878, 1979.
6. Hassler O: Microradiographic investigations of calcifications of the female breast, *Cancer* 23:1103, 1969.
7. Hickey RC et al: The detection and diagnosis of early, occult and minimal breast cancer, *Adv Surg* 10:287, 1976.
8. McLelland R: Mammography in the detection, diagnosis and management of carcinoma of the breast, *Surg Gynecol Obstet* 146:735, 1978.
9. Pollei SR et al: Occult breast cancer: prevalence and radiographic detectability, *Radiology* 163:459, 1987.
10. Rogers JV, Powell RW: Mammographic indications for biopsy of clinically normal breasts: correlation with pathologic findings in 72 cases, *Am J Roentgenol Radium Ther Nucl Med* 115:794, 1972.
11. Kopans DB et al: Positive predictive value of breast biopsy performed as a result of mammography: there is no abrupt change at age 50 years, *Radiology* 200:357, 1996.
12. Gallager HS: Breast specimen radiography: obligatory, adjuvant and investigative, *Am J Clin Pathol* 64:749, 1975.
13. Kolbenstvedt A, Heldaas O: Value of radiography of the remaining breast following mastectomy for carcinoma, *Acta Radiol Diagn (Stockh)* 14:435, 1973.
14. Block MA, Reynolds W: How vital is mammography in the diagnosis and management of breast carcinoma? *Arch Surg* 108:588, 1974.
15. Brobeil A et al: Medical-legal pitfalls for the breast surgeon: incomplete mammographic localization of suspicious lesions and the correlation between palpable and mammographic abnormalities, *Am Surg* 62:484, 1996.
16. Millis RR et al: Biopsy of the impalpable breast lesion detected by mammography, *Br J Surg* 63:346, 1976.
17. Schmidt RA: Stereotactic breast biopsy, *CA Cancer J Clin* 144:172, 1994.
18. Schwartz AM, Siegelman S: A technique for biopsy of nonpalpable breast tumors, *Surg Gynecol Obstet* 23:1321, 1966.
19. Seidman H et al: Survival experience in the Breast Cancer Detection Demonstration Project, *CA Cancer J Clin* 37:258, 1987.
20. Heywang-Kobrunner SH et al: International investigation of breast MRI: results of a multicentre study (11sites) concerning diagnostic parameters for contrast-enhanced MRI based on 519 histopathologically correlated lesions, *Eur Radiol* 11:531, 2001.

21. Bennett IC, Freitas R, Jr, Fentiman IS: Diagnosis of breast cancer in young women, *Aust NZ J Surg* 61:284, 1991.
22. Becker W: Stereotactic localization of breast lesions, *Radiology* 133:240, 1979.
23. Dietler PC, Wineland RE, Marolo NM: Localization of nonpalpable breast lesions detected by xeromammography, *Ann Surg* 42:810, 1976.
24. Hall FM, Frank HA: Preoperative localization of nonpalpable breast lesions, *AJR Am J Roentgenol* 132:101, 1979.
25. Homer MJ, Rangel DM, Miller HH: Pre- and transoperative localization of nonpalpable breast lesions, *Am J Surg* 139:889, 1980.
26. Horns JW, Arndt RD: Percutaneous spot localization of nonpalpable breast lesions, *Am J Roentgenol* 127:253, 1976.
27. Jensen SR, Luttenegger TJ: Wire localization of nonpalpable breast lesions, *Radiology* 132:484, 1979.
28. Kalisher L: An improved needle for localization of nonpalpable breast lesions, *Radiology* 128:815, 1978.
29. Libshitz HI, Feig SA, Fetouh S: Needle localization of nonpalpable breast lesions, *Radiology* 121:557, 1976.
30. Loh CK et al: An improved method for localization of nonpalpable breast lesions, *Radiology* 130:244, 1979.
31. Snyder RE: Specimen radiography and preoperative localization of nonpalpable breast cancer, *Cancer* 46(suppl 4):950, 1980.
32. Stephenson TF: Chiba needle–barbed wire technique for breast biopsy localization, *AJR Am J Roentgenol* 135:184, 1980.
33. Stevens GM, Jamplis RW: Mammographically directed biopsy of nonpalpable breast lesions, *Arch Surg* 102:292, 1971.
34. Bauermeister DE, Hall MH: Specimen radiography: mandatory adjunct to mammography, *Am J Clin Pathol* 59:782, 1973.
35. Koehl RH, Snyder RE, Hutter RVP: The use of specimen roentgenography to detect small carcinomas not found by routine pathologic examination, *Cancer* 21:2, 1971.
36. Moss JP, Voyles RG: Operative localization of the suspicious lesion on mammography, *J Ky Med Assoc* 76:324, 1978.
37. Rosen P et al: Detection of occult carcinoma in the apparently benign breast biopsy through specimen radiography, *Cancer* 26:944, 1970.
38. Rosen PP, Snyder RE, Robbins G: Specimen radiography for nonpalpable breast lesions found by mammography: procedures and results, *Cancer* 34:2028, 1974.
39. Snyder RE, Rosen P: Radiography of breast specimens, *Cancer* 28:1608, 1971.
40. Wallace TI: Radiographic identification of calcifications in breast specimens, *Cancer* 21:11, 1971.
41. Fischer U et al: MR imaging–guided breast intervention: experience with two systems, *Radiology* 195:533, 1995.
42. Homer MJ, Fisher DM, Sugarman HJ: Post-localization needle for breast biopsy of nonpalpable lesions, *Radiology* 140:241, 1981.
43. Muhlow A: A device for precision needle biopsy of the breast at mammography, *Am J Roentgenol Radium Ther Nucl Med* 121:843, 1974.
44. Dodd GD: Pre-operative radiographic localization of nonpalpable lesions. In Gallagher HS (ed): *Early breast cancer; detection and treatment*, New York, 1975, John Wiley & Sons.
45. Hasselgren PO, Hummel RP, Fieler MA: Breast biopsy with needle localization: influence of age and mammographic feature on the rate of malignancy in 350 nonpalpable breast lesions, *Surgery* 110:623, 1991.
46. Hasselgren PO et al: Breast biopsy with needle localization: accuracy of specimen x-ray and management of missed lesions, *Surgery* 114:836, 1993.
47. Frank HA, Hall FM, Steer ML: Preoperative localization of non-palpable breast lesions demonstrated by mammography, *N Engl J Med* 295:259, 1976.
48. Cox CE et al: Analysis of residual cancer after diagnostic breast biopsy: an argument for fine-needle aspiration cytology, *Ann Surg Oncol* 2:201, 1995.
49. Gisvold JJ et al: Breast biopsy: a comparative study of stereotaxically guided core and excisional techniques, *AJR Am J Roentgenol* 162:815, 1994.
50. Meyer JE et al: Evaluation of nonpalpable solid breast masses with stereotaxic large-needle core biopsy using a dedicated unit, *AJR Am J Roentgenol* 167:179, 1996.
51. Morrow M et al: Preoperative evaluation of abnormal mammographic findings to avoid unnecessary breast biopsies, *Arch Surg* 129:1091, 1994.
52. Parker SH et al: Percutaneous large-core breast biopsy: a multi-institutional study, *Radiology* 193:359, 1994.
53. Fine RE et al: Percutaneous removal of benign breast masses using a vacuum-assisted hand-held device with ultrasound guidance, *Am J Surg* 184:332, 2002.
54. Bender JS et al: Will stereotactic breast biopsy achieve results as good as current techniques? *Am Surg* 62:637, 1996.
55. Rubin E et al: Needle-localization biopsy of the breast: impact of a selective core needle biopsy program on yield, *Radiology* 195:627, 1995.
56. Fahy BN et al: Cost-benefit analysis of biopsy methods for suspicious mammographic lesions, *Arch Surg* 136:990, 2001.
57. Wallace JE et al: The role of stereotactic biopsy in assessment of nonpalpable breast lesions, *Am J Surg* 171:471, 1996.
58. Burak WE, Jr et al: Vacuum-assisted stereotactic breast biopsy: histologic underestimation of malignant lesions, *Arch Surg* 135:700, 2000.
59. Liberman L et al: Core needle biopsy of synchronous ipsilateral breast lesions: impact on treatment, *AJR Am J Roentgenol* 166:1429, 1996.
60. Dershaw DD et al: Nondiagnostic stereotaxic core breast biopsy: results of rebiopsy, *Radiology* 198:313, 1996.
61. Liberman L et al: Atypical ductal hyperplasia diagnosed at stereotaxic core biopsy of breast lesions: an indication for surgical biopsy, *AJR Am J Roentgenol* 164:1111, 1995.
62. Liberman L et al: Stereotaxic 14-gauge breast biopsy: how many core biopsy specimens are needed? *Radiology* 192:793, 1994.
63. Fine RE, Boyd BA: Stereotactic breast biopsy: a practical approach, *Am Surg* 62:96, 1996.
64. Parker SH, Burbank F: A practical approach to minimally invasive breast biopsy, *Radiology* 200:11, 1996.
65. Liberman L et al: To excise or to sample the mammographic target: what is the goal of stereotactic 11-gauge vacuum-assisted breast biopsy? *AJR Am J Roentgenol* 179:679, 2002.
66. Liberman L et al: Bracketing wires for preoperative breast needle localization, *AJR Am J Roentgenol* 177:565, 2001.
67. Yim JH et al: Mammographically detected breast cancer: benefits of stereotactic core versus wire localization biopsy, *Ann Surg* 223:688, 1996.
68. Price JG, Kortz AB, Clark DG: US-guided automated large-core breast biopsy, *Radiology* 187:507, 1993.
69. Frazier TG et al: The value of aspiration cytology in the evaluation of dysplastic breasts, *Cancer* 45:2878, 1980.

70. Ariga R et al: Fine-needle aspirations of clinically suspicious palpable breast masses with histopathologic correlation, *Am J Surg* 184:410, 2002.

71. Kline TS, Neal HS: Role of needle aspiration biopsy in diagnosis of carcinoma of the breast, *Obstet Gynecol* 46:89, 1975.

72. Krishnamurthy S et al: Role of ultrasound-guided fine-needle aspirations of indeterminate and suspicious axillary lymph nodes in the initial staging of breast cancer, *Cancer* 95:982, 2002.

73. Doyle AJ et al: Selective use of image-guided large-core needle biopsy of the breast: accuracy and cost-effectiveness, *AJR Am J Roentgenol* 165:281, 1995.

74. Cady B: How to perform breast biopsies, *Surg Oncol Clin North Am* 4:47, 1995.

75. Tafra L, Guenther JM, Giuliano AE: Planned segmentectomy: a necessity for breast carcinoma, *Arch Surg* 128:1014, 1993.

76. Khatri VP, Smith DH: Method of avoiding tunneling during needle-localized breast biopsy, *J Surg Oncol* 60:72, 1995.

77. Simkovich AH et al: Role of contralateral breast biopsy in infiltrating lobular cancer, *Surgery* 114:555, 1993.

78. Smith BL et al: Evaluation of the contralateral breast: the role of biopsy at the time of treatment of primary breast cancer, *Ann Surg* 216:17, 1992.

79. Spratt JS, Donegan WL: Surgical management. In Donegan WL, Spratt JS (eds): *Cancer of the breast,* ed 5, Philadelphia, 2002, WB Saunders.

80. Farley DR, Meland NB: Importance of breast biopsy incision in final outcome of breast reconstruction, *Mayo Clin Proc* 67:1050, 1992.

81. Warren HW et al: Should breast biopsy cavities be drained? *Ann R Coll Surg Engl* 76:39, 1994.

82. Goff JM et al: Long-term impact of previous breast biopsy on breast cancer screening modalities, *J Surg Oncol* 59:18, 1995.

83. Sickles EA, Herzog KA: Mammography of the postsurgical breast, *AJR Am J Roentgenol* 136:585, 1981.

84. Cox G et al: Choice of anesthetic technique for needle localized breast biopsy, *Am Surg* 57:414, 1991.

85. Grannan KJ, Lamping K: Impact of method of anesthesia on the accuracy of needle-localized breast biopsies, *Am J Surg* 165:218, 1993.

CHAPTER

39

General Principles of Mastectomy: Evaluation and Therapeutic Options

KIRBY I. BLAND

JOHN B. McCRAW

EDWARD M. COPELAND III

LUIS O. VASCONEZ

Chapter Outline

The treatment of a presumably surgically operable mammary carcinoma may be reinforced by two methods: radiation alone and combined radiation and operation. The outlook upon the adoption or otherwise of the reinforcing methods depends upon the experience and judgment of the surgeon.   G.L. Cheatle and M. Cutler (1933)

With pathologic confirmation of the diagnosis of breast cancer, a complete history, physical examination, and accurate clinical staging evaluation are requisite to therapy of the primary invasive neoplasm. Mammary adenocarcinoma that is 5 cm (T_2) or less (T_1) in transverse diameter and limited to the central or lateral aspect of the breast with the absence of pectoral fascia, skin fixation, and axillary lymphadenopathy can usually be treated with conservation surgery or total mastectomy with or without node dissection alone. Lesions smaller than 4 cm in diameter may be optionally treated with segmental mastectomy (partial mastectomy, lumpectomy, or tylectomy) and postoperative irradiation, with results comparable to those achieved with radical surgical techniques. Conservation approaches are discussed in Chapter 42. For cancers larger than 5 cm (T_3) in transverse diameter (stage IIIA or IIIB), a combination of radical surgery and radiation therapy, often following neoadjuvant therapy, is essential to achieve locoregional control of the breast, axilla, and chest wall (see Chapters 63, 65, and 66).

The significant contributions of investigators for breast cancer management in the twentieth century established the outcome results for conservation surgical techniques to be equivalent to those of radical approaches with regard to disease-free and overall survival. Thus the procedure to be completed and the anatomic site to receive irradiation for stages 0, I, and II disease depend on the location of the primary neoplasm in the breast, the presence or absence of axillary metastases, phenotype of the index cancer, and the growth characteristics of the index tumor (e.g., extension to musculature of chest wall, skin, axilla).[1]

Moreover, the increasing importance of the primary tumor characteristics and its phenotype relative to its natural history have been established in clinical trials as important criteria for procedure selection. The integration of cellular, biochemical, immunohistochemical, and molecular biologic features of the tumor phenotype will increasingly direct therapies for future decades.

Lesions in the *lateral aspect of the breast* drain principally through axillary lymphatic channels (see Chapter 2). Index tumor presentations in this location can be eradicated from the chest wall by using the modified radical mastectomy with sentinel lymph node biopsy (SLNB) (see Chapters 41, 51, and 52). This surgical

procedure is defined as a total mastectomy with preservation of the pectoralis minor/major muscles and includes dissection of level I and II axillary lymph nodes. These laterally placed neoplasms with histologically positive axillary lymph node metastases may be associated with internal mammary or supraclavicular lymph node metastases in as many as 25% to 30% of patients. Radiation therapy and chemotherapy are used for "grave" presentations of the tumors: skin fixation, nodularity, greater than 20% of nodes dissected histologically involved, more than three histologically involved nodes, and chest wall tumor fixation.[2]

Centrally located lesions that are fixed to the pectoralis major fascia or high-lying (superiorly located) lesions that are fixed to this fascia may be treated with radical mastectomy or with a combination of radical mastectomy and peripheral lymphatic and chest wall irradiation when palpable axillary lymph node metastases smaller than 2 cm are evident. These centrally placed lesions commonly metastasize through lymphatics that parallel the course of the neurovascular bundle medial to the pectoralis minor muscle. This medial neurovascular bundle that contains the lateral pectoral nerve and innervates the pectoralis major muscle is preserved in the modified radical mastectomy to ensure function of the pectoralis major muscle after mastectomy. In the radical mastectomy procedure, this neurovascular bundle, associated lymphatics, and areolar tissue are resected en bloc with the specimen to accomplish adequate surgical extirpation of regional disease.

For *medially located neoplasms*, the principal lymphatic drainage is through routes that course to lymph nodes near the ipsilateral internal mammary vessels. These medial lesions may be associated with metastasis to the internal mammary lymphatics in 10% to 30% of patients, as previously confirmed by Handley.[3] The presence of pathologically positive axillary metastasis with an associated medial lesion escalates this incidence of internal mammary metastasis to greater than 50%. In the absence of clinically positive axillary metastases, medially located cancers may be adequately treated with segmental (partial) mastectomy or with modified radical mastectomy and peripheral lymphatic irradiation.

Whether the surgeon chooses the conservation or radical approach depends on tumor size and characteristics, general medical status, patient choice, and desire for reconstruction. Regardless of the operative procedure selected, clearance of pathologically "free" margins about the neoplasm in three dimensions is paramount to enhancement of locoregional disease-free survival. Margins of the tumor resection that invade the costochondrium and periosteum of ribs or sternum or the intercostal musculature (as confirmed with magnetic resonance imaging or a chest computed tomography scan) require full-thickness chest wall resection with immediate myocutaneous flap reconstruction. With "clear" margins pathologically, radiation may be administered concomitant with the treatment regimen and depends on the presenting tumor characteristics and location and the presence (number) of metastatic lymph nodes (see Chapters 57, 59, and 60). Furthermore, it is common to include chest wall irradiation when axillary metastases are identified pathologically in more than 20% of the removed axillary lymphatics. This principle was originally established because of the high incidence of skin flap recurrence evident with metastatic disease that courses to the axilla through the subdermal lymphatics from medially located primary lesions.

The principal determinant of actuarial survival of the patient after therapy of the primary breast lesion is the pathologic stage of the tumor. As established by the American Joint Committee on Cancer (AJCC), the staging system most commonly used is the tumor, node, metastasis (TNM) system. It is the responsibility of surgeons and radiation therapists to jointly plan an operative procedure that encompasses, en bloc, the extent of the disease and provides the maximum probability for locoregional chest wall control of the tumor. It is also their responsibility to achieve this end result with minimal morbidity and mortality. These principles are best served by avoiding axillary irradiation after the Patey (complete) surgical dissection of level I to III axillary lymphatics; otherwise, the incidence of lymphedema of the extremity of the ipsilaterally irradiated axilla will be increased approximately sevenfold to tenfold. Following radical resection of lymphatic channels with en bloc dissection of levels I to III, the remaining lymphatics are destroyed with radiation therapy, thus increasing the incidence of lymphedema. In principle, operable breast cancer (stages I and II) treated with total mastectomy and axillary node removal with the radical or modified radical mastectomy should not require postoperative irradiation. Currently, control of the axilla can best be achieved with level I and II dissections; clearance of level III (Patey procedure) is required only if nodes are involved clinically at dissection.[4] In contradistinction, for the treatment of stage III disease with axillary metastases that clinically present with large, matted, or multiple nodes, the radiation therapist should plan the application of tangential fields to the apex of the axilla, including the peripheral lymphatics and chest wall after the extended simple (total) mastectomy. This therapeutic regimen is essential because level III (apical) lymphatics remain intact after a resection that includes only lymphatics lateral to the border of the pectoralis major and minor muscles. With the extended total mastectomy performed for stage III breast cancer, the primary cancer or lymphatics, or both, that are larger than 1 cm in diameter are unlikely to be sterilized with irradiation alone and require surgical extirpation.

Extension of the primary neoplasm into the axillary space with invasion of the axillary artery, vein, or brachial plexus does not technically allow complete surgical removal and is best treated with regional ionizing irradiation to the axilla, breast chest wall, and supraclavicular sites. Radiotherapy should also be added to low or central axillary nodes that are determined pathologically to have *extranodal capsular extension into axillary soft tissues*, because local and regional control rates are enhanced with this modality despite the significantly increased risk for lymphedema in the ipsilateral arm. In the absence of clinically palpable nodes with primary neoplasms that exceed 5 cm in diameter, neoadjuvant chemotherapy with or without preoperative irradiation often (>80%) induces regression of the primary lesion. Preferably, surgery is performed after neoadjuvant induction with tumor regimen to reduce tumor burden before radiotherapy. The selection of surgical technique depends on the extent (volume) of regression of the primary tumor, the presence or absence of fixation to pectoralis major fascia, location, and the presence or absence of local "grave" signs (ulceration, skin edema and fixation, or satellitosis).[5]

Surgeons should plan the operative procedure with the objective of achieving, at minimum, 1- to 2-cm skin margins with subcutaneous and parenchymal margins of 2 to 3 cm in all directions from the index tumor, which can be accomplished with a radical, modified radical, or extended simple mastectomy. Patients with distant metastases, including supraclavicular lymph node metastases, are best treated with systemic chemotherapy with or without locoregional irradiation. Again, it is the responsibility of surgeons and the radiotherapists to achieve locoregional control except when adequate surgical margins are unobtainable in the absence of tumor regression, thereby reducing the probability of radiotherapeutic responses. The choice of these operative procedures must be individualized for each patient following determination of the site, clinical stage, and histologic type of the primary neoplasm. Similar principles guide the management of inflammatory breast cancers, which may be large, fixed, or ulcerated (see Chapters 63, 65, and 66).

As indicated in Chapters 12, 21, and 24, estrogen receptor (ER) and progesterone receptor (PR) activity, ploidy and S-phase determination, *HER2/neu* status, and cytologic and nuclear grading indicators should be obtained for all pathologically invasive breast cancer specimens to aid the therapeutic planning of endocrine replacement or cytotoxic therapy in the event that adverse prognostic indicators are evident. Prospective data available for analysis suggest that mean survival rates for patients receiving either chemotherapy or hormonal manipulation are greater for patients possessing positive ER/PR activity and favorable biochemical and cellular growth phase indicators than those for patients who do not (negative ER/PR; positive *HER2/neu*). Regardless of the pathologic stage of the tumor or the receptor activity, the optimal chemotherapeutic regimen for patients with metastatic breast cancer continues to evolve (Section XX). Qualitative values for hormone receptor activity of the primary neoplasm and cellular/biochemical and molecular prognosticators are of significant value to the oncologist and should be obtained from the primary lesion and metastatic sites to prospectively guide subsequent therapy.

The proper technique for the processing of tissues that contain ER and PR activity is essential to the design and implementation of future chemotherapy protocols for specific patients; the surgeon's attention to the preservation and processing of biopsy tissue is essential. Despite the importance of the ER and PR activity and other cellular/biochemical and oncogene markers to guide future therapies, processing of neoplastic tissue for pathologic examination, in all cases, must take *precedence* over determination of steroid receptor activity, as well as the procurement of additional tissues to determine cellular, biochemical, and molecular prognostic characteristics that evaluate tumor phenotype (see Chapters 21, 22, and 24).

Immunohistologic methodologies have been extensively applied for the past decade with replacement of quantitative steroid receptor analyses with less problematic concern for receptor invalidation. However, surgeons should also be aware of the potential for electrocautery to diminish steroid receptor activity. This has been confirmed by Ellis and associates[6,7] and by Bland and colleagues[8] to be dependent on heat inactivation by the ambient temperature and by devascularization (Table 39-1). The procurement of primary breast cancer tissue for pathologic diagnosis and for determination of immunohistologic (qualitative) steroid receptor activity is best accomplished with the cold scalpel. This technique avoids the possibility of heat induction artifact, tissue necrosis, cellular death, and temperature-dependent inactivation of steroid receptor activity of the procured tissues. Nonetheless, tumor excision with cautery can be used if the operator avoids *direct contact* of tumor specimen with the cautery blade. The indications and techniques for biopsy of suspicious breast masses are comprehensively reviewed later in this chapter.

Topographical Surgical Anatomy

Chapter 2 provides a detailed review of the anatomy of the breast, including discussions of regional vasculature, neurologic structures, and lymphatic drainage. Hollingshead[9] observed that the fibrous and fatty components of breast tissue occupied that interval between the second or third rib superiorly, with extension to the sixth or seventh ribs inferiorly. The breadth of extension includes the parasternal to the midaxillary lines. The glandular portion of the breast rests largely on the pectoral fascia and the serratus anterior musculature; however, mammary tissue extends typically into the anterior axillary fold (tail of Spence) and may be visible as a well-defined superolateral extension from the upper outer quadrant of breast tissue. Extent of the mammary tissue is ill defined and varies considerably with patient habitus and lean muscle mass.

Parenchymal volume of the gland, with anterior and lateral projections, is variable and depends on lean body mass, habitus, age, and ovarian functional status. Because the ductal and lobular components are almost exclusively sensitive to the trophic effects of secretory estrogen and progestational hormones, the breast remains underdeveloped and rudimentary in the male. In men, short ducts with poorly developed acini are evident. Thus a deficiency of parenchymal fat and

| TABLE **39-1** | Steroid Hormone Receptor versus Ischemia Time* |

	ISCHEMIA TIME (min)				
RECEPTOR (*n*=11)	0	30	60	90	150
ER	100	79 ± 10[†]	67 ± 11[†]	54 ± 11[†]	56 ± 13[†]
PR	100	100 ± 21	101 ± 26	94 ± 14	84 ± 27
AR	100	57 ± 12[†]	53 ± 15[†]	28 ± 9[‡]	42 ± 12[†]

*Ischemia significantly decreased estrogen receptor (ER) levels within the first 30 minutes ($p = .05$). ER values had sustained decrease throughout 150 minutes of ischemia. Similarly, androgen receptor (AR) levels were significantly lower by 30 minutes of ischemia ($p = .002$) and remained so throughout 150 minutes of ischemia. The largest decrease in ER and AR levels occurred within the first 30 minutes of ischemia. In contrast, progesterone receptor (PR) levels were unchanged throughout 150 minutes of ischemia.
[†]$p < .005$ compared with baseline by analysis of variance.
[‡]Values are mean ± SEM, expressed as percent of control at baseline.

nipple/areola development are apparent and contribute to the nonspheroidal or flat appearance of the male breast.

Relative to the male breast, the nonparous breast is hemispheric and somewhat flattened above the nipple. The multiparous breast, on the other hand, is large and is replaced in part with fat, which accounts for its lax, soft appearance; it rarely regains its initial configuration until menopause, when atrophy of glandular tissue is initiated. The breast is circumscribed anteriorly by a superficial layer and posteriorly by a deep layer of the superficial investing fascia of the chest wall. The superficial layer of the superficial fascia of the chest wall derives its anterior boundaries from the fibrous tissue of the tela subcutanea. Haagensen[10] observed the deep layer of the superficial fascia to be contiguous with the pectoral fascia.

Following loss of estrogen influence on breast parenchyma and ductal structures, the postmenopausal breast is replaced by fat and is consistently noted to lack supportive parenchymal connective tissue and active (proliferative) glandular components. Spratt and Donegan[11] and Spratt and Tobin[12] note the nonlactating breast to weigh between 150 and 225 g, whereas the lactating organ may weigh as much as 500 g.

NEUROLOGIC INNERVATION OF THE PECTORAL MUSCLES*

As evident in major surgical texts, the anatomy of the medial/lateral pectoral nerves and the innervation of the pectoral muscles has evoked only minimal interest. Major textbooks of surgical anatomy have long considered the names of the medial pectoral and lateral pectoral nerves on the basis of *origin* from the *brachial plexus*. Therefore the names in classic anatomic teaching are *not* correlated with their medial or lateral anatomic positions found during surgery (Figure 39-1). Moosman,[13] however, completed a detailed study of the pectoral nerves by dissection of 100 adult fixed and fresh cadaver pectoral regions (56 male and 44 female), and transposed the names of the medial and lateral pectoral nerves according to their anatomic relationship to the pectoral muscles and to the anterior chest wall. These nerves, sometimes called *anterior thoracic nerves,*

*For purposes of clarity and consistency, the editors have retained the classic anatomic description and nomenclature for the pectoral (anterior thoracic) nerves and the accompanying neurovascular bundles (see Chapter 2, Section II). The name of the neurovascular bundle (lateral or medial) is synonymous with its course (position) in the axilla. Classic anatomy teaches that the pectoral nerves are named from the brachial cord (medial or lateral) from which they originate. In the technical description of operative procedures within this chapter and in anatomic descriptions elsewhere in this textbook (see Chapters 40 through 42), we have retained the classic nomenclature.

originate cephalad and posterior to the axillary vein from an anastomotic nerve loop of variable size between the medial and lateral brachial plexus cords.

Moosman[13] notes in his anatomic dissections that the *lateral pectoral nerve* arises anatomically from the lateral cord and in location is *medial* to the pectoralis minor muscle. In its course, it divides into two to four branches that pass downward and medial to supply the clavicular, manubrial, and sternal components of the pectoralis major muscle. Thereafter the nerve passes through the costocoracoid foramen with the thoracoacromial vessels and enters the interpectoral space to

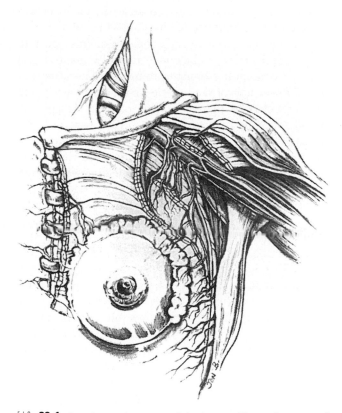

FIG. **39-1** Arteries and nerves of the breast. View of nerves of the axilla that provide innervation to the pectoral muscles and muscles of the chest wall and posterior axillary space. The long thoracic nerve is identified and protected at the juncture where the axillary vein passes over the second rib. Injury or division of this nerve will result in "winged scapula" as a result of paralysis of the serratus anterior. The thoracodorsal nerve is found in the posterior axillary space with origin medial to the thoracodorsal vessels. This nerve may accompany the thoracodorsal artery and vein en route to its innervation of the latissimus dorsi. Injury results in weakness of abduction; internal rotation of the shoulder also will result. The medial (anterior thoracic) pectoral nerve is superficial to the axillary vein and lateral to the pectoralis minor muscle, which it variably penetrates en route to its innervation of the pectoralis major muscle. The lateral (anterior thoracic) pectoral nerve lies at the medial edge of the pectoralis minor muscle and superficial to the axillary vein. With origin from the lateral cord of the brachial plexus, this nerve supplies major motor innervation to the pectoralis major.

mix with tributaries of vascular origin to the muscle. Moosman observed that this nerve is larger than the medial pectoral nerve because of the greater volume of muscle it innervates.

The *medial pectoral nerve* is smaller (approximately 1 to 2 mm in diameter and 10 to 15 cm in length) than the lateral pectoral nerve, and its origin is medial or posterior to the pectoralis minor. This nerve sends branches to the pectoralis minor and descends on its dorsal surface. Typically this nerve crosses the axillary vein and is accompanied by small tributaries from the axillary or thoracoacromial vessels. It enters the interpectoral space and supplies the lower third of the costoabdominal portion of the pectoralis major muscle. In an extensive review of the anatomy of the medial pectoral nerve, Moosman[13] observed the relationship of this nerve to the pectoralis minor to be one of several variants: (1) as a single descending branch around the lateral border of the lower half of the muscle (38%); (2) division into two branches, with one branch passing *through* the muscle and the other *around* its lateral margin (32%); (3) as a single descending branch that passed *through* the muscle (22%); and (4) as two or three descended branches of varying size, each of which passes through the muscle often at different levels (8%). He observed motor branches to the pectoralis major coursing through the pectoralis minor in 62% of cases.

In rare circumstances the medial pectoral nerve may pass through the medial muscular components of the pectoralis minor or, in other cases, may remain entirely on its medial surface. When numerous branches arise from the major trunks, a more diminutive size can be expected for branches that innervate the pectoralis major. The nerve remains relatively large when it is a single branch, whereas multiple branches passing through the muscle may be of thread size.[13]

Regardless of the anatomic nomenclature used, the surgeon must be cognizant of potential damage to the nerve supply to the pectoralis muscles at all levels of dissection. Manipulation, traction, electrocautery, or resection may destroy the lateral or medial pectoral nerves unless they are carefully separated from nerve branches of variable size.

VASCULAR DISTRIBUTION

Nutrient arterial supply to the skin and breast is through branches of the *lateral thoracic arteries*, the *acromiothoracic branch of the axillary artery*, and the *internal mammary artery*.[14] The venous drainage system includes the intercostal veins, which traverse the posterior aspect of the breast from the second or third through the sixth or seventh intercostal spaces to terminate and enter posteriorly into the vertebral veins. The intercostal veins may arborize centrally with the azygos system to terminate in the superior vena cava. The deep

venous drainage of the breast in large part parallels the pectoral branches of the acromiothoracic artery and the lateral thoracic artery.

The large epithelial and mesenchymal surface area of the superior, central, and lateral aspects of the breast is drained by tributaries that enter the *axillary vein*. Venous supply from the pectoralis major and minor muscles also drains into tributaries that enter the axillary vein. Perforating veins of the *internal mammary venous system* drain the medial aspect of the breast and the pectoralis major muscle. This large venous plexus can be observed to traverse the intercostal musculature and terminate in the innominate vein, providing a direct embolic route to the venous capillary network of the lungs. Each plexus of veins in the lateral and medial aspects of the breast is observed to have multiple, racemose anastomotic connections.

LYMPHATIC DRAINAGE AND ROUTES FOR METASTASES

The rich and elaborate lymphatic drainage generally parallels the arterial and venous supply of the breast. This lymphatic flow is primarily unidirectional except in subareolar and central aspects of the breast or in circumstances in which physiologic lymphatic obstruction occurs as a consequence of neoplastic, inflammatory, or developmental processes that initiate a reversal of flow with bidirectional egress of lymph.[15] This bidirectional lymphatic flow (see Figures 2-12 and 2-14) may account for metastatic proliferation in sites remote from the primary neoplasm (e.g., the opposite breast and axilla). The delicate lymph vessels of the corium are valveless and encircle the lobular parenchyma to enter each echelon of the regional lymphatic nodes in a progressive and orderly fashion (e.g., level I → level II → level III). As indicated in Chapter 2 (see Figures 2-14 through 2-16), multiple lymphatic capillaries anastomose and fuse to form fewer lymph channels that subsequently terminate in the large left thoracic duct or the smaller right lymphatic duct (see Figures 2-6 and 2-16). As a consequence of the predominant unidirectional flow of lymph, two accessory drainage routes exist for lymph en route to nodes of the apex of the axilla and include the *transpectoral* and the *retropectoral* routes, as defined by Anson and McVay.[14] First described by German pathologist Rotter, Rotter's nodes are lymphatics of the *transpectoral* or *interpectoral* routes that occupy the position between the pectoralis major and minor muscles. Cody and coworkers[16] and Netter[17] report Rotter's nodes to be present in up to 75% of individuals, with an average of two to three nodes per patient. Cody and colleagues[16] observed that 0.5% patients with negative nodes and 8.2% of patients who had positive axillary nodes had evidence of Rotter lymph node metastases. This observation was rarely reported by Haagensen.[10] Therefore, although the Patey axillary dissection, included in the Halsted radical[18] and in the modified radical mastectomy, removes the interpectoral Rotter group en bloc, this nodal group plays only a diminutive role in the diagnosis and therapy of breast cancer. The retropectoral lymphatics, however, may play a more important physiologic role in drainage of the breast because they are exposed to the superior and internal portions of the mammary glands. These lymphatics arborize lateral and posterior to the surface of the pectoralis major muscle and terminate at the apex of the axilla. To achieve an adequate en bloc resection of major axillary nodal groups, the surgeon must achieve a thorough conceptualization of breast lymphatic drainage. Familiarization with the anatomy of this area is essential for staging and for curative resection.

Section II, Chapter 2, deals with the *principal axillary nodal groups* as described by Anson and McVay.[14] Figure 39-2 topographically depicts anatomic levels I to III of the axillary contents with relation to the neurovascular bundle, the pectoralis minor, the latissimus dorsi, and the chest wall. The following axillary nodal groups are included in *level I*:

1. The *external mammary group* parallels the course of the lateral thoracic artery from the sixth or seventh rib to the axillary vein. This group occupies the loose areolar tissue inferior and lateral to the pectoralis major muscle in the medial distal axillary space.
2. The *subscapular group* is contiguous with thoracodorsal branches of the subscapular vessels. This group extends from the ventral surface of the axillary vein to the lateral thoracic chest wall and includes loose areolar tissue on the serratus anterior and subscapularis musculature.
3. The *lateral axillary vein group* is the most laterally placed nodal group of the axillary space. This group also contains the largest number of nodes in the axilla and is observed to be caudad and ventral to the surface of the axillary vein often lateral to the latissimus dorsi muscle. This nodal group is first encountered in the course of proximate dissection on the anterior-most surface of the latissimus dorsi muscle.

Level II, or the *central nodal group*, is immediately beneath the pectoralis minor muscle and is the most centrally located of the axillary lymphatic groups. This nodal group is located between the anterior and posterior axillary fold and occupies a superficial position beneath the skin and fascia of the midaxilla. The highest and most medially placed of the lymph node groups is the *subclavicular (apical group)*, designated as *level III*. This is the cephalomedial lymph nodal group that is

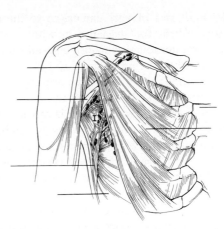

FIG. **39-2** Topographic anatomic depiction of levels I, II, and III of the axillary contents with relation to the neurovascular bundle, pectoralis minor, latissimus dorsi, posterior axillary space, and chest wall. Level I comprises three principal axillary nodal groups: the external mammary group, the subscapular group, and the axillary vein (lateral) group. Level II, the central nodal group, is centrally placed immediately beneath the pectoralis minor muscle. The subclavicular (apical) group is designated level III nodes and is superomedial to the pectoralis minor muscle.

located just proximate to the termination of the axillary vein at its confluence with the subclavian vein at the level of *Halsted's (costoclavicular) ligament* (condensation of the clavipectoral fascia). Figure 39-2 depicts the position of these nodes relative to the pectoralis minor muscle and the posterior axillary space. These nodal groups are described relative to topographic anatomic relationships with the pectoralis minor muscle and the medial, lateral, and posterior axillary space. These lymphatics may be different from the nodal groups described by pathologists to indicate the area of metastatic involvement within the axilla.

Evolution of Surgical Techniques for Mastectomy

In 1894, Halsted[18] and Meyer[19] simultaneously reported their radical operations for treatment of cancer of the breast. By demonstrating superior locoregional control rates using en bloc radical resection techniques, these eminent surgeons established the radical mastectomy as the "state-of-the-art" modality of that era to control cancer of the breast. Subsequently, many modifications of the original incision developed by Halsted have been reported and include those of Meyer, Kocher, Rodman, Stewart, Warren, Greenough, Orr, Gray and MacFee, to mention only a few variations of the incision.[20] Many of the original incisions were developed to permit multiple approaches for extirpation of the mamma and to allow access to the axillary contents.

The Halsted[18] and Meyer[19] radical mastectomies differed technically in the sequence in which the breast and nodes were removed. Halsted insisted on primary resection of the breast and pectoral muscles before dissection of the axillary contents. In contrast, the Meyer technique (modified Halsted incision) advised the axillary dissection first, which was followed in sequence by breast and pectoral muscle resections, respectively. As indicated in Figure 39-3, the result achieved and the final cosmetic appearance for the Halsted and Meyer mastectomies are similar. Both procedures use a vertical incision to facilitate detachment of the pectoralis major from the clavicle and humerus and removal of the pectoralis minor from the coracoid process of the scapula. Incisions subsequently adopted by various European and American surgeons are indicated in Figure 39-3 and represent incision modifications for operable breast cancer in each quadrant of the organ. It should be noted that Halsted[18] and Meyer[19] strongly advocated the necessity of en bloc resections for extirpation of the breast and the contents of the axilla but had little appreciation for clinical staging and the ultimate consequences of systemic disease. In their era, no adjuvant modalities (radiation/chemotherapy) existed to provide effective cytoreduction of the advanced primary lesion; thus advanced stages of disease could be extirpated only with the use of wider skin margins and larger flaps. For this reason, various incision modifications that incorporate breast resection and wound closure were developed.

Eminent breast surgeons of the late nineteenth and early twentieth centuries appreciated early in the formulation of therapeutic principles that the total mastectomy incision should incorporate both the nipple and the biopsy site to reduce the possibility of tumor implantation in the wound. In original dissections of the axilla, both Halsted[18] and Meyer[19] advocated complete axillary dissection of all three nodal levels from the latissimus dorsi muscle laterally to the thoracic outlet medially. Both surgeons routinely sacrificed the long thoracic nerve and the thoracodorsal neurovascular bundle en bloc with the axillary contents. Therefore it is not surprising that much of the initial criticism leveled at the radical mastectomy in the treatment of breast carcinoma concerned itself with the limitation of motion in the shoulder and the ipsilateral lymphedema that followed surgery. It also could be argued that survival rates for these patients, especially those with advanced locoregional disease, were not increased in proportion to the resultant disabilities (e.g., the "winged scapula" and shoulder fixation) evident with the procedures. Subsequently, Haagensen[10] advocated preservation of the long thoracic nerve to avoid the winged scapula disability and motor apraxia evident with loss of innervation to the serratus anterior. Furthermore, Haagensen[10]

advocated removal of the thoracodorsal neurovascular bundle (with neural innervation to the latissimus dorsi muscle) to allow clearance of the subscapular and external mammary lymphatics that follow the course of this neurovascular structure. However, the majority of breast surgeons currently preserve *both* the long thoracic and the thoracodorsal nerves in the absence of gross invasion by the neoplasm or nodal fixation to these nerves. These principles are strictly enforced to ensure function of the scapula and to preserve viability and motor innervation of the latissimus dorsi, such that myocutaneous breast reconstruction may be a future option.

It should be noted that contemporary modifications of the Halsted or Meyer radical mastectomy, with preservation of the long thoracic nerve, can be performed with little or no increase in morbidity compared with simple mastectomy.[15,21] In addition, any argument of the simple versus the radical procedure should be concerned with the long-term survival of the patient, which is the ultimate goal of therapy. To deny a patient the benefit of an adequate operative procedure on the basis of difficulty in placing cosmetic incisions or difficulty with wound closure is tantamount to disregard of an indisputable tenet that portends locoregional recurrence of disease.

The highly regarded and significant contributions of D. H. Patey[22,23] of the Institute of Clinical Research, Middlesex Hospital, London, should be recognized. His careful clinical development and scientific demonstration of the worth of the "modified radical mastectomy" technique are laudable. In Britain in the 1930s, only a small minority of physicians questioned the absolute necessity of radical mastectomy for carcinoma of smaller size (AJCC stage I/II) with absence of fixation to the pectoral muscles. Three major influences led Patey in the 1930s and 1940s to consider therapeutic alternatives; design of the modified radical mastectomy technique followed. The first and most important consideration was the development and application of modern radiation therapy. The second influence was the growing evidence of dissatisfaction with Sampson Handley's theory of "lymphatic permeation" as the primary process for the dissemination of carcinoma of the breast—a theory that, in its day, provided a logical pathologic basis for some of the technical details of the radical mastectomy.[22] Third, with newer techniques for the study of lymphatic anatomy, Patey was able to scientifically refute the unproven postulates on which the original radical operations were based.[11,15] Thereafter, Patey and his colleagues developed the technique for incontinuity removal of the breast and axillary contents (levels I, II, and III) with preservation of the pectoralis major muscle. This technique removes the pectoralis minor, like the standard radical operation, as the essential operative maneuver to provide access for complete

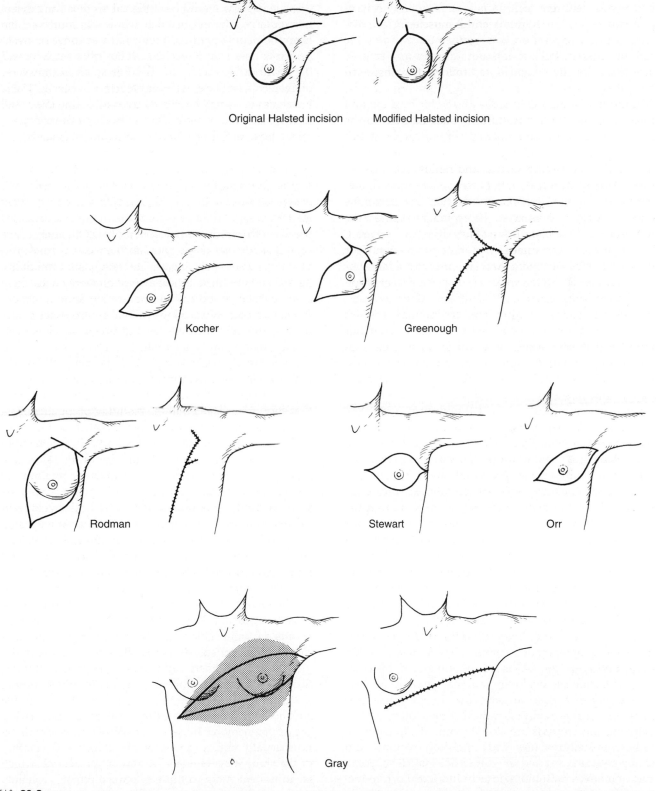

Original Halsted incision   Modified Halsted incision

Kocher   Greenough

Rodman   Stewart   Orr

Gray

FIG. **39-3** Variants of the radical mastectomy incision used in the therapy of primary carcinoma of the breast by various surgeons. The original Halsted incision was revised to avoid encroachment on the cephalic vein, which was preserved in subsequent procedures.

clearance of the axillary contents. Thereafter, objective demonstration of the efficacy for removal of axillary lymphatics with the technique was proven with lymphangiography by Kendall and associates[24] in 1963. Although this operation was performed by Patey for the first time in 1932, it was not adopted as a routine alternative to the standard radical mastectomy until late 1936.[11]

Although Patey is credited with the formulation and implementation of the modified radical mastectomy as a standard approach for operable breast cancer, it was Auchincloss[25] and Madden[26] who described and developed technical variants of the modified radical mastectomy. As described earlier, the Patey mastectomy differs from the Halsted mastectomy in that the pectoralis major muscle is preserved. Patey acknowledged the importance of the complete axillary dissection (levels I, II, and III) and appreciated the anatomic necessity for preservation of the medial and lateral pectoral (anterior thoracic) nerves, which may serve as dual innervation to the pectoralis major. In contrast, Madden[26] and Auchincloss[25] advocated modified radical mastectomies with preservation of *both* the pectoralis major and minor muscles. The similarities of the approaches were that these techniques required total mastectomy with at least *partial* axillary lymph node dissection. Because these approaches preserved the pectoralis minor, dissection of the apical (subclavicular, level III) nodes was restricted, and in all cases, nodal recovery was less complete than with the Patey modified technique. The advantage of the Auchincloss[25] and Madden[26] procedures may be the greater probability for preservation of the medial pectoral nerve, which courses in the lateral neurovascular bundle of the axilla and may course through the pectoralis minor to supply the lateral border of the pectoralis major muscle. Expectantly, the Madden and Auchincloss techniques dissect only level I and II nodes and preserve level III lymphatics. Even currently, some surgeons advocate preservation of the pectoralis minor and simply detach the tendinous portion of the muscle from the coracoid process of the scapula to allow near-complete dissection of level III nodes to Halsted's ligament. On completion of the nodal dissection, the tendon of the pectoralis minor was reapproximated to the coracoid with stainless steel wire or nonabsorbable suture.

Students of breast surgery quickly recognize that incisions for the modified radical mastectomy are less extreme, and wounds are closed primarily. In contrast, radical procedures use wide incision margins, and skin is routinely grafted to wound defects. The application of modern radiobiologic techniques and cytoreductive chemotherapy currently does not require primary incisions that totally ablate the skin of the breast (see Figure 39-3). Before the application of modern adjuvant techniques, incisions for large tumors that were considered locally advanced (because of ulceration, edema, and other "grave" signs) were designed to encompass these lesions with wide (3 to 5 cm) margins.

All skin flaps should be designed so that the incision incorporates skin and parenchyma at minimum of 1 cm from the periphery of the tumor in three dimensions. In principle, less skin is excised when lesions are located deep within the breast and T-size is small in transverse diameter (T_1 <2 cm). As indicated in Chapter 2, viable breast tissue is anatomically distributed on the chest wall from the sternum to the axilla and from the clavicle to the aponeurosis of the rectus abdominis tendon. Haagensen[10] demonstrated that small foci of glandular tissue could be histologically identified in close proximity to the dermis just beneath the superficial fascia. Halsted[18] and Haagensen[10] each considered that wide skin excision of at least 5 cm in all directions from the tumor was essential because of the rich superficial lymphatic channels of the central subareolar tissue and subcutaneous dermal lymphatic plexuses of the breast. The rationale of the classic radical and modified radical mastectomies is increasingly being challenged because of the availability of adjuvant modalities that enhance locoregional control with potential lengthening of disease-free and overall survival rates. These tenets form the anatomic and pathologic basis for the *skin-sparing mastectomy,* which is comprehensively discussed later in this chapter.

Debate continues regarding the *thickness* of skin flaps that should be elevated in the planning of the total mastectomy as part of the radical or modified radical procedure. Krohn and colleagues[27] report a two-arm study to evaluate the necessity of the "ultrathin" skin flap and the use of autogenous skin graft as methods to enhance local wound control with 5- and 10-year survival. A similar group of women who underwent radical mastectomy with narrow margins of skin excision with primary wound closure *without* ultrathin flaps had comparable 5- and 10-year survival and local recurrence rates. Wound complications, duration of hospital stay, and subsequent lymphedema, however, were significantly greater in the patients with thinner skin flaps. Most surgeons acknowledge that superior cosmetic results are achievable with well-vascularized flaps and the avoidance of split-thickness skin grafting. We maintain these basic tenets and avoid development of ultrathin flaps. Flaps developed at the plane of insertion of Cooper's ligament deep to the cutis reticularis with the subcutaneous fat ensure extirpation of the underlying breast parenchyma. In general, flaps of 6- to 8-mm thickness usually ensure generous vascularity and viability of the skin. Subcutaneous fat may be preserved, which is consistent with complete parenchymal resection. Although the deep layer of the superficial investing fascia that intervenes between the subcutaneous fat and the breast tissue is easily identified, the thickness of this well-vascularized flap varies considerably with the patient's habitus and lean body mass.

Total mastectomy for operable cancer that is not amenable to conservation surgical techniques has been addressed previously. In principle, advanced primary lesions (T_2 or T_3), with pectoralis major fixation, high-lying lesions, and perhaps some lesions with "grave" signs should be treated with radical or modified radical techniques. As discussed previously, the operations designed by Halsted, his predecessors, and his students reflect the necessity of designing wider flaps with large incisions for advanced primary cancers (T_3a, T_3b, T_4) to technically encompass the primary lesion by at least 5 cm. When considering the advanced primary lesions that were treated in that era without adjuvant techniques, the necessity of larger resections can be rationalized as surgery was the only option for locoregional control.

The design of incisions that allow removal of the entire mammary gland (total or simple mastectomy) must incorporate the nipple/areola complex with the primary tumor in a three-dimensional aspect such that deep and peripheral margins are free of disease.[28] Donegan and co-workers[29] previously determined that incisions that resect skin and breast parenchyma at a distance of more than 4 cm from any margin of the palpable tumor achieve no therapeutic success. Currently, many surgeons consider a 1- to 2-cm margin adequate to achieve local control without tumor implantation.

Intraoperative frozen section for marginal clearance is appropriate, especially margins 1 cm or less from the index neoplasm. As discussed earlier in Chapter 38, incisions placed in the breast for suspicious masses must be planned with consideration for the subsequent need for total mastectomy. Incisions should incorporate the primary biopsy scar, which should be well planned at the time of initial biopsy to allow complete extirpation of the neoplasm with the definitive mastectomy. When the primary breast lesion has been totally removed with the original biopsy as an excisional technique, incisions placed for total mastectomy should incorporate the skin and scar of the biopsy site by a minimal 1-cm margin in all three dimensions of the resection. We prefer incisions (Orr/modified Orr) that are slightly oblique from the transverse line and that extend cephalad toward the axilla. However, under no circumstance should the cosmetic design of an incision compromise the successful extirpation of the primary neoplasm. Split-thickness skin grafting has virtually been replaced with myocutaneous flap reconstruction following mastectomy for T_3 or T_4 primary neoplasms when wider margins and larger flaps are required for wound closure after neoadjuvant therapy.

Figures 39-4 through 39-10 depict the various locations of breast primaries in which adequate therapy,

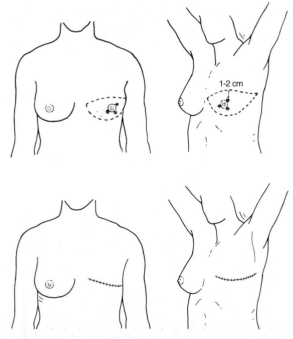

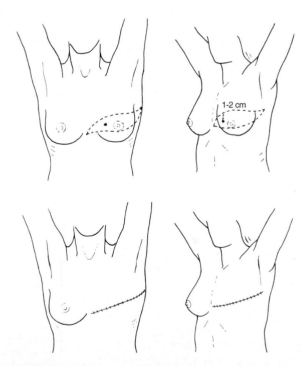

FIG. **39-4** Design of the classic Stewart elliptical incision for central and subareolar primary lesions of the breast. The medial extent of the incision ends at the margin of the sternum. The lateral extent of the skin incision should overlie the anterior margin of the latissimus dorsi. The design of the skin incision should incorporate the primary neoplasm en bloc with margins that are 1 to 2 cm from the cranial and caudal edges of the tumor.

FIG. **39-5** Design of the obliquely placed modified Stewart incision for cancer of the inner quadrant of the breast. The medial extent of the incision often must incorporate skin to the midsternum to allow a 1- to 2-cm margin in all directions from the edge of the tumor. Lateral extent of the incision ends at the anterior margin of the latissimus.

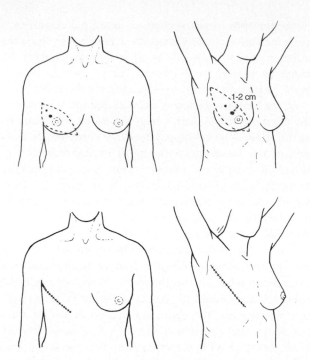

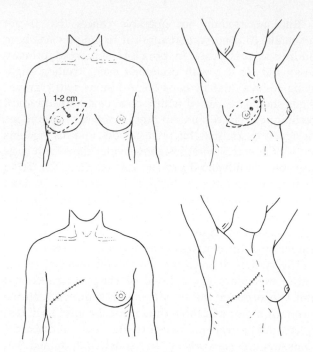

FIG. **39-6** Design of the classic Orr oblique incision for carcinoma of the upper outer quadrants of the breast. The skin incision is placed 1 to 2 cm from the margin of the tumor in an oblique plane that is directed cephalad toward the ipsilateral axilla. This incision is a variant of the original Greenough, Kocher, and Rodman techniques for flap development.

FIG. **39-8** Design of skin flaps for upper inner quadrant primary tumors of the breast. The cephalad margin of the flap must be designed to allow access for dissection of the axilla. With flap margins 1 to 2 cm from the tumor, variation in the medial extent of the incision is expectant and may extend beyond the edge of the sternum. On occasion, the modified Stewart incision can incorporate the tumor en bloc, provided that the cancer is not too high on the breast and craniad from the nipple/areola complex. All incision designs must be inclusive of the nipple/areola when total mastectomy is planned with primary therapy.

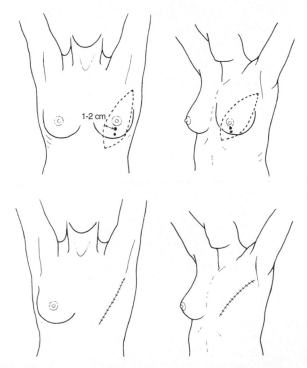

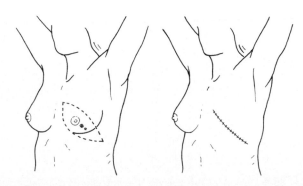

FIG. **39-7** Variation of the Orr incision for lower inner and vertically placed (6 o'clock) lesions of the breast. The design of the skin incision is identical to that of Figure 39-5, with attention directed to margins of 1 to 2 cm.

FIG. **39-9** Incisions for cancer of the lower outer quadrants of the breast. The surgeon should design incisions that achieve margins of 1 to 2 cm from the tumor with cephalad margins that allow access for dissection of the axilla. The medial extent is the margin of the sternum. Laterally, the inferior extent of the incision is the latissimus.

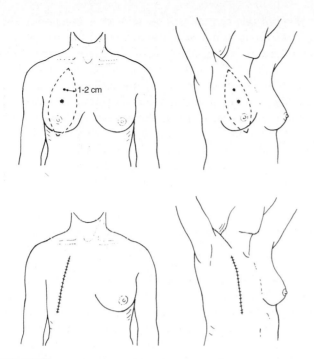

FIG. **39-10** Depiction of skin flaps for lesions of the breast that are high lying, infraclavicular, or fixed to the pectoralis major muscle. Fixation to the muscle and/or chest wall necessitates Halsted radical mastectomy with skin margins at least 2 cm. Skin grafting is necessary when large margins of skin are resected for T$_3$ and T$_4$ cancers. Primary closure for T$_1$ and some T$_2$ tumors is often possible.

with or without irradiation and chemotherapy, necessitates total mastectomy, which is completed with conventional technique in which reconstruction is not planned. For all mastectomy procedures, note that wide (radical) skin margin (>5 cm) excisions are not considered essential for locoregional disease control. However, skin margins of at least 1 to 2 cm from the gross index tumor or the surgical biopsy (excision) scar are necessary to ensure final pathology-free margins. Margins in excess of 2 cm are technically feasible for most total mastectomies in which reconstruction (early or delayed) will not be completed. Preoperative consideration should be given to the skin-sparing technique (see discussion later in this chapter) when the patient desires reconstruction.

Design of Incisions for Mastectomy in the Treatment of Breast Cancer

CENTRAL AND SUBAREOLAR PRIMARY LESIONS

Figure 39-4 depicts the design of the classic Stewart elliptical skin incision (see Figure 39-3) that is used for mastectomy of *subareolar or central* breast primaries.

The original biopsy preferably is done through a periareolar incision for lesions in this location. The residual scar should have precise measurements for the cephalad and caudad extents of the incision to include a minimal 1-cm margin. Availability of adequate skin to complete the primary closure is rarely difficult in the pendulous or large breast. For most patients with small breasts, the Stewart (transverse) incision will allow primary closure of skin except when more than 4 to 5 cm of skin are encompassed in the primary resection or if evidence of skin devascularization is apparent following completion of the procedure. Loss of skin secondary to loss of vascularity with ultrathin dissection planes or trauma to the flaps may necessitate even wider resections of skin margins.

Figure 39-5 shows an optional elliptical incision in the contour of the breast for an *inner quadrant* primary lesion. This incision would perhaps best be described as the *modified Stewart incision*, which has a predominant extension in a more oblique and cephalad direction toward the ipsilateral axilla. The Stewart incision is commonly preferred by plastic surgeons anticipating *delayed reconstruction* with myocutaneous flaps, especially when a contralateral simple mastectomy is planned for treatment of high-risk disease or as a prophylactic procedure. Furthermore, this technique is often the choice of oncologic surgeons when radiation to the chest wall is planned before reconstruction.

LESIONS OF THE UPPER OUTER OR LOWER INNER QUADRANTS

Figures 39-6 and 39-7 denote the incision design for operable breast cancer in the *upper outer* or *lower inner* quadrants. Minimal skin margins of 1 to 2 cm from the primary neoplasm are incorporated in a *modified Orr incision* that is slightly oblique from the transverse line with cephalad extension toward the axilla. Similar to the Orr and Stewart incisions, although somewhat more oblique, these incisions lend themselves to cosmetically satisfactory breast reconstruction results using myocutaneous or subpectoral augmentation breast implants.

LESIONS OF THE UPPER INNER QUADRANTS

Lesions of the *upper inner* quadrants of the breast are the most difficult to manage because of their anatomic location. Surgeons should recognize the inherent problems encountered with elevation of skin flaps that allow adequate surgical margins and provide cosmesis for wound closure and potential reconstruction. Surgeons should be able to develop a 1- to 2-cm margin for lesions that are in this quadrant, providing the lesion is not cephalad (infraclavicular). These lesions may be accessed through the modified Stewart incision. Commonly, surgeons encounter the dilemma of designing an elliptical incision that is widely based near the cephalomedial aspect of the breast to incorporate a 1- to 2-cm margin of the tumor with extension laterally and inferiorly such that the incision terminates at the anterior axillary line (Figure 39-8). Surgeons should plan the cephalic portion of the incision for the superior flap such that adequate access to the pectoralis major and to the axillary contents is ensured.

LESIONS OF THE LOWER OUTER QUADRANTS

Lesions of the *lower outer* quadrants of the breast should have an incision design similar to those of the upper inner quadrant, with margins of 1 to 2 cm around the primary lesion (Figure 39-9) and with maximum extension of the cephalad margin to provide access to flaps for dissection of the pectoralis major and the axillary contents.

HIGH-LYING (INFRACLAVICULAR) LESIONS

With large lesions (T_2, T_3, T_4) that are *high lying*, *infraclavicular*, or fixed to the pectoralis major, incisions designed to provide a minimal 1- to 2-cm margin will necessitate skin grafting of the defect or coverage with myocutaneous flaps. The original Halsted and Meyer incisions, with subsequent modifications by Greenough, Rodman, and Gray (see Figure 39-3), were used for treatment of primary lesions of T_2, T_3, and T_4 size.[21] For T_1 lesions in this position, design of an elliptical incision placed in a vertical dimension from the clavicle provides adequate access for axillary dissection and clearing of the pectoralis major muscle when indicated, but is unequivocally cosmetically deforming. Figure 39-10 depicts the design of this cosmetically inferior vertical, elliptical incision for these high-lying lesions and the vertical closure. Because these incisions are placed perpendicular to Langer's lines, cosmesis is minimized and the planes of cleavage for the medial breast are subsequently ablated.

Skin-Sparing Mastectomy

TOTAL MASTECTOMY WITH LIMITED SKIN EXCISION: RATIONALE AND TECHNIQUE OF THE "SKIN-SPARING" TOTAL MASTECTOMY

Wide skin excision is routinely used with every radical and modified mastectomy. A mastectomy with wide skin excision is often inclusive of an excision in excess of 30% to 50% of the breast skin. This is removed as an ellipse, usually measured 10 cm (width) by 20 cm (length), and is closed primarily. The elliptical excision facilitates removing the dog-ears that are technically created by the wide skin removal and subsequent tension of excessive tissue at the terminal points of skin closure.

Limited skin excision can be defined as excision of the nipple/areola complex, the skin around the biopsy site, and the skin within 1 to 2 cm of the tumor margin. This technique usually sacrifices 5% to 10% of the breast skin, which is either approximated primarily or closed with an autogenous myocutaneous flap that is used to replace the breast volume. Dog-ears do not occur with this technique, because the limited skin removal does not initiate skin contracture with closure.

Over the course of the twentieth century, the clinical guidelines for breast skin excision with mastectomy have developed anecdotally and have been applied by convention. Furthermore, the benefits of wide versus limited skin excision have not been subjected to prospective randomized trials. Because locoregional surgical control of breast cancer has improved over the last 60 years, the extent of the breast skin excision with mastectomy has decreased proportionally. Standards of practice have sequentially evolved as follows: (1) total excision of the breast skin, to (2) wide excision without primary closure, to (3) wide excision with primary closure, and finally to (4) the "skin-sparing total mastectomy." Indications and techniques for limited skin excision with mastectomy are reviewed here.

FACTORS AFFECTING LOCAL RECURRENCE

With the increasing acceptance and application of breast conservation techniques for the therapy of ductal carcinoma in situ and invasive neoplasms of lobular and ductal origin, it is essential that the surgeon determines whether adequate excision margins are achieved to confer long-term local control. Gilliland and co-workers[30] and Johnson and associates[31] determined the necessity of total mastectomy with and without node dissection; with the exception of advanced disease (T_3, T_4 tumors), immediate breast reconstruction can be completed without any effect on the quality or duration of survival. As noted by Johnson and colleagues, local recurrence is usually a harbinger of systemic disease and, predictably, factors for local recurrence also represent prognostic indicators of survival. The 1992 report by Kurtz[32] reviewed common host and histologic features that influence local failure following breast conservation and irradiation to the intact breast for clinical stage I and II disease. Kurtz determined that the significant features that correlate with increased risk are young age at time of primary therapy and the presence of an extensive intraductal component within the invasive index (primary) neoplasm. In addition, this clinical study determined that adequacy (volume) of the surgical excision, the use of systemic adjuvant therapy, and high-quality radiation therapy techniques all contribute to a reduction in the risk of locoregional recurrence.

Biologic Factors: Effect on Local Recurrence. Contemporary oncologic treatment planning necessitates the incorporation of biologic factors related to the tumor phenotype and cellular characteristics. Aside from nodal status, these parameters exceed all other considerations in assessing various treatment modalities, including total excision of the breast. With the increasing acceptance and application of breast conservation techniques for treatment of both in situ and invasive neoplasms of lobular and ductal origin, it is essential that the surgeon determine whether adequate excisional margins are achieved to confer long-term locoregional control. Many investigators[33-39] acknowledge the importance of patient selection to achieve optimal disease-free survival relative to locoregional recurrence within the ipsilateral mastectomy site. The large prospective analysis ($n = 1036$) by the German Breast Cancer Study Group for therapy of $T_1N_0M_0$ disease concluded that the width of the margin of excision (in centimeters) had no impact on prognosis.[40] However, this analysis of patients who were randomized between breast preservation and mastectomy did establish conclusively that poorer disease-free survival was associated with microscopically involved margins in the conservation technique when compared with the mastectomy study group (75% versus 90% at 3 years). Tumor size and tumor grade were also prognostic factors that accurately predicted recurrence. Age, ER/PR status, menopausal status, histologic tumor type, and type of therapy (mastectomy versus breast preservation) were not significant predictive factors of recurrence.

The full realization of the impact of contemporary developments in molecular and genetic markers as prognostic indicators of locoregional recurrences has not yet been fully assimilated into oncologic practice.[41] As these tests gain acceptance, recognition of patients with unfavorable disease will be facilitated at the outset following cellular, biochemical, and molecular-genetic analysis of the primary neoplasm. The current method, which uses one variant of the mastectomy for all patients, can then be improved through the design of individual treatment. Moreover, the comprehensive prospective analysis of the National Surgical Adjuvant Breast and Bowel Project (NSABP) by Fisher and associates[42] suggests that the extent (type) of mastectomy and regional node excision are not associated with significant differences in survival from more radical procedures.

Tumor Volume (Size): Effect on Local Recurrence. For patients who are *not* treated with irradiation after breast conservation surgery, tumor size is an important determinant of risk for local recurrence, as reported in data from the NSABP by Fisher and co-investigators.[43,44] Fowble and colleagues,[45] Stotter and associates,[46] and

Kurtz and co-workers[47] note that larger neoplasms (e.g., T_3, T_4) comprise most of these local failures. These findings are further amplified by the large, long-term study by Kurtz of operable T_1 and T_2 invasive breast cancers. Within the range of tumor diameter appropriate to breast conservation, Kurtz[32] determined that the size of the primary lesion had no apparent influence on the risk for local recurrence, provided that macroscopically complete resection was achieved (Table 39-2). Although the analysis by Kurtz[32] includes radiation of the intact breast with the goal of preserving the organ, other researchers[48,49] have come to similar conclusions in patients undergoing mastectomy alone. Kroll and colleagues[49] and Dao and Nemoto[48] reiterate that this reduction in the local recurrence rate is evident when the adequacy of resection is confirmed.

Of significance, Holland and co-workers[50] previously determined in serial subgross sectioning of mastectomy specimens that the percentage of breasts harboring residual foci 2 cm distal to the edge of the index tumor was similar for T_1 (T_1a, T_1b, T_1c) cancers (≤ 2 cm) and those between 2 and 5 cm (T_2) in transverse diameter. Data from virtually all large series designed to corroborate these findings determined that local failure is not more frequent in operable T_2 than in T_1 primary tumors. However, from a technical perspective, adequate local excision with macroscopically clear margins is more difficult to achieve in the T_2 lesion, especially for patients with diminutive native breast volume.

Breast Skin Excision: Effect on Local Recurrence. The 1963 study by Dao and Nemoto[48] confirmed that the risks associated with skin preservation in mastectomy are in effect more theoretical than actual. In a series of 135 consecutive cases of breast cancer, these

TABLE 39-2	Crude Rate of Local Recurrence in the Breast for 1350 Stage I and II Patients as a Function of Clinical Breast Tumor Size*

TNM STAGE	CLINICAL TUMOR SIZE (cm)	LOCAL RECURRENCE (%)	p VALUE
T_{1a}, T_{1b}	<1	29/255 (11.4)	NS
T_{1c}	1.1-2.0	45/438 (10.3)	NS
T_2	2.1-3.0	40/392 (10.2)	NS
T_2	3.1-4.0	21/179 (11.7)	NS
T_2	4.1-5.0	21/86 (13.9)	NS

Modified from Kurtz JM: *Eur J Cancer* 28:660, 1992.
NS, Nonsignificant; *TNM*, tumor, node, metastasis.
*Patients were treated at the Cancer Institute and associated clinics in Marseille between 1962 and 1981 (median follow-up 10 years).

investigators observed that skin recurrence was evident in 27.5% of locally advanced tumors, but the incidence was only 2% for patients with nonadvanced disease. Later, Kroll and associates[49] determined that a low recurrence rate (1.2%) could be achieved with conservation of the uninvolved breast skin. In this study, patients undergoing mastectomy with immediate autogenous breast reconstruction were treated with skin-sparing mastectomy. The limited breast skin excision included the nipple, areola, and a 1-cm margin around the previous biopsy scar. Significantly, this mixed group of T_1, T_2, T_3, and T_x TNM-staged cancers did not demonstrate any additional risk for local recurrence when treated with a 1-cm skin margin around the biopsy scar and even narrower cutaneous margins for deep or small tumors. Both of these studies, therefore, relate local recurrences to biologic aspects of the tumor more than to extirpative (technical) differences of the procedure. Moreover, Dao and Nemoto[48] concluded "skin recurrence is nothing more than metastasis at an additional site in patients with widespread disease." These authors further noted that "the frequency of skin recurrence is governed by the pathological stage of the disease, rather than by the amount of skin that is removed."

EVOLUTION OF BREAST SKIN EXCISION WITH MASTECTOMY

Radical Mastectomy. The Halstedian principles of complete mastectomy embodied an anatomic basis for cancer surgery, which presumed an improved survival rate with the more radical extirpative approach (see Chapter 40). Recurrences were usually interpreted as evidence of inadequate locoregional therapy, and therapy was rarely directed to systemic disease.[27] This premise dictated therapy of breast cancers managed in the halstedian era, because the majority were T_3 and T_4 neoplasms. Extremely wide excision of skin was established as an absolute dictum for the cancer cure; unfortunately, this concept prevailed for 80 years, well into the twentieth century. Before World War II, mastectomies for cancer were designed to remove *all* breast tissue and included the pectoralis major and minor muscles and the axillary lymph nodes. There was some variation, however, in the management of the volume and technique for breast skin excision (see Figure 39-3).

Near-Total Excision of the Breast Skin without Undermining to Develop Skin Flaps. In concurrent evolution of the technique of mastectomy, Halsted and Meyer advocated extremely wide skin excision because of the advanced presentation of disease at that time (T_3, T_4) for most patients.[18,19,51,52] Primary closure was rarely attempted, except by skin grafting. The wound was routinely allowed to granulate.

Wide Dissection of Skin Flaps with Extensive Skin Removal. Handley[53] popularized dissection of the breast

skin away from the breast tissue as a thin skin flap. Because the skin removal was much less radical, primary closure of the skin flaps was occasionally attempted.

Wide Dissection of Thin Skin Flaps with Less Extensive Skin Removal. Finney[20] also developed thin skin flaps, but with less extensive skin removal.[54] Primary closure of the skin flaps was usually attempted. After World War II the Finney modification of the Halsted-Meyer mastectomy evolved into the predominant method of radical mastectomy.

Modified Radical Mastectomy. With the evolution of less radical techniques, modified radical mastectomy was popularized by Patey and Dyson[23] in 1948 as an acceptable therapeutic option to the Halsted procedure (see Chapter 41). As stated earlier, Patey began using this method in 1932 and used it routinely after 1936. This conservative approach was a revolutionary departure from the previous time-honored and proven methods espoused by Halsted and Meyer and their surgical pupils in that it preserved the pectoralis major muscle. Patey based his method on the belief that locoregional dissemination of the breast cancer did not commonly involve the pectoralis muscle, unless the tumor was attached to the fascia and/or infiltrated this muscle. However, he did believe that wide skin excision was essential to cancer control because of the histologic proximity of the ductal tissue and the breast skin and their lymphatic-venous connections. In 1969, Handley and Thackray,[55] also from the Middlesex Hospital in London, confirmed the effectiveness of Patey's modified mastectomy. Although the procedure preserved the pectoralis major muscle, all of these surgeons were firmly convinced of the necessity of wide skin excision, as evidenced by the fact that more than 50% of their patients required skin grafting for closure. It was not until the 1960s that primary closure of the Patey mastectomy was routinely attempted. Auchincloss,[25] and later Madden,[26] preserved the pectoralis major and minor muscles and advocated low axillary node dissection (levels I and II) with less extensive skin resection. Auchincloss used a horizontal skin closure, whereas Madden used a vertical skin closure. The Auchincloss-Madden technique routinely allowed the surgeon to close the breast skin, with survival results comparable to those of the operations championed and advocated by Halsted, Meyer, and Patey. As noted by Bland and colleagues[56] (see Chapter 37), the contemporary modified radical mastectomy is essentially the same operation originally described by Moore[57] in 1867, more than a century before it became the worldwide standard of breast cancer therapy.

Currently, the modified radical mastectomy remains the most common surgical therapy for both invasive and in situ carcinoma of the breast, despite the eligibility of many women for breast conservation techniques or skin-sparing total mastectomy approaches. Furthermore, as of 1991, most patients with ductal carcinoma in situ still had axillary node dissections, despite the low nodal positivity rate that approximates 1% to 2%[4] (see Chapters 11, 47, 48, and 54). Although the 1995 report of the Commission on Cancer of the American College of Surgeons[58] suggests increasing use of breast-conserving surgery for in situ disease from 20.9% in 1985 to 35.4% in 1991, modified radical mastectomy represented the principal therapy of the disease and remained constant at 42%. Moreover, the use of radiation for patients with ductal carcinoma in situ following partial mastectomy without node dissection ranged from 24.2% in 1990 to 37.7% in 1985. These contemporary trends suggest an enlightened awareness of the design of the technical procedure to accommodate patient desires while achieving locoregional disease control equivalent to that seen with more radical approaches. However, similar reports emphasize the necessity of inculcation of various objective pathologic and radiologic criteria (e.g., cellular and biochemical variables, oncogenes, mammograms) to integrate risk parameters of the tumor phenotype. These various factors allow the clinician to more accurately determine risk for locoregional recurrence. Future prospective clinical trials will determine the specter of limitations for breast conservation. Regardless, the necessity of total mastectomy with or without regional nodal dissection will maintain primacy as the desired therapeutic modality for various stages of presentation.

Skin Preservation Procedures. With the introduction of the breast conservation treatments of lumpectomy radiation and quadrantectomy radiation, surgeons introduced the concept of minimal skin removal in the quadrant of the tumor and nipple/areola complex preservation, if the latter was clinically uninvolved.[59,60] Lumpectomy radiation was initially proposed by Mustakallio in 1954 for patients who refused radical mastectomy.[61] This new (but unconventional) treatment proved to be effective in providing disease-free survival, and it evolved as a consequence of the interest and the advocacy of a number of clinical investigators.[62,63] Fisher and co-workers[59] first experimentally introduced the new concept of systemic tumor cell dissemination that varied from the pure mechanical and anatomic factors previously espoused by Halsted and others. Fisher's concepts of "biological determinism" and hematogenous dissemination acknowledged the ineffectiveness of regional lymphatic systems as tumor "filters." Today, both lumpectomy and quadrantectomy are well-accepted variants of treatment options because of the theories developed by Fisher and colleagues[42-44,59,64] and by Veronesi and co-workers,[60] respectively.

In the late 1970s, the mammographic diagnosis of in situ disease and minimal breast cancer (T_{mic}, T_1a, T_1b) produced a new subset of patients with early-stage disease. In 1986, Bland and associates[65] described a skin preservation technique in which the nipple is resected and augmentation is achieved with subpectoral prosthetic implants. This procedure described a total "glandular" mastectomy with skin preservation of the entire breast. In 1991, Toth and Lappert[66] described a total mastectomy without extensive skin resection as an appropriate treatment for patients with minimal breast cancer and in situ disease. These authors were first to coin the term *skin-sparing mastectomy* (SSM), which was used primarily in patients with relatively favorable disease indicators. These patients had limited skin resection, which included the biopsy site, the nipple/areola complex, and any additional breast skin adjacent to the tumor needed to provide an adequate histologically free margin of tumor excision. In the skin-sparing mastectomy, skin resection is limited and all ductal tissue is completely extirpated, as would be completed for any total glandular mastectomy. The technical dictum of complete parenchymal resection is scrupulously observed in this method, including the posterior margins and the axillary tail of Spence. The uninvolved breast skin can be preserved without compromise of oncologic purpose of the procedure. The reconstruction and rehabilitation goal is to provide the patient with breast symmetry, form (cleavage), and contour, which often can be achieved without placement of incisions in medial and upper (infraclavicular) quadrants of the breasts.

The skin-sparing mastectomy has been used primarily for patients with AJCC–TNM stages 0, I, and early II disease requiring mastectomy when eligible for immediate autogenous breast reconstruction.[49,66-68] Most of the patients eligible for the technique of combined mastectomy-reconstruction were selected because they were *not* candidates for lumpectomy and postoperative radiation. The authors consider the following to be *indications for skin-sparing techniques:*

1. Multicentricity of disease (ductal in situ, any invasive histology)
2. Invasive carcinoma associated with an extensive intraductal component that is 25% or more of tumor volume
3. T_2 tumors (2 to 5 cm), especially those with unfavorable features on radiographic or physical examination that defy confidence in follow-up examination
4. A central tumor that would require removal of the nipple/areola complex

None of the aforementioned indications necessitates wide skin removal to achieve adequate extirpation of the neoplasm. Additional patients have been selected for limited skin resection because of *relatively favorable indications,* and include the following:

1. In situ cancers of lobular and ductal origin
2. Multifocal, minimal breast cancer (T_{mic}, T_1a, T_1b)
3. All T_1 and possibly T_2a tumors deep within the breast parenchyma, following neoadjuvant therapy, with significant cytoreduction of tumor volume
4. A positive family history (first-degree relatives) or genetically confirmed oncogene mutagenesis (e.g., *BRCA1, BRCA2*) together with worrisome histologic features such as atypical lobular or ductal hyperplasia
5. Patients with and without familial inheritable (genetic) disease when physical or radiographic features, or both, defy confidence in follow-up examination, especially when multiple biopsies are indicated

For the aforementioned patients, extensive removal of breast skin does *not* enhance treatment control by improving survival or decreasing local recurrences. Conversely, for patients with large tumors (e.g., ≥5 cm, T_3, T_4), particularly with attachment to the overlying skin and subcutaneous tissues, with or without ulceration, extensive skin removal is clearly justified and advisable; the SSM technique is inadvisable with this stage of presentation of disease.

To achieve total glandular mastectomy, some clinics advocate preservation of the areola by nipple-coring to enhance aesthetic appearance. Although this practice is acceptable, it may prove ill-advised for oncologic procedures that attempt total extirpation of mammary ducts of the nipple/areola complex, because this premise incorrectly assumes that the areola is devoid of mammary ductal tissue. Schnitt and associates[69] performed marginal excision of the nipple (nipple-coring) on eight consecutive mastectomy specimens, excised the areolas, and thereafter submitted all tissues for histologic analysis. Mammary ducts in the areola were extensive and were identical to those of extralobular ducts in the breast parenchyma. Schnitt and colleagues concluded that mammary ducts represent a normal histologic component of the areolar dermis and that nipple-coring alone does not result in complete removal of all mammary ductal tissue from the nipple/areola complex. However, areolar preservation may be an insignificant risk parameter relative to local recurrence, because residual breast tissue is evident in all viable skin flaps following total glandular mastectomy.

Technical Aspects of Skin-Sparing Mastectomy. It is unfortunate that total glandular mastectomy techniques with axillary lymph node dissection

(e.g., modified radical mastectomy) and without axillary lymph node dissection (e.g., simple [total] mastectomy), followed by immediate reconstruction in which skin preservation is a prominent feature of the mastectomy, have received little attention in the general surgical or surgical oncology literature. Resection of the previous biopsy scar and wound cavity with skin overlying the neoplasm, the nipple or the nipple/areola complex, and the entire breast parenchymal contents are cardinal technical caveats of the skin-sparing mastectomy (Table 39-3). Furthermore, Carlson[67] notes that breast symmetry with reconstruction will be enhanced with preservation of the native skin because of similar skin color and an improved shape. As indicated previously, technical access to the axilla for lymph node dissection is essential; planning of cosmetically acceptable incisions that allow partial access to sampling (levels I and II) or Patey dissection (levels I, II, and III) are critical to the technical design. Currently, we and others conduct SLNB with the skin-sparing approach. If possible, the SLNB is "frozen" for pathologic analysis by hematoxylin and eosin touch prep technique; axillary node dissection (level I/II) should be completed when the node is histologically positive. This approach is preferred rather than delay the axillary node dissection following transverse rectus abdominis myocutaneous (TRAM) or latissimus dorsi myocutaneous reconstruction. Reentry nodal dissections may injure the vascularity of the tissue transfer or create axillary hematomas with levels I/II node removal.

The anatomy of the breast with regard to skin-sparing mastectomy has been properly outlined by Carlson.[67] The glandular tissue, including the nipple and areola, is removed en bloc. When the tumor is located within 3 cm or less from the skin surface, the overlying skin is removed en bloc with the specimen. A 1- to 2-cm

TABLE 39-3	Technical Features of the Skin-Sparing Mastectomy

1. Skin excision (1-cm margins) of the previous biopsy site or scar overlying index neoplasm
2. Skin excision (marginal only) of nipple/areola complex
3. Total glandular mastectomy, which includes the index tumor or previous biopsy wound cavity en bloc with skin excisions 1 and 2
4. Skin incision design must ensure technical access to the axilla when lymph node dissection (sampling, levels I/II; Patey, levels I, II, III) is indicated
5. Sentinel lymph node biopsy as indicated; if histologically positive, lymph node dissection to be completed synchronously with skin-sparing mastectomy

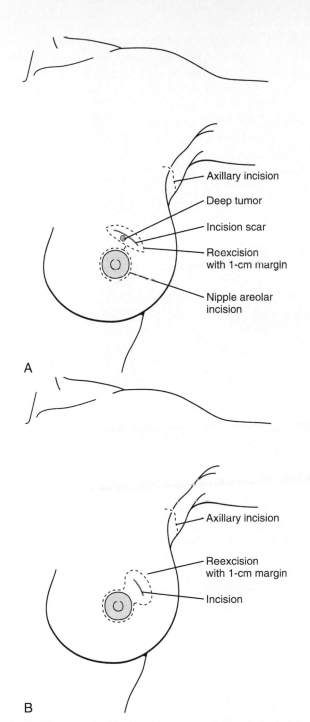

A

B

FIG. **39-11** A and B, Breast incisions when the biopsy site is contiguous with the areola. Note that axillary incision is remotely placed.

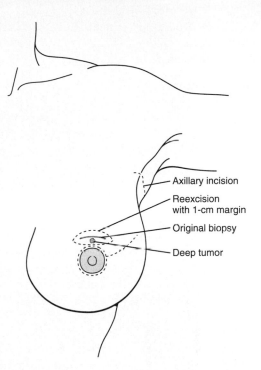

FIG. **39-12** Lateral extension of the periareolar incision to enhance exposure for dissection. Remote axillary incision may not be essential if incision is extended toward axilla.

technically more demanding than the ablative modi-fied/radical approach, this procedure is technically pos-sible in patients with small tumors or minimal breast cancer. This approach is also an option in patients after stereotactically placed core guidance biopsy, where often the cylinder of the needle does not provide com-plete excision of the tumor. The increasing application of SLNB is diminishing the need for formal axillary node dissections, thus avoiding separate (and deform-ing) axillary dissections.[70-74] When nodes are histolog-ically positive following sentinel mapping, level I/II dissection should be completed synchronously with the skin-sparing mastectomy.

Figures 39-11 through 39-25 depict the various therapeutic principles and their application that may exist for patients eligible for skin-sparing techniques. Figures 39-16, 39-18, 39-21, 39-23, and 39-25 show breast incision variants of skin-sparing mastectomy for all quadrants when the primary tumors and biopsy sites are located in a site *remote* from the nipple/areola complex. Essential to completion of the oncologic aspects of this technique are removal of the nipple or the nipple/areola complex and a 1-cm margin of skin about the biopsy site. Lesions that are juxtapositioned to the areola may be excised with a single skin island flap (Figures 39-26 through 39-36). Lesions with biopsy scars greater than 4 cm from the areola margin require *separate excisions* with attention to preservation of a well-vascularized intervening skin bridge. All excisions

margin of breast skin is typically removed around the biopsy scar; the remaining breast skin contour is preserved in its entirety.

Incision Design. Ideally, the entire mastectomy should be performed through a keyhole approach, circumscribing the sacrificed nipple and areola, which remain en bloc with the breast parenchyma. Although

Text continued on page 836

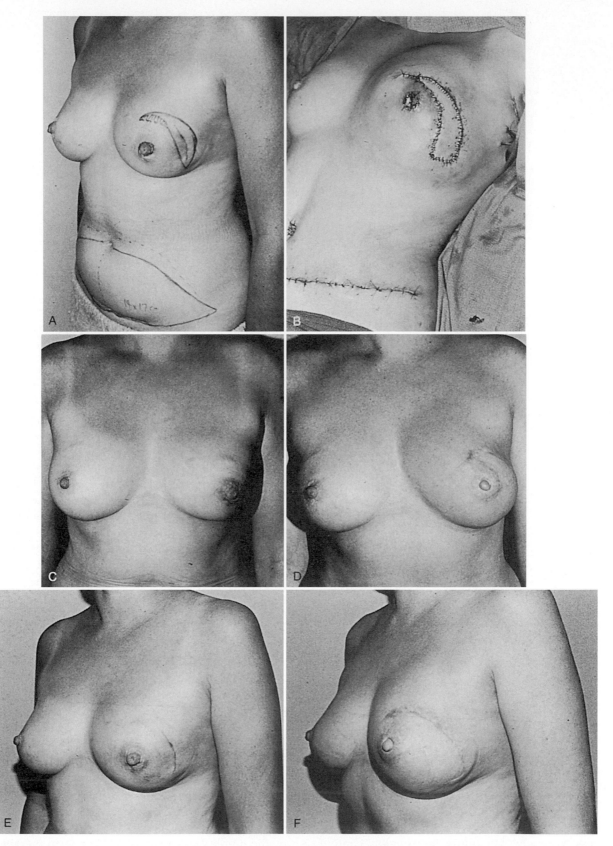

FIG. **39-13 A** and **B,** Preoperative markings of a conservation mastectomy and immediate transverse rectus abdominis myocuta-neous (TRAM) flap breast reconstruction. Intraoperative view of the skin replacement of the lateral breast in the area of the previous biopsy. The TRAM flap was used for volume, surface skin replacement, and immediate nipple reconstruction. Preoperative **(C)** and postoperative **(D)** views following completion of the left breast and nipple reconstruction. No procedure was completed in the right breast. Without the skin conservation mastectomy, it would not have been possible to match the normal right breast. Oblique preoperative **(E)** and postoperative **(F)** views.

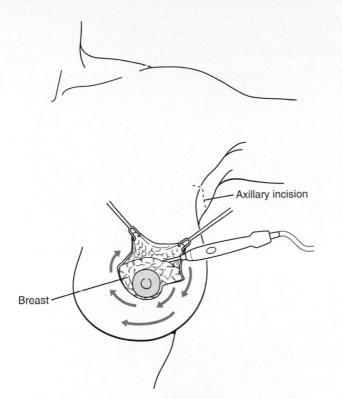

FIG. **39-14** Skin flap elevation is above the superficial fascia. Centripetal dissection enhances exposure. Flap contour with thickness of 7 to 8 mm ensures viability. Dissection should not enter breast parenchyma because margins are developed to chest wall en bloc.

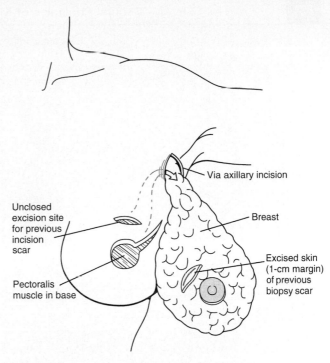

FIG. **39-15** After dissection of the flaps and breast parenchyma from the pectoralis major fascia and mammary bursae, the axillary contents are dissected en bloc and delivered through the axillary incision.

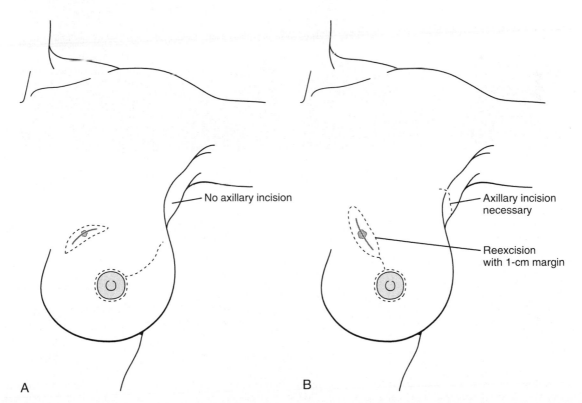

FIG. **39-16** Upper inner (medial) quadrant. **A,** One-centimeter excision that is remote from periareolar incision with lateral extension of modified Orr incision. No axillary incision is necessary because exposure with this approach is adequate for lymph node sampling. **B,** This figure depicts a primary tumor and biopsy site that are vertically placed and radial with 1-cm margins. Following incisions at margin of nipple/areola complex, continuous development of incision allows adequate breast parenchymal exposure. When axillary dissection is necessary, remote incision may be planned.

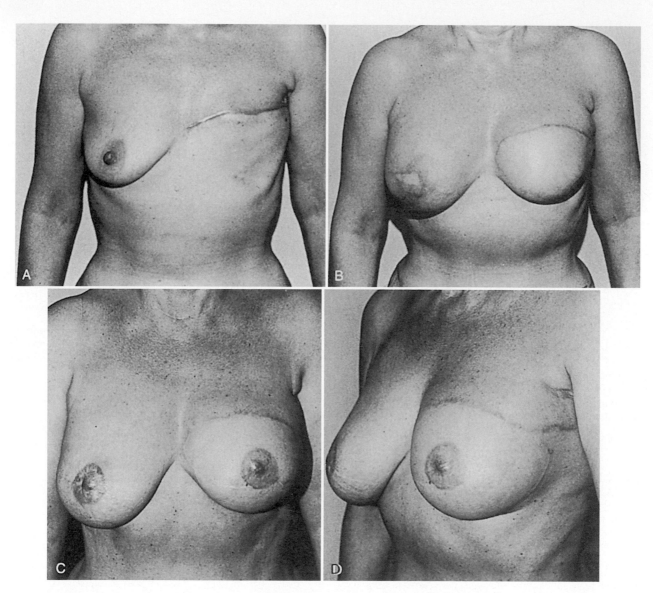

F I G. **39-17** Upper inner (medial) quadrant. **A,** Patient with a previous left modified mastectomy for stage I disease with no special reason for extensive skin removal. **B,** Bilateral transverse rectus abdominis myocutaneous (TRAM) flap breast reconstruction done at the time of the right skin conservation mastectomy. Note the difficult skin replacement in the left breast. It was necessary to replace all of the missing skin below the mastectomy scar with a TRAM flap. In the right breast, all of the TRAM flap was buried except for the part needed to form the nipple and areola. **C,** One year following the completion of the breast and nipple reconstructions. **D,** Achieving symmetry was difficult because of the radical skin excision of the left breast.

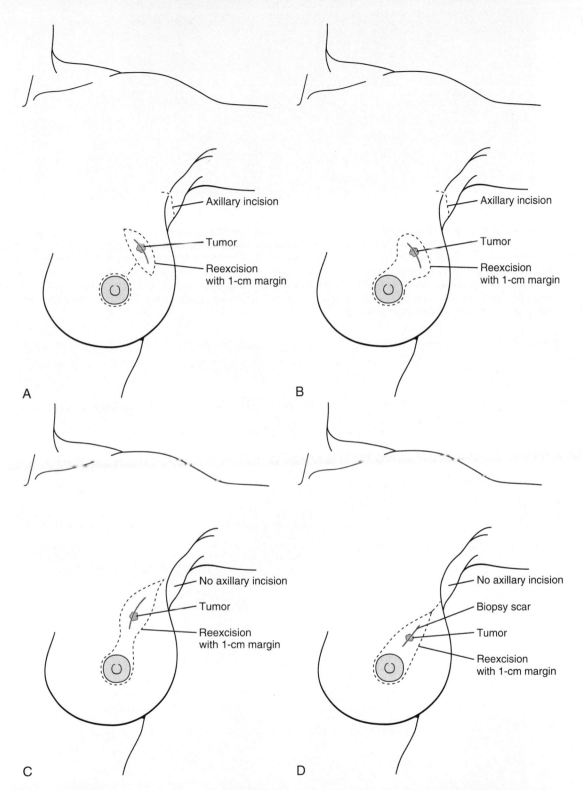

FIG. **39-18** Upper–outer (lateral) quadrant. **A,** Nonradial biopsy site excised with 1-cm margins; nipple/areola marginal incision becomes contiguous with biopsy site to give breast exposure for dissection. Remote axillary dissection incision may be essential for proper technical access to level I and II nodes. **B,** Nonradial biopsy site excised with 1-cm margins at the most lateral extension of incision with resection of contiguous skin intervening between nipple and areola. Remote axillary incision is usually necessary for adequate sampling exposure. **C,** Vertically placed (radial) biopsy site necessitates modified Orr skin flaps inclusive of the 1-cm margins of the biopsy site. Axillary exposure is adequate without remote incision. **D,** Has similar radial biopsy site to **C.** Periareolar incision in continuity with 1-cm margin of biopsy site gives excellent exposure to breast and axilla.

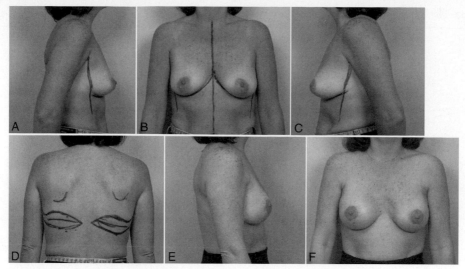

FIG. **39-19** This image series shows a 40-year-old woman with a history of familial, premenopausal breast cancer who before consultation had six breast biopsies, including three within the last year. This patient underwent bilateral mastectomies and immediate reconstruction using bilateral latissimus dorsi myocutaneous flaps with saline-filled silicone implants to add volume. **A, B,** and **C,** Preoperative markings from anterior and lateral views (note the midline, inframammary, and anterior axillary line markings). **D,** A skin island design based on underlying muscle. The skin island is designed as an ellipse to close primarily at the level of the brassiere line. The tips of the scapulae are marked denoting the cephalad extent of the latissimus dorsi muscle bilaterally. **E** and **F,** Postreconstruction anterior and lateral views.

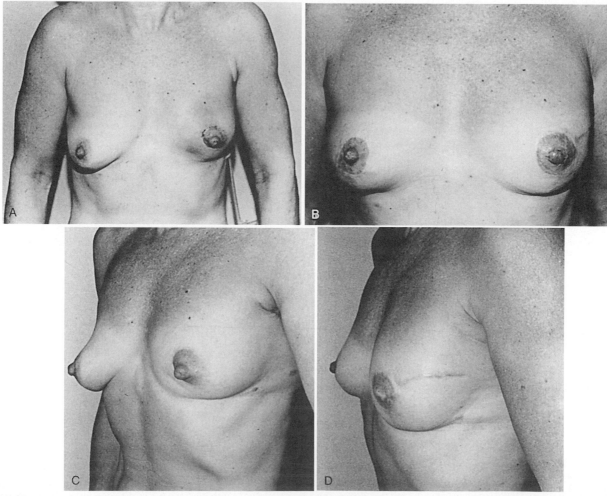

FIG. **39-20** Upper outer (lateral). Preoperative **(A)** and postoperative **(B)** views following left skin conservation mastectomy for stage I disease. The time of mastectomy, an immediate free transverse rectus abdominis myocutaneous (TRAM) flap breast and nipple reconstruction were performed in a single stage, with a right mastopexy for symmetry. Oblique preoperative **(C)** and postoperative **(D)** views at 1 year. No revision was needed. The areolar tattoo was performed in the office. Note the short lateral skin incision, which was used to encompass the previous biopsy sites.

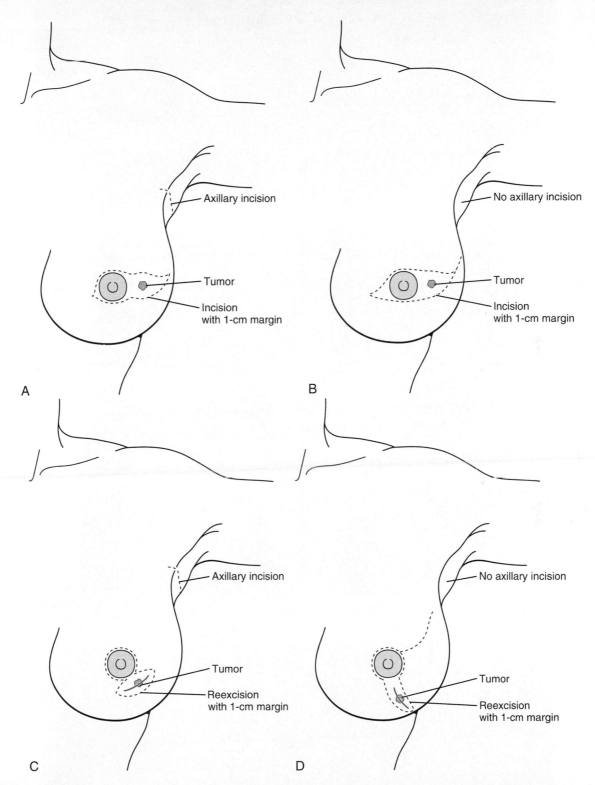

FIG. **39-21** Lateral and lower outer (lateral) quadrant. **A,** Incision around margin of areolar en bloc with 1-cm tumor margin completed as modified Stewart incision. Separate axillary incision may be required when nodal sampling is indicated. **B,** Similar to **A,** tumor is noncontiguous with the areola. A modification of the transverse Stewart incision with superolateral extension provides excellent access to breast flap dissection and mastectomy. The axillary dissection can be readily completed with this approach with no need for a separate incision. **C,** Nonradial biopsy incision continuous with areolar margin allows adequate breast exposure. Remote axillary incision is necessary. **D,** Radial biopsy incision contiguous with areolar. Superolateral extension is necessary to complete flap exposure to parenchyma of breast and axillary dissection.

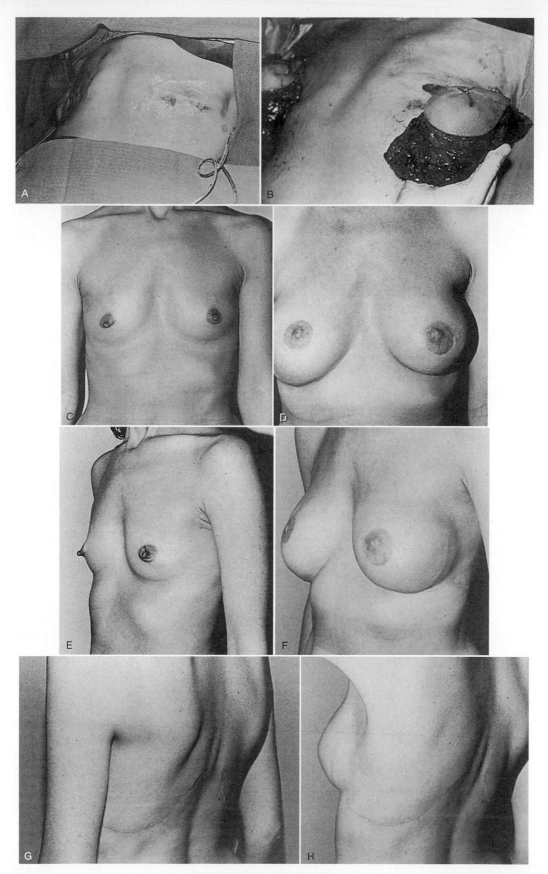

FIG. 39-22 A, Bilateral mastectomy for in situ disease using skin conservation technique through a 10-cm modified transverse (Stewart) incision. B, Bilateral latissimus flaps are brought out through the incisions before insetting in this immediate reconstruction. Preoperative (C) and postoperative (D) views following completion of nipple/areola reconstructions. Projection was enhanced with 100-ml implants. Oblique preoperative (E) and postoperative (F) views. The excellent result is directly attributable to the skin conservation and the immediate reconstruction. This reconstruction was a prerequisite to the mastectomy in this patient, and there was no reason to delay the reconstruction. Radical skin excision would not have enhanced the extirpation. G and H, Autogenous latissimus flap donor sites. The scar is usually inconspicuous if placed in the line of a posterolateral thoracotomy.

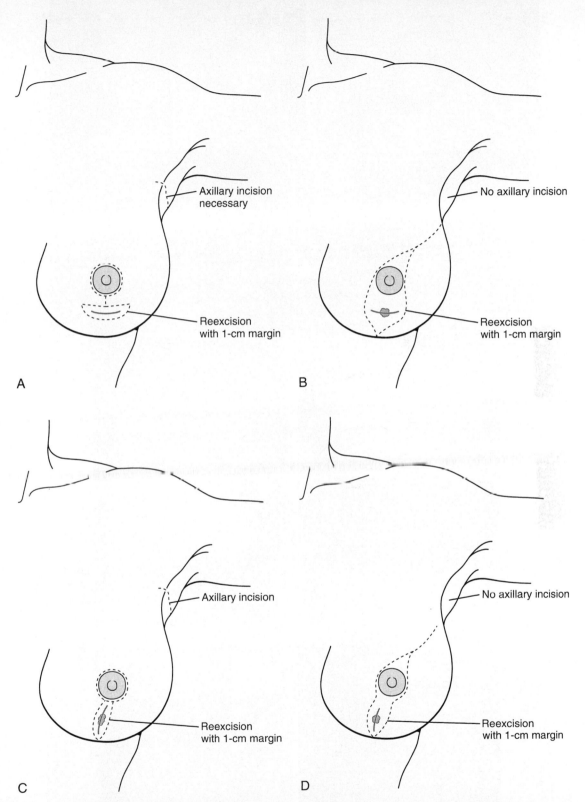

FIG. 39-23 Lower half (6 o'clock). **A,** Biopsy site may often be placed as a nonradial incision; skin-sparing requires 1-cm marginal excision continuous with periareolar incision. Remote axillary incision is necessary for adequate exposure and dissection. **B,** Biopsy site is nonradial in skin-fold contour. Similar to **A,** reexcision margins are 1 cm and are contiguous with skin bridge cephalad toward areola. Superolateral extension of incision allows total mastectomy and axillary dissection (when indicated). **C,** Biopsy site is radially placed. Excision of 1-cm biopsy site margin in continuity with areola allows proper breast exposure. Axillary access requires a separate incision. **D,** Radial biopsy site excised with tumor inclusion of 1-cm skin-sparing margin. Superolateral extension provides adequate exposure for total mastectomy and axillary dissection.

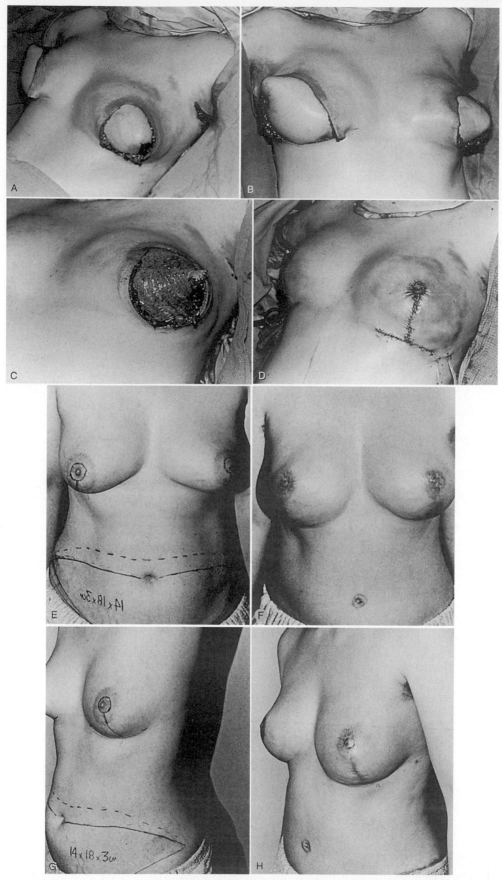

FIG. **39-24** **A** and **B,** Bilateral immediate transverse rectus abdominis myocutaneous (TRAM) flap reconstruction of skin conservation mastectomies for in situ disease. No breast skin was excised. **C,** View of the deepithelialized TRAM flap with an immediate nipple reconstruction the surface of the flap. **D,** The mastectomy flaps were closed in the lines of a Wise reduction pattern to remove redundant skin. Preoperative **(E)** and postoperative **(F)** views of the bilateral reconstructions. No revision was performed. **G,** Oblique views of the preoperative markings. **H,** The postoperative results of breast and nipple reconstructions. The areolas and nipples were tattooed in an office procedure.

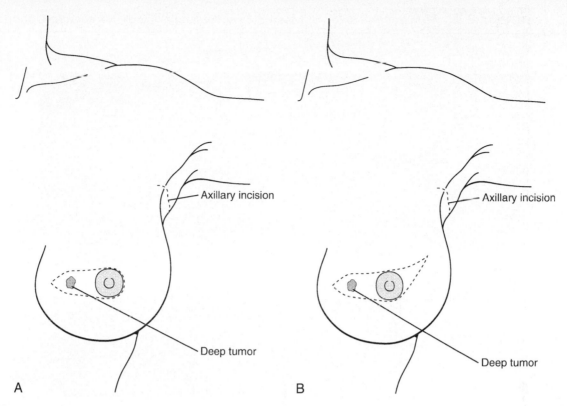

FIG. **39-25** Inner (medial) quadrant. **A,** Contiguous 1-cm excision of superficial tumor with areolar margin. Remote incision for axillary dissection is always necessary if node sampling is indicated. **B,** Similar to **A,** a 1-cm margin around superficial tumor with lateral and superior extension of incision is essential for breast exposure. Remote axillary incision is necessary when dissection is indicated.

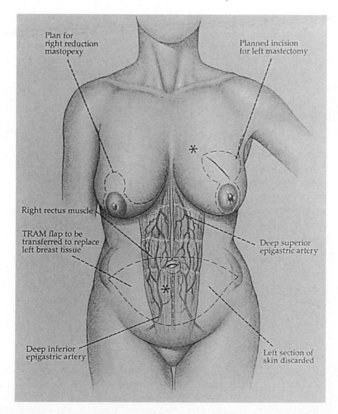

FIG. **39-26** The preoperative plan calls for a left modified radical mastectomy; reconstruction with a contralateral, single-pedicle, abdominal flap; and a matching mastopexy on the right. The asterisk indicates the position of the medial edge of the flap after its rotation and transfer to the chest. *TRAM,* Transverse rectus abdominus myocutaneous. *(From Copeland EM III, Yu LT: Surg Illus 1993.)*

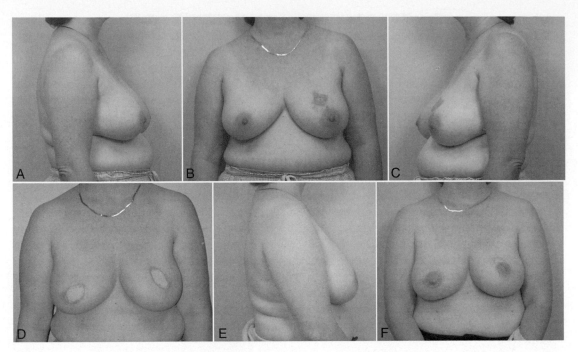

FIG. 39-27 This image series shows a 40-year-old woman with a history of a palpable mass in the left breast, which was shown by core biopsy to be invasive lobular carcinoma. Because of the high risk for bilaterality, left modified radical mastectomy in conjunction with prophylactic contralateral mastectomy was selected. Immediate bilateral reconstruction with ipsilateral transverse rectus abdominis myocutaneous (TRAM) flaps was performed. **A, B,** and **C,** Preoperative anterior and lateral views. **D, E,** and **F,** Postoperative results. **D,** Anterior view before nipple reconstruction and areolar tattooing. **E** and **F,** Lateral and anterior views, respectively, after nipple reconstruction and areolar tattooing.

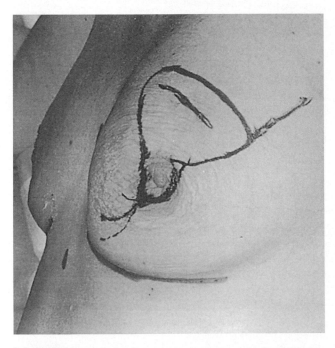

FIG. 39-28 General anesthesia has been induced, and the skin incision has been outlined on the left breast. (Nitrous oxide is not used for anesthesia because it could distend the bowel and increase intraabdominal pressure during closure.) The area to be resected includes the biopsy scar and the nipple. Both inframammary folds have been marked to guide the reconstruction and matching mastopexy. *(From Copeland EM III, Yu LT: Surg Illus 1993.)*

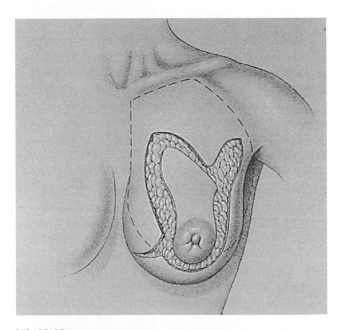

FIG. 39-29 The skin has been incised. Skin flaps are raised by electrocautery dissection, and breast tissue beneath the flaps is removed under direct vision. The subcutaneous margins of the flaps *(dashed line)* will extend superiorly to the medial half of the clavicle, superolaterally to the deltopectoral triangle and the cephalic vein, laterally to the anterior edge of the latissimus dorsi muscle, medially to the lateral border of the sternum, and inferiorly to the inframammary fold. *(From Copeland EM III, Yu LT: Surg Illus 1993.)*

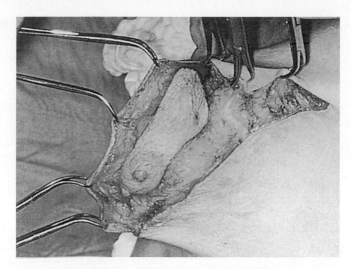

F I G. **39-30** For the skin-sparing mastectomy, the superior flap is elevated first by dissection in the plane between the subcutaneous tissue and the investing fascia of the breast. The skin edges are held with towel clips. *(From Copeland EM III, Yu LT: Surg Illus 1993.)*

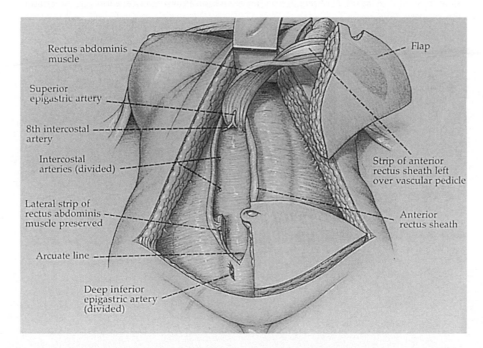

F I G. **39-31** Following skin-sparing modified radical mastectomy, formation of the transverse rectus abdominis myocutaneous (TRAM) flap and its pedicle is complete. The pedicle of rectus muscle includes sufficient deep epigastric vasculature to ensure the flap's viability. A narrower strip of anterior rectus sheath attached to the muscle helps protect the epigastric artery. A lateral segment of the muscle remains in place from the most inferior tendinous intersection to the arcuate line. *(From Copeland EM III, Yu LT: Surg Illus 1993.)*

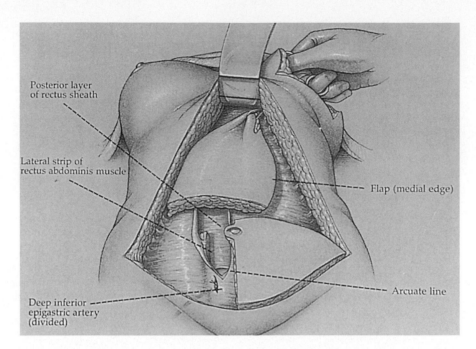

FIG. **39-32** The flap is passed through the tunnel into the mastectomy site. Counterclockwise rotation during passage ensures optimal drainage for the flap and avoids kinking of the pedicle. The pedicle is examined to ensure that it is not twisted. The flap will be allowed to perfuse while the abdomen is closed. The left wing of the skin flap is discarded. The right anterior rectus sheath is closed with a running 0 Prolene suture. An opening is left at the cephalad end of the closure to avoid constricting the muscular pedicle. The left sheath is imbricated to centralize the umbilicus. Two large Jackson Pratt drains are left anterior to the rectus sheath. *(From Copeland EM III, Yu LT: Surg Illus 1993.)*

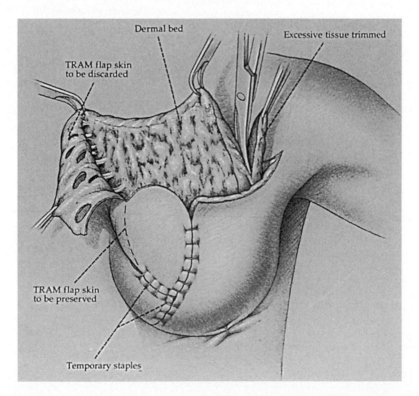

FIG. **39-33** Sections of poorly vascularized tissue have been excised from the transverse rectus abdominis myocutaneous *(TRAM)* flap, and the flap is temporarily stapled in place so that it can be trimmed and contoured. As the reconstruction proceeds, any excess skin is deepithelialized, leaving a well-vascularized dermal bed, which will be buried. *(From Copeland EM III, Yu LT: Surg Illus 1993.)*

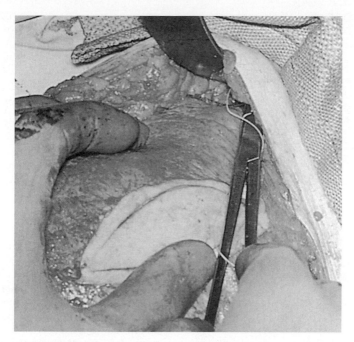

FIG. **39-34** To fill the infraclavicular hollow, the most superior edge of the flap is set onto the pectoralis major muscle. The buried, deepithelialized portions of the flap are rolled and positioned to create an appropriate degree of projection and ptosis. A symmetric inframammary fold is constructed by tacking the transverse rectus abdominis myocutaneous (TRAM) flap to the periosteum of a rib. *(From Copeland EM III, Yu LT: Surg Illus 1993.)*

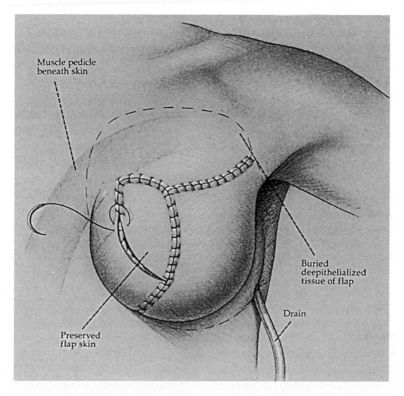

FIG. **39-35** The breast skin is closed with a single layer of continuous 5-0 Prolene suture. The axilla will be closed over a drain. *(From Copeland EM III, Yu LT: Surg Illus 1993.)*

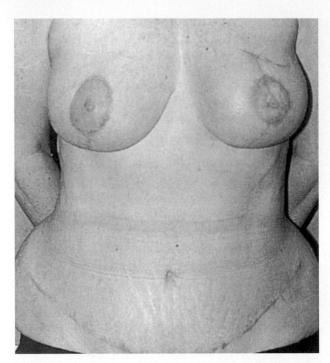

FIG. **39-36** Nipple/areola reconstruction has completed the procedure. The left nipple/areola is tattooed for color symmetry. (*From Copeland EM III, Yu LT: Surg Illus 1993.*)

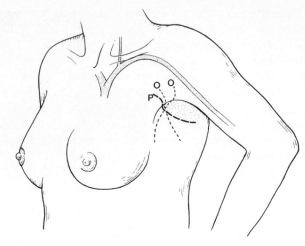

FIG. **39-37** Illustration of preferred *(P)* and optional *(O)* incisions used in axillary dissection. Ideally, incisions are placed in skin folds that parallel Langer's lines. Incisions are preferably curvilinear with placement just caudal to the hairline of the axilla. Optional incisions depicted are oblique or vertically placed with the chest wall. Because these optional incisions cross the lines of tension (Langer's lines), delay in wound repair and inferior cosmetic results may be observed.

for both upper and lower hemispheres of the breast are excised through 1-cm margins placed elliptically as nonradical incisions that typically parallel Langer's lines.

Placement of superolateral (modified Orr) incisions (see Figure 39-3) as an extension of the periareolar incision ensures comprehensive exposure for completion of the total mastectomy and axillary lymph node dissection. This incision has value for limited exposure in the course of flap elevation following incision around 1-cm margins of the biopsy scar and marginal excision of the nipple/areola complex. The 1-cm skin margins that circumvent the biopsy site are resected en bloc with the breast parenchyma and are inclusive of the undisturbed (intact) tumor or the biopsy cavity of the index neoplasm.

On occasion, separate axillary incisions designed as indicated in Figure 39-37 for level I and II nodal sampling or Patey dissection may be used to facilitate exposure with mastectomy. For all presentations of cancer in any quadrant or contiguous with the nipple/areola complex, the design of incisions is guided foremost by oncologic principles that place paramount the concern for locoregional disease control. Incision planning jointly by oncologic and plastic surgeons ensures optimal appearance and functional outcome with mastectomy techniques that enhance these disease control measures.

Exposure is gained through ample skin incisions, which are placed precisely parallel to the lines of skin tension. Incisions are placed below the level of the nipple, laterally and inferiorly, passing around the areola. The most satisfactory incisions, both from the standpoint of exposure and the quality of the final scar, extend from the areola at 2 to 3 o'clock and 6 to 8 o'clock. The lateral incision is contoured upward toward the axilla exactly in the lines of skin tension. If the incision is lengthened 10 to 12 cm lateral to the areola, the exposure of the axillary contents should be excellent. Alternatively, a separate 10-cm incision in the axillary hair-bearing skin can be used. The incision inferior to the nipple typically results in an discreet scar, even when it is not placed precisely in the lines of skin tension.

Flap Elevation. After circumscribing the nipple and areola, the skin flaps are elevated widely to reach the axilla and beyond the entire circumference of the peripheral boundaries of breast parenchyma. These anatomically distinct boundaries usually extend to the deltopectoral groove and below the clavicle to the subclavius muscle, to the lateral extent of the sternum, and to the anterior border of the latissimus dorsi muscle. Inferiorly, dissection should not extend below the inframammary line, which is tattooed with methylene blue or demarcated with sutures preoperatively. This advice should be heeded because there is no breast tissue below the inframammary line and the inframammary fold represents an important guideline for breast reconstruction.

Thereafter, skin flaps should be elevated at the subcutaneous tissue level, not at the subdermal level, to preserve the subcutaneous vascular plexus, which nourishes the overlying skin. If elevation is done at the correct level below the subcutaneous plexus, the dissection is bloodless. If profuse bleeding is encountered, the dissection has been conducted in a more superficial plane. It should be noted that the most likely complication of skin-sparing mastectomy is fat necrosis (18% to 20% in most series).[75-77]

Skin flap mobilization is commenced following elevation of periareolar tissues centrally and those continuous with margins of the excised biopsy scar. Although flap thickness depends on body habitus and fat content, typical thickness of the skin flap is 6 to 8 mm. Electrocautery scalpel using blended cut-coagulation mode may be used for flap elevation but is conducted with extreme caution. Uniform flap thickness that is well vascularized must be fastidiously sought and accomplished; if not, the sole remaining blood supply of the breast and skin—the subcutaneous plexus—will be injured. When the white undersurface of the dermis is exposed, the subcutaneous plexus will be injured and flap viability may be harmed distal to the surgical injury. Variation in flap thickness in the process of thinning may devascularize the flap and initiate disastrous wound repair problems.

With completion of flap elevation in superior and medial boundaries, attention is focused to the inferiormost extent of the boundary dissection. Preoperative marking of the inframammary fold or fixation with 2-0 silk sutures allows the oncologic surgeon to determine readily the caudad extent of mammary parenchymal resection. The mammary bursa facilitates mobilization of the breast off the pectoralis major fascia. With axillary dissection, when sentinel nodal sampling of levels I and II or Patey dissection (levels I to III) is indicated (see Chapters 53 through 55), preservation of the thoracodorsal neurovascular bundle and the long thoracic nerve are requisite to ensure intact motor innervation of the latissimus dorsi and serratus anterior muscles, respectively. Sensory innervation of the axilla and medial upper inner arm may be preserved when sacrifice of the traversing intercostobrachial cutaneous nerves is avoided. However, transection of these sensory branches creates little long-term morbidity because reinnervation occurs usually within 8 to 10 months. In addition, in the course of axillary lymph node dissection, avoidance of section of the medial pectoral neurovascular bundle ensures motor innervation and function of the pectoralis major and minor muscles. Moreover, it is most important to protect the subscapular vascular pedicle and its thoracodorsal branch, which supplies the latissimus dorsi muscle. Injury of these vessels eliminates the vascular supply and survival of the latissimus myocutaneous flap, which remains as one of the primary reconstructive options. In addition, the subscapular pedicle is an important recipient vessel for free flaps, which may be of value some time in the future to reconstruct radiation injuries of the chest wall and axilla. It is also helpful, but not essential, to protect the serratus anterior branch of the subscapular pedicle, because this represents the alternative vascular supply to the proximal latissimus dorsi muscle.

After the autogenous flap is inset, the breast skin flaps are used to shape the breast replacement volume. It is at this juncture in the procedure that the breast skin is so critical to provide a satisfactory contour for the reconstruction. The essential factor in breast reconstruction is symmetry between the normal breast and the reconstructed breast. Proper symmetry requires that the reconstructed breast shape and color "match" the normal appearance of the organ. In practice, it is usually necessary to alter the normal breast with either a mastopexy or reduction mammaplasty to obtain symmetry. An important tenet for the plastic surgeon to follow is the correction of any deformity of the opposite breast rather than to shape the reconstructed breast to match an unattractive, ptotic breast.

Finally, the importance of the skin color provided by the skin-sparing mastectomy should be emphasized. The native breast skin gives the best possible color match because it is identical to the opposite breast skin. A pale myocutaneous flap on the surface of the breast has the appearance of a "patch" and is remarkably detractive. Use of the autogenous flap on the surface to replace lost breast skin also diminishes the amount of flap that is available for shaping purposes. When implants are used, the breast skin is even more critical for coverage of the implant and subsequent shaping.

The most satisfactory reconstructions are evident in patients with skin-sparing mastectomies, particularly in those done bilaterally. The breast mound is replaced with autogenous tissue alone or with autogenous tissue and an implant to supplement volume. These techniques leave only the keyhole, left by resection of the nipple and areola, with different colored skin that is later tattooed to stimulate the areola. The molding of the breast is simplified in that almost the entire skin envelope is available and one needs only close the pocket to the envelope that corresponds with that of the contralateral breast from its superior extent to the preserved inframammary fold and anterior axillary line. The surgeon should be aware that in patients with small breasts and no abdominal laxity, the simple placement of an expander is usually unsatisfactory, producing a high rate (>50%) of complications. This occurs because it is difficult to obtain proper muscle coverage for the lower portion of the implant and the 6- to 8-mm skin flaps are relatively thin. For this group of patients, we plan additional padding with transposition of the latissimus dorsi myocutaneous flap, which provides muscle as well as the skin island for the keyhole of the nipple and the areola.[78,79] Increasing experience suggests that no increase in the risk for locoregional recurrence in the reconstituted breast exists; this locoregional failure rate approximates the recurrence rate of the modified radical mastectomies.[80]

Overview

With the common application of autogenous myocutaneous flap reconstruction in surgical practice, the majority of breast reconstructions are now completed synchronously with mastectomy rather than at subsequent intervals. A reconsideration of the placement of improper incisions and the unfounded tenet of extensive breast skin removal in these cases is a byproduct of the preoperative planning by the surgical oncologist together with the plastic surgeon. There are two reasons to consider skin conservation in this setting: (1) Little justification exists to remove the usual 10- by 20-cm ellipse of breast skin around the nipple, and (2) preservation of the native breast skin dramatically enhances the quality of the reconstruction.

This skin conservation approach appears to be justified in mastectomies when patients are ineligible for lumpectomy radiation. Many of these factors have little to do with a need for wide skin excision (e.g., invasive T_1, T_2 with an extensive intraductal component, a central tumor that would deform the breast, or multifocality). Favorable conditions for skin-sparing approaches include minimal cancers (T_1a, T_1b, ductal carcinoma in situ); diffuse microinvasive or multicentric cancers; benign conditions, such as familial (high-risk) breast cancer or difficult diagnostic breasts; and small breast cancers that are deep in the breast and remote from the overlying skin. Even in large tumors (T_2, T_3, T_4), the expected local recurrences virtually always represent failures together with systemic disease, rather than inadequate locoregional excision. In no immediate reconstructive series has there been any increase in local recurrence that can be related to the autogenous reconstruction.[49,66-68]

Surgical literature often purports that the purpose of the skin-sparing mastectomy is to improve "cosmesis." In actuality, the skin-sparing mastectomy provides a major advantage in the quality of every variant of the breast reconstructive procedure, particularly when implant augmentation is planned. Conversely, wide skin excision is the principal requirement for the complex TRAM flap in breast reconstruction; the skin deficit is so extensive that no other reconstruction method would be satisfactory. When limited skin excision has

been planned and implemented, simpler variants of reconstruction, such as the autogenous latissimus flap and tissue expanders, can be used because there will be no requirement for surface skin replacement. With increasing evidence that no deleterious outcome results from skin conservation in a broad range (stage presentations) of mastectomy patients, this technique has gained general acceptance as the conventional approach. It can be expected in the future that wide skin excision will have limited indications, such as direct skin invasion or a massive tumor.

FACTORS INFLUENCING IMMEDIATE/DELAYED POSTMASTECTOMY RECONSTRUCTION

The rapid advances in understanding of the fundamental biology of breast cancer in the twentieth and early twenty-first centuries, together with advances in surgical techniques following the advent and application of the vascularized myocutaneous flaps (TRAM and latissimus), have provided viable options for reconstruction after mastectomy. Until recently, little data were evident regarding the influences and attitudes of women who favor the reconstructive procedure. The National Cancer Data Base of the American College of Surgeons evaluated a large sample of women undergoing mastectomy between 1985 and 1990 ($n = 155,463$) and between 1994 and 1995 ($n = 68,348$). Reconstruction use and patient and tumor factors in these two time periods were evaluated and compared. The investigators determined that nationally only 3.4% of mastectomy patients of the 1985 to 1990 era selected early or immediate reconstruction; this group size increased to 8.3% in 1994 to 1995. Patient age, income, geographic locale, type of hospital providing treatment, and AJCC tumor stage all influenced the consideration and usage of reconstruction (in univariate analysis). Patients 50 years or younger had a 4.3 greater probability for favoring reconstruction than their older patient cohorts (Table 39-4).[81] Of interest, patients with ductal carcinoma in situ were twice as likely as those with invasive carcinoma to favor reconstruction. Thus breast reconstruction is an underused procedure that enhances postmastectomy patient satisfaction and self-esteem.

The principal deterrent for breast reconstruction consideration often follows anecdotal ill-advised consideration of the general oncologic surgeon; previous opinions for an increased probability of failed (and delayed) tumor detection with recurrent disease in the reconstructed breast were not supported by objective data. To answer this essential question, a large analysis of patients ($n = 540$) undergoing immediate reconstruction following modified radical mastectomy identified 50 patients within this database to have locally advanced breast cancer (LABC). Postoperative chemotherapy was given to all patients who underwent

TABLE 39-4 | Multivariate Analysis of Factors Influencing the Use of Reconstruction, 1994-1995 ($n = 55,728$)

VARIABLE	ODDS RATIO	95% CONFIDENCE INTERVAL
Age: ≤50 vs. ≥50 yr	4.3	4.2-4.4
PAJCC stage: 0 vs. I-IV	2.1	2.1-2.2
Family income: ≤$40,000 vs. ≥$40,000	2.0	2.0-2.1
Ethnicity: Non–African American vs. African American	1.6	1.5-1.7
Hospital type: NCI-recognized vs. other	1.4	1.3-1.7
Geographic region: Northeast, Southeast, Mountain, and Pacific vs. Midwest and South	1.3	1.2-1.3

From Morrow M et al: *J Am Coll Surg* 192:1, 2001.
NCI, National Cancer Institute; *PAJCC,* Pathologic American Joint Committee on Cancer.

immediate reconstruction; radiotherapy was used in 40% of this cohort, depending on tumor/nodal status. At median follow-up of 58.4 months, these patients treated at the University of Texas M.D. Anderson Cancer Center had no statistically significant differences in local or distant relapse compared with those patients treated with modified radical mastectomy *without* reconstruction. Furthermore, no differences were evident regarding treatment failure for patients with LABC who did or did not have immediate breast reconstruction (Table 39-5).[82] Thus immediate reconstruction can be performed with low surgical morbidity and also with acceptable recurrence rates similar to those for patients who did not pursue reconstruction.

In a more recent analysis, Nold and colleagues[83] note that only 20% to 50% of patients with early-stage disease choose breast conservation procedures. These authors further sought to determine the influences that were most important to select the ablative modified radical mastectomy with or without reconstruction versus breast conservation approaches; both cohorts were eligible for the skin-sparing procedure. Overall, the most influential factor for consideration of a procedure was the "fear of cancer." Women choosing conservation surgery indicated that their surgeon, the (expected) cosmetic result, and psychological issues were more influential in their decision than for those selecting modified radical mastectomy without reconstruction ($p < .02$) (Table 39-6).[83] Fear of cancer-related death remained a major factor influencing women selecting the modified radical *without* immediate reconstruction. In comparing those with the ablative mastectomy with

TABLE 39-5 | Outcome for Locally Advanced Breast Cancer Patients Undergoing Mastectomy with or without Immediate Breast Reconstruction*

OUTCOME	IMMEDIATE BREAST RECONSTRUCTION ($n = 50$)	NO RECONSTRUCTION ($n = 72$)	p VALUE
Interval to postoperative chemotherapy (range number postoperative wound complications percentage)	35 days (5-91)	21 days (8-145)	.05
Major	4/50 (8%)	3/72 (4.2%)	.23
Minor	3/50 (6%)	5/72 (6.9%)	.66
Local recurrence			
Stage IIB	1/23 (4.4%)	2/12 (16.7%)	.22
Stage III	4/27 (14.8%)	7/60 (11.7%)	.70
Distant relapse			
Stage IIB	5/23 (21.7%)	4/12 (33.3%)	.37
Stage III	11/27 (40.7%)	22/60 (36.7%)	.85

From Newman LA et al: *Ann Surg Oncol* 6:671, 1999.
*Median follow-up of 58.6 months (range, 15 to 116 months).

TABLE **39-6** Responses of Women Undergoing Breast-Conserving Surgery (BCS), Modified Radical Mastectomy with Reconstruction (MRN-R), or Modified Radical Mastectomy without Reconstruction (MRM-NR) Regarding Degree to which Various Factors Influenced Choice of Surgical Option

FACTOR*	BCS MEDIAN (25TH, 75TH PERCENTILES)[†]	MRM-R MEDIAN (25TH, 75TH PERCENTILES)[†]	MRM-NR MEDIAN (25TH, 75TH PERCENTILES)[†]	p VALUE
Number	43	14	39	
Family	3 (1,4)	1.5 (1,5)	2 (1,3)	0.5989
Primary care physician	1 (1,3)	1 (1,1)	1 (1,2)	0.8378
Surgeon	4.5 (3,5)	3 (1,4)	2 (1,5)	0.0009
Medical oncologist	1.5 (1,4)	1 (1,1)	1 (1,1)	0.0194
Previous (personal) history	1 (1,2)	1 (1,1)	1 (1,1)	0.7071
Family history	1 (1,3)	2.5 (1,5)	1 (1,3)	0.3099
Cosmetic appearance	3 (2,5)	4 (1,5)	1 (1,1)	0.0001
Fear of breast cancer	3 (2,5)	4.5 (4,5)	5 (3,5)	0.0420
Difficult cancer diagnosis	1.5 (1,3)	1 (1,3)	1 (1,3)	0.8581
Concern about radiation	2 (1,4)	4.5 (1,5)	3 (1,5)	0.2290
Travel for radiation	1 (1,1)	1 (1,1)	1 (1,1)	0.7236
Time for radiation therapy	1 (1,3)	1 (1,1)	1 (1,1)	0.7844
Psychological aspects	3 (2,5)	3 (1,4)	1 (1,2)	0.0001
Insurance	1 (1,2)	1 (1,1)	1 (1,1)	0.1363

From Nold RJ et al: *Am J Surg* 180:413, 2000.
*Superscripts within rows are used to identify significant treatment differences. Median responses within a row that share the same superscript are not significantly different, and those that have different superscripts are significantly different ($p <.05$).
[†]Median responses and 25th and 75th percentiles for responses regarding choice of surgical option: 1 = did not influence, 2 = minimally influenced, 3 = influenced, 4 = moderately influenced, and 5 = greatly influenced decision.

or without reconstruction, there was a similar fear of cancer-related deaths; predictably, those who selected reconstruction had greater concern with cosmetic appearance ($p = .0002$).

In summary, the surgeon's input (opinion) is of paramount concern and importance to the patient considering breast conservation versus an ablative approach with immediate reconstruction. Although proper counseling of the patient regarding equivalent outcomes for recurrence and survival for either ablative procedure is essential, the patient's fear of cancer (relapse and death) may overshadow the surgeon's proper and proactive advice.

INCISIONS FOR AXILLARY DISSECTION

The advent of SLNB and the early diagnosis of breast cancer (up to 30% of newly diagnosed breast cancers are ductal carcinoma in situ) have had an impact on the application of formal axillary node dissections. Nonetheless, one has to be cognizant of the need for axillary node dissections at the time of the mastectomy or in some instances at a later date. This need for reoperation occurs in as many as 40% of false-negative readings. There are few false-positive results in sentinel node sampling with use of the combined blue dye and isotope mapping techniques. When the former

occurs, and permanent pathology of histologically positive nodal disease is present, the surgeon must return to the axilla after breast reconstruction. Cooperation between the oncologic surgeon and the plastic surgeon is essential in these cases, particularly in microvascular free-tissue transfers.[74,84]

Figure 39-37 depicts the *preferred* incision and the *optional* incisions for axillary dissections performed synchronously with lumpectomy (segmental mastectomy, tylectomy). The surgeon is well advised to complete incisions placed parallel with Langer's lines and designed in a curvilinear fashion just caudal to the axillary hairline. These incisions are designed at the time of sentinel lymph node biopsy and must be enlarged when axillary dissection is indicated for the histologically confirmed positive sentinel node. Preferably, axillary incisions are made separately from incisions of the segmental mastectomy. Optional incisions indicated in Figure 39-37 obliquely cross Langer's lines and are not positioned in axillary skin folds. It is perhaps for this latter reason that delay in primary healing and inferior cosmetic results are obtained. Adequate skin exposure should be provided so that dissection of level I and level II nodes beneath the pectoralis minor is possible without undue traction on the pectoralis major or minor muscles. This principle prevents damage to the medial and lateral (anterior thoracic) pectoral nerves located in the lateral and medial neurovascular bundles, respectively. Incisions placed in a curvilinear transverse, oblique, or vertical fashion all allow adequate access to the axillary vein, the medial border of the pectoralis minor muscle, and the lateral aspect of the latissimus dorsi muscle. This exposure should permit visualization of the long thoracic nerve to the serratus anterior and the thoracodorsal nerve to the latissimus dorsi.

REFERENCES

1. Harris JR, Hellman S: Primary radiation therapy for early breast cancer, *Cancer* 52:2547, 1983.
2. Copeland EM III: Carcinoma of the breast. In Copeland EM III (ed): *Surgical oncology,* New York, 1983, John Wiley & Sons.
3. Handley RS: The conservative radical mastectomy of Patey: ten year results in 425 patients breasts, *Dis Breast* 2:16, 1976.
4. Kinne DW: Axillary clearance in operable breast cancer: still a necessity? *Cancer Res* 152:161, 1998.
5. Slavin SA, Love SM, Sadowsky NL: Reconstruction of the radiated partial mastectomy defect with autogenous tissues, *Plast Reconstr Surg* 90:854, 1992.
6. Ellis LM et al: Correlation of estrogen, progesterone, and androgen receptors in breast cancer: significance to the androgen receptor, *Am J Surg* 157:577, 1989.
7. Ellis LM et al: Lability of steroid hormone receptors following devascularization of breast tumors, *Arch Surg* 124:39, 1989.
8. Bland KI et al: The effects of ischemia on estrogen and progesterone receptor profiles in the rodent uterus, *J Surg Res* 42:653, 1987.
9. Hollingshead WH: The breast. In Hollingshead WH (ed): *Anatomy for surgeons,* vol 2, *Thorax, abdomen, and pelvis,* ed 2, New York, 1971, Harper & Row.
10. Haagensen CD: Anatomy of the mammary gland. In Haagensen CD (ed): *Diseases of the breast,* ed 2, Philadelphia, 1971, WB Saunders.
11. Spratt JS Jr, Donegan WL: Anatomy of the breast. In Donegan WL, Spratt JS Jr (eds): *Cancer of the breast,* ed 3, Philadelphia, 1979, WB Saunders.
12. Spratt JS, Tobin GJ: Gross anatomy of the breast. In Donegan WL, Spratt JS (eds): *Cancer of the breast,* ed 4, Philadelphia, 1995, WB Saunders.
13. Moosman DA: Anatomy of the pectoral nerves and their preservation in modified mastectomy, *Am J Surg* 139:883, 1980.
14. Anson BJ, McVay CB: Breast or mammary region. In Anson BJ, McVay CB (eds): *Thoracic walls: surgical anatomy,* vol 1, Philadelphia, 1971, WB Saunders.
15. Gray JH: The relation of lymphatic vessels to the spread of cancer, *Br J Surg* 26:462, 1939.
16. Cody HS, Egeli RA, Urban JA: Rotter's node metastases, *Ann Surg* 199:266, 1984.
17. Netter FH: *CIBA collection of medical illustrations, 7:6,* Summit, NJ, 1979, CIBA Pharmaceutical.
18. Halsted WS: Results of operation for cure of cancer of breast performed at Johns Hopkins Hospital from June 1889 to January 1894, *Ann Surg* 20:497, 1894.
19. Meyer W: An improved method of the radical operation for carcinoma of the breast, *Med Rec NY* 46:746, 1894.
20. Finney JMT: *Keen's surgery,* Philadelphia, 1924, WB Saunders.
21. Gray DB: The radical mastectomy incision, *Am Surg* 35:750, 1969.
22. Patey DH: A review of 146 cases of carcinoma of the breast operated upon between 1930–1943, *Br J Cancer* 21:260, 1967.
23. Patey DH, Dyson WH: Prognosis of carcinoma of the breast in relation to type of operation performed, *Br J Cancer* 2:7, 1948.
24. Kendall BE, Arthur JF, Patey DH: Lymphangiography in carcinoma of the breast: a comparison of clinical, radiological, and pathological findings in axillary lymph nodes, *Cancer* 16:1233, 1963.
25. Auchincloss H: Significance of location and number of axillary metastases in carcinoma of the breast: a justification for a conservative operation, *Ann Surg* 158:37, 1963.
26. Madden JL: Modified radical mastectomy, *Surg Gynecol Obstet* 121:1221, 1965.
27. Krohn IT, Cooper DR, Bassett JG: Radical mastectomy, *Arch Surg* 227:760, 1982.
28. Gray SW, Skandalakis JE: *Atlas of surgical anatomy for general surgeons,* Baltimore, 1985, Williams & Wilkins.
29. Donegan WL, Perez-Mesa CM, Watson FR: A biostatistical study of locally recurrent breast carcinoma, *Surg Gynecol Obstet* 122:529, 1966.
30. Gilliland MD, Barton RM, Copeland EM III: The implications of local recurrence of breast cancer as the first site of therapeutic failure, *Ann Surg* 197:284, 1983.
31. Johnson CH et al: Oncological aspects of immediate breast reconstruction following mastectomy for malignancy, *Arch Surg* 124:819, 1989.
32. Kurtz JM: Factors influencing the risk of local recurrence in the breast, *Eur J Cancer* 28:660, 1992.
33. Cheatle GL, Cutler M: *Tumours of the breast,* Philadelphia, 1933, JB Lippincott.
34. Copeland EM III, Yu LT: Skin-sparing mastectomy and immediate autologous flap reconstruction, *Surg Illus* 3, 1993.
35. Greco RJ et al: Two-staged breast reconstruction in patients with symptomatic macromastia requiring mastectomy, *Ann Plast Surg* 32:572, 1994.
36. Lebovic GS, Laub DR, Berkowitz RL: Aesthetic approach to simple and modified radical mastectomy, *Contemp Surg* 45:15, 1994.
37. Silverstein MJ et al: Can intraductal breast carcinoma be excised completely by local excision? *Cancer* 73:2985, 1994.
38. van Dongen JA et al: Long-term results of a randomized trial comparing breast-conserving therapy with mastectomy: European organization for research and treatment of cancer 10801 trial, *J Natl Cancer Inst* 92:1143, 2000.
39. Verhoef LCG et al: Breast-conserving treatment or mastectomy in early breast cancer: a clinical decision analysis with special reference to the risk of local recurrence, *Eur J Cancer* 27:1132, 1991.
40. Sauer R et al: Therapy of small breast cancer: a prospective study on 1036 patients with special emphasis on prognostic factors, *Int J Radiat Onc Biol Phys* 23:907, 1992.
41. Bland KI et al: Oncogene protein co-expression: value of Ha-*ras*, c-*myc*, c-*fos*, and p53 as prognostic discriminants for breast cancer, *Ann Surg* 221:706, 1995.
42. Fisher B et al: Ten-year results of a randomized trial comparing radical mastectomy and total mastectomy with or without radiation, *N Engl J Med* 312:674, 1985.
43. Fisher B et al: Significance of ipsilateral breast tumour recurrence after lumpectomy, *Lancet* 338:327, 1991.

44. Fisher ER et al: Pathologic findings from the National Surgical Adjuvant Breast Project (Protocol 6). II. Relation of local breast recurrence to multicentricity, *Cancer* 57:1717, 1986.

45. Fowble B et al: Breast recurrence following conservative surgery and radiation: patterns of failure, prognosis, and pathologic findings from mastectomy specimens with implications for treatment, *Int J Radiat Oncol Biol Phys* 19:833, 1990.

46. Stotter AT et al: Predicting the rate and extent of locoregional failure after breast conservation therapy for early breast cancer, *Cancer* 64:2217, 1989.

47. Kurtz JM et al: Inoperable recurrence after breast-conserving surgical treatment and radiotherapy, *Surg Gynecol Obstet* 172:357, 1991.

48. Dao TL, Nemoto T: The clinical significance of skin recurrence after radical mastectomy in women with cancer of the breast, *Surg Gynecol Obstet* 117:447, 1963.

49. Kroll SS et al: The oncologic risks of skin preservation at mastectomy when combined with immediate reconstruction of the breast, *Surg Gynecol Obstet* 172:17, 1991.

50. Holland R et al: Histologic multifocality of Tis, T1-2 breast carcinomas: implications for clinical trials of breast-conserving surgery, *Cancer* 56:979, 1985.

51. Halsted WS: The results of radical operation for the cure of cancer of the breast, *Trans Am Surg Assoc* 25:61, 1907.

52. Lewis D, Rienhoff WF Jr: Study of the results of operation for cure of cancer of breast performed at Johns Hopkins Hospital 1889 to 1931, *Ann Surg* 95:336, 1932.

53. Handley WS: *Cancer of the breast and its treatment*, ed 2, London, 1922, A Murray.

54. Brooks B, Daniel RA Jr: Present status of the "radical operation" for carcinoma of the breast, *Ann Surg* 3:688, 1940.

55. Handley RS, Thackray AC: Conservative radical mastectomy (Patey's operation), *Ann Surg* 170:880, 1969.

56. Bland KI et al: Primary therapy for breast cancer: surgical principles and techniques. In Bland KI, Copeland EM (eds): *The breast: comprehensive management of benign and malignant diseases*, Philadelphia, 1991, WB Saunders.

57. Moore CH: On the influence of inadequate operation on the theory of cancer, *J R Med Chir Soc Lond* 1:244, 1867.

58. Winchester DP et al: Treatment trends for ductal carcinoma in situ of the breast, *Ann Surg Oncol* 2:207, 1995.

59. Fisher B et al: Eight-year results of a randomized clinical trial comparing total mastectomy and lumpectomy with and without irradiation in the treatment of breast cancer, *N Engl J Med* 320:822, 1989.

60. Veronesi U et al: Quadrantectomy versus lumpectomy for small size breast cancer, *Eur J Cancer* 26:671, 1990.

61. Mustakallio S: Treatment of breast cancer by tumor extirpation and roentgen therapy instead of radical operation, *J Fac Radiol* 6:23, 1954.

62. Calle R et al: Conservative management of operable breast cancer: ten years' experience at the Foundation Curie, *Cancer* 42:2045, 1978.

63. Crile G Jr: Treatment of breast cancer by local excision, *Am J Surg* 109:400, 1965.

64. Fisher B: Lumpectomy and axillary dissection. In Bland KI, Copeland EM (eds): *The breast: comprehensive management of benign and malignant diseases*, Philadelphia, 1991, WB Saunders.

65. Bland KI et al: One-stage simple mastectomy with immediate reconstruction for high-risk patients: an improved technique: the biologic basis for ductal-glandular mastectomy, *Arch Surg* 121:221, 1986.

66. Toth BA, Lappert P: Modified skin incisions for mastectomy: the need for plastic surgical input in preoperative planning, *Plast Reconstr Surg* 87:1048, 1991.

67. Carlson GW: Skin sparing mastectomy: anatomic and technical considerations, *Am Surg* 62:151, 1996.

68. Sampaio Goes J: Mastectomy by periareolar approach with immediate breast reconstruction, *Rev Loc Bras Cir Estet Reconstr* 10:44, 1995.

69. Schnitt SJ, Goldwyn RM, Slavin SA: Mammary ducts in the areola: implications for patients undergoing reconstructive surgery of the breast, *Plast Reconstr Surg* 92:1290, 1993.

70. Hammond DC et al: Use of a skin-sparing reduction pattern to create a combination skin-muscle flap pocket in immediate breast reconstruction, *Plast Reconstr Surg* 110:206, 2002.

71. Kuerer HM, Krishnamurthy S, Kronowitz SJ: Important technical considerations for skin-sparing mastectomy with sentinel lymph node dissection, *Arch Surg* 137:747, 2002.

72. Shrotria S: The peri-areolar incision—gateway to the breast! *Eur J Surg Oncol* 27:601, 2001.

73. Skoll PJ, Hudson DA: Skin-sparing mastectomy using a modified Wise pattern, *Plast Reconstr Surg* 110:214, 2002.

74. Stradling BL et al: Skin-sparing mastectomy with sentinel lymph node dissection: less is more, *Arch Surg* 136:1069, 2001.

75. Foster RD et al: Skin-sparing mastectomy and immediate breast reconstruction: a prospective cohort study for the treatment of advanced stages of breast carcinoma, *Ann Surg Oncol* 9:462, 2002.

76. Losken A et al: Trends in unilateral breast reconstruction and management of the contralateral breast: the Emory experience, *Plast Reconstr Surg* 110:89, 2002.

77. Medina-Franco H et al: Factors associated with local recurrence after skin-sparing mastectomy and immediate breast reconstruction for invasive breast cancer, *Ann Surg* 235:814, 2002.

78. Beer GM et al: Incidence of the superficial fascia and its relevance in skin-sparing mastectomy, *Cancer* 94:19, 2002.

79. de la Torre JI et al: Reconstruction with the latissimus dorsi flap after skin-sparing mastectomy, *Ann Plast Surg* 46:229, 2001.

80. Carlson GW et al: Results of immediate breast reconstruction after skin-sparing mastectomy, *Ann Plast Surg* 46:222, 2001.

81. Morrow M et al: Factors influencing the use of breast reconstruction postmastectomy: a National Cancer Database Study, *J Am Coll Surg* 192:1, 2001.

82. Newman LA et al: Feasibility of immediate breast reconstruction for locally advanced breast cancer, *Ann Surg Oncol* 6:671, 1999.

83. Nold RJ et al: Factors influencing a woman's choice to undergo breast-conserving surgery versus modified radical mastectomy, *Am J Surg* 180:413, 2000.

84. Simmons RM et al: Analysis of nipple/areolar involvement with mastectomy: can the areola be preserved? *Ann Surg Oncol* 9:165, 2002.

INDEX

Page numbers followed by f indicate figures; t, tables.